METHODOLOGICAL AND BIOSTATISTICAL FOUNDATIONS OF CLINICAL NEUROPSYCHOLOGY AND MEDICAL AND HEALTH DISCIPLINES

STUDIES ON NEUROPSYCHOLOGY, DEVELOPMENT, AND COGNITION

Series Editor:

Linas Bieliauskas, Ph.D.
University of Michigan, Ann Arbor, MI, USA

METHODOLOGICAL AND BIOSTATISTICAL FOUNDATIONS OF CLINICAL NEUROPSYCHOLOGY AND MEDICAL AND HEALTH DISCIPLINES

second edition

Edited by

DOMENIC V. CICCHETTI

AND

BYRON P. ROURKE

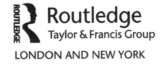

Routledge
Taylor & Francis Group

LONDON AND NEW YORK

Library of Congress Cataloging-in-Publication Data

Methodological and biostatistical foundations of clinical neuropsychology and medical
    and health disciplines / edited by Domenic V. Cicchetti and Byron P. Rourke.--2nd ed.
        p. ; cm. -- (Studies on neuropsychology, development, and cognition)
    Rev. ed. of: Methodological and biostatistical foundations of clinical neuropsychology /
edited by Byron P. Rourke ... [et al.]. c1991.
    "Selected articles published between 1992 and 2003 in the Journal of clinical and
experimental neuropsychology, The Clinical neuropsychologist, and ... Child
neuropsychology" -- Pref.
    Includes bibliographical references and index.
    ISBN 90-265-1964-8
        1. Neuropsychological tests–Statistical methods. 2. Clinical neuropsychology–
Research–Methodology. 3. Biometry. I. Cicchetti, Domenic V. II. Rourke, Byron P.
(Byron Patrick), 1939- III. Methodological and biostatistical foundations of clinical
neuropsychology. IV. Series.
    [DNLM: 1. Neuropsychology–methods–Collected Works.
2. Biometry–methods–Collected Works. 3. Data Interpretation, Statistical–Collected
Works. 4. Neuropsychological Tests–Collected Works. WL 103.5 M592 2004]
    RC386.6.N48M48 2004
    152–dc22

                                                                    2003070388

First published 2004 by Psychology Press

Published 2019 by Routledge
2 Park Square, Milton Park, Abingdon, Oxon OX14 4RN
52 Vanderbilt Avenue, New York, NY 10017

Routledge is an imprint of the Taylor & Francis Group, an informa business

Copyright © 2004 by Taylor & Francis

Cover design: Magenta Grafische Producties, Bert Haagsman
Typesetting: Charon Tec Pvt. Ltd, Chennai, India

This book contains reprints of earlier published journal articles. The original publication
data (journal title, volume and issue number, page numbers, year of publication) are
clearly indicated on the first page of each article.

ISBN 13: 978-90-265-1964-2 (hbk)

CONTENTS

FROM THE SERIES EDITOR

I am particularly proud of the addition of the contribution of Drs. Cicchetti and Rourke to our series. *Methodological and Biostatistical Foundations of Clinical Neuropsychology and Medical and Health Disciplines* fits in well with our general underlying theme of combining contemporary theoretical and scientific reviews and perspectives with their practical application. The volume's topics range from basic statistical and biostatistical concepts to direct determination of reliability and validity in research design. The volume is appropriate for a wide audience from advanced graduate students to senior scientists wishing a review or refresher for statistical methods and applications. The authors are well-known for their expertise and provide clearly written explanations to facilitate methodological and statistical understanding, also including contemporary articles from other contributors in the field. I believe the reader will thoroughly enjoy and appreciate this work, finding it a ready reference when approaching either the design, implementation, reporting, or consumption of research in psychology and all other health disciplines. I am confident that this volume will find a welcome place on the bookshelf of students and colleagues, contributing to increased understanding of research practices and their role in the advancement of our professions.

Linas A. Bieliauskas
Ann Arbor, January, 2004

PREFACE

The predecessor to this volume (Rourke, Costa, Cicchetti, Adams, & Plasterk, 1992) and the current volume were designed to function as a guide to and explanation of many of the major methodological and biostatistical components of both 'pure' and 'applied' aspects of clinical neuropsychology. Also, both have as their intended audience advanced graduate students, as well as more seasoned research scientists. We noted in the Introduction to Rourke et al. (1992) that the book was intended not only for professionals and students in clinical and experimental neuropsychology, but also for those in other fields of psychology, as well as neurology, psychiatry, speech pathology, and other related health areas. Hence the appropriate re-wording of the title to reflect this conceptualization of intended audience.

Given the complexity and interrelatedness of most of the areas of functioning that neuropsychologists have investigated over the years, it is quite difficult to conceive of many disorders or physical injuries that do not have neuropsychological issues to be addressed in order to provide state-of-the-art diagnosis and treatment. The neuropsychology of traumatic brain injury or the neuropsychology of Diabetes Mellitus are obvious examples of the types of injuries and major medical disorders that are of great interest to dedicated clinical and research neuropsychologists. Another area of interest that has been studied extensively over the past decade is the Nonverbal Learning Disability (NLD) syndrome, a disorder that impinges upon other health areas outside the realm of neuropsychology.

The papers in Rourke et al. (1992) were derived from selected articles published between 1979 and 1991 in the *Journal of Clinical Neuropsychology*, its successor, the *Journal of Clinical and Experimental Neuropsychology*, and *The Clinical Neuropsychologist*. The current volume includes selected articles published between 1992 and 2003 in the *Journal of Clinical and Experimental Neuropsychology*, *The Clinical Neuropsychologist*, and the more recent Swets & Zeitlinger journal, *Child Neuropsychology*, which appeared in 1995. Although the articles included in Rourke et al. (1992) are not contained in the current work, we refer to some of them whenever it is necessary to provide continuity of thought for concepts and contexts that are common to both volumes.

Finally, we are deeply indebted to the authors for permission to publish their original works in this new format. The text, needless to say, would not have been possible without their important contributions to clinical and experimental neuropsychology, and to science more generally.

We also wish to extend our warmest thanks and appreciation to Arnout Jacobs, Martin Scrivener, Leon Bijnsdorp, and the editorial staff at Swets & Zeitlinger for their prodigious efforts and extreme diligence in indexing and organizing all the papers and commentaries appearing in this work. We trust that these efforts by so many dedicated scientists, editors, and publishers serve to render the text readable and easily accessible to its intended audience. Any errors that may remain in the work are solely the responsibility of the Editors of this volume.

The Editors

REFERENCE

Rourke, B.P., Costa, L., Cicchetti, D.V., Adams, K.M., & Plasterk, K.J. (1992). *Methodological and biostatistical foundations of clinical neuropsychology.* Lisse, The Netherlands: Swets & Zeitlinger.

Chapter I

INTRODUCTION AND OVERVIEW

Our purpose in this volume is to introduce the advanced undergraduate or graduate student and more seasoned research scientists in clinical neuropsychology and other health sciences to a wide array of methodological and biostatistical issues, as they occur in the context of both published and ongoing research. As was the case in the earlier volume, our text is intended to serve the needs of both those who wish to contribute to the literature and those who wish to consume the literature in an intelligent manner.

While building upon a working knowledge and understanding of the basic univariate data analytic techniques and the research designs to which they apply, the approach to the more complex multivariate techniques are presented primarily at a conceptual and essentially non-mathematical level. It is felt that the researcher who desires a more thorough understanding of the mathematical underpinning of the various multivariate data analytic strategies will be motivated to consult the references we cite.

In keeping with this philosophy, we feel that it is very important for the research scientist to understand both the advantages and limitations of the various univariate and multivariate techniques. We hope that readers of this text will refrain from applying new multivariate techniques just because they happen to exist, but rather will obtain the necessary knowledge to know whether or when these might apply to a given research problem.

Although the issue of the complexity of some of the more recent and standard approaches to data analytic strategies and their important role in specific research designs is important to convey, there remains an even more fundamental issue of whether the results of *correctly* applied data analytic strategies make any practical or clinical sense, above and beyond their having reached levels of 'statistical significance.' These critical issues are addressed throughout various commentaries that we make at various points in the text.

As was the case in the earlier volume, we feel that the current material can also be used in courses in research methodology, but should not be regarded as a complete, integrated biostatistical text, in and of itself.

Chapter 1

INTRODUCTION

Chapter II

DISTINGUISHING BETWEEN STATISTICS AND BIOSTATISTICS

As noted recently by the late Alvan Feinstein (2002), in *Principles of Medical Statistics*, the term *statistics* dates back to two important events, one occurring during the 17th and part of the 18th century surrounding the interest of nations in assembling quantitative data pertaining to their wealth. This collection of information was referred to as "Political Arithmetic". The persons who assembled these data were called "statists" and the data themselves were referred to as *statistics*. It is interesting that two current journals in the field still bear witness to these early roots, namely, *Statist Inference for Stochastical Processes* and *Statist Methods in Medical Research*.

The second relevant event was documented later in the 18th century, and centered about the activity of gambling as a form of amusement practiced by royalty. These noblemen gave, in a matter of speaking, 'grants' to individuals in payment for ideas that served the purpose of improving the odds of winning bets. The resulting 'calculus of probabilities' was eventually applied well beyond the area of gambling per se. As Feinstein notes further, the theory that developed for use in estimating gambling probabilities served as the basis for making inferential decisions deriving from descriptive information based upon specific samples of data. This dual source of information, namely, descriptive and inferential, then became the basis for concepts such as ... "p values, confidence intervals, and other mathematical inferences that found their way into modern 'statistical analysis'" (Feinstein, 2002).

The distinction between statistics and biostatistics rests upon the added meaning that 'bio' brings to the differentiation. The meaning of biostatistics derives from the fact that 'bio' refers to life. Thus, biostatistics would refer to statistics applied to living organisms, as opposed to say, agricultural statistics that often focus upon the various crop yields of different plots of land. Because this text focuses on neuropsychology and related disciplines, such as neurology, clinical psychology, speech pathology, and medicine, the distinction seems apt.

Chapter III

DISTINGUISHING BETWEEN PARAMETRIC AND NONPARAMETRIC APPROACHES TO DATA ANALYSIS

A. Overview

As noted by Bradley (1968), the terms 'nonparametric' and 'distribution-free' are by no means synonymous because, in fact, a statistical test can be both parametric and distribution-free. Nonetheless, the two terms have been treated equally in popular usage to the extent that they are usually used interchangeably. Although we will adhere to this early recommendation, it would perhaps make more sense to refer to nonparametric techniques as assumption-free, as opposed, at least theoretically, to their parametric counterparts.

But the issue is still more complex. In addition to the basic assumption that each observation or data point is obtained independently before a statistical test can be validly applied, there are three further assumptions underlying the use of parametric tests: normality of distribution; equality of variances in the samples being compared; and equality of sample sizes. It has been shown extensively by computer simulation methodology and analyses of multiple data sets that any one of these assumptions can be violated, and the application of parametric and nonparametric techniques will nonetheless produce very similar probability levels when these tests are applied to the same data set (e.g., Boneau, 1960, 1962; Cicchetti, 1994a; Petrinovich & Hardyck, 1969; Sheskin, 2000).

That said, when any two or all three assumptions underlying parametric statistical tests are violated, parametric approaches to data analysis are no longer valid, and nonparametric techniques should be applied. Based upon the statistical literature, Cicchetti (1994b; pp. 601–607) provided guidelines to define what constitutes a meaningful departure from the underlying assumptions of a given parametric test. For a comparison of sample sizes, the criterion would be a difference of three times or more (e.g., sample size 1 is comprised of 20 individuals and the second sample contains 60 subjects). A meaningful difference in variances in this instance would be a factor of 4-to-1, or greater, for example, the variance of sample 1 is 4 and that of the second sample is 18. And a meaningful difference in sample distributions would be qualitative, such as one sample being normally distributed, the other following a distribution skewed heavily to the right.

This reasoning is similar to that of Jacob Cohen (1988) who noted the following:

> *In the formal development of the* t *distribution for the difference between two independent means, the assumption is made that the populations sampled are normally distributed and that they are of homogeneous (i.e., equal) variance. Moderate departures from these assumptions, however, have generally negligible effects on the validity of both Type I and Type II error calculations. This is particularly true for nondirectional tests and as sample sizes increase above 20 or 30 cases. The only noteworthy exception to the above is under the condition of substantially unequal variances together with substantially unequal sample sizes (whether small or large). Summaries of the evidence in regard to the 'robustness' of the* t *and (and F) test is provided by Scheffé (1959, Chapter 10), and in less technical terms, by Cohen (1965, pp. 114–115). See also Boneau 1960, 1962 (pp. 19–20).*

For more details on this issue, the interested reader is referred to Toothaker (1991, Chapter 4) on violations of assumptions underlying parametric tests and robustness in the context of appropriate and recommended multiple comparison methods.

One notable albeit unusual example of when nonparametric statistics should be chosen over their parametric analogues was given very recently by the late Alvan Feinstein.

In his last biostatistics textbook (Feinstein, 2002, pp. 285–286), presents data from two hypothetical groups whose mean values are being compared by both the parametric t test for independent groups and the nonparametric counterpart, the Mann–Whitney U test. The data shown below fit the condition of highly discrepant variances, coupled with a difference in the shape of the two sample distributions (Group A data is highly skewed because of an extreme outlying value and that deriving from Group B is much more evenly distributed and essentially non-skewed):

Group A: 15, 16, 16, 16, 17, 18, 19, 70   **Mean = 23.75;   Variance = 356.45**
Group B: 21, 23, 25, 27, 29, 32, 33, 37   **Mean = 28.375; Variance = 29.**

Application of the independent groups t test produces a nonsignificant t value of only 0.67, which does not even approach statistical significance at the conventional probability level of 0.05. However, the application of the Mann–Whitney U test (which converts the raw data into ranks) produces a two-tailed probability level of <0.05, and is, therefore, statistically significant.

Further, it should be noted that because these extreme examples rarely occur in most biomedical research applications, Sheskin (2000, p. 434), in his *Handbook of Parametric and Nonparametric Statistics* (see Cicchetti, 2002a, for a review) is correct when he states that ...

In the final analysis, the debate concerning whether one should employ a parametric or nonparametric test for a specific experimental design turns out to be of little consequence in most instances. The reason for this is that under most circumstances when a parametric test and its nonparametric analogue are employed to evaluate the same set of data, they lead to identical or similar conclusions.

B. Conceptual Links to Parametric Data Analytic Strategies

As noted by Borenstein (1998) tests of statistical significance can all be conceptualized as 'variations on the theme' that can be defined as:

$$\text{Test Statistic} = \frac{\text{Observed difference}}{\text{Dispersion of the difference}}$$

In the parametric case, as one example, the numerator might be the difference between two sample averages, or means; and the denominator might be a pooled average of the two sample standard errors of the mean difference. This would define the standard t test for independently derived means.

Swinscow applied this concept to a series of biostatistical articles that were published originally in the British Medical Journal (*BJM*) in 1976, and showed that other statistics follow the same form, namely, the differences between two percentages, two correlation coefficients, and so forth. Another general principle that applies here is that whatever the two entities that one is comparing, a value of 2 will always produce a level of statistical significance at the conventional probability level of 0.05, whether deriving from a t test (with $N > 60$) or Z test (with any size n).

The *BJM* series was then extended and revised in a medical statistical textbook entitled *Statistics at Square One*, by the same author, with revisions and new editions published between 1976 and 1996. Swinscow's simple numeric applications required only the availability of a hand calculator. The topics introduced, one short chapter at a time were: Tabulation and mean; Standard deviation; Populations and samples; Statements of probability; Differences between means; Percentages and paired alternatives; the t test; the χ^2 tests; Fisher's Exact Probability test; the Nonparametric Rank Sum tests; Correlation and Regression; Rank correlation; and finally, what Swinscow referred to as "Unwieldy numbers". For a recent extension of Swinscow's work, see Abbott's (2002) review of Campbell's (2001) text: *Statistics at square two: Understanding modern statistical applications in medicine*.

It is important to stress that the concept put forward by Swinscow and Borenstein can be further generalized to the analysis of variance (ANOVA) and its various and sundry models. The only conceptual difference is that the numerator now represents the overall differences *among three or more mean values* and the denominator is a pooled average of the variability or dispersion within the multiple groups. Finally, the same concept can be applied to multiple regression models that would include much more complex multivariate techniques, such as the following: standard ordinary least squares multiple regression, hierarchical regression, curvilinear regression, hierarchical linear modeling, individual growth curve analysis, and structural equation modeling.

Thus, parametric statistics, both univariate and multivariate in form can be understood and reduced conceptually to a simple ratio of the difference between or among two or more entities divided by the standard error of that difference. Whether that difference has any practical or clinical meaning in addition to having occurred beyond chance expectancy is quite another matter, and a topic that will be examined later in the text.

C. Conceptual Links to Nonparametric Data Analytic Strategies

Whereas the same general formula of Borenstein (1998) would also apply to nonparametric tests, Leach (1979) introduced a concept in the numerator that derives from a two column by two row, or so-called four-fold, contingency table containing the four cells, beginning with the upper left-hand corner, designated as cell a, the second cell in the same row, designated as b, the lower left hand cell, designated as c, and the last cell designated as cell d.

This *numerator* is the difference between the product of cells a and d and the corresponding product of cells b and c, which produces $(ad - bc)$. The denominator again represents an estimate of the dispersion about this difference.

Leach then equates this numerator to the symbol S. This becomes the numerator for a series of nonparametric tests, with the denominator being the differentiating property that separates one test from another. The concept of S, or its equivalent $(ad - bc)$, in the four-fold case, is then used to describe and apply a variety of nonparametric statistical tests, including: Chi square (d); Fischer's Exact test; other, less well-known tests of association, such as Delta and Gamma; the Wilcoxon Rank-Sum Test (the nonparametric analogue of the t test for independent groups), the Wilcoxon Signed-Rank Test (the nonparametric analogue of the paired t test), the Binomial test, the McNemar test for correlated proportions, the Gart test for order effects, and a number of nonparametric tests that compare more than two groups, having as their parametric counterpart some variant of the analysis of variance such as the Kruskal–Wallis test for comparing independent groups, the Friedman test (for correlated groups), several tests of correlation, the phi coefficient, the kappa statistic, Kendall's Tau (in its various forms), Spearman's rank-order statistic (Rho), and several tests of trend (the Gart test, the Mann test, and the Jonckheere test in its various forms). For further details about some of the more esoteric or arcane of these statistical tests, the interested reader is referred to Leach (1979), and to the scholarly and comprehensive text of Sheskin (2000).

Chapter IV

SCALES OF MEASUREMENT

A. Overview

The purpose of this chapter is to focus on the critical role of scales of measurement in biobehavioral research, in general, and clinical and experimental neuropsychology, in particular. In order to accomplish this objective, we first examine the seminal work of S.S. ('Smitty') Stevens' quadripartite classification of scales of measurement and then deal with the question of whether the underpinning or theoretical rationale behind their development is, in fact, feasible and valid.

B. The S.S. Stevens' Quadripartite System of Pure Scales of Measurement: Nominal, Ordinal, Equal Interval, and Equal Ratio Scales

In three now-classic publications, S.S. Stevens (1946, 1951, 1968) put forth his classification of scales of measurement into nominal, ordinal, equal interval, and equal ratio. The system was considered hierarchical at two levels: first, as a function of the increasing complexity of the scales, from nominal to ordinal, to equal interval, to equal ratio; and second, according to the putative corresponding increase in the quality of the scientific value of the information produced by each successive scale. The direct implication here is that variables measured on equal ratio scales produce the most reliable and valid information, followed in decreasing order by equal interval, ordinal, and nominal scales.

The first issue, that of the increasing complexity of the scales, can be conceptualized, as follows. Each successive scale incorporates all the classification features of each preceding scale, and then adds a unique defining feature of its own, thereby systematically increasing the structural complexity of the scale. The unique feature of ordinal scales is a ranking of the nominal categories. The next scale in the hierarchy adds the unique feature of equality of measured intervals, above and beyond its ordinal and nominal features. Finally, the most complex of the scales adds the unique feature of equal ratio of measurements, while also retaining its equal interval, ordinal, and nominal features.

The simplest of scales, the *nominal* scale, pertains to variables that measure a particular dimension that can be classified into two or more categories that are qualitatively different. The classic example used by Stevens is the assignment of arbitrary numbers to the jerseys that are worn by sports team players. Biobehavioral analogues would include the diagnoses of Autism or Nonverbal Learning Disabilities as present or absent. An early example deriving from the psychotherapy literature is the nominal classification of a given psychotherapist's voice quality as one of the following: Emotional, Focused, Externalizing, or Limited (Rice & Wagstaff, 1967).

Ordinal scales are next in the hierarchy of structural complexity. Variables measured on this type of scale incorporate the nominal classification procedure but, unlike the simplest form of scale, they add the defining feature of the classification categories bearing a rank-ordered relationship to each other. Stevens' classic example of ordinal scale measurement was a hardness scale for classifying rocks on the basis of a 'scratch' test that enables one to determine how the rocks compare, one to the other, in terms of degree of softness or hardness (e.g., very soft, somewhat soft, slightly soft, slightly hard, somewhat hard, very hard). This type of measurement deals with the issue of degrees of 'more' or 'less,' as applied to any possible pairing of two stones measured on such a scale. Specifically, the greatest difference would be between a 'very hard' and a 'very soft' rock; whereas those rocks classified into adjacent categories would vary the least among each other. A biobehavioral example of a variable measured on an ordinal scale might be the extent of Phobic Anxiety, classified as Slight, Moderate, or Severe.

Equal-interval scales retain both the nominal and ordinal classification features, and have as their unique defining characteristic that intervals that are the same distance apart can be treated as equal. The example given by Stevens is the Fahrenheit temperature scale. Thus, the 10-degree difference between 70° and 80° is equal to the difference between 50° and 40°, or 10° in each case. An example from biobehavioral research would be a total IQ score.

As implied from the preceding, *equal-ratio* scales retain the nominal, rank ordering, and equal-interval properties of the three previous scales, and add the defining feature of expressing scores at the various points on the scale in terms of ratios. An example given by Stevens and his disciples would be the variable 'length' (e.g., Bolanowski & Gescheider, 1991). Thus, it is accurate to state that a length of 60 inches is twice as long as one of 30 inches. Examples of well-known variables that are measured on an equal-ratio scale in biobehavioral research would be systolic or diastolic blood pressure, gestation age of newborn infants, and years of formal education.

Whereas the equal-interval/equal-ratio distinction is both theoretically and technically correct, one can, and should, question the distinction from a *practical* point of view. As Embretson and Hershberger (1999) correctly note:

> *Stevens distinguished ratios from intervals. But logarithms of ratios are intervals. And exponential intervals are ratios. If we have one, we have the other (p. 67).*

It is also the case that the distinction between interval and ratio-scaled variables is not necessary for choosing among data analytic strategies. One is as likely to apply the same parametric technique (e.g., t-test, ANOVA) in either case. What differs is the interpretation of the results. As one example, one would not interpret a mean IQ of 90 as twice as high as one of 45.

The second property of Stevens' scales of measurement is in terms of the putative scientific accuracy of variables measured on nominal, ordinal, and equal-interval scales. In Stevens' conceptualization, as the scale of measurement becomes more complex and inclusive, so does its scientific usefulness in terms of reliability and accuracy of the information that is produced.

To carry the concept further, scientific areas of inquiry have been classified and hierarchized according to the frequency with which their variables of study derived from these four scales. This meant that the natural sciences, such as Physics and Chemistry, that have a heavy reliance on the usage of equal-interval and equal-ratio scales, have often been viewed as the 'hard' sciences, as contrasted to the so-called 'soft' sciences of Education, Political Science, Sociology, and Psychology, whose variables are often measured on ordinal and nominal scales (Chase, 1970). This belief still holds sway in some scientific quarters. In the next section, we discuss the need for a revision of Stevens' conceptualizations of scales of measurement and science, more generally.

C. The Relevance and Place of Stevens' Conceptualization of Scales of Measurement in Biobehavioral Research

In this section we critically re-evaluate the role and relevance of Stevens' classification of scales of measurement in the current context of behavioral and medical research. There are a number of relevant facts and arguments that one can invoke to question seriously this quadripartite approach. These include, but are not limited, to the following: (1) There are more than four scales of measurement; (2) There is no basis for the belief that scales of measurement can be compared in terms of scientific usefulness; (3) There is no basis for the belief that so-called 'hard sciences' produce data that are inherently more reliable and valid than that produced by the so-called 'soft sciences'; and (4) The *same* variable can and will be defined on very *different* scales of measurement depending upon which scale will produce the more meaningful and valid results in a specific research context.

1. There are more than four scales of measurement
There are more than four scales of measurement, and this holds true whether or not one agrees with the Embretson and Hershberger (1999) insight that combines interval and ratio scales into the broader category of interval scales per se. More specifically, Embretson and Hershberger cite the philosophical literature to arrive at two levels of scientific awareness or consciousness that

precede Stevens' (1946) first level of measurement, namely, the nominal or naming scale of measurement. These both derive from the classification of Buchler (1940).

The first of these is referred to by Embretson and Hershberger (1999, p. 66) as ... "a private fancy, a flash of thought, a wild hypothesis ... It is the seed of creativity." In Buchler's six levels of classification of scientific level of awareness, it is referred to as a "possible ICON."

The second pre-nominal level of scientific awareness is one in which the previous 'wild idea' begins to acquire some level of meaning, in the specific sense that the idea is one that is thought about over and over again, and is one that has been thought about by others. However, it is not possible, at this stage of thought, to be able to point to the idea in a more concrete sense. As Embretson and Hershberger (1999), note ... 'It is still a quality.' This stage of scientific consciousness is designated as a "possible INDEX" (p. 66).

The third, fourth, and fifth levels of scientific awareness are designated as "factual INDEX", "possible SYMBOL", and "factual SYMBOL", and both predate and mirror, respectively, Stevens' (1946) nominal, ordinal, and interval/ratio scales of measurement.

A sixth scale of measurement derives from the bifurcation of ordinal scales into separate and distinct levels. Thus, Cicchetti (1976) demonstrated that there are two types of scales for measuring ordinal variables. This was explicated within the context of symptomatology scales but, as we shall see, has wider relevance for biobehavioral research in general. Specifically, one can differentiate between those ordinal variables that have three or more levels of 'presence' of a given entity (e.g., a patient's symptomatic level of anxiety) and those symptoms that have an 'absence' category, followed by two or more ordered categories of 'presence' of that same symptom.

To illustrate, suppose that a person's level of anxiety is being measured on the aforementioned ordinal scale, with specific criteria for distinguishing levels of 'slight,' 'moderate,' and 'severe.' Suppose further that multiple independent assessments are made on a group of subjects and we wish to examine the overall level of reliability of the scale. Examiner disagreements between 'slight' and 'moderate', it seems safe to say, are no more clinically serious than those between 'moderate' and 'severe.'

Let us contrast this with the diagnosis of extent of hallucinatory behavior, rank-ordered as 'None,' 'Slight,' 'Moderate,' and 'Severe.' Whereas the difference between 'Slight' and 'Moderate' still seems no more clinically serious than the difference between 'Moderate' and 'Severe,' the difference between 'None' and 'Slight' is far more serious clinically than the previous two differences, despite the fact that they are each one category apart. This is because it is much more serious to confuse presence of a symptom with its absence than to confuse degrees of presence of the symptom that are the same number of categories apart.

An example deriving from medicine further illustrates the point. Suppose two diagnosticians are examining the results of a patient's biopsy for presence of a particular type of cancer that can be classified as one of the following: 'Benign Tumor,' 'Malignant Tumor *in situ*' or 'Metastatic Cancer.' Clearly, a disagreement between 'Benign Tumor' and 'Malignant tumor *in situ*' is far more serious than a disagreement between 'Malignant Tumor *in situ*' and 'Metastatic Cancer' despite the fact that both disagreements are one category apart.

Cicchetti (1976) referred to the first type of scale (one without a point defining absence) as a Continuous-Ordinal scale of measurement and the latter as a Dichotomous-Ordinal scale, because of the dichotomy between presence and absence. Also, specific weighting systems were provided for reliability assessments so that a higher level of examiner agreement is assigned to degrees-of-presence discrepancies than to presence–absence discrepancies that are the same number of categories apart.

More broadly speaking, the dichotomous-ordinal scale of measurement can be classified as a 'mixed' scale of measurement, because it has both nominal (presence–absence) and ordinal (degrees of presence) features of a given symptom, trait, or other clinical entity. Cicchetti, Volkmar, Sparrow, Cohen, Fermanian, and Rourke (1992b) discuss how reliability assessment can be undertaken for variables deriving from mixed scales of measurement. An obvious example of such a mixed scale of measurement in clinical neuropsychology is the variable extent of brain damage or dysfunction that can be classified as none, mild, moderate, or severe. By adding the Cicchetti et al. (1992b) conceptualization of mixed scales of measurement to Buchler's classification of levels of scientific awareness, we now have six distinct levels of scientific awareness as reflected in scales of measurement.

Philosophically, one can ask the question: When does an ordinal variable, for all intents and purposes, function as an interval/ratio variable? This question was addressed empirically by Cicchetti, Showalter, and Tyrer (1985), who demonstrated that seven category ordinal scales were no less reliable than those containing many more categories or scale points (e.g., 10, 15, ..., 100). These results were corroborated by the more recent findings of Preston and Colman (2000).

Whereas Stevens' (1946) classification terminates at the level of interval and/or ratio scales, Buchler's classification adds a further level that is referred to as an "arguable SYMBOL." This is the 'final' stage in which variables are not treated on a mere unitary basis (as is true of the preceding six levels of scientific awareness), but in a relational context so that the development of theory can begin to occur. As Embretson and Hershberger (1999) query... "What good is one variable, if it does not lead to another?" (p. 68). Or, as Rourke has argued, and Cicchetti certainly agrees, science is often about questions, not answers.

In the context of relevant data analytic strategies, one can argue that the first six levels of scientific awareness pertain to single variables of classification and would be understood in terms of descriptive statistics that would include simple displays of means, medians, modes, and frequency distributions. The seventh level of scientific consciousness would lead to inferential statistics of one form or another, and would include the entire armamentarium of univariate and multi-variate data analytic strategies.

2. There is no basis for the belief that scales of measurement can be compared meaningfully in terms of their relative scientific usefulness

Stevens' stated belief (1946, 1951, 1968) was that for quality of scientific usefulness, specifically, reliability and accuracy of measurement, variables measured on equal-ratio scales are superior to those measured on equal-interval scales which, in turn, are superior to those deriving from ordinal scales, and, finally, that variables measured on nominal scales are the most useless of all from a scientific standpoint. Specifically, Stevens (1946) noted the following:

> *The nominal scale is a primitive form, and quite naturally there are many who will urge that it is absurd to attribute to this process of assigning numerals the dignity implied by the term measurement. Certainly there can be no quarrel with this objection, for the naming of things is an arbitrary business (p. 679).*

The early influence that this reasoning had upon other scientists is reflected in the words of Coombs (1953) who stated that the nominal "level of measurement is so primitive that it is not always characterized as measurement, *but it is a necessary condition for all higher levels of measurement*" (p. 473).

In a much more recent publication, Grimm and Yarnold (1995, p. 6) note their endorsement of the Stevens' and Coombs' disdain for nominal scale measurement.

Despite the sentiment just expressed, it is readily demonstrated that the level of reliability and/or validity of a given clinical variable cannot be distinguished on the basis of whether the variable was measured on a nominal, ordinal, equal interval, or equal-ratio scale. Thus, an expert's diagnosis of presence or absence of autism on the basis of DSM-IV or ICD-10 criteria can be more reliable than a total cholesterol reading, despite the fact that autism is measured on the simplest of scales (nominal-dichotomous) and cholesterol on the most complex of scales (equal-ratio). In fact, as Kraemer, Kazdin, Offord, Kessler, Jensen, and Kupfer (1997) have correctly noted, the most critical medical decisions tend to be binary (nominal-dichotomous in nature).

3. There is no basis for the belief that so-called 'hard sciences' produce data that are inherently more reliable and valid than those produced by the so-called 'soft sciences'

This is because the particular scale upon which a given variable is measured does not define its scientific usefulness, in terms of level of either reliability or validity. Indeed, in a recently terminated multicenter trial in the USA and Canada, the reliabilities of IQ measurements over a nine-year period were considerably higher than a number of 'hard' measurements such as fundus photographs and cholesterol levels.

4. The *same* variable can and will be defined on very *different* scales of measurement depending upon which scale will produce the more meaningful and valid results within a specific research or clinical context

As one specific example, if a physician wanted to know the meaning of the total cholesterol reading for a given patient, say one of 225 mg/dl, she/he would *not* be interpreting it on the basis of the equal-ratio scale upon which it was measured. Rather, the physician would use the tri-partite ordinal scale that classifies total cholesterol readings as one of the following: Ideal (<200 mg/dl); Borderline (200–239 mg/dl); or High (240 mg/dl and above). Thus, the patient's total cholesterol reading of 225 mg/dl would be classified as Borderline. It is of further interest that these clinical cut-points derive from research relating total cholesterol values to the probability of a myocardial infarct.

Suppose, instead, that a clinical investigator wished to study the association between total cholesterol level and age at first myocardial infarct in a representative sample of American males between the ages of 30 and 75. In this instance, it would not be prudent to measure the predictor variable on the aforementioned ordinal scale because this truncation would serve to attenuate the size of the correlation. In this instance the scale of measurement of choice would be an interval, here equal-ratio scale, defined in continuous increments of milligrams per deciliter.

As a third and much more complex usage of clinical scales in a form well suited to providing useful results, consider the clinical classification system (Cicchetti, 2001; pp. 662–667) for interpreting the strength of kappa and R_i and related indexes of interexaminer reliability: The percentage of observed agreement (PO) values use a four-category numeric ordinal scale (<70%, 70–79%, 80–89% and 90–100%). This ordinal scale derives from an equal-ratio scale ranging between 0% and 100%. The chance-corrected reliability coefficients are expressed on a second numeric ordinal scale that derives from another equal ratio scale, ranging essentially between -1 and $+1$. The levels of strength (Poor, Fair, Good, Excellent) are based on a verbal, or non-numeric ordinal scale. The name of the phenomenon that is being measured (Strength of K, K_w, and R_i Values) represents the very simplest of all measuring scales, namely, a single category nominal scale! Thus, it can be seen the extent to which scales of measurement will be altered in any given research context in order to provide clinical meaningfulness to the obtained results.

In summary, despite its enormous contribution to science, when re-evaluated according to today's level of scientific knowledge, Stevens' quadripartite classification of scales of measurement is incomplete. We have, in fact, shown that there are at least six or seven rather than the four scales of measurement identified by Stevens. It is also quite likely that additional scales of measurement will be identified and reported in the subsequent scientific literature. Further, there is no preferred or superior scale of measurement. It is further understood that without mixed scales of measurement (e.g., those having both nominal and ordinal features) many clinical phenomena could not be reliably or validly evaluated. The research context itself, rather than purely theoretical arguments and conjectures, dictates the scale upon which a variable is most appropriately measured. Finally, expressing clinical variables on appropriate scales of measurement enhances the probability of correctly designing and executing clinical research objectives, selecting appropriate biostatistical tests, and drawing reliable and valid study conclusions.

It should be noted that Stevens' fundamental arguments about scales of measurements continue to influence the leading psychophysicists of today, as exemplified by the opening statement made by Bolanowski and Gescheider (1991) in their introduction to the edited text *Ratio Scaling of Psychological Magnitude: In Honor of the Memory of S.S. Stevens:*

> *It is generally agreed that the highest form of measurement is achieved with ratio scales typified by the well-established scales used in the physical sciences such as those used for measuring length and mass (p. 1).*

For all of the reasons just presented, we do not agree with either S.S. Stevens or his present-day disciples in their evaluation of the utility of Stevens' classification of scales of measurement.

Chapter V

RELIABILITY

A. Definition

Reliability refers to the extent to which multiple independent assessments of the same (clinical) phenomena can be substituted, one for the other; or, put another way, the extent of replicability, or duplicability of independently derived measurements.

B. Types of Reliability Assessments/Research Designs

1. Measures of internal consistency and caveats for interpreting what they mean

Measures of internal consistency provide information about the extent to which items in a test, domain, or subdomain 'hang together' or are inter-correlated. Cronbach (1951) introduced two correlation coefficients, in the form of the Kuder–Richardson (KR-20) formula for dichotomous data and Coefficient Alpha for ordinally scaled data, to measure this degree of what we might term interrelatedness of items. The actual size of the resulting correlation is a function not only of the extent to which the items are inter-correlated, but also on the number of items in the test (Nunnally, 1978).

Caveat 1: These two statistics measure correlation or association, *not* agreement as is the case for actual reliability assessment. In this basic sense, the term, reliability, as measured by these two statistics, is a misnomer. Thus, if two independent examiners use a five-category ordinal scale to rate three subjects on a given trait and the paired ratings, respectively, for examiners A and B are 1–3, 2–4, and 3–5, the correlation will be perfect, giving a value of 1.00. This obtains despite the fact that the two examiners are consistently two categories apart. For further explication and differentiation between correlation and agreement, see Cicchetti (1994a) and Fleiss (1981, Chapter 13).

Caveat 2: Even taken and understood correctly as measures of correlation or association, measures of internal consistency will be *artifactually* lowered by the well known clinical phenomena of floor and ceiling effects.

Caveat 3: Because of the problems just cited, Coefficient Alpha cannot be meaningfully substituted for a true measure of reliability, such as the level of inter-examiner reliability. High internal consistency of test items is *not* synonymous with high inter-examiner reliability.

Taking into account the arguments just presented, when applied appropriately the size of the resulting Coefficient Alpha (or its KR-20 special case) can be evaluated in terms of its practical or clinical significance by the following set of criteria (Cicchetti, 1994a):

Criteria for Interpreting Internal Consistency Coefficients.

Size of coefficient	Clinical significance
<0.70	Poor
0.70–0.79	Fair
0.80–0.89	Good
0.90–1.00	Excellent

For a more comprehensive discussion of further conditions under which Coefficient Alpha and related statistics should be viewed as appropriate or inappropriate (and therefore invalid) measures in behavioral and biomedical research, the interested reader is referred to the recent work of Rubin (2002).

2. Intra-examiner (test–retest) reliability
The simplest form of reliability is the extent to which a given examiner agrees with her/his own previous assessment of a given phenomenon. Although this form of agreement is not a substitute for inter-examiner agreement, it has application for tests or clinical instruments that qualify as self-reports. Also, this form of reliability can be useful as a screening guide when a clinical investigator is in the market for choosing a test-examiner. As Detre, Wright, Murphy, and Takaro (1975) stated, if a given examiner fails to agree well with his/her own previous ratings, one can hardly expect him to agree with other independent examiners of the same phenomenon.

3. Inter-examiner reliability
This is the standard or prototypic reliability research design in which one assesses the level of agreement between two or more independent clinical examiners who investigate the same phenomenon.

4. Temporal reliability
Though not as frequently employed as either test–retest or inter-examiner agreement, this form of agreement is applicable to a reliability research design in which one is measuring both the extent of agreement among independent examiners at each of two or more time periods and the extent to which the assessments may vary over time. This usage of more than one examiner, at each assessment period,

is essential in order to distinguish between phenomena that are or are not expected to change over time. Providing a measure of inter-examiner agreement at each time period prevents the confounding of changes over time that are real, as opposed to those that may occur because of unreliable examiner ratings at any one of the assessment periods. Unfortunately, this design strategy is not often undertaken in research investigating temporal reliability or the stability of measurements over time.

5. Caveats for interpreting the correct meaning of intra-examiner, inter-examiner, and temporal reliability indices

Caveat 1: In designing either a *test–retest* or an *inter-examiner* reliability research design, it is important for the clinical investigator to understand the *phenomenon* being measured, as well as the study population, in order to be able to select test time intervals in an optimal manner. To the extent possible, one needs to rule out artifactually high levels of reliability that occur simply because the subject remembered at the second assessment the material to which she/he was exposed at the initial assessment.

Caveat 2: With respect to the assessment of temporal reliability, one needs to select either the same pair of examiners at each time point (preferably), or at least two different pairs of examiners who are trained to the same level of high reliability. This precaution again enables the investigator to distinguish changes over time that are real as opposed to those caused by the unreliability of the examiners.

C. Kappa Statistics as Chance-Corrected Reliability Coefficients

As Fleiss (1981) and, more recently, Fleiss, Levin, and Cho Paik (2003) have noted, whenever two or more independent judgments are made on the same person or object, one can expect a certain amount of agreement to occur on the basis of chance alone. Thus, if two examiners each apply a positive diagnosis to 10% of the cases and a negative one to each of the remaining 90%, it is easily shown that the two independent examiners will agree at a level of 82%, *by chance alone* (i.e., $[(0.9 \times 0.9) + (0.1 \times 0.1)] = 0.82 = 82\%$). In order to correct for this phenomenon, Scott (1955) developed a chance-corrected, inter-examiner reliability statistic that was designed to be used with nominal data.

Cohen (1960) built upon Scott's early work and developed a statistic that, without going into excessive detail, was an improvement with respect to the derivation of chance agreement. The statistic became known as Kappa. It has many variations to fit an array of differing reliability research designs and differing types of scales of measurement (Nominal, Ordinal, or Mixed). Despite the variations on the theme, all models of Kappa can be defined rather simply as the following:

Kappa = (PO − PC)/(1 − PC), in which:
PO = the Proportion of Observed Examiner Agreement (e.g., 0.90);
PC = the Proportion of Agreement by Chance Alone (e.g., 0.60); and

$(1 - PC)$ = the Maximum Amount of Chance-Corrected Agreement that is Possible.

Note: Here, Reliability = 0.30/0.40 = 0.75, which is Excellent by the criteria of both Cicchetti and Sparrow (1981) and Fleiss (1981).

In the final step of the process, the value of Kappa is divided by its standard error to produce a z test of the level of statistical significance of the Kappa value. As is true of the wide variety of statistics expressed as z, a value of 2 should be interpreted as having reached a level of statistical significance at the 0.05 level of probability, given an appropriately large sample size. Several biostatisticians working in the area of reliability assessment realized that just as is true with standard correlation coefficients, very small values of K (nominal variables), K_w (ordinal variables), or the intraclass correlation coefficient (R_i—ordinal or interval variables) will be highly statistically significant providing only that the sample size upon which they are based is sufficiently large. Because of this phenomenon, several researchers have put forth a set of criteria to be used to define levels of practical or clinical significance, or strength of agreement, above and beyond levels of mere statistical significance. The first was developed by Landis and Koch (1977) and later simplified by Fleiss (1981) and Cicchetti and Sparrow (1981). Because all three are quite consistent, we will utilize the one most recently developed (Cicchetti & Sparrow, 1981):

Size of K, K_w, R_i	Strength of agreement
<0.40	Poor
0.40–0.59	Fair
0.60–0.74	Good
≥0.75	Excellent

Caveat: The same K or K_w value can derive from a wide range of PO values (Cicchetti, 1988). Therefore, the Level of PO must also be part of the criteria for interpreting K or K_w.

This produces the following more comprehensive set of criteria (Cicchetti, 2001):

Level of K, K_w, R_i	% Agreement	Strength
<0.40	<70	Poor
0.40–0.59	70–79	Fair
0.60–0.74	80–89	Good
≥0.75	90–100	Excellent

D. Mathematical Relationships between Kappa and Kappa-Type Statistics

Fleiss (1975) demonstrated the conditions under which there is a mathematical equivalence between K and R_i for nominal-dichotomous variables and Fleiss and

Cohen (1973) showed the conditions under which there is a mathematical equivalence between K_w and R_i for ordinally scaled variables.

E. Kappa and Weighted Kappa in the Context of Single-Case Reliability Assessments

It has been amply documented in both the biostatistical and biomedical literature that major breakthroughs in scientific knowledge have often been accomplished through an in-depth study of a single case. As a frequently cited example in the field of biostatistics, Sir Ronald Fisher (1935) conducted a single-case experiment on a lady who claimed to be able to distinguish cups of tea within which the milk had been poured before the tea from those within which the milk was poured after the tea. From this now considered classical study in biostatistics, Fisher was able to derive the concepts of appropriate research design, randomization, sensitivity, and tests of statistical significance (Holschuh, 1980). For more information on this classic experiment and its importance to the development of the field of biostatistics, see Salsburg (2001).

In a second far-reaching single-case study, Broca, studying his patient 'Tan' discovered the area of the brain responsible for human speech, known eponymously as Broca's area. Broca's discovery is viewed as "heralding the beginning of modern neuropsychology" (Wilson, 1987).

In a series of recent studies, Cicchetti and colleagues have provided both the rationale and the means to determine levels of reliability when multiple examiners assess independently the same single case.

In the first of these studies, Cicchetti, Showalter, and Rosenheck (1997), outlined the methodology and applied it to a hypothetical case using a computer program reported in Cicchetti and Showalter (1997). In a second study, the method was applied to investigate inter-rater reliability levels among 39 clinical examiners who independently examined the same schizophrenic patient in three areas: quality of life, level of functioning, and level of psychiatric symptomatology (Cicchetti, Rosenheck, Showalter, Charney, & Cramer, 1999). In a third study, the method was applied to train 37 psychiatrists preparatory to participating in a clinical trial of the effects of antidepressant medication (Baca-Garcia, Blanco, Saiz-Ruiz, Rico, Diaz-Sastre, & Cicchetti, 2001).

Currently, the method is being used to produce Kappa or weighted Kappa values for the single case (Cicchetti, 2002b). This was made possible by using as chance agreement a value of 0.70, which Cicchetti and colleagues have defined as the minimally acceptable level of agreement that is clinically useful (Cicchetti, 1994b, 2001; Volkmar, Cicchetti, Dykens, Sparrow, Leckman, & Cohen, 1988). Using, again, a value of 0.40 as the minimal level of clinically acceptable chance-corrected agreement (e.g., Cicchetti, 2001), the minimally acceptable level of inter-examiner agreement would be 82%, since $(0.82 - 0.70)/0.30 = 0.40$.

For current updating of the role of Kappa and its many variations, the interested reader is referred to the scholarly tutorial on the role of Kappa coefficients in biomedical research by Kraemer, Periyakoil, and Noda (2002). For an explanation and resolution of the paradoxes that can occur when the level of inter-rater agreement is high (say, greater than 85%), but Kappa is very low (e.g., well below 0.40), the interested reader is referred to Cicchetti (1988), Cicchetti and Feinstein (1990), and Feinstein and Cicchetti (1990).

F. Computer Programs for Making Reliability Assessments

The programs consist of appropriate models of Kappa, weighted Kappa and the Intraclass correlation coefficient (R_i) and the aforementioned new technique for assessing the reliability or accuracy of independent clinical judgments when multiple examiners evaluate a single case. These programs enable the investigator to assess levels of intra- or inter-examiner reliability and examiner bias whether the data are measured on: nominal scales (Kappa—Cohen, 1960; Fleiss, 1981; Fleiss, Cohen, & Everrit, 1969; Fleiss, Nee, & Landis, 1979); ordinal or mixed scales (weighted Kappa—Cohen, 1968; Fleiss, 1981; Fleiss, Cohen, & Everitt, 1969) using appropriate standard errors reported in Cicchetti, 1981; Cicchetti and Fleiss, 1977; Fleiss and Cicchetti, 1978; or Continuous/Interval/Dimensional scales of measurement (Bartko, 1966, 1976; Fleiss, 1981).

Computer programs developed for these purposes are described in Cicchetti, Aivano, and Vitale (1976, 1977); Cicchetti, Lee, Fontana, and Dowds (1978); Cicchetti and Heavens (1979); and Heavens and Cicchetti (1978).

Specialized programs are also available to assess reliability when varying numbers of multiple examiners independently evaluate multiple subjects, and the data are measured on a nominal scale (Fleiss, 1971; Fleiss, Nee, & Landis, 1979) using a computer program described in Cicchetti, Heavens, Didriksen, and Showalter, 1984; as well as when one wishes to determine the significance of the difference between two independently derived Kappa or weighted Kappa values (Fleiss & Cicchetti, 1978) using a computer program described in Heavens and Cicchetti (1979). In addition, a specialized computer program has been developed to assess independently derived kappa or weighted Kappa values, on a subject-by-subject basis (Cicchetti, Showalter, & McCarthy, 1990).

Cicchetti and Showalter (1997) have described a computer program to assess levels of reliability and bias when multiple independent examiners evaluate a single case (Baca-Garcia et al., 2001; Cicchetti, Showalter, & Rosenheck, 1997; Cicchetti, Rosenheck, Showalter, Charney, & Cramer, 1999).

Concerning quantitative data, a program is available to assess inter-examiner reliability and systematic levels of examiner bias when the data are measured on continuous or interval scales (Cicchetti, Aivano, & Vitale, 1976; Cicchetti & Showalter, 1988). It uses models of the intra-class correlation coefficient that distinguish research designs in which the same examiners evaluate each subject from ones in which different sets of examiners are used. A specialized computer program was also developed to determine the reliability of interval-scale data when the numbers and specific sets of examiners may vary at each assessment (Cicchetti & Showalter, 1988).

G. Invalid Reliability Statistics: Kendall's Tau; Spearman's Rho; and the Pearson Product–Moment Correlation (PPMC)

The basic problem with each of these statistical approaches is that they involve the fundamental error of confusing agreements in *rank-orderings* of pairs of ratings with the level of agreement between the actual ratings (or scores) themselves. Whereas the aforementioned presentation of the work of Cicchetti (1994a) focuses upon the misuse of the PPMC, the same argument applies to the other two indices and their variations. A further problem is that once one converts a true assessment value (e.g., an IQ score) into a ranking, then much specific information is lost in the process. In effect, the variable no longer has meaning in terms of its actual numeric value. Thus, although Tau, Rho, and the PPMC are all *valid* measures of *correlation*, or *association*, they are *not* appropriate as measures of *agreement* and should therefore not be used for such purposes.

In the next section of the text, we introduce, with brief descriptions, 11 papers appearing in *JCEN, TCN,* and *CN* during the period 1992–2003. Each of these previous publications illustrates one or more important aspects of the reliability process, the problems posed, and the solutions that have been proposed.

... ...

Chapter VI

EDITORS' COMMENTARIES INTRODUCING SELECTED ARTICLES ON RELIABILITY ASSESSMENT PUBLISHED IN *JCEN*, *TCN*, AND *CN* BETWEEN 1992 AND 2003

Cicchetti, Volkmar, Sparrow, Cohen, Fermanian, and Rourke (1992b; pp. 27–36) is an illustration of how reliability can be assessed when the scales of interest have both nominal and ordinal features. Brown, Del Dotto, Fisk, Taylor, and Breslau (1993; pp. 37–44) examine the agreement among pediatric neuropsychologists when rating the functioning of normal and low birth-weight children in seven neuropsychological domains. Bowden, Whelan, Long, and Clifford (1995; pp. 45–48) deal with the issue of temporal stability. Franzen, Haut, Rankin, and Keefover (1995; pp. 49–52) and Franzen, Paul, and Iverson (1996; pp. 53–56) address the issue of alternate forms of reliability. Carter, Shore, Harnadek, and Kubu (1998; pp. 57–60) contains a simple demonstration of inter-rater reliability. Cicchetti, Rosenheck, Showalter, Charney, and Cramer (1999; pp. 61–73) address the issue of inter-rater reliability of a large number of raters for the single case. Demsky and Sellers (1995; pp. 74–77) demonstrate how reliability can be improved. Maassen (2000; pp. 78–87) addresses the issue of defining reliable change indices. McSweeny, Naugle, Chelune, and Lüders (1993; pp. 88–97) offer a somewhat different approach to the determination of the reliability of change in clinical neuropsychology. And finally, Winegarden, Yates, Moses, Benton, and Faustman (1998; pp. 98–100) develop an optimally reliable short form of a well-known neuropsychological test.

Journal of Clinical and Experimental Neuropsychology
1992, Vol. 14, No. 5, pp. 673–686

Assessing the Reliability of Clinical Scales When the Data Have Both Nominal and Ordinal Features: Proposed Guidelines for Neuropsychological Assessments*

Domenic V. Cicchetti[1], Fred Volkmar[2], Sara S. Sparrow[2], Donald Cohen[2],
Jacques Fermanian[3], and Byron P. Rourke[4]

[1]West Haven VA Medical Center and Yale University, [2]Yale Child Study Center,
[3]Necker Hospital, Paris, France and [4]University of Windsor

ABSTRACT

The purpose of this article is to present, for the first time, a comprehensive methodology for assessing the reliability of a clinical scale that is frequently utilized in neuropsychological research and in biomedical studies, more generally. The dichotomous-ordinal scale is characterized by a single category of "absence" and two or more ordinalized categories of "presence" of a symptom trait, state, or behavior, and it also has special properties that need to be understood in order for its reliability to be appropriately assessed. Using the Brief Psychiatric Rating Scale (BPRS) as a clinical example, we cover the principles of expressing scale reliability in terms of a dichotomy ("absence"-"presence" of a given BPRS symptom); as a trichotomy ("none"; "mild to moderate" symptomatology; and "severe" symptomatology); and as the full 7-category dichotomous-ordinal scale: "none," "very mild," "mild," "moderate," "moderately severe," "severe," and "extremely severe." Criteria are presented that can be used to evaluate which of these three formats produces the most reliable results. Finally, we address, with a second sample, the important issue of replication, or whether the original reliability findings generalize to other independent populations.

Ordinal scales are often used in neuropsychological research, and in biomedical research, more generally. As noted earlier (Cicchetti, 1976) one subset of such scales consists of a dichotomous-ordinal format such that the scale is anchored at one end by the "absence" of a symptom and at the other by "severe" symptomatology. Additional descriptors, such as "mild" and "moderate," are used to define the intervening gradient of symptomatology. For purposes of interexaminer reliability assessment, disagreements between the absence and mild expression of a symptom (e.g., visual hallucinations) is clinically much more serious than disagreements between either "mild" and "moderate" or between "moderate" and "severe" expressions of that same symptom. Examples of dichotomous-ordinal scales

abound in the neuropsychology literature (e.g., the Brief Psychiatric Rating Scale (BPRS) (Overall & Gorham, 1962; Overall & Klett, 1972); the Present State Examination (PSE) (Wing, Cooper, & Sartorius, 1974); the Behavior Inventory for Rating Development (BIRD–Sparrow & Cicchetti, 1984); the Vineland Adaptive Behavior Scales (Sparrow, Balla, & Cicchetti, 1984a; 1984b; 1985); the Childhood Autism Rating Scales (CARS–Schopler, Reichler, & Renner, 1986); the Personality Assessment Schedule (PAS–Tyrer, Alexander, Cicchetti, Cohen, & Remington, 1979; Cicchetti & Tyrer, 1988); the Hamilton Depression Rating Scale (Hamilton, 1960; Cicchetti & Prusoff, 1983; Williams, 1988); the Brief Scale of Anxiety (Tyrer, Owen, & Cicchetti, 1984); and

* Correspondence to be addressed to Domenic V. Cicchetti, Ph.D., Department of Veterans Affairs, Medical Center, 950 Campbell Avenue, West Haven, CT 06516, USA.
Accepted for publication: November 10, 1991.

the Structured Clinical Inter-view for DSM-III-R Dissociative Disorders (SCID-D–Steinberg, Rounsaville, & Cicchetti, 1990).

Prototypic dichotomous-ordinal scales in medicine would include the familiar Apgar scale for rating the clinical condition of a newborn infant (Apgar, 1953); and indices for classifying the severity of acute myocardial infarct (Horwitz, Cicchetti, & Horwitz, 1984; Killip & Kimball, 1967; Norris, Brandt, Caughey, Lee, & Scott, 1969). For a comprehensive and scholarly evaluation of the development, structure, and function of clinical rating scales, in general, the interested reader is referred to Feinstein (1987).

The purposes of this report are to describe, for the first time, a comprehensive set of guidelines for assessing the reliability of clinical rating scales fitting the DO classification. These guidelines will be applied to data deriving from the aforementioned BPRS, one of the most commonly utilized diagnostic instruments in behavioral science research. In order to accomplish study objectives, we will discuss (1) specific rater agreement weighting systems which distinguish dichotomous-ordinal clinical rating scales from more standard types of ordinal rating scales; (2) appropriate reliability statistics; and (3) available computer programs for performing the required reliability analyses.

EXAMINER AGREEMENT WEIGHTING SYSTEMS

Cicchetti (1976) – see also Cicchetti and Sparrow (1981) – introduced the concept of dichotomous-ordinal (DO) scales (such as the BPRS classification of visual hallucinations as "absent," "mild," "moderate" or "severe"). Such scales of measurement are to be differentiated from more standard clinical rating scales, or continuous-ordinal (CO) scales, such as the classification of levels of anxiety as "mild," "moderate" or "severe." From the point of view of assigning specific rater agreement weighting systems for a DO clinical rating scale, examiner confusion between "absent" and "mild" levels of hallucination is much more clinically serious than, say, confusion between "mild" and "moderate" levels of the same symptom. The critical clinical implication here is that examiner

disagreements about whether a given patient hallucinates or not ("absent" vs. "mild" in form) should be assigned *lower* agreement weights than those examiner disagreements over whether a given hallucination varies, to the same extent, in intensity only (e.g., "mild" vs. "moderate" or "moderate" vs. "severe" forms of the symptom). In stark contrast, the same phenomenon does not present for CO clinical rating scales. Thus, a disagreement between "mild" and "moderate" forms of anxiety seems no more clinically serious than that between "moderate" and "severe" forms.

A second major difference between CO and DO scales (not previously recognized in the neuropsychological or biomedical literature) is the critical distinction that DO (but *not* other types of ordinal scales) can be assessed for reliability (e.g., interexaminer agreement) at three basic levels of complexity:

1. As a simple dichotomy, in which a given symptom, trait, or behavior is classified by the two independent examiners as either 1 = "absent" or 2 = "present" (e.g., the extent to which the examiners agree or disagree that a patient does or does not hallucinate).
2. As a dichotomous-ordinal trichotomy (e.g., as 1 = "absent"; 2 = "mild to moderate"; or 3 = "severe") and, for scales of more than 3 cateogries.
3. As the full dichtomous-ordinal scale (e.g., the BPRS categories 1 = "absent"; 2 = "very mild"; 3 = "mild"; 4 = "moderate"; 5 = "moderately severe"; 6 = "severe"; and 7 = "extremely severe").

It should be noted further that data deriving from each one of these three scales of measurement can be assessed, for level of interexaminer agreement, at two levels: (1) as an *average* over the 2, 3, or more categories of classification; or (2) *separately* for each category of classification. It should be noted that this particular distinction is important for two basic reasons. The first is that even quite acceptable levels of agreement *averaged* over all categories of assessment can be associated with a wide range of levels of agreement of *specific* categories. The second is a more mathematical reason, namely, that overall agreement (averaged over all categories) is simply a weighted average over each of the various specific categories of classification (e.g., "none," "mild to moderate," "severe" symptomatology), thereby providing mathematical justification for separating overall examiner agreement from that on specific categories of classification.

CLINICAL EXAMPLES, USING THE BPRS

The data for this section of the report are based upon two sets of BPRS symptom ratings, one deriving from a U.S. sample and another deriving from a European (French) sample. Both sets of data were obtained prior to the availability of DSM-III or DSM-III-R diagnostic criteria for major psychiatric illnesses (American Psychiatric Association, 1987). Therefore, the extent to which the obtained results may or may not generalize to patients receiving such state-of-the-art diagnoses is unknown. However, this is not relevant to the focus of the paper, which is purely methodologic.

The full BPRS, consisting of 18 symptoms (Overall & Klett, 1972), was administered to 146 (U.S. sample) and 181 (French sample) adult patients of mixed psychiatric diagnoses by pairs of independent clinical examiners. (For purposes of analysis, these data will be treated as if the same two examiners were used to evaluate each patient.) The 18 symptoms, each rated on the previously defined 7-category dichotomous-ordinal scale, were as follows: (1) Somatic Concern; (2) Anxiety; (3) Emotional Withdrawal; (4) Conceptual Disorganization; (5) Guilt Feelings; (6) Suspiciousness; (7) Hallucinatory Behavior; (8)

Motor Retardation; (9) Uncooperativeness; (10) Unusual Thought; (11) Tension; (12) Mannerisms/Posturing; (13) Grandiosity; (14) Depressive Mood; (15) Hostility; (16) Blunted Affect; (17) Excitement; and (18) Disorientation.

The purpose of this section of the report is to explain, derive, and apply appropriate models of kappa statistics to, first, the U.S. sample, and then to examine whether the results generalize to the French sample. At appropriate places in the exposition, we will suggest specific criteria for addressing the statistical and clinical significance of the results.

In order to introduce the mathematical formulae required to undertake the three types of reliability assessment (dichotomy, trichotomy, full BPRS scale) we will utilize data deriving from both the U.S. and French samples, for one of the BPRS symptoms, "Hallucinatory Behavior."

Table 1 shows the full data for severity ratings of the 146 U.S. psychiatric patients on the BPRS symptom "Hallucinatory Behavior."

RELIABILITY BASED UPON A DICHOTOMY

Overall Agreement Levels
The most fundamental or basic question one can ask about the utility of a given diagnostic instrument is whether or not it can distinguish reliably between the "absence" and "presence" of a given disorder. The model for this dichotomy, as previously shown in Cicchetti (1988), is given in Table 2, and is expressed in numbers of cases for which two independent examiners are in agreement or disagreement

Table 1. Severity Ratings of Psychiatric Patients on the BPRS Symptom "Hallucinatory Behavior".

Examiner B	Examiner A							
	(1) None	(2) Very Mild	(3) Mild	(4) Moderate	(5) Moderately Severe	(6) Severe	(7) Extremely Severe	Totals
(1)	89	0	4	0	0	0	0	93
(2)	4	1	1	0	0	0	0	6
(3)	3	1	2	1	1	0	0	8
(4)	1	0	3	6	4	0	0	14
(5)	0	1	0	1	5	4	1	12
(6)	0	0	1	2	2	3	1	9
(7)	0	0	0	1	0	2	1	4
Total	97	3	11	11	12	9	3	146

Table 2. Interexaminer Agreement on the Absence or Presence of the BPRS Symptom "Hallucinatory Behavior".[1]

Diagnosis by Examiner B	Statistic	Diagnosis by Examiner A		Total $n_{i.}$
		Absent	Present	
Absent	W_{ij}	1.00	0.00	
	n_{ij}	89.00	4.00	93
	$(n_{i.}n_{.j})/n..$	61.79	31.21	
Present	W_{ij}	0.00	1.00	
	n_{ij}	8.00	45.00	53
	$(n_{i.}n_{.j})/n..$	35.21	17.79	
Total	$n_{.j}$	97	49	n.. 146

Note. [1]w_{ij} refers to the *agreement* (coded as 1.00) or *disagreement* (coded as 0.00) for each of the four cells (N-N, P-P, N-P, P-N); n_{ij} refers to the *proportion* of cases comprising each of the four cells; $n_{i.}$ refers to the diagnostic assignments (N or P) made by examiner B; $n_{.j}$ refers to the *corresponding* diagnostic assignments made by examiner A; and $n_{i.}n_{.j}$ refers to the *proportion* of cases, in each cell, which is to be expected by *chance* alone.

as to "absence" or "presence" (combined categories 2–7) of "Hallucinatory Behavior."

Applying the notation presented in Table 1 (see also, Cicchetti, 1988; Cicchetti, Lee, Fontana, & Dowds, 1978; Fleiss, Cohen, & Everitt, 1969):

$$PO = \sum_{i=1}^{r} \sum_{j=1}^{c} (w_{ij}n_{ij})/n.. \text{ in which} \quad (1)$$

PO = the *P*roportion (or *P*ercentage) of *O*bserved interexaminer agreement r and c refer to a given *r*ow or *c*olumn deriving from an examiner 1 by examiner 2 contingency table, w_{ij} refers to the examiner agreement weight applied to each r × c cell (between 0 and 1), n_{ij} refers to the observed number of cases in each possible r × c cell, and $n..$ refers to the total number of examined cases.

$$PC = \sum_{i=1}^{r} \sum_{j=1}^{c} (w_{ij}n_{i.}n_{.j})/n.. \text{ in which} \quad (2)$$

$n_{i.}$ refers to the numbers of cases the first examiner (i) assigns independently to each possible category of diagnostic classification,
$n_{.j}$ refers to the *corresponding* number of cases the second examiner (j) assigns independently to each possible category of diagnostic classification, and r, c, w_{ij}, n_{ij}, and $n..$ are defined as in formula [1].

Finally, kappa (due to Cohen, 1960) is defined as:

$$Kappa\ (\kappa) = \frac{PO - PC}{1 - PC}$$

(Cohen, 1960; Fleiss, Cohen, & Everitt, 1969), (3)

which, in words, means that kappa is defined, simply, as the difference between *observed* (PO) and *expected* (PC) interexaminer agreement, relative to the maximum difference that can possibly occur (1 − PC).

For purposes of evaluating the level of statistical significance of any given kappa value (and in a manner similar to the logic underlying application of the paired *t* test) kappa is divided by the standard error of kappa and the resulting normally distributed Z value is interpreted in the usual way. (Therefore, a Z of kappa value of ±1.96 is statistically significant at the .05 (two-tailed) level (e.g., Cicchetti & Fleiss, 1977; Fleiss, Cohen, & Everitt, 1969.)).

However, when sample sizes are very large (say N = 200 or more), even trivial levels of kappa (say .10 or less) will be highly statistically significant. Consequently, statistical workers in the field have proposed guidelines which evaluate the level of clinical or practical significance of a given kappa value, *above and beyond* its level of statistical significance. Consistent with the guidelines of Fleiss (1981), Cicchetti and Sparrow (1981) have proposed that kappa values be interpreted as follows: *below* .40 = POOR; .40–.59 = FAIR; .60–.74 = GOOD; and .75–1.00 = EXCELLENT. These guidelines, in turn, represent a simplified version of those presented previously by Landis and Koch (1977).

Applying formulae (1), (2), and (3) to the data deriving from Table 2, we obtain the following:

PO = [89 + 45]/146
    = .9178, or the *P*roportion of *O*bserved interexaminer agreement on the extent of hallucinatory behavior
PC = [61.79 + 17.79]/146
    = .5451, or the proportion of interexaminer agreement expected by *C*hance alone, and
Kappa (κ)
    = (PO − PC)/(1 − PC)
    = (.9178 − .5451)/(.4549)
    = .82, which according to the guidelines of Cicchetti and Sparrow (1981) and Fleiss (1981), represent EXCELLENT levels of *chance-corrected* interexaminer agreement for the symptom "hallucinatory behavior." Similarly, by the criteria of Landis and Koch (1977), this value of kappa represents "Almost Perfect" chance-corrected agreement.

Specific Agreement on Negative and Positive Cases (SO neg and SO pos)

The general formulae for determining the extent of specific category interexaminer agreement, for any given single *nominal* category of classification, are:

$$SO = \left(\sum_{i=1}^{r_i} n_{ij}w_{ij} + \sum_{j=1}^{c_i} n_{ij}w_{ij}\right)/(n_{i.} + n_{.j}), \quad (4)$$

in which r_i refers to a given category of classification for examiner i (e.g., the number of subjects classified into category 1 by examiner i); and c_i refers to the *corresponding* number of subjects classified into category 1 by examiner j (the second examiner).

$$SC = \left(\sum_{i=1}^{r_i} n_{i.}n_{.j}w_{ij} + \sum_{j=1}^{c_i} n_{i.}n_{.j}w_{ij}\right)/(n_{i.} + n_{.j})$$

$$(5)$$

and, finally

$$S_{Kappa} = (SO − SC)/(1 − SC) \quad (6)$$

The formulae for SO and SC can be simplified in the purely dichotomous case (e.g., "presence" or "absence" of a symptom) as follows:

$$SO_{(dichotomy)} = (2n_{ii})/n_{i.} + n_{.j}) \quad (7)$$

in which

n_{ii} = the number of cases of interexaminer agreement on any given k nominal categories of classification (here, joint *positive* or *negative* diagnoses)

$n_{i.}$ = the number of cases assigned independently to a given category k, by the *first* rater, i, and

$n_{.j}$ = the number of cases assigned independently to the same given category k, by the *corresponding* second rater, j.

Applying formula [4] to assess levels of interexaminer agreement on "negative" and "positive" diagnoses, we obtain, from the data given in Table 2:

$$SO_{neg} = 2(89)/190$$
$$= .9368$$

Analogously,

$$SO_{pos} = 2(45)/102$$
$$= .8824$$

It has been noted that, whenever a diagnosis, trait, or behavior is expressed as a *binary outcome*, the chance-corrected levels of both SO_{neg} and SO_{pos} will be *mathematically identical* to the overall kappa value, which in our case, was .82 (e.g., see Cicchetti & Feinstein, 1990; Feinstein & Cicchetti, 1990; Fleiss, 1981). It should be noted further that the high values of both SO_{neg} (94%) and SO_{pos} (88%) are quite consistent with the overall PO value of 92%. As shown in Cicchetti (1988), this degree of consistency between SO_{neg} and SO_{pos} is very strongly associated with correspondingly high values of kappa, such as the .82 found for these diagnostic data. (For mathematical explanations of this phenomenon, again, see Cicchetti & Feinstein, 1990; Feinstein & Cicchetti, 1990.)

Reliability Based Upon a Summing Over Each Ordinal Category of Classification

As shown by Cicchetti (1976), the number of linear agreement weights (W) for any given DO scale is given by the very simple algebraic formula

$$W = 2(k - 1), \qquad (8)$$

in which k refers to the number of categories or points on the ordinal scale.

For our 7-category DO scale,

$$W = 2(6) = 12.$$

Once W is obtained, its value can be substituted into formula (9), for determining the entire set of linear agreement weights. In our example,

$$DO_{(Linear\ Weights)} = \frac{W - 1}{W - 1}; \frac{W - 2}{W - 1}; \frac{W - 3}{W - 1}; \\ ...\frac{W - W}{W - 1}, \text{ for which} \qquad (9)$$

for which the specific DO linear weights beginning with complete interexaminer agreement, become:

1.00 (for Complete interexaminer agreement, or
1-1, 2-2, 3-3, 4-4, 5-5, 6-6, and 7-7 pairings)
.91 (for 2-3, 3-2, 3-4, 4-3, 4-5, 5-4, 5-6, 6-5, 6-7, 7-6 pairings)
.82 (for 1-2 and 2-1 pairings)
.73 (for 2-4, 4-2, 3-5, 5-3, 4-6, 6-4, 5-7, 7-5 pairings)
.64 (for 1-3 or 3-1 pairings)
.55 (for 2-5, 5-2, 3-6, 6-3, 4-7, 7-4 pairings)
.45 (for 1-4, 4-1 pairings)
.36 (for 2-6, 6-2, 3-7, 7-3 pairings)
.27 (for 1-5, 5-1 pairings)
.18 (for 2-7, 7-2 pairings)
.09 (for 1-6, 6-1 pairings)
0.00 (for 1-7, 7-1 pairings)

We will now apply formulae (1) through (6) to assess interexaminer reliability, first, treating the BPRS as a trichotomy and, finally as the full BPRS, using each of the seven categories of symptom classification.

Reliability Based Upon a Dichotomous-Ordinal Trichotomy–Overall Agreement Levels

Recall that the full BPRS is a 7-category dichotomous-ordinal symptom severity scale in which 1 = "none"; 2 = "very mild"; 3 = "mild"; 4 = "moderate"; 5 = "moderately severe"; 6 = "severe"; and 7 = "extremely severe." As noted earlier, such a scale can also be logically expressed, more simply, as a dichotomous-ordinal trichotomy, in which symptom severity is rank ordered from 1 = "none"; to 2 = "mild to moderate" (a combination of categories 2-4); and 3 = "severe" (which combines categories 5-7). These trichotomized data, which derive from combining appropriate symptom severity categories from the entries appearing in Table 1, are shown in Table 3.

Applying the *general* formula (1) for *overall* kappa, (and using the 12 DO linear weights just described), we obtain:

$$PO = \sum_{i=1}^{r}\sum_{j=1}^{c}(w_{ij}n_{ij})/n.. \\ = [(89 + 15 + 19)(1) + (5 + 6)(.6667) \\ + (4 + 8)(.3333) + 0(0)]/146 \\ = .9201$$

Table 3. Interexaminer Agreement on the BPRS Symptom "Hallucinatory Behavior," Expressed As a Dichotomous-Ordinal Trichotomy.

Examiner B	Statistic	Examiner A			Total
		None	Mild/Mod	Severe	
None	w_{ij}	1.00	.33	0.00	
	n_{ij}	89	4	0	93
	$(n_i.n_{.j})/n..$	61.79	15.92	15.29	
Mild/Mod	w_{ij}	.33	1.00	.67	
	n_{ij}	8	15	5	28
	$(n_i.p_{.j})/n..$	18.60	4.80	4.60	
Severe	w_{ij}	0	.67	1.00	
	n_{ij}	0	6	19	25
	$(n_i.p_{.j})/n..$	16.61	4.28	4.11	
Total		97	25	24	146

Using the *general* formula (2) to these same data, we obtain:

$$PC = \sum_{i=1}^{r} \sum_{j=1}^{c} (w_{ij} n_{i.} n_{.j})/n..$$

$$= [(70.70)(1) + (8.88)(.6667)$$
$$+ (34.52)(.3333)]/146$$

$$= .6036$$

$$Kappa_{(w)} = (PO - PC)/(1 - PC)$$
$$= (.9201 - .6036)/(.3964)$$
$$= .80 \text{ (or EXCELLENT chance-corrected agreement)}$$

Specific Category Agreement Levels

The formulae for any given specific category kappa were designated as (4), (5), and (6) for SO, SC, and S_{Kappa}, respectively.

Applying the formulae to our trichotomized version of the BPRS symptom, "Hallucinatory Behavior" we obtain, for the U.S. sample:

$SO_{(absent)} = .9579$; $SC_{(absent)} = .7110$;
$\quad kappa_{(absent)} = .85$ (excellent)
$SO_{(mild/mod)} = .7799$; $SC_{(mild/mod)} = .5099$;
$\quad kappa_{(mild/mod)} = .55$ (fair)
$SO_{(severe)} = .9252$; $SC_{(severe)} = .2886$;
$\quad kappa_{(severe)} = .89$ (excellent)

Reliability Based Upon the Seven Symptom Categories

Applying the same formulae (general and specific category, as required) produced the results shown in Table 4.

These data indicate that, at least for the symptom "Hallucinatory Behavior," the dichotomized, trichotomized, and full BPRS scale produce, in general, very reliable interexaminer agreement levels. It is nonetheless instructive that the average frequency of examiner usage for both the "very mild" and "mild" categories, which show "Poor" levels of kappa are only 4 and 10 cases respectively. While the "extremely severe" category is based upon even fewer cases (only 3), its kappa value of .82 falls into the "Excellent" range. At least two clinical or biostatistical phenomena seem to be operating here: first, the strain that low prevalence places on any reliability statistic (e.g., see Cicchetti, Sparrow, Volkmar, Cohen, & Rourke, 1991; Shrout, Spitzer, & Fleiss, 1987); and secondly, the fact that this strain or demand is alleviated, or mitigated by the stark presence of blatant symptomatology such as the manifestation of extremely severe hallucinatory behavior.

The broader question now becomes: Are the data, based upon the U.S. sample, similar to the results obtained when the BPRS is applied to another independently derived sample, here one comprised of French psychiatric patients?

These data are presented in Table 5 which compare the U.S. and French samples as a dichotomy, a trichotomy, and then as the full 7-category scale, for the BPRS "Hallucinatory Behavior" symptom.

As one can note, the results are strikingly similar and suggest: (a) that the BPRS symptom "Hallucinatory Behavior" can be measured quite reliably, both on an initial and replication sample; and

Table 4. Interexaminer Agreement on the BPRS Symptom "Hallucinatory Behavior," Expressed As the Full 7-Category Dichotomous-Ordinal Rating Scale.

BPRS Symptom (Hallucinatory Behavior)	Average Freq of Usage	Observed Agreement PO	Chance Agreement PC	Weighted Kappa k_w	Clinical Significance
1 = Absent	.65	.9799	.7841	.91	Excellent
2 = Very Mild	.03	.8485	.7570	.38	Poor
3 = Mild	.07	.7990	.6973	.34	Poor
4 = Moderate	.09	.9055	.5951	.77	Excellent
5 = Moderately Severe	.08	.9167	.4751	.84	Excellent
6 = Severe	.06	.8990	.3263	.85	Excellent
7 = Extremely Severe	.02	.8571	.2147	.82	Excellent
Summed Over all categories N (Total Scale Reliability)	1.00	.9446	.6935	.82	Excellent

Table 5. A Comparison of U.S. and French Samples on the Interexaminer Reliability of the BPRS Symptom "Hallucinatory Behavior".

DICHOTOMY

BPRS Symptom Category	Aver Freq of Usage		Observed Agreement		Chance Agreement		Kappa		Clinical Significance	
	US	France	US	France	US	France	US	France	US	France
1 = Absent	.65	.48	.94	.86	.65	.48	.82	.73	Excellent	Good
2 = Present	.35	.52	.88	.87	.35	.52	.82	.73	Excellent	Good
Total	1.00	1.00	.92	.87	.55	.50	.82	.73	Excellent	Good

TRICHOTOMY

BPRS Symptom Category	Aver Freq of Usage		Observed Agreement		Chance Agreement		Kappa		Clinical Significance	
	US	France	US	France	US	France	US	France	US	France
1 = Absent	.65	.48	.96	.89	.71	.56	.85	.76	Excellent	Excel
2 = Mild/ Moderate	.18	.22	.78	.82	.51	.58	.55	.57	Fair	Fair
3 = Severe	.17	.30	.93	.90	.29	.44	.89	.83	Excellent	Excel
Total	1.00	1.00	.92	.88	.60	.53	.80	.75	Excellent	Excel

FULL SCALE

BPRS Symptom Category	Aver Freq of Usage		Observed Agreement		Chance Agreement		Kappa		Clinical Significance	
	US	France	US	France	US	France	US	France	US	France
1 = Absent	.65	.48	.98	.94	.78	.67	.91	.81	Excellent	Excel
2 = Very Mild	.03	.09	.85	.89	.76	.71	.38	.61	Poor	Good
3 = Mild	.07	.07	.80	.87	.69	.68	.36	.60	Poor	Good
4 = Moderate	.09	.07	.91	.88	.60	.63	.77	.68	Excellent	Good
5 = Moderate/ Severe	.08	.10	.92	.90	.48	.55	.84	.78	Excellent	Excel
6 = Severe	.06	.12	.90	.86	.33	.44	.85	.74	Excellent	Good
7 = Extremely Severe	.02	.07	.86	.90	.21	.33	.82	.85	Excellent	Excel
Total	1.00	1.00	.94	.91	.69	.61	.82	.77	Excellent	Excel

(b) that this is true (with few exceptions) both for overall scale results and for each category of classification, whether it be based upon a dichotomy, a trichotomy, or the full 7-category DO scale.

Moreover, the guidelines presented in this paper can be used with any qualitative scale of measurement (nominal, CO, DO) and provide, for the first time, a set of carefully specified criteria for judging the level of reliability of any given clinical instrument. While the examples shown here focused upon decomposing a full scale of 7 categories into standard dichotomous and trichotomous classification systems, the methods provided here can easily be generalized to any other number of truncated categories depending upon the clinical exigencies presented by a given examiner reliability problem (e.g., the reexpression of a 7-category continuous ordinal (CO) scale into a 5-category (CO) scale by combining the two extreme categories at each end of the scale. In this regard the interested reader is referred to Cicchetti, Showalter, and Tyrer (1985) for an empirical study examining the effect that the number of categories of classification has on the reliability of a particular clinical scale.).

Computer programs for making all the reliability assessments discussed in this report are available upon request from one of the authors (DVC), e.g., Cicchetti, Aivano, and Vitale (1977); Cicchetti, Lee, Fontana, and Dowds (1978); Cicchetti and Heavens (1979); Cicchetti and Showalter (1988); and Heavens and Cicchetti (1978).

REFERENCES

American Psychiatric Association (1987). *Diagnostic and statistical manual of mental disorders* (3rd ed. rev.). Washington, DC.

Apgar, V.A. (1953). A proposal for a new method of evaluation of the newborn infant. *Anesthesia and Analgesia, 32*, 260–267.

Cicchetti, D.V. (1976). Assessing inter-rater reliability for rating scales: Resolving some basic issues. *British Journal of Psychiatry, 129*, 452–456.

Cicchetti, D.V. (1988). When diagnostic agreement is high, but reliability is low: Some paradoxes occurring in independent neuropsychological assessments. *Journal of Clinical and Experimental Neuropsychology, 10*, 605–622.

Cicchetti, D.V., Aivano, S.L., & Vitale, J. (1977). A computer program for assessing rater agreement and rater bias for qualitative data. *Educational and Psychological Measurement, 37*, 195–201.

Cicchetti, D.V., & Feinstein, A.R. (1990). High agreement but low kappa: II. Resolving the paradoxes. *Journal of Clinical Epidemiology, 43*, 551–568.

Cicchetti, D.V., & Fleiss, J.L. (1977). Comparison of the null distributions of weighted kappa and the C ordinal statistic. *Applied Psychological Measurement, 1*, 195–201.

Cicchetti, D.V., & Heavens, R. (1979). RATCAT (Rater Agreement/Categorical Data). *The American Statistician, 33*, 91.

Cicchetti, D.V., Lee, C., Fontana, A.F., & Dowds, B.N. (1978). A computer program for assessing specific category rater agreement for qualitative data. *Educational and Psychological Measurement, 38*, 805–813.

Cicchetti, D.V., & Prusoff, B.A. (1983). Reliability of depression and associated clinical symptoms. *Archives of General Psychiatry, 40*, 987–990.

Cicchetti, D.V., & Showalter, D. (1988). A computer program for determining the reliability of dimensionally scaled data when the numbers and specific sets of examiners may vary at each assessment. *Educational and Psychological Measurement, 48*, 717–720.

Cicchetti, D.V., Showalter, D., & Tyrer, P. (1985). The effect of number of rating scale categories upon levels of interrater reliability: A Monte Carlo investigation. *Applied Psychological Measurement, 9*, 31–36.

Cicchetti, D.V., Sparrow, S.S., Volkmar, F., Cohen, D., & Rourke, B.P. (1991). Establishing the reliability and validity of neuropsychological disorders with low base rates: Some recommended guidelines. *Journal of Clinical and Experimental Neuropsychology, 13*, 328–338.

Cicchetti, D.V., & Sparrow, S.S. (1981). Developing criteria for establishing interrater reliability of specific items: Applications to assessment of adaptive behavior. *American Journal of Mental Deficiency, 86*, 127–137.

Cicchetti, D.V., & Tyrer, P. (1988). Reliability and validity of personality assessment. In P.J. Tyrer (Ed.), *Personality disorders: Diagnosis, management and course* (pp. 63–73). London: Butterworth Scientific Ltd.

Cohen, J. (1960). A coefficient of agreement for nominal scales. *Educational and Psychological Measurement, 20*, 37–46.

Feinstein, A.R. (1987). *Clinimetrics.* New Haven, CT: Yale University Press.

Feinstein, A.R., & Cicchetti, D.V. (1990). High agreement but low kappa: I. The problems of two paradoxes. *Journal of Clinical Epidemiology, 43*, 543–549.

Fleiss, J.L. (1981). *Statistical methods for rates and proportions* (2nd ed.). New York: Wiley.

Fleiss, J.L., Cohen, J., & Everitt, B.S. (1969). Large sample standard errors of kappa and weighted kappa. *Psychological Bulletin, 72*, 323–327.

Hamilton, M. (1960). A rating scale for depression. *Journal of Neurological and Neurosurgical Psychology, 23*, 56–62.

Heavens, R.H., Jr., & Cicchetti, D.V. (1978). A computer program for calculating rater agreement and bias statistics using contingency table input. *Proceedings of the American Statistical Association* (Statistical Computing Section), 21, 366–370.

Horwitz, R.I., Cicchetti, D.V., & Horwitz, S.M. (1984). A comparison of the Norris and Killip Coronary Prognostic Indices. *Journal of Chronic Diseases, 37*, 369–375.

Killip III, T., & Kimball, J.T. (1967). Treatment of myocardial infarction in a coronary care unit. *American Journal of Cardiology, 20*, 457–464.

Landis, J.R., & Koch, G.G. (1977). The measurement of observer agreement for categorical data. *Biometrics, 33*, 159–174.

Norris, R.M., Brandt, P.W.T., Caughey, D.E., Lee, A.J., & Scott, P.J. (1969). A new coronary prognostic index. *Lancet, 1*, 274–278.

Overall, J.E., & Gorham, D.R. (1962). The Brief Psychiatric Rating Scale. *Psychological Reports, 10*, 799–812.

Overall, J.E., & Klett, C.J. (1972). *Applied multivariate analysis.* New York: McGraw-Hill.

Schopler, E., Reichler, R.J., & Renner, B.R. (1986). *The Childhood Autism Rating Scales (CARS) for diagnostic screening and classification of Autism.* New York: Irvington.

Shrout, P.E., Spitzer, R.L., & Fleiss, J.L. (1987). Quantification of agreement in psychiatric diagnosis revisited. *Archives of General Psychiatry, 44*, 172–177.

Sparrow, S.S., Balla, D.A., & Cicchetti, D.V. (1984a). The Vineland Adaptive Behavior Scales: A revision of the Vineland Social Maturity Scale by Edgar A. Doll. I. Survey Form. Circle Pines, MN: American Guidance Service.

Sparrow, S.S., Balla, D.A., & Cicchetti, D.V. (1984b). The Vineland Adaptive Behavior Scales: A revision of the Vineland Social Maturity Scale by Edgar A. Doll. II. Expanded Form. Circle Pines, MN: American Guidance Service.

Sparrow, S.S., Balla, D.A., & Cicchetti, D.V. (1985). The Vineland Adaptive Behavior Scales: A revision of the Vineland Social Maturity Scale by Edgar A. Doll. III. Classroom Edition. Circle Pines, MN: American Guidance Service.

Sparrow, S.S., & Cicchetti, D.V. (1984). The Behavior Inventory for Rating Development (BIRD): Assessments of reliability and factorial validity. *Applied Research in Mental Retardation, 5*, 219–231.

Steinberg, M., Rounsaville, B., & Cicchetti, D.V. (1990). The Structured Clinical Interview for DSM-III-R Dissociative Disorders: Preliminary report on a new diagnostic instrument. *American Journal of Psychiatry, 147*, 76–82.

Tyrer, P., Alexander, M.S., Ciccheti, D., Cohen, M.S., & Remington, M. (1979). Reliability of a schedule for rating personality disorders. *British Journal of Psychiatry, 135*, 168–174.

Tyrer, P., Owen, R., & Cicchetti, D.V. (1984). The Brief Scale for Anxiety: A subdivision of the Comprehensive Psychopathological Rating Scale. *Journal of Neurology, Neurosurgery and Psychiatry, 47*, 970–975.

Williams, J.B.W. (1988). A structured interview guide for the Hamilton Depression Rating Scale. *Archives of General Psychiatry, 45*, 742–747.

Wing, J.K., Cooper, J.E., & Sartorius, N. (1974). *The measurement and classification of psychiatric symptoms.* Cambridge: Cambridge University Press.

The Clinical Neuropsychologist
1993, Vol. 7, No. 2, pp. 179–189

CLINICAL ISSUES

Analyzing Clinical Ratings of Performance on Pediatric Neuropsychological Tests

Gregory G. Brown[1], Jerel E. Del Dotto[1], John L. Fisk[1],
H. Gerry Taylor[2], and Naomi Breslau[3]

[1]Neuropsychology Division, Department of Psychiatry, Henry Ford Hospital, [2]Department of Pediatrics,
Case Western Reserve University, and [3]Department of Psychiatry, Henry Ford Hospital

ABSTRACT

This project examined the agreement among pediatric neuropsychologists when rating the functioning of normal and low-birth-weight children in seven neuropsychological domains. In Phase 1, two neuropsychologists rated 154 children; in Phase 2, three neuropsychologists rated 41 children. Intraclass correlations of agreement in Phase 1 were: attention .39, intelligence .85, auditory/linguistic .82, haptic .70, visual perceptual/visuomotor .78, mnestic .72, and global .61. Intraclass correlations observed in Phase 2 were similar to those found in Phase 1 except that agreement in rating attention increased to .53. Linear modeling of global judgments revealed that two raters emphasized the auditory/linguistic, haptic, and visual perceptual/visuomotor domains in deriving global ratings, whereas the third emphasized the intellectual and attentional domains. In general, agreement among raters was sufficient to justify using clinical ratings to combine individual test scores into more general behavioral measures.

Research in clinical neuropsychology often requires the integration of data from multiple behavioral measures. The need to combine measures is most obvious when drawing conclusions about the global functioning of a particular patient. However, inferences about functioning in more specific behavioral domains, such as language, episodic memory, and attention, also typically require the combination of scores from several neuropsychological tests. The need to combine scores when assessing performance in specific domains results from the multifactorial structure of the measures involved. Factor-analytic studies show that scores on many commonly used neuropsychological tests reflect several different dimensions of performance (Francis, Espy, Rourke, & Fletcher,

1991; Swiercinsky & Howard, 1982). Therefore, functioning in specific behavioral domains is generally more accurately reflected in combinations of scores than in any single score. Also, inferences regarding the lateralization and localization of brain dysfunction are often based on configurations of test scores, which involve combining information across several tests. These configural relationships among neuropsychological tests appear in research on double dissociations (Teuber, 1955), in comparisons involving the left and right sides of the body (Reitan, 1966), and in patterns of test scores that define clinical syndromes (Goodglass & Kaplan, 1979). Developing useful methods to combine neuropsychological scores is especially challenging when no previously validated procedure to

This study was supported in part by National Institute of Mental Health grant MH45586 to Naomi Breslau. We gratefully acknowledge Patricia Andreski for performing the data analysis presented in this paper. Request for reprints should be sent to Gregory G. Brown, Neuropsychology Division (K-11), Psychiatry Department, Henry Ford Hospital, 2799 W. Grand Blvd., Detroit Mi. 48202, USA.
Accepted for publication: November 5, 1992.

combine scores is available and when no independent criterion exists to validate newly developed procedures.

One method of integrating results in the absence of an independent criterion is to have experienced clinicians rate the performance of individuals on neuropsychological domains of interest. This method has been used in studies of the neuropsychological effects of such adult onset disorders as chronic obstructive pulmonary disease (Grant, Heaton, McSweeny, Adams, & Timms, 1982), polydrug abuse (Grant et al., 1978), and stroke (Brown, Spicer, Robertson, Baird, & Malik, 1989). While the subjective nature of this method could lead to idiosyncratic ratings by a particular clinician, studies of agreement among clinicians rating adult protocols have found acceptable levels of agreement (Brown et al., 1989; Grant et al., 1978, 1982). Less research has focused on agreement involving tests used in neuropsychological research with children; one aim of the present study is to determine the extent of rater agreement in a pediatric sample.

A second aim of this study involves examining the cognitive activity of a clinician when rating a child's global level of neuropsychological functioning. Such an analysis would not only elucidate similarities and differences in the cognitive activity of clinical neuropsychologists, it would also suggest ways of improving agreement among clinicians. Our approach to this analysis involves the paramorphic modeling of clinical judgment (Hoffman, 1960), a method related to Brunswik's (1947) lens model of human judgment. Paramorphic representations of clinical judgments can be developed whenever a clinician uses a fixed set of specific cues to make a clearly defined decision. The cognitive activity of the clinician can be modeled by linear regression analysis, with the informational cues used as predictors and the decision the criterion (Wiggins, 1973, pp. 156–179). The square of the multiple correlation between the cues and the clinical judgment, corrected for shrinkage (Cohen & Cohen, 1983, pp. 106–107), measures the success of the model in describing the cognitive activity of the clinician. The regression weights (or related parameters) reflect the relative contribution of each cue to the prediction of clinical decisions. When more

than one judge is modeled by this approach, differences among judges in their weighing of evidence would appear as differences in the patterns of weights produced by their respective linear models. Further, differences in the intercept (constant) of the linear model would reflect how conservative or liberal judges are when making decisions. Linear regression analysis has been successful in modeling human judgments in general (Dawes, 1979) and clinical judgments in particular (Meehl, 1954; Wiggins, 1973).

The two aims of the study, (1) determining the degree of agreement among expert clinicians in rating the extent of impairment among children in six specific neuropsychological domains and (2) examining the cognitive activity of a clinician when rating a child's global level of neuropsychological functioning, were completed in two phases, permitting a test of the generalizability of the findings. In Phase 1, the ratings of two clinicians with similar training, whose clinical practice is at the same institution, are compared. In Phase 2, the ratings of these two clinicians are compared with the ratings of a third expert, who practices neuropsychology at a different facility.

METHOD

Subjects

One hundred fifty-four children, all 6 years old, were examined. Sixty-three children represented consecutive births of less than 2000 g (low birth weight, LBW) occurring at a large inner city hospital in 1982. The remaining 91 children represented a random sample of children born at greater than 2500 g (normal birth weight, NBW) at the same hospital in 1982. Findings describing the effects of low birth weight on neuropsychological functioning will be published when this ongoing study is completed. Fifty-three percent of the subjects were female; 70% were black. Mean maternal education was 12.5 years for the LBW children and 12.0 years for the NBW children.

Procedure

All children received a battery of neuropsychological tests comprised of the Wechsler Intelligence Scale for Children – Revised (WISC-R, Wechsler, 1974), Sentence Memory Test, Target Test, Verbal Fluency Test, Auditory Analysis Test, Formulated Sentences (Semel, Wiig, & Secord, 1980), Beery Visual Motor

Integration Test (Beery & Buktenica, 1967), Judgment of Line Orientation Test (Benton, Hamsher, Varney, & Spreen, 1983), Tactile Finger Recognition, Finger Tip Number Writing, Grooved Pegboard Test, Arm and Leg Coordination Tests (McCarthy, 1972), Name Writing, and Underlining Test. Description of tests not specifically referenced above appear in the appendix of Rourke, Bakker, Fisk, and Strang (1983). The clinical ratings were performed in two phases. In the *first phase*, two pediatric neuropsychologists, working at the same institution and trained at the same graduate program, used the neuropsychological test results to rate, on a 7 point scale, all children on the following seven behavioral domains: intelligence, auditory perceptual/ language functioning, visual perceptual/visuomotor functioning, haptic perceptual functioning, memory, attention, and global functioning. Ratings were based upon the standard scaled scores from the WISC-R, scaled and raw scores for both Formulated Sentences and the Visual Motor Integration Test, and upon the raw scores from the remaining tests. Additional detail about the exact scores used by the raters can be obtained from the authors. Although raters agreed upon what behavioral domains should be rated, they were blind to one another's ratings, to the subject's identity, and to birthweight status. In the *second phase*, a third pediatric neuropsychologist, trained in a different graduate program and working at a separate institution, rated a random sample of 41 subjects examined in Phase 1. In order to study naturally occurring differences among raters, there was no attempt to obtain a consensus about how ratings should be performed.

Analyses

To measure the degree of agreement between raters, we calculated intraclass correlations for ratings of each of the seven behavioral domains described above. The specific calculation of the intraclass correlation was based on Model III of Shrout and Fleiss (1979). This intraclass model measures agreement as the degree of interchangeability of independently derived, matched measurements, corrected for the degree of chance agreement (Brown, Rourke, & Cicchetti, 1989). The advantages of intraclass models of agreement over the Pearson-Product Moment Correlation are discussed in Brown et al. (1989).

Paramorphic modeling of each clinician's judgment of global impairment was performed by regressing the global rating onto the ratings of the six specific domains. Ratings for all six domains were entered simultaneously into the regression analysis. Domains of behavior important to each clinician's judgment of global impairment were identified initially by statistical tests of the six regression coefficients. While authors differ on the best method to use in determining the relative importance of predictors in a regression model,

Hoffman (1960) has recommended that the identification of important predictors be based on relative weights, which he defines as:

$$\frac{\beta_i * r}{R^2}$$

where β_i is the standardized partial regression weight for the ith predictor, and r is the simple correlation between the ith predictor and the criterion. Additionally, we examined the unstandardized regression weights and the semi-partial correlations. The square of the semi-partial correlation of a predictor is equal to the drop in R^2 associated with removing the predictor from the set of independent variables (Darlington, 1968).

RESULTS

Phase 1

Measuring agreement For all seven domains, the ratings of the two judges significantly correlated at $p = .0001$ or less. The corresponding intraclass correlations of agreement were: intelligence .85 (excellent), auditory perceptual/language .82 (excellent), visual perceptual/visuomotor .78 (excellent), haptic perceptual .70 (good), memory .72 (good), attention .39 (poor), and global .61 (good). The clinical significance of different levels of agreement, reported in parentheses, were based on the criteria of Cicchetti and Sparrow (1981).

Additional analyses were performed to identify the causes of the attenuated agreement in the attentional domain. Differences in either the means or standard deviations of the ratings of the two judges could reduce the intraclass measure of agreement (judge 1: mean rating of attention domain = 2.73, $SD = 1.00$; judge 2: mean rating = 2.25, $SD = 0.64$). A paired t test revealed that the mean rating of the first judge was significantly higher than the other, $t(153) = 6.78$, $p < .0001$. Also, a test for differences between standard deviations of correlated variables confirmed that the variation in the ratings of judge 1 was greater than judge 2, $t(153) = 6.02$, $p < .01$. These analyses indicate that some of the differences in agreement about performance in the attention domain was related to differences in how clinicians scaled this variable. To determine the degree of association between the two judges' ratings of the attention domain, when computationally adjusting for differences in mean and standard deviation, a Pearson-product moment correlation between ratings was calculated. The modest Pearson-product moment correlation of .50 indicated that factors other than differences in scaling decisions must be involved in the low agreement between raters on the attentional domain.

Other factors influencing agreement about attentional functioning, include differences in the selection or weighing of test scores used to operationalize the construct of attention. This hypothesis was tested further by asking both judges to independently select the 10 most important variables used to assess attention, from among the 43 variables measured on each subject. Each judge then rated each variable in terms of its usefulness in assessing attention, with a rating of 1 indicating 'useful, but barely' and a rating of 4 indicating a 'very useful' variable. The two judges selected similar variables. Both judges selected the total score for the Underlining Test and scores on Tactile Finger Recognition, Finger Tip Number Writing, Target Test and scores on the Arithmetic, Digit Span, and Coding subtests from the WISC-R. One judge selected the Sentence Memory test, whereas the other judge selected the Auditory Analysis Test and the Grooved Pegboard as useful measures of attention. With the exception of two measures, the judges rated the importance of these tests similarly, that is, they assigned them ratings that did not deviate by more than one point. However the exceptions were quite striking, with one judge rating scores on Tactile Finger Recognition and Finger Tip Number Writing as 'very useful', and the other judge rating both of these tests as 'useful, but barely'.

Modeling the clinician's cognitive activity. Similarities and differences in the selection and weighing of the six specific domains were examined in regard to the rating of *global* impairment. The global rating was regressed onto ratings of the six specific domains for each of the judges. The six domain-specific ratings correlated $R = .92$, $p < .0001$ with the global rating for judge 1, and .89 for judge 2. These multiple Rs are stable estimates of their respective population values; the R^2 corrected for shrinkage (Cohen &

Cohen, 1983, pp. 106–107) is only .006 less than the uncorrected value for judge 1, and only .008 less than the uncorrected value for judge 2.

Table 1 shows the importance of the six specific domains to each judge's global ratings. All measures of the importance of each domain in predicting global ratings suggested the same finding. Both judges weighted the auditory perceptual/language and visual perceptual/visuomotor domains more than the other domains, with the haptic perceptual domain weighted somewhat less. None of the remaining three domains appeared to contribute independent information to the judges' ratings. The haptic perceptual domain appeared to be slightly more useful to judge 2 than judge 1.

Although the two judges agreed on which domains were most important in the rating of global impairment, the intercept for rater 2 was significantly less than zero and no different from zero for rater 1. These findings suggest that the two raters differed in mean severity of their global rating. A paired *t* test directly confirmed this interpretation $t(153) = 10.33$, $p < .0001$. The negative intercept for judge 2 indicates that his rating of global impairment was less severe than what one would expect from the weighted mean severity of his ratings of the specific domains.

Phase 2

The intraclass correlations involving all three raters were: intelligence .88 (excellent), auditory perceptual/language .83 (excellent), visual perceptual/visuomotor .77 (excellent), haptic perceptual .72 (good), memory .73 (good), attention .53 (fair), and global .67 (good). With the exception of the improved attentional value, these intraclass correlations were very similar to those observed in Phase 1.

To provide for a more direct comparison with rater 3, we repeated the regression analysis of ratings of global impairment done by raters 1 and 2 on the smaller sample of 41 subjects. As with the larger sample, these two raters emphasized the importance of the domains of auditory perceptual/language functioning and visual perceptual/visuomotor functioning when rating global impairment. One rater's global rating was also significantly influenced by findings in the attentional domain,

Table 1. Importance of Specific Neuropsychological Domains to Rating of Global Impairment.

Neuropsychological domain	Judges		
	1	2	3
Unstandardized regression weights[a]			
Attention	.04	.06	.39[b]
Intelligence	−.05	.03	.41[b]
Memory	.05	.04	−.13
Auditory perceptual/language	.48[b]	.40[b]	.11
Haptic perceptual	.08[b]	.25[b]	.12
Visual perceptual/visuomotor	.46[b]	.37[b]	.07
Relative weights			
Attention	.02	.03	.46[b]
Intelligence	−.04	.02	.35[b]
Memory	.03	.03	−.10
Auditory perceptual/language	.47[b]	.42[b]	.11
Haptic perceptual	.05[b]	.16[b]	.10
Visual perceptual/visuomotor	.46[b]	.34[b]	.07
Squared semi-partial correlations			
Attention	.00	.00	.08[b]
Intelligence	.00	.00	.05[b]
Memory	.00	.00	.00
Auditory perceptual/language	.13[b]	.10[b]	.00
Haptic perceptual	.01[b]	.02[b]	.01
Visual perceptual/visuomotor	.12[b]	.06[b]	.00

Note. [a] Values of standardized weights were nearly identical to the unstandardized values.
[b] Domains contributed significantly to the prediction of global ratings.

although the contribution of the attentional domain was less than the contributions of the auditory perceptual/language functioning and visual perceptual/visuomotor functioning domains. In contrast, the regression weights, the relative weights, and the squared semi-partial correlations all revealed that rater 3 found information from the intelligence and attention domains to be more important than information from other domains. However, Table 2 shows that, generally, ratings of the language and visuospatial domains are moderately correlated with ratings of the attention and intelligence domains for all three judges. Furthermore, correlations with the global ratings indicate that judge 3 emphasized ratings of intelligence and attention only slightly more than ratings of linguistic and visuospatial functioning, whereas judges 1 and 2 showed a slight preference for the reverse emphasis. Given the similarities in the pattern of correlations of domain-specific and global ratings among all three judges, it is not

Table 2. Pearson Correlations for Behavioral Domains.

	Attention	Intelligence	Global
Judge 1			
Language	.61	.61	.78
Visuospatial	.38	.65	.88
Global	.52	.64	
Judge 2			
Auditory perceptual language	.69	.63	.85
Visuoperceptual	.65	.70	.87
Gobal	.77	.75	
Judge 3			
Auditory perceptual language	.75	.71	.81
Visuoperceptual	.73	.66	.78
Global	.87	.81	

surprising that the multiple correlation, corrected for shrinkage, of the linear model of judge 3's global ratings was .94, a value comparable to judges 1 and 2.

DISCUSSION

In general, good to excellent agreement can be obtained among clinical judges rating pediatric neuropsychological scores. The degree of agreement is sufficient to justify using clinical ratings to combine multiple test scores into measures of more general behavioral domains. Although the clinical combination of test scores might produce a less useful marker of the phenomena of interest than a cross-validated regression equation based on the same information as that used by the clinician (Wiggins, 1973), the clinical method is defensible, especially when alternative statistical approaches are impractical to use. Statistical rules for combining test scores are particularly difficult to develop when no independent criterion exists to validate the rules (as when a battery of neuropsychological tests is created to provide the outcome criterion for a specific treatment study), when the development and cross-validation of the statistical rule is expensive, or when the ratio of subjects to variables in a study is low.

The method of clinical rating presumably capitalizes on the clinician's experience in identifying patterns of test results. The subjective weights used by the clinician to combine test scores into a clinical judgement have, in a sense, been cross-validated through the clinician's previous experience with the tests. An obvious limitation of the method is that it cannot be used when the test battery contains unfamiliar measures. Another limitation is that the clinician might combine scores suboptimally, perhaps relying on an idiosyncratic weighing of test scores. Illusory correlations with little validity are a risk for research designs that rely exclusively upon the consensual validation of clinical ratings (Chapman & Chapman, 1967). However, studies validating clinical knowledge in the child neuropsychology literature typically involve correlating findings from neuropsychological tests with extratest criteria, such as electrophysiological or imaging findings, parental ratings, or school grades. Therefore, the methods of validating a clinical hypothesis in child neuropsychology reduce the risk of introducing illusory correlations into the field's corpus of knowledge.

The excellent agreement on ratings of intelligence was probably due to having a single, well-validated marker of intelligence, WISC-R performance, available to the raters. However, excellent agreement can be obtained even for domains, such as language, where clinicians must synthesize information from several measures. When differences among judges occur, they may reflect differences in how cautiously judges rate impairment. For example, the negative intercept of the regression equation modeling the cognitive activity of the judge with the lowest mean global rating indicates that he rated global impairment more conservatively than would be expected from his own ratings of the six specific domains. The global ratings of the other two judges were more in line with their ratings of specific domains.

In addition, disagreement among raters can go beyond differences involving conservative or liberal biases, as with the rating of the attentional domain. The relatively low level of agreement for the attentional domain was in part related to scaling discrepancies reflected in differences among judges in mean rating and in the range of ratings. Judges also differed in the importance that they attached to specific tests, especially the haptic-perceptual tests, in arriving at a judgment about the integrity of attentional functioning. A third factor that might have contributed to poor agreement in the rating of attention was suggested by independent interviews with the two raters of Phase 1. Both clinicians reported that they interpreted inconsistencies in performance as evidence of inattentiveness. However, in comparing protocols on which the two judges rated attention differently, it became clear that one judge used inconsistency as evidence of inattentiveness in more cases than did the other.

We developed a paramorphic model of the cognitive activity of each of the three neuropsychologists when making global ratings. This type of model has several known limitations. For example, Hoffman (1960) took the term, 'paramorph', from mineralogy, where it refers to two substances that are chemically identical, even though they differ in their crystalline structure. Whether or not paramorphs are considered identical depends upon the level of description at which the identity is sought. By analogy, a paramorphic model of an individual's cognitive function might perform identically to the individual, especially for a narrow set of judgments, even though the structural rules used by the model might not match those used by the individual. A more comprehensive study than the one we completed would be required to determine whether the structural rules used by each judge to combine information is adequately modeled by a linear regression equation. Nonetheless, studies on human decision making (Dawes, 1979) and our own results make the linear assumption plausible. In our study, the squared multiple-correlation coefficients, corrected for shrinkage, ranged from .79 to .89 for the three judges; most of the systematic variance in the global rating was accounted for by linear combinations of ratings of more specific domains. Still, these same judges might use nonlinear rules to combine neuropsychological scores in other contexts. Another limitation of linear paramorphic models is that there is disagreement about the best statistic to use to judge the importance of an independent variable in fitting the criterion (Darlington, 1968; Hoffman, 1960; Ward, 1962). Unstandardized regression weights, relative weights, and semipartial correlations can lead to a different ordering of the importance of variables in a regression equation (Darlington, 1968). In the present study, these three approaches produced the same pattern of findings.

The judges appeared to adopt one of two approaches in combining information from specific domains when rating global functioning. Two raters attached importance to domains of auditory perceptual/language functioning, visual perceptual/visuomotor functioning, and, to a lesser extent, haptic perceptual functioning. These domains are fundamental to a neuropsychologist's analysis of learning problems in childhood (Rourke, 1981; Spreen, Tupper, Risser, Tuokko, & Edgell, 1984, pp. 350–352). The third rater was not as likely to make interpretations from the perceptual, linguistic, and visuomotor domains used by the other two raters, relying instead on domains involving attention and psychometric intelligence. Even though judge 3 arrived at his global rating differently from the other two judges, agreement about the global functioning of subjects was good, perhaps due to the generally high intercorrelations among the domains of behavior rated. When discussing the differences in arriving at a global rating with

the raters, it became clear that the different approaches did not reflect a conscious, philosophical difference in how children should be assessed. Rather, common experience and the opportunity to collaborate appeared to lead to a greater consensus between the first two raters, who work together. Finally, there might have been a greater degree of consensus about what behavioral domains should be emphasized in a particular case, if a clinical history and parental interviews were available to guide decisions. More research needs to be done on how clinicians integrate information obtained from history and from parental reports with neuropsychological test scores.

REFERENCES

Beery, K., & Buktenica, N.A. (1967). *Developmental test of visual-motor integration.* Chicago: Follet Education Company.

Benton, A.L., Hamsher, Kerry deS., Varney, N.R., & Spreen, O. (1983). *Contributions to neuropsychological assessment: A clinical manual.* New York: Oxford University Press.

Brown, G.G., Spicer, K.B., Robertson, W.M., Baird, A.D., & Malik, G. (1989). Neuropsychological signs of lateralized arteriovenous malformations: Comparison with ischemic stroke. *The Clinical Neuropsychologist, 3,* 340–352.

Brown, S.J., Rourke, B.P., & Cicchetti, D.V. (1989). Reliability of neuropsychological measures in children. *The Clinical Neuropsychologist, 3,* 353–368.

Brunswik, P.J. (1947). *Systematic and representative design of psychological experiments.* Berkeley: University of California Press.

Chapman, L.J., & Chapman, J.P. (1967). The genesis of popular but erroneous psychodiagnostic observations. *Journal of Abnormal Psychology, 72,* 193–204.

Cicchetti, D.V., & Sparrow, S.S. (1981). Developing criteria for establishing the interrater reliability of specific items in a given inventory: Applications to assessment of adaptive behavior. *American Journal of Mental Deficiency, 86,* 127–137.

Cohen, J., & Cohen, P. (1983). *Applied multiple regression/correlation analysis for the behavioral sciences* (2nd ed.). Hillsdale, NJ: Lawrence Erlbaum Associates.

Darlington, R.B. (1968). Multiple regression in psychological research and practice. *Psychological Bulletin, 69,* 161–182.

Dawes, R.M. (1979). The robust beauty of improper linear models in decision modeling. *American Psychologist, 34,* 571–582.

Francis, D.J., Espy, K.A., Rourke, B.P., & Fletcher, J.M. (1991). Validity of intelligence test scores in the definition of learning disability: A critical analysis. In B.P. Rourke (Ed.), *Neuropsychological validation of learning disability subtypes* (pp. 15–44). New York: The Guilford Press.

Goodglass, H., & Kaplan, E. (1979). Assessment of cognitive deficit in the brain-injured patient. In M.S. Gazzaniga (Ed.), *Handbook of behavioral neurology,* Vol. 2 (pp. 3–22). New York: Plenum Press.

Grant, I., Adams, K.M., Carlin, A.S., Rennick, P.M., Judd, L.I., Schoof, K., & Reed, R. (1978). Organic impairment in polydrug users: Risk factors. *American Journal of Psychiatry, 135,* 178–184.

Grant I., Heaton, R.K., McSweeny, J., Adams, K.M., & Timms, R.M. (1982). Neuropsychologic findings in hypoxemic chronic obstructive pulmonary disease. *Archives of Internal Medicine, 142,* 1470–1476.

Hoffman, P.J. (1960). The paramorphic representation of clinical judgment. *Psychological Bulletin, 57,* 116–131.

McCarthy, D. (1972). *Manual of McCarthy Scales of Children Abilities.* New York: The Psychological Corporation.

Meehl, P.E. (1954). *Clinical versus statistical prediction: A theoretical analysis and a review of the evidence.* Minneapolis: University of Minnesota.

Reitan, R.M. (1966). In N.R. Ellis (Ed.), *International Review of Research in Mental Retardation, Vol. 1.* (pp. 153–218). New York: Academic Press.

Rourke, B.P. (1981). Neuropsychological assessment of children with learning disabilities. In S.B. Filskov & T.J. Boll (Eds), *Handbook of clinical neuropsychology, Vol. I.* (pp. 453–478). New York: John Wiley & Sons.

Rourke, B.P., Bakker, D.J., Fisk, J.L., & Strang, J.D. (1983). *Child neuropsychology: An introduction to theory, research, and clinical practice.* New York: The Guilford Press.

Semel, E., Wiig, E.H., & Secord, W. (1980). *Manual of clinical evaluation of language fundamentals – Revised.* New York: The Psychological Corporation.

Shrout, P.E., & Fleiss, J.L. (1979). Intraclass correlations: Uses in assessing rater reliability. *Psychological Bulletin, 86,* 420–428.

Spreen, O., Tupper, D., Risser, A., Tuokko, H., & Edgell, D. (1984). *Human developmental neuropsychology.* New York: Oxford University Press.

Swiercinsky, D.P., & Howard, M.E. (1982). Programmatic series of factor analyses for evaluating the structure of neuropsychological test batteries. *Clinical Neuropsychology, 4,* 147–152.

Teuber, H.L. (1955). Physiological psychology. *Annual Review of Psychology, 6,* 267–296.

Ward, J.H. Jr. (1962). Comments on "The paramorphic representation of clinical judgment." *Psychological Bulletin, 59,* 74–76.

Wechsler, D. (1974). *Wechsler Intelligence Scale for Children-Revised.* New York: The Psychological Corporation.

Wiggins, J.S. (1973). *Personality and prediction: Principles of personality assessment.* Reading, MA.: Addison-Wesley Publishing Company.

The Clinical Neuropsychologist
1995, Vol. 9, No. 2, pp. 194–197

VI

BRIEF REPORT

Temporal Stability of the WAIS-R and WMS-R in a Heterogeneous Sample of Alcohol Dependent Clients*

Stephen C. Bowden[1], Gregory Whelan[2], Caroline M. Long[1], and Christine C. Clifford[3]

[1]University of Melbourne, [2]St. Vincent's Hospital, Melbourne, and [3]University of Tasmania, Australia

ABSTRACT

We examined the temporal stability of WAIS-R IQs, factor scores, Profile Variability Indexes (PVIs), and WMS-R Index scores in a heterogeneous sample of 50 alcohol dependent clients. The average retest interval was approximately 4–5 months. Stability correlations for all scores were significant and high. These results replicate the well-known stability of WAIS-R IQs and confirm the stability of the PVIs and WAIS-R factor scores. WMS-R Index stability coefficients compared favourably with those reported in the manual for a shorter retest interval. Using the *standard error of prediction* to set a 95% confidence interval around the *predicted true score* at initial testing, most scores obtained at retest were found to fall within the predicted range.

The temporal stability of the WAIS-R is well-known, with typical figures averaging around .9 for Verbal, Performance, and Full Scale IQ (Atkinson et al., 1990; Shuerger & Witt, 1989). Currently, there is interest in clinical use of WAIS-R factor scores, which differ from the usual Verbal, Performance, and Full Scale IQ aggregates (Kaufman, 1990; Waller & Waldman, 1990).

McLean and colleagues (McLean, Reynolds, & Kaufman, 1990) recently described a method for testing the WAIS-R profiles for abnormality of subtest scatter using the so-called Profile Variability Index (PVI). If clinicians are to employ the PVI then it is important to establish the reliability of this method for testing hypotheses about the pattern of abilities observed on the WAIS-R.

The Wechsler Memory Scale-Revised (WMS-R: Wechsler, 1987) is used as a compliment to the WAIS-R in many clinical settings. However, apart from the study reported in the manual, which used a retest interval of 4–6 weeks (Wechsler, 1987), we are not aware of any further data bearing on the temporal stability of the WMS-R.

METHOD

Subjects

Data for this study were drawn from an initial random sample of 122 clients. The clients were recruited from an inner-city alcohol detoxification centre. All of the clients were seen for initial assessment while residing in the detoxification unit, were followed-up after discharge, and were invited back for reassessment, at least 3 months later. Thus the retest sample comprised 50 clients who were successfully recruited for reassessment. The remainder of the initial sample (72 subjects) declined reassessment or could not be contacted. The average retest interval was 137 days ($SD = 57.8$), with a median of 107 and range of 71–295 days. The retest interval was positively skewed because some clients, being homeless, were lost to follow-up for a

* This research was supported in part by a grant from the Victorian Health Promotion Foundation. We also acknowledge the generous assistance of the clients and staff at De Paul House, Fitzroy, Victoria, and Ms Marilyn Hage, ARBIAS Association, Victoria. A full report regarding this article is available from Stephen C. Bowden, Ph.D., Department of Psychology, University of Melbourne, Parkville, Victoria, 3052, Australia.
Accepted for publication: June 9, 1994.

time, contact being reestablished subsequent to the target retest date.

The mean age of this sample was 39.3 years ($SD = 10.0$), and clients had completed a mean of 9.9 years ($SD = 2.2$) of education. The average duration of the history of alcohol dependence was 17.6 years ($SD = 8.5$), and the typical quantity of alcoholic beverage consumed on a regular daily basis prior to admission was equivalent to 411.6 g of ethanol ($SD = 217.7$). Only 12% of the retest sample were currently employed and 38% were homeless at the time of initial admission. The retest sample was predominantly male (5 female, 45 male), which reflected the gender ratio of the client population.

Procedure

All clients were initially tested while in the treatment unit, on average 4.8 days ($SD = 1.7$, range 3–7 days) after cessation of drinking. At initial testing, clients were informed that participation in the study was voluntary and were asked to provide informed consent. Clients were assessed, as part of the larger study, with the WAIS-R and WMS-R which were administered according to the standard instructions (Wechsler, 1981, 1987). Subjects were tested by a trained examiner, and initial and follow-up testing occurred in the same treatment centre.

RESULTS

Seventy-three percent of the clients acknowledged drinking during the retest interval, but all subjects were asked to refrain from alcoholic beverages on the day of their retest interview. The demographic, drinking history, and ability scores obtained in the retest sample at initial testing ($n = 50$) were contrasted with scores from the other subjects seen only at initial testing ($n = 72$). None of the differences were significant (all p's $> .05$). Further, the scores on the WAIS-R and WMS-R at retest, in the subjects who reported drinking during the retest interval, were contrasted with scores in those subjects who reported remaining abstinent. Again none of these contrasts was significant, either at the first or second testing (all p's $> .05$).

WAIS-R IQs, factor scores, and PVIs, and WMS-R Index scores at initial testing and at retest are shown in Table 1. The three WAIS-R factor scores Verbal Comprehension (VC), Perceptual Organisation (PO), and Memory/Freedom from

Table 1. Mean Scores and Stability Correlations for the WAIS-R IQs, Factor Scores, PVIs and the WMS-R Index Scores in the Alcohol Dependent Sample ($N = 50$). Also Shown Are the Proportion of Cases at Retest Which Fell Within the 95% Confidence Interval Around Predicted True Scores at First Testing.

	First Test		Second Test		Pearson's	Predicted
	M	SD	M	SD	r	Proportion (%)
WAIS-R						
Verbal IQ	90.5	(11.5)	91.4	(11.5)*	.97[#]	97.8
Performance IQ	89.3	(11.1)	94.9	(13.0)**	.88[#]	93.6
Full Scale IQ	89.5	(11.2)	92.5	(12.2)**	.96[#]	95.5
VC	92.7	(12.5)	93.5	(12.1)	.96[#]	97.8
PO	91.6	(11.0)	96.7	(11.8)**	.82[#]	100
M/FD	89.4	(12.5)	90.3	(13.0)	.90[#]	97.8
Verbal PVI	3.28	(2.5)	3.44	(2.3)	.64[#]	
Performance PVI	3.49	(3.1)	4.86	(3.9)**	.68[#]	
Full Scale PVI	4.03	(2.3)	4.52	(2.3)	.71[#]	
WMS-R						
Verbal Memory	93.9	(14.3)	98.3	(15.0)**	.83[#]	95.5
Visual Memory	88.7	(14.3)	94.3	(15.6)**	.80[#]	90.7
General Memory	90.8	(15.7)	96.7	(17.2)**	.88[#]	93.0
Attention/Conc.	85.5	(16.7)	88.0	(18.2)	.82[#]	86.0[@]
Delayed Index	92.8	(15.0)	98.9	(17.2)**	.88[#]	83.3[@]

Note. $*p < .05$, $**p < .01$, using repeated measures t tests for difference between first and second assessments.
[#]$p < .01$, for correlations.
[@]$p < .01$, χ^2 test of difference from the expected proportion of 95%.

Distractibility (M/FD) were computed according to the method described by Kaufman (1990) which provides factor scores with a mean of 100 ($SD = 15$). As can be seen the factor scores were very similar in value to the IQ scores, both at initial testing and at retest.

There were significant differences on the WAIS-R IQ scores, the PO factor score, the Performance PVI, and most of WMS-R Index scores between testing occasions (Table 1). All of the differences on IQ, factor, and Index scores were in the direction of improvement at retest but the magnitude of differences was relatively modest (Table 1). Correlations between WAIS-R and WMS-R scores obtained at the first and second testing are also shown in Table 1. All correlations were significant and reflect a high degree of stability in scores across testing occasions. When the correlations were recomputed for clients who continued to drink versus those who did not, there were no differences on any test scores (all p's > .05).

Given the variation in the retest interval, we were concerned to ensure that there was no consistent trend in scores across the range of the retest interval. To this end, we correlated IQ scores, factor scores, PVIs, and Indexes with the number of days to retest for each subject. None of the correlations was significant (all p's > .05).

To determine the accuracy with which scores could be predicted at retest, we calculated *standard errors of prediction* (Dudeck, 1979) for the WAIS-R IQ and factor scores and WMS-R Indexes, using the stability coefficients reported in Table 1. We assumed that all scores had a mean of 100 and standard deviation of 15. We then used these standard errors to predict individual scores at retest, using the 95% confidence interval around each individual's *predicted true score* at initial testing (Atkinson, 1991; Dudeck, 1979). Table 1 shows the proportion of scores obtained at retest which fell within the predicted 95% confidence interval.

There was close conformity between the predicted scores and proportions observed to fall within the 95% confidence interval at retest (Table 1). Only the Attention/Concentration and Delayed Memory Indexes from the WMS-R showed significant deviations from the expected proportion of 95% (Table 1). The success of the predictions is noteworthy considering that we took no account of retest gains.

DISCUSSION

In terms of duration and severity of alcohol dependence, and in terms of demographics including age, our subjects were typical of hospitalised alcohol dependent clients seen in treatment centres throughout the world (Lishman, 1987; Parsons, Butters, & Nathan, 1987). Similarly, the subset of clients who were retested did not differ from the initial pool of subjects in terms of demographic and drinking history variables, nor in terms of the scores on the WAIS-R and WMS-R obtained at initial testing. Despite the high level of homelessness and unemployment in the sample and the high level of continued drinking, the retest correlations were large and indicated substantial common variance in WAIS-R and WMS-R scores between testing occasions (Table 1).

The stability coefficients observed for the WAIS-R IQ scores were typical of figures reported previously (Kaufman, 1990). We are aware of only one previous examination of the stability of WAIS-R factor scores (Atkinson et al., 1990), using factors which differed slightly from the factors used in the present study. We used the factor scores recommended by Kaufman, which provide a better coverage of the variance in the scale (Kaufman, 1990). Regarding the PVIs, the retest stabilities were somewhat lower but still highly significant (Table 1). The stability coefficients for the WMS-R obtained in our sample compare favourably with those reported in the manual over a shorter interval (Wechsler, 1987). All Index correlations were .80 or greater; the General Memory and Delayed Index correlations were both .88.

In our sample, most of the IQ, factor, and Index scores at the end of the retest interval were higher than at initial testing. However, the improvements in WAIS-R IQ scores were clearly within the range of typical retest gains (Kaufman, 1990). The average gain on the WMS-R Indexes ranged from 2–6 points (Table 1). To our knowledge, there has been no previous report of retest gains on the WMS-R. Clearly, further work is required to determine the magnitude of typical practice effects on the WMS-R.

Despite the consistent gains with retest, the proportion of scores obtained on second testing which fell within the range predicted from initial testing was very high (Table 1). When we have better information on typical retest gains on the WMS-R, it should be possible to predict scores even more accurately. To illustrate this point, we adjusted the confidence intervals for the WMS-R Indexes, which were based on the predicted true score at first testing, by the average retest gain observed in Full Scale IQ (3 points: Table 1). Not surprisingly, the predictions at retest improved, only the prediction for the Attention/Concentration Index remaining significantly different from chance ($p = .046$), at 88%. These figures suggest that, despite the less than optimal reliabilities in some scores, predictions based on the WAIS-R IQ scores, factor scores, and WMS-R Indexes can be made with a high degree of confidence, at least over equivalent retest intervals.

It is commonly assumed that a stable estimate of cognitive state in alcohol dependent clients cannot be obtained until several weeks of abstinence has elapsed (Parsons et al., 1987). However, review of the relevant studies suggests that this inference may be unduly cautious (Unkenstein & Bowden, 1991). Data from the present study provides further evidence that assessment in alcohol dependent clients toward the end of the first week of abstinence may permit predictions of cognitive state over ensuing months, whether or not clients remain abstinent.

REFERENCES

Atkinson, L. (1991). Three standard errors of measurement and the Wechsler Memory Scale-Revised. *Psychological Assessment, 3*, 136–138.

Atkinson, L., Bowman, T.G., Dickens, S., Blackwell, J., Vasarhelyi, J., Szep, P., Dunleavy, B., MacIntyre, R., & Bury, A. (1990). Stability of the Wechsler Adult Intelligence Scale-Revised factor scores across time. *Psychological Assessment, 2*, 447–450.

Dudeck, F.J. (1979). The continuing misinterpretation of the standard error of measurement. *Psychological Bulletin, 86*, 335–337.

Kaufman, A.S. (1990). *Assessing adolescent and adult intelligence.* Massachusetts: Simon & Schuster.

Lishman, W.A. (1987). *Organic psychiatry* (2nd ed.). Oxford: Blackwell Scientific Publications.

McLean, J.E., Reynolds, C.R., & Kaufman, A.S. (1990). WAIS-R subtest scatter using the profile variability index. *Psychological Assessment, 2*, 289–292.

Parsons, O.A., Butters, N., & Nathan P.E. (Eds.). (1987). *Neuropsychology of alcoholism: Implications for diagnosis and treatment.* New York: Guilford.

Shuerger, J.M., & Witt, A.C. (1989). The temporal stability of individually tested intelligence. *Journal of Clinical Psychology, 45*, 294–302.

Unkenstein, A.E., & Bowden, S.C. (1991). Predicting the course of neuropsychological status in recently abstinent alcoholics: A pilot study. *The Clinical Neuropsychologist, 5*, 24–32.

Waller, N.G., & Waldman, I.D. (1990). A reexamination of the WAIS-R factor structure. *Psychological Assessment, 2*, 139–144.

Wechsler, D. (1981). *Wechsler Adult Intelligence Scale-Revised manual.* New York: Psychological Corporation.

Wechsler, D.A. (1987). *Wechsler Memory Scale-Revised manual.* New York: Psychological Corporation.

The Clinical Neuropsychologist
1995, Vol. 9, No. 3, pp. 225–229

VI

Empirical Comparison of Alternate Forms of the Boston Naming Test*

Michael D. Franzen, Marc W. Haut*, Eric Rankin, and Robert Keefover*

Dept. of Behavioral Medicine and Psychiatry (*and of Neurology), WVU Medical Center, Morgantown, WV

ABSTRACT

Various short forms of the Boston Naming Test (BNT) are compared including an empirically derived 30-item form, odd and even items split-half forms, four 15-item forms, and a rationally derived 15-item form used in conjunction with the Consortium to Establish a Registry in Alzheimer's Disease (CERAD). The present analysis was conducted using a sample of 320 individuals with diagnoses including dementia ($n = 194$), thought disorder ($n = 46$), depression ($n = 16$), general neuropsychiatric disorders ($n = 12$), and cerebral tumors ($n = 52$). Results indicated that all forms possess adequate, although variable internal consistency, and correlations between forms were reasonable. Average item difficulty indices also differed with the CERAD version being least desirable. Finally, classification rates were different by forms, indicating limitations on the extent to which the forms may be used interchangeably.

The Boston Naming Test (BNT; Kaplan, Good-glass, & Weintraub, 1983) is probably the most frequently used assessment of confrontation naming. Originally, the BNT was comprised of 85 items, but the commercially available version contains 60 items. Standard instructions involve establishing a baseline and continuing until six consecutive errors are committed. The score is based on the total number of items that are spontaneously correct plus the number of correct items following a stimulus cue.

Williams, Mack, and Henderson (1989) investigated the use of three short forms of the BNT. Two of the forms were based on an odd-and even-numbered items split of the BNT. The third form was an empirically derived 30-item version. In evaluating 40 subjects with probable dementia diagnoses and 15 control subjects, the authors reported reasonable correlations between the forms ranging

from .99 for the empirical form and the full version to .94 for the even items version and the full version. Furthermore, the empirical 30-item version produced significantly lower scores for the Alzheimer's patients in their sample than did the odd or even items versions. There were no differences for the normal control subjects. There was no comparison of the long form of the BNT with the short forms.

Probably because some subjects may be so impaired that even a 30-item version may be burdensome, Mack, Freed, Williams, and Henderson (1992) developed four 15-item forms by assigning items alternately to the four forms. Additionally, the Consortium to Establish a Registry in Alzheimer's Disease (CERAD) has developed a 15-item form by choosing five items at each of the three levels of low, medium, and high frequency of word usage. Mack et al. (1992) investigated these five forms, comparing them to the full 60-item form and the

* Dr. Franzen is currently at Allegheny Neuropsychiatric Institute.

Portions of this paper were presented at the 22nd Meeting of the International Neuropsychology Society, Cincinnati, February, 1994.

Direct all correspondence to: Michael D. Franzen, Ph.D., Allegheny Neuropsychiatric Institute, 4 Allegheny Center, 8th Floor, Pittsburgh, PA, 15212 USA.

Accepted for publication: November 7, 1994.

three 30-item forms. The control subjects performed significantly better than subjects with probable Alzheimer's on each of the forms studied. The authors multiplied the 15-item forms' scores by 4 in order to compare the scores to the full form and there were no differences, except in the case of the CERAD version which performed less well than the other four short forms.

In neither of these two studies did the investigators report the internal consistency of the alternate forms. This is important because as a test is shortened, the internal consistency estimates are attenuated, lowering the reliability of the test. Furthermore, the reported analyses were conducted on samples that were limited both in terms of size and in terms of clinical diagnosis. Because the BNT is used in a wide range of clinical populations, there is a need to investigate the relations among these alternate forms in a larger, more diverse sample as well as a need to investigate the clinical utility of the forms by comparing classification rates.

METHOD

Subjects
A total of 320 subjects received the BNT as part of comprehensive neuropsychological evaluations. There were 124 males and 196 females. The average age of the total sample was 61.33 years ($SD = 20.91$). The subjects had an average level of education of 10.91 years ($SD = 3.27$). The majority of the subjects had been diagnosed with a dementing disease ($n = 194$). Of these 194 subjects, 43 were evaluated using the CERAD battery (Morris et al., 1989) and diagnosed with probable Senile Dementia of the Alzheimer's Type according to NINCDS/ADRDA criteria (McKhann et al., 1984). Of the other specifically diagnosed dementias, cerebrovascular disease was the most common etiology. Additional non-dementia neuropsychiatric diagnoses included thought disorders ($n = 46$), depression ($n = 16$), various neuropsychiatric disorders including head injury and seizure disorder ($n = 12$), and cerebral tumor ($n = 52$). The subjects were varied in their level of naming skill with scores ranging from 4 to 60. The mean BNT score was 38.44 ($SD = 13.47$).

Procedures
All subjects received each item of the BNT, and standard scoring was utilized. Scores for the various short forms were also calculated for each subject. Cronbach's coefficient alpha was calculated for each form as an index of internal consistency. Scores from the various forms were

correlated with each other. Subjects were classified as demonstrating normal performance if the scores were less than one standard deviation below average based on normative information in the research studies reported in the development of the scales. For the 60-item form of the BNT, the normative information contained in the manual (Kaplan et al., 1983) was used. Subjects were classified as borderline if their scores were between one and two standard deviations below average. Finally, the subjects were classified as impaired if their scores were at least two standard deviations below average. Classification rates for the various forms were compared. Analyses were conducted separately for each of the diagnostic groups. Because no statistically significant differences were detected among groups in terms of coefficient alpha or correlations among forms, the data were collapsed for purposes of reporting.

RESULTS

Overall, total scores on each of the short forms were strongly related to the full form. Correlations between the full and short forms ranged from .99 for the empirically derived 30-item version to .93 for the CERAD version. See Table 1 for a complete listing of correlation coefficients.

Additionally, internal consistency appeared to be good as Cronbach's coefficient alpha values ranged from .96 for the full version to .83 for the CERAD version. The range of internal consistency values by BNT form collapsed across samples is reported in Table 2.

Item difficulty indices were calculated for each of the items in each of the forms. The item difficulty index is the proportion of subjects who pass a given item (Anastasi, 1988). For the full 60-item form the mean item difficulty index was .65. For the empirical 30-item form, the mean index value was .51, for the odd items form the mean value was .64, and for the even items form the value was .66. The mean index values for the four short forms in Mack et al. (1992) were .66 (BNT4), .64 (BNT5), .67 (BNT6), and .62 (BNT7), respectively. The mean index value was .80 for the CERAD short form.

A test with discontinue rules generally progresses from easier items to more difficult items. Therefore, the sequence of item difficulty indices was examined for the entire group of subjects. In the full 60-item form, the sequence of item difficulty indices deviated from the optimal in a minority of

Table 1. Correlations Among Forms of the Boston Naming Test.

	BNT1	BNT2	BNT3	BNT4	BNT5	BNT6	BNT7	BNT8
BNT2	.97							
BNT3	.97	.94						
BNT4	.95	.96	.95					
BNT5	.95	.95	.94	.90				
BNT6	.93	.94	.94	.90	.88			
BNT7	.95	.94	.94	.89	.89	.87		
BNT8	.92	.91	.93	.91	.89	.90	.88	
BNT9	.99	.99	.98	.97	.96	.95	.95	.93

Note. $N = 320$, all correlations are significant at $p < .001$.
BNT1 = empirical 30-item form, BNT2 = odd items form, BNT3 = even items form, BNT4–BNT7 = Mack et al. (1992) 15-item form, BNT8 = CERAD 15-item form, BNT9 = 60-item full length form.

Table 2. Cronbach's Coefficient Alpha Values for the Various Forms.

	Coefficient Alpha
BNT1	.95
BNT2	.93
BNT3	.92
BNT4	.87
BNT5	.84
BNT6	.86
BNT7	.84
BNT8	.83
BNT9	.96

Note. BNT1 = empirical 30-item form, BNT2 = odd items form, BNT3 = even items form, BNT4–BNT7 = Mack et al. (1992) 15-item forms, BNT8 = CERAD 15-item form, BNT9 = 60-item full form.

cases. The three 30-item forms also had minimal deviations from a generally decreasing trend in item difficulty index values, and most deviations were on the order of a .10 value. The discontinue rules do not apply to the short forms; however, examination of the four short forms; however, examination of the four short forms from the Mack et al. (1992) article indicated decreasing trends in item difficulty index values. The CERAD form had larger deviations from this trend. For example, two of the items in the Medium word frequency level had item difficulty indices lower than those in the Low frequency level, and two of the items in the Low frequency level had item difficulty indices equivalent to the values found in the High frequency

level. Therefore, caution is recommended in interpreting errors based on the location of the item in the CERAD short form.

The important consideration in evaluating the clinical utility of these short forms is whether clinical decisions using the short forms are in agreement with clinical decisions made using the full form. For all 3×3 classification tables of pairwise comparisons with the full version, both the chi-square statistic and the kappa coefficient were significant, but the statistical significance may have been due to the large number of subjects involved. In examining the rates of disagreement, the empirically derived 30-item version fared best as only 26 subjects (8%) were misclassified when compared to the full version. The four 15-item versions ranged from 59 (18%) to 77 subjects (24%) misclassified. The CERAD version had 86 subjects (27%) misclassified when compared to the classifications from the full 60-item form.

The even and odd versions disagreed with each other 25% of the time. The four 15-item versions disagreed with each other ranging from 20% of the time for versions 1 and 2 as well as for versions 1 and 3 to 27% for versions 3 and 4. The CERAD version disagreed with the other 15-item forms ranging from 18% for BNT4 (version 1) to 27% for BNT7 (version 4). Examination of the contingency tables indicated that the disagreement was usually in cases where the CERAD misidentified subjects as normal who were otherwise classified as impaired. For example, in comparing the CERAD version to the full version, 34% of the subjects classified as normal by the CERAD were

Table 3. Means and Standard Deviations
for the Various Forms.

	M	SD
BNT1	16.15	8.80
BNT2	18.74	7.20
BNT3	20.20	6.45
BNT4	10.13	3.78
BNT5	9.90	3.35
BNT6	10.30	3.39
BNT7	9.20	3.13
BNT8	12.07	2.86
BNT9	38.94	13.46

Note. BNT1 = empirical 30-item form,
BNT2 = odd items form, BNT3 =
even items form, BNT4– BNT7 =
Mack et al. (1992) 15-item form,
BNT8 = CERAD 15-item form,
BNT9 = 60-item full form.

classified as borderline or impaired by the full version. Because the present sample is large, the obtained means and standard deviations are probably fairly stable for this population. Therefore, the means and standard deviations are presented in Table 3 for comparison purposes. No attempt was made to obtain a representative sample and these values should not be considered normative.

CONCLUSIONS

Overall, the results suggest that caution be exercised in attempting to utilize any of the short forms of the BNT. Earlier research (Mack et al., 1992; Williams et al., 1989) had indicated that these forms were interchangeable. However, that research was based solely upon correlational analyses. Our analyses indicate larger differences among the forms. The use of these forms as alternate forms requires further empirical work to establish accurate cut-off scores. In particular, the CERAD short form appears to be easiest for subjects and tends to misclassify as normal, subjects who would otherwise be classified as experiencing some impairment in naming ability. Use of the cut-off scores for the 15-item forms suggested in Mack et al. (1992) also resulted in misclassification.

The fact that coefficient alpha values were reasonably high indicates that the short forms are relatively homogeneous tests of naming skill. The fact that correlations between forms were high indicates that these forms may be interchangeable if generalizable cut-off scores can be determined. The differences in classification rates indicate that different cut-off scores are necessary for each of the short forms. This is particularly true of the CERAD version which generally had the smallest correlations with other forms and the lowest classification agreement with the full form. It should be noted that even though these correlation values were lower than for the other forms, they were still reasonably high. The most problematic finding is related to the differences in classification rates. Currently, the full form should be used whenever a classification question is being addressed. Comparison between the short forms should be made on the basis of standardized scores, optimally derived from a normal sample. Furthermore, the relative ability of the various forms to identify subjects classified on the basis of diagnosis needs to be investigated.

REFERENCES

Anastasi, A. (1988). *Psychological testing* (6th ed.) New York: Macmillan Publishing.

Kaplan, E., Goodglass, H., & Weintraub, S. (1983). *Boston Naming Test* (rev. ed.) Boston: Boston University.

Mack, W.J., Freed, D.M., Williams, B.W., & Henderson, V.W. (1992). Boston Naming Test: Shortened version for use in Alzheimer's Disease. *Journal of Gerontology: Psychological Sciences, 47,* 164–158.

McKhann, G., Drachman, D., Folstein, M., Katzman, R., Price, D., & Stadlan, E. (1984). Clinical diagnosis of Alzheimer's disease: Report of the NIN-CDS-ADRDA Work Group under the auspices of the Department of Health and Human Services Task Force on Alzheimer's disease. *Neurology, 34,* 939–944.

Morris, J.C., Heyman, A., Mohs, R.C., Hughes, J.P., van Belle, G., Fillenbaum, G., Mellits, E.D., Clark, C., and the CERAD investigators (1989). The Consortium to Establish a Registry for Alzheimer's Disease (CERAD). Part I: Clinical and neuropsychological assessment of Alzheimer's disease. *Neurology, 39,* 1159–1165.

Williams, B.W., Mack, W., & Henderson, V.W. (1989). Boston Naming Test in Alzheimer's disease. *Neuropsychologia, 27,* 1073–1079.

The Clinical Neuropsychologist
1996, Vol. 10, No. 2, pp. 125–129

VI

Reliability of Alternate Forms of the Trail Making Test

Michael D. Franzen[1], David Paul[2], and Grant L. Iverson[2]

[1]Department of Psychiatry and ANI, Medical College of Pennsylvania and Hahnemann University,
and [2]West Virginia University

ABSTRACT

Initial research in a limited sample of 15 closed-head-injury patients indicated reasonable reliability for alternate forms of the Trail Making Test, Parts A and B, called Form C and D, respectively. The present study examined the reliability of these alternate forms in a larger and more heterogeneous sample of 192 subjects with neurologic, psychiatric, or substance abuse diagnoses. The two forms correlated significantly, and there were no significant differences in mean scores for the two forms. The results indicate adequate reliability, although separate cut-off values for Form C may be necessary due to a nonsignificant tendency for scores on Form C to be lower than for the Trail Making Test, Part A.

The Trail Making Test is a frequently used and very sensitive indicator of cerebral dysfunction (Berg, Franzen, & Wedding, 1987; Reitan & Wolfson, 1985). Because of its brevity and sensitivity, the Trail Making Test is sometimes employed serially to evaluate cognitively impaired patients. The serial application of the Trail Making Test is problematic because of the existence of practice effects. The Trail Making Test shares this characteristic in common with other neuropsychological assessment instruments, many of which have practice effects and almost none of which have alternate forms.

For example, Dye (1979) reported significant improvements in scores on both Part A and Part B of the Trail Making Test (TMT) when normal control subjects were administered the test twice in the same day. Matarazzo, Wiens, Matarazzo, and Goldstein (1974) administered the Halstead Reitan Neuropsychological Battery twice to a sample of 29 medical students and reported modest correlation coefficient values; .46 for TMT Part A and .44 for TMT Part B. Lezak (1982) also administered the TMT to normal subjects on two occasions using a 6- and 12-month retest period.

The overall stability of scores using a coefficient of concordance (W) was .78 for TMT Part A and .67 for TMT Part B. The practice effect was significant for TMT Part A.

Because of these practice effects, previous researchers have attempted to develop alternate forms. Lewis and Rennick (1979) developed four alternate forms for TMT Part B, but none for Part A. A recent report (Kelland & Lewis, 1994) indicates that the original TMT Part B and a first alternate form correlate .74 in a sample of 20 control subjects. In another venture, desRosiers and Kavanaugh (1987) have developed alternate forms called TMT Parts C and D. These authors report alternate forms reliability coefficients of .66 for TMT Parts A and C, and .89 for TMT Parts B and D in a sample of 50 orthopedic patients. In a sample of 15 closed-head-injury patients the alternate forms reliability values were .79 for TMT Parts A and C and .88 for TMT Parts B and D. Independently, Charter, Adkins, Alekoumbides, and Seacat (1987) used an identical methodology to develop alternate forms of the Trail Making Test. These authors report alternate forms reliability coefficients

---

Address for correspondence: Michael D. Franzen, Ph.D., Department of Psychiatry and ANI, Allegheny General Hospital, Four Allegheny Center, Pittsburgh, PA 15212, USA.
Accepted for publication: May 15, 1995.

of .95 for TMT Parts A and Form C and .94 for TMT Parts B and Form D in a sample of over 300 subjects that included 123 normal control subjects. The test-retest interval was not specified.

Although these initial results are promising, extension of the methods to other clinical populations would help evaluate the generality of the results. In this study, the alternate forms reliability of the two forms of the Trail Making Test (Parts A and B vs. Forms C and D) were evaluated in a larger sample of neurologic, psychiatric, and substance abuse patients. A previous study using a different sample indicated that the alternate forms, Part A and Form C loaded on the same factor as did the alternate forms, Part B and Form D in a principal components analysis conducted on a variety of neuropsychological screening instruments (McCracken & Franzen, 1992).

METHODS

Subjects

Subjects were 192 patients referred for neuropsychological evaluation at a university medical center. There were 64 subjects in each of three groups. The first group consisted of patients with neurologic disorders including closed-head injury, seizure disorder, stroke, and cerebral tumor. All neurologic diagnoses were given by a board-certified neurologist. The second group consisted of patients with a psychiatric diagnosis including major affective disorder, schizophrenic disorders, and personality disorders. All psychiatric diagnoses were given by a board-certified psychiatrist. The third group consisted of patients who carried a primary diagnosis of substance abuse, typically alcohol abuse, although some subjects also abused marijuana, cocaine, or benzodiazepines. All substance abuse patients were detoxed and free of drug use for at least 1 week at the time of testing. Because of the homogeneity of subjects in the desRosiers and Kavanaugh (1987) study, an effort was made to collect data on a more heterogeneous group in order to better evaluate the generalizability of the findings.

There were no significant differences in age or education among groups. (See Table 1 for group means and standard deviations). The overall mean age was 42.8 years (SD = 16.59, range = 15–74 years) and the overall mean level of education was 11.8 years (SD = 2.81, range 4–20 years).

Procedures

All subjects were administered the original and alternate forms of the Trail Making Test in counter-balanced

Table 1. Means, Standard Deviations, and Ranges of Age and Education by Groups.

Group	Age	Education
Psychiatric	43.6 (17.9) range 15–79	11.7 (2.51) range 6–19
Neurologic	40.7 (16.7) range 15–79	11.5 (3.34) range 5–20
Substance Abuse	44.3 (15.02) range 18–70	12.1 (2.56) range 4–20

Note. Standard deviations in parentheses.

order (either TMT Parts A and B first or Forms C and D first). In each case, the alternate forms were administered consecutively in order to minimize the influence of time interval between administrations (the same procedure as used by desRosiers & Kavanaugh, 1987). The tests were administered as part of a neuropsychological evaluation conducted by trained psychometrists under the supervision of a licensed psychologist. All testing was conducted in the psychological assessment laboratory at a university medical center.

Statistical Analyses

Statistical analyses were conducted to accomplish two broad goals. First, traditional correlational reliability analyses were conducted in order to determine the extent to which scores on TMT Parts A and B co-varied with scores on TMT Forms C and D. Because traditional correlational analysis can result in high reliability estimates in situations where scores increase or decrease uniformly across the two sessions, an analysis of variance was also conducted in order to evaluate whether there was a difference in level as well as in distribution.

As an evaluation of the clinical reliability of the alternate forms, raw time scores were translated into the 6-point level of impairment scale suggested in Russell, Neuringer, and Goldstein (1970). The scaled scores for the alternate forms were then correlated. The Russell et al. (1970) scale was investigated because Trail Making Test scores frequently are translated to this scale before clinical interpretation. In this way we hoped to evaluate the clinical reliability of the alternate forms. As another method of evaluating the clinical reliability of the results, alternate Trail Making Test scores were translated into the scaled score equivalents devised by Heaton, Grant, and Matthews (1991) and these scores were then correlated.

RESULTS

A mixed analysis of variance was conducted in order to determine if there were significant differences in time score between TMT Parts A

Table 2. Mean Values for Time in Seconds.

	Trail Making Test			
	Part A	Form C	Part B	Form D
ORDER				
ABCD	47.3	41.4	147.5	140.4
	(13.6)	(15.9)	(48.3)	(51.2)
CDAB	39.8	41.3	132.3	143.1
	(14.1)	(13.9)	(50.7)	(48.3)
ABCD				
Psychiatric	49.9	44.3	151.4	137.8
	(14.7)	(14.9)	(59.6)	(75.8)
Neurologic	51.1	49.0	161.3	124.4
	(15.0)	(15.3)	(60.3)	(53.4)
Substance	34.8	30.9	129.8	124.4
Abuse	(13.3)	(13.7)	(61.4)	(58.6)
CDAB				
Psychiatric	38.0	43.0	117.6	128.2
	(14.2)	(14.2)	(58.6)	(68.7)
Neurologic	43.7	42.5	140.9	166.5
	(14.7)	(14.3)	(58.7)	(61.3)
Substance	37.5	38.5	138.5	134.5
Abuse	(15.1)	(14.6)	(69.3)	(64.1)

Note. Standard deviations in parentheses.

and C and between TMT Part B and Form D. The between-subjects independent variables were diagnosis and order of administration. The within-subjects independent variable was form (A vs. C and B vs. D). The dependent variables were the time scores. There were no significant effects for any of the independent variables. Mean values are presented in Table 2. Examination of the means reveals a trend for times to be faster for the form administered second (i.e., practice effects), however, this effect was not significant.

Initially, TMT Part A score was correlated with Form C, and TMT Part B was correlated with Form D separately for each diagnostic group. There were no significant differences among groups on the correlational analyses. Therefore, the analyses were collapsed across groups. Correlational analyses indicated good agreement in total time for TMT Part A and Form C ($r = .70$) as well as for TMT Part B and Form D ($r = .78$). Using the original classification system of impaired versus nonimpaired (Reitan & Wolfson, 1985) resulted in a significant chi-square statistic with continuity correction (chi square = 75.15, $p < .0001$) in

comparing the classification from TMT Part A and Form C. A similar analysis of the classification results for TMT Part B and Form D resulted in a significant association between these two forms (chi square = 84.97, $p < .0001$). The Russell, Neuringer, and Goldstein (1970) impairment scale scores correlated .67 for TMT Part A and Form C (contingency coefficient for 6×6 table = .68) and correlated .77 for TMT Part B and Form D (contingency coefficient for 6×6 table = .73). The Heaton, Grant, and Matthews (1991) scale scores also correlated well with a value of $r = .69$ for TMT Part A and Form C and a value of $r = .78$ for TMT Part B and Form D.

DISCUSSION

Initial research indicated that the desRosiers and Kavanaugh (1987) alternate forms of the Trail Making Test (Forms C and D) may have reasonable alternate forms reliability, at least in their limited sample of 15 closed-head-injury patients. The current research attempted to extend these results to larger sample sizes of neurologic, psychiatric, and substance abuse patients. It was found that there were no significant differences in subjects' overall level of performance between TMT Part A and Form C, and between TMT Part B and Form D. Therefore, patients' total time on the alternate forms are grossly comparable to the original forms. The alternate forms reliability estimates were $r = .70$ for TMT Part A and Form C and $r = .78$ for TMT Part B and Form D. The results indicate adequate reliability of the alternate forms.

The somewhat lower reliability coefficients produced in this study relative to the desRosiers and Kavanaugh (1987) study may reflect a difference in sample characteristics since their sample exclusively contained head-injured patients and orthopedic patients. However, the larger sample sizes used in the present study as well as the lack of significant differences among the substance abuse, psychiatric, and neurologic samples indicate that the reliability coefficients from this study may be more stable estimates. Charter et al. (1987) also reported higher correlation coefficients, although the relative values for TMT Parts A and B were consistent. Charter et al. (1987) analyzed data from a mixed sample including normal control subjects, and this may in part account for some of the difference between these two sets of results. Cross-validation in a separate sample of heterogeneous subjects as well as in separate samples of diagnostic groups would help address this issue. In the meantime, it appears that the reliability of the two forms is adequate to recommend clinical use. Although there was a tendency for scores on Form C to be lower than scores for TMT Part A, this difference was not significant even in this large sample, and the examination of clinical reliability did not result in differences either. The potential need for separate cut-off values for Form C will need to be addressed empirically. In the meantime, scores on Form C near the cut-off values for TMT Part A should be interpreted carefully.

REFERENCES

Berg, R.A., Franzen, M.D., & Wedding, D. (1987). *Screening for brain impairment.* New York: Springer.

Charter, R.A., Adkins, T.G., Alekoumbides, A., & Seacat, G.F. (1987). Reliability of the WAIS, WMS, and Reitan battery: Raw scores, and standardized scores corrected for age and education. *The International Journal of Clinical Neuropsychology, 9,* 28–32.

desRosiers, G., & Kavanaugh, D. (1987). Cognitive assessment in closed head injury: Stability, validity and parallel forms for two neuropsychological measures of recovery. *International Journal of Clinical Neuropsychology, 9,* 162–173.

Dye, O.A. (1979). Effects of practice on Trail Making Test performance. *Perceptual and Motor Skills, 48,* 206.

Heaton, R.K., Grant, I., & Matthews, C.G. (1991). *Comprehensive norms for an expanded Halstead-Reitan Battery.* Odessa, FL: Psychological Assessment Resources.

Kelland, D.Z., & Lewis, R.F. (1994). Evaluation of the reliability and validity of the Repeatable Cognitive-Perceptual-Motor Battery. *The Clinical Neuropsychologist, 8,* 295–308.

Lewis, R.F., & Rennick, P.M. (1979). *Manual for the Repeatable Cognitive–Perceptual–Motor Battery.* Grosse Pointe Park, MI: Axon Publishing.

Lezak, M.D. (1982). *The test-retest stability and reliability of some tests commonly used in neuropsychology.* Paper presented at the Fifth European Conference of the International Neuropsychological Society, Deauville, France.

Matarazzo, J.D., Wiens, A.N., Matarazzo, R.G., & Goldstein, S.G. (1974). Psychometric and clinical test-retest reliability of the Halstead–Reitan Impairment Index in a sample of healthy, young, normal men. *Journal of Nervous and Mental Disease, 158,* 37–49.

McCracken, L.M., & Franzen, M.D. (1992). Principal-components analysis of the equivalence of alternate forms of the Trail Making Test. *Psychological Assessment, 4,* 235–238.

Reitan, R.M., & Wolfson, D. (1985). *The Halstead-Reitan Neuropsychological Test Battery: Theory and clinical interpretation.* Tucson, AZ: Neuropsychology Press.

Russell, E.W., Neuringer, C., & Goldstein, G. (1970). *Assessment of brain damage: A neuropsychological key approach.* New York: John Wiley & Sons.

The Clinical Neuropsychologist
1998, Vol. 12, No. 4, pp. 531–534

VI

Normative Data and Interrater Reliability of the Design Fluency Test*

Sherri L. Carter[1], Douglas Shore[1], Michael C. S. Harnadek[2], and Cynthia S. Kubu[2]

[1]University of Windsor, Ontario, Canada and [2]London Health Sciences Centre, Ontario, Canada

ABSTRACT

This study generated normative data for the free and fixed conditions of the Design Fluency Test (DFT; Jones-Gotman & Milner, 1977) and investigated its interrater reliability. Three raters independently scored DFT protocols from 66 normal adults according to criteria that have only recently been published (Jones-Gotman, 1990; see Spreen & Strauss, 1998 for summary). Interrater reliability was good to excellent for novel output scores and perseverative errors, but nameable errors and designs with the incorrect number of lines yielded lower reliability coefficients. Overall, interrater reliability of the DFT appears to be relatively good, especially for the free condition and, therefore, clinical use with adequate normative data may be justified.

Until recently, only limited normative data were available on both the free and fixed conditions of the Design Fluency Test (DFT; Jones-Gotman & Milner, 1977). Woodard, Axelrod, and Henry (1992) have provided normative data for a group of older adults (M age = 69.4), as well as initial data regarding the interrater reliability of the DFT. Two independent raters scored the DFT protocols according to the original scoring rules outlined by Jones-Gotman and Milner (1977) and varying degrees of reliability for different scoring parameters, with fair to good interrater agreement, were obtained. Interrater agreement was 0.64 for novel output in the free condition and was 0.71 for novel output in the fixed condition (Woodard et al., 1992). Varney et al. (1996) investigated DFT performance in a group of 86 individuals with closed-head injury and a comparison group of 87 normal controls. These authors reported that "the judgments of two trained, independent raters agreed 90% of the time" (p. 347) on DFT scores for the free condition. For a sample of college students,

Ross and Axelrod (1996) reported that interrater agreement ranged from 0.21 for nameable errors to 0.98 for the total number of designs.

The present study sought to replicate and extend previous findings by generating additional normative data for both conditions of the DFT in a younger group of healthy adults. In addition, the interrater reliability of the DFT was investigated when scoring was in accordance with additional criteria provided by Jones-Gotman (1990; see Spreen & Strauss, 1998 for summary). These scoring criteria are stricter than those originally outlined by Jones-Gotman and Milner (1977) and may have a significant impact on the interrater reliability of the test.

METHOD

Participants

Participants were 66 unpaid volunteers (19 males, 47 females), primarily recruited from an introductory

* We gratefully acknowledge the assistance of Dr. Marilyn Jones-Gotman and the provision of her scoring guidelines.
Address correspondence to: Sherri L. Carter, Department of Psychology, University of Windsor, 401 Sunset, Windsor, Ontario, Canada, N9B 3P4. E-mail: carterm@server.uwindsor.ca.
Accepted for publication: July 21, 1998.

psychology course at the University of Windsor. The original sample consisted of 77 individuals recruited as part of a larger study. Eleven of these participants were excluded because they did not meet the following inclusion criteria: age 18–60 years, right-handed, English as a first or main language, no evidence of significant neurological, systemic, or psychiatric illness, and adequate intellectual ability (i.e., Wechsler Adult Intelligence Scale – Revised [WAIS-R] Full Scale IQ estimate greater than or equal to 80).

The mean age of the sample was 25.06 years ($SD = 7.83$; range 19–56) and the mean years of education was 15.21 ($SD = 1.60$; range 12–20). Tables published by Brooker and Cyr (1986) were used to derive WAIS-R (Wechsler, 1981) Full Scale IQ (FSIQ) estimates from scores on the Arithmetic, Block Design, Similarities, and Vocabulary subtests. The mean WAIS-R FSIQ estimate was 100.85 ($SD = 11.07$; range 81–124).

Procedure

Participants were administered the free and the fixed (four-line) conditions of the DFT according to administration guidelines provided by Jones-Gotman (see Spreen & Strauss, 1998 for summary). Three raters, two neuropsychologists from London Health Sciences Centre (London, Ontario), and one clinical neuropsychology graduate student from the University of Windsor (Windsor, Ontario), independently scored these DFT protocols according to their own understanding of Jones-Gotman's scoring criteria (see Spreen & Strauss, 1998 for summary). DFT protocols were scored strictly, as recommended by Jones-Gotman. Scores on the DFT included the total number of designs produced, the number of designs considered to be nameable, the number of perseverative designs, a novel output score (total output minus nameable errors and

perseverative errors), and the number of designs drawn with the incorrect number of lines (fixed condition only). For further information on the scores derived from DFT protocols, refer to Jones-Gotman and Milner (1977) or Jones-Gotman (1990; see Spreen & Strauss, 1998 for summary).

RESULTS AND DISCUSSION

For each of the three raters, mean scores for each scoring parameter of the DFT are presented in Table 1, together with the mean scores across raters for each scoring parameter. The mean novel output score for the free condition was 13.9 ($SD = 6.3$) designs, and the mean novel output score for the fixed condition was 16.7 ($SD = 6.1$) designs.

Intraclass correlation coefficients (ICC) were calculated as indices of interrater agreement and consistency according to formulae provided by Shrout and Fleiss (1979). The formula for interrater agreement considers raters to be random effects, and permits generalization from a particular set of raters to a population of potential raters. The formula for interrater consistency considers raters to be fixed effects and reflects the consistency of a particular set of raters. The ICC was used as a measure of interrater agreement because it takes into account more than one source of variance (Bartko, 1976; see Berk, 1979 for advantages of the ICC). Table 2 presents the ICC values

Table 1. Mean Scores on the Design Fluency Test for Three Raters.

Condition and scoring parameter	Rater 1		Rater 2		Rater 3		Across raters	
	M	(SD)	M	(SD)	M	(SD)	M	(SD)
Free condition								
Total designs	21.1	(10.4)	21.1	(10.5)	21.1	(10.4)	21.1	(10.4)
Novel output	12.5	(5.5)	15.3	(7.8)	13.9	(7.0)	13.9	(6.3)
Perseverative errors	8.5	(9.1)	5.7	(7.1)	7.1	(8.3)	7.1	(7.8)
Nameable errors	0.1	(0.4)	0.1	(0.4)	0.2	(0.5)	0.2	(0.4)
Fixed condition								
Total designs	26.0	(10.9)	26.0	(10.8)	26.0	(10.9)	26.0	(10.9)
Novel output	15.1	(6.1)	15.8	(6.5)	19.2	(7.5)	16.7	(6.1)
Perseverative errors	7.8	(7.5)	6.3	(5.6)	5.1	(4.8)	6.4	(5.5)
Nameable errors	0.3	(0.8)	0.5	(1.2)	0.4	(1.1)	0.4	(0.8)
Incorrect number of lines	2.9	(2.7)	3.3	(3.7)	1.2	(1.8)	2.5	(2.3)

Note. $N = 66$.

for each scoring parameter of the free and the fixed conditions of the DFT. Levels of clinical significance were determined according to criteria specified by Cicchetti and Sparrow (1981) and are also listed in Table 2.

ICC values ranged from good (fixed condition) to excellent (free condition) for novel output scores and perseverative errors. Novel output scores and perseverative errors appear to be more reliably scored across raters for the free versus the fixed condition of the test. Nameable errors and designs with the incorrect number of lines yielded lower reliability coefficients; this may be partly related to their less frequent occurrence in DFT protocols. Across scoring parameters, coefficients of interrater consistency were generally higher than were those of interrater agreement.

Although interrater reliability varied, the good to excellent coefficients for novel output scores and perseverative errors, especially in the free condition, provide support for clinical use of the test. Given that the novel output score may be the most sensitive clinical scoring parameter on the DFT, the good to excellent interrater reliability of this score supports its clinical utility, particularly with the addition of normative data based on scores from multiple raters.

In addition, interrater reliability coefficients for some scoring parameters, such as perseverative errors, are higher than those reported in pre-vious studies (e.g., Woodard et al., 1992).

This finding would suggest that stricter scoring criteria may improve scorer reliability. The availability of standardized administration and scoring guidelines (see Spreen & Strauss, 1998) for the DFT may also assist in reducing the discrepancies among raters.

REFERENCES

Bartko, J.J. (1976). On various intraclass correlation reliability coefficients. *Psychological Bulletin, 83,* 762–765.

Berk, R.A. (1979). Generalizability of behavioral observations: A classification of interobserver agreement and interobserver reliability. *American Journal of Mental Deficiency, 83,* 460–472.

Brooker, B.H., & Cyr, J.J. (1986). Tables for clinicians to use to convert WAIS-R short forms. *Journal of Clinical Psychology, 42,* 982–986.

Cicchetti, D.V., & Sparrow, S.A. (1981). Developing criteria for establishing interrater reliability of specific items: Applications to assessment of adaptive behavior. *Journal of Mental Deficiency, 86,* 127–137.

Jones-Gotman, M. (1990). *Design fluency scoring instructions.* Unpublished manuscript.

Jones-Gotman, M., & Milner, B. (1977). Design fluency: The invention of nonsense drawings after focal cortical lesions. *Neuropsychologia, 15,* 653–674.

Ross, T.P., & Axelrod, B.N. (1996). The interrater and test-retest reliability of the Design Fluency and Ruff Figural Fluency tests (Abstract). *Journal of the International Neuropsychological Society, 2,* 3.

Table 2. Interrater Reliability of the Design Fluency Test.

Condition and scoring parameter	Interrater agreement	Interrater consistency	Clinical significance
Free condition			
Total designs	0.99	0.99	Excellent
Novel output	0.77	0.80	Excellent
Perseverative errors	0.82	0.84	Excellent
Nameable errors	0.50	0.50	Fair
Fixed condition			
Total designs	0.99	0.99	Excellent
Novel output	0.66	0.73	Good
Perseverative errors	0.70	0.73	Good
Nameable errors	0.47	0.47	Fair
Incorrect number of lines	0.42	0.48	Fair

Note. Clinical significance levels are based on criteria outlined by Cicchetti and Sparrow (1981).

Shrout, P.E., & Fleiss, J.L. (1979). Intraclass correlations uses in assessing rater reliability. *Psychological Bulletin, 86*, 420–428.

Spreen, O., & Strauss, E. (1998). *A compendium of neuropsychological tests: Administration, norms, and commentary* (2nd ed.). New York: Oxford University Press.

Varney, N.R., Roberts, R.J., Struchen, M.A., Hanson, T.V., Franzen, K.M., & Connell, S.K.

(1996). Design fluency among normals and patients with closed-head injury. *Archives of Clinical Neuropsychology, 11*, 345–353.

Wechsler, D. (1981). *WAIS-R manual: Wechsler Adult Intelligence Scale – Revised*. San Antonio, TX: Psychological Corporation.

Woodard, J.L., Axelrod, B.N., & Henry, R.R. (1992). Interrater reliability of scoring parameters for the Design Fluency Test. *Neuropsychology, 6*, 173–178.

The Clinical Neuropsychologist
1999, Vol. 13, No. 2, pp. 157–170

Interrater Reliability Levels of Multiple Clinical Examiners in the Evaluation of a Schizophrenic Patient: Quality of Life, Level of Functioning, and Neuropsychological Symptomatology*

Domenic V. Cicchetti[1,3], Robert Rosenheck[2,3], Donald Showalter[2], Dennis Charney[2,3], and Joyce Cramer[2,3]

[1]Child Study Center, Yale University of Medicine, New Haven, CT, [2]Northeast Program Evaluation Center (NEPEC), West Haven, CT, and [3]Department of Psychiatry, Yale University School of Medicine, New Haven, CT

ABSTRACT

Sir Ronald Fisher used a single-subject design to derive the concepts of appropriate research design, randomization, sensitivity, and tests of statistical significance. The seminal work of Broca demonstrated that valid and generalizable findings can and have emerged from studies of a single patient in neuropsychology. In order to assess the reliability and/or validity of any clinical phenomena that derive from single subject research, it becomes necessary to apply appropriate biostatistical methodology. The authors develop just such an approach and apply it successfully to the evaluation of the functioning, quality of life, and neuropsychological symptomatology of a single schizophrenic patient.

The purpose of this research investigation is first to present arguments for the necessity of single-subject designs, both in statistics and in clinical and experimental neuropsychology; and then to discuss an important application of a recently published methodology for assessing the reliability of multiple clinical examiners in the evaluation of a schizophrenic patient, in terms of quality of life, level of functioning, and neuropsychological symptomatology.

Concerning the first issue, it has been well documented that the famous statistician, Sir Ronald A. Fisher (1935) launched his illustrious career on the basis of what he learned from his now classical single-subject research involving the lady tea drinker. Some will recall that the subject was presented, in random order, a number of cups of tea. To half of them (4 cups) tea (T) was added first and milk (M) thereafter (the TM condition); and

to the remaining 4 cups, milk was added first and tea thereafter (the MT condition). The subject claimed that she could reliably discriminate between these two conditions, and it was her task to do just that. As correctly noted by Holschuh (1980) "Fisher explains the notions of adequate design, tests of significance, randomization, and sensitivity, all through the lady tasting tea example." (p. 36)

Concerning the second point, there is also ample evidence that the single-case design has produced invaluable information in clinical and experimental neuropsychology. This includes the early work of Shallice (1979) who, after describing some of the problems deriving from the single-subject design, was able to argue that "the case study approach is the most promising neuropsychological technique for providing information on the functional organization of cognitive subsystems" (p. 183). Similarly, Marshall and Newcombe (1985)

---

* Address correspondence to: D. Cicchetti, Yale Child Study Center, Home Office, 94 Linsley Lake Road, North Branford, CT 06471, USA. E-mail: dom.cicchetti@yale.edu.
Accepted for publication: December 4, 1998.

develop the cogent argument that "there are no useful groups in neuropsychology: there are only groupings of individuals. And in order to be grouped in a rational, theoretically revealing fashion, the members must first be investigated in highly detailed single-case studies." (p. 89)

Finally, Barbara A. Wilson (1987) laments the disturbing fact that it is often difficult to convince members of the clinical and scientific communities that good research can be undertaken with single individuals. She stated specifically that: "Despite this general background of skepticism, it can be demonstrated quite readily within the field of neuropsychology that valid and generalizable results are obtainable from studies of individual patients." (pp. 112–113) Broca's study of his patient 'Tan', for example (1861), heralded the beginning of modern neuropsychology; and it can be demonstrated today that, with certain exceptions, damage to Broca's area consistently leads to expressive dysphagia. H.M., the amnestic patient of Scoville and Millner (1957), has probably been written about more than any other individual in the literature of psychology. Studies of H.M.'s memory disorder have contributed enormously to our understanding of normal human memory. Studies of individual patients such as 'Tan', H.M., and others allow us to test theoretical models of normal cognitive functioning.

It is within the setting of this historical backdrop that we wish to present the results of a single-case study, in which the authors apply a recently published statistical methodology to assess the reliability of 39 clinical examiners, who evaluated independently a single schizophrenic patient, in three broad areas of behavior, that would be of interest to both clinical and experimental neuropsychologists: quality of life, level of functioning, and extent of neuropsychological symptomatology.

The investigation distinguishes itself by dint of the fact that the major emphasis is on the relative success of multiple examiners evaluating only one patient, as compared to the much more prevalent research activity in which the emphasis is upon evaluating the level of interexaminer agreement, when a pair of independent examiners evaluates a large number of representative patients. In the typical interexaminer reliability study, whether in

behavioral or biomedical areas of assessment, the interest is on the psychometric properties (reliability, validity) of the measuring instrument. Thus, a group of investigators might be interested in the interexaminer (usually two independent examiners) and temporal reliability of a symptomatol-ogy scale (such as the Brief Psychiatric Rating Scale-BPRS), as applied in a particular clinical setting, say, in a chronic inpatient psychiatric hospital, over certain specified time periods, (e.g., 1 week, 2 weeks, and 1 month after current hospitalization) to a random sample of 100 schizophrenic patients. In this hypothetical example, the emphasis is clearly on the reliability of the BPRS for a very specialized sample, namely, hospitalized schizophrenics.

Suppose we contrast this with an investigation of interexaminer reliability (40 independent examiners) of the BPRS, on two separate occasions, of only one schizophrenic patient. Here the interest is more on the relative interchangeability of the 40 examiners, than on the BPRS per se. This reliability research design was used in the current investigation.

Research Questions

In this investigation, the major question we address is to what extent are multiple clinical examiners in agreement in their independent assessments of psychiatric symptomatology, interpersonal relationships, and quality of life of a schizophrenic male veteran patient?

A number of additional questions are also of interest. These include the following: (1) To what extent are the examiners' levels of reliability on global assessments similar or dissimilar to levels of agreement on domains or on individual items? (2) Are some areas of assessment, for example, extent of patient symptomatology, more reliable than others, such as quality of the patient's interpersonal relations? (3) Are there statistical and/or clinical differences in reliability among the multiple examiners in a reassessment, as compared to the assessment that was made initially? (4) Are there any statistically and/or clinically significant differences in patient assessments as a function of the type of clinical examiner, that is, psychiatrists, nurse-case managers, or psychology technicians?

METHOD

Source of Study Data

The data for this report derive from a VA Cooperative Study in Health Services 17 (CSHS #171): "The Clinical and Economic Impact of Clozapine Treatment on Refractory Schizophrenia," that was designed and executed by three of the authors RR, DC, and JC.

Briefly stated, the clinical trial was a multi-site comparison of Clozapine and Haloperidol in the treatment of refractory schizophrenia, on the basis of DSM-III-R criteria (American Psychiatric Association, 1987).

Patients were randomly assigned to one of the two treatment conditions and were assessed at baseline, at 6 weeks, and again at 3, 6, 9, and 12 months after the initiation of treatment. The detailed results of this clinical trial were recently published by Rosenheck et al. (1997).

Criteria for Subject Selection

The independent assessments were made by group-taught and self-trained clinical examiners who viewed and rated video-taped patients, initially at a training session and 1 year later. The 39 clinical examiners, or assessors, came from each of 15 VA Medical Centers participating in the clozapine trial and were divided, more or less equally, into 12 psychiatrist investigators, 13 nurse-case managers, and 14 psychology technicians. Each patient evaluation was made independently or blind to the ratings of all the remaining clinical examiners. A small number of patients was chosen to take part in reliability assessments. A single subject was selected, and his ratings provide the data for this report.

Subject Characteristics

The subject was a middle-aged patient, who was diagnosed with refractory schizophrenia on the basis of DSM-III-R criteria. He was selected for this case report as one who had complete information and also showed a wide range of responses on the various clinical rating scales that were employed.

Assessment Instruments

The four assessment instruments were: (1) The Heinrichs Carpenter Quality of Life (QOL) Scale; (2) the Strauss and Carpenter (1972) Level of Function (LOF) Scale; (3) the Brief Psychiatric Rating Scale (BPRS); and (4) the Structured Clinical Interview for the Positive and Negative Symptom Scale (SCI-PANSS). Each of these clinical rating instruments will now be discussed in more detail.

The Heinrichs-Carpenter Quality of Life (QOL) scale (Heinrichs, Hanlon, & Carpenter, 1989) consists of three areas: (1) Interpersonal Relations and Social Network (8 items, e.g., the quality of relations with friends); (2) Instrumental Role Functioning (4 items, e.g., in terms of level of adequacy); and (3) Intrapsychic Foundations and Common Objects and Activities (9 items, e.g., level of empathy). Each of the 21 items is rated, on a 7-category ordinal scale that ranges between "absent" (a score of 0) and "maximal" (a score of 6).

The Strauss-Carpenter LOF Scale (Strauss & Carpenter, 1972) is comprised of 9 items, each of which is rated on a 5-category ordinal scale, that ranges between 0 (lowest level) and 4 (highest level) of functioning. One item on this LOF scale pertains to the quality of useful work.

The BPRS (Overall & Klett, 1972) is comprised of 18 psychiatric symptoms, each of which is rated on a 7-category dichotomous-ordinal scale (Cicchetti, 1976). The absence of a given symptom, for example, "hallucinations" is scored as 0, whereas a score of 6 represents the symptom appearing in its most florid form.

Finally, the SCI-PANSS is a 30-item scale in which each psychiatric symptom is also given a rating that can vary between 0 denoting "absence" of symptomatology, and 6 indicating the "presence" of the symptom in its "extreme" form.

Recommended Reliability Statistics

In the prototypic reliability design, as described earlier, a very small number of raters (usually 2) assesses a relatively large sample of subjects (often somewhere between 30 and more than 100). For such applications a number of recommended statistical approaches, that cover a wide range of different designs, have been available for more than a decade (e.g., see Fleiss, 1981, Chapter 13; and, more recently, McGraw & Wong, 1996).

The situation is quite different for the type of reliability research design discussed here, namely, one in which multiple independent examiners (here there are 39) evaluate only one subject. Technical aspects of the recommended statistical approaches (e.g., relationship to kappa) can be found in Cicchetti, Showalter, and Rosenheck, 1997; and the availability of a computer program for applying the necessary statistics has also been reported recently (Cicchetti & Showalter, 1997).

Therefore, the emphasis in this report will be primarily on the conceptual aspects of an application of this methodology to a problem that should be of interest to both clinical and research neuropsychologists. The more technical aspects of the new methodology will be described in an Appendix, for the interested reader.

The recommended statistics will probably be familiar to many *JCEN* readers. However, as far as we are aware, they have not, until recently (Cicchetti, Showalter, & Rosenheck, 1997) been appropriately modified to fit a multi-rater-one-subject reliability research design. In broad terms, we are applying a measure of interexaminer agreement that takes into account all levels of partial agreement (e.g., Cicchetti & Fleiss, 1977) as well as whether the scale of focus has a category denoting absence (e.g., most symptom scales, as noted earlier in

Cicchetti, 1976; and, more recently, in this journal, by the first author and colleagues, i.e., Cicchetti et al., 1992).

Conceptually, we will, after determining an *average* level of agreement across all 39 clinical examiners, apply a familiar and standard Z statistic. This will allow us to determine whether a given examiner's rating (e.g., a score of 5 on a 6-category clinical scale) is either statistically higher or lower than the average examiner rating, to which it will be compared. We will also describe criteria for classifying what we shall refer to as the level of clinical significance of the percent agreement each independent examiner has with the remaining examiners. The specific criteria will be defined in one of four ways: (1) by whether the average level of agreement, for a given examiner, is clinically meaningful (70–100%), or not clinically meaningful (below 70%); (2) by whether the level of agreement for a given examiner is statistically lower (or higher) than the average level of agreement (e.g., a Z of 2.58; $p = .01$); but clinically quite meaningful, such as a level of 85.6%, compared to the average examiner level of agreement of 94.8%; (3) by whether a given examiner's agreement level with the remaining examiners is clinically low (e.g., 62.1%), compared to that of the average rating (e.g., 82.2%), but not statistically lower, as evidenced by a Z value of, for example, -1.50; and (4) by whether a given clinical examiner's rating is *both* clinically low (<70% in agreement with the average, or consensus diagnosis) as well as, statistically low or high (e.g., a Z of -2.86).

It now becomes important to detail the criteria we have applied for determining the levels of both statistical and clinical significance.

Statistical Criteria

The statistical criteria are quite standard. Specifically, Z scores below 1.645 ($p > .10$ are not statistically significant; one of 1.645 shows a trend at the .10 level of probability; a Z of 1.96 is statistically significant at the .05 level; one of 2.24 reaches the .025 level; one of 2.58, the .01 level; one of 2.81, the .005 level; and, finally, a Z value of 3.29 reaches statistical significance at the .001 level.

Clinical Criteria

Concerning levels of interexaminer agreement, expressed as a percentage, clinical criteria have recently been published that define below 70% as POOR; 70–79% as FAIR; 80–89% as GOOD; and 90–100% as EXCELLENT (Cicchetti, Volkmar, Klin, & Showalter, 1995, p. 33.). For an example of how the new statistical approach can be applied, the reader is referred to the Appendix.

RESULTS AND DISCUSSION

Results will now be presented and discussed, with respect to how the 39 examiners agreed with each other on each of the behavior scales, at three levels of focus, namely, in terms of global, domain, and individual items, as they might apply. The format we have chosen is to present tabular data, based on levels of agreement, averaged over the 39 clinical examiners. Next, we shall discuss the more specific findings that are not represented in the four tables, one representing each of the four clinical instruments, described earlier. The areas to be discussed are whether there are specific examiners whose reliability levels do not fit the more general pattern and whether there are consistent differences in average reliability levels between psychiatrists, nurses and psychology technicians both at initial evaluation and upon retest; and whether there are meaningful changes in reliability levels between test and retest conditions. The findings pertinent to each of the four clinical assessment instruments will be found in Tables 1–4, respectively.

The first set of results will focus on the Heinrichs-Carpenter Scale-Quality of Life (QOL) Scale. This scale consists of 21 items, grouped into three domains: Interpersonal Relations and Social Net-work; Instrumental Role Functioning; and Intrapsy-chic Foundations and Common Objects and Activities. The scale can be scored on an individual item basis, as one of three domain scores, and as an overall, total, or so-called global score.

Global Score, QOL Scale

The global score was determined for each examiner by averaging across the 21 items and rounding to the nearest whole number (in this case, a value that could range between 0 and 6). Results indicate the following: Levels of agreement, on both occasions of testing, were EXCELLENT (95.3%, at initial testing, and 96.2% at retest). For individual examiners, agreement levels ranged between GOOD and EXCELLENT (85.0%– 96.8%-initial Test; and 89.4%–98.1%-Retest). There were no clinically significant differences between the three types of examiners, either initially or at the follow-up assessment. Specifically, the ranges of agreement were between 94.9% and 95.3% initially and between 95.4% and 96.8% on the second assessment.

In terms of the initial ratings of individual examiners, one of them assigned a rating that was statistically lower than the overall rating averaged across the 39 examiners. The Z score was -4.48, with $p < .0001$. However, the percentage agreement of this "deviant" examiner with the remaining 38 examiners was a quite respectable 85%, which, by our stated criteria, is classified as falling midway into the GOOD range (80%–89%).

Similarly, on the second assessment, 4 of the 39 examiners had global Z scores that were significantly below the average for all the examiners. All 4 examiners had a Z score of -2.05. However, their level of average agreement with the remaining examiners was 89.4%, which falls just short of the EXCELLENT range. This underlines the importance of judging levels of reliability on a clinical as well as on a statistical basis.

To summarize: On average, the overall agreement levels among the 39 examiners on the GLOBAL score derived from the QOL scale were EXCELLENT at both initial testing and upon retesting, with the retest reliability levels being a few percentage points higher than at initial testing.

Domain Scores (QOL)

Interpersonal relations and social network
Analogous to the derivation of the global QOL score, each of the three domain scores was obtained, for a given examiner, by averaging the scores across all items in the domain and then rounding off to the nearest whole number. Because the range of possible responses to each item was the same, a given domain score could range between 0 and 6.

For the first domain, the levels of agreement among the 39 examiners ranged between 85.6% (GOOD) and 94.9% (EXCELLENT) at the first assessment; and between 81.4% (GOOD) and 94.1% (EXCELLENT) at the second assessment. The mean levels of agreement across the 39 examiners were 91.2% (Test) and 92.8% (Retest).

When divided on the basis of profession, levels of agreement were in the excellent range both at the first (90.5%–92.6% agreement) and the second assessment (92.3%–93.1%).

In terms of levels of statistical significance, the four examiners who averaged 81.4% agreement with the remaining examiners on the second assessment had values of -3.13, meaning that their ratings were significantly lower than the average rating at a probability level of .002. Because the average agreement level of each of these examiners (81.4%)

is in the GOOD range, this Z value can be classified as a statistically significant finding that is of little clinical importance.

Instrumental role functioning
As shown in Table 1, results deriving from the domain Instrumental Role Functioning illustrate that interexaminer agreement levels fell into the GOOD to EXCELLENT range, (i.e., 90.3% (Test) and 89.1% (Retest)). However, one examiner, at the initial assessment, assigned a rating that was significantly below the average rating, as evidenced by a Z value of -3.29 ($p = .001$), with an associated level of interexaminer agreement at the lower bounds of FAIR, specifically, 70.2%.

At the second assessment, 22 of the examiners had agreement levels with the remaining examiners that were in the EXCELLENT range, at 92.0%; another 16 were in the GOOD range, 1 examiner at 80.1%, and the remaining 15 at 87.3%; the last examiner had a rating that was significantly below the average rating, with a Z value of -5.43 ($p < .0001$), and an associated percentage of inter-examiner agreement, well into the POOR range of clinical significance at 62.4%. Because this result represents an examiner rating that is lower than the average rating, both at a statistical and clinical level, it takes on much more meaning than a rating that is statistically higher or lower than the average, but is associated with an acceptable level of interexaminer agreement, for example, in the GOOD or EXCELLENT range, as was true of a number of our previously discussed results.

As was true for the previous domain, differences in reliability levels between the three professions were trivial (i.e., between 89.8% and 91.2% on the first assessment and between 87.7% and 90.2% at retest).

Intrapsychic foundations and common objects and activities
As shown in Table 1, the overall levels of agreement at both the initial testing (98.3%) and at retesting (95.1%) were well into the EXCELLENT range. On the first assessment, 35 of the examiners had levels of agreement with the remaining examiners that were almost "perfect" at 98.9%. Nonetheless, 4 examiners had ratings that were statistically lower

than the average rating, as evidenced by three Z values of -2.67 and one at -2.89 with ($p = .008$ and $p = .004$, respectively). However, these scores were associated with very respectable interexaminer agreement levels of 90.5% and 89.9%, respectively.

These results etch in bold relief that Z scores need to be interpreted in the specific research context in which they occur. This particular set of findings shows that a level of interexaminer agreement as high as 90% or 91% can be associated with a Z score that is significantly lower (or higher) than that based on the average interexaminer rating. In our case, this occurred because the remaining 35 examiners had agreement levels that were almost perfect (99%). Because the group standard deviation that forms the denominator in the formula for Z is relatively quite small, even minor departures from the average rating will produce much higher Z scores than would otherwise occur.

On the second assessment, 16 of the examiners had agreement levels of 94.5%. The remaining 23 had levels of 96.2%. These excellent, and quite similar, levels of reliability, as one might predict, were associated with Z values that did not even approach statistical significance, the values being -1.19 and 0.82, respectively.

The interexaminer agreement levels of psychiatrists, nurses, and psychology technicians were in the EXCELLENT range both initially and at the second assessment (i.e., ranging between 97.5% and 98.3%, initially, and between 95.2% and 95.7%, on the follow-up assessment). Again, these differences are clinically meaningless.

Individual Items (QOL)

The general pattern of results for individual items was the same as for domains and the global QOL score, except that, as might be expected, the average levels of interexaminer agreement were both lower and wider in range, across the 21 items, than was true of either the global or domain scores. Specifically, the agreement levels on individual items, at pretest, ranged between a low of 37.2% and a high of 98.3%. Corresponding levels, at post-treatment assessment were between 29.4% and 97.0%.

Again, there were no discernible differences between the three groups of examiners, namely,

psychiatrists, registered nurses, and pysychology technicians.

Next, we shall discuss the extent of interexaminer agreement on items deriving from the Strauss-Carpenter Level of Function (LOF) Scale, in terms of the overall or global score and at the level of individual items.

Global Score (LOF Scale)

A global score was calculated for each patient, by averaging 8 of the 9 ratable items (duration of psychiatric disorder could not be determined from video-taped material) and then, as in the case of the Heinrichs-Carpenter Scale, by rounding to the nearest whole number. This produced a score that could range between a low of 0 and a high of 4.

Specific results demonstrated that the average global LOF at initial testing was in the EXCELLENT range, at 93.2%, with individual examiners' scores varying between 90.2% and 95.1%. At retest, the average score was 99.0%, with no variability at all ($SD = 0$).

Once again, there were no meaningful differences between psychiatrists, nurses and psychology technicians. For initial testing, the average global scores were virtually indistinguishable, with psychiatrists showing 92.4%, and both nurses and psychology technicians displaying agreement levels of 93.6%. The same phenomenon occurred on retest, namely, both psychiatrists and nurses showed average levels of agreement of 99.0%. Similarly, psychology technicians were at a level of reliability of 97.1%.

Individual Items (QOL)

As expected, scores on individual QOL items followed the same general pattern as did the global score, with most items showing an increase (usually no more than a few points) in reliability from test to retest. As shown in Table 2, these ranged between 37.3% and 97.9% at the initial assessment, and between 40.5% and 98.3% at treatment follow-up.

Again, there were no meaningful differences by profession with respect to reliability levels. For specific details, see Table 2.

The Brief Psychiatric Rating Scale (BPRS; Overall & Klett, 1972) is comprised of 18 symptom scales, three domains, or clusters of symptoms (1–8 constitutes the first cluster, symptoms 9–13

Table 1. Interexaminer Agreement Levels in the Evaluation of a Single Schizophrenic Patient on the Heinrichs-Carpenter Quality of Life Scale.

Area of Assessment	Initial Evaluation			Retest Evaluation		
	M	(SD)	% Range	M	(SD)	% Range
A. Global score	95.3	2.4	85.0–96.8	96.2	3.6	89.4–98.1
B. Domains						
1. Interpersonal Relations & Social Network	91.6	3.4	85.6–94.9	92.8	3.9	81.4–94.1
2. Instrumental Role Functioning	90.3	6.4	70.2–94.7	89.1	5.2	62.4–92.0
3. Intrapsychic Foundations & Common Objects and Activities	98.0	2.6	89.9–98.9	95.5	0.8	94.5–96.2
C. Individual Items						
1. Household member	83.9	8.3	60.0–89.2	85.5	8.6	64.7–90.3
2. Friends	83.5	9.9	54.5–90.3	78.9	12.0	29.4–85.4
3. Acquaintances	81.4	11.3	41.4–88.4	85.5	5.0	79.3–89.6
4. Activity	85.9	8.9	51.4–90.7	80.6	8.3	57.7–87.5
5. Social network	82.8	7.1	60.3–89.0	86.4	8.1	66.7–91.6
6. Social initiatives	86.9	8.3	49.7–91.8	85.1	6.1	62.8–89.2
7. Social withdrawal	89.4	5.5	76.7–93.4	89.9	6.0	69.6–93.2
8. Social-sexual relations	93.1	3.7	79.9–94.7	86.8	7.7	57.7–89.9
9. Extent	91.4	4.8	84.4–94.7	86.4	8.2	49.3–91.8
10. Adequacy	86.1	9.8	37.2–91.8	85.4	4.8	65.1–89.9
11. Underemployment	89.1	5.9	66.8–93.4	89.8	4.1	74.0–92.0
12. Satisfaction[a]	–	–	–	–	–	–
13. Sense of purpose	90.9	6.8	66.2–94.1	83.4	7.2	49.5–89.4
14. Motivation	92.6	8.2	64.9–96.2	90.6	4.5	72.1–94.1
15. Curiosity	91.1	8.5	44.4–93.7	86.9	8.9	42.9–92.0
16. Anhedonia	93.0	6.4	60.0–95.3	87.8	6.5	71.9–92.8
17. Time Utilization	89.1	7.0	71.5–93.7	87.0	8.3	64.9–91.1
18. Objects	97.6	2.0	91.8–98.3	94.6	6.6	75.5–97.0
19. Activities	93.3	10.9	47.6–96.0	95.1	4.7	74.4–97.3
20. Empathy	94.4	4.1	76.5–96.6	84.4	9.9	64.7–90.5
21. Interaction	92.7	5.2	68.5–95.6	81.0	7.7	62.2–87.1

Note. Items 1–8 comprise the Interpersonal Relations & Social Network domain; items 9–12 derive from the Instrumental Role Functioning domain, and the remaining items, 13–21 form the Intrapsychic Foundations and Common Objects and Activities Domain. [a] It was not possible to rate patient on this item from the information provided in the videotape.

the second cluster, and 14–18 the third) and an overall or global symptom score. The same averaging and rounding process was used to derive both the cluster scores and the global scores. This resulted in a BPRS cluster or global score that could range, theoretically, between 0 and 6.

BPRS Global Scores

BPRS results, shown in Table 3, indicate that the mean level of interexaminer agreement was in the EXCELLENT range, both at the initial testing, which produced a value of 94.7% and again, at retest, as evidenced by a value of 96.1%.

Again, the average examiner agreement levels were very similar for psychiatrists, nurses, and psychology technicians. They were, respectively, values of 95.3%, 95.2% and 93.7%, initially, and values of 96.0%, 95.9% and 96.4%, respectively, at retest.

BPRS Domain Scores

The first cluster, consisting of responses to BPRS symptoms 1–8, the second cluster comprised of symptoms 9–13, and the third, of the remaining symptoms, 14–18, were all highly reliable and virtually interchangeable. The mean levels of

Table 2. Interexaminer Agreement Levels in the Evaluation of a Single Patient on the Strauss-Carpenter Level of Function Scale.

Area of Assessment	Initial Evaluation			Retest Evaluation		
	M	(SD)	% Range	M	(SD)	% Range
A. Global score	93.2	2.4	90.2–95.1	98.3	2.9	86.4–99.0
B. Individual Items						
1. Duration of psychiatric disorder[a]						
2A. Frequency of social contacts	90.4	7.2	60.6–94.4	80.6	15.7	40.5–88.0
2B. Quality of social contacts	92.8	3.8	76.7–94.8	83.8	5.6	69.4–87.7
3A. Quantity of useful work	95.9	6.9	72.8–97.9	87.3	10.9	51.2–92.7
3B. Quality of useful work	80.4	8.4	37.3–83.3	84.3	3.5	63.8–85.0
4. Absence of symptoms	84.0	9.0	40.8–90.6	88.0	8.8	64.8–92.7
5. Ability to meet basic needs	83.5	9.9	48.4–89.5	88.6	5.3	71.1–90.4
6. Fullness of life	90.3	7.8	65.5–93.7	96.5	5.8	69.4–98.3
7. Overall level of function	87.4	5.7	73.5–90.9	89.2	8.4	68.8–94.0

Note. [a] It was not possible to obtain information for this item from videotapes.

inter-examiner agreement averaged approximately 93% initially, and about 95% at retest.

This narrow range of differences also typified the average agreement levels for psychiatrists, nurses, and psychology technicians. Again, differences between the three professions were trivial and of no clinical significance.

Individual BPRS Symptoms

There was more variability and lower, though quite acceptable levels of interexaminer agreement on individual BPRS symptoms. The average levels of examiner agreement ranged between 75.3% (Hostility, FAIR range) and 92.7% (Anxiety, EXCELLENT range), at initial evaluation; and, similarly, between 81% (Hallucinatory Behavior and Conceptual Disorganization), and 96% (Disorientation), at reassessment. The range of values across the individual symptoms was much broader. For initial assessment, the range was between 41% (Hostility) and 94% (Anxiety, Conceptual Disorganization, and Unusual Thought Content). Similarly, the corresponding range of agreement levels at the second evaluation was between 42% (Hallucinatory Behavior) and 97% (Disorientation).

Agreement levels among the three professions parallel the overall findings just presented. Once again, there were no appreciable differences between psychiatrists, nurses, and psychology technicians.

The next section of the report will focus on interexaminer agreement levels on the Positive and Negative Syndrome Scale (PANSS; Kay, Fizbein, and Opler, 1992). For a comparison of the reliability levels of the PANSS and the BPRS, see Bell, Milstein, Beam-Goulet, Lysaker, and Cicchetti, (1992).

The PANSS is comprised of 30 symptoms, each ratable on a 7-category dichotomous-ordinal scale, in the same manner as the BPRS. Possible scores range between a score of 0, denoting absence of the symptom, to 6, indicating the presence of a given symptom in extreme form.

The PANSS can also be interpreted by averaging symptom scores that comprise three domains or subscales, namely, a POSITIVE, a NEGATIVE, and a GENERAL PSYCHOPATHOLOGY subscale. The POSITIVE subscale score is derived by averaging scores on seven symptom scales, namely: Delusions, Conceptual Disorganization, Hallucinatory Behavior; Excitement; Grandiosity; Suspiciousness/Persecution; and Hostility. The NEGATIVE scale is also comprised of seven symptoms. These are: Blunted Affect, Emotional Withdrawal, Poor Rapport, Passive/Apathetic Social Withdrawal, Difficulty in Abstract Thinking, Lack of Spontaneity and Conversation Flow, and Stereotyped Thinking. The third and last subscale of the PANSS, the GENERAL PSYCHOPATHOLOGY scale is composed of the

Table 3. Interexaminer Agreement Levels in the Evaluation of a Single Schizophrenic Patient on the Brief Psychiatric Rating Scale.

Area of Assessment	Initial Evaluation			Retest Evaluation		
	M	*(SD)*	% Range	*M*	*(SD)*	% Range
A. Global score	94.7	3.3	86.1–96.8	96.1	2.6	86.3–97.5
B. Domains						
1. Items 1–8	93.9	3.6	87.7–96.5	95.3	3.1	86.5–97.3
2. Items 9–13	92.7	3.5	84.4–95.2	94.8	3.6	77.2–96.6
3. Items 14–18	93.1	4.1	71.9–94.2	95.3	0.0	95.3–95.3
C. Individual Items						
1. Somatic concern	89.4	4.9	77.7–92.9	90.3	4.5	71.9–94.3
2. Anxiety	92.7	3.5	80.7–93.7	88.2	3.5	78.2–90.3
3. Emotional withdrawal	83.3	6.7	72.7–88.7	87.8	8.0	49.7–92.6
4. Conceptual disorganization	90.5	4.5	72.5–94.4	81.2	6.5	71.7–87.1
5. Guilt feelings	89.1	6.6	70.6–92.6	79.6	7.6	64.9–87.1
6. Tension	84.3	3.3	79.7–88.3	92.4	7.1	57.9–95.8
7. Mannerisms and posturing	84.6	4.8	63.6–88.7	86.5	8.4	48.0–92.2
8. Grandiosity	80.5	9.4	55.0–86.6	88.5	5.1	74.4–91.1
9. Depressive mood	85.7	9.7	55.4–90.9	86.1	6.6	71.9–91.8
10. Hostility	75.3	11.5	41.1–84.4	83.9	3.2	79.5–87.9
11. Suspiciousness	83.6	8.4	64.9–89.8	93.0	8.3	67.2–96.2
12. Hallucinatory behavior	89.9	4.9	80.3–92.5	81.4	10.4	41.6–87.9
13. Motor retardation	82.1	5.1	72.7–88.1	90.8	4.4	78.6–93.5
14. Uncooperativeness	89.9	6.0	71.9–93.1	92.2	7.4	51.4–94.7
15. Unusual thought content	90.4	5.1	77.2–93.6	91.3	4.4	78.2–94.1
16. Blunted affect	82.8	8.8	65.8–89.4	87.3	6.3	75.3–92.2
17. Exitement	85.3	5.3	75.8–88.7	89.1	3.9	82.2–92.6
18. Disorientation	87.5	5.1	78.6–91.3	95.7	3.9	84.4–97.0

remaining 16 symptoms, as follows: Somatic Concern, Anxiety, Guilt Feelings, Tension, Mannerisms and Posturing, Depression, Mental Retardation, Uncooperativeness, Unusual Thought Content, Disorientation, Poor Attention, Lack of Judgment and Insight, Disturbance of Volition, Poor Impulse Control, Preoccupation, and Active Social Avoidance.

Finally, a GLOBAL scale score can be derived from the PANSS. As for the other three clinical research instruments, it is obtained as an average across each of the 30 individual symptom scores. As previously, each averaged subscale or domain score and the averaged GLOBAL score is rounded to the nearest whole number. For the PANSS, this will produce summary symptomatology scores that can range between a minimum score of 0 to a maximum score of 6. PANSS reliability results will now be discussed, for global, subscale, and individual symptom scores.

PANSS Global Score

As shown in Table 4, and, consistent with average interexaminer agreement levels for the three previously discussed scales, the PANSS global score reached an average level of agreement at initial testing of 96.1%, and one of 98.7% at retest. The corresponding ranges of scores were between 87.9% and 97.9% (initial assessment) and between 90.9% and 99.2% (at retest).

Again, there were no substantive differences in the average agreement levels between psychiatrists, nurses, or psychology technicians, at either the initial testing (respective levels of 96.0%, 96.3%, and 96.0%) or at retesting (respective levels of 98.5%, 99.2%, and 98.5%).

PANSS Subscale Scores

As also shown in Table 4 the average agreement levels for each of the three subscales of the PANSS, namely, the Positive, Negative, and the

General Psychopathology subscales, were virtually interchangeable with the results just discussed for the PANSS Global score.

Consistent with these data, the average interexaminer reliability levels for psychiatrists, nurses, and psychology technicians varied within the narrow ranges of 94% and 97% at initial evaluation and between 95% and 97%, at retest.

The last set of results pertains to the reliability levels of the 30 individual PANSS symptom scores.

PANSS Individual Symptom Scores

As expected, and consistent with the results obtained on the previous three clinical research instruments, the overall levels of interexaminer agreement on individual PANSS symptom scores were, in the main, both lower and more variable than the corresponding levels of examiner agreement on the PANSS domain or global scores. More specifically, whereas PANSS global and subscale scores showed typical levels of agreement in the EXCELLENT range, or between GOOD and EXCELLENT, the analogous levels of average agreement on individual PANSS symptom scores, ranged between a low of 51.7% (Passive/apathetic withdrawal) and a high of 96.5% (Depression) at initial assessment, and between 41.4% (Passive/apathetic withdrawal) and 97.7% (Tension) at reassessment.

SUMMARY AND CONCLUSIONS

This report addresses the question of how to determine both the average and individual levels of reliability when multiple independent clinical examiners assess only one subject on one or more occasions. In our particular application: (1) the 39 clinical examiners were rather evenly divided between psychiatrists, nurses, and psychology technicians; (2) the subject was a veteran schizophrenic adult male patient; and (3) the four assessment instruments were: (a) the Heinrichs-Carpenter Quality of Life (QOL) Scale; (b) the Strauss-Carpenter Level of Function Scale (LOF); (c) the Brief Psychiatric Rating Scale (BPRS); and (d) the Structured Clinical Interview for the Positive and Negative Symptom Scale (SCI-PANSS). Patient

evaluations were examined, as appropriate, at three levels of analysis: on a global, domain, and individual score basis.

Levels of reliability were consistently in the EXCELLENT range (93%–99%) when averaged across the 39 examiners. As expected, however, reliability levels became progressively lower and more variable as based on global, domain, and individual symptom scores, respectively. The three groups of clinical examiners were virtually indistinguishable from each other in terms of the reliability of their patient assessments. Finally, there was a tendency for examiner agreement levels to increase, very slightly (i.e., clinically negligible), from the initial to the retest assessment.

Although our interest was in the assessment of psychiatric symptomatology in one schizophrenic patient, the methodology has relevance for a very broad range of assessments, when multiple examiners evaluate independently the responses of only one person. In the present application, we were interested in determining the reliability of multiple examiners who applied the same complement of well-known reliable and valid clinical instruments to the assessment of one psychiatric patient. The generally high levels of interexaminer reliability for global, domain, and most of the individual items would be of use to clinicians and other mental health professionals in care of the patient under assessment.

A second application is one in which each examiner's clinical rating of a given subject is compared to a best clinical rating or expert judgment. This comes close to what one would regard as the validity of multiple examiners' ratings. This paradigm would be applicable, for example, in screening for clinical examiners to be selected for a given reliability research investigation.

Another application is to use this methodology to train multiple examiners to reach a standard or best clinical rating across a number of clinical instruments.

A very different application would be one in which there is interest in either revising a standard clinical rating scale or creating a new one, at a stage in the development of the instrument that is too rudimentary to warrant the design and execution of a comprehensive reliability study. At this stage, rather, there is a need to have multiple clinical

Table 4. Interexaminer Agreement Levels in the Evaluation of a Single Schizophrenic Patient on the Positive and Negative Syndrome Scale.

Area of Assessment	Initial Evaluation			Retest Evaluation		
	M	(SD)	% Range	M	(SD)	% Range
A. Global score	96.1	3.3	87.9–97.9	98.7	1.9	90.9–99.2
B. Domains						
1. Positive Scale	95.9	3.2	87.4–97.7	95.6	2.5	85.4–97.0
2. Negative Scale	94.6	3.7	88.8–97.0	95.7	2.7	85.8–97.3
3. General Psychopathology Scale	95.6	3.5	88.1–97.7	96.3	2.9	87.1–97.9
B. Individual items						
1. Conceptual disorganization	89.4	5.3	72.3–93.7	90.1	8.3	50.1–94.3
2. Poor rapport	87.1	6.7	64.3–91.6	91.1	3.4	84.4–94.1
3. Lack of spontaneity & flow of conversation	84.7	9.1	58.0–90.2	92.8	6.6	59.4–95.8
4. Anxiety	89.7	4.4	73.7–92.1	87.7	3.6	77.8–89.6
5. Delusions	89.0	5.3	71.6–93.5	87.7	8.1	49.3–92.6
6. Unusual thought content	80.6	7.0	52.7–87.4	81.4	7.9	66.2–88.4
7. Suspiciousness/persecution	90.3	5.7	67.6–94.2	84.5	5.4	68.7–89.6
8. Passive/apathetic withdrawal	80.1	6.2	51.7–86.7	79.2	10.8	41.4–86.9
9. Active social avoidance	82.8	6.8	61.1–86.5	88.2	5.3	72.3–92.2
10. Poor impulse control	88.8	5.3	71.1–93.0	85.9	3.7	82.7–90.5
11. Hallucinatory behavior	85.4	7.9	61.8–91.8	83.0	7.7	58.4–88.8
12. Somatic concern	91.7	7.8	63.2–95.6	94.4	2.3	84.6–96.0
13. Depression	95.5	1.4	93.5–96.5	81.7	4.5	65.8–86.7
14. Guilt feelings	82.4	6.4	73.9–87.6	86.1	10.2	61.9–91.5
15. Grandiosity	90.3	4.7	69.9–94.2	87.9	8.5	45.0–93.2
16. Disorientation	87.4	3.8	80.9–91.1	91.5	4.2	77.0–94.7
17. Difficulty in abstract thinking	91.1	6.9	62.2–94.9	85.9	8.4	70.4–91.5
18. Lack of judgement and insight	93.4	3.8	78.3–95.6	88.1	5.6	78.4–92.8
19. Blunted affect	78.6	7.3	64.3–85.8	85.2	4.2	78.0–88.4
20. Emotional withdrawal	79.5	6.8	63.9–86.5	94.4	6.1	67.4–96.6
21. Stereotyped thinking	93.4	3.2	83.4–95.3	84.1	6.0	60.7–87.3
22. Excitement	87.4	7.0	56.6–91.6	90.9	7.0	70.4–94.1
23. Hostility	85.7	8.1	61.8–91.6	87.0	8.4	51.0–91.3
24. Tension	91.0	3.4	84.1–93.9	96.0	3.4	87.9–97.7
25. Mannerisms and posturing	86.2	8.4	67.4–92.1	77.4	7.2	64.7–85.0
26. Motor retardation	86.7	4.9	78.1–91.4	94.3	2.3	84.8–95.8
27. Uncooperativeness	85.8	7.2	72.0–90.2	84.5	9.8	60.7–90.1
28. Poor attention	90.3	7.7	69.7–93.7	90.8	9.1	66.6–95.1
29. Disturbance of volition	89.0	8.9	61.8–93.9	85.8	8.0	69.1–90.9
30. Preoccupation	86.6	8.2	64.1–92.5	90.7	5.0	67.9–93.7

examiners assess the responses of a more or less "typical" subject of interest to a wide range of potential items across which the subject can be expected to vary considerably. Such a strategy, in the early stages of test development can be justified by the fact that, beyond a certain point, reliability levels are increased faster by increasing the number of examiners rather than the number of subjects.

More specifically, Donner and Eliasziw (1987) have demonstrated convincingly, by the application of exact power curves, that a decrease in the number of examiners below 10 results in a steep rise in the number of subjects required to maintain power at the conventional desideratum of 80%. Rather than increasing the number of subjects dramatically, the same level of power can be achieved by a very modest increase in the number of independent clinical examiners. The particular combination of the number of examiners and the number of subjects to employ will depend largely upon the objectives of the specific reliability study. More-over, the work of Donner and Eliasziw indicates clearly that when such prudent decisions are, in fact, undertaken, they can prove to be quite cost-efficient.

As another important comment, it should be noted that extensive computer simulation studies have confirmed that the new statistical methodology is distribution-free, meaning that it can be validly applied whether the data derive from symmetric or extremely skewed distributions, providing the minimum number of independent examiners is 30. When the number of clinical examiners falls below this level, the examiner ratings and rankings should be based on a t test, *rather* than a Z test (Cicchetti, Showalter, & Rosenheck, 1997). The rationale behind this strategy is that the statistic t will approximate a Z, or normal distribution, when the number of examiners, or raters reaches 30. It is instructive, in this regard, that, while the t value for statistical significance at the conventional $p = .05$ level is the well-known value of 1.96, when the sample size is extremely large (or infinite), the corresponding t value, at the .05 level, when the sample size is 30, is quite similar, at 2.04. The user-friendly computer software (described in Cicchetti & Showalter, 1997), including detailed documentation that is required to perform these specialized types of reliability assessments, can be obtained free of charge by writing to the first author.

REFERENCES

American Psychiatric Association (1987). *Diagnostic and Statistical Manual of Mental Disorders* (3rd ed., rev.) Washington, DC: Author.

Bell, M., Milstein, R., Beam-Goulet, J., Lysaker, P., & Cicchetti, D.V. (1992). The Positive and Negative Syndrome Scale and the Briel Psychiatric Rating Scale: Reliability, comparability and predictive validity. *Journal of Nervous and Mental Disease, 1180*, 723–728.

Broca, P. (1861). Nouvelle observation d'aphemie produite par une lesion de la moitie' posterieure des deuxieme et troiseme circonvolutions frontales. *Bulletin de la Societé Anatomique de Paris, 6*, 398–407.

Cicchetti, D.V. (1976). Assessing inter-rater reliability for rating scales: Resolving some basic issues. *British Journal of Psychiatry, 129*, 452–456.

Cicchetti, D.V., & Fleiss, J.L. (1977). Comparison of the null distributions of weighted kappa and the C ordinal statistic. *Applied Psychological Measurement, 1*, 195–201.

Cicchetti, D.V., & Showalter, D. (1997). A computer program for assessing interexaminer agreement when multiple ratings are made on a single subject. *Psychiatry Research, 72*, 65–68.

Cicchetti, D.V., Showalter, D., & Rosenheck, R. (1997). A new method for assessing interexaminer agreement when multiple ratings are made on a single subject: Applications to the assessment of neuropsychiatric symptomatology. *Psychiatry Research, 72*, 51–63.

Cicchetti, D.V., & Sparrow, S.S. (1981). Developing criteria for establishing interrater reliability of specific items: Applications to assessment of adaptive behavior. *American Journal of Mental Deficiency, 86*, 127–137.

Cicchetti, D.V., Volkmar, F., Klin, A., & Showalter, D. (1995). Diagnosing autism using ICD-10 criteria: A comparison of neural networks and standard multivariate procedures. *Child Neuropsychology, 1*, 26–37.

Cicchetti, D.V., Volkmar, F., Sparrow, S.S., Cohen, D., Fermanian, J., & Rourke, B.P. (1992). Assessing the reliability of clinical scales when the data have both nominal and ordinal features: Proposed guidelines for neuropsychological assessments. *Journal of Clinical and Experimental Neuropsychology, 14*, 673–686.

Donner, A., & Eliasziw, M. (1987). Sample size requirements for reliability studies. *Statistics in Medicine, 6*, 441–448.

Fisher, R.A. (1935). *The design of experiments*. Edinburgh, Scotland: Oliver & Boyd.

Fleiss, J.L. (1981). *Statistical methods for rates and proportions* (2nd ed.). New York: Wiley.

Heinrichs, D.W., Hanlon, T.E., & Carpenter, W.T. (1989). The Quality of Life Scale: An instrument for rating the schizophrenic deficit syndrome. *Schizophrenic Bulletin, 10*, 388–398.

Holschuh, N. (1980). Randomization and design. In S.E. Feinberg & D.V. Hinkley (Eds.), *R.A. Fisher: An appreciation.* (pp. 35–45). New York: Springer-Verlag.

Kay, S.R., Fiszbein, A., & Opler. L.A. (1992). The Positive and Negative Syndrome Scale (PANSS) for schizophrenics. *Schizophrenic Bulletin, 13*, 261–276.

Marshall, J.C., & Newcombe, F. (1984). Putative problems and pure progress in neuropsychological single-case studies. *Journal of Clinical Neuropsychology, 6*, 65–70.

McGraw, K.O., & Wong, S.P. (1996). Forming inferences about some intraclass correlation coefficients. *Psychological Methods, 1*, 30–46.

Overall, J.E., & Gorham, D.R. (1962). The Brief Psychiatric Rating Scale. *Psychological Reports, 10*, 799–812.

Overall, J.E., & Klett, C.J. (1972). *Applied multivariate analysis*. New York: McGraw-Hill.

Rosenheck, R., Cramer, J., Weichun. X., Thomas, J., Henderson, W., Frisman, L., Fye, C. & Charney, D. (1997). A comparison of clozapine and haloperidol in hospitalized patients with refractory schizophrenia. *New England Journal of Medicine, 337*, 809–815.

Scoville, W.B., & Milner, B. (1957). Loss of recent memory after bilateral hippocampal lesions. *Journal of Neurology, Neurosurgery, and Psychiatry, 20*, 11–21.

Shallice, T. (1979). Case study approach in neuropsychological research. *Journal of Clinical Neuropsychology, 1*, 183–211.

Strauss, J.S., & Carpenter, W.T. (1972). The prediction of outcome in schizophrenics. *Archives of General Psychiatry, 27*, 739–746.

Wilson, B.A. (1987). Single-case experimental designs in neuropsychological rehabilitation. *Journal of Clinical and Experimental Neuropsychology, 9*, 527–544.

APPENDIX

Determining Reliability Levels When Multiple Clinical Examiners Evaluate One Subject

Suppose 40 clinical examiners evaluate independently a single schizophrenic patient, on the Positive and Negative Syndrome Scale, (PANSS) and there is interest in assessing the overall reliability of these evaluations. Suppose, further, that the results present as follows:

Rating: 0 1 2 3 4 5 6
No. of Raters: 0 1 13 22 4 0 0

With 40 clinical examiners, there are $(40 \times 39)/2 = 780$ examiner pairings. Applying the weighting system from Cicchetti (1976) and Cicchetti and Sparrow (1981), we can calculate the overall level of agreement, among the multiple examiners (ME), as:

Agreement (ME)
 = [315(1.00) + 387(0.9091)
 + 74(0.7273) + 4(0.5454)]/780
 = .9267
 = 92.67%, or about 93%.

In this application, there are 315 rater pairings in complete agreement, therefore, receiving a weight of 1.00, or 100%; another 387 pairings are one scale category apart, and receive a weight of .9091 or 90.91%; 74 pairs of ratings are 2 categories apart and receive a weighting of .7273, or 72.73% and the remaining 4 pairs of ratings are 3 categories apart and receive a weighting of .5454 or 54.54%.

Using the same formula, each of the 22 clinical examiners whose average global PANSS rating was a 3, received a level of agreement, with the remaining examiners, of 95%; the 13 examiners with a global rating of 2 were 92% in agreement with the remaining examiners; the 4 clinical examiners with a global rating of 4 were in 85% agreement with the other raters; and the remaining clinical examiner, with a global rating of 1, was in 77% agreement with the remaining 39 examiners.

Finally, the average global ratings of 1, 2, 3, and 4, respectively, had a mean of 2.725 and a standard deviation (*SD*) of 0.6789. Using the standard formula for *Z*, namely, $(X - \text{Mean})/SD$ showed that the clinical examiner whose PANSS global score was 1, received a *Z* score of -2.54. Consulting a table of areas under the normal curve, shows that this score of 1 is significantly lower than the average clinician rating of 2.725 at $p = .007$. Moreover, the level of agreement, 77%, is in the FAIR range while the average ratings of the remaining examiners are in the GOOD (i.e., 85%) or EXCELLENT range (i.e., 92% and 95%, respectively). For a more technical description of this new biostatistical methodology, as well as its mathematical underpinning, as confirmed by extensive computer simulation studies, the interested reader is again referred to Cicchetti, Showalter, and Rosenheck (1997) and Cicchetti and Showalter (1997).

The Clinical Neuropsychologist
1995, Vol. 9, No. 1, pp. 079–082

BRIEF REPORT

Improving Examiner Reliability on the Visual Memory Span Subtest of the Wechsler Memory Scale – Revised

Yvonne I. Demsky and Alfred H. Sellers

Nova University, Fort Lauderdale, Florida

ABSTRACT

Standard administration and scoring of the Visual Memory Span (VMS) subtest of the Wechsler Memory Scale – Revised is problematic because accuracy depends upon the experience and concentration abilities of the examiner. The standard administration method was contrasted with a new method that enables the examiner to rely on cue cards. Comparisons showed the cue-card method to be superior in ease of administration and scoring accuracy to the standard method. Results suggest that cue cards help both novices and veterans obtain more accurate VMS assessments; their use also significantly improves interexaminer reliability.

Most Wechsler Memory Scale – Revised (WMS-R; Wechsler, 1987) subtests are well standardized and easy to administer. Because the majority of the subtests are objective, interscorer reliability on the WMS-R has only been computed for Logical Memory and Visual Reproduction (Franzen, 1989). Accurate administration and scoring of the Visual Memory Span (VMS) subtest is highly dependent upon the examiner's memory and concentration abilities. Scoring errors committed by the examiner can degrade the reliability, and hence the validity, of the test (Anastasi, 1988).

Cue cards were developed in an effort to improve the reliability by enabling examiners to receive immediate feedback while administering and scoring a subject's responses (Demsky & Sellers, 1993). For an examiner, this eliminates the need to depend solely on memory and concentration abilities.

Two studies were undertaken. Study 1 compared scoring errors committed by naive undergraduates who either administered the test in the standard manner or with the assistance of cue cards. Study 2 also compared scoring errors, but in a within-subject design with participants who were advanced graduate students formally trained in the standard administration of the WMS-R. In both studies it was hypothesized that more scoring errors would be committed by examiners using standard administration procedures than those using the cue cards. It was also hypothesized that reliability coefficients would be higher for the card-assisted administration than for the standard administration.

STUDY 1

METHOD

Subjects

Fourteen second-year college students (mean age = 26.61, SD = 7.33) enrolled in an introductory psychology course served as subject-examiners in this study. All were given extra credit for their participation. None had prior experience administering psychological tests. One-half of these subject-examiners (Group 1) were

Correspondence to: Yvonne I. Demsky, Ph.D., Center for Psychological Studies, Nova University, 3301 College Ave., Ft. Lauderdale, FL 33314 U.S.A.
Accepted for publication: March 8, 1994.

randomly assigned to the standard VMS administration condition and one-half (Group 2) were assigned to the experimental card administration condition. There were no differences between the two groups in age ($p > .2$) or gender ($p > .2$).

Cue Cards

Fourteen 4 in. × 2.5 in. laminated cards representing the forward tapping series were prepared with a computer graphics program and laser printer. Each card was a reduced facsimile of the red-and-white forward tapping stimulus card contained in the kit. Each card was labeled with the item and trial number it represented. The correct tapping sequence was indicated on the actual cue cards by numbering sequentially the squares that were to be tapped. For example, Trial 1 of Item 1 squares 2 and 6 were labeled "1" and "2," respectively. Thus, the subject had to tap square "1" first, then square "2" second, and so on.

An additional twelve 4 in. × 2.5 in. laminated cards representing the backward tapping series were used. Each of these cue cards contained two side-by-side reduced facsimiles of the green-and-white backward stimulus card. The left side of each card indicated the order in which to administer the item, and the right side indicated the correct order in which the examinee's response should be given. Examples of forward and backward cue cards are shown in Figures 1 and 2.

Procedures

All subject-examiners were initially trained to administer the VMS subtest according to the procedures specified in the WMS-R manual. Following training, each was given 30 min to practice administering the test, and then directed to proceed to an examination room to evaluate an examinee. No one was yet aware of the cue-card administration method. Upon entering the examination room, each subject-examiner was seated opposite a research confederate who served as an examinee. The confederate possessed a separate set of cue cards with planted errors. These were held out of the view of the subject-examiner. The same errors were committed by the confederate for each test administration by each subject-examiner. Errors were committed in such a way that the confederate should have achieved a score of 16 on the VMS for every administration.

Those subject-examiners assigned to Group 1 administered the VMS to the confederate in the standard manner for which they had been trained. However, just prior to test administration, the subject-examiners assigned to the experimental condition were directed to use the cue cards that, until then, they had not seen. Group 2 subject-examiners were instructed to tap the corresponding boxes on the stimulus card in the sequential order that appeared on the cue cards. They

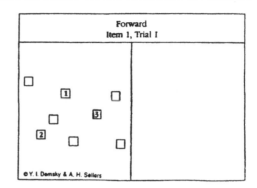

Fig. 1. Example of a forward tapping series cue card.
Note. Pattern of squares is from *Wechsler Memory Scale – Revised* by D. Wechsler, 1987. Copyright 1987 by Psychological Corporation. Reproduced by Permission.

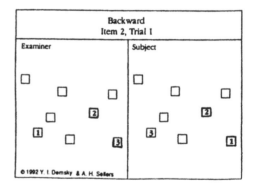

Fig. 2. Example of a backward tapping series cue card.

were further instructed to glance back and forth from the cue card to the stimulus card while administering and scoring each of the items. All subject-examiners in both groups were asked to record either a "P" (for Pass) or "F" (for Fail) on each trial of each item. The number of scoring errors (i.e., scoring a "P" when the confederate committed an error, or scoring an "F" when the confederate actually performed a sequence correctly) and the item scores served as the dependent measures for the analyses.

RESULTS

Subject-examiners who administered the VMS with the cue cards made significantly fewer scoring errors (Mean = 2, $SD = 1.29$) than did those who administered the test in the standard fashion (Mean = 5.57, $SD = 2.64$), $t = 3.22$, $p < .01$. Reliability coefficients were computed for the two administration methods by correlating the item scores recorded by the subject-examiners with each other for each of the groups. Individual correlations were converted to Fisher Z values that were averaged and compared by way of z tests (Hays, 1988). The mean Fisher Zs were transformed back into correlation coefficients to serve as reliability measures of the two methods (Anastasi, 1988). The mean Fisher Zs were transformed back into correlation coefficients to serve as reliability measures of the two methods (Anastasi, 1988). Reliabilities for both the forward ($r = .989$) and backward ($r = .969$) cue-card administrations were significantly higher ($p < .05$) than for those of the standard administration ($r = .589$ and .507, respectively).

STUDY 2

METHOD

Subjects
Seven female and four male doctoral level clinical psychology students (mean age = 33.9 years, $SD = 7.9$; mean years of education = 19.1, $SD = 1.2$) served as subject-examiners. All had received formal doctoral training in the administration of the WMS-R. On average, each had administered and scored 14.4 WMS-R protocols (range = 2 to 30).

Procedures
Each participant administered the VMS subtest to a confederate examinee twice in a randomized counterbalanced order (i.e., once in the standard fashion, followed by the cue-card method or vice versa). Cue cards prepared for Study 1 were again used. In each case, the confederate used a special set of cue cards with consistent planted performance errors to achieve an expected score of 16 on each examination. Subject-examiners were instructed to follow the standard administration of the VMS with or without the cue cards, depending on their order of assignment. All subject-examiners were asked to record either a "P" or "F" on each trial of each item. No subject-examiners received practice using the cue cards. Thus, as for Group 2 in Study 1, all subjects were instructed to use the cards for the first time during the actual experimental administration.

RESULTS

The subject-examiners made significantly fewer errors (Mean = .82, $SD = 1.08$) during the cue-card administration than during the standard administration of the VMS (Mean = 2.64, $SD = 1.91$), dependent $t = 5.16$, $p < .001$. Also, fewer deviations from the expected total score of 16 resulted when the subject-examiners used the cue cards (Mean = .54, $SD = .69$) versus when they did not use them (Mean = 2.36, $SD = 1.36$), dependent $t = 5.16$, $p < .001$.

As in Study 1, examiner reliability for each method was investigated by correlating the item scores recorded by each subject-examiner with each other for each of the administrations. Individual correlations were transformed to Fisher Z values, which were then averaged. Since these means were derived from the same subjects, and hence were dependent, a method described by Steiger (1980) was used to compare them. The mean Fisher Zs were then transformed back into correlation coefficients. Cue-card administration reliabilities for the forward ($r = .999$), backward ($r = .950$), and total series ($r = .966$) were significantly higher ($p < .01$, $p < .05$, and $p < .001$, respectively) than those for the standard administration ($rs = .985, .684$, and $.662$, respectively).

DISCUSSION

As can be seen from these results, the standard administration method is subject to a significantly greater number of examiner errors, thus reducing examiner reliability. These errors are drastically reduced when using the cue cards. Comparisons between the two administration methods showed the cue card method to be superior in ease of administration and scoring to the standard method. Thus, use of the cue-card method of administration is a more reliable and effective method of assessment for both experienced and inexperienced examiners.

REFERENCES

Anastasi, A. (1988). *Psychological testing* (6th ed.). New York: Macmillan.

Demsky, Y.I., & Sellers, A.H. (1993, February). *Improving examiner reliability on the Visual Memory Span subtest of the WMS-R.* Paper presented at the annual meeting of the International Neuropsychological Society, Galveston, TX.

Franzen, M.D. (1989). *Reliability and validity in neuropsychological assessment.* New York: Plenum Press.

Hays, W.L. (1988). *Statistics* (4th ed.). New York: Holt, Rinehart, & Winston.

Steiger, J.H. (1980). Tests for comparing elements of a correlation matrix. *Psychological Bulletin, 87,* 245–251.

Wechsler, D. (1987). *Wechsler Memory Scale-Revised Manual.* San Antonio: The Psychological Corporation.

Journal of Clinical and Experimental Neuropsychology
2000, Vol. 22, No. 5, pp. 622–632

Principles of Defining Reliable Change Indices

Gerard H. Maassen

Utrecht University, Faculty of Social Sciences, Department of Methodology and Statistics,
Utrecht, The Netherlands

ABSTRACT

In this article, several salient measures for determining reliable change are scrutinized. The classic null hypothesis method is compared with more recent procedures based on interval estimation of the true change, including Kelley's formula. The latter category of methods are shown to entail serious drawbacks. If Kelley's formula is expanded to a null hypothesis method (including a correct treatment of the stochastic character of the sample information), the classic method reveals itself as a large sample approximation. We conclude that the classic method is undeservedly regarded inferior by the authors who proposed new indices.

The determination of change in a person subjected to an intervention is an important element of many studies. Usually, the researcher is interested in progress or improvement, for instance as a result of a psychotherapy, although such areas as deterioration of mental functioning, e.g., as a consequence of a medical intervention, may also be a focus of attention. There are various means of characterizing change (see for example, Plewis, 1985). This article does not aim to compare or even discuss the various procedures, but focuses on just one mode of establishing change, i.e., the situation where one attempts to ascertain change, improvement or deterioration, by means of two test assessments, a pretest and a post-test, without the use of a control group.

The difference observed between pretest and post-test is an obvious measure of change. However, only when variables perfectly measure the phenomenon they are supposed to measure is the observed difference really dependable. Unfortunately, the assessment of mental status is always contaminated by effects that preclude a perfect measurement. An observed difference may be partly or even totally due to measurement errors,

practice effects, or sample fluctuations. Such influences may also conceal true changes. Naturally, researchers are not interested in changes which can be explained by trivial effects. They are concerned in the first place with the question of whether an observed change is of substantive importance, or has *clinical significance* (Jacobson, Follette, & Revenstorf, 1984). However, clinical significance is only a matter for discussion if the observed change is *statistically reliable*. How clinical relevance should be established has often been disputed, but at the same time there has been a quest for methods and measures for the determination of statistical reliability of an observed change. These measures, which we, following Jacobson et al. (1984), refer to as *Reliable Change Indices (RC)*, are the topic of this article.

A *RC* is always a ratio. The numerator contains the observed change for a given participant, corrected for the nuisance effects mentioned above if so desired. A measure which calibrates the disturbance effects has been placed in the denominator. This denominator operates as a criterion: If the numerator exceeds the denominator sufficiently, the nuisance effect can be ruled out with high

Address correspondence to: G.H. Maassen, Utrecht University, Faculty of Social Sciences, Department Methodology and Statistics, P.O.Box 80140, 3508 TC Utrecht, The Netherlands. Tel.: 030-2534765. Fax: 030-2535797.
E-mail: g.maassen@fss.uu.nl.
Accepted for Publication: January 20, 2000.

probability as an alternative explanation for the observed change. Usually, the ratio is regarded as (or transformed into) a standardized normally distributed quantity. If the *RC* exceeds a chosen percentile in the normal distribution, the observed change is taken to be *reliable*.

More recently proposed *RC*'s have become increasingly complicated. This is a consequence of attempts to take the different disturbance effects into account. Initially, only measurement unreliability was dealt with (Christensen & Mendoza, 1986; McNemar, 1962, 1969). In subsequent variants, adjustments were also made for regression to the mean. Hsu (1989), Nunnally and Kotsche (1983), and Speer (1992) all proposed a measure in which the pretest score was replaced by a regression estimate for the true pretest score (from the observed pretest score). This means that information on the group (population or sample) to which the person in question belongs, is also required. These measures can be distinguished according to the delineation of the group, or the standard error used in the denominator.

Hageman and Arrindell (1993), and Zegers and Hafkenscheid (Bruggemans, Van de Vijver. & Huysmans, 1997; Hafkenscheid, 1994; Zegers & Hafkenscheid, 1994) adopt a regression estimate of the true difference from the observed difference. The indices of these authors, too, differ with respect to the criterion in the denominator. Chelune, Naugle, Lüders, Sedlak, and Awad (1993), and McSweeny, Naugle, Chelune, and Lüders (1993) proposed measures in which the practice effect resulting from repetition of measurements has been taken into account. Recently, Bruggemans et al. (1997) proposed a *RC*, which combines this correction with the index of Zegers and Hafkenscheid.

Different *RC*'s may lead to different conclusions concerning the effect of an intervention on a given person, a cause of much confusion. In this article, we demonstrate that this confusion is partly the result of the essentially different principles underlying the *RC*'s. Both principles and their practical consequences are discussed. The drawbacks entailed by the way some of the *RC*'s are constructed will be demonstrated. Several salient *RC*'s are central to our argument, but our reasoning and our remarks apply to other measures as well.

Null Hypothesis Model and Estimation Interval Model

The classic approach

An obvious estimator for the true intra-individual change of a given person i is the observed difference D_i between the pretest score X_i and the post-test score Y_i. In terms of classical test theory (CTT), an observed difference D_i can be split into a true difference and a component containing measurement error:

$$D_i = Y_i - X_i = \Delta_i + E_{D_i}$$

Usually it is assumed that, for all participants, the error components are normally distributed with zero mean and standard deviation equal to σ_{ED} (Lord & Novick, 1968, p. 159). We note that the observed difference score, then, is an unbiased estimator of the true difference. Under the null hypothesis that the treatment has no effect,

$$D_i / \sigma_{ED} \qquad (1)$$

has a standardized normal distribution. According to McNemar (1962, 1969), an observed difference score is considered *dependable* – the term reliable change had not yet been introduced – if this quantity exceeds a chosen critical value, for instance 1.96. Thus, the procedure can be characterized as a statistical test for the null hypothesis H_0: "The true change of the given individual equals 0". There is always a risk that rejection of H_0 is purely an artifact of an unreliable measurement instrument. If alpha is set at .05, the probability of committing a type I error is .05. If a change is called reliable only in the case of improvement ($Y > X$), or in the case of deterioration ($Y < X$), this probability is .025. The objective of this procedure is to rule out measurement error as an explanation for an observed change with a known but low risk of drawing a wrong conclusion.

It should be noted that this procedure may reflect clinical practice in a simplified way. Firstly, the assumptions of zero mean of error components and equal standard error of measurement of the difference score may be violated in clinical situations. For instance, when a therapeutic client is selected for a low pretest score, the assumption of zero mean of error components is no longer valid. The method is obviously not suitable for such situations. Secondly, this method, as well as the other methods discussed in this article, has to depart from the assumption that effects which may jeopardize the validity of conclusions, such as a practice effect due to repeated measurement, are zero. The procedures that are central to this article cannot be experimentally controlled and there is no way of circumventing this assumption.

This simple procedure, based on statistical testing of a null hypothesis, is central to this article and will be referred to as the *classic approach*. The procedure has been rediscovered by Christensen and Mendoza (1986), and Jacobson and Truax (1991). In both publications, the authors also assume that the standard errors of measurement of pretest and post-test are equal, which is not relevant to our discussion.

The Regressed Score Method
Several authors held that the *RC* could be sharpened by replacing the observed change by an improved estimate for the true change in the numerator. The observed difference is an unbiased estimate of the true change, but other estimates may be worth considering for other reasons. For instance, Nunnally and Kotsch (1983), Hsu (1989), and Speer (1992) emphasized that when estimating the true difference score of person *i*, regression to the mean should be taken into account. Hsu (1989) states, "Given assumptions of the reliability model, regression toward the mean can be interpreted as the difference between pretreatment and post-treatment scores which would be expected in the absence of treatment effect, because of unreliability of the response measure" (p. 462). These authors propose to estimate the post-test score which would be expected in the absence of a treatment effect:

$$\hat{Y}_i = \varrho_{XX} \left(X_i - \mu_X \right) + \mu_X$$

Here μ_X and ϱ_{XX}, respectively, are the mean and the reliability of the pretest score in a relevant population, called the *reliability group* (Hsu, 1989). Such an estimate for the final score has also been referred to as the *regressed score* (McNemar, 1958, 1969). Then, the improved estimate of the true difference score is taken to be the difference

between this estimate for the post-test score and the observed post-test score:

$$\hat{\Delta}_i = Y_i - \hat{Y}_i = D_i + \left(X_i - \mu_X \right)\left(1 - \varrho_{XX}\right). \quad (2)$$

The standard error of estimate of this estimation is:

$$\sigma_X \sqrt{1 - \varrho_{XX}^2} \quad (3)$$

where σ_X denotes the standard deviation of the pretest score in the reliability group. The *RC* proposed by Hsu (1989) is the ratio with Equation 2 in the numerator and Equation 3 in the denominator, and, in fact, is applied as follows: "If the estimation interval

$$D_i + \left(X_i - \mu_X \right)\left(1 - \varrho_{XX}\right) \pm 1.96 \, \sigma_X \sqrt{1 - \varrho_{XX}^2}$$

does not contain 0, the observed change is called *reliable*." The factor 1.96 suggests that this conclusion has a reliability of 95%.

This procedure suffers from the shortcoming that the estimate according to Equation 2 is generally a biased estimate for the true difference. This is revealed by:

$$E\left(\hat{\Delta}_i \mid \xi_i, \Delta_i\right) = \Delta_i + (\xi_i - \mu_\xi)(1 - \varrho_{XX}), \quad (4)$$

where ξ_i denotes the true pretest score of person *i*, and μ_ξ denotes the population mean of the true pretest scores. To express that a given person *i* is not characterized by his or her observed pretest score, which is stochastic, but by the true score, the expectation in Equation (4) is conditioned on the true pretest score as well.

The estimate is only unbiased if $\xi_i = \mu_\xi$ or $\varrho_{XX} = 1$. If Δ_i and $\xi_i - \mu_f$ have a different sign, then Δ_i and the expected value of the estimate can have a different sign. If the bias of the estimate is sufficiently large, it may be expected that a reliable change in the wrong direction will be concluded. This is the case if:

$$|\xi_i - \mu_\xi| \, (1 - \varrho_{XX}) - |\Delta_i| > 1.96 \, \sigma_X \sqrt{1 - \varrho_{XX}^2}.$$

If there is no real change, it may be expected that nevertheless the conclusion 'reliable change' will be drawn if:

$$\left|\frac{\xi_i - \mu_\xi}{\sigma_X}\right| > 1.96 \sqrt{\frac{1 + \varrho_{XX}}{1 - \varrho_{XX}}}. \quad (5)$$

The classic approach and the method under consideration are based on different principles. The latter can not boast a uniform probability distribution that the researcher can rely on to indicate the probability of making a type I error. In the method in question, an estimation interval is used for the true difference score, based on the regressed score estimate of the true pretest score. Hence, we call this method an *estimation interval method*. At most, the interval that contains the true difference score with high probability is roughly indicated. In the majority of the cases, the decision of reliable change will be justified. However, the estimation of the true difference score is biased, and for patients with an extreme true pretest score (see Equation 5) the bias can be so great that there is a high probability of making a wrong decision. The lower the reliability of the pretest score, the greater is this threat. Hsu (1989) shows in his Table 1, how in such cases the criteria for the decisions in the classic approach and the regressed score method may diverge. If the population mean and variance of the pretest scores are unknown, and if they are estimated with the help of a sample, the regressed score method entails the additional drawback that sample fluctuations may also be conducive to a wrong decision. The regressed score estimate may be attractive as an estimate, but as a basis for the assessment of reliable change it entails shortcomings compared with the null hypothesis model, with no clear advantages.

Reliable Change Indices Based on Kelley's Formula

Hageman and Arrindell's RCID
Several authors have held the view that the *RC* could be improved by sharpening even more the estimate of the true difference in the numerator. Hageman and Arrindell (1993) were the first to employ Kelley's formula (Kelley, 1947, p. 409) as the improved estimate and as the basis of a *RC*.

Kelley's estimate, also known as the *weighted reliability measure*, is:

$$\hat{\Delta}_i = \varrho_{DD} D_i + \left(1 - \varrho_{DD}\right) \overline{D} \quad (6)$$

It is a regression estimate of the true change and thus it has the advantage that, on the whole, the estimation errors are minimized in the sense of least squares (Rogosa, Brandt, & Zimowski, 1982). We note in this context that various regression estimates are eligible. A regressed score estimate was discussed earlier which only employs the pretest score. Kelley's formula is based on the observed difference. Even more precise are estimates which employ observed initial and final scores separately (see Cronbach & Furby, 1970; Lord, 1956; McNemar, 1958), but as far as we know, these have never been used as a basis for a *RC*.

The question is now: Which denominator fits Kelley's formula? Hageman and Arrindell (1993) proposed the standard error of measurement of the difference score:

$$\sigma_{E_D} = \sqrt{\sigma_{E_X}^2 + \sigma_{E_Y}^2}$$

The *RC* with this standard error in the denominator and Equation 6 in the numerator was named RC_{ID} by Hageman and Arrindell (1993), who simply state that their formula is "the most appropriate way of combining (a) the benefits of the original formulas of Jacobson et al. (1984) and Christensen and Mendoza (1986), and (b) the search for a better approximation of the true difference score" (p. 697). Thus, their choice is hardly justified statistically. Nevertheless, Hageman and Arrindell's RC_{ID} seems to have become established in the research literature. It has already been applied by several researchers (Debats, 1996; De Haan et al., 1997; Rudy, Turk, Kubinski, & Zaki, 1995; Van Oppen et al., 1995; Wykes, 1998) or at least mentioned as a serious alternative (Barkham et al., 1996; Taylor, 1995).

The RC of Zegers and Hafkenscheid
As a sequel to Hageman and Arrindell's index, Zegers and Hafkenscheid (1994) proposed the following standard error:

$$\sigma_{\Delta.D} = \sigma_\Delta \sqrt{1 - \varrho_{DD}} = \sigma_D \sqrt{\varrho_{DD}} \sqrt{1 - \varrho_{DD}}$$
$$= \sigma_{E_D} \sqrt{\varrho_{DD}}. \quad (7)$$

This expression has been known for some time as the *standard error of estimate* belonging to Kelley's formula (Lord & Novick, 1968; McNemar, 1958). Once again, within the context of reliable change indices an old formula has been rediscovered. The index of reliable change with Equation 6 in the numerator and Equation 7 in the denominator was christened RC_{URCI} by Zegers and Hafkenscheid. The authors did not succeed in publishing their RC officially and RC_{URCI} found its way into the literature circuitously (see Bruggemans et al., 1997). Recently, Hageman and Arrindell (1999), however, did publish the same index (accompanied by the condition $\varrho_{DD} > .40$), now referred to as RC_{INDIV}. They seem to recognize their error as they state: "RC_{INDIV} may also be considered an improved version of the RC_{ID} index (...) Though under standard conditions, RC_{ID} could be considered superior to RC in terms of correct classification of individuals, the present authors now recommend its even more precise successor RC_{INDIV}." (p. 1175). As it seems only fair, throughout this article the new index will be denoted by RC_{URCI}.

Due to its history, RC_{URCI} has hardly been applied yet. Nevertheless, this index deserves more attention, because it certainly has statistical foundation. The method of Zegers and Hafkenscheid is a regression estimate method, where Kelley's formula is (correctly) regarded as an estimate of the true change of person i, given his or her observed difference, and where the standard error of estimate in Equation 7 is appropriate. We will now elaborate on the features of this method.

If Zegers and Hafkenscheid choose Equation 7 as the denominator for their RC, then in fact they are proposing to use Kelley's formula as a criterion for *reliable change* in the following way:

"The true value of the difference of person i is comprised with probability .95 by the interval:

$$\varrho_{DD} D_i + (1 - \varrho_{DD}) \overline{D} \pm 1.96 \, \sigma_{\Delta.D}$$

and if 0 lies outside this interval the observed difference is denominated *reliable*."

With regard to this approach, we observe the following. Firstly, the procedure has the attractive characteristic that the standard error in Equation 7 is smaller than the standard error of measurement of the difference scores in Equation 1. This can be explained by the fact that when estimating the true

difference extra information is used in Equation 6, namely the reliability and the group average of the difference score (see Lord & Novick, 1968, p. 68). However, less attractively, the stochastic character of this information has not been taken into account.

Secondly, if the mean true effect of the intervention in the population (μ_Δ) is known, then one should obviously take

$$\hat{\Delta}'_i = \varrho_{DD} D_i + (1 - \varrho_{DD}) \mu_\Delta$$

as the estimate of the true change of person i rather than Equation 6. This is the estimate with which, on the whole, the errors of estimation are minimized. It is also known that this estimate is generally biased (Willett, 1988), since its mean (expected) value is:

$$E\left(\hat{\Delta}'_i | \Delta_i\right) = \varrho_{DD} \Delta_i + (1 - \varrho_{DD}) \mu_\Delta$$
$$= \Delta_i + (1 - \varrho_{DD}) (\mu_\Delta - \Delta_i). \quad (9)$$

The estimate is only unbiased when the true change of person i equals the average true change in the population, or when the difference has been perfectly assessed. Usually, neither will be the case. Our comments here are comparable to those regarding the regressed score method. If Δ_i and $\mu_\Delta - \Delta_i$ have different signs, Δ_i and the expected value of the estimate can have different signs. If the bias of the estimate is sufficiently large, it can be expected that the reliable change is assessed in the wrong direction. This is the case if:

$$|\Delta_i - \mu_\Delta| (1 - \varrho_{DD}) - |\Delta_i|$$
$$> 1.96 \, \sigma_D \sqrt{\varrho_{DD}} \sqrt{1 - \varrho_{DD}}.$$

If no true change of person i has taken place, it can nevertheless be expected that the observed change will be taken as reliable if:

$$\left|\frac{\mu_\Delta}{\sigma_D}\right| > 1.96 \sqrt{\frac{\varrho_{DD}}{1 - \varrho_{DD}}}. \quad (10)$$

The lower the reliability of the difference scores, and the more that the true change of person i and the average true change in the population differ, the higher is the probability of drawing a wrong conclusion (see Equation 10). The interval of Zegers and Hafkenscheid may be useful as an estimation interval for the true gain of person i. However, instead of ruling out trivial explanations for an observed difference, such as the unreliability of the measurements, the procedure opens the possibility that the denomination of an observed difference as reliable may in fact be explicable by other trivial factors.

The classic approach and the approach of Zegers and Hafkenscheid are similar in the sense that both methods are based on the observed change of person i. However, the principles underlying the two methods are different and this may even lead to contrary conclusions in practice. In order to demonstrate this, we write RC_{URCI} as follows:

$$\left|\frac{\varrho_{DD}\,D_i + (1-\varrho_{DD})\overline{D}}{\sigma_{E_D}\sqrt{\varrho_{DD}}}\right| > 1.96. \qquad (11)$$

We apply the following reparametrization:

$$D_i = A_i * 1.96 \quad \text{and} \quad \overline{D} = B * 1.96 * \varrho_{E_D}$$

(Thus $A_i > 1$ implies that in the classic approach an observed difference is designated a reliable change.) Now Equation 11 reduces to:

$$\left|A_i * \sqrt{\varrho_{DD}} + \frac{B}{\sqrt{\varrho_{DD}}} * (1 - \varrho_{DD})\right| > 1.$$

Table 1 shows, for given values of B and ϱ_{DD}, the minimum values of A that lead to the assessment of a reliable change according to RC_{URCI}. The table shows only the A values for positive values B. This will do, since the full Table is symmetric: If one changes the sign of B, then the sign of A also changes. The table covers a realistic value range of B (0.5 through 3.0), which can be demonstrated

as follows. Incorporating Cohen's d reflecting effect size (Cohen, 1977, pp. 20, 48) and assuming equal variances S_X and reliabilities ϱ_{XX} of pre- and post-test scores (for the sake of simplicity), the following formula can be derived:

$$B = \frac{\overline{D}}{1.96\sigma_{E_D}} = \frac{dS_X}{1.96\sqrt{2\sigma_E^2}} = \frac{d}{1.96\sqrt{2(1 - \varrho_{XX})}}.$$

The largest average effect size of a psychotherapy reported by Smith, Glass, and Miller (1980, p. 89) is 2.38 (averaged over 57 effects of cognitive psychotherapy for an unknown number of studies). If Cohen's d equals 2.38 and, for instance, $\varrho_{XX} = .92$, then, under the assumptions mentioned, B is equal to 3.0.

The section of Table 1 where $A < -1$, draws special attention, for then, in the classic approach, the observed change will be interpreted as a reliable deterioration. (The section where $B < 0$ and $A > 1$, not shown in the table, of course, is of equal importance.) From the table we see, for instance, that when $B = 1.5$ and $\varrho_{DD} = .35$ (which is the case when, say, $\varrho_{XX} = .85$, $\varrho_{XY} = .77$, and $d = 1.61$) following the classic method, the researcher will interpret a negative difference score as a reliable deterioration of person i and, at the same time, according to RC_{URCI} as a reliable improvement!

The Reliability-Stability Index Based on RC_{URCI}

Recently, Bruggemans et al. (1997) proposed a RC in which a correction for practice effects is

Table 1. Minimum Values of A Leading to the Designation of Reliable Change According to the RC of Zegers and Hafkenscheid, For Given Values of B and ϱ_{DD}.

ϱ_{DD}	B					
	0.5	1.0	1.5	2.0	2.5	3.0
.25	.50	−1.00	−2.50	−4.00	−5.50	−7.00
.30	.66	−.51	−1.67	−2.84	−4.01	−5.17
.35	.76	−.17	−1.10	−2.02	−2.95	−3.88
.40	.83	.08	−.67	−1.42	−2.17	−2.92
.45	.88	.27	−.34	−.95	−1.56	−2.18
.50	.91	.41	−.09	−.59	−1.09	−1.59
.55	.94	.53	.12	−.29	−.70	−1.11
.60	.96	.62	.29	−.04	−.38	−.71
.65	.97	.70	.43	.16	−.11	−.38
.70	.98	.77	.55	.34	.12	−.09
.75	.99	.82	.65	.49	.32	.15

combined with the method of Zegers and Hafkenscheid. Basically, the change in every patient of the sample is compared with the mean change in a matched control group. Then, RC_{URCI} is applied to such a control group:

$$RC_{mc} = \frac{D_{mc}\varrho_{DD} + D_c(1 - \varrho_{DD})}{\sigma_D \sqrt{\varrho_{DD}} \sqrt{1 - \varrho_{DD}}},$$

where D_{mc} and D_c respectively denote the observed change in the matched control group and in the control group as a whole. If RC_{URCI} is also applied with respect to patient i (and the result is denoted by RC_i), then the reliability-stability index based on RC_{URCI} is defined as follows:

$$RST_{\text{new}} = RC_i - RC_{mc}.$$

Bruggemans et al. argue that "because RST_{new} is the difference between two z-scores, like for the other z-score indices, its absolute value had to be larger than 1.645 in order to indicate significant cognitive deterioration" (p. 548). (The authors were interested in the negative effects of a medical intervention.) This procedure compounds several mistakes. First, it has been shown above that neither component should be regarded as a z-score if the change in patient i differs from the average changes in the population. Secondly, the difference of two z-scores generally is not a z-score. This is only the case when the correlation between the two components equals .5. If this correlation is higher, then the standard deviation of the difference is smaller than 1. Thirdly, the stochastic character of the results in the control group(s) is not taken into account. It should not be surprising that the conclusions drawn with RST_{new} differ strongly from the conclusions resulting from other criteria. Bruggemans et al. report relatively many reliable changes on the basis of their RST_{new}. A trivial explanation for this finding may be the correlation between both components. It will be clear that the use of RST_{new} is not to be recommended.

Kelley's Formula as the Basis for a Null Hypothesis Method

We have shown that the null hypothesis method is clear in the sense that the appropriate null hypothesis "$\Delta_i = 0$" is put to a statistical test. In this way, measurement unreliability can be ruled out with high

probability as an explanation for the observed difference score. It was emphasized that Kelley's formula has its advantages as an estimate, but the way it has been expanded into a RC has serious drawbacks.

These observations raise the question of whether Kelley's formula can serve as the basis of a null hypothesis method with the concomitant advantages. In answering this question, we distinguish two situations. First, we start from the practical situation that the average true change in the population μ_Δ is unknown. In the second situation, it will be assumed that the researcher knows this quantity.

Average true change in the population unknown
In the form of Equation 6, also, Kelley's formula is a biased estimate of the true change of person i (Maassen, 1998, 2000; Rogosa et al., 1982). Again, the mean (expected) value is given by Equation 9. If the fact that the sample information is stochastic is taken into account, the standard error of estimate of the predicted true score is not the correct denominator for the RC. The variance of Kelley's estimate should be adopted, with the sample information treated as a random element. We have calculated this variance elsewhere (Maassen, 1998, 2000):

$$\text{Var}\left(\hat{\Delta}_i \,|\, \Delta_i\right)$$
$$= \sigma_{E_D}^2 \left(\varrho_{DD}^2 + \frac{(1 + 2\varrho_{DD})(1 - \varrho_{DD})}{n} \right). \quad (12)$$

(Here it is assumed that person i belongs to the sample whose information is used in Kelley's formula.) In order to yield a standardized normally distributed variable, Equation 9 is subtracted from Equation 6 and the result is divided by the square root of Equation 12. If, finally, the null hypothesis "$\Delta_i = 0$" is implemented, the following expression results:

$$\frac{\varrho_{DD} D_i + (1 - \varrho_{DD})(\overline{D} - \mu_\Delta)}{\sigma_{E_D} \sqrt{\varrho_{DD}^2 + \dfrac{(1 + 2\varrho_{DD})(1 - \varrho_{DD})}{n}}}. \quad (13)$$

Under the null hypothesis, this expansion of Kelley's estimate has a standardized normal distribution and can be regarded as a RC in the shape of a test statistic. Equation 13, however, is of theoretical interest rather than practical importance.

On the one hand, it offers the same advantages as the classic approach, such as the testing of an appropriate null hypothesis and a limited chance of committing a Type I error. Moreover, the bias of Kelley's estimate and the stochastic character of the sample information are adequately treated (which inevitably entails a certain loss of power). On the other hand, application of this *RC* requires information on the effect of the intervention in the population (μ_Δ), which above was assumed to be unknown. The researcher then has to estimate μ_Δ by means of a large sample. Let us assume that the sample size is sufficiently large for the sample statistics to be a good approximation of the population values. Then, from Equation 12 follows:

If $n \rightarrow \infty$, then $\overline{D} - \mu_\Delta \rightarrow 0$ and

$$\text{Var}\left(\widehat{\Delta}_i \mid \Delta_i\right) \rightarrow \varrho_{DD}^2 \ \sigma_{E_D}^2.$$

This implies a return to the start: The classic method. Consequently, the classic approach can be regarded as the large sample approximation for the properly composed *RC* based on Kelley's formula.

Average true change in the population known
When the average true change in the population is already known, Kelley's formula takes the shape of Equation 8. The expected value of this statistic can also be found in Equation 9, and since the second term on the right of Equation 8 is a constant, its conditional variance is:

$$\text{Var}\left(\widehat{\Delta}_i' \mid \Delta_i\right) = \varrho_{DD}^2 \ \sigma_{E_D}^2.$$

Standardization of the estimator yields the following standardized normally distributed statistic:

$$\frac{\varrho_{DD}\left(D_i - \Delta_i\right)}{\varrho_{DD}\sigma_{E_D}} = \frac{D_i - \Delta_i}{\sigma_{E_D}},$$

which under "H_0: $\Delta_i = 0$" boils down to Equation 1, the classic approach. Again, we return to our starting point, which should not surprise the reader.

SUMMARY AND DISCUSSION

Scrutinizing the reliable change indices proposed in the clinical psychology literature over the past twenty years does not encourage confidence in the progress of science. One observes a series of proposals that merely repeat pre-existing knowledge, faulty proposals that have had to be corrected, or erroneous proposals that have not yet been corrected. This has happened in spite of the peer review system. The present author was amazed to find that even when reviewers agree that a previously proposed index is wrong, they may give low priority to an adjustment. Paraphrasing Churchill, it would seem that "the peer review system is the worst, save all other systems."

Explanations for the lack of continuous progress in the development of methods for the assessment of reliable change are not difficult to find. A lack of statistical knowledge and an uncritical zeal to demonstrate the efficacy of an intervention, which should require constant refining of the criteria employed, are undoubtedly conductive to the current situation.

In this article, a number of previously proposed reliable change indices (*RC*'s) are examined. According to the principle which underlies them, they can be categorized as a null hypothesis testing or an estimation interval method. The only representative of the former category discussed here is based on the ratio of the observed difference and the standard error of measurement of the difference scores. With this method, which we have named the classic approach, the probability that observed changes erroneously will be designated reliable is limited by a low level of significance.

Most of our attention has been devoted to various estimation interval methods. These methods originate in the view that the estimate of the true change should be improved. We have elaborated on the two representatives of this category that possess an appropriate standard error in the denominator, namely *the regressed score method*, proposed among others by Hsu, and the *RC of Zegers and Hafkenscheid*. In the majority of the cases, all the methods mentioned will probably lead to the same interpretation of the observed change, but in this article it has been shown that, with regard to the estimation interval methods, no uniform upper limit exists for the probability of an incorrect conclusion. This probability depends on the relative position of the patient within the population to which he or she belongs, either with respect to the true initial score (in the regression estimate method) or the true difference score (in the method of Zegers and Hafkenscheid). The probability of committing a type I error may be high if the participant in question takes an extreme position in the population. Only a few participants will be the victim of a type I error or an interpretation in the wrong direction, but for deviant individuals a faulty interpretation may have particularly important consequences. Whereas the classic method rules out with high probability measurement errors as a possible explanation for an observed change, the qualities of the estimation interval methods are less clear. Trivial effects may possibly lead to an observed change (or an observed zero change) being designated reliable, or an observed change interpreted as reliable change in the wrong direction. Such trivial effects also include sample fluctuations, if the RC comprises sample information.

Recently, various estimation interval-based RC's have been proposed, which depart from Kelley's estimate of the true change of a given person. The RC_{URCI} of Zegers and Hafkenscheid is the most salient example. We observe that some individuals run the risk that the classic approach and RC_{URCI} can lead to the designation of reliable change in opposite directions. Considering our earlier observations, we put our trust in the results of the classic approach rather than the estimation interval method.

Finally, we have examined whether Kelley's estimate may be the basis of a null hypothesis method. This led us to the following conclusions: (1) If Kelley's formula is correctly expanded to a RC, the researcher is confronted with the problem that, in principle, population information is required; this information is generally not available; (2) If the researcher has a large sample from the population at his or her disposal, the sample or population information turns out to be superfluous. The classic approach reveals itself as the large sample approximation for correctly composed RC's based on Kelley's formula.

All in all, in our view there are strong arguments for preferring the classic approach to the estimate interval method. This method has been undeservedly regarded inferior by the authors who recently proposed new indices in the clinical psychology literature.

REFERENCES

Barkham, M., Rees, A., Stiles, W.B., Shapiro, D.A., Hardy, G.E., & Reynolds, S. (1996). Dose-effect relations in time-limited psychotherapy for depression. *Journal of Consulting and Clinical Psychology, 64*, 927–935.

Bruggemans, E., Van de Vijver, F.J.R., & Huysmans, H.A. (1997). Assessment of cognitive deterioration in individual patients following cardiac surgery: Correcting for measurement error and practice effects. *Journal of Clinical and Experimental Neuropsychology, 19*, 543–559.

Chelune, G.J., Naugle, R.I., Lüders, H., Sedlak, J., & Awad, I.A. (1993). Individual change after epilepsy surgery: Practice effects and base-rate information. *Neuropsychology, 7*, 41–52.

Christensen, L., & Mendoza, J.L. (1986). A method of assessing change in a single subject: An alternation of the RC index. *Behavior Therapy, 12,* 305–308.

Cohen, J. (1977). *Statistical power analysis for the behavioral sciences.* New York: Academic Press.

Cronbach, L.J., & Furby, L. (1970). How we should measure "change" – or should we? *Psychological Bulletin, 74*, 68–80.

Debats, D.L. (1996). Meaning in life: Clinical relevance and predictive power. *British Journal of Clinical Psychology, 35*, 503–516.

De Haan, E., Van Oppen, P., Van Balkom, A.J.L.M., Spinhoven, P., Hoogduin, K.A.L., & Van Dyck, R. (1997). Prediction of outcome and early vs. late improvement in OCD patients treated with cognitive-behavior therapy and pharmacotherapy. *Acta Psychiatrica Scandinavica, 96*, 354–361.

Hafkenscheid, A.J.P.M. (1994). *Rating scales in treatment efficacy studies: Individualized and normative use.* Unpublished doctoral dissertation, Rijksuniversiteit Groningen. Groningen, The Netherlands.

Hageman, W.J.J.M., & Arrindell, W.A. (1993). A further refinement of the reliable change (RC) index by improving the pre-post difference score: Introducing RC_{ID}. *Behaviour Research and Therapy, 31*, 693–700.

Hageman, W.J.J.M., & Arrindell, W.A. (1999). Establishing clinically significant change: Increment of precision and the distinction between individual and group level of analysis. *Behaviour Research and Therapy, 37*, 1169–1193.

Hsu, L.M. (1989). Reliable changes in psychotherapy: Taking into account regression toward the mean. *Behavioral Assessment, 11*, 459–467.

Jacobson, N.S., Follette, W.C., & Revenstorf, D. (1984). Psychotherapy outcome research: Methods for reporting variability and evaluating clinical significance. *Behavior Therapy, 15*, 336–352.

Jacobson, N.S., & Truax, P. (1991). Clinical significance: A statistical approach to defining meaningful change in psychotherapy research. *Journal of Clinical and Consulting Psychology, 59,* 12–19.

Kelley, T.L. (1947). *Fundamentals of statistics.* Cambridge: Harvard University Press.

Lord, F.M. (1956). The measurement of growth. *Educational and Psychological Measurement, 16,* 421–437.

Lord, F.M., & Novick, M.R. (1968). *Statistical Theories of Mental Test Scores.* Reading, MA: Addison-Wesley.

Maassen, G.H. (1998). The reliability weighted measure of individual change as an indicator of reliable change. *Kwantitatieve Methoden, 19,* nr. 58, 29–40.

Maassen, G.H. (2000). Kelley's formula as a basis for the assessment of reliable change. *Psychometrika, 65,* 187–197.

McNemar, Q. (1958). On growth measurement. *Educational and Psychological Measurement, 18,* 47–55.

McNemar, Q. (1962). *Psychological Statistics (4th ed.).* New York: Wiley.

McNemar, Q. (1969). *Psychological Statistics (4th ed.).* New York: Wiley.

McSweeny, A.J., Naugle, R.I., Chelune, G.J., & Lüders, H. (1993). "T Scores for change": An illustration of a regression approach to depicting change in clinical neuropsychology. *The Clinical Neuropsychologist, 7,* 300–312.

Nunnally, J.C., & Kotsch, W.E. (1983). Studies of individual subjects: Logic and methods of analysis. *British Journal of Clinical Psychology, 22,* 83–93.

Rogosa, D., Brandt, D., & Zimowski, M. (1982). A growth curve approach to the measurement of change. *Psychological Bulletin, 92,* 726–748.

Rudy, T.E., Turk, D.C., Kubinski, J.A., & Zaki, H.S. (1995). Differential treatment responses of TMD patients as a function of psychological characteristics. *Pain, 61,* 103–112.

Smith, M.L., Glass, G.V., & Miller, T.I. (1980). *The Benefits of Psychotherapy.* Baltimore: Johns Hopkins University Press.

Speer, D.C. (1992). Clinically significant change: Jacobson and Truax (1991) revisited. *Journal of Consulting and Clinical Psychology, 60,* 402–408.

Taylor, S. (1995). Assessment of obsessions and compulsions: Reliability, validity and sensitivity to treatment effects. *Clinical Psychology Review, 15,* 261–296.

Van Oppen, P., de Haan, E., Van Balkom, A.J.L.M., Spinhoven, P., Hoogduin, K., & Van Dyck, R. (1995). Cognitive therapy and exposure in-vivo in the treatment of obsessive-compulsive disorder. *Behaviour Research and Therapy, 33,* 379–390.

Willett, J.B. (1988). Questions and answers in the measurement of change. In E.Z. Rothkopf (Ed.): *Review of research in education, 15 (1988–89),* 345–422. Washington: American Educational Research Association.

Wykes, T. (1998). What are we changing with neurocognitive rehabilitation. Illustrations from 2 single cases of changes in neuropsychological performance and brain systems as measured by SPECT. *Schizophrenia Research, 34,* 77–86.

Zegers, F.E., & Hafkenscheid, A.J.P.M. (1994). The ultimate reliable change index: An alternative to the Hageman & Arrindell approach. Groningen: *Universiteit van Groningen, Heymans Bulletin HB-94-1154-EX.*

The Clinical Neuropsychologist
1993, Vol. 7, No. 3, pp. 300–312

COMPUTERIZING THE CLINICIAN

"T Scores for Change": An Illustration of a Regression Approach to Depicting Change in Clinical Neuropsychology

A. John McSweeny[1], Richard I. Naugle[2], Gordon J. Chelune[3], and Hans Lüders[4]

[1]Department of Psychiatry, Medical College of Ohio, [2]Department of Psychiatry and Psychology, Cleveland Clinic Foundation, [3]Department of Psychiatry and Psychology, Cleveland Clinic Foundation, and [4]Department of Neurology, Cleveland Clinic Foundation

ABSTRACT

The interpretation of change scores in neuropsychological assessment is of increasing importance. In order to illustrate a regression approach to depicting change, 50 patients with chronic seizure disorders were assessed twice with the WAIS-R and the Wechsler Memory Scale-Revised over an average interval of 7.8 months. Regression analysis was employed to develop norms for change that were converted into standardized scores. These T Scores for Change were analyzed with a MANOVA to compare the effects of epilepsy surgery on cognition and memory in 50 right-temporal lobectomy and 47 left-temporal lobectomy patients. Significant group, test, and interaction effects were found. A profile of the T Scores for Change permitted quick and accurate appreciation of the major findings. The characteristics of the regression-derived T Score approach are compared with a recently suggested reliability approach.

The measurement of change over time using repeated assessments is becoming increasingly important in clinical neuropsychology. The increased significance of measuring change in neuropsychology was evident in recent symposia sponsored by Division 40 (Clinical Neuropsychology) of the American Psychological Association (Chelune & Goldstein, 1991) and the International Neuropsychological Society (Kay & Kane, 1991), as well as in recent articles (e.g., McCaffery, Ortega, Orsillo, Nelles, & Haase, 1992), reflecting the changing emphasis of the field as it enters its "dynamic" phase (Rourke, 1982). According to Rourke, the major focus of neuropsychology during its early development was on discovering psychological correlates of localized brain lesions. This

research interest had immediate clinical application in the form of neurodiagnosis and provided evidence that clinical neuropsychology was a legitimate professional enterprise. Recent improvements in neuroradiologic techniques have led to a decline in the practical need for the use of neuropsychological assessment in locating discrete lesions and a concomitant increase in the importance of neuropsychological assessment in other areas.

The increased role of neuropsychology in rehabilitation has been particularly impressive. Neuropsychological assessments are used to judge the course of recovery from brain injury and to evaluate the effects of various training programs and assistive devices designed to address the cognitive deficits associated with such injuries (Benedict,

This research was supported by a Faculty Improvement Leave from the Medical College of Ohio to the first author and by a grant from the Epilepsy Foundation of America to the other authors.
The authors would like to thank the anonymous reviewers for their helpful suggestions.
Reprints may be obtained from A. John McSweeny, Ph.D., Department of Psychiatry, Medical College of Ohio, P.O. Box 10008, Toledo, OH 43699-0008, USA.
Accepted for publication: January 20, 1993.

1989; Franzen & Haut, 1991; Matthews, Harley, & Malec, 1990; Meier, Benton, & Diller, 1987). Similarly, neuropsychological assessment has taken a central role in the evaluation of medical and surgical treatments for epilepsy (Chelune, Naugle, Lüders, Sedlak, & Awad, 1993; Dodrill & Willensky, 1990; Seidenberg, O'Leary, Giordani, Berent, & Boll, 1981), Alzheimer's Disease (Davis & Thal, in press; Eagger, Levy, & Sahakian, 1991), hypertension (Goldstein, 1991) and other disorders.

The evaluation of interventions inherently involves the evaluation of change over time and, in clinical neuropsychology, over repeated assessments. The use of repeated assessments can also be important in certain diagnostic applications. The diagnosis of the dementias, particularly the progressive dementias, can best be done with serial neuropsychological assessments (Cummings & Benson, 1983; Mortimer, Ebbit, & Jun, 1991; Saxton, Smith, & Boller, 1991). Thus, the importance of neuropsychological assessment in the diagnosis of dementia has increased in importance even as other diagnostic uses (e.g., lesion localization) have become less important.

Several issues confront neuropsychologists when considering how to assess change. First, most of the instruments in current neuropsychological batteries, including the Halstead-Reitan Battery (HRB), were chosen because of their utility in the identification of brain dysfunction rather than for assessing change in those functions over time. Validity has been established by investigating group differences rather than intraindividual changes. As noted in a review by Fremouw, McSweeny, Fabry, and Trout (1982), instruments that have established criterion validity based on group differences are not necessarily sensitive to intervention effects and, therefore, not necessarily good measures of change. Additional research will be necessary to establish that current neuropsychological measures are sensitive to intraindividual changes as well as to group differences.

A second issue relates to normative information that can be used to judge the amount of change in individuals and groups. While norms are available for assessing individuals at one point in time, norms for change over time in neuropsychology do not exist (Bieliauskas & McSweeny, 1991). A common practice in the clinical situation is to consider any

change as significant. As Chelune et al. (1993), and Hermann et al. (1991) have noted, this approach is fraught with difficulties, given the less than perfect test-retest reliability inherent in neuropsychological measures, which results in the phenomenon of regression toward the mean, as well as practice effects.

In this context, Chelune et al. have suggested an application of the "Reliable Change Index" (RCI) described by Jacobson and Truax (1991). This approach uses known data about practice effects and the standard error of the difference (S_{diff}) between the baseline and follow-up test scores to decide whether an observed individual change is significant. In brief, an individual's test–retest change score is divided by S_{diff} and then corrected by subtracting a constant that represents the practice effect. A change score is considered significant if (after correction for practice) it lies outside ± 1.64 S_{diff} (i.e., a 90% confidence interval). Chelune et al. illustrated this reliability-based approach with a sample of seizure disorder patients undergoing left- or right-temporal lobectomies, using a sample of nonsurgical seizure patients to establish S_{diff} and the constant for practice effects for the WAIS-R and the Wechsler Memory Scale-Revised (WMS-R).

Related to the issue of developing norms for change is the issue of how to present this information. Chelune et al. used a categorical approach to display their results; temporal lobectomy patients were judged as significantly improved, significantly worse, or having not changed on each of the WAIS-R and WMS-R indices. While this categorical scheme may be adequate for many clinical situations, it might be advantageous to use a continuous approach in others. Ideally, norms for change would be population-specific and in a format that is familiar to neuropsychologists and other clinicians. Such norms do not exist currently in neuropsychology. This paper is offered as a means of illustrating how norms for change can be developed and presented.

We illustrate a regression approach to present norms for change using the samples described in the article by Chelune et al. (1993). Regression analysis is used to predict WAIS-R and WMS-R performance at posttest with the pretest score as the predictor. The predicted scores are then converted to standardized T scores with $M = 50$ and

SD = 10. Statistical analyses and graphic presentations demonstrate the advantages of the approach.

METHOD

Subjects

The samples in this study are expanded versions of those employed in the study by Chelune et al. (1993). Two basic samples are included. Fifty seizure patients (31 males, 19 females) from the Cleveland Clinic Foundation who were being treated medically served as the control population used to develop the change norms. The second group consisted of 97 patients (60 males, 37 females) whose seizure disorders were refractory to medication and had undergone either left-temporal lobectomy (LTL; $n = 47$) or right-temporal lobectomy (RTL; $n = 50$). The control sample contains 10 additional subjects recruited since the study by Chelune et al. and the RTL sample contains 1 additional subject; the LTL samples in the two studies are identical.

The basic demographic characteristics of the samples are included in Table 1. Statistical tests using either analysis of variance or Chi-square revealed no significant differences between the controls, LTL, and RTL groups except for the test-retest interval where the control group did have a significantly shorter test-retest interval than the seizure patients ($F = 10.28$, $p < .001$). As will be seen below, subsequent investigation of the relationship of test-retest interval length to outcome using regression analysis indicated that it was noncontributory.

Assessment Procedures

All subjects received two comprehensive neuropsychological test batteries. For purposes of brevity, this study will focus on the results on the WAIS-R (Wechsler, 1981) and WMS-R (Wechsler, 1987).

The surgical patients were evaluated before and after surgery. Mean baseline-to-surgery time was 4.7 months and mean surgery-to-follow-up interval was 6.2 months. The nonsurgical epileptic control subjects were volunteers who received financial compensation for their participation.

Data Analytic Procedures

Change-score norm development. We employed regression analysis to develop norms for change for the three IQ scores associated with the WAIS-R (VIQ, PIQ, FSIQ) and the five Memory Indices associated with the WMS-R: Verbal Memory (VMI), Visual Memory (VISMI), General Memory (GMI), Delayed Recall (DRI), and Attention/Concentration (ACI). Standard IQ scores were used in the data analyses. However, we employed raw score totals for the Memory Indices rather than the standardized scores because the WMSR norms result in restricted ranges of scores at the lower end. Comparison of the results from regression analyses using raw versus standardized Memory Index scores revealed essentially equivalent results but slightly better fit when the raw scores were used. One could argue that we should have used raw scores to develop our change norms for the WAIS-R as well as for the WMS-R. We preferred the use of IQ scores given their greater familiarity to clinicians and the availability of WAIS-R norms with adequate range to encompass all of the subjects in our sample. Thus, using WAIS-R raw scores would have resulted in a loss of familiarity without providing any statistical advantages.

The basic strategy of the regression analysis was to determine those factors that might affect performance at follow-up in the control group. Initial variables tested included age, education, duration of illness, test-retest

Table 1. Presurgical Demographic Characteristics of Study Sample.

Variable	Group					
	Controls ($n = 50$)		LTL ($n = 47$)		RTL ($n = 50$)	
	M	SD	M	SD	M	SD
Age	31.6	8.2	29.4	7.6	29.2	7.6
Education (years)	12.8	2.3	12.7	1.8	13.3	2.5
Seizure onset age	13.5	8.5	12.5	9.2	13.7	9.1
Seizure duration	18.6	8.8	17.1	8.8	15.8	8.0
Full scale IQ	90.9	11.4	87.3	9.1	91.8	13.8
Retest interval (mos.)	7.8	2.8	11.0	4.3	11.1	4.9
Sex (males/females)	31/19		31/16		29/21	
Preferred hand (R/L)	44/6		39/8		44/6	

Key: LTL = Left Temporal Lobectomy Group. RTL = Right Temporal Lobectomy Group.

Table 2. Regression Coefficients and Indices of Significance for Equations
Predicting Posttest WAIS-R IQs and WMS-R Indices (Raw Scores).

Variable	β^a	C^b	$SEest^c$	F^d	$r_{1,2}^e$
VIQ	0.94	6.19	3.92	419.4	.95
PIQ	1.09	−3.73	7.01	141.5	.86
FSIQ	1.04	−1.26	4.36	359.2	.94
VMI	0.78	22.29	10.96	98.4	.82
VISMI	0.88	7.08	10.50	100.5	.82
GMI	0.83	28.25	12.76	141.6	.86
DRI	0.78	17.66	10.82	102.6	.83
ACI	0.83	11.49	9.56	51.8	.72

Note: [a] Unstandardized beta (slope)
[b] Constant
[c] Standard error of the estimate
[d] All $p < .001$
[e] Test–retest correlation

Key: VIQ = WAIS-R Verbal IQ. PIQ = Performance IQ. FSIP = Full Scale
IQ. VMI = WMS-R Verbal Memory Index. VISMI = Visual Memory
Index. GMI = General Memory Index. DRI = Delayed Recall Index.
ACI = Attention/ Concentration Index.

interval, and the baseline score, including nonlinear components of the relationship of the baseline score to the follow-up score. The baseline score was entered first and the remaining variables were entered according to size of their partial correlation with the criterion (i.e., the follow-up score) using a step-wise procedure. The probability level necessary to enter or remove a variable at each step was set at .15. When regression analysis was conducted with each of the WAIS-R IQs and WMS-R Indices, we discovered that, after baseline performance was entered, none of the remaining variables consistently demonstrated significance levels below .15 and in no case below .05. Therefore, the final regression model used to develop the change norms for each of the variables of interest was:

$$Y_p = \beta X + C$$

where Y_p is the predicted follow-up score, β is the regression coefficient (slope), X is the observed baseline score, and C is a constant (intercept). The regression coefficients and significance indices for each WAIS-R and WMS-R variable are listed in Table 2.

The final step in the development of the change-score norms was to convert them to standardized T scores having a mean of 50 and a standard deviation of 10 using the following formula:

$$T = 50 + [10 * (Y_o - Y_p)/SE_{est}]$$

where Y_o is the observed follow-up score, Y_p is the predicted score (from the regression equation), and SE_{est} is

the standard error of the estimate from the regression equation.

The approach illustrated here could be used to produce a variety of standard scores including Z scores or Wechsler ($M = 100$, $SD = 15$) scores. We decided to use T scores because of their familiarity to psychologists and because they are not likely to be confused with the Wechsler scores used with the WAIS-R IQs and WMS-R Memory Indices.

RESULTS

Table 3 contains the Ms and SDs for the WAIS-R IQs and WMS-R Indices (raw scores) at baseline and at follow-up. Group comparisons and practice (test-retest) effects using the WAIS-R and WMS-R variables are addressed in detail in the article by Chelune et al. (1993). We repeated the raw-score analyses performed by Chelune et al. and found shifts in significance levels on some specific comparisons with the expanded samples used in the present study. However, the major effects were essentially the same.[1] In brief, significant Practice effects but no Group effects were noted for the IQ scores.

Analysis of the memory indices revealed significant Group and Group x Practice interaction effects for GMI and VMI, with the control group

Table 3. Mean and Standard Deviations at Baseline and Follow-Up.

Variable	Baseline group					
	Controls (n = 50)		LTL (n = 47)		RTL (n = 50)	
	M	SD	M	SD	M	SD
VIQ	91.9	12.2	87.8	9.0	91.6	12.5
PIQ	91.5	10.9	89.0	10.5	93.9	15.8
FSIQ	90.9	11.4	87.2	9.7	91.8	13.8
VMI	67.8	20.0	61.8	14.3	63.4	16.7
VISMI	51.6	8.5	51.7	8.1	52.3	9.2
GMI	119.3	26.2	113.5	19.7	115.9	22.1
DRI	67.3	20.1	61.9	15.7	64.4	20.6
ACI	65.6	11.8	66.2	10.4	66.9	12.9

Variable	Follow-up group					
	Controls (n = 50)		LTL (n = 47)		RTL (n = 50)	
	M	SD	M	SD	M	SD
VIQ	92.5	12.1	88.7	11.0	93.1	12.4
PIQ	96.4	13.8	95.3	12.4	96.7	15.7
FSIQ	93.3	12.6	90.4	11.4	93.9	13.6
VMI	75.1	18.9	51.3	16.4	65.9	15.8
VISMI	52.4	9.1	52.7	7.4	52.8	11.2
GMI	127.2	25.1	104.1	20.5	118.6	22.4
DRI	70.0	19.0	59.8	17.2	67.2	19.1
ACI	66.1	13.6	67.2	10.1	69.5	12.1

improving, the LTL group declining, and the RTL group showing no change over the test–retest interval. A significant Practice effect only was found for ACI; significant effects were not found for VISMI or DRI.

The "T Scores for Change" for the two surgical groups are presented in Table 4. T-score profiles for the LTL and RTL groups are shown in Figure 1. The control group, having been used to construct the T scores for change, assumes a straight line at 50 in Figure 1. Scores above 50 indicate better than expected performance at posttest; scores below 50 indicate poorer than expected performance.

The T scores for change for the WAIS-R and the WMS-R, with the exception of FSIQ and GMI, were entered into a MANOVA. Because they are composites of other scores, FSIQ and GMI were examined in a separate analysis (see below) to avoid multicollinearity error. The MANOVA revealed significant effects for Group ($F = 3.66$, $p = .028$), IQ/Memory Index

Table 4. T Scores for Change in Right- and Left Temporal Lobe-Surgery Patients.

Variable	Group			
	LTL (n = 47)		RTL (n = 50)	
	M	SD	M	SD
VIQ	50.2	16.4	52.4	11.9
PIQ	52.3	9.8	46.8	2.8
FSIQ	52.0	12.2	49.1	13.8
VMI	32.6	12.1	44.7	9.6
VISMI	50.4	9.1	49.7	13.8
GMI	35.7	11.9	45.9	10.2
DRI	44.4	11.2	49.5	10.7
ACI	50.6	7.9	52.5	8.4

($F = 16.21, p < .001$), and Group x Scale interaction ($F = 8.31, p < .001$). Post hoc testing with Tukey HSD tests demonstrated that the LTL group showed more positive change than did the

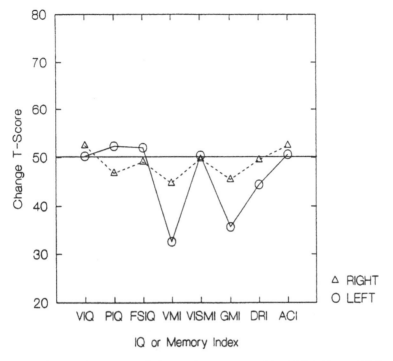

Fig. 1. Profiles of *T* Scores for Change for Left-Temporal Lobectomy (LTL) and Right-Temporal Lobectomy (RTL) Groups.

RTL group on PIQ ($p = .033$), but neither surgical group differed significantly from the control group. No significant group differences were found for VIQ. When WMS-R Indices were examined, both the RTL group ($p = .035$) and the LTL group ($p < .001$) declined significantly relative to the controls on VMI. In addition, the LTL group declined more significantly than did the RTL group ($p < .001$) on VMI using the Tukey HSD test. The LTL group also showed a greater decline than did the controls on DRI ($p = .027$) and a similar difference with RTL group approached significance ($p = .050$). No significant differences were found for ACI or VISMI.

Comparisons of the *T* scores for change for the different scales using the surgical groups only were conducted using dependent *t* tests (df = 96). Verbal memory (VMI) declined to a greater degree than VIQ ($t = 7.83, p < .001$); PIQ ($t = 5.66, p < .001$), VISMI ($t = 7.43, p < .001$), and DRI ($t = 7.73, p < .001$), and ACI ($t = 8.53, p < .001$). Delayed

Recall (DRI) was noted to decline significantly when compared to VIQ ($t = 2.70, p = .008)^2$, VISMI ($t = 2.31, p = 0.23)^2$, and ACI ($t = 3.28, p = .001$). No other significant differences were found.

The MANOVA with the FSIQ and GMI using *T* scores for change also produced a significant Group ($F = 5.76, p = .004$), Scale ($F = 30.25, p < .001$), and Group x Scale interaction ($F = 17.26, p < .001$) effects. Post hoc testing revealed no significant group differences for FSIQ. The LTL group declined on GMI relative to the RTL group ($p = .001$) and the control ($p < .001$). The latter two groups did not differ significantly.

DISCUSSION

The major focus of this paper was to illustrate an approach to presenting change data in clinical neuropsychology, the advantages of which are apparent in Figure 1. The T scores for change incorporate information about expected change or practice effects using prediction equations resulting from regression analyses. The reliability of such predictions is manifested in the Standard Error of the Estimate. Thus, the T scores for change address the concerns about measuring change and regression toward the mean raised by Chelune and Goldstein (1991), Kay and Kane (1991), Hermann et al. (1991), and others.

The T-score format is very familiar to psychologists and other clinicians and has the advantage of using a common metric for all scales. This allows for visual comparisons of groups and scales (i.e., visual profile analysis). Indeed, even a brief glance at Figure 1 permits appreciation of the major findings of the study. The major effect is clearly the decline in memory, particularly Verbal Memory. This effect is most dramatic for the LTL group but it is also evident in the RTL group. A decline in Delayed Recall in the LTL group is also obvious, although less striking than for Verbal Memory or immediate General Memory. The reader can also easily see that the RTL and LTL groups do not differ from each other in change for Visual Memory or Attention/Concentration, and that both groups perform according to expectations for unoperated seizure controls.

When the IQ scores are examined, the effects are more subtle than for memory. Only PIQ clearly separates the LTL and RTL groups. Finally, Figure 1 makes clear that neither the LTL or RTL group benefitted from surgery in terms of memory and intellectual functioning; all scale means are approximately 50 or less, indicating that in no case did the surgical groups exceed expectations on those variables included in the study. This would appear to contradict the concept of "release of function" (Rausch & Crandall, 1982; c.f. Novelly et al., 1984) which would lead to the prediction that patients should show gains in cognitive functions mediated by unoperated areas of the brain following the removal of a seizure focus. Of course, we do recognize that the essential function of surgery in epilepsy is to control seizures rather than to improve cognition and memory.

The findings of this study are also consistent with those of Hermann et al. (1991) in two respects. First, of the various predictors of posttest scores

employed, only the baseline scores consistently demonstrated significant relationships. Second, the effect of laterality of resection on basic verbal cognitive skills, represented by VIQ in the present study, was not as dramatic as on verbal memory (VMI). However, inconsistent with Hermann et al. was the present finding of a significant laterality effect for nonverbal cognitive skills (PIQ). Hermann et al. did not assess nonverbal memory.

The development of change norms and T scores for change could be especially useful for conducting research where a suitable control group is not readily available, as is often the case in clinical practice. While not without problems, such quasi-experimental research can be very useful for evaluating treatment programs (Cook & Campbell, 1979). What is needed is change norms for different diagnostic groups and for normal individuals across the age span. In order for the norms to have some generalizability they should be based on data supplied by several investigators. Heaton, Grant, and Matthews (1991) have provided an example of how this can be accomplished with their publication of norms for the Halstead-Reitan Neuropsychological Test Battery (Reitan & Wolfson, 1985).

In addition to being useful for research and program evaluation, change norms and T scores for change could be useful for evaluating change in the individual case. As noted above, judging change relative to expectations could have diagnostic or prognostic value, and may be helpful in patient counseling and rehabilitation planning as well as measuring response to treatment.

Two case examples that illustrate this approach are presented in Figure 2. Both cases are similar demographically and surgically. Case One is a 47-year-old right-handed woman with 14 years of education and a presurgical Full Scale IQ of 93. Case Two is a 43-year-old left-handed woman with 15 years of education and a presurgical Full Scale IQ of 94. Both individuals underwent right-temporal lobectomies. One key difference between the two women is that Case One demonstrated left-hemisphere dominance for language while Case Two demonstrated right-hemisphere dominance upon Wada testing.

Figure 2 shows that the two women experienced very different outcomes from surgery.

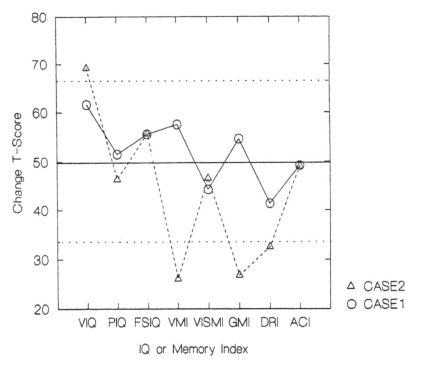

Fig. 2. Profiles of *T* Scores for Change for Case Examples with 90% Confidence Interval Indicated by Dotted Lines.

Case One might be considered a typical right-temporal lobectomy case. Although some variability in response is apparent across the different scales, none of the scores falls outside the 90% confidence interval (50 ± 16.4) suggested by Chelune et al. for judging the significance of change. Parenthetically, it might be noted that raw score gains were present on all three IQ scores as well as on GMI and VMI; losses were present for DRI and VISMI; no change was present on ACI. A naive interpretation of the raw score changes might lead a clinician to conclude that intelligence, General Memory, and Verbal Memory improved following surgery whereas Visual Memory and Delayed Recall declined.

Case Two, in contrast to Case One, is atypical. She demonstrated significant gains in terms of Verbal IQ and significant losses in Verbal Memory, General Memory, and Delayed Recall. In many respects, her profile is more similar to the mean profile for the LTL cases than to the profile for the RTL cases.

Some discussion of the similarities and differences between the present approach and the reliability approach to judging change, recently suggested by Chelune et al., is in order. Both approaches are designed to incorporate information about expected change and reliability. An essential difference between the approaches is that the use of *T* scores provides results with continuous data whereas the method described by Chelune et al. provides categorical information (i.e., individuals are categorized as showing a gain, a loss or no change). Chelune et al. also suggest adjusting the mean practice effect size to produce a distribution as close as possible to a theoretical normal distribution in the unoperated sample when deriving norms for reliable change. Thus, the reliability approach of Chelune et al. might be most useful in situations involving non-normally distributed data for change, whereas the present approach appears more appropriate for use with parametric data. Of course, it would be possible to convert ranges of *T* scores into discrete categories if this is desired.

Perhaps future studies will explore further the relative advantages of the two methods of presenting change in neuropsychological status.

Finally, while this paper has been primarily concerned with the depiction of change in neuropsychology over two assessments, it should be considered in the context of the broader literature on statistical models of change. For example, an alert reviewer led us to early papers by Benjamin (1963) and Lacey (1956) that discuss recommendations for measuring change in autonomic research that are statistically equivalent to some of the methods in this paper. The reader also may wish to consult the classic paper by Cronbach and Furby (1970) as well as the more recent book edited by Collins and Horn (1991) to gain a full appreciation of the statistical issues in assessing the significance of change and modeling growth over repeated assessments.

NOTES

1. For the purposes of this article we have focussed on the use of the T scores for change to describe the effects of surgery on cognition and memory. A complete description of the raw-score analyses, including comparisons of the results from the original samples used by Chelune et al. (1993) and the expanded samples used in this study, intercorrelations among each of the predictor variables for the RTL, LTL and control groups separately, and the correlation of baseline scores with change, may be obtained by writing the first author.
2. This comparison is nonsignificant if the Bonferroni correction for multiple tests is applied.

REFERENCES

Benedict, R.H.B. (1989). The effectiveness of cognitive remediation strategies for victims of traumatic head injury: A review of the literature. *Clinical Psychology Review, 9*, 605–626.

Benjamin, L.S. (1963). Statistical treatment of the law of initial values (LIV) in autonomic research: A review and recommendation. *Psychosomatic Medicine, 25*, 556–566.

Bieliauskas, L.A., & McSweeny, A.J. (1991). *Development of norms for assessment of cognitive status in the elderly.* Unpublished grant proposal.

Chelune, G.J., & Goldstein, G. (1991). Interpreting test-retest changes in neuropsychological practice. *The Clinical Neuropsychologist, 5*, 262–264.

Chelune, G.J., Naugle, R.I., Lüders, H., Sedlak, J., & Awad, I.A. (1993). Individual change following epilepsy surgery: Practice effects and baserate information. *Neuropsychology, 7*, 41–52.

Collins, L.M., & Horn, J.L. (Eds.) (1991). *Best methods for the analysis of change: Recent advances, unanswered questions, future directions.* Washington, DC: American Psychological Association.

Cook, T.D., & Campbell, D.T. (1979). *Quasi-experimentation: Design and analysis issues for field settings.* Chicago: Rand-McNally.

Cronbach, L.J., & Furby, L. (1970). How should we measure "change" – or should we? *Psychological Bulletin, 74*, 68–80.

Cummings, J.L., & Benson, D.F. (1983). *Dementia: A clinical approach.* Boston: Butterworth.

Davis, K.L., & Thal, L.J. (in press). Tacrine in patients with Alzheimer's Disease. *New England Journal of Medicine.*

Dodrill, C.B., & Willensky, A.J. (1990). Intellectual impairment as an outcome of Status Epilepticus. *Neurology, 40*(Suppl. 2), 23–27.

Eagger, S.A., Levy, R., & Sahakian, B.J. (1991). Tacrine in Alzheimer's Disease. *Lancet, 337*, 989–992.

Franzen, M.D., & Haut, M.W. (1991). The psychological treatment of memory impairment: A review of empirical studies. *Neuropsychology Review, 2*, 29–64.

Fremouw, W.J., McSweeny, A.J., Fabry, B.D., & Trout, B.A. (1982). Evaluation of short-term outcomes. In A.J. McSweeny, W.J. Fremouw, & R.P. Hawkins (Eds.), *Practical program evaluation in youth treatment* (pp. 164–202). Springfield, IL: Thomas.

Goldstein, G. (1991). Practice effect phenomena in a national hypertension study. *The Clinical Neuropsychologist, 5*, 263.

Heaton, R.K., Grant, I., & Matthews, C.G. (1991). Norms for the Halstead-Reitan *Neuropsychological Test Battery.* Odessa, FL: Psychological Assessment Resources.

Hermann, B.P., Wyler, A.R., VanderZwagg, R., LeBailly, R.K., Whitman, S., Sommes, G., & Ward, J. (1991). Predictors of neuropsychological change following anterior temporal lobectomy: Role of regression toward the mean. *Epilepsy, 4*, 139–148.

Jacobson, N.S., & Truax, P. (1991). Clinical significance: A statistical approach to defining meaningful change in psychotherapy research. *Journal of Consulting and Clinical Psychology, 59*, 12–19.

Kay, G., & Kane, R.L. (1991). Repeated measures in neuropsychology: Use of serial testing to measure changes in cognitive functioning. *Journal of Clinical and Experimental Neuropsychology, 13*, 49–50.

Lacey, J.I. (1956). The evaluation of autonomic responses: Toward a general solution. *Annals of the New York Academy of Sciences, 67*, 125–163.

Matthews, C.G., Harley, J.P., & Malec, J.F. (1990). *Guidelines for computer assisted neuropsychological rehabilitation and cognitive remediation.* (Division 40 Task Force Report). Washington, DC: American Psychological Association.

McCaffery, R.J., Ortega, A., Orsillo, S.M., Nelles, W.B., & Haase, R.F. (1992). Practice effects in repeated neuropsychological assessments. *The Clinical Neuropsychologist, 6*, 32–42.

Meier, M.J., Benton, A.L., & Diller, L. (1987). *Neuropsychological rehabilitation.* New York: Guilford.

Mortimer, J.A., Ebbitt, B.J., & Jun, S.P. (1991). Neuropsychological and behavioral predictors of decline in Alzheimer's Disease. *Journal of Experimental and Clinical Neuropsychology, 13*, 109.

Novelly, R.A., Augustine, E.A., Mattson, R.H., Glaser, G.H., Williamson, P.D., Spenser, D.D., & Spenser, S.S. (1984). Selective memory improvement and impairment in temporal lobectomy for epilepsy. *Annals of Neurology, 15*, 64–67.

Rausch, R., & Crandall, P.H. (1982). Psychological status related to surgical control of temporal lobe seizures. *Epilepsia, 23*, 191–202.

Reitan, R.M., & Wolfson, D. (1985). *The Halstead-Reitan Neuropsychological Test Battery: Theory and clinical interpretation.* Tucson, AZ: Neuropsychology Press.

Rourke, B. (1982). Central processing deficiencies in children: Toward a developmental neuropsychological model. *Journal of Clinical Neuropsychology, 4*, 1–18.

Saxton, J., Smith, P., & Boller, F. (1991). Cognitive decline in Alzheimer's Disease. *Journal of Experimental and Clinical Neuropsychology, 13*, 109.

Seidenberg, M., O'Leary, D.S., Giordani, B., Berent, S., & Boll, T.J. (1981). Test-retest IQ changes of epi-lepsy patients. *Journal of Clinical Neuropsychology, 3*, 237–255.

Wechsler, D. (1981). *Wechsler Adult Intelligence Scale-Revised* [manual]. New York: Psychological Corporation.

Wechsler, D. (1987). *Wechsler Memory Scale-Revised* [manual]. New York: Psychological Corporation.

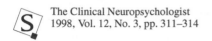
The Clinical Neuropsychologist
1998, Vol. 12, No. 3, pp. 311–314

Development of an Optimally Reliable Short Form for Judgment of Line Orientation*

Babbi J. Winegarden[1], Barbara L. Yates[2], James A. Moses, Jr.[1,3], Arthur L. Benton[4],
and William O. Faustman[1,3]

[1]Stanford University School of Medicine, CA, [2]University of California-San Francisco, [3]Veterans Affairs Palo Alto Health Care System, CA, and [4]Departments of Neurology and Psychology, The University of Iowa, Iowa City

ABSTRACT

Standard and short forms of Judgment of Line Orientation-Form V (JLO; Benton, Sivan, Hamsher, Varney, & Spreen, 1994) were examined for internal consistency (coefficient alpha) in a diagnostically mixed neuropsychiatric sample ($N = 230$). Equivalence of internally consistent short forms was assessed by correlating them with the full form of the test. Internal consistency for the full 30-item form of JLO (alpha = .84) approximated the optimal level of .80 (Nunnally, 1978). Two 20-item short forms of JLO (items V1–V20 and items V11–V30) also reached comparable alpha levels (alpha = .75 and .80, respectively). These two JLO short forms correlated .90 and .97, respectively, with the full 30-item form. We recommend the JLO short form based on items V11–V30 for clinical use in situations in which employment of the full form may not be advisable and offer a short-to-long-form conversion table for clinical use.

Judgment of Line Orientation (JLO; Benton, Sivan, Hamsher, Varney, & Spreen, 1994) is a quantitative assessment tool that is designed to measure visual–spatial perceptual ability. It was normed on a mixed sample of persons ($N = 137$), who were demographically crossclassified by age and gender. Internal consistency was determined by corrected split-half reliability estimates. For Forms H and V, the corrected split-half reliability values were .94 and .89, respectively. When these two forms were combined (the items differ only by order of presentation), the split-half reliability was .91. In a critique of the JLO test, Moses (1994) suggested that Cronbach's coefficient alpha statistic would be the optimal estimate of internal reliability (cf. Nunnally, 1978). Cronbach's coefficient alpha is the mean of all possible split-half values, and therefore it provides an unbiased estimate of internal consistency.

Using a mixed clinical sample of 386 patients, Woodard et al. (1996) found the coefficient alpha of the full form to be .85, which is comparable to Benton et al.,'s (1994) report of a split-half reliability estimate of .89.

In an attempt to address the concerns regarding the length of the 30-item test, particularly when used with elderly persons or with patients of limited endurance, researchers have begun to explore short-form versions of the JLO (Duis, Schefft, & Wood, 1996; Woodard et al., 1996). The optimal short form would be internally consistent and also would correlate highly with the full form of the JLO test. Woodard et al. provided evidence that the coefficient alpha values of the even- and odd-numbered items of the JLO full form approximated the .80 cutoff (.72 and .75, respectively) that was recommended by Nunnally (1978). Duis, Schefft, and

* This work was supported by the Department of Veterans Affairs and grant MH-30854 from the National Institute of Mental Health. We also would like to thank Martha Losch, M.D. for assistance in gathering archival data. Address correspondence to: Babbi J. Winegarden, New College of California, 741 Valencia Street, San Francisco, CA 94110, USA. E-mail: babbi@ncgate.newcollege.edu
Accepted for publication: August 18, 1997.

Wood and Woodard et al. found high correlations between the even- and odd-item short forms and the long form of JLO.

This study was designed to provide further evidence of the reliability of the full form of JLO and to determine whether an optimal short form could be developed from the full form of the JLO. This optimal short form should be more internally consistent than those described above; thus, it should be more in line with Nunnally's (1978) recommendation of a .80 coefficient alpha level. The optimal short form also should have reliability estimates closer to those of the full form. In addition, should a more optimal short form be developed, short-form-to-long-form score conversions would be necessary to guide the clinical examiner with regard to interpretation of the short-form scores.

METHOD

Subjects/Procedures

Neuropsychological clinical files of the third author (JAM) were reviewed to provide archival data on which the current study is based. Institutional Review Board approval was granted for the use of these archival testing data. All files contained diagnostic and demographic information on neurologic, psychiatric, and diagnostically mixed Veteran's Administration patients who were evaluated with the JLO as part of a thorough clinical neuropsychological evaluation. All available cases of individuals who had completed JLO ($N = 230$) were included in the study. The persons were almost exclusively male (97.4%). Their ages ranged from 21 to 84 years ($M = 48.89$, $SD = 14.43$) and their average educational level was 13.26 years ($SD = 2.33$). The persons sampled were predominantly right-handed (88.7%). The majority of the persons were Anglo-American (83.5%). There were 47 cases who presented with primary neurologic disorder, 101 cases with primary psychiatric disorder, 71 cases with mixed neuropsychiatric syndromes, and 11 cases without a definitive diagnosis.

Statistical Analyses

Coefficient alpha was computed for the full sample based on the complete, 30-item version of the JLO, Form V. This statistic also was computed on five shortened forms of the JLO items: items V1–V10, items V1–V20, items V11–V30, the odd-numbered items of JLO-Form V, and the even-numbered items of JLO-Form V. Summary scores for each of these JLO short forms also were correlated with the total score for the 30-item JLO, Form

Table 1. Internal Reliability and Consistency of Standard and Short Forms of the JLO.

	Alpha	Correlation with full form
Full form (V1–V30)	.84[a]	
JLO short form (V1–V10)	.61	.73
JLO short form (V1–V20)	.75	.90[b]
JLO short form (V11–V30)	.80[a]	.97[b]
JLO short form (Evens)	.69	.94[b]
JLO short form (Odds)	.72	.95[b]

Note. JLO = Judgment of Line Orientation. Form V. ($N = 230$).
[a]Coefficient alpha achieves optimal value of .80.
[b]Correlation $\geq$ .75.

Table 2. JLO Short-form (V11–V30) to Full-Form Score Conversions.

JLO short form (V11–V30)	JLO long form (V1–V30)	JLO short form (V11–V30)	JLO long form (V1–V30)
0	3	11	19
1	5	12	20
2	6	13	22
3	7	14	23
4	9	15	24
5	10	16	25
6	11	17	26
7	13	18	28
8	15	19	29
9	17	20	30
10	18		

Note. JLO = Judgment of Line Orientation. Form V. ($N = 230$).

V. Values for these internal consistency and short-form versus long-form correlations are presented in Table 1.

After determining the optimal short-form version of JLO, short-form scores were equated with long-form scores by use of the equipercentile method (Lindquist, 1951). Short-to-long-form score conversions are presented in Table 2.

RESULTS

Inspection of Table 1 shows that the correlation of four of the JLO short forms with the full form exceeded .90; the only short form that failed to reach this criterion value was the V1–V10 short form. The two short forms with 15 items (the even- and odd-item forms) and the two short forms with 20 items (forms V1–V20 and V11–V30) met this global performance-level criterion.

Consideration of the internal consistency values provides a basis for choosing among the four JLO short forms that correlated highly with the full form. Similar to the findings of Woodard et al. (1996), our results show that the full JLO form has a coefficient alpha value of .84, which exceeds the .80 value that is recommended by Nunnally (1978). At this internal consistency level the error of measurement due to item sampling inaccuracy is reduced to a practical minimum. The odd- and even-short forms are close to the .70 level of internal consistency, and are comparable to the Woodard et al. (1996) results, whereas the V1–V20 and the V11–V30 short forms rank in the .75–.80 co-efficient alpha range.

We recommend adoption of the V11–V30 JLO short form as the best alternative based on these data because it provides the highest level of internal consistency (.80), meets Nunnally's reliability standard, and it also provides a near-perfect estimate of the JLO total score. Table 2 provides the short-form-to-long-form conversions for the recommended JLO short form (V11–V30). This table will assist the clinician in normative interpretation of these short-form scores.

DISCUSSION

When there is a need for brevity in the administration of the JLO, the V11–V30 version of the test appears to be a suitable alternative to the full form of the test for neuropsychiatric patients. Suggestions for future research include replication of this study with the use of diagnostically homogeneous samples and with a sample composed primarily of women, in order to assess the generalizability of these findings across gender. Further, the use of this short form should be validated, as it is difficult to assess what change might be incurred with the adoption of item 11 as the starting item.

REFERENCES

Benton, A.L., Sivan, A.B., Hamsher, K., Varney, N.R., & Spreen, O. (1994). *Contributions to neuropsychological assessment: A clinical manual* (2nd ed.). New York: Oxford.

Duis, C., Schefft, B., & Wood, K. (1996, November). *Classification accuracy of short forms of Benton's Judgment of Line Orientation and Visual Form Discrimination in an epilepsy population*. Poster presented at the 16th Annual Meeting of the National Academy of Neuropsychology, New Orleans, LA.

Lindquist, E.F. (1951). *Educational measurement*. Washington DC: American Council on Education.

Moses, J.A. Jr. (1994). Judgment of line orientation. In D.J. Keyser & R.C. Sweetland (Eds.), *Test critiques* (Vol. X, pp. 327–339). Austin, TX: Pro-Ed.

Nunnally, J.C. (1978). *Psychometric theory* (2nd ed.). New York: McGraw-Hill.

Woodard, J.L., Benedict, R.H.B., Roberts, F.C., Kinner, K.M., Capruso, D.X., & Clark, A.N. (1996). Short-form alternatives to the Judgment of Line Orientation Test. *Journal of Clinical and Experimental Neuropsychology, 18*, 898–904.

Chapter VII

VALIDITY

A. Definition

The acid test of whether a particular concept is valid is the extent to which it measures what it was intended to measure. In the specific arena of the development of clinical instruments, Kaufman and Kaufman (1993) expand the definition as the following: "The validity of a test is defined as the degree to which it accomplishes what it was designed to do" (p. 84).

Our definition of validity is intended to apply to both of these aspects of the concept.

B. Types of Validity Assessments: Content-Related, Face, Concurrent, Differential/Discriminant, Predictive or Criterion/Sensitivity–Specificity, Factorial, and Construct

We share the view of the late Samuel Messick (1980) that although validity assessments may assume many forms, they can all be logically subsumed under the rubric of Construct Validity. Thus, we review the different types of validity from this perspective.

1. *Content validity* refers to the extent to which a test represents the content that it is meant to reflect. Thus, a spelling test would be valid to the extent that it contains words-to-be-spelled that the student was asked to study. 'Content-related' validity is a concept coined by Anne Fitzpatrick (1983) to convey the idea that it is virtually impossible to cover entirely the full range of content areas that are designated by the concept under investigation. In the area of test construction, and more generally, there are a number of major sources that the clinical scientist utilizes to satisfy this criterion of validity: a comprehensive review of the relevant clinical research and biostatistical literature; the investigators' own clinical, educational, administrative, and research experiences; and pilot testing of preliminary ideas and or large pools of test items that are purported to measure key aspects of the concept under investigation. The concept is then measured on whatever appropriate scales most accurately reveal the more manifest and subtler aspects of the concept such as: nominal–dichotomous; nominal–polychotomous; dichotomous–ordinal; continuous–ordinal; interval/ratio.

2. *Face validity*. Once the concept is content-defined, it should have easily passed the test of face validity, namely, a yes response to the question: Does the concept/item look as though it measures what it was supposed to measure? In the context of the Vineland Adaptive Behavior Scales (Sparrow, Balla, & Cicchetti, 1984), for example, an item deriving from the Receptive subdomain of the Communication domain is intended to measure "what the individual understands." Any such item would never be confused with one derived from either the Expressive subdomain ("what the individual says") or the Written subdomain ("what the individual reads and writes").

3. *Concurrent validity*. This concept concerns the extent to which two measures of a given construct, taken at the same point in time, are correlated with one other. The size of the correlation is the criterion, and does involve a certain degree of subjectivity of interpretation. Certainly, if one were developing a new measure of cognition, and were to compare IQ assessments of one instrument with those derived from performance, for example, on a standard test in the field, one would not wish either to have a perfect correlation approaching +1.00 or a correlation approaching 0. In the first instance, one would be criticized for having developed little more than a clone of an already existing standard in the field. In the latter case, one would seriously question whether the new test was measuring the construct of IQ at all. Depending upon the objectives underlying the development of the new instrument, the desired level of correlation would vary. If, for example, the goal were to develop a short form of an already existing test, then one would want and expect the correlation to be somewhat high, for example, ≥ 0.85. If, on the other hand, the new test incorporated as a large component a measure of creativity that was not part of the underpinning of the standard test, then one might be satisfied with a somewhat lower correlation between scores deriving from the two instruments, for example, one of 0.70.

In clinical neuropsychology, the classic example of concurrent validity is the extent to which a test (or tests) correlates with the state of the brain. Just as one would have confidence in a blood test that signifies the presence of diabetes, so too one would have confidence in a test that signifies the presence, extent, and/or absence of brain dysfunction.

4. *Differential (discriminant) validity*. When a clinical investigator purposefully selects two distinct groups, one expected to be characterized by the investigated concept (e.g., Aspergers' Syndrome) and the other not to be so characterized, and then demonstrates empirically that this is indeed the case, that investigator could be said to have satisfied the criterion for discriminant or differential validity of the syndrome.

5. *Predictive validity (sometimes referred to as criterion validity)* can be measured in several different ways and by several different data analytic strategies that vary widely in levels of complexity. In perhaps the simplest case, this would involve predicting the later performance of those individuals manifesting high as opposed to low levels of the concept under study. As one example, those scoring lower on a test of early reading comprehension would be expected to obtain poorer levels of reading comprehension five years later, than would their peers who scored higher on the same test.

A more complex model for testing predictive validity derives from the Sensitivity–Specificity model, which might also be viewed as a form of Criterion Validity. This type of validity has special application in the identification of confirmed positive and negative cases that characterize specific diseases, disorders, or syndromes.

6. *Criterion validity: the Sensitivity–Specificity model.* The Sensitivity (Se)–Specificity (Sp) model is comprised of several components: Sensitivity (Se), the percentage of confirmed positive cases that test positive for the trait or disorder in question; Specificity (Sp) the percentage of confirmed negative cases that test negative for it; Overall Accuracy (OA), the combined percentage of confirmed positive and confirmed negative cases that test positive *or* negative; Predicted Positive Accuracy (PPA), the percentage of test-positive cases that are confirmed positive cases; and Predicted Negative Accuracy (PNA), the percentage of test-negative cases that are confirmed negatives.

Finally, two possible errors that are a result of the misclassification of positive and negative cases are referred to, respectively, as False Positives and False Negatives. These errors can be calculated relative to either the number of confirmed cases or to the number of test cases.

An extension of the Predicted Positive Accuracy (PPA) component of the Se–Sp model is discussed briefly in a later section of the text.

Caveat 1: Even when Se and Sp are high, large imbalances between true positive and true negative cases can lower/raise the value of PPA and/or PNA (Feinstein, 1977). Because the number of negative cases in most given areas of investigation is much larger than the corresponding numbers of positive cases, this becomes a matter for concern. As an example of this phenomenon, suppose that our original data are spread in a 2 × 2 contingency table as follows:

Best or Confirmatory Diagnosis.

Test	(+)	(−)	Total
(+)	45	5	50
(−)	5	45	50
Total	50	50	100

Note. OA, Se, Sp, PPA, and PNA, all = 90%.

Now suppose that we quadruple the number of true negative cases and then examine its effect upon the five components of diagnostic accuracy. The data in the revised table will be spread as follows:

Best or Confirmatory Diagnosis.

Test	(+)	(−)	Total
(+)	45	20	65
(−)	5	180	185
Total	50	200	250

Now, OA, Se and Sp still = 90%, but PPA falls to 69% and PNA rises to 97%, with both representing obvious artifactual effects caused by quadrupling the number of negative cases.

A sensible solution to this dilemma is to simply sample randomly from the usually much larger number of negative cases to reach an n (sample size) that is identical to the number of true positive cases. This will resolve the problem.

Caveat 2: It has been noted that Se and Sp can also vary according to the comparison or control group that is chosen by the clinical investigator (Feinstein, 1977).

As an example of this phenomenon, when the diagnostic accuracy of schizophrenic patients is compared to that of normal controls, Se and Sp can be expected to be higher than when the comparison is made with another psychiatric disorder. In other contexts, Se can also be lowered dramatically when the number of negative cases is highly predominant. An example would be the study of the validity of the diagnosis of rare disorders in the community such as autism (e.g. see Cicchetti, Sparrow, Volkmar, Cohen, & Rourke, 1991).

Caveat 3: False negative errors are much more serious than false positive errors. The reason for this phenomenon is that false negatives represent cases of an *undetected* disorder or disease, but false positives will remain and will be detected by a best or confirmatory diagnosis. Therefore, in developing a screener it becomes critical to *minimize* the false negative error.

Caveat 4: While much less serious, false positive errors can still be of some concern. The reason for this is that if the percentage of false positives is very high, then the time required to re-examine all these cases may result in too little in the saving of time and expense to make a given screener worthwhile.

The clinical or practical implication of all of this is that the clinical researcher, in the development of a new diagnostic instrument or in the evaluation of an already existing test in the field, needs to strike a clinically meaningful balance between an allowable maximal false negative and false positive error rate. Whereas this critical decision is purely clinical, rather than biostatistical, at least a rough set of criteria should be considered, with the understanding that it may and should be revised as appropriate depending upon the clinical seriousness of a test's failing to identify a positive case. With this contingency in mind, criteria have been published in Cicchetti, Volkmar, Klin, and Showalter (1995; pp. 322–332), using the principle of setting a maximum False Negative error of 10%, and a maximum False Positive error of 30%. By this rule-of-thumb, we imply that a False Negative error is three times as serious as a False Positive error, and that this forms the basis for the following set of criteria, that apply to each of the previously defined five components of diagnostic accuracy that are generated by the Se–Sp model: <70% = Poor, 70–79% = Fair, 80–89% = Good, and 90–100% = Excellent.

These guidelines have been applied to various diagnostic classification systems. For example, Nelson and Cicchetti (1991) tested the predictive power of the MMPI as a potential screener for clinical depression. Results showed that OA = 77%; Se = 78%; Sp = 75%; PPA = 93%; and PPN = 43%. With a

False Negative error of 22%, carrying a risk of potential suicide, we concluded that the MMPI should not be used as a screen for clinical depression.

As a second application, Cicchetti et al. (1995; pp. 322–332) showed that ICD-10 criteria for the diagnosis of autism produced the following results: OA = 81–83%; Se = 77–86%; Sp = 77–86%; PPA = 76–83%; and PNA = 81–87%.

In an earlier medical application, the Se–Sp model was applied to examine the accuracy of a series of radiological signs considered diagnostic of mega-colon, or Hirschsprung Disease, among neonates and young children (Rosenfield, Ablow, Markowitz, DiPietro, Seashore, Touloukian, & Cicchetti, 1984). Not unexpectedly, the signs were less diagnostically accurate in neonates than they were in young children. In addition, some signs were highly sensitive (i.e., sensitivity and predicted positive accuracies between 90% and 100%); others were highly specific (88–100%); and still others were poor diagnostic indicators for both positive and negative diagnoses.

It should be noted here that one of the indexes deriving from the Se–Sp model, namely, Predicted Positive Accuracy (PPA) can be extended beyond the dichotomous case by application of a special form of the Jonckheere test of trend for assessing predictive validity when the predictor or independent variable is ordinal and the dependent, outcome, or response variable is dichotomous. As an example of a medical application, Garcia, Rosenfield, Markowitz, Seashore, Touloukian, and Cicchetti (1987) applied the test to investigate the predictive validity of the Barium Enema examination (ordinalized as Negative, Equivocal, or Positive) upon the probability of acute appendicitis in children and adolescents. As the Barium test results varied from negative to equivocal to positive, the *corresponding* proportions of confirmed cases of acute appendicitis increased from 0% to 50% to 92%. Application of Jonckheere's test of ordinal trend with a dichotomous outcome (Cicchetti, Showalter, Rourke, and Fuerst, 1992a, pp. 123–126; Jonckheere, 1970; Leach, 1979) produced a z value of 2.06, which was statistically significant at the 0.02 level of probability. As another application, it was shown that level of grade school education (Kindergarten, Grades 1, 2, 3, 4, 5, 6) is linearly related to the percentage of children having a conceptual understanding of AIDS (Shoemaker, Schonfeld, O'Hare, Showalter, & Cicchetti, 1996).

7. *Factorial validity*. Kaufman and Kaufman (1993) argue persuasively and convincingly that "factor structure is probably the most important evidence of a theory-based, multiscale test's construct validity." Applying both exploratory and confirmatory factor analyses to data deriving from their 1993 *Kaufman Adolescent And Adult Intelligence Test (KAIT)*, the test authors demonstrated impressive results showing: (1) that the two factors that emerged from their analyses coincided very closely to the two subtests defining the KAIT, namely, Fluid and Crystallized Scales of Adult Intelligence; and (2) that these same two factors emerged consistently across age groups.

Similarly, Sparrow et al. (1984) applied principal component and principal factor analyses to demonstrate that the type of adaptive behavior derived from the three subdomains (interpersonal relationships, play and leisure time, and coping skills) were the subdomains most highly correlated with the Vineland Socialization Domain, which consists precisely of just these three subdomains.

8. *Construct validity: the 'unifying concept.'* We began this section on validity assessment by referring to Messick's (1980) treatise, entitled: "Test Validity and the Ethics of Assessment." We should like to elaborate more on what we referred to then as Messick's contention that the basic forms or components of validity can probably best be subsumed under the single rubric of construct validity. These were encompassed in a pithy set of relevant statements made by Messick (1980):

> *Others have similarly argued that "any reference relative to prediction and ... all inferences relative to test scores, are based upon underlying constructs" (Tenopyr, 1977, p. 48). Guion (1977, p. 410) concluded that "all validity is at its base some form of construct validity." I will argue, building on Guion's (1976) conceptual groundwork, that construct validity is indeed the unifying concept of validity that integrates criterion and content considerations into a common framework for testing rational hypotheses about theoretically relevant relationships. The bridge or unifying theme that permits this integration is the meaningfulness or interpretability of the test scores, which is the goal of the construct validation process. This construct meaning provides a rational basis both for hypothesizing predictive relationships and for judging content relevance and representativeness (p. 1015).*

We agree that this earlier contention is still valid.

Thus far, we have defined, reviewed, and given examples of the basic forms of validity assessment that are discussed in biobehavioral and medical research areas of clinical investigation. Having now completed our discussions of some of the more fundamental issues concerning reliability and validity assessments, we present a short section that acts as a unifying concept in relating these two basic psychometric components. This is the issue of the mathematical equivalence between reliability and validity assessments, in the specific context of the Kappa statistic and the Sensitivity and Specificity indexes.

C. The Mathematical Relationship Between Reliability and Validity Assessments

The relationship holds under the following condition: When two clinical examiners independently identify the same percentage of cases as positive or negative, then the exact value of Kappa (the reliability statistic of choice for dichotomously scaled data) can be derived solely on the basis of one's knowledge of the Sensitivity (Se) and Specificity (Sp) of the diagnostic test that has been applied, according to the following simple formula:

Kappa = [(Sensitivity (Se) + Specificity (Sp) − 1]
(Cicchetti, Sparrow, Volkmar, Cohen, & Rourke, 1991; pp. 64–73; Kraemer, 1982; Youden, 1950).

For example, suppose two independent clinical examiners each diagnose 80% of a group of children with Pervasive Developmental Disorders as Non-Autistic with the remaining 20% being diagnosed as Autistic. Further, with Examiner A considered the one to represent a criterion diagnosis, assume Se at 90% and Sp at 92%. Then

$$\text{Kappa} = [0.90 + 0.92 - 1] = 1.82 - 1.00 = 0.82$$

Note: Consistent with the clinical criteria suggested in Cicchetti (2001), both the reliability and validity assessments can be considered excellent.

Next, we discuss more elaborate applications and extensions of the critical concept of validity or accuracy of measurement in the context of some of the basic univariate and multivariate procedures that are utilized to measure them as these present in a series of articles originally appearing in the *The Journal of Clinical and Experimental Neuropsychology*, *The Clinical Neuropsychologist*, and *Child Neuropsychology*, between 1992 and 2003. This wide array of publications covers the following diverse content areas: numerous further applications of predictive and construct validity utilizing diverse methodological techniques, namely, the odds ratio, common factor analysis, structural equation modeling, and sub-type analysis. Another series of articles focuses upon aspects of validity assessment that though of great clinical importance have not been widely investigated. These include the following: post-diction to estimate levels of premorbid intelligence; examining aspects of validity through the implementation of meta-analysis and the study of the effects of moderator variables on selected outcome measures; using patients' base rates to investigate the validity of brain–behavior relationships; understanding issues of validity through the invocation of Bayesian theory; controlling for practice effects acting as threats to the reliability and validity of study results; controlling statistically for threats to reliability and validity assessments; application of reliability and validity procedures to the development of new or existing clinical tests; and validity assessment in the larger context of null-hypothesis significance testing (NHST), and in power and precision decisions. The final section of the text includes articles on the critical role of model building as a validity procedure in clinical neuropsychology and biobehavioral research more generally.

Chapter VIII

EDITORS' COMMENTARIES PRECEDING ARTICLES ON VALIDITY ASSESSMENT PUBLISHED IN *JCEN*, *TCN*, AND *CN* BETWEEN 1992 AND 2003

A. Predictive Validity

Fuerst, Fisk, and Rourke (1990) posed the question: To what extent might the degree of children's neuropsychological symptomatology be linearly related to a clinically meaningful difference of 10 points or more, favoring Wechsler Intelligence Scale Scores (WISC) of Verbal IQ (VIQ) over Performance IQ (PIQ)? Symptom severity was based upon a tripartite classification of children's Personality Inventory for Children (PIC) scores into 'None/Very Mild,' 'Mild/ Moderate,' or 'Severe.' This application, as well as the availability of a computer program to perform the aforementioned Jonckheere test is described, in detail, in Cicchetti, Showalter, Rourke, and Fuerst (1992a; pp. 123–126).

In other applications of predictive validity, this time in the context of the Sensitivity (Se)–Specificity (Sp) model, Receiver Operating Curve (ROC) Methodology (deriving from Signal–Detection methodology) has been utilized, in a number of research investigations (e.g., Hsiao, Bartko, & Potter, 1989; Pepe, 2000). It is especially useful for identifying optimal levels of Sensitivity and Specificity for a given diagnostic area. Examples include the diagnoses of: Autism (Volkmar, Carter, Sparrow, & Cicchetti, 1993) and Dissociative Disorders (Steinberg, Rounsaville, & Cicchetti, 1991), as well as the accurate assessment of defense mechanisms in mothers and their children (Laor, Wolmer, & Cicchetti, 2001). ROC analysis is also highlighted in a *JCEN* publication by Drake and Hannay (1992; pp. 127–131).

The assessment of predictive validity has also varied widely over content domains and data analytic techniques. This will be illustrated by seven publications deriving from *JCEN*, *TCN*, and *CN* publications between 1995 and 1998.

In a novel and informative application, Bieliauskas and colleagues (1997) demonstrated the utility of the Odds-Ratio well beyond its usual risk probability implications. Specifically, Bieliauskas, Fastenau, Lacy, and Roper (1997; pp. 316–321) compared the odds ratio (OR) to ordinary *t*-tests, *p* values, effect sizes and sensitivity and specificity for diagnosing the presence or absence of Alzheimer's Disease.

As demonstrated by Bieliauskas and colleagues, the OR compared favorably only to the sensitivity and specificity assessments.

More generally, when accuracy in classification is the primary research objective, then the Se–Sp model is recommended, because it is quite possible to obtain a statistically significant odds-ratio in the presence of clinically unacceptable sensitivity, specificity, and other components of diagnostic accuracy.

As an example, consider the following hypothetical data on 100 infants who are being screened for presence or absence of Autism, with the results occurring, as shown:

Criterion Clinical Diagnosis.

Screener	Autistic	Non-autistic
Autistic	31	19
Non-autistic	19	31

For these data, the Odds-Ratio = 2.61. This is a quite respectable value and statistically significant at $p < 0.05$. Yet, when the Se–Sp Model is applied to the same data, it produces sensitivity, specificity, overall accuracy, predicted positive accuracy, and predicted negative accuracy levels, each at only 62%, which is Poor by the criteria of Cicchetti, Volkmar, Klin, and Showalter (1995; pp. 322–332).

A second potential problem with the indiscriminate application of the odds-ratio was pointed out some decades ago by Berkson (1958) and Feinstein (1973), and reported later by Fleiss (1981): In applying the odds-ratio, the level of the rates is lost. As Fleiss (1981) states: "... a tenfold increase over a rate of one per million would be considered equivalent to a tenfold increase over a rate of one per thousand" (p. 91).

The take-home message from all of this is that the odds-ratio, *like any other biostatistical technique*, must be applied with wisdom in order to produce results that make clinical or practical sense as well as purely statistical sense.

Cicchetti, Volkmar, Klin, and Showalter (1995; pp. 322–332) applied a number of multivariate techniques, in order to examine the sensitivity, specificity, overall accuracy, and the predicted positive and negative accuracy of the diagnosis of autism, based upon 15 ICD-10 criteria. A comparison of logistic regression, linear and quadratic discriminant function analysis, and neural networks analysis revealed that although the first three methods were indistinguishable, neural networks produced initially impressive classification results that were lost upon cross-validation. This and other apparent disadvantages of neural networks (compared to its multivariate competitors) are discussed in some detail by the authors.

Lest one believe that this article settles the matter, one has only to read the recent commentary of Tryon (2002) who believes that "... network theories and models are also helping to unify cognitive and social neurosciences" and further that "... network theories and models address how mind and behavior emerge from the brain by examining how psychological and behavioral phenomena emerge from networks and simulated neurons. This approach is making discernible progress on the mind-body problem" (p. 728). Should this be seen as a cerebral stretch or carefully reasoned scientific theorizing? May future empirical research be the arbiter!

B. Examining Construct Validity Using Factor Analysis

A number of investigators have addressed the issue of construct validity, using a number of varying multivariate techniques: Fuchs, Hannay, Huckeba, and Espy (1999; pp. 333–343) applied Principal Factor Analysis to investigate the construct validity of the Continuous Recognition Memory Test.

C. Examining Construct Validity Using Structural Equation Modeling (SEM)

Francis (1988; reprinted in Rourke et al., 1992, pp. 326–342) provided a lucid description of SEM in our earlier volume. This same article was cited most favorably in a later publication by Bentler and Stein (1992). For an excellent edited text that focuses heavily on SEM in the context of analyzing longitudinal data, the interested reader is referred to Little, Schnabel, and Baumert (2000). We have recently applied SEM modeling and found it to be quite helpful for predicting the frequency of mothers' utilization of medical resources during their children's acute illnesses (McCarthy, Walls, Cicchetti, Mayes, Rizzo, López-Benitez, Salloum, Baron, Fink, Anderson, Little, LaCamera, & Freudigman, 2003).

Several investigators have applied SEM to examine the construct validity of the Wide Range Assessment of Memory and Learning Test (WRAML), utilizing data from the standardization sample. Burton, Donders, and Mittenberg (1996; pp. 344–351) utilized SEM to assess the construct validity of the (WRAML), using data deriving from the standardization sample, whereas Francis, Fletcher, Rourke, and York (1992; pp. 352–361) utilized SEM in a five-factor model for a number of tests used in the neuropsychological assessment of children.

It should be noted that SEM has some distinct advantages over other models, as noted by prominent devotees in the field, such as Hoyle and Smith (1994): SEM "does improve over traditional techniques such as analysis of covariance (ANCOVA) or multiple regression because it provides maximum flexibility in modeling the effects of extraneous variables" (p. 438).

Also, the large sample size problem has been obviated by the development of new statistical procedures for SEM models (see Chin & Newsted, 1999; Oud, Jansen, & Haughton, 1999).

This said in its defense, a major limitation of SEM is that its application is not as likely to prove causality, as would be true of results deriving from a well-designed clinical trial. This is because of the *lack* of random assignment to treatment and control groups that characterizes SEM (Bentler & Stein, 1992; Hoyle & Smith, 1994; the National Research Council—Coyle, Boruch, & Turner, 1991).

It is interesting from a methodological standpoint that application of clinical trials in neuropsychological research is noticeable mainly by its absence. In large part, this may well be due to the fact that neuropsychologists are interested primarily in the brain–behavior relationships of diseases, disorders, and syndromes, rather than in an assessment and comparison of the relative efficacy of various types of treatment for these afflictions. However, it should be stressed that clinical trials, when designed appropriately with adequate controls, can and should be applied to a wide range of problems having little or nothing to do with treatment issues. In one clinical trial, mothers were successfully trained to reliably and validly evaluate, by observation, the level of illness of febrile infants (McCarthy, Sznajderman, Lustman-Findling, Baron, Fink, Czarkowski, Bauchner, & Cicchetti, 1990), toward the broader goal of reducing unnecessary mother–child office visits during the course of acute pediatric illnesses. In a second investigation, a randomized clinical trial was utilized to measure the efficacy of a three-week, multifaceted HIV/AIDS education intervention program upon the level of conceptual understanding of factual knowledge and fears about AIDS among students in grades kindergarten through sixth grade. It too was quite successful (Schonfeld, O'Hare, Perrin, Quackenbush, Showalter, & Cicchetti, 1995).

D. Conceptual Relationships Between Structural Equation Modeling (SEM), Hierarchical (or Multi-Linear) Modeling (HLM)/(MLM) and Individual Growth Curve Analysis (IGCA)

HLM is a valuable multivariate technique that is applicable when one wishes to study nested effects, such as the effects of a school and classroom climate upon children's reading abilities. Here, children are nested within classrooms, and classrooms are nested within schools. HLM would make it possible to assess the main effects of school and classroom, as well as the effects of the interaction between the two, upon reading ability. An entire issue of the *Journal of Educational and Behavioral Statistics* was devoted to HLM in 1995: *20, Special Issue*, pp. 109–240. A useful, comprehensive, and very popular text on HLM was written by Bryk and Raudenbush (1992). The text was very recently revised and updated by Raudenbush and Bryk (2002). Whereas earlier applications of HLM have focused upon outcome or dependent variables measured on interval, or continuous scales of measurement, Chapter 10 of the revised text discusses HLM applications for which the outcome variable is ordinal or dichotomous, or even multinomial (several nominal categories of classification). A number of recently developed and revised computer programs are currently available for performing HLM. These include PROC MIXED, deriving from SAS; and both HLM and MLWin. Those interested in HLM would be well advised to consult this text primarily for its incorporation of state-of-the-art HLM methodology, as well as to benefit from what the Series Editor of the 2002 revision and HLM expert Jan de Leeuw (2002) refers to, rather candidly, in the Introduction (p. xxiv), as "hundreds of corrections and additions to the earlier chapters" of the 1992 text. It should also be noted (Raudenbush & Bryk, 2002, p. 159) that there is a website available that focuses on a wide range of HLM issues, including the availability of computer programs and updates, one of which can be used to calculate, among other things, power analyses for individual growth curve analysis research designs. We conclude this brief section on HLM with an important caveat expressed by de Leeuw (2002, p. xxiv) in his strong recommendation of the new and revised test: "Reading this book will not make you an expert in all these different areas, but hopefully it will teach you what these options are, where to find your expert, and which questions to ask her or him."

This sage caveat is very much in keeping with the current authors' emphasis on the realization that each technique must first be understood conceptually in terms of what it can and cannot accomplish, and then be applied very judiciously.

Individual Growth Curve Analysis (IGCA), which may be a more familiar technique to biobehavioral scientists in general, and neuropsychologists in particular, is a multivariate technique for measuring change over time. It is a multiple regression technique in which subjects are nested within repeated measurements. IGCA is also the simplest of the HLM models (Kreft, de Leeuw, & van der Leeden, 1994). IGCA has a number of advantages over Repeated Measures ANOVA with a linear or curvilinear trend component to measure change over time: It adjusts for unequal intervals between repeated assessments; it can provide growth curves on a subject-by-subject basis; it does not require a balanced design or one without missing data follow-up points; and it can adjust for subjects-lost-to-follow-up (albeit under somewhat restricted assumptions). However, IGCA and Repeated Measures ANOVA with a linear or curvilinear trend analysis component are mathematically equivalent when the following conditions hold: the time intervals between repeated measurements (assessments) are equal; correlations between measurements taken closer in time are not appreciably higher than those taken farther apart; and there are no missing data (Francis, Fletcher, Steubing, Davidson, & Thompson, 1991). Finally, in their discussion of HLM and SEM procedures, Little, Schnabel, and Baumert (2000) note that … "both approaches yield exactly or approximately the same results" (p. 12). In a recent article, Mayes, Cicchetti, Acharyya, and Zhang (2003) applied IGCA to compare the developmental trajectories of cocaine and other types of drug exposed children. Finally Coscia, Ris, Succop, and Dietrich (2003; pp. 362–373) applied growth curve analysis to study the effects of lead exposure in children ranging in age between 6 and 15 years of age.

Caveat: IGCA requires the assumption of random attrition rates in order to produce valid results. Specifically, IGCA fails to adjust for non-random or systematic loss of subjects to follow-up assessments (e.g., Littell, Milliken, Stroup, & Wolfinger, 1996). Because this state of affairs poses potential threats to the reliability and validity of the results produced by IGCA, it is the responsibility of the clinical investigator to test for the extent to which the subjects lost to follow-up may bias study results and their interpretation. The aforementioned method of Cicchetti and Nelson (1994; pp. 611–615) (see also Mayes & Cicchetti, 1995; pp. 616–627) compares attrited and maintained cohorts on all independent, demographic, and outcome variables at each assessment point to reveal the level of bias introduced by the systematic loss of subjects to follow-up assessments. For further approaches to this problem, the interested reader is referred to the work of Little, Lindenberger, and Maier (2000).

When IGCA becomes the data analytic strategy of choice, other conditions must be considered and resolved in the design of the clinical investigation.

1. One needs to classify the variables of interest (as one would with ordinary Repeated Measures ANOVA) into Fixed Effects (limits generalization of findings to populations under investigation); Random Effects (permits generalization to samples deriving from populations other than the ones under study); or Mixed Effects (some variables are fixed; others are random).

2. One needs to decide upon the minimal number of assessments (baseline plus follow-up) to investigate in order to best satisfy the key questions or test the relevant hypotheses that are being investigated. For example, choosing only two assessment points (Baseline and Endpoint) poses a problem, because connecting two data points will always produce a straight line indicating a linear trend. This means that if the independent variables being studied bear a curvilinear relationship with the outcome variable, this relationship will be masked, thereby completely invalidating the reported results of the investigation. Bearing directly upon this point, Venter, Maxwell, and Bollig (2002) demonstrate the value of adding a single intermediate time point to a standard pretest–posttest design.

3. The investigator needs a minimum of three assessments to analyze for a linear trend; and a minimum of four assessments, in order to analyze for either a quadratic or cubic trend.

   Until recently, research investigators tended to base sample-size estimates deriving from Power Analyses for IGCA on ordinary Least Squares (OLS) models (e.g., Personal Communication, David Francis). This is because to date there were no general-purpose power tables that are IGCA-specific. However, some preliminary work has been published. As one example, Hedeker, Gibbons, and Waternaux (1999) provided sample size estimations for a limited number of possible IGCA designs (two independent groups and four, six, or eight repeated assessments).

4. More recently, Raudenbush and Bryk (2002) made available a free Windows-based computer program for determining optimal sample designs and power for a number of IGCA study designs. The program was developed by Stephen Raudenbush and Xiao-Feng Liu.

All this said, it is expected that problems of this genre will be resolved, in the quite foreseeable future, not only for IGCA, but also for other multivariate techniques. For example, Hoyle (1999) discusses a number of small sample strategies for both SEM and Confirmatory Factor Analysis that have been tested for validity by computer simulation methodology.

E. Examining Construct Validity Using Subtype Analysis

As examples of this phenomenon, we present four studies that have utilized sub-type analysis and the development of typologies for examining the construct validity (internal and external validity) levels of both psychosocial functioning and Alzheimer's Disease: Butler, Rourke, Fuerst, and Fisk (1997; pp. 374–407); Fisher, Rourke, Bieliauskas, Giordani, Berent, and Foster (1996; pp. 408–429); Fisher, Rourke, and Bieliauskas (1999; pp. 430–457); Fuerst and Rourke (1995; pp. 458–473).

A fifth and very recent investigation by Ralston, Fuerst, and Rourke (2003; pp. 474–492) uses subtype analysis to compare the psychosocial typology of children with below average IQ to that of children diagnosed with learning disabilities. The investigation provides insights into methods for assessing the reliability or internal validity of subtype groupings when sample size limitations render it impossible to apply a given subtyping technique to two different groups or sets of subjects. The authors also stress the importance of a theory-driven, hypothesis generating approach to the development of subtype analysis, since clusters that statistically separate groups can and will occur on a completely random basis. Such sage advice is consonant with the caveats put forth by knowledgeable and prominent cluster analysts in the field, such as John Hartigan (personal communication).

F. Post-Diction: A Special Type of Validity Assessment

Post-Diction, as a validity assessment, occurs whenever currently measured 'independent' variables are used to estimate previously occurring but not measured 'dependent' variables. This interesting phenomenon is illustrated by the following five publications that appeared in *JCEN* and *TCN*: Basso, Bornstein, Roper, and McCoy (2000; pp. 493–505); Crawford and Allan (1997; pp. 506–510); Graves (2000; pp. 511–518); Snitz, Bieliauskas, Crossland, Basso, and Roper (2000; pp. 519–524); Yeates and Taylor (1997; pp. 525–536).

G. Examining Aspects of Validity through Meta-Analysis and the Effects of Moderator Variables

Some investigators have used meta-analytic techniques to examine the reliability and validity of reported findings across multiple studies in which investigators asked the same research question. In one such application, Wexler and

Cicchetti (1992) showed that contrary to a widespread scientific belief, a combination of psychotherapy and pharmacotherapy is no more effective for treating outpatient clinical depression than is either treatment administered alone. A computer program that can be applied to perform such meta-analytic techniques was reported in Cicchetti, Showalter, and Wexler (1993; pp. 537–540).

For a recently published computer program for performing meta-analyses, more generally, the interested reader is referred to Borenstein and Rothstein's (1999) Comprehensive Meta-Analysis program that was developed in collaboration with Larry Hedges and Jesse Berlin.

It should be noted that in most applications of meta-analysis, the goal is to discover whether the evidence establishes a consistent relationship between two variables. In the case just presented, this would be between type of treatment and its effect upon level of depression. However, this is not always the case. Sometimes the goal is not to confirm or disconfirm the putative relationship between an independent and a dependent variable but as Rosenthal (1991) describes it, "to determine the factors ... associated with variations in the magnitudes of the relationships between the two variables. Such factors are known as moderator variables because they moderate or alter the magnitude of a relationship" (p. 7).

The authors of two articles appearing in *The Clinical Neuropsychologist* reported on the role of moderator variables in clinical neuropsychological research. Sweet, Suchy, Leahy, Abramowitz, and Nowinski (1999; pp. 541–552) investigated the moderating role of age in the relationship between orientation and memory; and Uchiyama, D'Elia, Dellinger, Selnes, Becker, Wesch, Chen, Satz, Van Gorp, and Miller (1994; pp. 553–559) reported how demographic variables functioned as moderators affecting the Symbol Digit Modalities Test (SDMT) performance.

It should be noted at this point that the aforementioned Borenstein and Rothstein (1999) computer program also allows for investigating the role of moderator variables in meta-analytic research.

H. Using Base Rates to Study the Validity of Brain–Behavior Relationships

In this type of scientific inquiry, the focus of study differs from the traditional interest in the relationship between an independent and a dependent variable. Fox, Lees-Haley, Earnest, and Dolezal-Wood (1995; pp. 560–563) used patients' base rates to investigate the etiology of post-concussive symptoms.

I. Invoking Bayesian Theory to Examine Validity

Elwood (1993; pp. 564–570) appealed to Baysian theory to investigate clinical discriminations in neuropsychological tests. His imaginative work harmonizes well with our discussion of the sensitivity–specificity model on pp. 103–105.

J. Controlling for Practice Effects Acting as Threats to the Reliability and Validity of Study Results

A number of researchers investigated the role of practice effects in brain–behavior relationships: Basso, Bornstein, and Lang (1999; pp. 571–580) in the study of executive function; Bruggemans, Van de Vijver Hair, and Huysmans (1997; pp. 581–595) in cognitive deterioration following cardiac surgery; and Rapport, Brines, Axelrod, and Theisen (1997; pp. 596–600) in the assessment of IQ.

K. Controlling Statistically for Threats to the Reliability and Validity of Study Results

There are a number of ways to control statistically, rather than experimentally, for threats to the reliability and validity of reported study results. One of the most widely known sets of procedures is aimed at the necessity to control for the extent to which a reported result could have occurred by chance but was mistakenly interpreted as statistically valid. But, as we are aware, there are investigators who tend to treat the $p = 0.05$ level of statistical significance, whether legitimately or illegitimately obtained, as the Holy Grail of scientific achievement. Abelson (1995) paints a mocking picture of such an individual as he poses the following:

> *What devices are available to the desperate researcher for arguing that the results look good, when a dispassionate observer would say they are marginal or worse? There are at least five:*
> 1. *Use a one-tailed test.* [Editors' Note: *This alone will increase the probability two-fold that one has obtained a statistically significant result*]
> 2. *When there is more than one test procedure available, use the one producing the most significant result(s).*
> 3. *Either include or exclude "outliers" from the data, depending upon which works better.*
> 4. *When several outcomes are tested simultaneously, focus on the one(s) with the best* p *value-the "hocus focus" trick.*
> 5. *State the actual* p *value, but talk around it.*

As Abelson concludes, research investigators who employ these five 'devices' invite 'skepticism' and 'disfavor' (p. 55).

Cicchetti (1994a; pp. 601–607) presents guidelines for *appropriately* applying multiple comparison methods in order to obviate the problem of claiming statistical significance when none can be legitimately claimed. This article also reviews the principles of a method that increases the power of multiple comparisons deriving from statistically significant interactions based upon a factorial analysis of variance (i.e., the method developed by Cicchetti, 1972; and recommended by multiple comparison specialists, such as Toothaker, 1991, pp. 124–126).

As described in a publication appearing in our earlier text, Adams, Brown, and Grant (1985; reprinted in Rourke et al., 1992, pp. 157–174) used the results of computer simulation methodology to argue against the application of ANCOVA to equate groups mismatched on relevant demographic variables.

In the current volume, Berman and Greenhouse (1992; p. 608) question the logic of the Adams et al. (1985) arguments, and Adams, Brown, and Grant (1992; pp. 609–610) offer counter-arguments as refutation of their conclusions.

Cicchetti and Nelson (1994; pp. 611–615) describe a new method for assessing the potential biasing effects of subjects lost to follow-up upon the reliability and validity of reported study results. The authors then apply the method to a longitudinal investigation of changes in personality following right and left hemisphere stroke. Mayes and Cicchetti (1995; pp. 616–627) apply the same method to investigate the extent to which subjects lost to follow-up threaten the reliability and validity of the reported relationship between prenatal cocaine exposure and neurobehavioral development in neonates and young children.

In a recent investigation Cicchetti, Kaufman, and Sparrow (*in press*) develop and apply a more comprehensive set of six methodologic criteria to evaluate the accuracy of a large body of literature focusing upon the association between prenatal and postnatal exposure to polychlorinated biphenyls (PCBs), on the one hand, and putative cognitive, neuropsychological, and behavioral deficits, on the other. These six fundamental scientific criteria involved a critical examination of: (1) the levels of reliability and validity of assessment instruments; (2) the appropriateness of the reliability and validity assessments themselves; (3) the adequacy of controlling for chance findings when multiple comparisons are made; (4) the necessity to distinguish between clinically and merely statistically significant results; (5) the level of success in controlling for fundamental confounding variables; and (6) the extent to which studies are appropriately designed and analyzed when the outcome variables are repeated measurements across time.

In commenting upon these criteria Hebben (*in press*) notes that: "these criteria are crucial in the design of sound scientific studies and in the appropriate analysis of study results. Errors in design and analysis weaken, and in some cases, eliminate the reliability and validity of scientific data. Such data when published has far reaching effects in the clinic and the scientific world, and, in some instances, the courts and legislature. Unfortunately the effect of this is that clinicians will make unwarranted inferences of causality based on unreliable and invalid conclusions contained in an article published in a peer-reviewed journal."

L. Application of Reliability and Validity Procedures to the Development of New or Existing Clinical Tests

Several groups of researchers have applied reliability and validity procedures to the development of clinical tests: Byrne, Dywan, and Connolly (1995; pp. 628–639), in the assessment of children's receptive vocabulary; Schretlen, Bobholz, and Brandt (1996; pp. 640–648), in the development of the Brief Test of Attention; and Schretlen, Brandt, and Bobholz (1996; pp. 649–654), in the validation of the same test on a patient sample.

M. Validity Assessment in the Context of Null-Hypothesis Significance Testing (NHST), Power, and Precision Decisions

In a provocative text that covers a number of fundamental issues surrounding power analysis, Helena Kraemer and Sue Thiemann (1987) provide a quick, easy, and accurate way to de-mystify the process of deciding appropriate sample sizes in bio-behavioral research. The basic questions they answer are as follows: "How large a sample size must I have?"; "Which approach should I take in designing my experiment?"; "Which measure should I use, and which test to analyze my data?"; "Will I have enough power with only the 20 (or 50 or 100) subjects available to me?" (p. 16). The authors are also careful to stress that ... "power calculations yield approximations, not exact values, both because of the nature of the calculation and the estimates of effect sizes involved in the calculation" (p. 39).

Power, precision, and Null Hypothesis Significance Testing (NHST) in the more general context of distinguishing between statistical and clinical or practical levels of significance has been widely discussed in the research literature (e.g., Borenstein, 1998; Borenstein, Rothstein, & Cohen, 1997; Hoenig & Heisey, 2001; Rosenthal, 1991; Rosenthal & Rubin, 1979, 1982).

In a thoughtful and scholarly publication dedicated to the memory of the renowned biostatistician Jacob Cohen, one of his colleagues and research collaborators (Borenstein, 1998) discussed the shift in research emphasis over the past several years from relying on levels of statistical significance ($p \leq 0.05$) alone to the size of the obtained effect or effect size (ES) estimation, or level of practical or clinical significance. This, in turn, serves as the gold standard for deciding on whether a given scientific conclusion is important enough to be considered meaningful or of practical usefulness.

Prior to this important shift in reasoning, the emphasis was solely on whether the result, say, of the success of a new treatment for a particular neuropsychological or medical disorder, could have occurred beyond chance expectancy. In fact, as Borenstein notes, the problem was even more serious than what it appears to be on the surface: There was widespread belief among scientists that high levels of statistical significance were synonymous with high levels of practical or clinical significance.

Thus, if a new treatment were shown in one study to be significantly more successful than standard treatment of the disorder under investigation, at, say, the nominal $p = 0.05$ level of probability, then a result that favored the new treatment at $p < 0.001$ would be falsely interpreted to reflect a higher (and therefore, scientifically more meritorious) level of practical or clinical significance of the treatment effect, even if the actual difference between the two treatments were identical in the two investigations, merely reflecting the fact that the sample size in the second study was, say, three times as large as the one resulting in $p = 0.05$. This is compounded by the fact that scientific journals today still use as an important criterion for publication whether a particular study produced statistically significant results. This unfortunate and widespread editorial policy is even more of a threat to the validity of conclusions when they derive from a *series* of published results of a study of the same phenomenon.

As one example, let us assume that a new treatment has been developed for anxiety disorder in teen-age children. Assume further that the ten best conceived, designed, and executed studies that have been published produce the following results. Five produce statistically significant results favoring the new treatment over the standard treatment. The remaining five studies show the same result, except that they do not reach a commonly accepted level of statistical significance. As Borenstein (1998) notes, the conclusion that would have been reached here is that the study results do not favor the new treatment, and it should therefore be removed from the market. Further analysis reveals a power issue. The sample sizes in the negative studies were all quite small, strongly suggesting the need for further investigations with appropriately powered sample sizes. This would be an example of how invalid scientific reasoning can lead unwittingly to the denial of appropriate treatment to patients who are in need of it. In a word, statistical significance may gain priority over clinical or practical significance, in spite of the fact that it is the latter that needs to be the driving force of research in clinical and experimental neuropsychology and in biobehavioral research more generally.

But what, in fact, is the relationship between statistical and practical significance? This relationship can be discussed in the framework of a four-part classification system, as follows.

1. *When they are one and the same.* This is usually not discussed in the literature, but would certainly obtain, for example, in the search for the location of specific genes for specific disorders. One identifies with a certain p value (say, <0.001) the location of one or more of such genes. If this finding successfully replicates, one has demonstrated an 'equivalence' between statistical and clinical significance, in the context of a valid and valuable scientific finding.

2. *When very small effect sizes (ES) have high clinical or practical significance.* This would be exemplified by the numerous large-scale randomized trials of treatment effects (e.g., the relationship between aspirin therapy and myocardial infarct, as reported in Rosenthal [1991]). This trial showed that the proportion of variance accounted for outcome (presence/absence) of heart attack, based on presence/absence of aspirin treatment, was a paltry 0.1%! Yet, as Rosenthal notes, the aspirin trial, on the basis of these results, was discontinued because it was concluded ... "that aspirin was so effective in preventing heart attacks (and deaths) that it would be unethical to continue to give half the physician subjects a placebo" (p. 135).

An even more dramatic example would be in the field of politics where a candidate can win an election by obtaining a single vote more than her/his opponent! In this case, what could not be less meaningful statistically turns out to be of the highest practical or substantive significance!

3. *When a very small ES has very low or poor clinical meaning.* For example, a test–retest kappa value of 0.10 based on 200 subjects becomes highly statistically significant at $p < 0.001$, but at a level of practical significance that must be viewed as trivial or having little or no validity. Finally, the most readily understood condition is the following.

4. *When both the ES and level of statistical significance are very high.* An example here would be the sensitivity, specificity, predicted positive, and predicted negative accuracy levels of the diagnosis of, say, Asperger's Syndrome that all exceed 90%.

Three Methodologic Commentaries (Cicchetti, 1998, pp. 655–657; 1999, pp. 658–661; 2001, pp. 662–667) appeared in *JCEN*. The first discusses the role of NHST in neuropsychological research; and the other two challenge the assumption that at least 400 subjects are required for determining precise split-half, coefficient alpha, test–retest, alternate forms, and inter-examiner reliability assessment results.

In addition to the broad set of arguments on the issues of NHST put forth by Borenstein (1998), a number of authors have studied more specific aspects of these areas of scientific inquiry. Very brief introductions to some topics that have appeared in the recent literature follow for the interested reader to pursue further.

1. Hoenig and Heisey (2001) discuss a number of inappropriate uses of power analysis, including the large body of literature that advocates performing power analyses whenever a research result turns out to be less than statistically significant.

2. Wainer (1999) provides examples of when a result occurring at the lowest level of statistical significance, with a chance probability of the nominal five times in 100, would nonetheless make a substantial scientific contribution. Six examples are given. These are drawn from a diverse number of fields of inquiry, namely, physics, cosmology, psychology, geophysics, career counseling and theology.

3. Krantz (1999) provides a critical examination of the NHST controversy in psychological research and emphasizes the importance of placing confidence intervals around specific research results.

4. Chow (1998) presents a comprehensive target article dealing with arguments to limit the role of NHST. This is followed by the critical commentaries of a number of scientists, and then an Author's Response. Two more recent commentaries, also followed by Chow's response, were written by Haig (2000) and Sohn (2000).

5. Consistent with the suggestions of Cohen (1994, 1997), Krueger (2001) emphasizes the role of replication of research results, a critical phenomenon that does not play a major role in NHST. In a more recent series of commentaries that appeared in the *American Psychologist* (2002), Brand; Schmidt and Hunter; Guenther; Marcus; and Hofman comment on some of Krueger's positions, and Krueger replies.

Still on the topic of replication, it seems important to correct a frequent misconception of the concept in the context of power analysis. It is often thought that if one obtains a result that is statistically significant at a particular level (e.g., a probability level of 0.05), at a given sample size (e.g., $n = 50$), then this result can be expected to replicate at the same level of p, using the same sample size. Abelson (1995) refers to this as the "replication fallacy." In his words:

> "*Imagine an experimenter who has run a two-group study, and has found by t test the result* p = .05. *What is the chance that if she exactly repeated the study with a new sample of subjects (and the same* n *per group) that she would again get a significant result at the .05 level?*" (p. 75).

Abelson (1995) provides the following counter-intuitive solution to the problem: Half the time, the observed effect size from the second study ought to be bigger than that of the first study, and half the time, smaller. Because the first observed effect size was just big enough to obtain a p value of 0.05, anything smaller would yield a nonsignificant $p > 0.05$. This analysis thus yields an expected repeatability of 50–50, much lower than the usual intuition (p. 75).

A logical question that arises is what minimal level of p is required to insure replicability at $p = 0.05$? The work of Greenwald, Gonzalez, Harris, and Guthrie (1993) shows that a p of 0.005 will replicate at $p < 0.05$ approximately 80% of the time.

6. Cortina and Dunlap (1997) argue that confidence intervals cannot nor should not replace tests of statistical significance, "... but that instead they should be done in conjunction with significance tests" (p. 169).

Before completing this section on power analysis, it should be mentioned that an update of an earlier power and precision computer program by Borenstein, Rothstein, and Cohen (1997) is now available. The updated program, due to Borenstein, Rothstein, and Cohen (2001) is very user-friendly and will enable the researcher to compute power and precision estimates for means, proportions, correlations, ANOVA/ANCOVA, multiple regression, and has the added features (not appearing in the 1997 version) of power analysis and precision options for survival analysis, logistic regression, and bio-equivalence tests. This latter feature applies whenever a research scientist has interest in whether two means or treatments are similar to each other rather than statistically and/or practically different. This would apply when two treatments appear to produce similar effects but one of them has more serious side effects than the other. If it can, indeed, be shown that this conjecture is true, then one would have empirical data for choosing the treatment that has the less serious side effects.

In the final section, we discuss the critical role of model building and model testing as demonstrated in a number of applications in clinical neuropsychology with direct implications for other areas of biobehavioral research.

N. Validity Assessment in the Context of Model Building and Model Testing

The final round of nine publications consists of a series of papers in clinical neuropsychology that appeared between 1995 and 2003 with a specific focus upon model building and model testing. These illustrate how a variety of methodological approaches can be employed to focus on a single goal—such as the validation of a particular theory regarding the neurological and neurodevelopmental basis of the syndrome of nonverbal learning disabilities: Brouwers, Van der Vlugt, Moss, Wolters, and Pizzo (1995; pp. 668–679); Buono, Morris, Morris, Krawiecki, Norris, Foster, and Copeland (1998; pp. 680–692); Don, Schellenberg, and Rourke (1999; pp. 693–707); Fisher and DeLuca (1997; pp. 708–713); Fletcher, Bohan, Brant, Beaver, Thorstad, Brookshire, Francis, Davidson, and Thompson (1993; p. 714); Hepworth and Rovet (2000; pp. 715–726); Ryan, Crews, Cowen, Goering, and Barth (1998; pp. 727–734); Swillen, Vandeputte, Cracco, Maes, Ghesquière, Devriendt, and Fryns (1999; pp. 735–745); Rapport, Millis, and Bonello (1998; pp. 746–754).

The Clinical Neuropsychologist
1992, Vol. 6, No. 4, pp. 458–463

COMPUTERIZING THE CLINICIAN

A Computer Program for Analyzing Ordinal Trends With Dichotomous Outcomes: Application to Neuropsychological Research

Domenic V. Cicchetti[1], Donald Showalter[1], Byron P. Rourke[2], and Darren Fuerst[2]

[1]West Haven VA Medical Center and Yale University and [2]University of Windsor

ABSTRACT

This computer program analyzes for trend when the classification (independent) variable is ordinal and the outcome (dependent) variable is dichotomous. The test statistic, developed earlier by Jonckheere, is expressed as a standard Z score, and under certain specific conditions, bears mathematical equivalency to the more familiar chi-square (d), Fisher's Exact Probability, and Wilcoxon Rank Sum Tests. The statistic appears to have wide applicability in both the behavioral and medical sciences. In this particular application, the authors were interested in testing whether the extent of children's neuropsychological symptomatology might be linearly related to clinically meaningful differences favoring Verbal (VIQ) over Performance (PIQ) scores.

The question of whether linear trends are apparent in any given set of data is one of considerable scientific interest. A special subset of this general phenomenon occurs when the classification, explanatory, or independent variable is measured on an ordinal scale and the outcome, response, or dependent variable is dichotomous. Some examples follow:

1. In the recent past, there has been interest in whether the proportion of children diagnosed with acute appendicitis increases linearly as the results of a Barium Enema examination vary between negative, equivocal, and positive. In fact, it has been demonstrated that this is, indeed, the case (Garcia et al., 1987).

2. It has been demonstrated that there is a statistically significant linear trend between severity of class of myocardial infarct and the proportion of patients who survive this acute incident (Horwitz, Cicchetti, & Horwitz, 1984).

3. Fuerst, Fisk, and Rourke (1990) were interested in whether the degree of children's neuropsychological symptomatology might be linearly related to a clinically meaningful difference of 10 points or more, favoring Verbal (VIQ) over Performance (PIQ) intelligence test scores.

The severity of symptomatology ("none," "mild to moderate," or "severe") was based upon a tripartite classification of the scores of 132 children on the Personality Inventory for Children (PIC;-Wirt, Lachar, Klinedinst, & Seat, 1977). The IQ data were provided by administering the Wechsler Intelligence Scale for Children (WISC; Wechsler, 1944).

Address correspondence to: Domenic V. Cicchetti, Ph.D., VA Medical Center, 950 Campbell Avenue, West Haven, CT 06516, USA.
Accepted for publication: August 13, 1992.

These results are presented in tabular form as follows:

PIC Symptom Severity:	VIQ > PIQ: Yes	No	TOTALS:	PCT. YES (5)
None/Very Mild	1(a)	17(b)	18 t_1	5.6
Mild/Moderate	21(c)	51(d)	72 t_2	29.2
Severe	22(e)	20(f)	42 t_3	52.4
Total	44 u_1	88 u_2	132 n	

These data demonstrate quite clearly that the degree of PIC symptom severity ("none/very mild" to "mild/moderate" to "severe") is directly proportional to the percentage of children showing higher levels of VIQ than PIQ, namely, 5.6, 29.2 and 52.4, respectively. The Jonckheere (1970) statistic is the test of choice to answer whether, indeed, this linear trend is statistically significant.

The Jonckheere Test (1970) is mathematically identical, in reverse application, to the familiar nonparametric Wilcoxon Rank Sum Test (also known as the Mann-Whitney Test). As we have seen, the *classification* (or independent) variable is ordinal and the *outcome* (or dependent) variable is dichotomous when the Jonckheere test of linear trend is applicable. In distinct contrast, the Wilcoxon Rank Sum Test is applicable when the classification variable is dichotomous (a comparison of two independent groups), but the response variable is ordinal (the ranks which represent the outcome scores of individual subjects – e.g., Leach, 1979, p. 179).

When both the classification and outcome variables are dichotomies, the Jonckheere Test is mathematically equivalent to the Fisher's Exact Probability Test and the even more familiar Chi-square (d) Test, providing the required correction for continuity is employed (as recommended by Fleiss, 1981), and the total sample size is large, i.e., $n \geq 40$ cases.

Jonckheere's Z Test of linear trend can be defined, in both the general and specific case as:

$$Z_{(Jonckheere)} = \frac{Sc}{S.D.} \quad (1)$$

in which:
S   (in the simplest or 2 × 2 case) can be defined as the difference in the cross-products

(ad − bc), which comprise the four cells of the table. In the case of interest here, when the classification variable is ordinal, S is a simple, straight-forward generalization in which all possible cross-products of the form (ad − bc) are summed.

c   refers to the required correction for continuity and

S.D. refers to the square root of the variance of S.

The ratio (Sc)/(S.D.) is normally distributed as a Z statistic with mean of zero and unit variance. Thus, for a 2-tailed test, a Z of ±1.96 is significant at the .05 level; for a 1-tailed test, a Z of ±1.645 is also significant at the .05 level, and would be applicable whenever a linear trend in a specified direction (positive or negative) can be predicted a priori.

In our example, the 3 × 2 contingency table is comprised of the six respective cells a, b, c, d, e, and f.

The formula for the correction for continuity is defined by Leach (1979, p. 179) as:

$$c = \frac{(2n - t_1 - t_k)}{(2(k-1))},$$

in which:
n refers to the total number of cases
t_1 refers to the **first row total**
t_k refers to the **last row total** and
k refers to the **number of ordinal categories** comprising the independent, or classification variable.

Finally, the standard deviation of S can be defined as the **square root** of its Variance (V):

$$V = \frac{u_1 u_2 \left(n^3 - \sum t_i^3 \right)}{3n (n - 1)},$$

in which:
u_1 refers to the **first column total** and
u_2 refers to the **second column total**, and the remaining terms are defined, as previously.

Applying these three formulae to our data, we obtain the following results:

$$S = (ad - bc) + (cf - de) + (af - be),$$

which simplifies to:

$$S = (a (d + f) + cf) - (b (c + e) + de)$$

For our example:

$$
\begin{aligned}
S &= (1 (51 + 20) + 21 (20)) - (17 (21 + 22) \\
&\quad + 51 (22)) \\
&= (491 - 1853) \\
&= -1362 \\
c &= \frac{(2n - t_1 - t_k)}{(2(k-1))} \\
&= (2 (132) - 18 - 42) / (4) \\
&= 51
\end{aligned}
$$

Therefore,

$$S_c = (-1362 + 51) = -1311$$

$$
\text{Variance (V)} = \frac{u_1 u_2 \left(n^3 - \sum t_i^3\right)}{3n (n - 1)}
$$

$$
= \frac{(44) (88) (132^3 - (18^3 + 72^3 + 42^3))}{3 (132)(131)}
$$

$$= 137,844.2748$$

Therefore,

$$\text{S.D.} = \sqrt{137,844.2748} = 371.2739$$

Finally,

$$Z_{(Jonckheere)} = \frac{Sc}{\text{S.D.}} = \frac{-1311}{371.2739} = -3.53$$

Referring to a table of standard normal distribution, this value is statistically significant at beyond the .001 level whether one considers a two- ($p = .0004$) or one-tailed ($p = .0002$) test. Thus, the results of the Jonckheere Test inform one that there is evidence for a significant linear trend between level of neuropsychological symptomatology and increasing elevations in VIQ over PIQ.

As an important caveat, it needs to be stressed that the Jonckheere statistic answers only whether a linear trend occurs beyond chance expectation (usually taken to mean the .05 level or beyond). It does **not** inform as to the **strength** (based on size of correlation) of the linear trend.

The statistic of choice for determining the level of **correlation** when one variable is ordinal and the other is dichotomous is Kendall's (1962) Tau_c statistic, which is applicable when the numbers of rows and columns are dissimilar or unequal.

Application of the Kendall (1962) Tau_c statistic to our data produces an r value of .31 which, by Cohen's (1988) cut-off points, would define an "effect size" (ES) or strength of association of "medium." Thus, while there is evidence of a significant linear trend between level of PIC symptom severity and increasing proportions of VIQ-PIQ differences, the size of the correlation informs the clinical investigator that it would be unwise to predict VIQ-PIQ differences solely on the basis of severity of PIC scores. The guidelines provided by Cohen (below .10 = "trivial"; .10 = "small"; .30 = "medium"; and .50 = "large" effect size) are useful, both to keep the results of a given test of linear tend in proper perspective, and to prevent the confusion of statistical significance with clinical relevance.

PROGRAM FEATURES

It should be stressed that, with large sample sizes and large 2 × k contingency tables, the calculation of the Jonckheere Z statistic, because of the need to obtain cubed numbers, becomes prohibitive without the aid of a computer program, such as the one herein described.

Input to this computer program, (names of independent and dependent variables, numbers in each cell of a given k × 2 contingency table) is provided by the user. The program currently functions in the hard drive of any IBM PC computer and its compatibles, using C language. However, it is easily adaptable to other PCs, other computer languages, and also to applications using floppy discs. The program has been designed to accommodate up to 25 ordinal variables and an unlimited number of cases.

Output includes: the labeled 2 × k contingency table, showing the percentage of subjects scoring positively on the dichotomous outcome variable (e.g., percentage Yes responses) for each of the k ordinal categories; the Z value of the

Jonckheere test; and the exact corresponding p value for a two-tailed test of significance. For a one-tailed test, one simply halves this p value.

AVAILABILITY

A listing of the C source code, complete documentation, a set of sample problems and a program listing are available from Dr. Domenic V. Cicchetti, Senior Research Psychologist and Biostatistician, VA Medical Center and Yale University, 950 Campbell Avenue, West Haven CT 06516, USA.

REFERENCES

Cohen, J. (1988). *Power analysis for the behavioral sciences*. (2nd ed.). Englewood Cliffs NJ: Erlbaum Associates.

Fleiss, J.L. (1981). *Statistics for rates and proportions* (2nd ed.). New York: Wiley.

Fuerst, D.R., Fisk, J.L., & Rourke, B.P. (1990). Psychosocial functioning of learning-disabled children: Relations between WISC verbal IQ-performance IQ discrepancies and personality types. *Journal of Consulting and Clinical Psychology*, 58, 657–660.

Garcia, C., Rosenfield, N.S., Markowitz, R.I., Seashore, J.H., Touloukian, R.J., & Cicchetti, D.V. (1987). Appendicitis in children: Accuracy of the barium enema. *American Journal of Diseases of Children*, *141*, 1309–1312.

Horwitz, R.I., Cicchetti, D.V., & Horwitz, S.M. (1984). A comparison of the Norris and Killip Coronary Prognostic Indices. *Journal of Chronic Diseases*, *37*, 369–375.

Jonckheere, A.R. (1970). Techniques for ordered contingency tables. In J.B. Riemersma & H.C. van der Meer (Eds.), *Proceedings of the NUFFIC International Summer Session in Science "Het Oude Hof"*, The Hague.

Kendall, M.G. (1962). *Rank correlation methods.* (3rd ed.) New York: Hafner.

Leach, C. (1979). *Introduction to statistics: A nonparametric approach for the social sciences*. New York: Wiley.

Wechsler, D. (1949). *Manual for the Wechsler Intelligence Scale for Children*. New York: Psychological Corporation.

Wirt, R.D., Lachar, D., Klinedinst, J.K., & Seat, P.D. (1977). *Multidimensional description of child personality: A manual for the Personality Inventory for Children*. Los Angeles: Western Psychological Services.

Journal of Clinical and Experimental Neuropsychology
1992, Vol. 14, No. 4, pp. 539–544

Continuous Recognition Memory Tests: Are the Assumptions of the Theory of Signal Detection Met?*

Angela I. Drake[1] and H. Julia Hannay[2]

[1]San Diego Veterans Affairs Medical Center and [2]University of Houston

ABSTRACT

Two continuous recognition memory tests were administered to 20 males and 20 females using the confidence rating procedure to determine if the underlying assumptions of the theory of signal detection (TSD) are met by these tasks. Z-score transformed ROC curves proved to be straight lines parallel to the positive diagonal of the ROC graph. These findings suggest that the distributions of familiarity for old and new stimuli are normal and of equal variance for the Continuous Recognition Memory and Continuous Visual Memory Tests. TSD interpretation of test data appears to be justified.

Continuous recognition memory tests have proved to be useful in research on patients with closed-head injury (Brooks, 1972; 1974a,b; Hannay & Levin, 1989; Hannay, Levin, & Grossman, 1979), dementia (Cutting, 1978; Miller & Lewis, 1977), alcoholic Korsakoff's disease (Cutting, 1978; Riege, 1977), aphasia (Riege, Klane, Metter, & Hanson, 1982), and unilateral temporal-lobe lesions (Cutting, 1978; De Renzi, 1968; Kimura, 1963; Trahan & Larrabee, 1985). These tests are useful because they examine recognition memory while making minimal demands on verbal or visuomotor skills. Essentially, recognition memory is assessed by presenting a series of stimuli in which some of the stimuli reappear several times in the series. The rest of the stimuli, though in some cases perceptually similar to the recurrent items, appear only once. The subject simply states whether each stimulus is "new", that is, it is appearing for the first time in the series, or "old", that is, it is reappearing. Thus, there are four stimulus/response categories analogous to those in a signal detection experiment. The new stimuli constitute noise and

the old stimuli constitute signal which the subject is trying to detect. Calling an old stimulus "old" is a hit; calling an old stimulus "new" is a miss. Referring to a new stimulus as "old" is a false alarm; referring to a new stimulus as "new" is a correct rejection. Signal detection theory parameters d', c, and B can be calculated, as well as the more traditional measure of number of correct responses.

Although there are a number of recognition memory tests commercially available, only two such tasks provide normative data for calculating signal detection theory parameters in their manuals (Hannay & Levin, 1988; Trahan & Larrabee, 1988). The Continuous Recognition Memory Test (Hannay et al., 1979; Hannay & Levin, 1988) consists of 120 line drawings of living things and was designed as a nonlateralizing test of memory sensitive to the effects of head injury. The Continuous Visual Memory Test (Trahan & Larrabee, 1988) consists of 116 drawings of polygons, nonsense figures, complex line drawings, checkerboards and stick figures and was developed as a measure of nonverbal memory.

---

* This research was conducted as part of the doctoral dissertation of the first author at Auburn University. Reprint requests should be sent to A.I. Drake, Ph.D., Department of Psychology-116B, VAMC, 3500 La Jolla Village Dr, San Diego, CA 92122, USA.
Accepted for publication: October 30, 1991.

These continuous recognition memory tasks purport to meet the assumptions of TSD, and a number of articles have been published which report memory performance in terms of signal detection theory parameters (Hannay & Levin, 1988; Hannay et al., 1979; Trahan & Larrabee, 1985; Trahan, Larrabee, & Levin, 1986). However, no research has been conducted to determine whether these two tests actually meet the underlying assumptions of TSD and, thus, to justify such interpretations. First, in a detection task a subject is assumed to be continually receiving sensory input, some of which comes from a signal, in this case, the old drawings. The rest of the sensory input comes from noise, in this case the new stimuli, other environmental stimuli, and the nervous system itself. This assumption appears to be met by these memory tasks. Secondly, the amount of sensory input from noise is assumed to vary randomly over time and as such, the distribution of sensory input produced by noise is normal in shape. This assumption may or may not be met. Thirdly, when a signal does occur in a TSD experiment, it is of a fixed magnitude. Thus, the signal adds a fixed amount of sensory input to the level of noise present on that trial. Therefore, the distribution of sensory input for signal plus noise trials is also normal in shape. It is not clear that this assumption is met in continuous recognition memory tests since there are several signals of possibly different but fixed magnitudes. Finally, it is assumed that sensory input from signal plus noise is sometimes indistinguishable from noise because the distributions for the two variables overlap. In other words, the amount of sensory input produced on signal plus noise trials, must sometimes be the same as that produced on noise only trials. Since the stimulus situation is then ambiguous for the subject, it is assumed that the subject must adopt a level of sensory input as a response criterion. If the sensory input on any trial is above this criterion, the subject says that a signal was present. If the level of sensory input on a trial is below this criterion, the subject says that noise was present. The subjects will thus make errors, false alarms and misses. In continuous recognition memory tasks this assumption appears to be met, since several noise stimuli are created that are perceptually similar to each of the signals.

In trying to remember what has been presented, the subject sometimes calls a new stimulus "old" and an old stimulus "new", making both false alarms and misses respectively.

The present study was designed to determine whether these two continuous recognition memory tests meet the assumptions of TSD, despite variations from a traditional yes-no task just outlined. The outcome of a TSD experiment is completely specified by the rate of hits and the rate of false alarms (Hannay, 1986). The outcome can be conveniently plotted in terms of the probabilities of hits and false alarms on a two-dimensional graph known as the ROC or receiver operating characteristic graph. To obtain the graph, a series of experiments is conducted in which the signal remains constant in value throughout, but the subject is induced to change his/her response criterion across experiments. Each curve represents the way in which the subject responds under the same stimulus conditions but with different response criteria (Green & Swets, 1966; Hannay, 1986; McNicol, 1972). The ROC curves can be used to determine whether the underlying assumptions of TSD are met. When performance is plotted in terms of probabilities of hits P(S/s) and false alarms P(S/n), a symmetric bow-shaped curve results when the underlying distributions are normal and have equal variance. If performance is then plotted in terms of Z[P(S/s)] and Z[P(S/n)], straight lines will result. These lines are parallel to the positive diagonal if the distributions have equal variance (McNicol, 1972).

Continuous recognition memory tests, when administered in their usual detection format, can generate only one point on an ROC curve. Administering them several times with instructions designed to change the subject's response criterion would not only take a lot of time, but would also likely change sensitivity (d') as well, because subjects would remember particular signal and noise stimuli from one administration to another. Fortunately, it is possible to generate an ROC curve from a single set of trials by using a confidence rating procedure (Green & Swets, 1966; Hannay, 1986; McNicol, 1972). Essentially, the subject is given a scale on which to rate his/her confidence that a signal or noise is present on each trial. The scale must consist of at least four categories from which the minimal three points are generated for fitting a straight line. In the current experiment the categories included definitely old, probably old, probably new, and definitely new. Each of these categories represents a particular response criterion, and the number of hits and false alarms can be determined for responses falling in each of these categories. From these data is possible to determine whether performance on a continuous recognition memory test meets the underlying assumptions of TSD as just outlined.

METHOD

Subjects

Twenty females between the ages of 18–27 years ($M = 20.9$, $SD = 2.3$) and 20 males aged 18–30 years ($M = 20.1$, $SD = 2.6$) who were enrolled in introductory psychology classes at Auburn University received extra credit for their participation. Subjects denied a history of previous head injury, neurological or psychiatric disorder, alcohol or drug abuse.

Stimuli

The Continuous Recognition Memory Test (CRM; Hannay et al., 1979; Hannay & Levin, 1988) and the Continuous Visual Memory Test (CVM) (Trahan & Larrabee, 1988) were employed.

Procedure

In the present study the CRM and CVM tests were administered individually to each subject according to the instructions in their respective manuals. However, on each trial the subject not only stated whether a stimulus was "old" or "new" but how confident he/she was in each decision by pointing to one of the aforementioned categories on a rating scale placed directly below the stimuli and in front of the subject.

The order of test administration was counterbalanced to determine whether taking one test first resulted in a change in the willingness to use the various confidence rating categories on the other task. Half of the males and half of the females were given either the CRM or the CVM test first.

RESULTS

Initial analyses were completed on the rating scale data from each task to determine if the frequency with which rating scale categories were used by subjects varied with the order in which the tests were given and whether gender affected the use of the rating scale categories. Three-factor mixed analyses of variance of the frequencies with which each category was used were completed on the CRM and CVM test rating scale data. Order of test administration and gender were the between-subjects factors and rating scale category was the within-subjects factor. Neither the main effect of Order [$F_{(1,154)} = 0$, $p = .98$], the Order × Category interaction [$F_{(3,154)} = .79$, $p = .49$], nor the Order × Category × Gender [$F_{(3,144)} = .36$, $p = .78$], were significant for the analysis of data from the CRM test. Neither the main effect of Order [$F_{(1,154)} = .50$, $p = .82$], the Order × Category interaction [$F_{(3,154)} = 1.6$, $p = .19$], nor the Order × Category × Gender interaction [$F_{(3,144)} = .23$, $p = .88$], were significant for the analysis of data from the CVM test. Since order of test administration did not affect the use of the rating scale categories, the data for the two orders were thus combined for each of the tests for further analyses. Neither the main effect of Gender [$F_{(1,144)} = .00$, $p = $], nor the Gender × Category interaction, [$F_{(3,144)} = .63$, $p = .60$], were significant for the CRM data. Neither the main effect of Gender [$F_{(1,144)} = .00$, $p = .95$], nor the Gender × Category interaction [$F_{(3,144)} = 1.98$, $p = .12$], were significant for the CVM test data. Thus the data for males and females was also combined for subsequent analyses.

The confidence rating procedure outlined by McNicol (1972) was used to generate the points on an ROC curve for each test. The actual number of points obtained equals the number of categories minus one, which, in this case, was three. Hits and false alarms for each rating scale category for both tests were then converted to P(S/s) and P(S/n) respectively for each subject. These values were then converted to Z[P(S/s)] and Z[P(S/n)] respectively, and averaged across subjects to produce the data plotted in Figures 1a and 1b. The method of least squares was used to determine the best fit straight line to these data (Figures 1a & 1b).

The slope of the best fit line was 1.23 for the CRM test and .98 for the CVM test when predicting Y from X. These slopes are not significantly

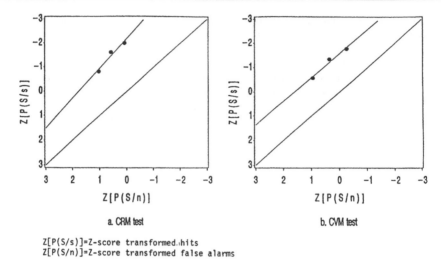

Z[P(S/s)]=Z-score transformed hits
Z[P(S/n)]=Z-score transformed false alarms

Fig. 1. Z-Score transformed ROC curves for data from a. CRM test and b. CVM test.

different from the slope of 1.0 for the positive diagonal as determined by a one sample t test for either the CRM ($t = .348$) or the CVM ($t = .026$) tests.

DISCUSSION

In detection experiments which use a TSD paradigm and parameters, a measure of sensitivity is obtained which is theoretically independent of the subject's response criterion. When applied to recognition memory the measure of sensitivity is referred to as memory efficiency. A separate measure of response criterion is also calculated. Such TSD analyses can be very useful in understanding memory deficits displayed by patients. For instance, two patients might demonstrate a similar number of correct responses, but for different reasons, i.e., differences in memory efficiency, willingness to make a particular response or both. The current research supports the use of TSD analyses and TSD interpretation of continuous recognition memory data, at least for the CRM and CVM tests, by demonstrating that the underlying assumptions of a yes-no task in which the distributions of noise and signal plus noise are normal and have equal variance are not violated.

REFERENCES

Brooks, D.N. (1972). Memory and head injury. *Journal of Nervous and Mental Disease, 155*, 350–355.

Brooks, D.N. (1974a). Recognition memory after head injury: A signal detection analysis. *Cortex, 10,* 224–230.

Brooks, D.N. (1974b). Recognition memory and head injury. *Journal of Neurology, Neurosurgery, and Psychiatry, 37,* 794–801.

Cutting, J. (1978). Patterns of performance in amnesic subjects. *Journal of Neurology, Neurosurgery and Psychiatry, 41,* 278–282.

De Renzi, E. (1968). Nonverbal memory and hemispheric side of lesion. *Neuropsychologia, 6,* 181–189.

Green, D.M., & Swets, J.A. (1966). *Signal detection theory and psychophysics.* New York: Wiley.

Hannay, H.J. (1986). Psychophysical measurement techniques and their application to neuropsychology. In H.J. Hannay (Ed.), *Experimental techniques in human neuropsychology,* (pp. 45–94). New York: Oxford University Press.

Hannay, H.J., & Levin, H.S. (1988). *The Continuous Recognition Memory Test. A manual.* Houston: Neuropsychological Resources.

Hannay, H.J., & Levin, H.S. (1989). Visual continuous recognition memory in normal and closed head-injured adolescents. *Journal of Clinical and Experimental Neuropsychology, 11,* 444–460.

Hannay, H.J., Levin, H.S., & Grossman, R.C. (1979). Impaired recognition memory after head injury. *Cortex, 15,* 269–283.

Kimura, D. (1963). Right temporal lobe damage. *Archives of Neurology, 8,* 264–271.

McNicol, D. (1972). *A primer of signal detection theory.* London: George Allen & Unwin.

Miller, E., & Lewis, P. (1977). Recognition memory in elderly patients with depression and dementia: A signal detection analysis. *Journal of Abnormal Psychology, 86,* 84–86.

Riege, W.H. (1977). Inconstant non-verbal recognition in Korsakoff patients and controls. *Neuropsychologia, 15,* 269–276.

Riege, W.H., Klane, L.T., Metter, E.J., & Hanson, W.R. (1982). Decision speed and bias after unilateral stroke. *Cortex, 18,* 345–355.

Trahan, D.E., & Larrabee, G.J. (1985). An examination of visual recognition memory in patients with unilateral vascular lesions. Paper presented at the 13th Annual Meeting of the International Neuropsychological Society, San Diego, CA.

Trahan, D.E., & Larrabee, G.J. (1988). *Continuous Visual Memory Test.* Odessa, FL: Psychological Assessment Resources.

Trahan, D.E., Larrabee, G.J., & Levin, H.S. (1986). Age-related differences in recognition memory for pictures. *Experimental Aging Research, 12,* 147–150.

Journal of Clinical and Experimental Neuropsychology
1998, Vol. 20, No. 5, pp. 755–762

Regression Equations in Clinical Neuropsychology: An Evaluation of Statistical Methods for Comparing Predicted and Obtained Scores*

J.R. Crawford[1] and David C. Howell[2]

[1]University of Aberdeen, UK and [2]University of Vermont, Burlington

ABSTRACT

Regression equations are widely used in clinical neuropsychology, particularly as an alternative to conventional normative data. In neuropsychological applications the most common method of making inferences concerning the difference between an individual's test score and the score predicted by a regression equation is to multiply the standard error of estimate by an appropriate value of z to form confidence limits around the predicted score. The technically correct method is to calculate the standard error of a new individual Y and multiply it by the value of t corresponding to the desired limits (e.g., 90% or 95%). These two methods are compared in data sets generated to be broadly representative of data sets used in clinical neuropsychology.

The former method produces confidence limits which are narrower than the true confidence limits and fail to reflect the fact that limits become wider as scores on the predictor deviate from the mean. However, for many of the example data sets studied, the differences between the two methods were trivial, thereby providing reassurance for those who use the former (technically incorrect) method. Despite this, it would be preferable to use the correct method particularly with equations derived from samples with modest Ns, and for individuals with extreme scores on the predictor variable(s). To facilitate use of the correct method a computer program is made available for clinical practice.

Regression equations can serve a number of useful functions in clinical neuropsychology. Perhaps their most common role is as an alternative to the use of conventional normative data. For example, if it is found that age, years of education, and gender are related to performance on a memory test then a regression equation can be built (in a healthy sample) which uses these demographic variables as predictors. Thus, an individual's predicted score reflects his/her particular combination of demographic characteristics. Such an approach is in keeping with the emphasis placed on individual versus normative comparison standards in neuropsychological assessment (Crawford, 1996; Heaton, Grant, Ryan, & Matthews, 1996; Lezak, 1995).

Even with a single predictor, such as age, the regression approach is to be preferred over conventional normative data. It provides what Zachary and Gorsuch (1985) have termed "continuous norms" rather than the discrete norms formed by creating arbitrary age bands; in the latter case, the relative standing of an individual can change dramatically as they move from one band to another.

A second common application of regression is in the assessment of change in neuropsychological functioning in the individual case. Here, a regression equation can be built (normally using healthy participants) to predict an individual's level of performance on a neuropsychological instrument at retest from their score at initial testing.

* Address correspondence to: John R. Crawford, Department of Psychology, King's College, University of Aberdeen, Aberdeen AB24 3HN, UK. E-mail: crawford@abdn.ac.uk.
Accepted for publication: July 27, 1998.

This approach simultaneously factors in the effects of practice (typically scores will be higher on retest) and regression to the mean (extreme scores on initial testing will, on average, be less extreme at retest).

In both of the foregoing examples, regression equations are used to generate a *predicted* or *expected* level of performance for an individual patient against which her/his *obtained* level of performance can be compared. A large discrepancy from the predicted score raises the suspicion of acquired cognitive deficit. The remainder of this paper is concerned with the statistical methods used to make inferences about the difference between an individual's predicted and obtained score. Before outlining the technically correct procedure, two methods commonly used in clinical neuropsychology will be described.

Using the Standard Error of Estimate ($S_{y.x}$) to Obtain a Confidence Interval

The standard error of estimate is a measure of the variability of observations about the regression line. As such, it reflects the precision of our estimation procedure. We can define the standard error of estimate ($S_{y.x}$) as

$$S_{y.x} = SD_y \sqrt{(1 - r^2) \frac{N - 1}{N - 2}}, \qquad (1)$$

where SD_y = the standard deviation of the criterion variable, r^2 = the squared correlation between the predictor and criterion variables and $S_{y.x}$ = the sample size. A more familiar (approximate) formula for $S_{y.x}$ is given as

$$S_{y.x} = SD_y \sqrt{1 - r^2}, \qquad (2)$$

and is a simplification of [1]. This formula yields a close approximation when the sample size is large, because $(N - 1)/(N - 2)$ rapidly approaches one as sample size increases.

Both formulae for the standard error of estimate make it clear that the precision of our estimate when we take other variables into account ($S_{y.x}$) is greater than the precision when we look only at raw scores on the criterion variable, which is

given by SD_y. This difference increases as the correlation between the measure of interest and the predictor variable(s) increases. Without considering predictor variables, for large samples we would expect 90% of the sample to lie within 1.64 standard deviations of the mean of Y. Similarly, if we use X to predict Y, and if the assumptions underlying the use of regression are met, then one would expect that 90% of the sample in which a regression equation was built would lie within 1.64 $S_{y.x}$ units of the regression line.

It is important to note that this statement is cast in terms of the sample used to build the equation. However, researchers often present confidence limits based on $S_{y.x}$ as a means by which the clinician can evaluate the scores of individuals who were not in the original sample (Crawford, Moore, & Cameron, 1992; Knight & Shelton, 1983; McSweeny, Naugle, Chelune, & Lüders, 1993; Paolo, Ryan, Tröster, & Hilmer, 1996).

For example, McSweeny et al. (1993) built a regression equation in a sample of 50 patients with epilepsy to predict scores on the Wechsler Memory Scale – Revised (WMS-R, Wechsler, 1987) and Wechsler Adult Intelligence Scale – Revised (WAIS-R, Wechsler, 1981) from scores at initial testing. They created a 90% "confidence interval" by multiplying $S_{y.x}$ by 1.64 and recommended that the difference between an individual's predicted and obtained score should be considered "significant" if it exceeded this interval (some authors would prefer the phrase "prediction interval," or "tolerance interval" because the term "confidence interval" is generally reserved for intervals on parameters. However, in common with McSweeny et al., the present authors have chosen to use the term "confidence interval" because it is more commonly referenced in that way). Similarly, Knight and Shelton (1983) used data from previously published reports of repeat testing with the Wechsler Adult Intelligence Scale (WAIS, Wechsler, 1955) to generate regression equations. They multiplied $S_{y.x}$ by 1.64 and 1.96 to obtain what were referred to as the critical values required to achieve "statistical significance" at the .05 and .01 levels (one-tailed) when comparing an individual's predicted retest score with her/his obtained retest score.

Tabulating Frequency Distribution of Discrepancies Between Predicted and Observed Scores

Another way of examining extreme deviations from predicted performance is to examine the frequency distribution of discrepancies between observed and predicted scores, tabulated for the sample used to build the equation. By referring to this table the clinician can observe the size of discrepancy required to exceed a given percentage of the sample. Provided that the assumptions underlying the use of regression are met, and the original sample is sufficiently large, this approach will yield 'critical values' that closely resemble those produced by the foregoing method; in the former case, the rarity of a discrepancy is estimated statistically, in the present case, it is empirically derived.

This technique has been commonly used with methods designed to estimate premorbid intelligence; for reviews see Crawford and O'Carroll. For example, Nelson (1982) built a regression equation using the National Adult Reading Test (NART, Nelson, 1982) to estimate premorbid WAIS IQs. The NART manual presents a table which records the frequency distribution in the standardization sample of discrepancies between obtained WAIS scores and scores predicted from the NART. The same approach was used when the NART was standardised against the WAIS-R (Nelson & Willison, 1991) and has also been used with approaches to the estimation of premorbid ability that are based on demographic variables (see Crawford & Allan, 1997).

Using Standard Error of a New Individual $\hat{Y}$ to Form Confidence Intervals

The foregoing methods take account of error in predicting an individual's score from the regression of the dependent variable on the independent variable(s), and are, therefore, a reasonable way of drawing inferences concerning the score of an individual drawn from the sample used to generate the equation. However, they ignore the error arising from using sample regression coefficients to estimate population regression coefficients. This has two consequences; first, the confidence limits will be too narrow and second, the true confidence limits will be wider as the score on the predictor deviates from the predictor mean. For an intuitive understanding of this latter effect, consider what would happen to the predictions for different values of X if we rotated the regression line slightly around the mean of X. A further issue is that, in the earlier examples of the use of the $S_{y.x}$ method, $S_{y.x}$ was multiplied by a value of z rather than t (with df of $N - 2$). The t statistic should be used because the estimates are based on sample statistics rather than parameters. Although this will have a negligible effect with large samples, it constitutes another factor which will produce an underestimation of the true confidence limits.

The correct method of drawing inferences concerning an individuals' predicted score is to use the standard error of a new individual $\hat{Y}$ ($SE_{yo-\hat{Y}o}$) to form confidence limits on Y (Howell, 1997). When there is a single predictor, a formula for the $SE_{yo-\hat{Y}o}$ is as follows:

$$SE_{yo-\hat{Y}o} = S_{y.x}\sqrt{1 + \frac{1}{N} + \frac{(X_o - \overline{X})^2}{SD_x^2(N-1)}}, \quad (3)$$

where $S_{y.x}$ is as defined previously, $\overline{X}$ = the mean score on the predictor variable, X_o = the individual's score on the predictor, and SD_x = the standard deviation of the predictor variable (there are a number of equivalent formula for $SE_{yo-\hat{Y}o}$, the present one is used because it is the simplest). Having calculated the $SE_{yo-\hat{Y}o}$, confidence limits on Y can be obtained from the following formula:

$$CI(Y) = \hat{Y} \pm (t_{\alpha/2})(SE_{yo-\hat{Y}o}), \quad (4)$$

where $t_{\alpha/2}$ = the value of t (with $df = N - 2$) corresponding to the required confidence limits. Thus, as a simple example, if $N = 52$, $SE_{yo-\hat{Y}o} = 10$, and 90% (two-sided) confidence limits were required, 10 would be multiplied by 1.676. If an individual's predicted score ($\hat{Y}$) was 50 then the 90% upper confidence limit for Y would be 66.76 and the lower limit would be 33.24.

To our knowledge no study in clinical neuropsychology has adopted this latter approach. In contrast, statistical, psychometric, and biometric texts advocate it consistently (Armitage & Berry, 1994; Cohen & Cohen, 1983; Daly, Hand, Jones, Lunn, & McConway, 1995; Daniel, 1983; Draper & Smith, 1981; Gardner & Altman, 1989; Howell,

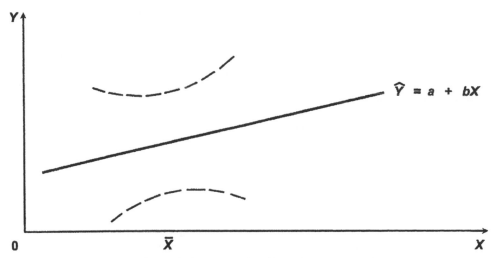

Fig. 1. A generic illustration of the elliptical nature of confidence intervals for an individual's score based on an illustration by Wittink (1988).

1997; Pedhazur, 1982; Sokal & Rohlf, 1981; Wittink, 1988; Zar, 1984, 1996). Moreover, some of these texts explicitly warn against using confidence intervals based on $S_{y.x}$. Zar (1984), for example, urges researchers to avoid the practice of following a regression equation with "$\pm S_{y.x}$", in order to, "keep the reader from inferring that this is an equation for determining a confidence interval for $\hat{Y}$" (p. 271).

The present authors do not dispute that the above procedure is the correct one and that the two commonly employed methods are technically incorrect. However, it is legitimate to explore the extent to which the choice of method makes a difference in *practical terms*. Many of the graphical representations used to depict the elliptical nature of confidence intervals suggest that the methods will yield very divergent results. For example, Figure 1 is adapted from Wittink (1988) and implies a dramatic difference in the magnitude of the confidence interval as scores on the predictor variable diverge from their mean. However, there may be an element of exaggeration for effect in such representations.

Comparison of Confidence Intervals Based on $S_{y.x}$ and $SE_{yo-\hat{y}o}$

In this section the methods are compared in hypothetical data sets designed to be reasonably typical

of those found in clinical neuropsychology in terms of sample size, the precision of measurement of the criterion variable, and the explanatory power of the predictor variable(s). For simplicity, the illustrative data sets are all limited to the case of one predictor variable and scores on the criterion and predictor variables are expressed as T scores. T scores were selected because they are familiar to clinicians and are often used when test scores are converted to a common metric (Crawford, 1996; Lezak, 1995). Additionally, most scales used in clinical neuropsychology express scores as integers with only two or three significant digits, for example, percentiles, Wechsler subtest scaled scores, IQs, and Memory Quotients (MQs). Therefore, there is no loss in generality from using T scores for these calculations.

The sample sizes of the data sets vary from 25 to 500. An N of 25 may seem modest but samples of this size, and smaller, have been used to generate equations for clinical use (Knight & Shelton, 1983). It can be seen from formula (1) that $S_{y.x}$ shrinks as sample size increases. Therefore, sample size will exert an effect on both methods as both incorporate $S_{y.x}$ in their computations. However, sample size will exert an additional, unique, effect on $SE_{yo-\hat{y}o}$ because the error in estimating the population regression coefficient will shrink as sample size increases.

For each of the selected sample sizes, the results from both methods are compared for two values of the correlation (r_{xy}) between predictor and criterion (0.50 and 0.75). Because the predictor and criterion variables have the same mean and SD in these examples, the regression coefficient (b) takes the same value as the corresponding r_{xy}. These values of r_{xy} are not atypical in neuropsychological applications. Although regression equations based on data with an r (or multiple R) below 0.5 would still have advantages over conventional normative data, such equations are rarely published or used. Correlations above .75 are less rare, particularly when scores on initial testing are used to predict scores at retest. However, preparatory work for this paper revealed that the results for higher rs (e.g., $r = .85$) were similar to those for $r = .75$. Therefore, in the interests of brevity such data are not presented.

Table 1 records 90% (two-sided) confidence intervals generated by applying the common and correct methods. The third column of Table 1 records $S_{y.x}$; multiplying $S_{y.x}$ by 1.64 produced the width of the confidence intervals in column four. The remaining columns record the widths of the confidence intervals generated from $SE_{yo-\hat{y}o}$ and critical values from the t distribution. As noted, these confidence intervals become wider as scores on the predictor variable(s) diverge from the mean of the predictor variable. Confidence interval widths are presented for scores which are 0, 0.5, 1, 1.5, 2, 3, and 4 SD units from the mean; as scores on the predictor variables are expressed as T scores, these correspond to T scores of 50, 55, 60, 65, 70, 80, and 90. (We have chosen to present scores which are above the mean, however the confidence interval widths would be identical for scores which were the equivalent number of SD units below the mean). The predicted scores from the regression equations when $b = 0.5$ and $b = 0.75$ are presented above their corresponding confidence intervals; these predicted scores are rounded to the nearest T score. To illustrate this table, take the specific example of a regression equation based on a sample with an N of 50 and an r and b of 0.5. If an individual's score on the predictor variable was 65 then it can be seen that the predicted score ($\hat{Y}$) would be 58. The 90% confidence limits based on $SE_{yo-\hat{y}o}$ in this example is 58 + 15.15 (15 when rounded to the nearest

Table 1. Comparison of 90% (Two-Sided) Confidence Intervals.[a]

b/r	N	$S_{y.x}$	$S_{y.x}$ 90%CI	90% Confidence Interval for $\hat{Y}$ based on $SE_{yo-\hat{y}o}$						
				X = 50	X = 55	X = 60	X = 65	X = 70	X = 80	X = 90
b = 0.50				$\hat{Y} = 50$	$\hat{Y} = 53$	$\hat{Y} = 55$	$\hat{Y} = 58$	$\hat{Y} = 60$	$\hat{Y} = 65$	$\hat{Y} = 70$
	25	8.85	14.51	15.46	15.54	15.77	16.15	16.66	18.04	19.81
	50	8.75	14.35	14.82	14.86	14.97	15.15	15.40	16.10	17.03
	100	8.70	14.28	14.53	14.54	14.60	14.69	14.81	15.17	15.65
	200	8.68	14.24	14.38	14.39	14.42	14.46	14.53	14.70	14.95
	500	8.67	14.22	14.30	14.30	14.31	14.33	14.36	14.43	14.53
b = 0.75				$\hat{Y} = 50$	$\hat{Y} = 54$	$\hat{Y} = 58$	$\hat{Y} = 61$	$\hat{Y} = 65$	$\hat{Y} = 73$	$\hat{Y} = 80$
	25	6.76	11.08	11.81	11.87	12.04	12.33	12.72	13.78	15.13
	50	6.68	10.96	11.32	11.35	11.43	11.57	11.77	12.30	13.00
	100	6.65	10.90	11.09	11.11	11.15	11.22	11.31	11.58	11.95
	200	6.63	10.88	10.99	10.99	11.01	11.05	11.10	11.23	11.42
	500	6.62	10.86	10.92	10.93	10.95	10.97	10.99	11.02	11.10

Note. [a]The confidence intervals were obtained from $S_{y.x}$ and from $SE_{yo-\hat{y}o}$ for varying sample sizes and two values of r/b (the examples are based on predictor and criterion variables that are expressed as T scores). Confidence intervals based on $S_{y.x}$ do not vary as a function of scores on the predictor and are presented in column four. Confidence intervals based on the use of $SE_{yo-\hat{y}o}$ are presented in the subsequent columns for each of seven values of the predictor (X), ranging from a predictor score that is at the mean (X = 50), to a score that is very extreme (X = 90). The *predicted* scores ($\hat{Y}$) are presented above each of the two sets of confidence intervals; the two sets of confidence intervals and predicted scores differ as a function of the correlation (r)/regression coefficient (b).

T score). Thus, if the discrepancy between an individual's obtained score on the criterion variable and the predicted score exceeded 15, it would exceed the 90% confidence limits, that is, the probability is less than 10% that this size of discrepancy would arise by chance. Alternatively, if the $S_{y.x}$ were used to construct the confidence limits, then the discrepancy would have to exceed 14.35 (14 when rounded to the nearest *T* score).

Table 1 demonstrates that the confidence limits based on $S_{y.x}$ underestimate those generated by the correct method for *all* values of the predictor variable. It can also be seen that the magnitude of the difference between these confidence intervals increases as the score on the predictor deviates from the mean. However, a notable feature of the present examples is that, for many of the entries in Table 1, the difference between these two methods is modest. For example, if the intervals were rounded to the nearest *T* score, then in many cases the two methods either yield the same interval or differ by only one *T*-score unit. Thus, in the present examples, the differences between the confidence intervals based on $S_{y.x}$ and $SE_{yo-\hat{y}o}$ only become substantial when the sample size is relatively modest ($\leqslant 100$) and an individual's score on the predictor variable is extreme ($\geqslant 2$ *SD*s). In practice, it would often be inappropriate to use a regression equation when these circumstances hold, because the individual's score on *X* may lie beyond the range of the values of *X* in the sample used to create the regression equation (the relationship between predictor and criterion may become nonlinear for scores that lie beyond the range of scores observed in the sample). We occasionally have to make such predictions, but considerable care should be taken in their interpretation, and particularly in the interpretation of a substantial deviation from this prediction.

The illustrative data were selected to be reasonably typical of those found in clinical neuropsychology in terms of sample size, the precision of measurement of the criterion variable, and the explanatory power of the predictor variable. Thus, the results provide some reassurance for those clinicians who use confidence limits based on $S_{y.x}$ when drawing inferences regarding an individual's score. As noted, the use of tabulated frequency distributions of discrepancies between observed and predicted scores will normally yield very similar results to the use of confidence limits based on $S_{y.x}$; therefore, the present data also provide reassurance for those using this latter method.

The present observations appear to be at odds with the conclusion that could be drawn from inspection of many of the graphical representations of the elliptical nature of confidence intervals (i.e., see Fig. 1). The reason for this apparently dramatic disparity arises because many graphical representations do not provide a scale for the abscissa (*X* axis). It may not be inappropriate to exclude a scale, given that such illustrations are intended to be generic. However, the result is that they obscure the fact that confidence intervals based on $SE_{yo-\hat{y}o}$ become *heavily* elliptical only at very extreme values of the predictor variable (i.e., >4 *SD*s). Such extreme values are rare with neuropsychological data and, as noted, when they occur often preclude (or make problematic) the use of a regression prediction for that individual in any case.

Computer Programs for Confidence Intervals Based on SE$_{yo-\hat{y}o}$

The present examples suggest that, in many circumstances, substituting confidence intervals based on $S_{y.x}$ for the correct method does not seriously compromise the validity of inferences concerning an individual's score. However, it remains the case that the use of $S_{y.x}$ to generate confidence limits is technically incorrect and will *systematically* yield confidence limits which are *narrower* than those obtained by using the correct method. Therefore, it would be preferable to use the correct method, particularly when sample size is relatively modest and scores are relatively extreme. On the other hand, it is undeniably more complicated and time-consuming to generate confidence limits using $SE_{yo-\hat{y}o}$ than $S_{y.x}$. To address this, the first author has written a computer program for PCs that automates the process. The program prompts the user for *b* (the regression coefficient), *a* (the intercept), the mean and *SD* of the predictor variables, and $S_{y.x}$. This information can be saved to file for future use. The user then enters an individual's score on the predictor and the desired confidence interval (e.g., 85% or 95% etc.). The output consists of the predicted score and confidence limits.

In clinical practice there will often be a need for *one*-sided confidence intervals. For example, if a regression equation is being used in place of conventional norms, the clinician may have hypothesised that an individual's obtained score will be significantly below that predicted by the equation (i.e., the hypothesis is directional). To deal with this situation, the program can generate one-sided intervals; it will be appreciated that this option should not be used post hoc.

Aside from saving time, use of this program reduces the chance of clerical error. Furthermore, it can also provide an exact probability (one- or two-tailed) for the discrepancy between an individual's predicted and obtained scores. This is achieved by dividing the discrepancy between an individual's predicted and obtained score by $SE_{yo-\hat{y}o}$. This yields a t statistic with degrees of freedom equal to $N - 2$ for which an exact p is then calculated (i.e., in essence this procedure simply rearranges the terms in the formula for a confidence interval (4) to solve for t).

In the interests of simplicity the examples and related discussion have, to this point, been limited to the case of a single predictor variable. However, the authors have also written a computer program to generate confidence limits for use with multiple regression equations. The computations are considerably more complicated when there are multiple predictor variables, to the extent that it is not realistic to generate them by hand or calculator. This program prompts for a (the intercept), the regression coefficients (bs), the means and SDs of the predictor variables, and $S_{y.x}$. The intercorrelations of the predictor variables is also required. After entering these data they can be saved to file for future use. Finally, an individual's scores on the predictor variables are entered and the required confidence interval specified. The program transforms the individual's scores on the predictors to z scores and inverts the correlation matrix. The $SE_{yo-\hat{y}o}$ is then obtained by implementing the following formula, which, with minor changes in notation, is taken from Cohen and Cohen (1983):

$$SE_{yo-\hat{y}o} = \frac{S_{y.x}}{\sqrt{n}} \sqrt{n + 1 + \Sigma r^{ii} \cdot z_{io}^2 + 2\Sigma r^{ij} \cdot z_{io} \cdot z_{jo}} \quad (5)$$

where r^{ij} identifies off-diagonal elements of the inverted correlation matrix, r^{ii} identifies elements in the main diagonal, and z identifies the individual's scores on the predictor variables in z-score form. The first summation is over the k diagonal elements and the second is over the $k(k - 1)/2$ off-diagonal elements below (or above) the diagonal. This program offers the same options as those outlined for the case of a single predictor.

Although the APA Publication Manual (American Psychological Association, 1994) recommends that authors reporting multiple regression analyses should include the correlation matrix as a table, this is not always done. Therefore, it will not always be possible to use this latter program to generate confidence intervals. Compiled versions of the two programs can be downloaded from the first author's website at the following address: http://www.psyc.abdn.ac.uk/homedir/jcrawford/clreg.htm.

REFERENCES

American Psychological Association (1994). *Publication manual of the American Psychological Association* (4th ed.) Washington, DC: Author.

Armitage, P., & Berry, G. (1994). *Statistical methods in medical research*. Oxford, UK: Blackwell.

Cohen, J., & Cohen, P. (1983). *Applied multiple regression/correlation analysis for the behavioural sciences* (2nd ed.). Hillsdale, NJ: Lawrence Erlbaum.

Crawford, J.R. (1992). Current and premorbid intelligence measures in neuropsychological assessment. In J.R. Crawford, D.M. Parker, & W.W. McKinlay (Eds.), *A handbook of neuropsychological assessment* (pp. 21–49). London: Lawrence Erlbaum.

Crawford, J.R. (1996). Assessment. In J.G. Beaumont, P.M. Kenealy, & M.J. Rogers (Eds.), *The Blackwell dictionary of neuropsychology* (pp. 108–116). London: Blackwell.

Crawford, J.R., & Allan, K.M. (1997). Estimating premorbid IQ with demographic variables: Regression equations derived from a U.K. sample. *The Clinical Neuropsychologist, 11*, 192–197.

Crawford, J.R., Moore, J.W., & Cameron, I.M. (1992). Verbal fluency: A NART-based equation for the estimation of premorbid performance. *British Journal of Clinical Psychology, 31*, 327–329.

Daly, F., Hand, D.J., Jones, M.C., Lunn, A.D., & McConway, K.J. (1995). *Elements of statistics*. Wokingham, UK: Addison-Wesley.

Daniel, W.W. (1983). *Biostatistics: A foundation for analysis in the health sciences*. New York: Wiley.

Draper, N.R., & Smith, H. (1981). *Applied regression analysis* (2nd ed.). New York: Wiley.

Gardner, M.J., & Altman, D.G. (1989). *Statistics with confidence – confidence intervals and statistical guidelines*. London: British Medical Journal.

Heaton, R.K., Grant, I., Ryan, L., & Matthews, C.G. (1996). Demographic influences on neuropsychological test performance. In I. Grant & K.M. Adams (Eds.), *Neuropsychological assessment of neuropsychiatric disorders* (2nd ed.) (pp. 141–163). New York: Oxford University Press.

Howell, D.C. (1997). *Statistical methods for psychology* (4th ed.). Belmont, CA: Duxbury Press.

Knight, R.G., & Shelton, E.J. (1983). Tables for evaluating predicted retest changes in Wechsler Adult Intelligence Scale scores. *British Journal of Clinical Psychology, 22,* 77–81.

Lezak, M.D. (1995). *Neuropsychological assessment* (3rd ed.). New York: Oxford University Press.

McSweeny, A.J., Naugle, R.I., Chelune, G.J., & Lüders, H. (1993). "T scores for change": An illustration of a regression approach to depicting change in clinical neuropsychology. *The clinical Neuropsychologist, 7,* 300–312.

Nelson, H.E. (1982). *National Adult Reading Test (NART): Test manual.* Windsor, UK: NFER-Nelson.

Nelson, H.E., & Willison, J. (1991). *National Adult Reading Test manual* (2nd ed.). Windsor, UK: NFER-Nelson.

O'Carroll, R. (1995). The assessment of premorbid ability: A critical review. *Neurocase, 1,* 83–89.

Paolo, A.M., Ryan, J.J., Troster, A.I., & Hilmer, C.D. (1996). Demographically based regression equations to estimate WAIS-R subtest scaled scores. *The Clinical Neuropsychologist, 10,* 130–140.

Pedhazur, E.J. (1982). *Multiple regression in behavioural research: Explanation and prediction* (2nd ed.). New York: Holt, Rinehart & Winston.

Sokal, R.R., & Rohlf, J.F. (1981). *Biometry.* San Francisco, CA: W.H. Freeman.

Wechsler, D. (1955). *Manual for the Wechsler Adult Intelligence Scale.* New York: Psychological Cor-poration.

Wechsler, D. (1981). *Manual for the Wechsler Adult Intelligence Scale-Revised.* New York: Psychological Corporation.

Wechsler, D. (1987). *Manual for the Wechsler Memory Scale-Revised.* San Antonio, TX: Psychological Corporation.

Wittink, D.R. (1988). *The application of regression analysis.* Boston: Allyn & Bacon.

Zachary, R.A., & Gorsuch, R.L. (1985). Continuous norming: Implications for the WAIS-R. *Journal of Clinical Psychology, 41,* 86–94.

Zar, J.H. (1984). *Biostatistical analysis* (2nd ed.), Englewood Cliffs, NJ: Prentice-Hall.

Zar, J.H. (1996). *Biostatistical analysis* (3rd ed.), London: Prentice-Hall.

Journal of Clinical and Experimental Neuropsychology
2002, Vol. 24, No. 5, pp. 605–614

METHODOLOGICAL COMMENTARY

Payne and Jones Revisited: Estimating the Abnormality of Test Score Differences Using a Modified Paired Samples t Test*

J.R. Crawford[1], David C. Howell[2], and Paul H. Garthwaite[3]

[1]University of Aberdeen, UK, [2]University of Vermont, Burlington, and [3]Department of Mathematical Sciences,
University of Aberdeen, UK

ABSTRACT

Payne and Jones (1957) presented a useful formula for estimating the abnormality of differences between an individual's scores on two tests. Extending earlier work by Sokal and Rohlf (1995) and Crawford and Howell (in press), we developed a modified paired samples t test as an alternative to this formula. Unlike the Payne and Jones formula, the new method treats data from a normative or control sample as sample statistics rather than as population parameters. Technically, the new method is more appropriate for any comparison of an individual's difference score against normative data. However, it is most useful when the normative data is derived from samples with modest Ns; in these circumstances the Payne and Jones method overestimates the abnormality of differences. We suggest that the modified t test can be a useful tool in clinical practice and in single-case research. A computer program is made available that automates the calculations involved and can be used to store relevant data for future use.

In the assessment of acquired cognitive deficits, normative comparison standards have limitations because of the large individual differences in premorbid competencies. For example, an average test score can represent a marked decline from the premorbid level for a gifted individual whereas a low score can represent an entirely normal level of functioning for someone with modest premorbid abilities. Thus, considerable emphasis is placed on *intra*-individual comparisons when attempting to detect and quantify acquired deficits (Crawford, 1992; Lezak, 1995; Walsh, 1991). In the simplest case the clinician may wish to compare an individual's scores on two tests; a fundamental

consideration in assessing the clinical significance of any discrepancy between scores on the tests is the extent to which it is rare or abnormal.

USES OF THE PAYNE AND JONES (1957) FORMULA FOR THE ABNORMALITY OF DIFFERENCES

Payne and Jones (1957) presented a formula for the abnormality of a difference between scores on two tests; the formula estimates the percentage of the population that will equal or exceed a given discrepancy. A number of authors have noted

*Address correspondence to: John R. Crawford, Department of Psychology, King's College, University of Aberdeen, Aberdeen AB24 2UB, UK. E-mail: crawford@abdn.ac.uk
Accepted for publication: July 30, 1998.

the usefulness of this formula for assessment in clinical psychology and clinical neuropsychology (Crawford, 1996; Jones, 1970; Ley, 1972; Miller, 1993; Neufeld, 1977; Silverstein, 1981). Applications of the formula include estimation of the abnormality of discrepancies between Verbal and Performance IQs (Grossman, Herman, & Matarazzo, 1985), and factor scores (Atkinson, 1991) on the Wechsler Adult Intelligence Scale Revised (WAIS-R; Wechsler, 1981), and estimation of the abnormality of discrepancies between memory indices (Mittenberg, Thompson, & Schwartz, 1991) on the Wechsler Memory Scale-Revised (Wechsler, 1987).

Although the formula has mainly been used as an aid in clinical practice it is also a useful research tool. In recent years there has been a resurgence of interest within academic neuropsychology in single-case studies (Ellis & Young, 1996; McCarthy & Warrington, 1990; Shallice, 1988). A principal aim of this work is to fractionate the cognitive system into its constituent parts by attempting to establish the presence of double dissociations of function. Miller (1993) draws a distinction between studies in which patients are selected a priori on the basis of an independent criterion (normally anatomical localisation of lesion), and studies in which patients showing a contrasting pattern of preserved and impaired performance are identified serendipitously from among large samples of patients with impairment in the general area of interest. He argues that, in the latter case, it is incumbent upon investigators to demonstrate that the dissociations observed were unlikely to have arisen from chance variations in performance. Miller (1993) suggests that the Payne and Jones formula can be used to estimate the rarity of an observed discrepancy and provides examples that suggest the *normal* range of variability may often be larger than investigators commonly suppose.

Although Miller emphasised that investigators may overestimate the rarity of a given discrepancy, there is also the opposite danger that clinicians may dismiss a discrepancy that appears modest but is, in fact, highly abnormal (this latter situation is liable to arise when the two tests are highly correlated in the healthy population).

PSYCHOMETRIC ASPECTS OF THE PAYNE AND JONES FORMULA

There are a number of variants on the generic Payne and Jones (1957) formula but the simplest version, both conceptually and computationally, requires that an individual's raw scores on the two tests of interest are first converted to z scores (Z_X and Z_Y) based on a normative sample. The difference between the two component scores is in turn expressed as a z score (Z_D); this z score can then be referred to a table of the area under the normal curve to estimate the percentage of the population which would exhibit a difference as large as that observed. The formula is presented below:

$$Z_D = \frac{Z_X - Z_Y}{\sqrt{2 - 2r_{xy}}} \qquad (1)$$

where r_{xy} represents the correlation between the two tests and all other terms are as defined above. Like any z score, Z_D is obtained by dividing a deviation score (which in the present instance is the difference score between two component deviation scores) by the standard deviation of deviation score (the denominator in Equation (1)). A formal derivation for this formula can be found in Ley (1972).

To illustrate its use take the example of an individual who has been administered tests of verbal and spatial short-term memory, and suppose that the correlation between these tests is 0.75. For simplicity assume that both tests are expressed as T scores (i.e., they have a mean of 50 and a SD of 10). If the scores obtained on the verbal and spatial tests were 55 and 40, respectively, these would correspond to z scores of 0.5 and -1.0. Entering the relevant data into the formula yields the following:

$$Z_D = \frac{0.5 - (-1.0)}{\sqrt{2 - 2(0.75)}} = \frac{1.5}{\sqrt{0.5}} = 2.12$$

Referring the Z_D of 2.12 to a table of the area under the normal curve yields a p of .017; thus it is estimated that 3.4% of the population would exhibit a discrepancy, in either direction, as large as that observed; 1.7% would be expected to exhibit a discrepancy in the *direction* observed (i.e., a discrepancy in favour of verbal memory).

The Payne and Jones formula assumes that scores on the two tests are normally distributed. This should be borne in mind when using the formula although, for many tests used in clinical practice (particularly fully standardized instruments), the assumption will not be an unreasonable one. However, another feature of the formula is that the data used in the computations are treated as if they were *population parameters* rather than as *sample statistics*. The effect of this is that the formula will systematically overestimate the abnormality of the difference between an individual's test scores. When the sample used to generate the statistics has a large N, this effect will be minimal.

However, situations arise where the only available data come from a small sample but a clinician nevertheless wishes to estimate the abnormality of a discrepancy between test scores. For example, most clinicians use tests derived from a variety of sources so that, although the individual standardization samples for any particular pair of tests may both have large Ns, the tests may only have been administered *together* in a much smaller sample. Even when the tests have been standardized together it may still be necessary to rely on a smaller sample for the necessary data because the test manual may not report the correlation between them.

The sample size issue is particularly relevant to single-case studies where, as noted, the principal aim is to establish dissociations of functions. In many of these studies the theoretical questions posed cannot be addressed using existing instruments and therefore novel instruments are designed specifically for the study. The sample size of the control or normative group recruited for comparison purposes in such studies is typically very modest (N is often <10 and sometimes <5).

The remainder of this paper is concerned with developing a method of estimating the abnormality of test score differences which treats the sample statistics as statistics rather than population parameters.

DEVELOPMENT OF A MODIFIED PAIRED SAMPLES *t* TEST FOR THE ABNORMALITY OF TEST SCORE DIFFERENCES

Sokal and Rohlf (1995), writing for biometricians, described a modification to the independent samples *t* test which can be used to compare a single specimen with a sample. In this modification the individual specimen (or person!) is treated as a sample of $N = 1$ and, therefore, does not contribute to the estimate of the within-group variance. Crawford and Howell (in press) have recently illustrated the use of this procedure in clinical practice to compare an individual with norms derived from samples with modest Ns. They contrast this approach with the standard procedure in which the sample statistics are treated as parameters; that is, the individual's score is converted to a z score and evaluated using tables of the area under the normal curve (Howell, 1997; Ley, 1972). Using Crawford and Howell's (in press) notation, Sokal and Rohlf's (1995) formula is as follows:

$$\frac{X_1 - \overline{X}_2}{S_2\sqrt{\dfrac{N_2 + 1}{N_2}}}, \tag{2}$$

where, for our purposes, $X_1 = $ the individual's score, $\overline{X} = $ the mean of the normative sample, $S_2 = $ the standard deviation of the normative sample, and $N_2 = $ the sample size. The degrees of freedom for t are $N_2 = N_1 - 2$ which reduces to $N_2 - 1$. Although this method can be used to determine if an individual's score is significantly different from that of the normative or control sample (and, thus, may be useful in single-case studies), Crawford and Howell (in press) emphasised that its value was primarily in providing an unbiased estimate of the *abnormality* of the individual's score (i.e., if the *p* value for *t* was calculated to be 0.03 then it can be estimated that only 3% of the healthy population would exhibit a score as extreme as that observed).

The above formula is for comparison of an individual's score on a *single* test with the mean of a normative sample. However, we can extend the approach to a paired *t* test and use it to compare the *difference* between an individual's scores on *two* tests with the mean difference between these tests in a normative sample. To achieve this we follow Payne and Jones and transform the individual's scores, and the scores of the normative sample, to z scores based on the mean and standard deviation of the normative sample. In the following formula the subscripts 1 and 2 identify the individual and normative sample, respectively, and X and Y identify the two tests (derivation of the formula is given in Appendix 1):

$$t = \frac{\left(Z_{X_1} - Z_{Y_1}\right) - \left(\overline{Z}_{X_2} - \overline{Z}_{Y_2}\right)}{\sqrt{2 - 2r_{xy}}\sqrt{\frac{N_2 + 1}{N_2}}} \quad (3)$$

The left-hand term in the denominator represents the standard deviation of the differences in the normative or control sample and is multiplied by the right-hand term to obtain the standard error of the difference. The right-hand term in the numerator drops out because, from centering, $\overline{Z}_{X_2}$ and $\overline{Z}_{Y_2}$ are both zero, and we can gather together terms in the denominator to obtain the following:

$$t = \frac{Z_{X_1} - Z_{Y_1}}{\sqrt{\left(2 - 2r_{xy}\right)\left(\frac{N_2 + 1}{N_2}\right)}} \quad (4)$$

This Equation (4) resembles the original Payne and Jones Equation (1) but differs in that the statistics of the normative or control sample are now treated as *statistics* rather than as *population parameters*. In Appendix 1 we show that the quantity in Equation (4) has a t distribution with $N_2 - 1$ degrees of freedom (rather than the standard normal distribution). This should be used to evaluate the abnormality of the difference between the individual's scores. Returning to the worked example of verbal and spatial memory tests used earlier; suppose that the normative data had been obtained from a small healthy, control group in which $N = 10$. Entry of these data into the formula for the modified t test (Equation (4)) yields the following:

$$t = \frac{1.0 - (-0.5)}{\sqrt{(2 - 2(0.75))\left(\frac{10 + 1}{10}\right)}}$$

$$= \frac{1.5}{\sqrt{(2 - 1.5)(1.1)}}$$

$$= \frac{1.5}{\sqrt{0.55}} = 2.023$$

The p value for a t of 2.023 with 9 $df = 0.037$. Therefore, it is estimated that, 7.4% of the population would exhibit a discrepancy, in either direction, as large as that observed; 3.7% would be expected to exhibit a discrepancy in the *direction* observed (i.e., a discrepancy in favor of verbal memory). This estimate of the abnormality of the patient's score would be preferred over the exaggerated estimate provided by the Payne and Jones formula (for which the corresponding figures were 3.4% and 1.7%), because the latter treats the control data as parameters.

Table 1 provides further data comparing the Payne and Jones formula with the modified t-test procedure. For consistency, the correlation between tests in this example was also taken as 0.75. Table 1 records the value that an individual's difference score must exceed to be significantly different from a normative or control sample at the 0.05 level, one-tailed; these difference scores correspond to the numerator in Equations (1) and (4). It can be seen that if $N = 20$ in the normative sample then an individual's difference score $(Z_{X_1} - Z_{Y_1})$ would have to exceed 1.25 to have a probability of less than 0.05; for example, if an individual's score on Test X was 0.1 (marginally above the normative sample mean) and was −1.1 on Test Y, the difference (−1.2) would not be large enough to be significantly different from the normative sample. The results from the t-test procedure can be compared with those from the Payne and Jones formula which, as noted, ignores the size of the normative sample and treats the sample statistics as parameters. The results from the Payne and Jones formula are presented in bold in the last row of Table 1.

The examples in Table 1 are intended to further illustrate that the Payne and Jones formula systematically overestimates the abnormality of an individual's difference score when used with data from samples with modest Ns. To this end we took

Table 1. Cutoff Values to Attain Significance.[a]

N_2	$Z_{X_1} - Z_{Y_1}$
5	1.65
7	1.47
10	1.36
15	1.29
20	1.25
25	1.23
30	1.22
50	1.20
70	1.19
120	1.18
–	1.16

Note. [a]Table shows the difference ($Z_{X_1} - Z_{Y_1}$) between an individual's scores on two tests required to be significantly different at the .05 level (one-tailed) when compared against normative samples of varying Ns. For
comparison purposes the last row records the values that would be required if the sample statistics were
treated as population parameters, that is, if the Payne and Jones formula were applied. This specific example is based on a correlation of 0.75 between the two tests.

a significance testing approach and demonstrated
that the critical values required for the Payne and
Jones approach are smaller than those required
with the modified t test. This inferential use of the
modified t test may be appropriate for single-case
studies in which there will be a legitimate concern
with rejecting the null hypothesis. However, it
should be stressed that we primarily see the value
of the modified t test as simply providing the clinician with a less biased estimate of the abnormality
of an individual's difference score.

Technically, the modified t test introduced in the
present paper is more appropriate than the original
Payne and Jones formula for *any* comparison of an
individual's difference score against norms for
difference scores. This is because the normative
data with which we work are always derived from
samples rather than populations. However, with
large samples (e.g., >250) the difference between
the value of t and z becomes vanishingly small
and, thus, the estimates of the abnormality of a
difference score also converge. Further, even with
more moderate sample sizes (e.g., $N = 50$), the
difference between the two are relatively trivial.
Thus, we would suggest that the modified t test
procedure be used with $N < 50$. With larger sample sizes the Payne and Jones formula approxi-
mates the technically more correct method, thus,
either method could be used. However, by using
the computer program accompanying this paper

the t-test procedure can be run in under 30 seconds. Thus the bias inherent in the Payne and
Jones method is not necessarily offset by any savings in time.

One of the assumptions underlying any form of
t test is that the data is normally distributed.
Monte Carlo simulations have revealed that t tests
are surprisingly robust in the face of moderate
violation of this assumption (Boneau, 1960;
Howell, 1997). However, especially given the
small Ns with which we are concerned, the t test
procedure and the Payne and Jones z procedure
are best avoided when it is known or suspected
that the normative data are markedly skewed.

When referring to discrepancies between an
individual's scores on two tests, it may be best to
reserve the term "significantly different" to describe
the case in which the scores are *reliably* different.
In that context a significant difference is taken to
mean that the difference is unlikely (e.g., $p < .05$)
to have occurred because of measurement error in
the tests concerned. If the tests have very high
reliabilities, it is quite possible that the majority of
healthy individuals would exhibit reliable differences between their scores. Thus, the issue of the
reliability of a difference should not be confused
with the topic of the present paper which is primarily concerned with the *rarity* or *abnormality* of
a patient's difference score; see Crawford, (1996),
Crawford, Sommerville, and Robertson, (1997),

Crawford, Venneri, and O'Carroll (1998), and Silverstein (1981) for related discussion of the distinction between reliable and abnormal differences.

COMPUTER PROGRAM FOR THE ABNORMALITY OF A DIFFERENCE BETWEEN A PAIR OF TEST SCORES

The calculations involved in the aforementioned procedure are relatively straightforward. However, a statistics package would be required to obtain the exact p corresponding to a given t. In view of this, and because of an awareness of the time pressures under which many of us operate, we have written a program for PCs that automates the process. Apart from saving time, use of this program reduces the chance of clerical and arith-metic errors. The user enters the mean and SD for the two tests of interest in the normative or control sample, followed by the tests' intercorrelation and the sample size. These data can be saved to a file (as can equivalent data for other pairs of tests) so that they need not be reentered each time the clinician wishes to use the procedure with future clients. Finally, the individual client's scores on the two tests are entered. The output consists of the original scores and the difference score in z-score form, and the estimate of the percentage of the population that will exceed the observed discrepancy (in either direction and in the observed direction). A compiled version of the program can be downloaded from the first author's website at the following address: http://www.psyc.abdn.ac.uk/homedir/jcrawford/pairabno.htm

CONCLUSION

There is much evidence that human judges are poor at estimating the rarity of differences involving correlated components (Hogarth, 1975; Slovic & Lichtenstein, 1971). Therefore, clinicians should, where possible, use a quantitative method to help them interpret an individuals' apparent neuropsychological strengths and weaknesses rather than rely solely on clinical intuition. The present method for estimating the abnormality of differences between an individual's test scores should assist in

this process. Unlike the Payne and Jones method, it does not systematically overestimate the rarity of differences when the normative or control data has been derived from samples with modest Ns.

REFERENCES

Atkinson, L. (1991). Some tables for statistically based interpretation of WAIS-R factor scores. *Psychological Assessment, 3*, 288–291.

Boneau, C.A. (1960). The effect of violation of assumptions underlying the t-test. *Psychological Bulletin, 57*, 49–64.

Crawford, J.R. (1992). Current and premorbid intelligence measures in neuropsychological assessment. In J.R. Crawford, D.M. Parker, & W.W. McKinlay (Eds.), *A handbook of neuropsychological assessment* (pp. 21–49). London: Lawrence Erlbaum.

Crawford, J.R. (1996). Assessment. In J.G. Beaumont, P.M. Kenealy, & M.J. Rogers (Eds.), *The Blackwell dictionary of neuropsychology* (pp. 108–116). London: Blackwell.

Crawford, J.R., & Howell, D.C. (in press). Comparing an individual's test score against norms derived from small samples. *The Clinical Neuropsychologist.*

Crawford, J.R., Sommerville, J., & Robertson, I.H. (1997). Assessing the reliability and abnormality of subtest differences on the Test of Everyday Attention. *British Journal of Clinical Psychology, 36*, 609–617.

Crawford, J.R., Venneri, A., & O'Carroll, R.E. (1998). Neuropsychological assessment of the elderly. In A.S. Bellack & M. Hersen (Eds.), *Comprehensive clinical psychology, vol. 7: Clinical geropsychology* (pp. 133–169) Oxford, UK: Pergamon.

Ellis, A.W., & Young, A.W. (1996). *Human cognitive neuropsychology: A textbook with readings.* Hove, UK: Psychology Press.

Grossman, F.M., Herman, D.O., & Matarazzo, J.D. (1985). Statistically inferred vs. empirically observed VIQ–PIQ differences in the WAIS-R. *Journal of Clinical Psychology, 41*, 268–272.

Hogarth, R.M. (1975). Cognitive processes and the assessment of subjective probability distributions. *Journal of the American Statistical Association, 70*, 271–294.

Howell, D.C. (1997). *Statistical methods for psychology* (4th ed.). Belmont, CA: Duxbury Press.

Jones, H.G. (1970). Principles of psychological assessment. In P.J. Mittler (Ed.). *The psychological assessment of mental and physical handicaps* (pp. 1–25). London: Tavistock.

Ley, P. (1972). *Quantitative aspects of psychological assessment.* London: Duckworth.

Lezak, M.D. (1995). *Neuropsychological assessment* (3rd ed.). New York: Oxford University Press.

McCarthy, R.A., & Warrington, E.K. (1990). *Cognitive neuropsychology: A clinical introduction.* San Diego, CA: Academic Press.

Miller, E. (1993). Dissociating single cases in neuropsychology. *British Journal of Clinical Psychology*, *32*, 155–167.

Mittenberg, W., Thompson, G.B., & Schwartz, J.A. (1991). Abnormal and reliable differences among Wechsler Memory Scale – Revised subtests. *Psychological Assessment*, *3*, 492–495.

Neufeld, R.W.J. (1977). *Clinical quantitative methods.* New York: Grune & Stratton.

Payne, R.W., & Jones, G. (1957). Statistics for the investigation of individual cases. *Journal of Clinical Psychology*, *13*, 115–121.

Shallice, T. (1988). *From neuropsychology to mental structure.* Cambridge, UK: Cambridge University Press.

Silverstein, A.B. (1981). Reliability and abnormality of test score differences. *Journal of Clinical Psychology*, *37*, 392–394.

Slovic, P., & Lichtenstein, S. (1971). Comparison of Bayesian and regression approaches to the study of information processing in judgment. *Organisational Behaviour and Human Performance*, *6*, 649–744.

Sokal, R.R., & Rohlf, J.F. (1995). *Biometry* (3rd ed.). San Francisco, CA: W.H. Freeman.

Walsh, K.W. (1991). *Understanding brain damage* (2nd ed.). Melbourne, Australia: Churchill Livingstone.

Wechsler, D. (1981). *Manual for the Wechsler Adult Intelligence Scale-Revised.* New York: Psychological Corporation.

Wechsler, D. (1987). *Manual for the Wechsler Memory Scale-Revised.* San Antonio, TX: Psychological Corporation.

APPENDIX 1

Distribution of the test statistic in Equation (4)

Assume the centres and scales of X and Y have been so chosen that both their sample means are 0 in the normative sample and their sample variances are both 1. Let x_i and y_i denote the values of X and Y for the ith individual in the normative sample $(i = 1, \dots, N_2)$. Then

$$r_{xy} = \frac{1}{N_2 - 1} \sum_{i=1}^{N_2} x_i y_i$$

and

$$\frac{1}{N_2 - 1} \sum_{i=1}^{N_2} (x_i - y_i)^2 = 2 - 2r_{xy}$$

Define $d = X - Y$ and assume it is normally distributed. In the normative sample the mean and sample variance of d are 0 and $(2 - 2r_{xy})$, respectively. Hence analogous to Equation (2),

$$\frac{d - 0}{\sqrt{(2 - 2r_{xy}) \left(\dfrac{N_2 + 1}{N_2} \right)}}$$

follows a t-distribution of $N_2 - 1$ degrees of freedom. With the given choice of centres and scales, $Z_{X_1} - Z_{Y_1} = d$, so the quantity in Equation (4) has a t distribution on $N_2 - 1$ degrees of freedom.

Child Neuropsychology
1996, Vol. 2, No. 3, pp. 227–232

Validity of a Short Form of the WISC-III in Children with Traumatic Head Injury*

Jacques Donders[1] and Seth Warschausky[2]
[1]Mary Free Bed Hospital and [2]University of Michigan

ABSTRACT

The concurrent, construct, and criterion validities of Donders' (in press) short form of the Wechsler Intelligence Scale for Children – Third Edition (WISC-III) were evaluated in a sample of 171 children with traumatic head injury (THI). Correlations between the short-form deviation quotients and their full-length counterparts were statistically significant. Confirmatory factor analysis revealed that a four-factor model (composed of Verbal Comprehension, Perceptual Organization, Freedom from Distractibility, and Processing Speed) fit the data relatively well. The short-form deviation quotients also had statistically significant correlations with length of coma. It is concluded that this short form is an accurate and valid alternative to the full-length WISC-III in children with THI.

Measures of psychometric intelligence are routinely included in most pediatric neuropsychological evaluations. However, time constraints can sometimes be a concern because most standard intelligence tests take more than one hour to administer (Silverstein, 1990). Also, such tests do not necessarily yield data that are more sensitive to cerebral impairment as compared to specific neuropsychological measures (Fletcher, Levin, & Butler, 1995). Recently, a short form was developed for the Wechsler Intelligence Scale for Children – Third Edition (WISC-III; Wechsler, 1991) that allowed computation of estimates of the Full Scale IQ as well as all four factor index scores (Donders, 1996). The purpose of the present investigation was to evaluate the validity of this short form in children with traumatic head injury (THI).

The validity of the four-factor structure of the WISC-III has been confirmed in independent samples of normal children (Roid, Prifitera, & Weiss, 1993) and children with THI (Donders &

Warschausky, 1996). Therefore, using the standardization sample, one of the criteria for the selection of the eight subtests for the WISC-III short form developed by Donders (in press) was that it should maintain this four-factor structure in addition to yielding significant time savings. It included Similarities and Vocabulary as measures of Verbal Comprehension (VC), and Picture Completion and Block Design as measures of Perceptual Organization (PO). In addition, the Freedom from Distractibility (FD) subtests, Arithmetic and Digit Span, and the Processing Speed (PS) subtests, Coding and Symbol Search, were included. Six of these subtests (excluding Digit Span and Symbol Search, which are not typically included in the calculation of Full Scale IQ for the full-length WISC-III) were also used for construction of a Full Scale (FS) index of this short form. Reliability and validity coefficients of the Deviation Quotients (DQ) of this short form ranged from .85 to .94, and standard errors of estimation ranged from 3.45 to 4.57; these were

* This research was supported by a grant from the Campbell Foundation.
Address correspondence to: Dr. Jacques Donders, Mary Free Bed Hospital, 235 Wealthy SE, Grand Rapids, MI 49503, USA. E-mail: jdonders@mfbrc.com.
Accepted for publication: October 15, 1996.

considered to be quite acceptable. In addition, confirmatory factor analysis indicated that the proposed four-factor structure fit the data of the short form better than any competing model in the WISC-III standardization sample (Donders, in press).

This short form has not yet been validated in specific clinical samples. The purpose of the present investigation was to evaluate the validity of this short form in a sample of children with THI. It has been well documented that THI in children is often accompanied by deficits in attention, speed of processing, and other cognitive domains (for reviews, see Dalby & Obrzut, 1991; Donders & Kuldanek, in press; Fletcher et al., 1995). There is also evidence that some of the WISC-III indexes have significant sensitivity to length of coma and other measures of injury severity in children with THI (Donders, 1995). A reliable and valid short form of the WISC-III could be of value in the clinical assessment of children with THI, especially when time constraints are an issue.

It was determined a priori that, in order to be clinically useful, this short form should meet several specific criteria, as follows. Criterion 1: There should be statistically significant correlations (corrected for spurious elements due to shared error variance) between the short-form deviation quotients and their full-length WISC-III counterparts. Criterion 2: There should be direct psychometric support for the validity of the four-factor structure of this form, as evaluated through confirmatory factor analysis. Criterion 3: The short-form deviation quotients should have statistically significant relationships with measures of injury severity.

METHOD

Participants
The 171 participants for this investigation were selected from a 4-year series of consecutive referrals to two Mid-Western regional rehabilitation facilities. The procedures for the selection of participants have been described in detail elsewhere (Donders & Warschausky, in press). All children had sustained a nonpenetrating THI through an external accelerating or decelerating force, with documented alteration of consciousness. They ranged in age from 6.0 to 16.11 years and had completed the entire WISC-III (excluding Mazes) as part of a psychometric evaluation within 12 months after injury.

No children with premorbid neurological, psychiatric, or special education histories were included. Injury severity was classified on the basis of Glasgow Coma Scale (Teasdale & Jennett, 1974) and on neuroradiological findings, using the classification criteria described by Williams, Levin, and Eisenberg (1990). Demographic and injury variables are presented for the complete sample in Table 1.

Procedure
The WISC-III was administered and scored according to standardized test procedures as part of neuropsychological evaluations that were requested by attending physicians during the rehabilitation of these children. All protocols were then rescored to derive the VCDQ, PODQ, and FSDQ short-form estimates according to

Table 1. Patient Characteristics for 171 Children with Traumatic Head Injury.

Gender (%)	
Female	48
Male	52
Ethnicity (%)	
African	6
Asian	2
Caucasian	85
Hispanic	7
Parental occupational status (%)	
Executive/professional	22
Semi-professional/clerical	29
Skilled/semi-skilled	36
Unskilled/unemployed	13
Injury circumstances (%)	
MVA – passenger	41
MVA – pedestrian/cyclist	35
Falls & recreation	21
Other	3
Injury severity (%)	
Mild	27
Moderate	32
Severe	41
Length of coma (days)	
M	2.73
SD	6.34
Injury-testing interval (days)	
M	81.84
SD	71.34
Age at testing (months)	
M	142.99
SD	37.96

Note. MVA = Motor vehicle accident.

the procedures described by Donders (in press). For the FD and PS factor indexes, Table A.7 of the WISC-III manual was used (Wechsler, 1991), and no additional procedures were necessary. Scaled subtest scores ($M = 10$, $SD = 3$) and standard factor index scores ($M = 100$, $SD = 15$) were used in all statistical analyses.

RESULTS

The average deviation quotients of the full-length and short-form versions of the WISC-III are presented in Table 2 as are correlations between the respective measures, which were computed to evaluate concurrent validity of the short form. These correlations were modified with Levy's (1967) correction formula to remove error variance that is shared between the short and long forms. As seen in Table 2, the corrected correlations were still statistically significant. To evaluate how accurately the short-form estimates could predict the full-length WISC-III standard scores, independent t tests for paired observations were also performed. VCDQ over-estimated the VC index by an average of less than one standard score point ($M = .66$, $SD = .43$; $t(169) = 1.54$, ns), whereas FSDQ underestimated the FSIQ by an average of less than one standard score point ($M = .29$, $SD = .35$; $t(169) = .83$, ns). The difference between PODQ and the PO index reached statistical significance ($t(169) = 3.54$, $p < .001$) with this large sample, but the average amount of overestimation was still less than two standard score points ($M = 1.84$, $SD = .52$).

The eight subtests of the short form were then subjected to confirmatory factor analysis by calculating sets of maximum-likelihood structural equations for each of six hypothetical models, using the SAS CALIS procedure (SAS, 1993) to evaluate construct validity of the short form. The first four of these models were evaluated previously as part of the standardization and validation of the WISC-III (Wechsler, 1991). The fifth model represented a variant of the three-factorial model that has been suggested for both the WISC-R (Kaufman, 1975) and the WISC-III (Reynolds & Ford, 1994). The sixth model was suggested as an alternative possibility by Kaufman (1994). These six models, that were also previously evaluated for the full-length WISC-III with this sample (Donders & Warschausky, 1996), can be summarized as follows:

Model 1 :	General Intelligence (eight
(one factor)	subtests)
Model 2 :	Verbal Intelligence (four subtests)
(two factors)	and Performance
	Intelligence (four subtests)
Model 3 :	Verbal Intelligence (four subtests),
(three factors)	Perceptual Organization
	(two subtests), and Processing
	Speed (two subtests)
Model 4 :	Verbal Comprehension (two
(four factors)	subtests),
	Perceptual Organization (two
	subtests), Freedom from
	Distractibility (two
	subtests), and Processing Speed
	(two subtests)
Model 5 :	Verbal Comprehension (two
(three factors)	subtests),
	Performance Intelligence (four

Table 2. Deviation Quotients for the Complete and Short Forms of the WISC-III, and Corrected Correlations (r) Between the Respective Measures.

	Complete		Short		r
	M	SD	M	SD	
Full Scale	91.31	14.71	91.02	15.77	.90*
Verbal Comprehension	93.91	13.35	94.56	13.28	.82*
Perceptual Organization	91.36	16.21	93.20	15.85	.80*
Freedom from Distractibility	95.64	14.27	–	–	–
Processing Speed	91.74	19.49	–	–	–

Note. Freedom from Distractibility and Processing Speed indexes are identical across forms.
    *$p < .0001$

subtests), and Freedom from Distractibility (two subtests)

Model 6 : Verbal Comprehension (two
(three factors) subtests), Perceptual Organization (two subtests), and Executive Ability (four sub-tests)

The statistical indexes for each of the six models are presented in Table 3. As seen in Table 3, Model 4 was the only one that had a statistically nonsignificant value of chi-square (χ^2). In addition, it had the lowest value of Akaike's Information Criterion (AIC) and the highest values of the Adjusted Goodness of Fit Index (AGFI) and of the Comparative Fit Index (CFI), all of which have been suggested to reflect better model fit (Akaike, 1987; Bentler, 1989; Hatcher, 1994). A chi-square test of the difference between this model and the apparently next best one (Model 3) suggested that the addition of a fourth factor yielded a statistically significant increase of predictive validity over the three-factor model ($\chi^2(3) = 12.88$, $p < .005$). For all of these reasons, Model 4 was considered to be the most psychometrically accurate model.

Finally, criterion validity of this short form was evaluated, using two types of analyses. The first involved computation of Pearson product-moment correlations between each short-form deviation quotient and length of coma for the complete sample. The second involved multivariate analysis of variance with post hoc comparisons to compare the subgroups of children with Mild ($n = 46$), Moderate ($n = 55$), and Severe ($n = 70$) injuries on the short-form deviation quotients. These data are presented in Table 4. For both the correlations and the post hoc subgroup comparisons, alpha was corrected to .003 (.01/3) because multiple computations might inflate Type I error rate, particularly with this large sample.

As seen in Table 4, the correlations between the short-form deviation quotients and length of coma all met the a priori specified level of statistical significance. The overall MANOVA main effect of groups was also statistically significant ($F(3,167) = 21.87$, $p < .0001$). Post hoc comparisons revealed that the group differences in PODQ ($F(2,168) = 27.44$, $p < .0001$) and FSDQ ($F(2,168) = 18.70$, $p < .0001$) met the a priori specified level of statistical significance;

Table 3. Goodness of Fit Statistics for Six Hypothetical Models.

Model	χ^2	df	p	AIC	AGFI	CFI
1	119.41	20	.0001	79.41	.70	.81
2	48.66	19	.0002	10.66	.86	.94
3	31.89	17	.02	−2.11	.90	.97
4	19.01	14	.17	−8.99	.93	.99
5	37.54	17	.003	3.54	.88	.96
6	76.69	17	.0001	45.69	.76	.88

Note. See text for details regarding statistical indexes.

Table 4. Short-Form Deviation Quotients for the Mild, Moderate, and Severe Injury Severity Groups and Correlations with Length of Coma (r) for the Complete Sample.

	Mild		Moderate		Severe		r
	M	SD	M	SD	M	SD	
Verbal comprehension	97.46	10.52	95.30	11.83	92.07	15.52	−.26*
Perceptual organization	100.44	12.43	99.11	14.08	83.81	14.50	−.35**
Full scale	97.00	10.02	96.27	13.33	82.97	17.23	−.40**

* $p < .001$.
** $p < .0001$.

however, the group difference in VCDQ ($F(2,168) = 2.45$, $p < .10$) fell short of statistical significance. As inspection of Table 4 may indicate, the Mild and Moderate groups were very similar on all variables, whereas the Severe group had much lower values of PODQ and FSDQ than did the Mild and Moderate groups.

DISCUSSION

The purpose of this investigation was to evaluate the validity of Donders' (in press) short form of the WISC-III in a clinical sample of children with THI. It was specified a priori that this short form should meet three criteria pertaining to concurrent, construct, and criterion validity. The results indicate that all three criteria were met.

Concurrent validity was demonstrated because the corrected correlations between the short-form deviation quotients and their full-length WISC-III counterparts were statistically significant. All of these correlations equaled or exceeded .80, the recommended magnitude for tests used for clinical decision making (Anastasi, 1988; Salvia & Ysseldyke, 1988; Sattler, 1988). Furthermore, the average amount of difference between the respective scores was consistently less than one or two standard score points, which is well within the standard error of measurement of either the short form (Donders, 1996) or the long form (Wechsler, 1991).

Construct validity was demonstrated in that when using confirmatory factor analysis, the four-factor (VC, PO, FD, PS) model out-performed all other evaluated models in terms of fit to the data. These findings are consistent with confirmatory factor analysis findings that have been described for the full-length WISC-III with the same group of children with THI (Donders & Warschausky, 1996).

Criterion validity was demonstrated because the short-form deviation quotients all had statistically significant correlations with length of coma. Two of these measures (PODQ and FSDQ) were also able to discriminate between groups with severe versus mild or moderate injuries. The finding that VCDQ was not as sensitive to

measures of injury severity as were the other measures is consistent with the results of a previous evaluation with the full-length WISC-III (Donders, 1995). This probably reflects the fact that the VC subtests primarily measure overlearned skills that are known to be relatively more resilient to the effects of THI (Dalby & Obrzut, 1991; Donders & Kuldanek, in press; Fletcher et al., 1995).

CONCLUSIONS

Our short form offers clinicians the opportunity to save more than a quarter of administration time while still obtaining the same crucial range of information (in terms of factor index scores). Analyses using the WISC-III standardization sample suggest quite acceptable reliability of this short form (Donders, in press). The current results also suggest acceptable validity in a large sample of children with THI. A possible limitation of this investigation is that the short-form deviation quotients were extracted from completed administrations of the full-length WISC-III. Therefore, there remains a slight possibility that the psychometric properties of this short form may change when it is administered in isolation, rather than extracted from the long form. There is also a need for additional validation of this short form in other clinical samples because this investigation was limited to children with THI.

With these reservations in mind, the current results suggest that interpretation of WISC-III factor and full scale indexes, derived from this short form, may provide reliable and valid information. However, such data should never be interpreted in isolation and should always be corroborated by independent results from specific neuropsychological tests before drawing conclusions about children's cognitive deficits or their associated cerebral integrity. Furthermore, as has been suggested previously (Donders, in press), clinicians should not rely on this short form for decision making purposes when calculation of the deviation quotients may be ill-advised because of an extraordinary amount of scatter between the two VC component subtests (i.e., >4 scaled points) or between the two PO component subtests (i.e., >5 scaled points). Under such circumstances, it would be advisable to administer the remaining subtests of the scale and calculate the usual index scores.

REFERENCES

Akaike, H. (1987). Factor analysis and AIC. *Psychometrika*, *52*, 317–332.

Anastasi, A. (1988). *Psychological testing* (6th ed.). New York, NY: MacMillan Publishing Company.

Bentler, P.M. (1989). *EQS structural equation program*. Los Angeles, CA: BMDP Statistical Software.

Dalby, P.R., & Obrzut, J.E. (1991). Epidemiological characteristics and sequelae of closed head-injured children and adolescents: A review. *Developmental Neuropsychology*, *7*, 35–68.

Denckla, M.B. (1995). Foreword. In S.H. Broman & M.E. Michel (Eds.), *Traumatic head injury in children* (pp. v–vii). New York, NY: Oxford University Press.

Donders, J. (1995). Validity of the Kaufman Brief Intelligence Test (K-BIT) in children with traumatic brain injury. *Assessment*, *2*, 219–224.

Donders, J. (in press). A short form of the WISC-III for clinical use. *Psychological Assessment*.

Donders, J., & Kuldanek, A.S. (in press). Traumatic brain injury. In R.T. Ammerman & J.V. Campo (Eds.), *Handbook of pediatric psychology and psychiatry*. Needham Heights, MA: Allyn & Bacon.

Donders, J., & Warschausky, S. (1996). A structural equation analysis of the WISC-III in children with traumatic head injury. *Child Neuropsychology*, *2*, 185–192.

Fletcher, J.M., Levin, H.S., & Butler, I.J. (1995). Neurobehavioral effects of brain injury on children: Hydrocephalus, traumatic brain injury, and cerebral palsy. In M.C. Roberts (Ed.), *Handbook of pediatric psychology* (2nd ed.), (pp. 362–383). New York, NY: Guilford Press.

Hatcher, L. (1994). *A step-by-step approach to using the SAS system for factor analysis and structural equation modeling*. Cary, NC: SAS Institute.

Kaufman, A.S. (1975). Factor analysis of the WISC-R at 11 age levels between 6½ and 16½ years. *Journal of Consulting and Clinical Psychology*, *43*, 135–147.

Kaufman, A.S. (1994). *Intelligent testing with the WISC-III*. New York, NY: John Wiley & Sons.

Levy, P. (1967). The correction for spurious correlation in the evaluation of short-form tests. *Journal of Clinical Psychology*, *23*, 84–86.

Reynolds, C.R., & Ford, L. (1994). Comparative three-factor solutions of the WISC-III and WISC-R at 11 age levels between 6½ and 16½ years. *Archives of Clinical Neuropsychology*, *9*, 553–570.

Roid, G.H., Prifitera, A., & Weiss, L.G. (1993). Replication of the WISC-III factor structure in an independent sample. In B.A. Bracken & R.S. McCallum (Eds.), *Journal of Psychoeducational Assessment monograph series, advances in psychoeducational assessment: Wechsler Intelligence Scale for Children – Third Edition* (pp. 6–21). Germantown, TN: Psychoeducational Corporation.

Salvia, J., & Ysseldyke, J.E. (1988). *Assessment in special and remedial education* (4th ed.). Boston, MA: Houghton Mifflin Company.

SAS (1993). *SAS/STAT user's guide* (4th ed., vol. 1). Cary, NC: SAS Institute.

Sattler, J.M. (1988). *Assessment of children* (3rd ed.). San Diego, CA: Author.

Silverstein, A.B. (1990). Short forms of individual intelligence tests. *Psychological Assessment*, *2*, 3–11.

Teasdale, G., & Jennett, B. (1974). Assessment of coma and impaired consciousness: A practical scale. *Lancet*, *2*, 81–84.

Wechsler, D. (1991). *Wechsler Intelligence Scale for Children – Third Edition*. San Antonio, TX: Psychological Corporation.

Williams, D.H., Levin, H.S., & Eisenberg, H.M. (1990). Mild head injury classification. *Neurosurgery*, *27*, 422–428.

The Clinical Neuropsychologist
1996, Vol. 10, No. 2, pp. 130–140

Demographically Based Regression Equations to Estimate WAIS-R Subtest Scaled Scores*

Anthony M. Paolo[1], Joseph J. Ryan[2], Alexander I. Tröster[1], and Craig D. Hilmer[3]

[1]University of Kansas Medical Center, [2]Dwight D. Eisenhower Department of Veterans Affairs, Medical Center, Leavenworth, Kansas, and [3]The Psychological Corporation, San Antonio, Texas

ABSTRACT

The WAIS-R (Wechsler, 1981) and elderly WAIS-R standardization samples (Ryan, Paolo, & Brungardt, 1990) were combined to develop demographically based regression equations to predict subtest scaled scores. Equations generated from a development sample cross-validated well and final equations were generated from the entire sample. The equations demonstrated adequate ability to suggest possible subtest decline in a sample of 247 persons with brain dysfunction. Examination of the difference between the estimated and obtained scaled scores also provided information beyond that of the typical normative and ipsative subtest comparisons. Confidence intervals at the 90% and 95% levels of abnormality were provided to assist clinicians in the detection of possible decline in subtest scaled scores.

Interpretation of the Wechsler Adult Intelligence Scale – Revised (WAIS-R; Wechsler, 1981) begins with an analysis of the Full Scale IQ, Verbal-Performance IQ discrepancy, and, if appropriate, factor-based Deviation Quotients. Attention is then focused on the individual subtests. Clinicians can perform normative interpretation of each subtest score as well as an examination of relative strengths and weakness within the profile. The entire process is designed to generate hypotheses that may be integrated with additional test and non-test information to answer a referral question and lead to practical recommendations concerning further assessment and/or treatment.

During the interpretative process, it is often informative to compare a patient's premorbid intellectual level with current intelligence test performance in order to determine the existence and extent of possible cognitive loss. In many cases, clinicians can only estimate pre-illness ability because information about actual premorbid functioning is not available. There is a growing body of literature available to clinicians to assist in the estimation of premorbid WAIS-R intelligence. Demographically based regression equations (Barona, Reynolds, & Chastain, 1984; Barona & Chastain, 1986) have been found, in general, to provide useful information concerning the possibility of intellectual decline (Eppinger, Craig, Adams, & Parsons, 1987; Paolo & Ryan, 1992; Paolo, Ryan, Tröster, & Hilmer, in press; Silverstein, 1987; Sweet, Moberg, & Tovian, 1990) and tend to have more predictive power than clinician's judgments (Kareken & Williams, 1994).

Another major aspect of the WAIS-R interpretive process is the examination of the subtest scaled scores. Current procedures for evaluating subtests consist of normative and ipsative methods. The normative procedure compares the current subtest score to the average of the normative sample ($M = 10$; $SD = 3$); any subtest falling outside ± 1 SD of the mean is a normative strength or weakness.

* Address for correspondence: Anthony M. Paolo, Ph.D., Department of Neurology, University of Kansas Medical Center, 3901 Rainbow Blvd., Kansas City, KS, 66160-7314, USA.
Accepted for publication: May 24, 1995.

The ipsative procedure compares the subtest score with the mean of the Verbal or Performance subtest scaled scores (if there is a significant IQ discrepancy) or of all 11 subtests (if there is no significant Verbal-Performance IQ difference) to determine relative strengths and weaknesses. Any subtest 3 or more points above or below the average is considered a relative strength or weakness, respectively (Kaufman, 1990).

These methods, while useful for describing current abilities, do not address the issue of whether a subtest has evidenced decline from a previously higher ability level for any particular patient. A subtest score, whether it is a strength or weakness, may also evidence deterioration. Kaplan, Fein, Morris, and Delis (1991) point out that a subtest score that is lower than that expected, based on educational and occupational attainment, suggests possible impairment in the cognitive domains measured by the subtest. However, there are no objective methods available to assist in the estimation of premorbid subtest scores as there are for estimating premorbid IQ. Therefore, clinicians are left to use their best judgment in determining whether a subtest score, be it a strength, weakness, or neither, might reflect an impairment.

One purpose of this study was to develop demographically based regression equations for the estimation of premorbid subtest scaled scores and to determine their utility in a sample of brain-damaged persons. A second purpose was to evaluate whether the estimated premorbid subtest scaled scores provide information not readily suggested by normative and ipsative subtest score comparisons.

METHOD

Participants

The 1880 individuals from the WAIS-R standardization sample (Wechsler, 1981) and the 130 elderly persons from the old age WAIS-R standardization sample (Ryan, Paolo, & Brungardt, 1990) served as the normal participants. Briefly, the WAIS-R standardization sample consists of persons 16 to 74 years of age, stratified on the basis of age, education, race, occupation, urban-rural residence, and geographic region. Equal numbers of males and females were included at each age level. The old age WAIS-R sample consists of persons 75 to 96 years of age, stratified on the basis of age, education, gender, and race. Therefore, the total normal sample consisted of 2010 persons ranging in age from 16 to 96 years.

A sample with brain damage referred for neuropsychological assessment was collected from a midwestern Veterans Affairs Medical Center and a university-based outpatient clinic. This group consisted of 221 males and 26 females ranging from 16 to 95 years of age. Means for age and education were 58.12 years $(SD = 12)$ and 11.91 years $(SD = 2.83)$, respectively. The sample consisted of 229 Whites, 17 Blacks, and 1 Hispanic whose primary language was English. Diagnoses included stroke $(n = 58)$, closed-head injury $(n = 46)$, Alzheimer's disease $(n = 40)$, alcohol dementia $(n = 20)$, dementia of unknown etiology $(n = 19)$, epilepsy $(n = 18)$, Parkinson's disease $(n = 16)$, cerebral tumor $(n = 10)$, Huntington's disease $(n = 6)$, cerebral anoxia $(n = 4)$, multiple sclerosis $(n = 4)$, hydrocephalus $(n = 4)$, neurotoxin exposure $(n = 1)$, and progressive supranuclear palsy $(n = 1)$.

Procedure

The WAIS-R manual contains a thorough description of the data collection procedures used with normal participants 16 to 74 years of age (Wechsler, 1981). For persons 75 years and older, each was screened with a medical history questionnaire, a medication review, and the Geriatric Depression Scale (Yesavage et al., 1983) prior to inclusion in the study. All were considered free from neurologic disease or disorder, major systemic illness, past and current psychiatric disturbance, including significant depression. Each possessed adequate vision and hearing, although most individuals wore glasses and some required hearing aids. Persons with controlled age-related conditions (e.g., senile diabetes, essential hypertension, mild neurosensory hearing loss, etc.) were not excluded. After screening, each subject was scheduled for an interview and standard WAIS-R administration by one of four qualified examiners.

The persons with brain damage were referred for evaluation and completed the WAIS-R as part of a comprehensive neuropsychological work-up. All were required to be at least 16 years of age and have medically diagnosed or documented brain damage or dysfunction.

The obtained WAIS-R Verbal, Performance, and Full Scale IQ scores for individuals younger than 75 were computed according to the procedures outlined in the WAIS-R manual (Wechsler, 1981). For persons older than 74 years, IQ scores were calculated using the norms provided by Ryan et al. (1990). Scaled scores for all ages were computed in the standard fashion and based on Wechsler's 20- to 34-year-old reference group. It should be noted that the estimation of age-corrected subtest scores would also be clinically relevant, but these data were not available for persons 16 to 74 years of age from the WAIS-R standardization sample.

Analyses

The total normative sample of 2010 persons was randomly divided into two equal-sized groups. One group was used to develop the regression equations and the second for cross-validation. Separate stepwise multiple regression analyses were employed to determine which demographic variables best predicted each of the 11 WAIS-R subtest scores for the development sample. These regression equations were then used to predict the scaled scores of the cross-validation sample. Inspection of changes in the multiple correlations between the development and cross-validation samples was used to determine the generalizability of the equations. With successful cross-validation of the original equations, a new set of equations based on the combined development and cross-validation samples was generated. Equations based on larger sample sizes yield more stable estimates. The clinical utility of the final equations was evaluated in the sample of persons with confirmed brain damage or dysfunction. The codes used for the demographic variables for the analyses are presented in Table 1. Some clarification concerning the coding of occupation is warranted. In general, the examiner codes the current occupation of the person. If the person is retired, the occupation code should reflect the highest ranking pre-retirement occupation achieved.

Table 1. Demographic Codes Used for the Regression Analyses.

Age:	1 = 16–17	7 = 55–64
	2 = 18–19	8 = 65–69
	3 = 20–24	9 = 70–74
	4 = 25–34	10 = 75–79
	5 = 35–44	11 = 80–84
	6 = 45–54	12 = 85+
Education:	1 = 0–7	4 = 12
	2 = 8	5 = 13–15
	3 = 9–11	6 = 16+
Gender:	1 = Female	2 = Male
Race:	0 = Nonwhite	1 = White
Job:	1 = Unskilled	4 = Skilled
	2 = Semi-Skilled	5 = Manager/ Clerical/Sales
	3 = Not Working	6 = Professional/ Technical
Region:	1 = Southern	3 = Western
	2 = North Central	4 = Northeast
Residence:	1 = Rural	2 = Urban

Note. These codes were adapted from the WAIS-R (Wechsler, 1981). Standardization data of the Wechsler Adult Intelligence Scale – Revised. Copyright © 1981 by the Psychological Corporation. Used by permission. All rights reserved.

RESULTS

Since independence of predictor variables is an underlying assumption of multiple regression analysis, all independent variables were inter-correlated. The highest relationship was .40 between education and occupation. Since the magnitude of this coefficient was well below the recommended cut-off of .70 for possible multi-collinearity (Tabachnick & Fidell, 1989), it was concluded that the predictor variables were generally independent.

Table 2 presents the actual and estimated scaled score means and standard deviations for the development sample as well as the multiple correlation (R) coefficients and the standard error of estimates for the initial regression analyses. All multiple Rs were significant and ranged from .48 on Digit Span to .69 on Digit Symbol. In addition, there were no significant differences between actual and estimated subtest scaled scores (all paired t test $ps > .05$). When these equations were used to predict the scaled scores for the cross-validation sample, there was minimal shrinkage with a maximum drop of .03 in the multiple correlation on Digit Span. According to paired t tests, there were no significant differences between the actual and estimated subtest scaled scores. The good cross-validation reflects, in part, the large size of the development sample ($n = 1005$) as well as the lack of statistically significant differences between the development and cross-validation groups in terms of age, education, gender, race, occupational classification, region, residence, and overall ability level as measured by the Verbal, Performance, and Full Scale IQ scores. The successful cross-validation allows the development and cross-validation samples to be combined in order to generate more stable regression equations based on a larger sample of 2010 individuals.

Table 3 presents the actual and estimated scaled score means and standard deviations as well as the multiple Rs and the standard errors of estimate (SEe) for the final regression analyses based on the combined sample. All multiple correlations were significant and ranged from .47 on Digit Span to .69 for Digit Symbol. Moreover, there were no statistically reliable differences between the actual and estimated subtest scaled scores (all paired t test $ps < .05$). It should be noted that for all subtests,

Table 2. Summary of Results for the Predicted and Actual Scores for the Development Sample ($n = 1005$).

Subtests	Actual		Predicted			
	M	SD	M	SD	R	SEe
Information	9.27	2.86	9.24	1.77	.61	2.27
Digit Span	9.27	2.84	9.27	1.41	.48	2.49
Vocabulary	9.27	2.97	9.27	1.91	.64	2.29
Arithmetic	9.20	2.90	9.26	1.76	.58	2.36
Comprehension	9.35	3.03	9.37	1.82	.59	2.45
Similarities	8.74	3.13	8.71	1.87	.59	2.54
Picture Completion	8.68	3.17	8.69	1.71	.53	2.69
Picture Arrangement	8.51	3.14	8.50	1.81	.57	2.59
Block Design	8.65	3.04	8.67	1.89	.61	2.42
Object Assembly	8.63	2.95	8.64	1.50	.50	2.56
Digit Symbol	8.27	3.37	8.24	2.35	.69	2.44

Note. Standardization data of the Wechsler Adult Intelligence Scale – Revised. Copyright © 1981 by the Psychological Corporation. Used by permission. All rights reserved.

Table 3. Summary of Results for the Predicted and Actual Scores for the Final Equations Based on the Combined Development and Cross-Validation Samples ($N = 2010$).

Subtests	Actual		Predicted			
	M	SD	M	SD	R	SEe
Information	9.31	2.97	9.29	1.89	.63	2.31
Digit Span	9.30	2.88	9.32	1.39	.47	2.54
Vocabulary	9.29	2.99	9.29	1.96	.65	2.28
Arithmetic	9.29	2.98	9.31	1.80	.58	2.44
Comprehension	9.41	3.06	9.41	1.81	.59	2.48
Similarities	8.84	3.22	8.82	1.90	.58	2.61
Picture Completion	8.67	3.21	8.69	1.85	.56	2.66
Picture Arrangement	8.51	3.16	8.51	1.81	.57	2.60
Block Design	8.62	3.03	8.63	1.88	.60	2.42
Object Assembly	8.60	3.04	8.60	1.58	.51	2.61
Digit Symbol	8.28	3.42	8.26	2.36	.69	2.47

Note. Standardization data of the Wechsler Adult Intelligence Scale – Revised. Copyright © 1981 by the Psychological Corporation. Used by permission. All rights reserved.

less than 50% of the variance was explained by the demographic variables. Table 4 provides the final regression equations that can be used to predict WAIS-R subtest scaled scores for persons 16 to 96 years of age.

The accuracy of the equations to predict scaled scores within ±3 points (i.e., one standard deviation) for the normal sample was calculated. The accuracy rates was 76% on Arithmetic, 82% on Similarities and Picture Completion, 83% on Digit Span and Object Assembly, 85% on Comprehension, Picture Arrangement, and Digit Symbol,

86% on Block Design, 88% on Information, and 89% on Vocabulary. In general, these findings reveal good estimation of the actual subtest scaled scores for normal persons.

Table 5 presents means and standard deviations of the actual and estimated scaled scores for the sample with brain damage. Paired t tests revealed that, on the average, the estimated scaled scores were significantly greater than the actual scaled scores on the 11 subtests (all $ps < .001$). In everyday practice, the examiner calculates the difference between the estimated and obtained

Table 4. Demographic Regression Equations to Predict WAIS-R Subtest Scaled Scores.

Information	=	age (0.131) + educ (1.184) + sex (0.854) + race (1.084) + job (0.247) + 1.174.
Digit Span	=	age (−0.092) + educ (0.795) + race (0.744) + job (0.235) + 5.36.
Vocabulary	=	age (0.184) + educ (1.23) + race (1.341) + job (0.271) + 1.669.
Arithmetic	=	educ (0.981) + sex (0.945) + race (1.448) + job (0.254) + 2.09.
Comprehension	=	age (0.107) + educ (1.125) + race (1.344) + job (0.27) + 2.568.
Similarities	=	age (−0.138) + educ (1.156) + race (1.163) + job (0.21) + 3.531.
Picture Completion	=	age (−0.388) + educ (0.84) + sex (0.508) + race (1.468) + 5.531.
Picture Arrangement	=	age (−0.409) + educ (0.757) + sex (0.385) + race (0.775) + job (0.148) + region (0.139) + 5.733.
Block Design	=	age (−0.355) + educ (0.71) + sex (0.655) + race (1.765) + job (0.21) + region (0.185) + 4.127.
Object Assembly	=	age (−0.382) + educ (0.641) + race (1.461) + 6.923.
Digit Symbol	=	age (−0.599) + educ (0.856) + sex (−0.947) + race (0.877) + job (0.251) + 7.971.

Note. Equations based on WAIS-R standardization sample. Standardization data of the Wechsler Adult Intelligence Scale – Revised. Copyright © 1981 by the Psychological Corporation. Used by permission. All rights reserved.

Table 5. Estimated and Actual WAIS-R Subtest Scores for the Brain-Damaged Sample.

Subtests	Actual		Estimated		
	M	SD	M	SD	t(246)*
Information	7.94	2.68	10.12	1.86	14.00
Digit Span	7.30	2.77	9.14	1.44	11.41
Vocabulary	7.85	2.72	9.87	1.96	12.86
Arithmetic	7.28	2.73	9.87	1.67	15.08
Comprehension	7.54	2.77	9.80	1.84	13.32
Similarities	6.43	2.89	8.77	1.90	15.03
Picture Completion	6.07	3.17	8.28	1.66	12.88
Picture Arrangement	5.77	2.69	7.93	1.62	14.99
Block Design	5.96	3.14	8.16	1.66	12.62
Object Assembly	5.71	3.16	7.98	1.49	13.35
Digit Symbol	4.10	2.69	6.74	2.20	18.18

*All paired t tests significant at $p < .001$.

scaled score and decides if that difference is clinically meaningful. The standard errors of estimate provided in Table 3 can assist in this process.

One-tailed confidence intervals at the 90% and 95% levels were computed from the SEe and rounded to the nearest whole number. One-tailed intervals are appropriate because the purpose of these estimation procedures is to assist in the determination of possible decline in subtest scores. For all 11 subtests, the rounded 90% interval is 3 points and the rounded 95% interval is 4 points. If the obtained scaled score is more than 3 points lower than the estimated scaled score, it falls below the 90% confidence limit, suggesting that the obtained score is beyond that expected from

measurement error for 90% of the normal persons in the standardization sample and is likely meaningful. For a more conservative estimate, the examiner can choose at 4-point discrepancy which is at the 95% confidence limit.

Table 6 presents the percentage of normal and brain-damaged persons whose obtained scaled score fell below the 90% and 95% confidence limit of the estimated scaled score. Proportional analyses using a Bonferroni corrected alpha level (i.e., $p < .002$), revealed that significantly more persons with brain dysfunction exceeded the 90% and 95% limits than did normal individuals for all subtests. Inspection of the participants that fell below the 90% and 95% confidence limits, showed

Table 6. Percentage of Normal and Brain-Damaged Persons whose Obtained Scaled Score Exceeded the 90% and 95% Confidence Limits.

Subtests	90% Confidence limit (>3 points)		95% Confidence limit (>4 points)	
	Normal	Neurologic	Normal	Neurologic
Information	6	27	2	16
Digit Span	8	28	3	14
Vocabulary	4	26	1	14
Arithmetic	6	38	3	22
Comprehension	6	30	3	16
Similarities	8	34	3	18
Picture Completion	9	33	4	19
Picture Arrangement	6	29	2	14
Block Design	7	31	3	21
Object Assembly	9	33	4	23
Digit Symbol	7	38	2	22

Note. Between-group proportional analyses all significant at the Bonferroni corrected alpha level of $p < .002$.

that at least 70% of these persons obtained scaled scores of 6 or less for both the normal and brain-damaged groups. Further, no normal or brain-impaired person who obtained a scaled score of 14 or more points evidenced possible decline on any subtest. These findings demonstrate that level of ability is important when interpreting the difference between estimated and obtained scaled scores.

Interpreting deterioration for individual subtests can provide useful information concerning the construct that is measured by the subtest under investigation. Another important issue is the total number of subtests that evidence possible deterioration. If it is common for normal persons to display only one or two subtests that fall below the selected confidence limit, then interpretation of only a single subtest that demonstrated decline may be inappropriate for any particular individual. Table 7 provides the frequency distribution of the number of subtests that evidenced possible decline at the 90% and 95% confidence limits. Using the 90% confidence limit, it can be seen that the majority (91%) of normal subjects had no more than two subtests showing possible decline, while 49% of the brain-damaged individuals evidenced decline in two or less subtests. Considering the 95% confidence limit, 94% of the normal subjects had at most one subtest showing possible decline, while 59% of the neurologic group evidenced a similar finding.

To determine whether comparing the estimated and obtained subtest scores provides information in addition to that of normative and ipsative subtest analyses, the number of brain-damaged persons that demonstrated strengths and weaknesses for the normative and ipsative procedures was cross-tabulated with the number of persons evidencing possible decline from the estimated subtest scores. For the normative analyses, obtained subtest scores from 1 to 6 were weaknesses, 7 to 13 were average, and 14 or more were strengths. Table 8 presents the number and percentage of brain-damaged persons who displayed unusual decline at the 90% confidence limit by normative subtest ability level classifications. As the data reveal, 12% of persons with average Vocabulary scaled scores evidenced possible decline on this subtest. In contrast, 52% of the individuals with a normative weakness on Block Design did not demonstrate potential decline from their estimated ability on this subtest. Overall, comparisons between the estimated and actual sub-test scaled scores seems to provide additional infor-mation about subtest performance that cannot be gleaned from simple normative analysis alone.

For the ipsative procedure, the average of all 11 subtests was used for comparison because less than 10% of the brain-damaged persons evidenced an abnormal Verbal-Performance IQ discrepancy of ±21 points (Ryan, Paolo, & Van Fleet, 1994).

Table 7. Cumulative Distribution of the Number of Subtests that Displayed Possible Decline at the 90% and 95% Confidence Limits for Normal and Brain-Damaged Persons.

Number of subtests evidencing decline	90% Confidence limit (>3 points)				95% Confidence limit (>4 points)			
	Normal		Brain damaged		Normal		Brain damaged	
	n	cum %	n	cum %	n	cum %	n	cum %
0	1314	65	53	22	1690	84	99	40
1	378	84	34	35	201	94	46	59
2	133	91	35	49	56	97	25	69
3	68	94	25	60	28	98	18	76
4	52	97	19	67	13	99	18	83
5	22	98	13	73	4	99	15	90
6	13	99	19	80	6	99	10	94
7	4	99	12	85	2	99	4	95
8	10	99	14	91	4	99	5	97
9	9	99	12	96	6	100	4	99
10	3	99	4	97	0	100	1	99
11	4	100	7	100	0	100	2	100

Table 8. Number and Percentage of Brain-Damaged Subjects Exceeding the 90% Confidence Limit by Normative Subtest Ability Levels.

Subtests	Scaled score range and classification					
	1 to 6 (weakness)		7 to 13 (average)		14 or more (strength)	
	n	%	n	%	n	%
Information	47	55	19	12	4	0
Digit Span	55	55	13	9	4	0
Vocabulary	45	54	18	12	8	0
Arithmetic	77	70	16	12	2	0
Comprehension	54	62	20	13	7	0
Similarities	75	56	8	7	0	0
Picture Completion	82	54	0	0	3	0
Picture Arrangement	70	44	2	2	1	0
Block Design	77	48	0	0	7	0
Object Assembly	82	54	0	0	2	0
Digit Symbol	94	44	1	3	1	0

Table 9 presents the proportion of persons with brain damage that displayed abnormal subtest decline according to the 90% confidence limit by ipsative classification (i.e., strength, weakness, or not significant). It can be seen that any subtest may evidence decline from the estimated premorbid scaled score, regardless of whether that subtest is also an ipsative weakness or not significantly different from the average of the subtest scaled scores. Further, some subtests evidenced possible

decline from the estimated premorbid scaled score even though they were considered an ipsative strength. For instance, on the Vocabulary subtest 6 persons displayed a relative weakness and 3 (50%) of these also demonstrated an abnormal decline from their estimated premorbid Vocabulary subtest score. Similarly, 57 individuals evidenced a relative strength on Vocabulary and 5 (9%) of these also demonstrated an unusual discrepancy from the estimated score. Further inspection

Table 9. Percentage of Brain-Damaged Persons that Evidenced Subtest Decline at the 90% Confidence Limit by Ipsative Analysis Classification.

Subtests	Ipsative classification		
	Weakness	NS	Strength
Information	83	31	10
Digit Span	94	31	0
Vocabulary	50	30	9
Arithmetic	82	42	3
Comprehension	40	36	8
Similarities	79	32	0
Picture Completion	90	27	0
Picture Arrangement	64	25	0
Block Design	75	26	0
Object Assembly	84	22	0
Digit Symbol	53	22	0

Note. NS = Not significantly different from the average of the 11 scaled scores.

reveals that when a subtest is a weakness, it usually displays abnormal decline from the estimated subtest score, but not in all cases. Thus, these tabulations reveal that comparisons between the estimated and obtained scaled scores provide additional information about subtest performance not necessarily evident from ipsative comparisons alone.

Another important issue concerning whether a clinician might wish to spend additional time to calculate the estimated subtest scores refers to whether or not estimated subtest scores yield information beyond that provided by estimated IQ values. The difference between the estimated and obtained scaled scores was correlated with the difference score between the estimated (Barona et al., 1984) and obtained IQs for the normal and brain-damaged groups. The coefficients for the normal group ranged from .58 on Digit Span and Digit Symbol to .77 on Vocabulary, with a median correlation of .70. For persons with central nervous system dysfunction, the coefficients ranged from .62 on Digit Span to .81 on Object Assembly, with a median correlation of .76. These coefficients reveal substantial overlap in the rank ordering of persons according to the differences between estimated subtest and IQ scores and their respective obtained values.

Similar rank ordering, however, does not necessarily reflect similarity in classification of persons

as evidencing potential deterioration. To assess the relationship between the IQ and subtest procedures in terms of classifying persons as displaying possible decline, the number of persons with brain damage demonstrating meaningful decline in Verbal IQ [i.e., the difference between the estimated and obtained IQ exceeded the 90% cut-off scores presented by Paolo et al., (in press)] was cross-tabulated with those showing potential decline on the six Verbal subtests. A similar procedure was followed for the Performance Scale. Table 10 presents the percentage of brain-damaged persons that evidenced a possible decline in subtest scores by those with and without corresponding decline in IQ.

Although many of the persons who displayed deterioration in IQ also showed decline in subtest performance, there was variability across subtests. Of the 85 individuals who evidenced decline in Verbal IQ, 72% also demonstrated decline on Arithmetic, but only 45% showed decline on Voca-bulary. Conversely, of the persons who did not show a decline in Verbal intelligence, 15% to 20% evidenced possible decline on at least one Verbal subtest. Similar results occurred for the Performance Scale. These findings reveal that the com-parison between estimated and obtained subtests scaled scores provides information not conveyed by demographically based IQ prediction equations.

DISCUSSION

This project developed demographically based regression equations to predict WAIS-R subtest scaled scores. The initial regression equations cross-validated successfully and, therefore, final regression equations were generated on a large sample of normal persons ranging from 16 to 96 years of age. There were no significant differences between estimated and obtained scaled scores for normal subjects and in about 80% or more of the cases, the estimated and obtained scaled scores fell within one standard deviation of each other. Significant mean differences emerged between the estimated and actual scaled scores for persons with brain dysfunction. Thus, the prediction equations may yield useful information for the detection of possible deterioration in subtest

Table 10. Percentage of Brain-Damaged Subjects Demonstrating Possible Decline in Subtest Scores by Those With and Without Possible Deterioration in IQ.

Subtests	Verbal IQ		Performance IQ	
	No decline (n = 162)	Decline (n = 85)	No decline (n = 154)	Decline (n = 93)
Information	15	49		
Digit Span	17	48		
Vocabulary	15	45		
Arithmetic	20	72		
Comprehension	17	55		
Similarities	17	66		
Picture Completion			18	58
Picture Arrangement			9	62
Block Design			12	63
Object Assembly			18	58
Digit Symbol			15	77

performance of persons with suspected or confirmed central nervous system damage.

In clinical practice, the examiner would likely subtract the obtained scaled score from the estimated score and decide if the difference is meaningful. If it is, the discrepancy should be explained. To assist clinicians in the decision of whether a difference score is meaningful, 90% and 95% confidence limits based on the SEe are provided. Persons who fall below the selected confidence limit demonstrate a difference between the estimated and obtained scaled score that is not due to measurement error and as such, may reflect a meaningful difference.

The clinical utility of the estimated premorbid equations to suggest possible decline in subtest ability was evaluated in a sample of persons with confirmed brain damage or dysfunction. Overall, one-fourth to one-third of the persons with neurologic dysfunction evidenced possible deterioration in at least one subtest. However, level of ability must be considered when interpreting the difference between estimated premorbid and obtained scaled scores. Consistent with other research that has employed demographic characteristics to estimate premorbid ability (Barona et al., 1984; Eppinger et al., 1987, Paolo & Ryan, 1992; Paolo et al., in press), the current equations tend to underestimate ability at the high end and overestimate ability at the low end. In the clinical setting, this phenomena may manifest itself as identifying relatively low scaled scores (i.e., 6 or less) as reflecting deterioration when in fact it may not be, while categorizing obtained scaled scores of 14 or more as normal, when they may actually be a decline for some persons with high abilities.

It is clear that the decision of whether an obtained scaled score represents deterioration from a previously higher level will require corroborating information. Such information may include specific educational and occupational attainment, family report, leisure activities, and so forth. In addition, the current results revealed that many normal persons may have one or two subtests that evidence possible decline. Thus, interpretation of a single subtest or only two subtests may not be warranted unless there is additional supportive information concerning the possible deterioration of the construct being measured.

Comparisons between the present procedure for determining possible subtest decline and established methods of describing current subtest abilities revealed that the difference between the estimated and obtained subtest scores yields information concerning subtest performance beyond that provided by the usual normative and ipsative evaluation methods. Individual subtests may constitute normative and/or ipsative strengths or weaknesses and also evidence possible decline from a previously higher ability level. In addition, the

Verbal and Performance IQ scores may evidence possible decline, but the subtests on which the IQ is based may or may not demonstrate decline. The latter suggests the possibility of a new method of profile analysis using the estimated subtest scaled scores for comparison. It should be noted that the relationships between IQ and subtest deterioration were examined using a sample of individuals with mostly chronic and diffuse cerebral pathology. It is possible that, in cases of acute and/or more localized pathology, subtest and IQ scores might be even less congruent. That is, in acute cases, one might expect subtest scaled scores to provide more information about specific cognitive decline than overall IQ.

In everyday practice, the traditional normative and ipsative subtest analyses should be conducted to describe current abilities. The calculation of estimated premorbid subtest scores will likely be most helpful for cases in which cognitive impairment is suspected or if the referral question is to rule out cognitive dysfunction. In such cases, the calculation of estimated premorbid subtest scores will likely provide additional information beyond that of the usual normative and ipsative WAIS-R subtest analyses.

The fact that less than 50% of the variance in subtest scaled scores can be predicted by demographic variables, suggests that information from additional sources (i.e., family, friends, work records, school records, etc.) must be sought to clarify any potentially meaningful discrepancies between the estimated premorbid subtest scores and a person's obtained score. One issue that deserves discussion is the choice of a single cross-validation method over the more elaborate and innovative double cross-validation procedure (Kerlinger & Pedhauzer, 1974; Peduzzi, Detre, Chan, Oberman, & Cutter, 1982). The double cross-validation method allows for a more thorough evaluation of the generalizability of the equations in order to determine if the two normal groups can be combined. The single cross-validation method was chosen for this study because of the large size of the development sample ($n = 1005$) and the equivalence of the development and cross-validation samples in terms of age, education, gender, race, region, residence, and overall ability level as measured by the Verbal, Performance, and Full Scale IQ scores. Because of the similarity of the two groups, it is highly likely that a double cross-validation procedure would have suggested (as did the single cross-validation procedure) that the development and cross-validation samples should be combined in order to generate more stable equations. Finally, it must be noted that the brain-impaired group was from the Midwest region of the USA and comprised of few females (11%) and non-Whites (7%). Since it has been reported that region, gender, and race can significantly impact WAIS-R subtests scores (Kaufman, McLean, & Reynolds, 1988), additional studies from different regions with larger groups of females and racial minorities should be conducted before routine application of these procedures is performed with such persons.

REFERENCES

Barona, A., Reynolds, C.R., & Chastain, R. (1984). A demographically based index of premorbid intelligence for the WAIS-R. *Journal of Consulting and Clinical Psychology, 52*, 885–887.

Barona, A., & Chastian, R.L. (1986). An improved estimate of premorbid IQ for Blacks and Whites on the WAIS-R. *International Journal of Clinical Neuropsychology, 8*, 169–173.

Eppinger, M.G., Craig, P.L., Adams, R.L., & Parsons, O.A. (1987). The WAIS-R index for estimating premorbid intelligence: Cross-validation and clinical utility. *Journal of Consulting and Clinical Psychology, 55*, 86–90.

Kaplan, E., Fein, D., Morris, R., & Delis, D.C. (1991). *WAIS-R as a neuropsychological instrument.* San Antonio, TX: The Psychological Corporation.

Kareken, D.A., & Williams, J.M. (1994). Human judgment and estimation of premorbid intellectual function. *Psychological Assessment, 6*, 83–91.

Kaufman, A.S. (1990). *Assessing adolescent and adult intelligence.* Boston: Allyn & Bacon.

Kaufman, A.S., McLean, J.E., & Reynolds, C.R. (1988). Sex, race, residence, region, and education differences on the 11 WAIS-R subtests. *Journal of Clinical Psychology, 44*, 231–247.

Kerlinger, F.N., & Pedhauzer, E.J. (1974). *Multiple regression in behavioral research.* New York: Holt, Rinehart, & Winston.

Paolo, A.M., & Ryan, J.J. (1992). Generalizability of two methods of estimating premorbid intelligence in the elderly. *Archives of Clinical Neuropsychology, 7*, 135–143.

Paolo, A.M., Ryan, J.J., Tröster, A.I., & Hilmer, C.D. (in press). Utility of the Barona demographic equations to estimate premorbid intelligence: Information from the WAIS-R standardization sample. *Journal of Clinical Psychology.*

Peduzzi, P.N., Detre, K.M., Chan, Y.K., Oberman, A., & Cutter, G.R. (1982). Validation of a risk function to predict mortality in a VA population with coronary artery disease. *Controlled Clinical Trials, 3,* 47–60.

Ryan, J.J., Paolo, A.M., & Brungardt, T.M. (1990). Standardization of the WAIS-R for persons 75 years and older. *Psychological Assessment: A Journal of Consulting and Clinical Psychology, 2,* 404–411.

Ryan, J.J., Paolo, A.M., & Van Fleet, J.N. (1994). Neurodiagnostic implications of abnormal verbal-performance IQ discrepancies on the WAIS-R: A comparison with the standardization sample. *Archives of Clinical Neuropsychology, 9,* 251–258.

Silverstein, A.B. (1987). Accuracy of estimates of premorbid intelligence based on demographic variables. *Journal of Clinical Psychology, 43,* 493–495.

Sweet, J.J., Moberg, P.J., & Tovian, S.M. (1990). Evaluation of Wechsler Adult Intelligence Scale-Revised premorbid IQ formulas in clinical populations. *Psychological Assessment: A Journal of Consulting and Clinical Psychology, 2,* 41–44.

Tabachnick, B.G., & Fidell, L.S. (1989). *Using multivariate statistics* (2nd ed.). New York: Harper Collins.

Wechsler, D. (1981). *WAIS-R Manual.* New York: The Psychological Corporation.

Yesavage, J.A., Brink, T.L., Rose, T.L., Lum, O., Huang, V., Adey, M., & Leirer, V.O. (1983). Development and validation of the Geriatric Depression Scale. *Journal of Psychiatric Research, 17,* 31–49.

Journal of Clinical and Experimental Neuropsychology
1995, Vol. 17, No. 6, pp. 909–917

Predicting Cognitive Impairment in Epilepsy: Findings from the Bozeman Epilepsy Consortium*

Esther Strauss[1], David Loring[2], Gordon Chelune[3], Michael Hunter[1], Bruce Hermann[4], Kenneth Perrine[5], Michael Westerveld[6], Max Trenerry[7], and William Barr[8]

[1]University of Victoria, [2]Medical College of Georgia, [3]Cleveland Clinic, [4]Baptist Memorial Hospital, [5]New York University, [6]Yale University, [7]Mayo Clinic, and [8]Long Island Jewish Medical Center

ABSTRACT

We examined the contribution of age of seizure onset, seizure duration, seizure laterality, seizure location, gender, handedness, and cerebral speech representation to cognitive attainment in 1,141 patients with medically refractory seizures. The combined influence of the predictor variables was modest. Age of seizure onset was the best single indicator of Full Scale IQ (partial r = .23) and General Memory (partial r = .20). Laterality and location of dysfunction, and cerebral speech dominance were also relevant and independent indicators of aspects of cognition. Except for age of onset of seizures (early onset was associated with poorer cognitive attainment), however, the magnitude of the effects was limited.

Seizure disorders are associated with an increased frequency of intellectual impairment (e.g., Aldenkamp, Alpherts, Dekker, & Overweg, 1990; Seidenberg & Berent, 1992; Tarter, 1972; Trimble, 1990). Although many potential risk factors of cognitive impairment have been investigated, there are few firm conclusions.

Age of seizure onset is an important predictor of cognitive ability, with early age of seizure onset linked to lower intellectual status (e.g., Dam, 1990; Dikmen, 1980; Dodrill, 1991; Dodrill & Mathews, 1992; Lennox & Lennox, 1960; Tarter, 1972). Dodrill and Mathews (1992) reported that Full Scale IQ (FSIQ) scores on the Wechsler Adult Intelligence Scale (WAIS) increased linearly with age of seizure onset from a mean of 83 when seizure onset began during the first year of life, to a mean of 102 for adult seizure onset. Preliminary data on a relatively small (n = 121) sample of patients (Strauss, Hunter, & Wada, in press) suggest that age of seizure onset emerges as an important predictor of intellectual functioning, even when the influences of other potentially important factors are controlled.

The unique contribution of other variables is less certain. *Seizure duration* may also be associated with intellectual attainment, with longer seizure duration associated with poorer intellectual ability (Delaney, Rosen, Mattson, & Novelly 1980; Dikmen, 1980; Dikmen & Mathews, 1977; Singhi, Bansal, & Singhi, 1992; Tartar, 1972). The predictive power of seizure duration, however, appears weaker than age at seizure onset. Dodrill and Mathews (1992) found that the correlation between mental ability (FSIQ) and duration of disorder, although reliable, is smaller in magnitude

* This work was supported in part by grants from NSERC and The March of Dimes to E. Strauss. We thank Dr. Lou Costa for his helpful comments. The order of the second through to the eighth author was determined randomly. Drs. William Barr, Gordon Chelune, Bruce Hermann, David Loring, Ken Perrine, Esther Strauss, Max Trenerry, and Michael Westerveldt are all members of the Bozeman Epilepsy Consortium.
Author's address for reprints: Esther Strauss Ph.D., Department of Psychology, University of Victoria, P.O.Box 3050, Victoria, British Columbia, Canada V8W 3P5.
Accepted for publication: May 30, 1995.

$(r = -.13)$ than the relation between cognition and age at seizure onset $(r = .29)$. Seizure duration, however, is related to other predictors of intellectual attainment, including age at seizure onset, which are themselves also related to intellectual status. When these other important factors are controlled for, the unique contribution of seizure duration to the prediction of intellectual ability may be negligible (Strauss et al., in press).

The influence of seizure location (e.g., temporal, extratemporal) is also controversial. Milner (1975) reported that general indices of intelligence are generally insensitive to location of disturbance. In contrast, we (Strauss et al., in press) observed that location of dysfunction is as potent a predictor of intellectual status as age of seizure onset. Extratemporal dysfunction, typically frontal lobe, was associated with lower FSIQ.

The effect of laterality of disturbance is also not clear. Some have suggested that laterality expresses itself in differential Verbal-Performance IQ discrepancies (e.g., Meier & French, 1966; Milner, 1958), although the effect tends to be weak (Dikmen, 1980; Jones-Gotman, Smith, & Zatorre, 1992). Stronger effects involving specific neuropsychological deficits have been reported in association with dysfunction to particular hemispheric sites. Thus, material-specific memory deficits vary with the side of temporal lobe dysfunction (Delaney et al., 1980), although the nonverbal memory deficits associated with right temporal lobe dysfunction are less consistent than the verbal memory impairment seen with left temporal lobe disturbance (Barr, 1995; Dikmen, 1980). Laterality of dysfunction associated with frontal lobe disturbance has also been reported, although the effect is less striking than that observed from temporal lobe disturbance (B. Milner cited in Kolb & Whishaw, 1990, p. 469).

Other variables also may be linked to cognitive functioning. For example, in epilepsy populations, males may be at greater risk than females for intellectual difficulties (Stores, 1978; Strauss, Wada, & Hunter, 1992), especially when verbal abilities are considered (Seidenberg et al., 1986; Strauss et al., in press). Left-handed patients are also likely to show a general cognitive impairment (Satz, Strauss, Hunter, & Wada, 1994; Strauss et al., in press), and people with atypical cerebral

speech dominance show a general cognitive retardation, with particular devastation to nonverbal functions (Milner, 1974; Satz et al., 1994; Strauss, Satz, & Wada, 1990; Strauss et al., in press). Both left-handedness and atypical speech dominance may figure as prominent risk factors because they reflect markers of gross disturbance to the left hemisphere during neuronal development.

To summarize, a number of risk factors for cognitive functioning have been suggested; however, there are few firm conclusions. The inconsistencies likely stem in part from the fact that investigators typically base their findings on relatively small samples (less than 200 cases) drawn from a single institution. Thus, results may reflect chance/sample specific fluctuations. Moreover, there is a dearth of research that has systematically investigated both the combined and unique contributions of these variables to cognitive ability in epilepsy patients. Finally, most of the attention regarding risk factors has been devoted to global indicators of neuropsychological status (e.g., Full Scale IQ, Halstead Impairment Index), and few studies have examined other areas, such as verbal and nonverbal memory. The latter omission is particularly striking given the high incidence of memory complaints in epilepsy populations, particularly those with temporal lobe epilepsy (TLE) (Chelune, Bornstein, & Prifitera, 1990; Jones-Gotman et al., 1992).

We undertook a detailed evaluation of the predictive power of several of the major neurocognitive variables (age of onset of seizures, duration, location and laterality of dysfunction, sex, handedness, cerebral speech pattern) associated with intellectual attainment in epilepsy. We expanded on previous studies in the following ways. First, our pool of potential subjects represents the largest group of epilepsy patients studied to date and comes from the Bozeman Epilepsy Consortium, a collaboration among eight epilepsy surgery centers in the United States and Canada. Second, statistical techniques were used to determine the *combined* and *unique* contribution of the variables for cognitive outcome. In this way, the relative explanatory power of the variables could be determined. Third, we studied two broad domains of functioning: general intellectual status (Full Scale IQ, Verbal IQ, Performance IQ) and memory

(General Memory, Verbal Memory, Visual Memory, Delayed Memory)[1]. Finally, we examined consistency of these predictors across both of these domains (intellectual status, memory).

Based on a review of the literature, the following general predictions were made:

1. We expected age of seizure onset to be the single best predictor of general intellectual status. Specifically, the earlier the age of onset, the worse the cognitive performance.
2. Duration of seizure disorder was also hypothesized to correlate with overall intellectual level, although its unique predictive power was expected to be smaller than that of seizure onset age. A greater degree of intellectual impairment was expected to be associated with disorders of longer duration.
3. Location of disturbance was expected to emerge as a strong correlate of general intellectual ability, with extratemporal dysfunction associated with poorer cognitive attainment.
4. Conventional measures of intelligence were expected to be relatively insensitive as indicators of lateralized dysfunction. When more specialized material-specific memory tasks were used, lateralized patterns of performance were expected to emerge. Because the left hemisphere is typically specialized for language related functions, and the right hemisphere is specialized for nonverbal functions, we anticipated that laterality of disturbance would be manifested, at least weakly, in predictable patterns of asymmetry in cognitive performance: left hemisphere dysfunction was expected to be associated with relative impairment in verbal abilities (viz., verbal memory) whereas right hemisphere disturbance was expected to be linked to nonverbal dysfunction (viz., nonverbal memory).
5. We hypothesized that gender would be related to cognitive status, with females outperforming males, particularly with respect to verbal functions.

6. Handedness was expected to be linked to general cognitive status, with poorer overall cognition in left-handers.
7. Cerebral speech pattern was also expected to be associated with intellectual attainment. Atypical speech was expected to be related to poorer overall cognition, and in particular, deficits in nonverbal ability.

METHOD

Subjects

The subject pool was patients with medically refractory seizures from the Bozeman Epilepsy consortium, a collaboration among eight epilepsy surgery centers (Cleveland Clinic, Long Island Jewish Medical Center, Mayo Clinic, Epi-Care Center, Yale University, New York University/Hospital for Joint Diseases, Medical College of Georgia and University of British Columbia (and University of Victoria)[2]. The current database consists of more than 1500 patients, most with temporal lobe dysfunction, who have been evaluated for possible surgical treatment. Patients were considered for inclusion in this study if they met the following criteria: (a) neurophysiological evidence of dysfunction to either the right or the left hemisphere from lateralized partial seizures; (b) information was available regarding age at onset of recurrent seizures, duration (computed as age at time of examination minus age at seizure onset) and location (temporal, extratemporal) of dysfunction, gender, hand preference and cerebral language dominance (left, atypical) and (c) they had received neuropsychological evaluation including the Wechsler Intelligence Scale – Revised (Wechsler, 1974; 1981) and/or the Wechsler Memory Scale-Revised (Wechsler, 1987).

The final sample consisted of 1,185 people: 590 men and 595 women. Carotid amytal testing revealed that the majority (1065 or 89.9%) had speech exclusively mediated by the left hemisphere whereas the remainder (120 or 10.1%) had atypical speech representation (right = 63; bilateral = 57). Most patients ($n = 1023$ or 86.3%) were right-handed. The remainder were left-handers or ambidextrals. The seizures tended to originate in the temporal lobes for most patients ($n = 1097$ or 92.6%). Approximately half of the cases ($n = 569$ or 48%) had their seizures lateralized to the right hemisphere whereas the remainder ($n = 616$ or 52%) had left-sided

---

[1] This study is in part a replication of some of the findings from an earlier study (Strauss, Hunter, & Wada, in press) pertaining to predictors of general intellectual attainment. However, it adds to the Strauss, Hunter, and Wada paper by focusing on a relatively neglected domain, memory.

[2] 121 cases from Strauss et al. (in press) were included for analysis. Additional analyses revealed that the results reported here for the entire group were identical to those obtained when these cases were deleted.

Table 1. Characteristics of the Sample.

N = 1,185

Gender	590 Men	595 Women
Speech	1065 Left	63 Right
Dominance		57 Bilateral
Handedness	1023 Right	162 Non-Right
Location	1097 Temporal	88 Extra-Temporal
Laterality	569 Right-Sided	616 Left-Sided
Age Sz Onset	11.91 Yrs (9.78)	
Age at Test	30.93 Yrs (9.65)	
Sz Duration	18.97 Yrs (10.79)	

seizure origin. In general, seizures began in childhood (mean = 11.91 years, SD = 9.78). At the time of cognitive testing, patients averaged 30.93 years of age (SD = 9.65) and had endured their seizure disorders for 18.97 years (SD = 10.79). The distribution of IQ scores was negatively skewed, with the average IQ falling in the low end of the average range (FSIQ mean = 88.61, SD = 12.33).

Materials and Procedure

Subjects were administered a battery of neuropsychological tests, including measures of general intellectual functioning and memory. The Wechsler Intelligence Scale (WAIS-R or WISC-R) (Wechsler, 1974, 1981) was administered according to standard instructions and Full Scale IQ (FSIQ), Verbal IQ (VIQ), and Performance IQ (PIQ) scores were computed. similarly, the Wechsler Memory Scale-Revised (WMS-R) (Wechsler, 1987) was given according to standard instructions and the following indexes were calculated: General Memory, Visual Memory, Verbal Memory, and Delayed Memory.

RESULTS

Table 2 presents the means and standard deviations for the patients on each dependent measure. As might be expected, mean scores for this sample of patients with medically refractory epilepsy tend to be lower than those for healthy individuals on all measures.

Analyses were directed at two issues: (1) We first examined the relationship of our predictor variables to the summary neuropsychological measures reflected by FSIQ, VIQ, and PIQ; (2) In addition, we examined the combined and unique contributions of the predictor variables to memory measures.

Table 2. Mean Performance on Cognitive Tasks (SD in Parentheses).[1]

Test	Patients	n
FSIQ	88.61 (12.33)	1084
VIQ	89.54 (12.67)	939
PIQ	89.84 (13.50)	939
GM	87.23 (17.72)	402
VRB Mem	88.01 (15.74)	439
VIS Mem	91.73 (16.77)	438
DEL Mem	85.09 (18.42)	273

Note. [1]Data for some subjects are missing since some centers do not give the particular test or all portions of the test. For example, in some centers FSIQ is estimated from a short form of the Wechsler test. In such cases, VIQ and PIQ are not calculated. Similarly, some centers do not give the WMS-R or all portions of the test.

IQ (FSIQ, VIQ, PIQ)

Three regression analyses were employed to evaluate whether FSIQ, VIQ, and PIQ were related to the predictor variables combined, and if so, to particular variables within the predictor set. For these analyses, a standard simultaneous multiple-regression analysis was computed for each IQ measure separately. The predictor variables included were age at chronic seizure onset, duration of disorder, location of dysfunction (temporal, extratemporal), laterality of disturbance (left, right), gender, speech dominance (left, atypical) and handedness (right, left).

FSIQ

An overall multiple correlation coefficient of .28 was obtained between the complete set of predictor variables and FSIQ [$F(7,1076)$ = 13.47, $p < .001$]. All variables together therefore accounted for 8% (R^2) of the variance in overall IQ (See Table 3). As expected, the individual variable most highly predictive of overall outcome was age of seizure onset (partial r = .23, $p < .001$). Early age of seizure onset was associated with poorer overall intellectual status. Full Scale IQ (FSIQ) scores increased in a linear fashion from age at onset during the first year of life (mean FSIQ = 84.4) to adult onset (i.e., age 20 years and above: mean FSIQ = 93.4).

Table 3. Relation of Neuropsychological Measures to Variables.[1]

	All	Duration	Onset	Sex	Speech	Hand	Lat	Loc
FSIQ	.28***		.23***				−.09**	.07*
VIQ	.28***		.20***				−.13***	
PIQ	.23***		.16***		.07*			.07*
GM	.25***		.20***					
VRB M	.28***		.22***					
VIS M	.15							
DEL M	.27*		.23***					

Note. [1]$p < .05 = *; p < .01 = **; p < .001 = ***$.
    All: [2]All predictors simultaneously; values in this column are multivariate R^2. Values in other columns are partial r.

Statistically significant contributions were also noted for laterality (partial $r = -.09, p < .005$) and location (partial $r = .07, p < .05$). Left-sided seizures were associated with poorer overall intellectual status when compared to right-sided seizures (mean FSIQ 87.4 vs. 89.9). Further, patients with extratemporal disturbances performed more poorly than those with temporal lobe dysfunction (mean FSIQ 85.60 vs 88.85).

The hypothesis regarding the relation of seizure duration to intellectual status was not supported. Seizure duration did not add a unique contribution.

VIQ

The predictor variables also generated a statistically significant multiple correlation coefficient of .28 for VIQ [$F(7,931) = 11.41, p < .001$], indicating that all variables taken together accounted for 8% of the variance in VIQ scores. The individual predictor variables most highly predictive of VIQ were age at seizure onset (partial $r = .20, p < .001$), and laterality (partial $r = -.13, p < .001$). VIQ was lower in those with an earlier age of seizure, and in those with a left-sided seizure focus.

PIQ

When PIQ was examined, the predictor variables yielded a statistically significant multiple correlation value of .23 [$F(7,931) = 7.30, p < .001$] and all variables together accounted for 5% of the variance. Of the individual predictor variables, age at seizure onset (partial $r = .16, p < .001$), location of dysfunction (partial $r = .07, p < .05$) and cerebral speech dominance (partial $r = .07, p < .05$), were reliable. Early age of seizure onset, extratemporal lobe dysfunction, and atypical speech were associated with poor non-verbal reasoning, as measured by PIQ.

Memory Measures (GM, Verbal Memory, Visual Memory, Delay Memory)

Four regression analyses were employed to evaluate whether GM, Visual, Verbal, and Delayed Memory were related to the predictor variables combined, and if so, to particular variables within the set. For these analyses, a standard simultaneous multiple-regression analysis was computed for each memory measure separately. The predictor variables were the same as those employed above and included age at seizure onset, duration of disorder, location of dysfunction (temporal, extratemporal), laterality of disturbance (left, right), gender, speech dominance (left, atypical) and handedness (right, left).

Correlates of General Memory

The regression of GM on the set of predictors revealed a statistically significant multiple correlation coefficient of .25 [$F(7,394) = 3.77, p < .001$], indicating that all variables together accounted for 6% of the variance in overall memory. Within the set of variables, only age at seizure onset was a significant predictor (partial $r = .20, p = .001$). Poor memory function tended to occur principally in those with early onset of seizures.

Correlates of Verbal Memory

An overall multiple correlation coefficient of .28 was obtained between Verbal Memory and the set of predictors [$F(7,431) = 5.39, p < .001$] and all variables together accounted for 8% of the variability in scores. Within the set, age at seizure onset (partial $r = .22, p < .001$) proved uniquely related to verbal ability. The relation between laterality and verbal memory approached significance (partial $r = -.09, p = .06$).

Correlates of Visual Memory
The overall relation of Visual Memory to the set of predictors was not significant [$F(7,430) = 1.3$, $p = .24$].

Correlates of Delayed Memory
The overall relation of Delayed Memory to the set of predictors was significant [$F(7,265) = 2.98$, $p = .005$]. The multiple correlation coefficient was .27, indicating that all variables together accounted for 7% of the variance in scores. Within the set, age at seizure onset (partial $r = .23$, $p < .001$) was a significant predictor of delayed recall. The relation between laterality (partial $r = -.11, p = .07$) and delayed memory approached significance. Poor delayed memory tended to occur in those with early age at seizure onset and, to some extent, in those with left-sided seizure origin.

DISCUSSION

This study profits from a database consisting of a very large sample of patients from diverse medical centers. The analyses focused on determining the relations between seizure-related factors and background characteristics (age at onset of seizures, duration, location and laterality of disturbance, handedness, sex and speech dominance) and general intellectual status and memory. The findings partially confirm and extend previous findings in the literature regarding predictors of cognitive ability in individuals with partial seizure disorders.

The combined influence of all the variables in predicting intellectual attainment was modest, the magnitude of the relations varying somewhat depending upon the target areas and accounting for between 5 and 10% of the variance. One way to put these findings into perspective is to classify patients into those whose general intellectual level is low average or better (e.g., Full Scale IQ 80 and above) and those whose level is borderline or worse (e.g., Full Scale IQ below 80), then using logistic regression analysis, determine the odds of being intellectually impaired as a function of age at seizure onset, duration, location, laterality,

handedness, gender, and cerebral speech dominance. The results of such an analysis on the current Full Scale IQ data showed that the odds of intellectual impairment for patients with extratemporal lobe disturbance were 1.35 times higher than those with temporal lobe disturbance ($z = 1.96$, $p < .05$), that patients with left-sided seizure origin were 1.60 times more likely to be intellectually impaired compared to patients with right-sided seizures ($z = 1.97$, $p < .05$), and that the odds of impairment decreased by .58 for each year increase in age at seizure onset ($z = -5.29$, $p < .001$).[3] Thus, although the variances accounted for were modest, they translate into meaningful classification indices. Moreover, the variances accounted for and the odds ratios would likely increase if the full ranges of both brain integrity and intelligence were present in the data rather than the restricted ranges on both dimensions that occur when epilepsy samples alone are considered.

Our findings confirm that age at seizure onset is the strongest single correlate of intellectual attainment. Full Scale IQ increased in a linear fashion from age of onset before 1 year of age (mean IQ = 84.4) to adult onset (mean IQ = 93.4). Similar differences between early and late onset cases have been reported by others (Dodrill, 1991; Dodrill & Mathews, 1992; Lennox & Lennox, 1960; Strauss et al., in press). This may reflect a multifactorial relationship due to greater disruption of neuronal processes during certain critical phases of neurodevelopment, tendency to use medications that have adverse cognitive and behavioral effects, lifetime total number of seizures, years of education, and etiology. Since these factors are also affected by age at onset, our result likely reflects several sources of variation (Dodrill & Mathews, 1992; Holmes, 1991).

Laterality also proved a reliable predictor of intellectual ability, and in particular, of verbal functions. Thus, verbal reasoning and verbal memory deficits tended to occur in the context of left hemisphere dysfunction. Our effect, however,

---

[3] Similar analyses were carried out on the remaining intelligence and memory measures. The results agreed with the corresponding regression analyses and produced odds ratios in magnitude similar to those reported for Full Scale IQ.

appeared quite small. The weak findings in this area, as well as their limited scope (relating largely to verbal, as opposed to nonverbal, abilities) may be a reflection, at least in part, of the lack of sensitivity of the measures used (Loring, 1990). They are, however, consistent with previous work employing a wide variety of test instruments (Barr, 1995; Chelune et al., 1990; Dikmen, 1980; Jones-Gotman et al., 1992). It is also worth pointing out that the strongest effects in the literature are seen postoperatively, and that it is more difficult to find specificity of effects in non-operated patients (Jones-Gotman et al., 1992; Milner, 1975).

Location of dysfunction also influenced psychological abilities, albeit weakly. Kolb and Whishaw (1990) report that lesions in the frontal lobe affect intellectual status less than lesions in posterior parts of the brain although there is some conflicting evidence that IQ may be depressed in patients with frontal disturbance (Kaufman, 1990; Strauss et al., in press). In the current study, extratemporal dysfunction (typically frontal lobe) was associated with lower IQ, regardless of the laterality of the disturbance. The explanation for this effect is not certain. Longstanding disturbances in extratemporal regions may interfere with the sort of abilities required for adequate performance on standard IQ tests, particularly those aspects that require non-verbal reasoning or fluid intelligence. Alternatively, patients with extratemporal disturbances may have more extensive underlying pathology or a more severe seizure disorder. Prospective investigation is needed to sort out these and other possibilities.

Cerebral speech dominance also correlates with intelligence, at least nonverbal reasoning, although the effect is subtle. The apparent deficit in certain nonlanguage perceptual domains associated with atypical speech is well known (e.g., Lansdell, 1969; Milner, 1974; Satz et al., 1994; Strauss et al., 1990; Teuber, 1974) and has been termed "the crowding phenomenon". Crowding refers to transfer of language to the right hemisphere following left hemisphere insult: while verbal functions are relatively spared, nonverbal functions are depressed. The reason that cerebral speech dominance correlates with intellectual status is not certain, but it may reflect limitations in brain capacity associated with brain reorganization induced by early injury (Satz et al., 1994).

Table 4. Zero-order Correlations Between Predictor Variables and FSIQ, GM.[1]

	FSIQ	General Memory
Duration	−.11***	−.13**
Handedness	−.06*	−.01
Laterality	−.11***	−.09*
Gender	−.02	−.01
Speech	.05*	.01
Onset	.26***	.23***
Location	−.07**	−.04

Note. [1]$p < .05 =$ *; $p < .01 =$ **; $p < .001 =$ ***; two-tailed significance.

Duration of seizure disorder showed no consistent relation with cognitive status, a finding generally consistent with earlier work (Dodrill & Mathews, 1992; Strauss et al., in press). One reason that seizure duration has little direct impact on intellectual attainment is that many patients go for years without an attack whereas others have seizures frequently (Dodrill & Mathews, 1992). Farwell, Dodrill, and Batzel (1985) have suggested that the number of years with seizures may be a more potent variable. Unfortunately, these data were not available for our patients. Interestingly, if we had only considered zero-order correlations, as in most of the previous research, then duration of seizures does emerge as a significant predictor of both general intellectual status and memory. As Table 4 shows, the zero-order correlations between FSIQ and age at seizure onset was .26 ($p < .001$), followed by seizure duration at −.11 ($p < .001$), laterality at −.11 ($p < .001$), location at −.07 ($p < .01$), speech at .05 ($p < .05$), handedness at −.06 ($p < .05$) and gender at −.02 ($p = .26$). However, after partialling out the effects of other predictors, the unique contribution of seizure duration was not reliable.

Some investigators (Satz et al., 1994; Seidenberg et al., 1986; Stores, 1978; Strauss et al., in press) have reported that handedness and gender impact on cognitive functioning. Our current experience, based on this large population of patients, is that the direct influence of these variables is minimal, at least when general intellectual status and memory are considered.

Our study also revealed a diverse pattern of relationships among neuropsychological measures and predictor variables when each measure was considered individually. Deficits on verbal reasoning and verbal memory tasks were associated with early age at seizure onset and left-sided dysfunction. By contrast, nonverbal reasoning deficits, while linked to early age at seizure onset, were also correlated with extratemporal dysfunction and atypical cerebral speech dominance. Except for age at seizure onset, however, the effects were generally limited in magnitude.

A practical conclusion that can be drawn from our study is that in patients with medically refractory seizures, the unique contributions of gender, handedness, and seizure duration appear negligable. Age of seizure onset is the single best predictor of overall cognitive status (FSIQ, VIQ, PIQ) and memory. Laterality and location of dysfunction as well as speech dominance also provide some relevant information, although their effects are quite subtle and relate to particular aspects of cognition. Finally, it is worth bearing in mind that these variables, considered as a set or individually, are relatively modest at predicting later cognitive status in epilepsy patients, underscoring the need for caution when making clinical inferences based solely upon these factors.

REFERENCES

Aldenkamp, A.P., Alpherts, W.C.J., Dekker, M.J.A., & Overweg, J. (1990) Neuropsychological aspects of learning disabilities in epilepsy. *Epilepsia, 31,* S9–S20.

Barr, W.B. (1995). *The right temporal lobe and memory: A critical reexamination.* Paper presented to the International Neuropsychological Society Seattle.

Chelune, J.G., Bornstein, R.A., & Prifitera, A. (1990). The Wechsler Memory Scale-Revised: Current status and applications. In J. Rosen, P. McReynolds, & G. Chelune (Eds.), *Advances in psychological assessment, Vol. 7,* (pp. 65–100). New York: Plenum Press.

Dam, M. (1990). Children with epilepsy: The effect of seizures, syndromes, and etiological factors on cognitive functioning. *Epilepsia, 31,* S26–S29.

Delaney, R.C., Rosen, A.J., Mattson, R.H., & Novelly, R.A. (1980). Memory function in focal epilepsy: A comparison of non-surgical, unilateral temporal lobe and frontal lobe samples. *Cortex, 16,* 103–117.

Dikmen, S. (1980). Neuropsychological aspects of epilepsy. In B.P. Hermann (Ed.), *A multidisciplinary*

handbook of epilepsy (pp. 38–73). Illinois: Charles C. Thomas.

Dikmen, S., & Mathews, C. G. (1977). Effect of major motor seizure frequency upon cognitive-intellectual functions in adults. *Epilepsia, 18,* 21–29.

Dodrill, C.B. (1991). Neuropsychological aspects of epilepsy. *Psychiatric Clinics of North America, 2,* 383–394.

Dodrill, C.B., & Matthews, C.G. (1992). The role of neuropsychology in the assessment and treatment of persons with epilepsy. *American Psychologist, 47,* 1139–1142.

Farwell, J.R., Dodrill, C.B., & Batzel, L.W. (1985). Neuropsychological abilities of children with epilepsy. *Epilepsia, 26,* 395–400.

Holmes, G.L. (1991). The long-term effects of seizures on the developing brain: Clinical and laboratory issues. *Brain and Development, 13,* 393–409.

Jones-Gotman, M., Smith, M.L., & Zatorre, R.J. (1992). *Neuropsychological testing for localizing and lateralizng the epileptogenic region.* Paper presented at Palm Desert Epilepsy Surgery Conference, Palm Desert.

Kaufman, A.S. (1990). *Assessing adolescent and adult intelligence.* Boston: Allyn & Bacon.

Kolb, B., & Whishaw, I.Q. (1990). *Fundamentals of human neuropsychology.* New York: W.H. Freeman & Co.

Lansdell, H. (1969). Verbal and nonverbal factors in right-hemisphere speech: Relation to early neurological history. *Journal of Physiological and Comparative Psychology, 69,* 734–738.

Lennox, W.G., & Lennox, M.A. (1960). *Epilepsy and related disorders.* Boston: Little, Brown.

Loring, D.W. (1990). The Wechsler Memory Scale – Revised, or the Wechsler Memory Scale – Revisited? *Clinical Neuropsychologist, 3,* 59–69.

Meier, M.J., & French, L.A. (1966). Longitudinal assessment of intellectual functioning following unilateral temporal lobectomy. *Journal of Clinical Psychology, 22,* 22.

Milner, B. (1958). Psychological defects produced by temporal-lobe excision. *Research Publication of the Association for Research of Nervous and Mental Disorders, 36,* 244–257.

Milner, B. (1974). Hemispheric specialization: Scope and limits. In F.O. Schmitt & F.G. Worden (Eds.), *The neurosciences: Third study program* (pp. 75–89). Cambridge: MIT Press.

Milner, B. (1975). Psychological aspects of focal epilepsy and its neurosurgical management. In D.P. Purpura, J.K. Penry, & R.D. Walter (Eds.), *Advances in neurology* (pp. 299–321). New York: Raven Press.

Satz, P., Strauss, E., Hunter, M., & Wada, J. (1994). Re-examination of the crowding hypothesis: Effects of age of onset. *Neuropsychology, 8,* 255–262.

Seidenberg, M., & Berent, S. (1992). Childhood epilepsy and the role of psychology. *American Psychologist, 47,* 1130–1133.

Seidenberg, M., Beck, N., Geisser, M., Giordani, B., Sackerellas, J.C., Berent, S., Dreifuss, F.E., & Boll, T.J. (1986). Academic achievement of children with epilepsy. *Epilepsia, 27,* 753–759.

Singhi, P.D., Bansal, U., & Singhi, S. (1992). Determinants of IQ profile in children with idiopathic generalized epilepsy. *Epilepsia, 33,* 1106–1114.

Stores, G. (1978). Schoolchildren with epilepsy at risk for learning and behavior problems. *Developmental Medicine and Child Neurology, 20,* 502–508.

Strauss, E., Satz, P., & Wada, J. (1990). An examination of the crowding hypothesis in epileptic patients who have undergone the carotid amytal test. *Neuropsychologia, 28,* 1221–1227.

Strauss, E., Wada, J., & Hunter, M. (1992). Sex-related differences in the cognitive consequences of early left-hemisphere lesions. *Journal of Clinical and Experimental Neuropsychology, 14,* 738–748.

Strauss, E., Hunter, M., & Wada, J. (in press). Risk factors for cognitive impairment in epilepsy. *Neuropsychologia.*

Tartar, R.E. (1972). Intellectual and adaptive functioning in epilepsy. *Diseases of the Nervous System, 33,* 763–770.

Teuber, H.L. (1974). Why two brains? In F.O. Schmitt & F.G. Worden (Eds.), *The neurosciences: Third study program.* (pp. 71–74). Boston: MIT Press.

Trimble, M.R. (1990). Antiepileptic drugs, cognitive function, and behavior in children: Evidence from recent studies. *Epilepsia, 31,* S30–S34.

Wechsler, D. (1974). *WISC-R Manual.* New York: Psychological Corporation.

Wechsler, D. (1981). *WAIS-R Manual.* New York: Psychological Corporation.

Wechsler, D. (1987). *Manual for the Wechsler Memory Scale-Revised.* New York: Psychological Corporation.

The Clinical Neuropsychologist
1997, Vol. 11, No. 3, pp. 258–265

Behavioral Dyscontrol Scale: Criterion and Predictive Validity in an Inpatient Rehabilitation Unit Population*

Yana Suchy, Andy Blint, and David C. Osmon
University of Wisconsin-Milwaukee

ABSTRACT

The Behavioral Dyscontrol Scale (BDS) was administered to inpatient rehabilitation patients to examine (a) the cognitive correlates of factors found by previous research ($N = 68$), and (b) the ability of the BDS to predict patients' independence after discharge ($N = 46$). First, stepwise forward multiple regression using three BDS factors as criterion variables yielded three different models and led to relabeling the factors as Motor Programming factor, Fluid Intelligence factor, and Environmental Independence factor. Second, the BDS was found to be superior to the Mini-Mental State Exam (MMSE) in predicting living situation (independent vs. assisted) and Functional Independence Measure (FIM) scores 3 months after discharge.

The prediction of independent functioning of patients after discharge from a hospital is an important role of a clinical neuropsychologist. Such prediction has traditionally been difficult, partly because of the multitude of cognitive and behavioral determinants of independent functioning (Katz & Stround, 1989). For example, memory measures have been shown to predict success in a self-medication program (Palmer & Dobson, 1994). Executive functioning and memory portions of the Dementia Rating Scale (DRS) have been shown to be related to a variety of areas of independent functioning, such as hygiene, safety, and community utilization (Nadler, Richardson, Malloy, Marran, & Hostetler-Brinson, 1993). Finally, the Behavioral Dyscontrol Scale (BDS) has been shown to predict executive aspects of independent functioning, in particular, apathy and disinhibition (Kaye, Grigsby, Robbins, & Korzun, 1990).

The BDS is a new instrument created specifically for the purpose of assessing individuals' ability to engage independently in activities of daily living (ADLs) (Grigsby & Kaye, 1992; Grigsby, Kaye, & Robbins, 1990, 1992). The BDS is a 10-minute measure based primarily on simple cognitive and motor tasks used by Alexander Luria (1980) in his studies of frontal lobe functioning. Although deficits detected by this measure are often associated with lesions in the prefrontal cortex, they can also be common to a number of other lesions as well as to normal aging (Grigsby et al., 1990).

The construct and criterion validity of the BDS were demonstrated by several initial studies conducted by its creators. First, the BDS has been shown to predict difficulties with ADLs, whereas the Mini-Mental State Exam (Folstein, Folstein, & McHugh, 1975), a brief working memory measure (Luria, 1976), and the WAIS-R Similarities subtest failed to do so. Second, the BDS has been shown to be unrelated to depression or apraxia (Kaye et al., 1990). Finally, factor analysis of the BDS items yielded three factors, corresponding to

---

*A portion of the data used in this study was collected as part of the first author's Master's Thesis, and contributed to a study entitled "Milwaukee Card Sorting Test: A measure of forming, switching, and maintaining mental set" (under review). The structure of the BDS and its factors is not discussed in the above article. The results in Study 1 were presented at the Midwestern Psychological Association meeting in Chicago in May, 1995.
Address correspondence to: David Osmon, Ph.D., Dept. of Psychology, University of Wisconsin-Milwaukee, PO Box 413, Garland Hall, Milwaukee, WI 53201, USA.
Accepted for publication: October 31, 1996.

(1) "the ability to use intention and guide behavior"; (2) "the ability to use feedback"; and (3) "the capacity for inhibition" (Grigsby et al., 1992). These studies demonstrate (a) the ability of the BDS to tap into different executive functions, and (b) the relationship between individual aspects of executive functioning and the ability to engage in ADLs.

The purpose of the research presented in this paper was to examine the validity of the BDS. Toward this end, two studies were conducted: The first study examined the construct validity by focusing on the BDS factors and their cognitive correlates, whereas the second study focused on criterion validity by examining the ability of the BDS to predict patients' outcome after discharge from the hospital.

STUDY 1

This study explored the cognitive correlates of the individual BDS factors. The specific purposes were (a) to examine the clinical and theoretical usefulness of these factors by identifying differences in cognitive structure among the factors, and (b) to examine the appropriateness of the BDS factor labels by gaining additional information about the underlying cognitive abilities associated with each factor.

METHOD

Participants

Subjects were 68 mostly geriatric patients (47 females and 21 males) with orthopedic or neurological insult treated in the rehabilitation unit of Community Memorial Hospital in Menomonee Falls, Wisconsin. Patients with moderate to severe aphasia, unilateral neglect, perceptual dysfunction, color blindness, or psychiatric diagnosis were excluded from the study. Diagnoses for patients in Study 1 included: 33 patients with orthopedic insult or generalized weakness, 15 patients with right middle cerebral artery cerebrovascular accident (CVA), 13 patients with left middle cerebral artery CVA, 3 patients with multiple bilateral CVAs, and 1 each of patients with right hemisphere neoplasm, multiple sclerosis, Parkinson's disease, and cerebellar dysfunction of unknown origin. The mean age of the subjects was 72.31 years (range 31

to 91, $SD = 12.89$). Mean estimated premorbid Full Scale IQ (Barona, Reynolds, & Chastain, 1984) was 100.02 (range 80 to 118, $SD = 7.73$). Mean Mini-Mental State Exam score was 23.97 (range 11 to 30, $SD = 4.73$). IQ estimate was available only on 66 subjects because of missing demographic data.

Apparatus

The following tests were administered as part of a larger neuropsychological battery:

Behavioral Dyscontrol Scale (BDS)

The BDS consists of nine items. The first factor includes four motor learning and motor programming tasks (e.g., tapping twice with one hand, once with the other; fist-edge-palm task; piano exercise). The second factor included one alpha-numeric sequencing task (i.e., oral version of Trail Making Test, Part B; Reitan & Wolfson, 1993), one non-mirroring task (i.e., copying without mirroring), one measure of insight rating (i.e., awareness of errors and their significance). The third factor includes two go/no-go tasks (i.e., tapping twice when experimenter taps once and vice versa; squeezing experimenter's hand when the experimenter says "red" and doing nothing when the experimenter says "green"). Participants are trained on each task so that purely motor deficits (e.g., hemiparesis) or purely comprehension deficits (e.g., aphasia) would not affect the performance.

Milwaukee Card Sorting Test (MCST)

The MCST is a modification of the Wisconsin Card Sorting Test (WCST) (Osmon & Johnson, 1992; Osmon & Suchy, 1996). The main change in the MCST administration from the WCST format is the requirement that subjects verbalize the sorting principle before the placement of the cards. The perseverative response (PR) score (used as an independent measure in this study) was scored according to Heaton, Chelune, Talley, Kay, and Curtiss (1993).

Controlled Oral Word Association (COWA)

Subjects were asked to generate as many words as they could think of that began with each given letter. Letters C, F, and L of form # 1 were used (Benton, Hamsher, Varney, & Spreen, 1983). The total number of words for all three trials constituted a raw score, which was used as an independent measure in the present study. This test has been shown to be sensitive to both bilateral and unilateral prefrontal damage (Janowsky, Shimamura, Kritchevsky, & Squire, 1989).

Stroop Color and Word Test Part C (STPC)

The STPC was administered using materials and instructions obtained from Golden (1978). Frontal-lobe-damaged patients perform more poorly on this task (Stuss,

Kaplan, & Benson, 1982), and functional imaging studies have linked this task to activation in the medial prefrontal region (Pardo, Pardo, Janer, & Raichle, 1990).

WAIS-R Information (INFO)

INFO was administered according to standard procedures (Wechsler, 1981). It correlates moderately with Full Scale IQ ($r = .76$) (Sattler, 1992). Declines in this score can occur due to left hemisphere lesions (Spreen & Benton, 1965) or may reflect an Alzheimer's patients' breakdown in the ability to make accurate responses to verbal stimuli (Lezak, 1983). This score tends to be relatively unaffected by age or focal brain lesions, in particular, those located in the frontal lobes (O'Brien & Lezak, 1981).

WAIS-R Similarities (SIMIL)

SIMIL was administered according to standard procedures (Wechsler, 1981). The SIMIL subtest correlates moderately with Full Scale IQ ($r = .75$) (Sattler, 1992). Decline in this score is associated with aging (Lezak, 1983) as well as with left frontal and temporal lesions (McFie, 1975).

Mini-Mental State Exam (MMSE)

MMSE was administered using standard procedures. This test is considered to be sensitive to general cognitive efficiency (Folstein et al., 1975).

Procedure

The above battery was administered to participants in the conference room or empty dining room of the rehabilitation unit during normal daytime hours. The testing was done in 1 to 2 sessions, no more than 1 week apart, and took between 1 to 2 hr.

Data were analyzed with the use of forward stepwise multiple regression, using the BDS factor scores as criterion variables and the remaining tests in the battery as predictors. In addition, two random subsamples of equal size ($n = 34$ each) were generated from the original sample and subjected to the same analysis as the original sample in order to test the robustness of the results.

RESULTS

Using the BDS Factor 1 as the criterion variable, a stepwise forward multiple regression of the entire sample yielded MMSE and STPC as significant predictors, $F(2,65) = 26.14, p < .0001$, Adjusted Squared Multiple $R = .429$. Analyses conducted with random subsamples of the original sample also yielded MMSE and STPC as significant predictors, $F(2,31) = 14.91, p < .0001$, Adjusted Squared

Multiple $R = .457$ (subsample 1) and $F(2,31) = 10.52, p < .0001$, Adjusted Squared Multiple $R = .366$ (subsample 2).

Using the BDS Factor 2 as the criterion variable, the entire sample yielded MMSE, STPC, and SIMIL as predictors, $F(3,64) = 20.89, p < .0001$, Adjusted Squared Multiple $R = .471$. Random sub-samples yielded models that, though not identical, were consistent with the original model. Specifically, these analyses yielded MMSE and STPC (subsample 1) and STPC and SIMIL (subsample 2) as significant predictors, $F(2,31) = 16.71, p < .0001$, Adjusted Squared Multiple $R = .488$, and $F(2,31) = 13.90, p < .0001$, Adjusted Squared Multiple $R = .439$, respectively.

Using the BDS Factor 3 as the criterion variable, the entire sample yielded MMSE, STPC, and MCST PR score as significant predictors, $F(3,64) = 15.84, p < .0001$, Adjusted Squared Multiple $R = .399$. Random subsamples again yielded models that, though not identical, were consistent with the original model. Specifically, these analyses yielded MMSE and STPC (subsample 1) and STPC and MCST PR score (subsample 2) as significant predictors, $F(2,31) = 11.76, p < .0001$, Adjusted Squared Multiple $R = .395$, and $F(2,31) = 8.61, p < .001$, Adjusted Squared Multiple $R = .316$, respectively.

DISCUSSION

The results suggest that the models are relatively robust, with STPC being the most consistent predictor for all three factors across samples, confirming the test's strong executive load. The model for Factor 1 showed the greatest consistency, yielding identical results with all three samples. Factor 2 and 3 subsample models, though not identical, were highly consistent with the original models. The failure of some of the variables from the original models to enter into the subsample models may be due to the smaller sample size ($n = 34$). Given the overall consistency, the remainder of the discussion will be focused on the interpretation of the original models generated from the entire sample.

The results suggest that the three BDS factors represent different aspects of executive functioning, superimposed over a common "cognitive/executive core" that reflects the ability to orient, attend, and follow directions (MMSE), as well as the abilities to inhibit overlearned responses and to maintain a mental set (STPC). Because of this common core, it is imperative that specific abilities beyond those described above be identified and used for factor labels.

Factor 1 analysis did not yield any predictors beyond the core. However, Factor 1 items seemed to rely heavily on volitionally generated motor responses, suggesting that abilities unique to motor programming and motor learning may be needed for performance of Factor 1 items. Because no such specific predictors were used in the study Factor 1 was labeled in somewhat general terms the Motor Programming factor.

Factor 2 was related to the Similarities subtest of the WAIS-R, performance of which declines with age (Lezak, 1983), a hallmark of fluid intelligence. Thus, this factor was labeled the Fluid Intelligence factor, consistent with the nature of its items, but only partly consistent with previous interpretation.

Factor 3 was related to the PR score of the MCST. Because perseveratory responding is complex and can result from a breakdown in a variety of processes (Osmon & Suchy, 1996), it can, and does, underpin faulty performance on Factor 1 as well. Because Factor 3 items challenge the ability to volitionally generate appropriate behaviors in a rapidly changing environment, perseveration here seems to be related to the inability to maintain flexible interaction between the internal and the external motor systems (Goldberg, 1987). Such inability may lead to the "environmental dependency" syndrome (Lhermitte, 1986). For this reason, this factor was labeled Environmental Independence factor. This label is only partially consistent with the previous interpretation of this factor.

STUDY 2

The purpose of the present study was to explore the predictive validity of the BDS and the predictive utility of the BDS factor scores. Specifically, it was hypothesized that the BDS would (a) predict independence of patients after discharge from a hospital, and (b) be more closely associated with

outcome than would the Mini-Mental State Exam (MMSE).

METHOD

Participants
Forty-six patients (32 females and 14 males) were selected from among those participating in Study 2 on the basis of the availability of 3-month discharge follow-up information. Diagnoses for patients in Study 2 included: 25 patients admitted for orthopedic insult or generalized weakness, 8 patients with right middle cerebral artery cerebrovascular accident (CVA), 10 patients with left middle cerebral artery CVA, 3 patients with multiple bilateral CVAs, and 1 each of patients with right hemisphere neoplasm, multiple sclerosis, Parkinson's disease, and cerebellar dysfunction of unknown origin. The mean age was 73.96 years (range 43 to 91, $SD = 11.17$). Mean estimated premorbid Full Scale IQ was 100.15 (range 80 to 117, $SD = 8.06$). Mean Mini-Mental State Exam score was 24.37 (range 12 to 30, $SD = 4.03$).

Apparatus
In addition to the BDS and MMSE, the *Functional Independence Measure* (FIM) was used. FIM is an assessment instrument developed by Uniform Data System for Medical Rehabilitation that provides, through a ranking system, an indication of severity of a person's disability and dependence at admission to the rehabilitation unit, at discharge, and at 3-month follow-up. FIM affords a cognitive subtotal, a motor subtotal, and a grand total reflecting the sum of the two subtotals. Information regarding the patients' living and work settings, and the identity of the phone interviewee for follow-up information is also collected. FIM scores have been demonstrated to have test–retest reliability of .95 and intraclass correlation of .88 (Fiedler, 1993).

Procedure
Participants were administered the BDS in the manner described in Study 1. Three months after discharge, the rehabilitation unit social worker, who was blind to the hypotheses of the study, conducted structured phone interviews with former patients or their caretakers to obtain FIM follow-up data as a routine procedure of the rehabilitation unit.

A set of stepwise forward multiple regressions were conducted using (a) living setting (home vs. assisted living, such as a nursing home) at discharge; (b) living setting at 3-month follow-up; and (c) follow-up FIM scores (cognitive and motor subtotals, and the grand total) as criterion variables. The three BDS factor scores, the total BDS score, and the MMSE score were used as predictors. When FIM scores were used, the source of information (i.e., patient or other) was forced into the equation first to control for subjective versus objective reports.

RESULTS

When living setting (home vs. assisted living) at discharge was used as a measure of outcome, the Fluid Intelligence factor of the BDS was the only predictor that entered into the model, $F(1,44) = 14.44$, $p < .0001$, Adjusted Squared Multiple $R = .230$. When living setting at 3-month follow-up was used as a measure of outcome, the Motor Programming factor of the BDS emerged as the only predictor, $F(1,44) = 15.58$, $p < .0001$, Adjusted Squared Multiple $R = .245$. Means and standard deviations of the MMSE and the BDS and its factors for the entire sample, for patients discharged to home, those discharged to a nursing home temporarily, and those discharged to a nursing home (or other assisted living setting) permanently can be found in Table 1.

When total FIM score at 3 months after discharge was used as a measure of outcome, the total BDS score emerged as the only significant predictor, $F(2,43) = 17.65, p < .0001$, Adjusted Squared Multiple $R = .425$. When cognitive FIM score at 3 months after discharge was used as a measure of outcome, the MMSE and the BDS Fluid Intelligence factor emerged as predictors, $F(3,42) = 7.41$, $p < .0001$, Adjusted Squared Multiple $R = .299$. Finally, when motor FIM score at 3 months after discharge was used as a measure of outcome, then the total BDS score emerged as the sole predictor,

$F(2,43) = 16.91$, $p < .0001$, Adjusted Squared Multiple $R = .414$.

Zero-order correlations between the outcome measures and the predictor variables show that whereas the BDS is more strongly related to living settings, the MMSE is more strongly related to the FIM scores, particularly those from the cognitive subscale (see Table 2).

Table 1. Means and Standard Deviations for the MMSE, the BDS, and the BDS Factor Scores for Patients Discharged to Home, to a Nursing Home Temporarily, and to a Nursing Home Permanently.

| | Living setting | | | |
	Home ($n = 29$)	Home/NH ($n = 13$)	NH ($n = 4$)	Total sample ($N = 46$)
BDS total	18.53	14.23	7.00	16.32
	(5.02)	(4.92)	(4.90)	(5.99)
Factor 1	8.53	6.65	2.75	7.52
	(2.37)	(2.28)	(3.10)	(2.91)
Factor 2	5.62	3.73	2.25	4.79
	(1.88)	(2.07)	(1.50)	(2.20)
Factor 3	4.35	3.85	2.00	4.00
	(1.74)	(1.41)	(.82)	(1.70)
MMSE	25.52	23.39	19.00	24.37
	(3.29)	(4.13)	(4.24)	(4.03)

Note. Standard Deviations are presented in parentheses. Home = Discharged to home; Home/NH = Temporarily discharged to nursing home, living at home within 3 months; NH = Permanently discharged to nursing home (or other assisted living setting), still living there after 3 months. BDS = Behavioral Dyscontrol Scale; MMSE = Mini-Mental State Exam.

Table 2. Correlation Coefficients Between Outcome Measures and Predictor Variables.

| | Living setting | | | FIM | |
	Discharge	Follow-up	Total	Motor	Cognitive
BDS total	.489*	.485*	.441	.425	.379
Factor 1	.475*	.511*	.397	.399	.288
Factor 2	.497*	.361	.436	.409	.417
Factor 3	.268	.367	.309	.289	.304
MMSE	.387	.416	.447	.413	.450*

Note. Follow-up = 3-month follow-up; FIM = Functional Independence Measure; BDS = Behavioral Dyscontrol Scale; MMSE = Mini-Mental State Exam.
* <.05, Bonferroni correction was applied.

DISCUSSION

The results show that, as hypothesized, the BDS scores are moderately related to patients' independence after discharge. Consistent with the findings of Kaye et al. (1990), the BDS total score was superior to the MMSE in its ability to predict independence. This superiority of the executive measures to general cognitive measures in predicting ADLs is consistent with the results of Nadler et al. (1993) which show that the executive area of the DRS is more strongly related to ADLs than are the areas that measure other cognitive abilities.

Patients' functioning in the area of cognitive abilities (cognitive FIM score) was most strongly associated with the BDS Fluid Intelligence factor. MMSE also entered into this model probably because of its memory and language components. The Fluid Intelligence factor also emerged as the single predictor of living setting at discharge, but not of eventual regaining of independence 3 months later (which was predicted by the BDS Motor Programming factor). The fact that those patients who were discharged to home care immediately exhibited better fluid intelligence than those who were discharged to home care after an intermediate period in an assisted living setting (such as a nursing home or a subacute rehabilitation unit) suggests that perhaps the former group was better at adapting to new situations. On the other hand, living at home 3 months after the initial discharge from the hospital perhaps no longer placed high demands on fluid intelligence, as by that point the patients had either had ample time to adapt to their new situation or had recovered. Thus, for returning home after 3 months, the abilities of the Motor Programming factor may be sufficient. These interpretations need to be viewed as tentative because of the small size of the group of patients who remained in nursing homes even after 3 months. In addition, the importance of fluid intelligence for independence needs to be further validated with a larger sample and a more comprehensive battery of executive function tests.

The importance of fluid intelligence in particular and executive abilities in general for independence can also be gleaned from correlation coefficients presented in Table 2. Specifically, the fact that the BDS and its factors are most strongly related to the living setting suggests that these executive skills are necessary for the ability to function *independently* (i.e., live alone). On the other hand, the fact that the MMSE scores are most strongly related to the FIM scores suggests that general cognitive efficiency affects the ability to *function* (i.e., to perform the various tasks assessed by the FIM), whether independently or in a structured institutional setting.

Finally, the Environmental Independence factor did not prove to be superior to the total BDS score in predicting any of the outcome measures.

CONCLUSIONS

First, results support the assertion by Kaye et al. (1990) that the BDS is a measure of executive functions. This is particularly evident in the strong relationship of all three BDS factors with STPC, and the lack of relationship with the INFO score.

Second, results support the notion that the BDS factors represent different aspects of executive functioning as related to ADLs.

Finally, the most important contribution of this study is its replication of previous results regarding the ability of the BDS to predict ADLs. This replication is particularly useful because it uses different dependent measures than previous research while using a similar sample, thus supporting the validity of the BDS as a predictor of functional autonomy in a predominantly geriatric population.

REFERENCES

Barona, A., Reynolds, C.R., & Chastain, R. (1984). A demographically based index of premorbid intelligence for the WAIS-R. *Journal of Consulting and Clinical Psychology*, 52, 885–887.

Benton, A.L., Hamsher, K. deS., Varney, N.R., & Spreen O. (1983). *Contributions to neuropsychological assessment: A clinical manual*. New York: Oxford Press.

Fiedler, R. (1993). Progress in medical rehabilitation: Issues in measurement conference: Article IV – Statistical standard for measurement in medical rehabilitation. *UDS Update*, 7, 3–4.

Folstein, M.F., Folstein, S.W., & McHugh, P.R. (1975). Mini mental state: A practical method of grading the cognitive state of patients for the clinician. *Journal of Psychiatric Research*, 12, 189.

Goldberg, G. (1987). From intent to action: Evolution and function of the premotor systems of the frontal lobe. In A. Perecman, (Ed.), *The frontal lobes revisited* (pp. 273–306). New York: IRBN Press.

Golden, C.J. (1978). *Stroop Color Word Test: A manual for clinical and experimental use.* Chicago: Stoelting.

Grigsby, J., & Kaye, K. (1992). *The Behavioral Dyscontrol Scale: Manual.* Denver, CO: Authors.

Grigsby, J., Kaye, K., & Robbins, L.J. (1990). Frontal lobe disorder, behavioral disturbance, and independent functioning among the demented elderly. *Clinical Research, 38,* 81A.

Grigsby, J., Kaye, K., & Robbins, L.J. (1992). Reliabilities and factor structure of the Behavioral Dyscontrol Scale. *Perceptual and Motor Skills, 74,* 883–892.

Heaton, R.K., Chelune, G.J., Talley, J.L., Kay, G.G., & Curtiss, G. (1993). *Wisconsin Card Sorting Test Manual: Revised and expanded.* Odessa, FL: Psychological Assessment Resources.

Janowsky, J.S., Shimamura, A.P., Kritchevsky, M., & Squire, L.R. (1989). Cognitive impairment following frontal lobe damage and its relevance to human amnesia. *Behavioral Neuroscience, 103,* 548–560.

Katz, S., & Stroud, M.W. (1989). Functional assessment in geriatrics: A review of progress and directions. *Journal of American Geriatric Society, 37,* 267–271.

Kaye, K., Grigsby, J. Robbins, L.J., & Korzun, B. (1990). Prediction of independent functioning and behavior problems in geriatric patients. *Journal of American Geriatrics Society, 38,* 1304–1310.

Lezak, M.D. (1983). *Neuropsychological assessment.* New York: Oxford University Press.

Lhermitte, F. (1986). Human anatomy and the frontal lobes. Part II. Patient behavior in complex and social situations: The "environmental dependency syndrome." *Annals of Neurology, 19,* 335–343.

Luria, A.R. (1976). *The neuropsychology of memory.* Washington, DC: V. H. Winston & Sons.

Luria, A.R. (1980). *Higher cortical functions in man.* (2nd ed.). New York: Basic Books.

McFie, J. (1975). *Assessment of organic intellectual impairment.* London: Academic Press.

Nadler, J.D., Richardson, E.D., Malloy, P.F., Marrran, M. E., & Hostetler-Brinson, M. E. (1993).

The ability of Dementia Rating Scale to predict everyday functioning. *Archives of Clinical Neuropsychology, 8,* 449–460.

O'Brien, K., & Lezak, M.D. (1981, July). *Long-term improvement in intellectual function following brain injury.* Paper presented at the Fourth European Conference of the International Neuropsychological Society, Bergen, Norway.

Osmon, D.C., & Johnson, N. (1992, May). *Fractionating executive functions: Evidence from the Milwaukee Card Sorting Test.* Paper presented at the meeting of the Midwest Neuropsychology Group, Rochester, MN.

Osmon, D.C., & Suchy, Y. (1996). Fractionating frontal lobe functions: Factors of the Milwaukee Card Sorting Test. *Archives of Clinical Neuropsychology, 11,* 541–552.

Palmer, H.M., & Dobson, K.S. (1994). Self-medication and memory in an elderly Canadian sample. *Gerontologist, 34,* 658–664.

Pardo, J.V., Pardo, P.J., Janer, K.W., & Raichle, M.E. (1990). The anterior cingulate cortex mediates processing selection in the Stroop attentional conflict paradigm. *Proceedings of the National Academy of Sciences, 87,* 256–259.

Reitan, R.M., & Wolfson, D. (1993). *Halstead-Reitan neuropsychological test battery: Theory and clinical interpretation* (2nd ed.). Tuscon, AZ: Neuropsychology Press.

Sattler, J.M. (1992). *Assessment of children.* San Diego: Author.

Spreen, O., & Benton, A.L. (1965). Comparative studies of some psychological tests for cerebral damage. *Journal of Nervous and Mental Disease, 140,* 322–333.

Stuss, D.T., Kaplan, E.F., & Benson, D.F. (1982). Long-term effects of prefrontal leucotomy: Cognitive functions. In R.N. Malatesha & L. Hartlage (Eds.), *Neuropsychology and cognition,* Vol. 2. (pp. 252–271). The Hague: Martinus Nijhoff.

Weschsler, D. (1981). *Weschler Adult Intelligence Scale-Revised: Manual.* San Antonio, TX: The Psychological Corporation.

SPECIAL ISSUE:

Normative Data from the Canadian Study of Health and Aging

Editors:

Holly Tuokko
Todd S. Woodward

Journal of Clinical and Experimental Neuropsychology
1996, Vol. 18, No. 2, pp. 479–616

Development and Validation of a Demographic Correction System for Neuropsychological Measures Used in the Canadian Study of Health and Aging*

H. Tuokko and Todd S. Woodward

Centre on Aging, University of Victoria, and Elderly Outreach Service, Province of British Columbia,
Ministry of Health and Ministry Responsible for Seniors, and Department of Psychology, University of Victoria

INTRODUCTION

The influence of demographic variables on neuro-psychological test performance is typically neglected or, at best, the means and standard deviations of test scores may be presented for predefined age or education groups. The result is that the normative standard is much more appropriate for some patients than for others. Careful scrutiny of normative standards is of particular importance when demographic variables are known to correlate highly with neuropsychological test performance. For example, changes in certain aspects of cognitive functioning are a normal consequence of aging (Poon, 1985), and it is inappropriate to compare a person above age 80 to "normal expectations" for younger samples.

The need for age-specific norms on all psychological tests has been identified as one of the most pressing needs facing clinicians who work with the elderly (Lezak, 1987). Although age is a major known influence on neuropsychological test performance, education, gender and other demographic variables may also be related. Moreover, different adjustments for one demographic variable may be necessary for persons who have different levels of another demographic variable. That is, interaction effects may exist in normative data sets and may require more complex corrections.

The purpose of the present project was to develop and validate a demographic correction system on measures appropriate for use with the elderly. These data were obtained from the Canadian Study of Health and Aging (CSHA). The procedure used in developing and validating the demographic correction system was adapted from the work of Heaton, Grant and Matthews (1991).

DATA COLLECTION FOR THE NORMATIVE PROJECT

Subject Samples

The data for this project were obtained from the CSHA, a nation-wide study of the epidemiology of dementia, and specifically Alzheimer's disease,

* The authors would like to thank Sophia Wang, Sandra Rae, Dale Robertson, and Jocelyn Robinson for their assistance in the preparation of this document. The data reported in this document were collected as part of the Canadian Study of Health and Aging (CSHA). This was funded by the Seniors Independence Research Program, administered by the National Health and Research Development Program of Health and Welfare Canada. The study was coordinated through the University of Ottawa and the Canadian government's Laboratory Centre for Disease Control. We thank Drs. A. Kosma, J. Fiske, E. Leblanc, M. Ruckman, J. Doyon, B. Ska, G. Forest, R. Steenhuis, W. G. Snow, R. Carbotte, S. Denburg, A. Tellier, J. Rallo, M. Crossley, G. Jason, A. Dobbs, I. Kiss, L. Costa, and O. Spreen, Ms. B. Collins, Mr. J. Woodrow, and Mme. L. Ladoucer who contributed to the development and implementation of the neuropsychological component of the CSHA. The authors would also like to thank all of the participants and staff from across Canada who were involved in the Canadian Study of Health and Aging. In particular, the support and assistance of Betsy Kristjansson from the CSHA Ottawa Coordinating Centre was greatly appreciated.

Address correspondence to: H. Tuokko, Centre on Aging, University of Victoria, P.O. Box 1700, MS 6369, Victoria, Canada V8W 2Y2.

Accepted for publication: February 10, 1996

in Canada. The CSHA involved two distinct populations of persons aged 65 years and older in Canada: (1) community-dwelling individuals; and (2) residents of institutions (see the Canadian Study of Health and Aging Working Group, 1994 for details). All participants were required to be fluent in either English or French and were assessed in their preferred language.

For the *community sample*, a two-phase approach to the identification of persons with dementia was taken. First, a screening interview was conducted on an age-stratified random sample of persons from five geographically defined regions (i.e., Maritimes, Quebec, Ontario, Prairies, and British Columbia; $n = 9008$). As part of this screening interview, the Modified Mini-Mental State Examination (3MS; Teng & Chui, 1987) was administered. All participants scoring below 78/100 on the 3MS[1] and a subsample of persons scoring 78 or greater were invited to attend the clinical component of the CSHA (total $n = 2339$). Those who could not complete the 3MS ($n = 59$) were sent for clinical evaluation. For the *institutional sample*, all randomly selected residents ($n = 1817$) were invited to take part in the clinical component of the CSHA without undergoing the screening examination. This approach was adopted because the high prevalence of dementia in institutions made screening unnecessary (Bland, Newman, & Orn, 1988; Robertson, Rockwood, & Stolee, 1989).

The clinical component was designed to confirm the presence of cognitive impairment in those who screened positive (<78 on 3MS) and to allow for a further differential diagnosis if cognitive impairment was confirmed. This process consisted of four parts: nurse's evaluation, physical examination, laboratory blood work, and neuropsychological assessment.

The *nurse's evaluation* included a re-administration of the 3MS, rudimentary measures of vision and hearing, recordings of vital signs, height, weight, and medication use. Information on the participant's medical history, cognitive and functional status was obtained from a collateral informant (usually a family member) using Section H of the Cambridge Examination for Mental

Disorders (CAMDEX; Roth, Huppert, Tym, & Mountjoy, 1988).

During the *physical examination*, the physician evaluated general appearance of the participant, examined the head, neck, limbs, chest, and cardiovascular system and evaluated the primitive and central reflexes, peripheral neuromuscular responses, and coordination. *Laboratory blood work* was done for participants suspected of having dementia or delirium. Those attaining 3MS scores of 50 or above during the nurse's evaluation were administered a standardized *neuropsychological battery* by a trained psychometrician (i.e., technician trained in test administration). In case conferences, typically attended by physicians, psychologists, nurses, and/or psychometricians, a consensus diagnosis was derived taking into account all clinically relevant information. Participants were classified using a three-stage process: confirmation of cognitive impairment, diagnosis of dementia using DSM-III-R criteria (American Psychiatric Association, 1987), and differential diagnosis based on DSM-III-R, NINCDS-ADRDA (McKhann et al., 1984), and ICD-10 (World Health Organization, 1987) criteria for depression, Alzheimer Disease, and other dementias, respectively. The clinical assessment resulted in classification of participants into the following categories:

No cognitive loss
Cognitive loss but no dementia
Dementia:
    Alzheimertype (possible, probable)
    Vascular
    Mixed vascular + Alzheimer
    Other specific dementia (specify)
    Unclassifiable dementia.

A total of 2914 people participated in the clinical examination: 1659 community-dwelling individuals and 1255 residents from institutions. Of these, 789 attained scores lower than 50 on the 3MS and were, therefore, not given the neuropsychological battery. An additional 246 participants did not complete the neuropsychological assessment, and thus, received no neuropsychological diagnosis. The resulting sample of 1879 participants seen for neuropsychological evaluation, in the context of the larger prevalence study, is a biased sample, selected on the basis of performance on the 3MS (i.e., scores falling between 50 and 78). A smaller proportion of

---

[1] Roughly equivalent to 22 or below on Mini-Mental State Examination (MMSE).

participants included (467/1879 = 24.9%) scored 78 or above on the 3MS.

Subjects selected for this project were English-speaking persons residing in the community who scored 78 or above on the 3MS in the screening examination, and received a diagnosis of No Cognitive Loss after clinical examination. These participants completed all of the neuropsycholog-ical measures identified below ($N = 274$).

To check the adequacy of the norms, 50 subjects were randomly selected to serve as a validation sample. The remaining 224 subjects formed the original normative, or base, sample. At a later stage of the analyses, 9 subjects were discarded as resid-ual outliers resulting in the final base sample of 215 subjects.

While the focus of this project was on the neuro-logically normal subjects, some limited compar-isons of the data with a sample of 187 persons who received diagnoses of dementia identified in the CSHA were conducted. Table 1 contains demo-graphic information for the three samples used in this project: the validation sample, the base sample, and the dementia sample.

Neuropsychological Testing

A detailed description of the development of and diagnostic findings from the neuropsychological component of the CSHA is provided elsewhere (Tuokko, Kristjansson, & Miller, 1995). The fol-lowing section summarizes the procedures and describes the measures selected from the CSHA neuropsychological component for the present project. All test administration was performed by examiners who were trained and/or supervised by psychologists involved in the CSHA. A videotape illustrating the administration sequence and lay-out of the test materials was produced as a training aid. The order of administration was designed to vary the task demands so as to maintain the inter-est of the participant (see Table 2) and to ensure that a core group of measures (i.e., those given first) would be administered to every participant. As a rule, each test protocol was first scored by the examiner who administered the tests, and the scoring was then checked independently by a second experienced examiner.

Measures were selected to reflect the constructs described in the Diagnostic and Statistical Manual

for Mental Disorders, Revised third edition (DSM-III-R) criteria for dementia (see Table 3). Measures of memory included a modified version of the Cued Recall paradigm of Buschke (Buschke, 1984; Tuokko, Vernon-Wilkinson, Weir, & Beattie, 1991), the Auditory Verbal Learning Test (AVLT; Bleecker & Bolla-Wilson, 1988; Rey, 1964; Taylor, 1959), the Information subtest from the Wechsler Memory Scale (Wechsler, 1975), the multiple choice form of the Benton Visual Retention Test (BVRT; Benton, 1974) and a digit span task invol-ving the forward repetition of digit sequences of increasing length.

The AVLT included a recognition trial that required the participant to indicate whether or not each of 30 words was presented in List A. This took place immediately following the sixth trial of List A. The BVRT multiple choice form F (15 items) was administered with a 10-s stimulus expo-sure followed immediately by the presentation of a response card depicting four different designs. The participant was asked to point to or name by letter (A, B, C, or D) the design that was shown on the stimulus card.

The Digit Symbol subtest of the Wechsler Adult Intelligence Scale-Revised (WAIS-R; Wechsler, 1981) and short forms (Satz & Mogel, 1962) of the Similarities, Block Design, and Comprehension subtests of the WAIS-R were administered to assess other areas of cognitive functioning. The Token Test (Benton & Hamsher, 1989) was abbreviated to an 11-item form for this study. This abbreviated Token Test and measures of the generation of words in response to letters (Spreen & Benton, 1977) and semantic (animal names) (Rosen, 1980) cuing were used to assess language skills.

The scores derived from each measure that were used in the development and validation of the demo-graphic correction system are described in Table 3. The maximum scores for each measure are also indicated on Table 3.

DEVELOPMENT AND VALIDATION
OF THE DEMOGRAPHIC CORRECTION
SYSTEM

Procedure

The specific goal of this project was to develop a system for converting raw scores on the various test measures to demographically corrected T scores. The success of the demographic corrections was examined in an independent subject sample as were the distributions of T scores. The following is a description of the analyses completed to accomplish these goals. All analyses were carried out using SPSS for Windows version 5.0.

Development of the T-Score Conversion System
The random assignment of subjects to the Base and Validation samples has been discussed above. The development of the T-score conversion system was done using only the data from the Base sample.

Step 1. The first step in the development of the T-score system was to normalize each test score distribution, converting raw scores to scaled scores having means of 10 and standard deviations of 3. The raw to scaled score conversions were done so that higher scaled scores always reflected better test performance. Note that the raw scores used in this transformation for the Similarities, Comprehension, and Block Design subtests of the WAIS-R were from the short forms (i.e., only half of the items administered, see Satz & Mogel, 1962) of these measures. The raw score to scaled score conversions are listed in Tables 4.1–4.4.

Step 2. Next, each test scaled score was regressed separately on the three demographic variables (age, years of education, gender). These three variables were chosen because it is well known that performances on many neuropsychological measures are strongly related to age and education, and that gender differences may also be observed (Lezak, 1995). The three independent variables were entered in a single step. This regression analysis determined the variable weightings by which combinations of age, years of education, and/or gender optimally predicted the subject's scaled scores. These weights were then used to calculate a predicted scaled score, based on the demographic characteristics.

The following variables were dropped at this point due to non-normality of regression residuals: Wechsler Memory Scale – Information subtest; Buschke Acquisition; Buschke Retention; Rey Auditory Verbal Learning Test – Recognition: True Positives and True Negatives; and the Token Test. For these tests, the vast majority of respondents in the base sample made very few errors, resulting

in negatively skewed regression residuals. Table 5 summarizes the raw score results of the Base sample on each of the 24 measures in the battery. Additional information concerning the 7 variables that were dropped from the regression analyses is contained in Appendix A.

The predicted scores resulting from the multiple regression are presented in Tables 6.1–31.2. For each age and gender combination, a predicted scaled score table for all measures and years of education (from 0 to 30 years) is presented. The variance accounted for by the demographic variables ranged from 26% to 63%, with a median of 44.5%. This regression-based approach to norm development allows more precise prediction of expected normal performance than do the traditional methods of collapsing into age and education groups.

Step 3. In the next step, the subjects' predicted scaled scores were subtracted from their actual scaled scores. The resulting differences, or residual scores, indicate how much better or worse the subjects did on the test as compared to what would be predicted on the basis of their demographic characteristics. Finally, these residual scores were converted to T scores using the following formula:

$$T \text{ score} = \{[\text{residual score divided by the standard deviation of the residual scores}) \times 10] + 50\}$$

Theoretically, the T score derived from the preceding steps should have several important characteristics. At least for neurologically normal subjects, the T scores should be normally distributed and should have a mean of 50 and a standard deviation of 10. The T scores should also show no gender differences and should be unrelated to age and education. However, these characteristics cannot be assumed without verification, and the validation sample was used to examine the integrity of the transformations.

Validation Process
The validation process was also carried out in several steps, which were done separately for the Base and Validation samples.

Step 1. First, the above-noted tables were used to convert the raw scores to T scores for the validation sample.

Step 2. Next, multivariate analyses were used to determine whether the T scores showed significant age, education, gender, or interaction effects. To correct for the inflated Type I error rate associated with multiple tests of significance, multivariate multiple regression was used. An alpha level of 0.05 was used for all multivariate tests. For the Base sample, the analysis using the main effects of age, years of education, and gender and the 4 additional interaction effects (i.e., Age × Education, Age × Gender, Education × Gender, Age × Education × Gender) as independent variables with the 17^2 dependent variables yielded a nonsignificant multivariate test (Wilks Lambda = 0.715, $df = 119, p = 1.0$). This indicates that there were no significant main effects of age, gender, and education on the 17 measures, and no significant interactions between these demographic variables.

For the validation sample, the multivariate test was significant (Wilks Lambda = 0.001, $df = 119$, $p < 0.01$). The univariate regression main effects and interactions were then examined, and their significance assessed at an alpha level of 0.01. Four significant effects were found: (1) Gender accounted for significant variance over and above age and education on Animal Naming $F(1,46) = 14.02$, $p < 0.001$; (2) Education accounted for significant variance over and above gender and age on Animal Naming $F(1,46) = 9.52$, $p < 0.01$; (3) The interaction between age and gender accounted for significant variance over and above that accounted for by the main effects on List A3 of the Rey Auditory Verbal Learning Test $F(1,45) = 11.04$, $p < 0.01$; and (4) The interaction between age and education accounted for significant variance over and above that accounted for by the main effects on List B1 of the Rey Auditory Verbal Learning Test $F(1,45) = 9.20, p < 0.01$.

The proportion of error reduced by the variable of interest was assessed over and above effects of the same (for main effects) or higher (for interaction effects) hierarchical importance. The order of importance for the independent variables was as follows: main effects, two-way interactions, then three-way interactions. The effects sizes for the significant univariate effects are considered small (Cohen, 1969). Thus, although the validation sample was not completely free from the effects of age, gender, and education, the influence of these demographic variables was substantially reduced, if not virtually eliminated, for most variables.

Step 3. The Base and Validation samples were then compared with respect to age, education, gender, and T scores on the 17 tests. Multivariate analysis of variance (MANOVA) was used to compare the Base and Validation samples on T scores. The multivariate omnibus test yielded nonsignificant results (Wilks Lambda = 0.925, $df = 20$, $p = 0.477$), indicating that there were no significant differences between the two groups for age, education, gender, or T-score means. Table 32 contains the T-score means and standard deviations for the Base and Validation samples (of particular interest were the T-score means and standard deviations in the Validation sample).

Step 4. Table 33 contains the percentage of subjects who would be predicted to score within seven T-score ranges, assuming a perfectly normal distribution, and then presents the actual percentages for the total subject group on each test measure. Also, Kolmogorov–Smirnov tests were performed to determine whether or not the actual cumulative frequencies across these seven T-score ranges differed significantly from the predictions for a normal distribution; this was done separately for the Base and Validation samples. In all, 36 T-score distributions were checked in this way; one, the WAIS-R Similarities subtest, differed significantly from normal at the 0.01 level (Kolmogorov-Smirnov $Z = 1.7, p < 0.01$).

Defining Impairment

A final issue to be addressed is a tentative proposal of T-score categories for use in clinical interpretation. The most important question in this regard is the selection of a cutoff score to define "impairment." One feature of the T scores is that, whatever the cutoff score one chooses, the resulting false positive rate (percentage of normals called "impaired") can be specified. The cutoff scores chosen by individual clinicians will probably vary in consideration of additional factors, such as the base rates of cerebral disorders in various clinical

---

[2] Only 17 of the 18 test scores described earlier were used in these analyses. Total for the Auditory Verbal Learning Test (AVLT) is a linear combination of the five AVLT learning trials so was dropped.

settings and the perceived costs of making false positive and false negative errors.

Heaton et al. (1991) suggested the following T-score categories for clinical use: 1–19 = severe impairment; 20–24 = moderate-to-severe impairment; 35–39 = mild impairment; 40–44 = below average/borderline impairment; 45–54 = average; 55+ = above average. In using this classification system, a false positive rate of up to 15% is accepted. Moreover, for any given T score under 40, the clinician can specify his or her likelihood of being wrong in calling the test result abnormal. To assist in this process, Table 33 lists the percentage of normals who would be predicted to score in each of the clinical T-score ranges; this is followed by a listing of actual frequencies for the total normal group on each test measure.

Dementia. In the preceding paragraph and in Table 33 the likelihood of normals being correctly classified (i.e., specificity) by various T-score cutoff points has been considered. The equally important topic of sensitivity (true positive classification rate with people who have dementia) needs to be addressed. If the distribution of scores for each measure were plotted for normals and our sample of 187 persons with dementia, the primary difference would be that the distribution of the dementia cases would be shifted to the left (direction of impairment). In addition, there would be a fair amount of overlap between the two distributions such that no cutoff score would correctly classify all subjects in both groups.

Table 34 contains the cutoff point for each measure that results in the optimal balance between sensitivity and specificity. As noted above, each clinician may wish to use different levels of sensitivity and specificity depending on the circumstances.

Tables 35 and 36 contain the resulting sensitivity (Table 35) and specificity (Table 36) for each measure for cutoff points ranging from 2 points below the optimal cutoff score to 2 points above the optimal cutoff point. Determining the performance of these T-score cutoff points for identifying different clinical populations requires further investigation.

Cognitively Impaired with No Dementia. A group of subjects of particular interest with respect to the early identification of dementia are those diagnosed as exhibiting cognitive impairment with no dementia (CIND) in the CSHA. Diagnoses for members of the community sample who underwent a clinical examination were approximately evenly distributed between the classifications of normal (approximately 38%), dementia (approximately 32%), and CIND (approximately 30%). Subjects who did not meet criteria for dementia but who were judged by clinicians as exhibiting some form of cognitive impairment were captured in this group. The clinicians were asked to identify the source (etiology) of the cognitive impairment, where possible.

Table 37 contains the approximate distribution of subclassifications within the CIND group. It must be noted that these classifications were not made according to predetermined criteria but were derived from available clinical information, in some instances on an ad hoc basis. Although criteria were available for Age-associated Memory Impairment (AAMI: Crook et al., 1986), these were not strictly applied in the CSHA and so this group cannot be viewed as AAMI as defined by Crook et al.

It may be that the CIND group contains individuals early in the course of a dementing disorder as well as individuals with more stable cognitive impairments. However, only in longitudinal follow-up it will be possible to identify those subjects who do and do not progress to dementia. The CIND classification implies mild or circumscribed cognitive impairment (i.e., not severe enough or not extensive enough to meet criteria for dementia). We compared the performance of the English-speaking CIND sample who had completed all neuropsychological tests ($N = 375$; 245 in the community and 130 from institutions) to the normal samples and the dementia sample to examine these assumptions in a number of ways.

Table 38 shows the percentage of subjects falling below the optimal cutoff score for identifying dementia, as determined above (see Table 34), for the validation, CIND, and dementia samples. In all instances but one (Digit Span), the percentage of CIND subjects performing below the cutoff falls between the normal (small percentage) and dementia (large percentage) samples. Depending on the measure, between 38% and 69% of the CIND subjects performed below the optimal cutoff score for dementia. If a T-score cutoff of 40 is used to identify dementia (see Table 39), the percentage of CIND subjects performing below the cutoff continues to fall between the normal and dementia samples (except on Digit Span), with a range of 23% to 60% depending on which measure is examined.

When measures were examined within the DSM-III-R criteria for dementia, the CIND group again performed between the normal and dementia samples on the number of memory measures falling below the optimal cutoff score (see Table 40). Approximately 89% of the normal subjects performed below the cutoff on one or fewer memory measures. Approximately 64% of the CIND performed below the cutoff score on two or more memory measures, and approximately 85% of dementia cases performed below the cutoff on three or more memory measures. In all instances, the percentage of CIND subjects performing below the optimal cutoff points for dementia fell between the normal and dementia samples, with a larger percentage of CIND than normals exhibiting impairment on multiple measures within a domain.

When the distribution of scores on each measure was examined for the CIND group, it was apparent that the data were skewed to the left (see Table 41) in relation to the normal subjects (see Table 33), but not as far to the left as the dementia sample (see Table 42) for most measures.

A stepwise logistic regression analysis was performed to determine the battery of tests that maximally discriminate between normal and demented subjects in this data set. The T-score variables that were found to contribute significantly (at the $p < 0.01$ alpha level) to the discrimination were: Buschke Cued Recall Retrieval (sum of Free Recall1 + Free Recall2 + Free Recall3), Rey Auditory Verbal Learning Test Recall on Trial 1, Rey Auditory Verbal Learning Test Recall on Trial 6 (i.e., List A recall following List B recall), Correct score on the multiple choice version of the Benton Visual Retention Test, Controlled Oral Word Association Test (i.e., Verbal Fluency), and the Digit Symbol subtest of the Wechsler Adult Intelligence Scale-Revised (correct overall classification of 93.14%). The tests assigned the largest logistic regression weights were the Retrieval score from Buschke's Cued Recall paradigm and Recall of List A on the Rey Auditory Verbal Learning Test following the presentation of List B (i.e. REYA6). When these two tests were entered into the logistic

regression equation alone, they together produced an overall correct classification of 91.15%.

When the weights from the logistic regression analysis were applied to the performance on the CIND subjects, a bimodal distribution for the probability that members of the CIND group would be identified as demented emerged (see Table 43). Approximately 18% showed less than a 10% probability of being demented whereas approximately 36% were classified as likely (>90% probability) to be demented. In contrast, the dementia sample showed 77% as likely to be demented (>90% probability), whereas the remainder were more or less equally distributed across lesser probability levels. Needless to say, the vast majority of normal subjects in both the base (80.5%) and validation (74.0%) samples were highly unlikely (<10%) to be classified as demented.

USE OF THE DEMOGRAPHIC CORRECTION SYSTEM

Converting Raw Scores to T Scores

The conversion of raw scores to demographically corrected T scores is accomplished by using Tables 4.1–4.4 and 6.1–31.2. Because exact age and education values are used, this conversion process is more precise than are systems which use age and education ranges.

To facilitate using Tables 4.1–4.4 and 6.1–31.2 to derive T scores, profile sheets have been developed. The profile sheet contains a list of variables and spaces for recording raw scores, scaled scores, predicted scores, and T scores. The profile sheet also contains a profile grid for plotting T scores for the measures grouped in accordance with the DSM-III-R criteria for dementia. The resulting T scores for each measure can then be plotted on the grid sheet which has optimal cutoff points indicated.

Using the Tables

Step 1. Record all of the raw scores for the measures that were administered. Care should be taken to ensure that the raw score units are the ones specified for each measure (e.g., WAIS-R subtest raw scores from short forms).

Step 2. Find and record the corresponding scaled scores in Tables 4.1–4.3. In addition to providing the data in standard units needed for the next step in the T-score conversion process, scaled scores may be clinically useful in their own right.

Step 3. Find, in Tables 6.1–31.2, the predicted score for each variable using the person's age, gender, and level of education (i.e., number of years of formal education completed).

Step 4. Subtract the predicted score from the scaled score and divide by the standard deviation of the residuals for that measure.

Step 5. The resulting value is then multiplied by 10 and added to 50 to yield the T-score value.

Review of Interpretive Issues

The use of the demographically corrected T scores is most straightforward when considering level of performance on individual test measures. The T scores can be applied to determine the likelihood that an individual of a particular age, gender, and education would obtain the achieved score. In other words, how abnormal is the obtained score for this particular individual? However, even in interpreting level of performance, a number of features and limitations of the T-score system that the clinician needs to take into consideration have been identified by Heaton et al. (1991).

First, not all demographic characteristics are corrected by the present system. Race and culture are potentially important factors in neuropsychological test interpretation (Barona et al., 1984; Wilson et al., 1979), but these were not considered because the subject sample included insufficient numbers of subjects from any specific ethnic minority group. Also, all subjects in the sample were English-speaking. It is unknown how well or whether their results would generalize to persons with other cultural/language backgrounds.

Second, a strictly statistical approach to interpreting T scores is particularly precarious for measures that were initially designed to assess pathognomic signs of cerebral dysfunction (e.g., aphasia, constructional dyspraxia). On most of these tests, normal individuals typically achieve the best possible raw score and rarely make more than one or two errors (e.g., Acquisition Score on Cued Recall). In these cases, even a trivial deviation from a perfect performance can place a person (statistically) within the impaired range. Great care should be taken when interpreting such impairments, particularly when slight deviations from a perfect performance can result from nonspecific factors such as brief inattention or carelessness. On these and other tests, it is also possible to obtain the same score in ways that are qualitatively quite different. Whereas these scores do have some limited uses (e.g., group data for research comparisons), clinical interpretation of results on these tests requires a qualitative analysis of the patient's performances (Reitan, 1984).

Third, it is a serious mistake to assume that one or more test scores beyond the accepted cutoff scores always indicate the presence of an acquired cerebral disorder. As demonstrated in Table 33, a T score in the impaired range (<40) on any given test measure is expected to occur in no more than 15% of neurologically normal older persons. However, in the context of the entire battery of measures, only 12% of the total sample of normal subjects had no T scores in the impaired range, and the group median was 3 abnormal scores (out of a possible 18) with a mode of 1.

In distinguishing the performance of normal individuals from the performance of persons with dementia, it is not just the number or even the severity of deficits, but also the nature and pattern of those deficits which needs to be considered. T scores are useful for identifying a person's poor performances within the context of demographic characteristics. However, the clinician must determine the *significance* of those deficits by considering a variety of additional factors.

These factors may include information about the person's school performance, vocational history, medical and psychiatric history, current medications, and behaviour during testing. For example, occasionally an adult patient's level of formal education appears to be a poor estimate of his or her premorbid abilities. A person in this age cohort may have left high school because of the outbreak of World War II and may then have excelled in vocational or other achievements typical of someone with much more education. Some current ability indicators (e.g., Wide Range Achievement Test Reading Recognition) might also suggest a level of premorbid functioning that is atypical for the educational level achieved.

Alternatively, a person may have some college background, but may never have done well either academically or vocationally. Historical information of this type should be considered when interpreting the T scores. For example, a person with a poor academic record would be expected to have more T scores in the below average range.

Heaton et al. (1991) noted that, whereas the clinical interpretation of T scores on individual test measures may be complex, analyses of T-score *patterns* is even more complex. To the extent that the T-score conversions remove the effects of demographic factors on patterns of test results, they should facilitate identification of patterns that are attributable to focal and diffuse disorders. T-score conversion systems, such as the one presented herein, hold specificity essentially constant at about 85% for all test measures, at all levels of age and education. By holding specificity constant, the T-score system also permits more direct comparisons of the sensitivities of different test measures to brain disorders involving different etiologies and cerebral locations. Future studies may elucidate the patterns of T-score results associated with Alzheimer disease and other forms of dementia.

Although specific T-score patterns may emerge, it must be acknowledged that distributional properties of raw scores and T scores can be quite different, and converting raw scores to T scores with constant standard deviations can have major effects on pattern features. This is particularly true for test measures in which the raw scores have either very low or very high variability in normals. For low variability measures, a small change in raw score (and in actual test performance) can translate into a relatively large T-score change. Furthermore, in measures for which raw score variability is quite high in normals, very large differences in test performances (e.g., in the number of errors made) would be required to cause an appreciable T-score shift. It is also the case that patterns of scores in the T-score conversion process may be altered because different test measures require different magnitudes of correction for age, education, and gender.

Patterns of demographically corrected T scores may eventually prove more informative than raw score patterns for neurodiagnostic purposes. Patterns of raw scores and T scores are different, and most previous clinical and research experience in neuropsychology has been restricted to raw scores. Therefore, at least until more is known about the relative merits of the different types of scores for different purposes, clinicians should find it useful to consider all three (raw, scaled, and T scores) in the interpretive process.

REFERENCES

American Psychiatric Association (1987). *Diagnostic and statistical manual of mental disorders* (3rd ed. rev.) Washington, DC: Author.

Barona, A., Reynolds, C.R., & Chastain, R. (1984). A demographically based index of premorbid intelligence for the WAIS-R. *Journal of Consulting and Clinical Psychology, 52*, 885–887.

Benton, A.L. (1974). *Revised Visual Retention Test: Clinical and experimental applications.* New York: Psychological Corporation.

Benton, A.L., & Hamsher, K. (1989). *Multilingual Aphasia Examination: Manual of instructions.* Iowa City, IA: AJA.

Bland, R.C., Newman, S.C., & Orn, H. (1988). Prevalence of psychiatric disorders in the elderly in Edmonton. *Acta Psychiatrica Scandinavica, 77 (suppl. 338)*, 57–63.

Bleecker, M.L., & Bolla-Wilson, K. (1988). Age-related sex differences in verbal memory. *Journal of Clinical Psychology, 44*, 403–411.

Buschke, H. (1984). Cued recall in amnesia. *Journal of Clinical Neuropsychology, 6*, 433–440.

Canadian Study of Health and Aging Working Group (1994). Canadian Study of Health and Aging: Study methods and prevalence of dementia. *Canadian Medical Association Journal, 150* (6), 899–913.

Cohen, J. (1969). *Statistical power analysis for the behavioral sciences.* New York: Academic Press.

Crook, T., Bartus, R.T., Ferris, S.H., Whitehouse, P., Cohen, G.D., & Gershon, S. (1986). Age-associated memory impairment: Proposed diagnostic criteria and measures of clinical change – Report of a National Institute of Mental Health Work Group. *Developmental Neuropsychology, 2*, 261–276.

Heaton, R.K., Grant, I., & Matthews, C.G. (1991). *Comprehensive norms for an expanded Halstead-Reitan battery: Demographic corrections, research findings and clinical applications.* Odessa: Psychological Assessment Resources.

Hosmer, D.W., & Lemeshow, S. (1989). *Applied logistic regression.* New York: Wiley.

Lezak, M.D. (1987). Norms for growing older. *Developmental Neuropsychology, 3* (1), 1–12.

Lezak, M.D. (1995). *Neuropsychological assessment.* (3rd ed.) New York: Oxford University Press.

McKhann, G., Drachman, D.A., Folstein, M.F., Katzman, R., Price, D., & Stadlan, E.M. (1984).

Clinical diagnosis of Alzheimer's Disease: Report of the NINCDS-ADRDA work group under the auspices of the Department of Health and Human Services task force on Alzheimer's Disease. *Neurology, 34*, 939–944.

Poon, L. (1985). Difference in human memory with aging: Nature, causes, and clinical implications. In J.E. Birren & K.W. Schaie (Eds.), *Handbook of the psychology of aging* (2nd ed.) (pp. 427–462). New York: Van Nostrand Reinhold.

Reitan, R. (1984). *Aphasia and sensory-perceptual deficits in adults.* Tuscon, AZ: Neuropsychology Press.

Rey, A. (1964). *L'examen clinique en psychologie.* Paris: Presses Universitaires de France.

Robertson, D., Rockwood, K., & Stolee, P. (1989). The prevalence of cognitive impairment in an elderly Canadian population. *Acta Psychiatrica Scandinavica, 80*, 303–309.

Rosen, W.G. (1980). Verbal fluency in aging and dementia. *Journal of Clinical Neuropsychology, 2*, 135–146.

Roth, M., Huppert, F.A., Tym, E., & Mountjoy, C.Q. (1988). *CAMDEX. The Cambridge examination for mental disorders of the elderly.* Cambridge: Cambridge University Press.

Satz, P., & Mogel, S. (1962). An abbreviation of the WAIS for clinical use. *Journal of Clinical Psychology, 18*, 77–79.

Spreen, O., & Benton, A.L. (1977). *Neurosensory Center Comprehensive Examination for Aphasia: Manual of instructions.* Victoria, BC: University of Victoria.

SPSS for Windows version 5.0 [Computer software]. (1992). Chicago: SPSS.

Taylor, E.M. (1959). *The appraisal of children with cerebral deficits.* Cambridge, MA: Harvard University Press.

Teng, E.L., & Chui, H.C. (1987). The modified Mini-Mental State (3MS) Examination. *Journal of Clinical Psychiatry, 48*, 314–318.

Tuokko, H., Kristjansson, E., & Miller, J. A. (1995). The neuropsychological detection of dementia: An overview of the neuropsychological component of the Canadian Study of Health and Aging. *Journal of Clinical and Experimental Neuropsychology, 17*, 352–373.

Tuokko, H., Vernon-Wilkinson, R., Weir, J., & Beattie, B.L. (1991). Cued recall and early identification of dementia. *Journal of Clinical and Experimental Neuropsychology, 13*, 871–879.

Wechsler, D. (1975). *Wechsler Memory Scale.* New York: Psychological Corporation.

Wechsler, D. (1981). *Wechsler Adult Intelligence Scale-Revised.* New York: Psychological Corporation.

Wilson, R., Rosenbaum, G., & Brown, G. (1979). The problem of premorbid intelligence in neuropsychological assessment. *Journal of Clinical Neuropsychology, 1*, 49–54.

World Health Organization (1987). Tenth revision of the International Classification of Diseases 1987 draft of chapter V, categories F00-F99, mental, behavioural and developmental disorders. In *Clinical Descriptions and Diagnostic Guidelines* (MNH/MEP/87.1 rev. 1), Geneva.

Table 1. Demographic Characteristics of the Subject Samples.

	Base Normal Sample	Validation Normal Sample	Total Normal Sample	Dementia Sample
n	215	50	265	187
Age				
Mean	78.30	79.02	78.43	81.42
SD	6.32	5.79	6.22	6.36
Education				
Mean	11.31	11.16	11.28	9.34
SD	3.62	2.92	3.50	3.80
Sex				
% Male	36.7	36.0	36.6	35.8
% Female	63.3	64.0	63.4	64.2
Diagnosis				
Probable Alzheimer Disease				36.4
Possible Alzheimer Disease				21.9
Vascular Dementia				19.8
Other Dementias				8.6
Unclassifiable Dementia				13.4

Table 2. Order of Test Administration.

Measure
Wechsler Memory Scale-Information Subtest
Buschke Cued Recall
WAIS-R Block Design
WAIS-R Similarities
Token Test
Digit Span
WAIS-R Comprehension
Rey Auditory Verbal Learning Test
Word Fluency
Benton Visual Retention Test-Multiple Choice
Animal Naming
WAIS-R Digit Symbol

Table 3. Neuropsychological Measures Grouped According To DSM-III-R Criteria.

DSM-III-R Criteria	Tests
Memory	Wechsler Memory Scale – Information (WECHSLER; max = 6)
	Buschke's Cued Recall Paradigm for Memory Assessment
	Immediate Recall (FR1) (BUSCHFR1; max = 12)
	Retrieval (sum of FR1 + FR2 + FR3) (BRETRIE; max = 36)
	Acquisition (sum of TR1 + TR2 + TR3) (BACQUIS; max = 36)
	Retention (TR on delayed recall) (BUSCHTR; max = 12)
	Rey Auditory Verbal Learning Test
	A1 (REYA1; max = 15)
	A2 (REYA2; max = 15)
	A3 (REYA3; max = 15)
	A4 (REYA4; max = 15)
	A5 (REYA5; max = 15)
	A Total (REYTOT; max = 75)
	B1 (REYB1; max = 15)
	A6 (REYA6; max = 15)
	Recognition: True Positives (TRUEPOSI; max = 15)
	True Negatives (TRUENEGA; max = 15)
	Benton Visual Retention Test – Multiple Choice Format (CORRECT; max = 15)
	Digit Span (DIGITSPA; max = 8)
B1. Abstract Thinking	WAIS-R[1] Similarities (WAISIMIL; max = 14)
B2. Judgement	WAIS-R[1] Comprehension (WAISJUDG; max = 16)
B3. Aphasia	Token Test (TOKENTES; max = 22)
	Verbal Fluency (VERBAL; max = 64)
	Animal Naming (ANIMAL; max = 30)
Construction	WAIS-R[1] Block Design (WAISBLOC; max = 30)
Other	WAIS-R[1] Digit Symbol (DIGIT; max = 93)

Note. [1] Wechsler Adult Intelligence Scale – Revised Similarities subtest short form raw score (items # 1, 3, 5, 7, 9, 11, 13).

[2] Wechsler Adult Intelligence Scale – Revised Comprehension subtest short form raw score (items # 1, 3, 5, 7, 9, 11, 13, 15).

[3] Wechsler Adult Intelligence Scale – Revised Block Design subtest short form raw score (items # 1, 3, 5, 7, 9).

[4] Wechsler Adult Intelligence Scale – Revised Digit Symbol subtest short form raw score.

Table 4.1. Raw to Scaled Score Conversions.

RAWSCORE	BUSCHFR1	BRETRIE	RAWSCORE
0.00	−5.06	−10.17	0.00
1.00	−3.19	−9.42	1.00
2.00	−1.32	−8.66	2.00
3.00	0.55	−7.91	3.00
4.00	2.42	−7.15	4.00
5.00	4.29	−6.40	5.00
6.00	6.16	−5.64	6.00
7.00	8.03	−4.89	7.00
8.00	9.90	−4.13	8.00
9.00	11.76	−3.38	9.00
10.00	13.63	−2.62	10.00
11.00	15.50	−1.87	11.00
12.00	17.37	−1.11	12.00
13.00		−0.36	13.00
14.00		0.40	14.00
15.00		1.15	15.00
16.00		1.91	16.00
17.00		2.66	17.00
18.00		3.42	18.00
19.00		4.17	19.00
20.00		4.93	20.00
21.00		5.68	21.00
22.00		6.44	22.00
23.00		7.19	23.00
24.00		7.95	24.00
25.00		8.70	25.00
26.00		9.46	26.00
27.00		10.21	27.00
28.00		10.97	28.00
29.00		11.72	29.00
30.00		12.48	30.00
31.00		13.23	31.00
32.00		13.99	32.00
33.00		14.74	33.00
34.00		15.50	34.00
35.00		16.25	35.00
36.00		17.01	36.00

Table 4.2. Raw to Scaled Score Conversions.

RAWSCORE	REYA1	REYA2	REYA3	REYA4	REYA5	REYA6	REYB1	REYTOT	RAWSCORE
0.00	2.26	−0.07	−0.97	−1.68	−2.83	2.29	3.50	−3.13	0.00
1.00	4.01	1.40	0.33	−0.45	−1.59	3.28	5.19	−2.80	1.00
2.00	5.76	2.88	1.63	0.78	−0.34	4.27	6.88	−2.47	2.00
3.00	7.50	4.35	2.93	2.00	0.90	5.26	8.58	−2.13	3.00
4.00	9.25	5.83	4.24	3.23	2.15	6.25	10.27	−1.80	4.00
5.00	11.00	7.30	5.54	4.46	3.40	7.24	11.96	−1.47	5.00
6.00	12.75	8.78	6.84	5.69	4.64	8.23	13.65	−1.14	6.00
7.00	14.49	10.25	8.14	6.92	5.89	9.23	15.34	−0.80	7.00
8.00	16.24	11.73	9.44	8.15	7.13	10.22	17.04	−0.47	8.00
9.00	17.99	13.20	10.74	9.38	8.38	11.21	18.73	−0.14	9.00
10.00	19.74	14.68	12.04	10.61	9.62	12.20	20.42	1.19	10.00
11.00	21.49	16.16	13.34	11.83	10.87	13.19	22.11	0.53	11.00
12.00	23.23	17.63	14.64	13.06	12.11	14.18	23.80	0.86	12.00
13.00	24.98	19.11	15.94	14.29	13.36	15.17	25.50	1.19	13.00
14.00	26.73	20.58	17.24	15.52	14.61	16.16	27.19	1.52	14.00
15.00	28.48	22.06	18.54	16.75	15.85	17.15	28.88	1.86	15.00
16.00								2.19	16.00
17.00								2.52	17.00
18.00								2.85	18.00
19.00								3.19	19.00
20.00								3.52	20.00
21.00								3.85	21.00
22.00								4.18	22.00
23.00								4.52	23.00
24.00								4.85	24.00
25.00								5.18	25.00
26.00								5.51	26.00
27.00								5.85	27.00
28.00								6.18	28.00
29.00								6.51	29.00
30.00								6.84	30.00
31.00								7.17	31.00
32.00								7.51	32.00
33.00								7.84	33.00
34.00								8.17	34.00
35.00								8.50	35.00
36.00								8.84	36.00
37.00								9.17	37.00
38.00								9.50	38.00
39.00								9.83	39.00
40.00								10.17	40.00
41.00								10.50	41.00
42.00								10.83	42.00
43.00								11.16	43.00
44.00								11.50	44.00
45.00								11.83	45.00
46.00								12.16	46.00
47.00								12.49	47.00
48.00								12.83	48.00
49.00								13.16	49.00

Table continues.

Table 4.2. Raw to Scaled Score Conversions (continued).

RAWSCORE	REYA1	REYA2	REYA3	REYA4	REYA5	REYA6	REYB1	REYTOT	RAWSCORE
50.00								13.49	50.00
51.00								13.82	51.00
52.00								14.16	52.00
53.00								14.49	53.00
54.00								14.82	54.00
55.00								15.15	55.00
56.00								15.49	56.00
57.00								15.82	57.00
58.00								16.15	58.00
59.00								16.48	59.00
60.00								16.82	60.00
61.00								17.15	61.00
62.00								17.48	62.00
63.00								17.81	63.00
64.00								18.15	64.00

Table 4.3. Raw to Scaled Score Conversions.

RAWSCORE	CORRECT	DIGITSPA	WAISIMIL	WAISJUDG	WAISBLOC	DIGIT	RAWSCORE
0.00	−7.12	−8.01	3.20	−0.65	2.80	1.20	0.00
1.00	−5.72	−4.99	4.00	0.41	3.45	1.49	1.00
2.00	−4.32	−1.98	4.81	1.47	4.10	1.77	2.00
3.00	−2.92	1.04	5.62	2.52	4.75	2.05	3.00
4.00	−1.53	4.05	6.42	3.58	5.40	2.33	4.00
5.00	−0.13	7.07	7.23	4.64	6.05	2.62	5.00
6.00	1.27	10.08	8.04	5.69	6.70	2.90	6.00
7.00	2.67	13.10	8.84	6.75	7.35	3.18	7.00
8.00	4.06	16.11	9.65	7.81	8.00	3.46	8.00
9.00	5.46		10.46	8.86	8.65	3.75	9.00
10.00	6.86		11.26	9.92	9.30	4.03	10.00
11.00	8.26		12.07	10.98	9.95	4.31	11.00
12.00	9.66		12.88	12.03	10.61	4.59	12.00
13.00	11.05		13.69	13.09	11.26	4.88	13.00
14.00	12.45		14.49	14.15	11.91	5.16	14.00
15.00	13.85			15.20	12.56	5.44	15.00
16.00				16.26	13.21	5.72	16.00
17.00					13.86	6.01	17.00
18.00					14.51	6.29	18.00
19.00					15.16	6.57	19.00
20.00					15.81	6.85	20.00
21.00					16.46	7.14	21.00
22.00					17.11	7.42	22.00
23.00					17.76	7.70	23.00
24.00					18.41	7.99	24.00
25.00					19.07	8.27	25.00
26.00					19.72	8.55	26.00
27.00					20.37	8.83	27.00
28.00					21.02	9.12	28.00
29.00					21.67	9.40	29.00

Table continues.

Table 4.3. Raw to Scaled Score Conversions (continued).

RAWSCORE	CORRECT	DIGITSPA	WAISIMIL	WAISJUDG	WAISBLOC	DIGIT	RAWSCORE
30.00						9.68	30.00
31.00						9.96	31.00
32.00						10.25	32.00
33.00						10.53	33.00
34.00						10.81	34.00
35.00						11.09	35.00
36.00						11.38	36.00
37.00						11.66	37.00
38.00						11.94	38.00
39.00						12.22	39.00
40.00						12.51	40.00
41.00						12.79	41.00
42.00						13.07	42.00
43.00						13.35	43.00
44.00						13.64	44.00
45.00						13.92	45.00
46.00						14.20	46.00
47.00						14.48	47.00
48.00						14.77	48.00
49.00						15.05	49.00
50.00						15.33	50.00
51.00						15.61	51.00
52.00						15.90	52.00
53.00						16.18	53.00
54.00						16.46	54.00
55.00						16.75	55.00
56.00						17.03	56.00
57.00						17.31	57.00
58.00						17.59	58.00
59.00						17.88	59.00
60.00						18.16	60.00
61.00						18.44	61.00
62.00						18.72	62.00
63.00						19.01	63.00
64.00						19.29	64.00

Table 4.4. Raw to Scaled Score Conversions.

RAWSCORE	VERBAL	ANIMAL	RAWSCORE
0.00	1.23	−1.59	0.00
1.00	1.51	−0.84	1.00
2.00	1.79	−0.09	2.00
3.00	2.07	0.66	3.00
4.00	2.34	1.41	4.00
5.00	2.62	2.17	5.00
6.00	2.90	2.92	6.00
7.00	3.18	3.67	7.00
8.00	3.46	4.42	8.00
9.00	3.74	5.17	9.00
10.00	4.02	5.92	10.00
11.00	4.30	6.67	11.00
12.00	4.58	7.42	12.00
13.00	4.86	8.18	13.00
14.00	5.14	8.93	14.00
15.00	5.42	9.68	15.00
16.00	5.70	10.43	16.00
17.00	5.98	11.18	17.00
18.00	6.26	11.93	18.00
19.00	6.53	12.68	19.00
20.00	6.81	13.43	20.00
21.00	7.09	14.19	21.00
22.00	7.37	14.94	22.00
23.00	7.65	15.69	23.00
24.00	7.93	16.44	24.00
25.00	8.21	17.19	25.00
26.00	8.49	17.94	26.00
27.00	8.77	18.69	27.00
28.00	9.05		28.00
29.00	9.33		29.00
30.00	9.61		30.00
31.00	9.89		31.00
32.00	10.17		32.00
33.00	10.45		33.00
34.00	10.72		34.00
35.00	11.00		35.00
36.00	11.28		36.00
37.00	11.56		37.00
38.00	11.84		38.00
39.00	12.12		39.00
40.00	12.40		40.00
41.00	12.68		41.00
42.00	12.96		42.00
43.00	13.24		43.00
44.00	13.52		44.00
45.00	13.80		45.00
46.00	14.08		46.00
47.00	14.36		47.00
48.00	14.64		48.00
49.00	14.91		49.00
50.00	15.19		50.00

Table continues.

Table 4.4. Raw to Scaled Score Conversions (continued).

RAWS CORE	VERBAL	ANIMAL	RAWS CORE
51.00	15.47		51.00
52.00	15.75		52.00
53.00	16.03		53.00
54.00	16.31		54.00
55.00	16.59		55.00
56.00	16.87		56.00
57.00	17.15		57.00
58.00	17.43		58.00
59.00	17.71		59.00
60.00	17.99		60.00
61.00	18.27		61.00
62.00	18.55		62.00
63.00	18.83		63.00
64.00	19.10		64.00

Table 5. Raw Score Means and Standard Deviations for Subject Samples.

Test Measure	Base Sample	Validation Sample	Total Sample
WECHSLER			
Mean	5.34	5.60	5.39
SD	0.88	0.64	0.84
BUSCHFR1			
Mean	8.06	7.90	8.03
SD	1.61	1.71	1.62
BRETRIE			
Mean	26.72	26.36	26.65
SD	3.97	4.19	4.01
BACQUIS			
Mean	35.81	35.66	35.78
SD	0.61	1.22	0.76
BUSCHTR			
Mean	11.94	11.88	11.93
SD	0.27	0.48	0.32
REYA1			
Mean	4.43	4.68	4.48
SD	1.72	1.67	1.71
REYA2			
Mean	6.83	6.72	6.81
SD	2.03	1.92	2.01
REYA3			
Mean	8.43	8.10	8.37
SD	2.31	2.30	2.30
REYA4			
Mean	9.51	8.78	9.37
SD	2.44	2.22	2.41
REYA5			
Mean	10.30	9.98	10.24
SD	2.41	2.44	2.41

Table continues.

Table 5. Raw Score Means and Standard Deviations for Subject Samples (continued).

REYTOT			
Mean	39.50	38.26	39.26
SD	9.02	8.41	8.91
REYB1			
Mean	3.84	4.20	3.91
SD	1.77	1.64	1.75
REYA6			
Mean	7.78	7.54	7.74
SD	3.03	3.11	3.04
TRUEPOSI			
Mean	13.82	13.82	13.82
SD	1.37	1.53	1.40
TRUENEGA			
Mean	14.31	14.62	14.37
SD	1.99	1.85	1.97
CORRECT			
Mean	12.25	11.68	12.14
SD	2.15	2.00	2.13
DIGITSPA			
Mean	5.97	6.12	6.00
SD	0.99	1.10	1.02
WAISIMIL			
Mean	8.43	8.38	8.42
SD	3.72	3.51	3.67
WAISJUDG			
Mean	10.07	10.04	10.07
SD	2.84	2.88	2.84
VERBAL			
Mean	31.40	31.44	31.41
SD	10.74	9.32	10.47
ANIMAL			
Mean	15.43	15.06	15.36
SD	3.99	3.67	3.93
TOKEN			
Mean	39.65	40.00	39.71
SD	5.19	4.39	5.05
WAISBLOC			
Mean	11.07	11.08	11.07
SD	4.61	4.72	4.62
DIGIT			
Mean	31.13	32.28	31.35
SD	10.62	10.33	10.64

Table 6.1. Age 65 – Male.

EDUCATION	BUSCHFR1	BRETRIE	REYA1	REYA2	REYA3	REYA4	REYA5	REYTOT	REYB1	REYA6
0 YRS	10.49	10.80	9.45	9.22	8.44	8.34	7.34	9.81	8.96	8.16
1 YRS	10.55	10.91	9.57	9.34	8.67	8.57	7.65	9.95	9.18	8.41
2 YRS	10.61	11.02	9.70	9.46	8.90	8.79	7.96	10.09	9.40	8.67
3 YRS	10.68	11.13	9.83	9.58	9.14	9.02	8.26	10.23	9.62	8.92
4 YRS	10.74	11.24	9.95	9.70	9.37	9.25	8.57	10.37	9.84	9.18
5 YRS	10.80	11.35	10.08	9.82	9.60	9.47	8.88	10.50	10.06	9.43
6 YRS	10.87	11.46	10.20	9.94	9.84	9.70	9.18	10.64	10.28	9.68
7 YRS	10.93	11.57	10.33	10.06	10.07	9.93	9.49	10.78	10.51	9.94
8 YRS	10.99	11.68	10.45	10.18	10.30	10.15	9.80	10.92	10.73	10.19
9 YRS	11.06	11.79	10.58	10.30	10.54	10.38	10.11	11.06	10.95	10.45
10 YRS	11.12	11.90	10.70	10.42	10.77	10.61	10.41	11.19	11.17	10.70
11 YRS	11.18	12.01	10.83	10.54	11.00	10.84	10.72	11.33	11.39	10.95
12 YRS	11.25	12.12	10.96	10.66	11.24	11.06	11.03	11.47	11.61	11.21
13 YRS	11.31	12.23	11.08	10.78	11.47	11.29	11.33	11.61	11.83	11.46
14 YRS	11.37	12.34	11.21	10.90	11.70	11.52	11.64	11.75	12.05	11.72
15 YRS	11.44	12.45	11.33	11.02	11.94	11.74	11.95	11.89	12.27	11.97
16 YRS	11.50	12.56	11.46	11.14	12.17	11.97	12.25	12.02	12.49	12.22
17 YRS	11.56	12.67	11.58	11.26	12.40	12.20	12.56	12.16	12.72	12.48
18 YRS	11.63	12.78	11.71	11.38	12.63	12.43	12.87	12.30	12.94	12.73
19 YRS	11.69	12.89	11.83	11.50	12.87	12.65	13.17	12.44	13.16	12.99
20 YRS	11.75	13.00	11.96	11.62	13.10	12.88	13.48	12.58	13.38	13.24
21 YRS	11.82	13.11	12.08	11.75	13.33	13.11	13.79	12.71	13.60	13.49
22 YRS	11.88	13.22	12.21	11.87	13.57	13.33	14.09	12.85	13.82	13.75
23 YRS	11.94	13.33	12.34	11.99	13.80	13.56	14.40	12.99	14.04	14.00
24 YRS	12.01	13.44	12.46	12.11	14.03	13.79	14.71	13.13	14.26	14.25
25 YRS	12.07	13.55	12.59	12.23	14.27	14.01	15.01	13.27	14.48	14.51
26 YRS	12.13	13.66	12.71	12.35	14.50	14.24	15.32	13.41	14.70	14.76
27 YRS	12.20	13.77	12.84	12.47	14.73	14.47	15.63	13.54	14.93	15.02
28 YRS	12.26	13.88	12.96	12.59	14.97	14.70	15.93	13.68	15.15	15.27
29 YRS	12.32	13.99	13.09	12.71	15.20	14.92	16.24	13.82	15.37	15.52
30 YRS	12.39	14.10	13.21	12.83	15.43	15.15	16.55	13.96	15.59	15.78

EDUCATION	CORRECT	DIGITSPA	WAISIMIL	WAISJUDG	VERBAL	ANIMAL	WAISBLOC	DIGIT
0 YRS	9.30	8.25	6.14	6.94	6.34	8.94	9.25	8.39
1 YRS	9.54	8.50	6.57	7.33	6.70	9.24	9.51	8.77
2 YRS	9.78	8.74	7.00	7.73	7.06	9.54	9.77	9.15
3 YRS	10.02	8.99	7.43	8.12	7.42	9.85	10.03	9.53
4 YRS	10.26	9.24	7.86	8.51	7.78	10.15	10.29	9.90
5 YRS	10.50	9.49	8.29	8.90	8.14	10.45	10.55	10.28
6 YRS	10.74	9.74	8.73	9.30	8.50	10.75	10.81	10.66
7 YRS	10.98	9.98	9.16	9.69	8.86	11.06	11.07	11.04
8 YRS	11.22	10.23	9.59	10.08	9.22	11.36	11.33	11.42
9 YRS	11.46	10.48	10.02	10.47	9.58	11.66	11.59	11.80
10 YRS	11.70	10.73	10.45	10.87	9.94	11.97	11.85	12.17
11 YRS	11.93	10.97	10.88	11.26	10.30	12.27	12.10	12.55
12 YRS	12.17	11.22	11.32	11.65	10.66	12.57	12.36	12.93
13 YRS	12.41	11.47	11.75	12.04	11.02	12.88	12.62	13.31
14 YRS	12.65	11.72	12.18	12.44	11.38	13.18	12.88	13.69
15 YRS	12.89	11.97	12.61	12.83	11.74	13.48	13.14	14.07
16 YRS	13.13	12.21	13.04	13.22	12.10	13.79	13.40	14.44
17 YRS	13.37	12.46	13.47	13.62	12.46	14.09	13.66	14.82
18 YRS	13.61	12.71	13.91	14.01	12.82	14.39	13.92	15.20
19 YRS	13.85	12.96	14.34	14.40	13.18	14.69	14.18	15.58
20 YRS	14.09	13.21	14.77	14.79	13.54	15.00	14.44	15.96
21 YRS	14.33	13.45	15.20	15.19	13.90	15.30	14.70	16.34
22 YRS	14.57	13.70	15.63	15.58	14.26	15.60	14.96	16.71
23 YRS	14.80	13.95	16.06	15.97	14.62	15.91	15.22	17.09
24 YRS	15.04	14.20	16.49	16.36	14.99	16.21	15.48	17.47
25 YRS	15.28	14.44	16.93	16.76	15.35	16.51	15.74	17.85
26 YRS	15.52	14.69	17.36	17.15	15.71	16.82	16.00	18.23
27 YRS	15.76	14.94	17.79	17.54	16.07	17.12	16.26	18.61
28 YRS	16.00	15.19	18.22	17.93	16.43	17.42	16.52	18.98
29 YRS	16.24	15.44	18.65	18.33	16.79	17.73	16.78	19.36
30 YRS	16.48	15.68	19.08	18.72	17.15	18.03	17.04	19.74

Table 6.2. Age 65 – Female.

EDUCATION	BUSCHFR1	BRETRIE	REYA1	REYA2	REYA3	REYA4	REYA5	REYTOT	REYB1	REYA6
0 YRS	10.49	10.80	9.45	9.22	8.44	8.34	7.34	9.81	8.96	8.16
1 YRS	10.55	10.91	9.57	9.34	8.67	8.57	7.65	9.95	9.18	8.41
2 YRS	10.61	11.02	9.70	9.46	8.90	8.79	7.96	10.09	9.40	8.67
3 YRS	10.68	11.13	9.83	9.58	9.14	9.02	8.26	10.23	9.62	8.92
4 YRS	10.74	11.24	9.95	9.70	9.37	9.25	8.57	10.37	9.84	9.18
5 YRS	10.80	11.35	10.08	9.82	9.60	9.47	8.88	10.50	10.06	9.43
6 YRS	10.87	11.46	10.20	9.94	9.84	9.70	9.18	10.64	10.28	9.68
7 YRS	10.93	11.57	10.33	10.06	10.07	9.93	9.49	10.78	10.51	9.94
8 YRS	10.99	11.68	10.45	10.18	10.30	10.15	9.80	10.92	10.73	10.19
9 YRS	11.06	11.79	10.58	10.30	10.54	10.38	10.11	11.06	10.95	10.45
10 YRS	11.12	11.90	10.70	10.42	10.77	10.61	10.41	11.19	11.17	10.70
11 YRS	11.18	12.01	10.83	10.54	11.00	10.84	10.72	11.33	11.39	10.95
12 YRS	11.25	12.12	10.96	10.66	11.24	11.06	11.03	11.47	11.61	11.21
13 YRS	11.31	12.23	11.08	10.78	11.47	11.29	11.33	11.61	11.83	11.46
14 YRS	11.37	12.34	11.21	10.90	11.70	11.52	11.64	11.75	12.05	11.72
15 YRS	11.44	12.45	11.33	11.02	11.94	11.74	11.95	11.89	12.27	11.97
16 YRS	11.50	12.56	11.46	11.14	12.17	11.97	12.25	12.02	12.49	12.22
17 YRS	11.56	12.67	11.58	11.26	12.40	12.20	12.56	12.16	12.72	12.48
18 YRS	11.63	12.78	11.71	11.38	12.63	12.43	12.87	12.30	12.94	12.73
19 YRS	11.69	12.89	11.83	11.50	12.87	12.65	13.17	12.44	13.16	12.99
20 YRS	11.75	13.00	11.96	11.62	13.10	12.88	13.48	12.58	13.38	13.24
21 YRS	11.82	13.11	12.08	11.75	13.33	13.11	13.79	12.71	13.60	13.49
22 YRS	11.88	13.22	12.21	11.87	13.57	13.33	14.09	12.85	13.82	13.75
23 YRS	11.94	13.33	12.34	11.99	13.80	13.56	14.40	12.99	14.04	14.00
24 YRS	12.01	13.44	12.46	12.11	14.03	13.79	14.71	13.13	14.26	14.25
25 YRS	12.07	13.55	12.59	12.23	14.27	14.01	15.01	13.27	14.48	14.51
26 YRS	12.13	13.66	12.71	12.35	14.50	14.24	15.32	13.41	14.70	14.76
27 YRS	12.20	13.77	12.84	12.47	14.73	14.47	15.63	13.54	14.93	15.02
28 YRS	12.26	13.88	12.96	12.59	14.97	14.70	15.93	13.68	15.15	15.27
29 YRS	12.32	13.99	13.09	12.71	15.20	14.92	16.24	13.82	15.37	15.52
30 YRS	12.39	14.10	13.21	12.83	15.43	15.15	16.55	13.96	15.59	15.78

EDUCATION	CORRECT	DIGITSPA	WAISIMIL	WAISJUDG	VERBAL	ANIMAL	WAISBLOC	DIGIT
0 YRS	9.30	8.25	6.14	6.94	6.34	8.94	9.25	8.39
1 YRS	9.54	8.50	6.57	7.33	6.70	9.24	9.51	8.77
2 YRS	9.78	8.74	7.00	7.73	7.06	9.54	9.77	9.15
3 YRS	10.02	8.99	7.43	8.12	7.42	9.85	10.03	9.53
4 YRS	10.26	9.24	7.86	8.51	7.78	10.15	10.29	9.90
5 YRS	10.50	9.49	8.29	8.90	8.14	10.45	10.55	10.28
6 YRS	10.74	9.74	8.73	9.30	8.50	10.75	10.81	10.66
7 YRS	10.98	9.98	9.16	9.69	8.86	11.06	11.07	11.04
8 YRS	11.22	10.23	9.59	10.08	9.22	11.36	11.33	11.42
9 YRS	11.46	10.48	10.02	10.47	9.58	11.66	11.59	11.80
10 YRS	11.70	10.73	10.45	10.87	9.94	11.97	11.85	12.17
11 YRS	11.93	10.97	10.88	11.26	10.30	12.27	12.10	12.55
12 YRS	12.17	11.22	11.32	11.65	10.66	12.57	12.36	12.93
13 YRS	12.41	11.47	11.75	12.04	11.02	12.88	12.62	13.31
14 YRS	12.65	11.72	12.18	12.44	11.38	13.18	12.88	13.69
15 YRS	12.89	11.97	12.61	12.83	11.74	13.48	13.14	14.07
16 YRS	13.13	12.21	13.04	13.22	12.10	13.79	13.40	14.44
17 YRS	13.37	12.46	13.47	13.62	12.46	14.09	13.66	14.82
18 YRS	13.61	12.71	13.91	14.01	12.82	14.39	13.92	15.20
19 YRS	13.85	12.96	14.34	14.40	13.18	14.69	14.18	15.58
20 YRS	14.09	13.21	14.77	14.79	13.54	15.00	14.44	15.96
21 YRS	14.33	13.45	15.20	15.19	13.90	15.30	14.70	16.34
22 YRS	14.57	13.70	15.63	15.58	14.26	15.60	14.96	16.71
23 YRS	14.80	13.95	16.06	15.97	14.62	15.91	15.22	17.09
24 YRS	15.04	14.20	16.49	16.36	14.99	16.21	15.48	17.47
25 YRS	15.28	14.44	16.93	16.76	15.35	16.51	15.74	17.85
26 YRS	15.52	14.69	17.36	17.15	15.71	16.82	16.00	18.23
27 YRS	15.76	14.94	17.79	17.54	16.07	17.12	16.26	18.61
28 YRS	16.00	15.19	18.22	17.93	16.43	17.42	16.52	18.98
29 YRS	16.24	15.44	18.65	18.33	16.79	17.73	16.78	19.36
30 YRS	16.48	15.68	19.08	18.72	17.15	18.03	17.04	19.74

Table 7.1. Age 66 – Male.

EDUCATION	BUSCHFR1	BREFTRIE	REYA1	REYA2	REYA3	REYA4	REYA5	REYTOT	REYB1	REYA6
0 YRS	10.37	10.64	9.35	9.11	8.29	8.19	7.20	9.66	8.80	8.00
1 YRS	10.43	10.75	9.48	9.23	8.52	8.42	7.50	9.80	9.02	8.25
2 YRS	10.50	10.86	9.60	9.35	8.75	8.64	7.81	9.94	9.24	8.51
3 YRS	10.56	10.97	9.73	9.47	8.99	8.87	8.12	10.08	9.46	8.76
4 YRS	10.62	11.08	9.85	9.59	9.22	9.10	8.42	10.22	9.68	9.02
5 YRS	10.69	11.19	9.98	9.71	9.45	9.33	8.73	10.35	9.90	9.27
6 YRS	10.75	11.30	10.11	9.83	9.69	9.55	9.04	10.49	10.12	9.52
7 YRS	10.81	11.41	10.23	9.95	9.92	9.78	9.34	10.63	10.34	9.78
8 YRS	10.88	11.52	10.36	10.08	10.15	10.01	9.65	10.77	10.56	10.03
9 YRS	10.94	11.63	10.48	10.20	10.39	10.23	9.96	10.91	10.79	10.29
10 YRS	11.00	11.74	10.61	10.32	10.62	10.46	10.27	11.04	11.01	10.54
11 YRS	11.07	11.85	10.73	10.44	10.85	10.69	10.57	11.18	11.23	10.79
12 YRS	11.13	11.96	10.86	10.56	11.08	10.91	10.88	11.32	11.45	11.05
13 YRS	11.19	12.07	10.98	10.68	11.32	11.14	11.19	11.46	11.67	11.30
14 YRS	11.26	12.18	11.11	10.80	11.55	11.37	11.49	11.60	11.89	11.56
15 YRS	11.32	12.29	11.23	10.92	11.78	11.60	11.80	11.74	12.11	11.81
16 YRS	11.38	12.40	11.36	11.04	12.02	11.82	12.11	11.87	12.33	12.06
17 YRS	11.45	12.51	11.49	11.16	12.25	12.05	12.41	12.01	12.55	12.32
18 YRS	11.51	12.62	11.61	11.28	12.48	12.28	12.72	12.15	12.77	12.57
19 YRS	11.57	12.73	11.74	11.40	12.72	12.50	13.03	12.29	12.99	12.83
20 YRS	11.64	12.84	11.86	11.52	12.95	12.73	13.33	12.43	13.22	13.08
21 YRS	11.70	12.95	11.99	11.64	13.18	12.96	13.64	12.56	13.44	13.33
22 YRS	11.76	13.05	12.11	11.76	13.42	13.18	13.95	12.70	13.66	13.59
23 YRS	11.83	13.16	12.24	11.88	13.65	13.41	14.25	12.84	13.88	13.84
24 YRS	11.89	13.27	12.36	12.00	13.88	13.64	14.56	12.98	14.10	14.09
25 YRS	11.95	13.38	12.49	12.12	14.12	13.87	14.87	13.12	14.32	14.35
26 YRS	12.02	13.49	12.62	12.24	14.35	14.09	15.17	13.26	14.54	14.60
27 YRS	12.08	13.60	12.74	12.36	14.58	14.32	15.48	13.39	14.76	14.86
28 YRS	12.14	13.71	12.87	12.48	14.82	14.55	15.79	13.53	14.98	15.11
29 YRS	12.21	13.82	12.99	12.60	15.05	14.77	16.09	13.67	15.20	15.36
30 YRS	12.27	13.93	13.12	12.72	15.28	15.00	16.40	13.81	15.43	15.62

EDUCATION	CORRECT	DIGITSPA	WAISIMIL	WAISJUDG	VERBAL	ANIMAL	WAISBLOC	DIGIT
0 YRS	9.15	8.18	6.04	6.88	6.28	8.82	9.13	8.17
1 YRS	9.39	8.43	6.47	7.27	6.64	9.12	9.39	8.55
2 YRS	9.63	8.68	6.90	7.66	7.00	9.43	9.65	8.93
3 YRS	9.87	8.93	7.34	8.05	7.36	9.73	9.91	9.31
4 YRS	10.11	9.17	7.77	8.45	7.72	10.03	10.17	9.68
5 YRS	10.34	9.42	8.20	8.84	8.08	10.33	10.43	10.06
6 YRS	10.58	9.67	8.63	9.23	8.44	10.64	10.69	10.44
7 YRS	10.82	9.92	9.06	9.63	8.80	10.94	10.95	10.82
8 YRS	11.06	10.17	9.49	10.02	9.16	11.24	11.21	11.20
9 YRS	11.30	10.41	9.93	10.41	9.52	11.55	11.47	11.58
10 YRS	11.54	10.66	10.36	10.80	9.88	11.85	11.73	11.95
11 YRS	11.78	10.91	10.79	11.20	10.24	12.15	11.99	12.33
12 YRS	12.02	11.16	11.22	11.59	10.60	12.46	12.25	12.71
13 YRS	12.26	11.40	11.65	11.98	10.96	12.76	12.51	13.09
14 YRS	12.50	11.65	12.08	12.37	11.32	13.06	12.77	13.47
15 YRS	12.74	11.90	12.52	12.77	11.68	13.37	13.03	13.85
16 YRS	12.98	12.15	12.95	13.16	12.05	13.67	13.29	14.22
17 YRS	13.22	12.40	13.38	13.55	12.41	13.97	13.55	14.60
18 YRS	13.45	12.64	13.81	13.94	12.77	14.27	13.81	14.98
19 YRS	13.69	12.89	14.24	14.34	13.13	14.58	14.07	15.36
20 YRS	13.93	13.14	14.67	14.73	13.49	14.88	14.33	15.74
21 YRS	14.17	13.39	15.10	15.12	13.85	15.18	14.59	16.12
22 YRS	14.41	13.64	15.54	15.51	14.21	15.49	14.85	16.49
23 YRS	14.65	13.88	15.97	15.91	14.57	15.79	15.11	16.87
24 YRS	14.89	14.13	16.40	16.30	14.93	16.09	15.36	17.25
25 YRS	15.13	14.38	16.83	16.69	15.29	16.40	15.62	17.63
26 YRS	15.37	14.63	17.26	17.09	15.65	16.70	15.88	18.01
27 YRS	15.61	14.87	17.69	17.48	16.01	17.00	16.14	18.39
28 YRS	15.85	15.12	18.13	17.87	16.37	17.31	16.40	18.76
29 YRS	16.09	15.37	18.56	18.26	16.73	17.61	16.66	19.14
30 YRS	16.33	15.62	18.99	18.66	17.09	17.91	16.92	19.52

Table 7.2. Age 66 – Female.

EDUCATION	BUSCHFRI	BRETRIE	REYA1	REYA2	REYA3	REYA4	REYA5	REYTOT	REYB1	REYA6
0 YRS	10.37	10.64	9.35	9.11	8.29	8.19	7.20	9.66	8.80	8.00
1 YRS	10.43	10.75	9.48	9.23	8.52	8.42	7.50	9.80	9.02	8.25
2 YRS	10.50	10.86	9.60	9.35	8.75	8.64	7.81	9.94	9.24	8.51
3 YRS	10.56	10.97	9.73	9.47	8.99	8.87	8.12	10.08	9.46	8.76
4 YRS	10.62	11.08	9.85	9.59	9.22	9.10	8.42	10.22	9.68	9.02
5 YRS	10.69	11.19	9.98	9.71	9.45	9.33	8.73	10.35	9.90	9.27
6 YRS	10.75	11.30	10.11	9.83	9.69	9.55	9.04	10.49	10.12	9.52
7 YRS	10.81	11.41	10.23	9.95	9.92	9.78	9.34	10.63	10.34	9.78
8 YRS	10.88	11.52	10.36	10.08	10.15	10.01	9.65	10.77	10.56	10.03
9 YRS	10.94	11.63	10.48	10.20	10.39	10.23	9.96	10.91	10.79	10.29
10 YRS	11.00	11.74	10.61	10.32	10.62	10.46	10.27	11.04	11.01	10.54
11 YRS	11.07	11.85	10.73	10.44	10.85	10.69	10.57	11.18	11.23	10.79
12 YRS	11.13	11.96	10.86	10.56	11.08	10.91	10.88	11.32	11.45	11.05
13 YRS	11.19	12.07	10.98	10.68	11.32	11.14	11.19	11.46	11.67	11.30
14 YRS	11.26	12.18	11.11	10.80	11.55	11.37	11.49	11.60	11.89	11.56
15 YRS	11.32	12.29	11.23	10.92	11.78	11.60	11.80	11.74	12.11	11.81
16 YRS	11.38	12.40	11.36	11.04	12.02	11.82	12.11	11.87	12.33	12.06
17 YRS	11.45	12.51	11.49	11.16	12.25	12.05	12.41	12.01	12.55	12.32
18 YRS	11.51	12.62	11.61	11.28	12.48	12.28	12.72	12.15	12.77	12.57
19 YRS	11.57	12.73	11.74	11.40	12.72	12.50	13.03	12.29	12.99	12.83
20 YRS	11.64	12.84	11.86	11.52	12.95	12.73	13.33	12.43	13.22	13.08
21 YRS	11.70	12.95	11.99	11.64	13.18	12.96	13.64	12.56	13.44	13.33
22 YRS	11.76	13.05	12.11	11.76	13.42	13.18	13.95	12.70	13.66	13.59
23 YRS	11.83	13.16	12.24	11.88	13.65	13.41	14.25	12.84	13.88	13.84
24 YRS	11.89	13.27	12.36	12.00	13.88	13.64	14.56	12.98	14.10	14.09
25 YRS	11.95	13.38	12.49	12.12	14.12	13.87	14.87	13.12	14.32	14.35
26 YRS	12.02	13.49	12.62	12.24	14.35	14.09	15.17	13.26	14.54	14.60
27 YRS	12.08	13.60	12.74	12.36	14.58	14.32	15.48	13.39	14.76	14.86
28 YRS	12.14	13.71	12.87	12.48	14.82	14.55	15.79	13.53	14.98	15.11
29 YRS	12.21	13.82	12.99	12.60	15.05	14.77	16.09	13.67	15.20	15.36
30 YRS	12.27	13.93	13.12	12.72	15.28	15.00	16.40	13.81	15.43	15.62

EDUCATION	CORRECT	DIGITSPA	WAISIMIL	WAISJUDG	VERBAL	ANIMAL	WAISBLOC	DIGIT
0 YRS	9.15	8.18	6.04	6.88	6.28	8.82	9.13	8.17
1 YRS	9.39	8.43	6.47	7.27	6.64	9.12	9.39	8.55
2 YRS	9.63	8.68	6.90	7.66	7.00	9.43	9.65	8.93
3 YRS	9.87	8.93	7.34	8.05	7.36	9.73	9.91	9.31
4 YRS	10.11	9.17	7.77	8.45	7.72	10.03	10.17	9.68
5 YRS	10.34	9.42	8.20	8.84	8.08	10.33	10.43	10.06
6 YRS	10.58	9.67	8.63	9.23	8.44	10.64	10.69	10.44
7 YRS	10.82	9.92	9.06	9.63	8.80	10.94	10.95	10.82
8 YRS	11.06	10.17	9.49	10.02	9.16	11.24	11.21	11.20
9 YRS	11.30	10.41	9.93	10.41	9.52	11.55	11.47	11.58
10 YRS	11.54	10.66	10.36	10.80	9.88	11.85	11.73	11.95
11 YRS	11.78	10.91	10.79	11.20	10.24	12.15	11.99	12.33
12 YRS	12.02	11.16	11.22	11.59	10.60	12.46	12.25	12.71
13 YRS	12.26	11.40	11.65	11.98	10.96	12.76	12.51	13.09
14 YRS	12.50	11.65	12.08	12.37	11.32	13.06	12.77	13.47
15 YRS	12.74	11.90	12.52	12.77	11.68	13.37	13.03	13.85
16 YRS	12.98	12.15	12.95	13.16	12.05	13.67	13.29	14.22
17 YRS	13.22	12.40	13.38	13.55	12.41	13.97	13.55	14.60
18 YRS	13.45	12.64	13.81	13.94	12.77	14.27	13.81	14.98
19 YRS	13.69	12.89	14.24	14.34	13.13	14.58	14.07	15.36
20 YRS	13.93	13.14	14.67	14.73	13.49	14.88	14.33	15.74
21 YRS	14.17	13.39	15.10	15.12	13.85	15.18	14.59	16.12
22 YRS	14.41	13.64	15.54	15.51	14.21	15.49	14.85	16.49
23 YRS	14.65	13.88	15.97	15.91	14.57	15.79	15.11	16.87
24 YRS	14.89	14.13	16.40	16.30	14.93	16.09	15.36	17.25
25 YRS	15.13	14.38	16.83	16.69	15.29	16.40	15.62	17.63
26 YRS	15.37	14.63	17.26	17.09	15.65	16.70	15.88	18.01
27 YRS	15.61	14.87	17.69	17.48	16.01	17.00	16.14	18.39
28 YRS	15.85	15.12	18.13	17.87	16.37	17.31	16.40	18.76
29 YRS	16.09	15.37	18.56	18.26	16.73	17.61	16.66	19.14
30 YRS	16.33	15.62	18.99	18.66	17.09	17.91	16.92	19.52

Table 8.1. Age 67 – Male.

EDUCATION	BUSCHFR1	BRETRIE	REYA1	REYA2	REYA3	REYA4	REYA5	REYTOT	REYB1	REYA6
0 YRS	10.25	10.47	9.25	9.01	8.14	8.04	7.05	9.51	8.63	7.84
1 YRS	10.32	10.58	9.38	9.13	8.37	8.27	7.36	9.65	8.85	8.09
2 YRS	10.38	10.69	9.51	9.25	8.60	8.50	7.66	9.79	9.08	8.35
3 YRS	10.44	10.80	9.63	9.37	8.84	8.72	7.97	9.93	9.30	8.60
4 YRS	10.51	10.91	9.76	9.49	9.07	8.95	8.28	10.07	9.52	8.86
5 YRS	10.57	11.02	9.88	9.61	9.30	9.18	8.58	10.20	9.74	9.11
6 YRS	10.63	11.13	10.01	9.73	9.54	9.40	8.89	10.34	9.96	9.36
7 YRS	10.70	11.24	10.13	9.85	9.77	9.63	9.20	10.48	10.18	9.62
8 YRS	10.76	11.35	10.26	9.97	10.00	9.86	9.50	10.62	10.40	9.87
9 YRS	10.82	11.46	10.38	10.09	10.23	10.08	9.81	10.76	10.62	10.13
10 YRS	10.89	11.57	10.51	10.21	10.47	10.31	10.12	10.89	10.84	10.38
11 YRS	10.95	11.68	10.64	10.33	10.70	10.54	10.42	11.03	11.06	10.63
12 YRS	11.01	11.79	10.76	10.45	10.93	10.77	10.73	11.17	11.29	10.89
13 YRS	11.08	11.90	10.89	10.57	11.17	10.99	11.04	11.31	11.51	11.14
14 YRS	11.14	12.01	11.01	10.69	11.40	11.22	11.35	11.45	11.73	11.40
15 YRS	11.20	12.12	11.14	10.81	11.63	11.45	11.65	11.59	11.95	11.65
16 YRS	11.26	12.23	11.26	10.93	11.87	11.67	11.96	11.72	12.17	11.90
17 YRS	11.33	12.34	11.39	11.05	12.10	11.90	12.27	11.86	12.39	12.16
18 YRS	11.39	12.45	11.51	11.17	12.33	12.13	12.57	12.00	12.61	12.41
19 YRS	11.45	12.56	11.64	11.29	12.57	12.36	12.88	12.14	12.83	12.67
20 YRS	11.52	12.67	11.77	11.42	12.80	12.58	13.19	12.28	13.05	12.92
21 YRS	11.58	12.78	11.89	11.54	13.03	12.81	13.49	12.41	13.27	13.17
22 YRS	11.64	12.89	12.02	11.66	13.27	13.04	13.80	12.55	13.49	13.43
23 YRS	11.71	13.00	12.14	11.78	13.50	13.26	14.11	12.69	13.72	13.68
24 YRS	11.77	13.11	12.27	11.90	13.73	13.49	14.41	12.83	13.94	13.93
25 YRS	11.83	13.22	12.39	12.02	13.97	13.72	14.72	12.97	14.16	14.19
26 YRS	11.90	13.33	12.52	12.14	14.20	13.94	15.03	13.11	14.38	14.44
27 YRS	11.96	13.44	12.64	12.26	14.43	14.17	15.33	13.24	14.60	14.70
28 YRS	12.02	13.55	12.77	12.38	14.66	14.40	15.64	13.38	14.82	14.95
29 YRS	12.09	13.66	12.90	12.50	14.90	14.63	15.95	13.52	15.04	15.20
30 YRS	12.15	13.77	13.02	12.62	15.13	14.85	16.25	13.66	15.26	15.46

EDUCATION	CORRECT	DIGITSPA	WAISIMIL	WAISJUDG	VERBAL	ANIMAL	WAISBLOC	DIGIT
0 YRS	8.99	8.12	5.95	6.81	6.22	8.70	9.02	7.95
1 YRS	9.23	8.36	6.38	7.21	6.58	9.01	9.28	8.33
2 YRS	9.47	8.61	6.81	7.60	6.94	9.31	9.54	8.71
3 YRS	9.71	8.86	7.24	7.99	7.30	9.61	9.80	9.09
4 YRS	9.95	9.11	7.67	8.38	7.66	9.91	10.06	9.46
5 YRS	10.19	9.36	8.10	8.78	8.02	10.22	10.32	9.84
6 YRS	10.43	9.60	8.54	9.17	8.38	10.52	10.58	10.22
7 YRS	10.67	9.85	8.97	9.56	8.75	10.82	10.84	10.60
8 YRS	10.91	10.10	9.40	9.95	9.11	11.13	11.10	10.98
9 YRS	11.15	10.35	9.83	10.35	9.47	11.43	11.36	11.36
10 YRS	11.39	10.60	10.26	10.74	9.83	11.73	11.61	11.73
11 YRS	11.63	10.84	10.69	11.13	10.19	12.04	11.87	12.11
12 YRS	11.87	11.09	11.13	11.52	10.55	12.34	12.13	12.49
13 YRS	12.10	11.34	11.56	11.92	10.91	12.64	12.39	12.87
14 YRS	12.34	11.59	11.99	12.31	11.27	12.95	12.65	13.25
15 YRS	12.58	11.83	12.42	12.70	11.63	13.25	12.91	13.62
16 YRS	12.82	12.08	12.85	13.09	11.99	13.55	13.17	14.00
17 YRS	13.06	12.33	13.28	13.49	12.35	13.85	13.43	14.38
18 YRS	13.30	12.58	13.71	13.88	12.71	14.16	13.69	14.76
19 YRS	13.54	12.83	14.15	14.27	13.07	14.46	13.95	15.14
20 YRS	13.78	13.07	14.58	14.67	13.43	14.76	14.21	15.52
21 YRS	14.02	13.32	15.01	15.06	13.79	15.07	14.47	15.89
22 YRS	14.26	13.57	15.44	15.45	14.15	15.37	14.73	16.27
23 YRS	14.50	13.82	15.87	15.84	14.51	15.67	14.99	16.65
24 YRS	14.74	14.07	16.30	16.24	14.87	15.98	15.25	17.03
25 YRS	14.98	14.31	16.74	16.63	15.23	16.28	15.51	17.41
26 YRS	15.21	14.56	17.17	17.02	15.59	16.58	15.77	17.79
27 YRS	15.45	14.81	17.60	17.41	15.95	16.89	16.03	18.16
28 YRS	15.69	15.06	18.03	17.81	16.31	17.19	16.29	18.54
29 YRS	15.93	15.30	18.46	18.20	16.67	17.49	16.55	18.92
30 YRS	16.17	15.55	18.89	18.59	17.03	17.79	16.81	19.30

Table 8.2. Age 67 – Female.

EDUCATION	BUSCHFR1	BRETRIE	REYA1	REYA2	REYA3	REYA4	REYA5	REYTOT	REYB1	REYA6
0 YRS	10.25	10.47	9.25	9.01	8.14	8.04	7.05	9.51	8.63	7.84
1 YRS	10.32	10.58	9.38	9.13	8.37	8.27	7.36	9.65	8.85	8.09
2 YRS	10.38	10.69	9.51	9.25	8.60	8.50	7.66	9.79	9.08	8.35
3 YRS	10.44	10.80	9.63	9.37	8.84	8.72	7.97	9.93	9.30	8.60
4 YRS	10.51	10.91	9.76	9.49	9.07	8.95	8.28	10.07	9.52	8.86
5 YRS	10.57	11.02	9.88	9.61	9.30	9.18	8.58	10.20	9.74	9.11
6 YRS	10.63	11.13	10.01	9.73	9.54	9.40	8.89	10.34	9.96	9.36
7 YRS	10.70	11.24	10.13	9.85	9.77	9.63	9.20	10.48	10.18	9.62
8 YRS	10.76	11.35	10.26	9.97	10.00	9.86	9.50	10.62	10.40	9.87
9 YRS	10.82	11.46	10.38	10.09	10.23	10.08	9.81	10.76	10.62	10.13
10 YRS	10.89	11.57	10.51	10.21	10.47	10.31	10.12	10.89	10.84	10.38
11 YRS	10.95	11.68	10.64	10.33	10.70	10.54	10.42	11.03	11.06	10.63
12 YRS	11.01	11.79	10.76	10.45	10.93	10.77	10.73	11.17	11.29	10.89
13 YRS	11.08	11.90	10.89	10.57	11.17	10.99	11.04	11.31	11.51	11.14
14 YRS	11.14	12.01	11.01	10.69	11.40	11.22	11.35	11.45	11.73	11.40
15 YRS	11.20	12.12	11.14	10.81	11.63	11.45	11.65	11.59	11.95	11.65
16 YRS	11.26	12.23	11.26	10.93	11.87	11.67	11.96	11.72	12.17	11.90
17 YRS	11.33	12.34	11.39	11.05	12.10	11.90	12.27	11.86	12.39	12.16
18 YRS	11.39	12.45	11.51	11.17	12.33	12.13	12.57	12.00	12.61	12.41
19 YRS	11.45	12.56	11.64	11.29	12.57	12.36	12.88	12.14	12.83	12.67
20 YRS	11.52	12.67	11.77	11.42	12.80	12.58	13.19	12.28	13.05	12.92
21 YRS	11.58	12.78	11.89	11.54	13.03	12.81	13.49	12.41	13.27	13.17
22 YRS	11.64	12.89	12.02	11.66	13.27	13.04	13.80	12.55	13.49	13.43
23 YRS	11.71	13.00	12.14	11.78	13.50	13.26	14.11	12.69	13.72	13.68
24 YRS	11.77	13.11	12.27	11.90	13.73	13.49	14.41	12.83	13.94	13.93
25 YRS	11.83	13.22	12.39	12.02	13.97	13.72	14.72	12.97	14.16	14.19
26 YRS	11.90	13.33	12.52	12.14	14.20	13.94	15.03	13.11	14.38	14.44
27 YRS	11.96	13.44	12.64	12.26	14.43	14.17	15.33	13.24	14.60	14.70
28 YRS	12.02	13.55	12.77	12.38	14.66	14.40	15.64	13.38	14.82	14.95
29 YRS	12.09	13.66	12.90	12.50	14.90	14.63	15.95	13.52	15.04	15.20
30 YRS	12.15	13.77	13.02	12.62	15.13	14.85	16.25	13.66	15.26	15.46

EDUCATION	CORRECT	DIGITSPA	WAISIMIL	WAISJUDG	VERBAL	ANIMAL	WAISBLOC	DIGIT
0 YRS	8.99	8.12	5.95	6.81	6.22	8.70	9.02	7.95
1 YRS	9.23	8.36	6.38	7.21	6.58	9.01	9.28	8.33
2 YRS	9.47	8.61	6.81	7.60	6.94	9.31	9.54	8.71
3 YRS	9.71	8.86	7.24	7.99	7.30	9.61	9.80	9.09
4 YRS	9.95	9.11	7.67	8.38	7.66	9.91	10.06	9.46
5 YRS	10.19	9.36	8.10	8.78	8.02	10.22	10.32	9.84
6 YRS	10.43	9.60	8.54	9.17	8.38	10.52	10.58	10.22
7 YRS	10.67	9.85	8.97	9.56	8.75	10.82	10.84	10.60
8 YRS	10.91	10.10	9.40	9.95	9.11	11.13	11.10	10.98
9 YRS	11.15	10.35	9.83	10.35	9.47	11.43	11.36	11.36
10 YRS	11.39	10.60	10.26	10.74	9.83	11.73	11.61	11.73
11 YRS	11.63	10.84	10.69	11.13	10.19	12.04	11.87	12.11
12 YRS	11.87	11.09	11.13	11.52	10.55	12.34	12.13	12.49
13 YRS	12.10	11.34	11.56	11.92	10.91	12.64	12.39	12.87
14 YRS	12.34	11.59	11.99	12.31	11.27	12.95	12.65	13.25
15 YRS	12.58	11.83	12.42	12.70	11.63	13.25	12.91	13.62
16 YRS	12.82	12.08	12.85	13.09	11.99	13.55	13.17	14.00
17 YRS	13.06	12.33	13.28	13.49	12.35	13.85	13.43	14.38
18 YRS	13.30	12.58	13.71	13.88	12.71	14.16	13.69	14.76
19 YRS	13.54	12.83	14.15	14.27	13.07	14.46	13.95	15.14
20 YRS	13.78	13.07	14.58	14.67	13.43	14.76	14.21	15.52
21 YRS	14.02	13.32	15.01	15.06	13.79	15.07	14.47	15.89
22 YRS	14.26	13.57	15.44	15.45	14.15	15.37	14.73	16.27
23 YRS	14.50	13.82	15.87	15.84	14.51	15.67	14.99	16.65
24 YRS	14.74	14.07	16.30	16.24	14.87	15.98	15.25	17.03
25 YRS	14.98	14.31	16.74	16.63	15.23	16.28	15.51	17.41
26 YRS	15.21	14.56	17.17	17.02	15.59	16.58	15.77	17.79
27 YRS	15.45	14.81	17.60	17.41	15.95	16.89	16.03	18.16
28 YRS	15.69	15.06	18.03	17.81	16.31	17.19	16.29	18.54
29 YRS	15.93	15.30	18.46	18.20	16.67	17.49	16.55	18.92
30 YRS	16.17	15.55	18.89	18.59	17.03	17.79	16.81	19.30

Table 9.1. Age 68 – Male.

EDUCATION	BUSCHFR1	BRETRIE	REYA1	REYA2	REYA3	REYA4	REYA5	REYTOT	REYB1	REYA6
0 YRS	10.13	10.31	9.16	8.90	7.99	7.89	6.90	9.36	8.47	7.68
1 YRS	10.20	10.42	9.28	9.02	8.22	8.12	7.21	9.50	8.69	7.93
2 YRS	10.26	10.53	9.41	9.14	8.45	8.35	7.52	9.64	8.91	8.19
3 YRS	10.32	10.64	9.53	9.26	8.69	8.57	7.82	9.78	9.13	8.44
4 YRS	10.39	10.75	9.66	9.38	8.92	8.80	8.13	9.92	9.35	8.70
5 YRS	10.45	10.86	9.79	9.50	9.15	9.03	8.44	10.05	9.58	8.95
6 YRS	10.51	10.97	9.91	9.62	9.38	9.26	8.74	10.19	9.80	9.20
7 YRS	10.58	11.08	10.04	9.75	9.62	9.48	9.05	10.33	10.02	9.46
8 YRS	10.64	11.19	10.16	9.87	9.85	9.71	9.36	10.47	10.24	9.71
9 YRS	10.70	11.30	10.29	9.99	10.08	9.94	9.66	10.61	10.46	9.97
10 YRS	10.77	11.41	10.41	10.11	10.32	10.16	9.97	10.74	10.68	10.22
11 YRS	10.83	11.52	10.54	10.23	10.55	10.39	10.28	10.88	10.90	10.47
12 YRS	10.89	11.63	10.66	10.35	10.78	10.62	10.58	11.02	11.12	10.73
13 YRS	10.96	11.74	10.79	10.47	11.02	10.84	10.89	11.16	11.34	10.98
14 YRS	11.02	11.85	10.92	10.59	11.25	11.07	11.20	11.30	11.56	11.24
15 YRS	11.08	11.96	11.04	10.71	11.48	11.30	11.50	11.44	11.79	11.49
16 YRS	11.15	12.07	11.17	10.83	11.72	11.53	11.81	11.57	12.01	11.74
17 YRS	11.21	12.18	11.29	10.95	11.95	11.75	12.12	11.71	12.23	12.00
18 YRS	11.27	12.29	11.42	11.07	12.18	11.98	12.43	11.85	12.45	12.25
19 YRS	11.34	12.40	11.54	11.19	12.42	12.21	12.73	11.99	12.67	12.51
20 YRS	11.40	12.51	11.67	11.31	12.65	12.43	13.04	12.13	12.89	12.76
21 YRS	11.46	12.62	11.79	11.43	12.88	12.66	13.35	12.27	13.11	13.01
22 YRS	11.53	12.73	11.92	11.55	13.12	12.89	13.65	12.40	13.33	13.27
23 YRS	11.59	12.84	12.05	11.67	13.35	13.11	13.96	12.54	13.55	13.52
24 YRS	11.65	12.95	12.17	11.79	13.58	13.34	14.27	12.68	13.77	13.77
25 YRS	11.72	13.06	12.30	11.91	13.81	13.57	14.57	12.82	14.00	14.03
26 YRS	11.78	13.17	12.42	12.03	14.05	13.80	14.88	12.96	14.22	14.28
27 YRS	11.84	13.28	12.55	12.15	14.28	14.02	15.19	13.09	14.44	14.54
28 YRS	11.91	13.39	12.67	12.27	14.51	14.25	15.49	13.23	14.66	14.79
29 YRS	11.97	13.50	12.80	12.39	14.75	14.48	15.80	13.37	14.88	15.04
30 YRS	12.03	13.61	12.92	12.51	14.98	14.70	16.11	13.51	15.10	15.30

EDUCATION	CORRECT	DIGITSPA	WAISIMIL	WAISJUDG	VERBAL	ANIMAL	WAISBLOC	DIGIT
0 YRS	8.84	8.05	5.85	6.75	6.17	8.59	8.90	7.73
1 YRS	9.08	8.30	6.28	7.14	6.53	8.89	9.16	8.11
2 YRS	9.32	8.55	6.71	7.53	6.89	9.19	9.42	8.49
3 YRS	9.56	8.79	7.15	7.93	7.25	9.49	9.68	8.86
4 YRS	9.80	9.04	7.58	8.32	7.61	9.80	9.94	9.24
5 YRS	10.04	9.29	8.01	8.71	7.97	10.10	10.20	9.62
6 YRS	10.28	9.54	8.44	9.10	8.33	10.40	10.46	10.00
7 YRS	10.52	9.79	8.87	9.50	8.69	10.71	10.72	10.38
8 YRS	10.75	10.03	9.30	9.89	9.05	11.01	10.98	10.76
9 YRS	10.99	10.28	9.74	10.28	9.41	11.31	11.24	11.13
10 YRS	11.23	10.53	10.17	10.68	9.77	11.62	11.50	11.51
11 YRS	11.47	10.78	10.60	11.07	10.13	11.92	11.76	11.89
12 YRS	11.71	11.03	11.03	11.46	10.49	12.22	12.02	12.27
13 YRS	11.95	11.27	11.46	11.85	10.85	12.53	12.28	12.65
14 YRS	12.19	11.52	11.89	12.25	11.21	12.83	12.54	13.03
15 YRS	12.43	11.77	12.32	12.64	11.57	13.13	12.80	13.40
16 YRS	12.67	12.02	12.76	13.03	11.93	13.43	13.06	13.78
17 YRS	12.91	12.26	13.19	13.42	12.29	13.74	13.32	14.16
18 YRS	13.15	12.51	13.62	13.82	12.65	14.04	13.58	14.54
19 YRS	13.39	12.76	14.05	14.21	13.01	14.34	13.84	14.92
20 YRS	13.62	13.01	14.48	14.60	13.37	14.65	14.10	15.30
21 YRS	13.86	13.26	14.91	14.99	13.73	14.95	14.36	15.67
22 YRS	14.10	13.50	15.35	15.39	14.09	15.25	14.62	16.05
23 YRS	14.34	13.75	15.78	15.78	14.45	15.56	14.87	16.43
24 YRS	14.58	14.00	16.21	16.17	14.82	15.86	15.13	16.81
25 YRS	14.82	14.25	16.64	16.56	15.18	16.16	15.39	17.19
26 YRS	15.06	14.50	17.07	16.96	15.54	16.47	15.65	17.57
27 YRS	15.30	14.74	17.50	17.35	15.90	16.77	15.91	17.94
28 YRS	15.54	14.99	17.94	17.74	16.26	17.07	16.17	18.32
29 YRS	15.78	15.24	18.37	18.14	16.62	17.37	16.43	18.70
30 YRS	16.02	15.49	18.80	18.53	16.98	17.68	16.69	19.08

Table 9.2. Age 68 – Female.

EDUCATION	BUSCHFR1	BRETRIE	REYA1	REYA2	REYA3	REYA4	REYA5	REYTOT	REYB1	REYA6
0 YRS	10.13	10.31	9.16	8.90	7.99	7.89	6.90	9.36	8.47	7.68
1 YRS	10.20	10.42	9.28	9.02	8.22	8.12	7.21	9.50	8.69	7.93
2 YRS	10.26	10.53	9.41	9.14	8.45	8.35	7.52	9.64	8.91	8.19
3 YRS	10.32	10.64	9.53	9.26	8.69	8.57	7.82	9.78	9.13	8.44
4 YRS	10.39	10.75	9.66	9.38	8.92	8.80	8.13	9.92	9.35	8.70
5 YRS	10.45	10.86	9.79	9.50	9.15	9.03	8.44	10.05	9.58	8.95
6 YRS	10.51	10.97	9.91	9.62	9.38	9.26	8.74	10.19	9.80	9.20
7 YRS	10.58	11.08	10.04	9.75	9.62	9.48	9.05	10.33	10.02	9.46
8 YRS	10.64	11.19	10.16	9.87	9.85	9.71	9.36	10.47	10.24	9.71
9 YRS	10.70	11.30	10.29	9.99	10.08	9.94	9.66	10.61	10.46	9.97
10 YRS	10.77	11.41	10.41	10.11	10.32	10.16	9.97	10.74	10.68	10.22
11 YRS	10.83	11.52	10.54	10.23	10.55	10.39	10.28	10.88	10.90	10.47
12 YRS	10.89	11.63	10.66	10.35	10.78	10.62	10.58	11.02	11.12	10.73
13 YRS	10.96	11.74	10.79	10.47	11.02	10.84	10.89	11.16	11.34	10.98
14 YRS	11.02	11.85	10.92	10.59	11.25	11.07	11.20	11.30	11.56	11.24
15 YRS	11.08	11.96	11.04	10.71	11.48	11.30	11.50	11.44	11.79	11.49
16 YRS	11.15	12.07	11.17	10.83	11.72	11.53	11.81	11.57	12.01	11.74
17 YRS	11.21	12.18	11.29	10.95	11.95	11.75	12.12	11.71	12.23	12.00
18 YRS	11.27	12.29	11.42	11.07	12.18	11.98	12.43	11.85	12.45	12.25
19 YRS	11.34	12.40	11.54	11.19	12.42	12.21	12.73	11.99	12.67	12.51
20 YRS	11.40	12.51	11.67	11.31	12.65	12.43	13.04	12.13	12.89	12.76
21 YRS	11.46	12.62	11.79	11.43	12.88	12.66	13.35	12.27	13.11	13.01
22 YRS	11.53	12.73	11.92	11.55	13.12	12.89	13.65	12.40	13.33	13.27
23 YRS	11.59	12.84	12.05	11.67	13.35	13.11	13.96	12.54	13.55	13.52
24 YRS	11.65	12.95	12.17	11.79	13.58	13.34	14.27	12.68	13.77	13.77
25 YRS	11.72	13.06	12.30	11.91	13.81	13.57	14.57	12.82	14.00	14.03
26 YRS	11.78	13.17	12.42	12.03	14.05	13.80	14.88	12.96	14.22	14.28
27 YRS	11.84	13.28	12.55	12.15	14.28	14.02	15.19	13.09	14.44	14.54
28 YRS	11.91	13.39	12.67	12.27	14.51	14.25	15.49	13.23	14.66	14.79
29 YRS	11.97	13.50	12.80	12.39	14.75	14.48	15.80	13.37	14.88	15.04
30 YRS	12.03	13.61	12.92	12.51	14.98	14.70	16.11	13.51	15.10	15.30

EDUCATION	CORRECT	DIGITSPA	WAISIMIL	WAISJUDG	VERBAL	ANIMAL	WAISBLOC	DIGIT
0 YRS	8.84	8.05	5.85	6.75	6.17	8.59	8.90	7.73
1 YRS	9.08	8.30	6.28	7.14	6.53	8.89	9.16	8.11
2 YRS	9.32	8.55	6.71	7.53	6.89	9.19	9.42	8.49
3 YRS	9.56	8.79	7.15	7.93	7.25	9.49	9.68	8.86
4 YRS	9.80	9.04	7.58	8.32	7.61	9.80	9.94	9.24
5 YRS	10.04	9.29	8.01	8.71	7.97	10.10	10.20	9.62
6 YRS	10.28	9.54	8.44	9.10	8.33	10.40	10.46	10.00
7 YRS	10.52	9.79	8.87	9.50	8.69	10.71	10.72	10.38
8 YRS	10.75	10.03	9.30	9.89	9.05	11.01	10.98	10.76
9 YRS	10.99	10.28	9.74	10.28	9.41	11.31	11.24	11.13
10 YRS	11.23	10.53	10.17	10.68	9.77	11.62	11.50	11.51
11 YRS	11.47	10.78	10.60	11.07	10.13	11.92	11.76	11.89
12 YRS	11.71	11.03	11.03	11.46	10.49	12.22	12.02	12.27
13 YRS	11.95	11.27	11.46	11.85	10.85	12.53	12.28	12.65
14 YRS	12.19	11.52	11.89	12.25	11.21	12.83	12.54	13.03
15 YRS	12.43	11.77	12.32	12.64	11.57	13.13	12.80	13.40
16 YRS	12.67	12.02	12.76	13.03	11.93	13.43	13.06	13.78
17 YRS	12.91	12.26	13.19	13.42	12.29	13.74	13.32	14.16
18 YRS	13.15	12.51	13.62	13.82	12.65	14.04	13.58	14.54
19 YRS	13.39	12.76	14.05	14.21	13.01	14.34	13.84	14.92
20 YRS	13.62	13.01	14.48	14.60	13.37	14.65	14.10	15.30
21 YRS	13.86	13.26	14.91	14.99	13.73	14.95	14.36	15.67
22 YRS	14.10	13.50	15.35	15.39	14.09	15.25	14.62	16.05
23 YRS	14.34	13.75	15.78	15.78	14.45	15.56	14.87	16.43
24 YRS	14.58	14.00	16.21	16.17	14.82	15.86	15.13	16.81
25 YRS	14.82	14.25	16.64	16.56	15.18	16.16	15.39	17.19
26 YRS	15.06	14.50	17.07	16.96	15.54	16.47	15.65	17.57
27 YRS	15.30	14.74	17.50	17.35	15.90	16.77	15.91	17.94
28 YRS	15.54	14.99	17.94	17.74	16.26	17.07	16.17	18.32
29 YRS	15.78	15.24	18.37	18.14	16.62	17.37	16.43	18.70
30 YRS	16.02	15.49	18.80	18.53	16.98	17.68	16.69	19.08

Table 10.1. Age 69 – Male.

EDUCATION	BUSCHFR1	BRETRIE	REYA1	REYA2	REYA3	REYA4	REYA5	REYTOT	REYB1	REYA6
0 YRS	10.02	10.15	9.06	8.80	7.83	7.74	6.76	9.21	8.31	7.52
1 YRS	10.08	10.26	9.19	8.92	8.07	7.97	7.06	9.35	8.53	7.77
2 YRS	10.14	10.37	9.31	9.04	8.30	8.20	7.37	9.49	8.75	8.03
3 YRS	10.21	10.48	9.44	9.16	8.53	8.43	7.68	9.63	8.97	8.28
4 YRS	10.27	10.59	9.56	9.28	8.77	8.65	7.98	9.77	9.19	8.54
5 YRS	10.33	10.70	9.69	9.40	9.00	8.88	8.29	9.90	9.41	8.79
6 YRS	10.40	10.81	9.81	9.52	9.23	9.11	8.60	10.04	9.63	9.04
7 YRS	10.46	10.92	9.94	9.64	9.47	9.33	8.90	10.18	9.86	9.30
8 YRS	10.52	11.03	10.07	9.76	9.70	9.56	9.21	10.32	10.08	9.55
9 YRS	10.59	11.14	10.19	9.88	9.93	9.79	9.52	10.46	10.30	9.81
10 YRS	10.65	11.25	10.32	10.00	10.17	10.01	9.82	10.59	10.52	10.06
11 YRS	10.71	11.36	10.44	10.12	10.40	10.24	10.13	10.73	10.74	10.31
12 YRS	10.78	11.47	10.57	10.24	10.63	10.47	10.44	10.87	10.96	10.57
13 YRS	10.84	11.58	10.69	10.36	10.87	10.70	10.74	11.01	11.18	10.82
14 YRS	10.90	11.69	10.82	10.48	11.10	10.92	11.05	11.15	11.40	11.08
15 YRS	10.97	11.80	10.94	10.60	11.33	11.15	11.36	11.29	11.62	11.33
16 YRS	11.03	11.91	11.07	10.72	11.57	11.38	11.66	11.42	11.84	11.58
17 YRS	11.09	12.02	11.19	10.84	11.80	11.60	11.97	11.56	12.06	11.84
18 YRS	11.16	12.13	11.32	10.96	12.03	11.83	12.28	11.70	12.29	12.09
19 YRS	11.22	12.24	11.45	11.09	12.26	12.06	12.58	11.84	12.51	12.35
20 YRS	11.28	12.35	11.57	11.21	12.50	12.29	12.89	11.98	12.73	12.60
21 YRS	11.35	12.46	11.70	11.33	12.73	12.51	13.20	12.12	12.95	12.85
22 YRS	11.41	12.57	11.82	11.45	12.96	12.74	13.51	12.25	13.17	13.11
23 YRS	11.47	12.68	11.95	11.57	13.20	12.97	13.81	12.39	13.39	13.36
24 YRS	11.54	12.79	12.07	11.69	13.43	13.19	14.12	12.53	13.61	13.61
25 YRS	11.60	12.90	12.20	11.81	13.66	13.42	14.43	12.67	13.83	13.87
26 YRS	11.66	13.00	12.32	11.93	13.90	13.65	14.73	12.81	14.05	14.12
27 YRS	11.72	13.11	12.45	12.05	14.13	13.87	15.04	12.94	14.27	14.38
28 YRS	11.79	13.22	12.58	12.17	14.36	14.10	15.35	13.08	14.50	14.63
29 YRS	11.85	13.33	12.70	12.29	14.60	14.33	15.65	13.22	14.72	14.88
30 YRS	11.91	13.44	12.83	12.41	14.83	14.56	15.96	13.36	14.94	15.14

EDUCATION	CORRECT	DIGITSPA	WAISIMIL	WAISJUDG	VERBAL	ANIMAL	WAISBLOC	DIGIT
0 YRS	8.69	7.99	5.76	6.68	6.11	8.47	8.79	7.51
1 YRS	8.93	8.23	6.19	7.08	6.47	8.77	9.05	7.89
2 YRS	9.16	8.48	6.62	7.47	6.83	9.07	9.31	8.27
3 YRS	9.40	8.73	7.05	7.86	7.19	9.38	9.57	8.64
4 YRS	9.64	8.98	7.48	8.26	7.55	9.68	9.83	9.02
5 YRS	9.88	9.22	7.91	8.65	7.91	9.98	10.09	9.40
6 YRS	10.12	9.47	8.35	9.04	8.27	10.29	10.35	9.78
7 YRS	10.36	9.72	8.78	9.43	8.63	10.59	10.61	10.16
8 YRS	10.60	9.97	9.21	9.83	8.99	10.89	10.86	10.54
9 YRS	10.84	10.22	9.64	10.22	9.35	11.20	11.12	10.91
10 YRS	11.08	10.46	10.07	10.61	9.71	11.50	11.38	11.29
11 YRS	11.32	10.71	10.50	11.00	10.07	11.80	11.64	11.67
12 YRS	11.56	10.96	10.93	11.40	10.43	12.11	11.90	12.05
13 YRS	11.80	11.21	11.37	11.79	10.79	12.41	12.16	12.43
14 YRS	12.04	11.46	11.80	12.18	11.15	12.71	12.42	12.81
15 YRS	12.27	11.70	12.23	12.57	11.52	13.01	12.68	13.18
16 YRS	12.51	11.95	12.66	12.97	11.88	13.32	12.94	13.56
17 YRS	12.75	12.20	13.09	13.36	12.24	13.62	13.20	13.94
18 YRS	12.99	12.45	13.52	13.75	12.60	13.92	13.46	14.32
19 YRS	13.23	12.69	13.96	14.15	12.96	14.23	13.72	14.70
20 YRS	13.47	12.94	14.39	14.54	13.32	14.53	13.98	15.08
21 YRS	13.71	13.19	14.82	14.93	13.68	14.83	14.24	15.45
22 YRS	13.95	13.44	15.25	15.32	14.04	15.14	14.50	15.83
23 YRS	14.19	13.69	15.68	15.72	14.40	15.44	14.76	16.21
24 YRS	14.43	13.93	16.11	16.11	14.76	15.74	15.02	16.59
25 YRS	14.67	14.18	16.54	16.50	15.12	16.05	15.28	16.97
26 YRS	14.91	14.43	16.98	16.89	15.48	16.35	15.54	17.35
27 YRS	15.15	14.68	17.41	17.29	15.84	16.65	15.80	17.72
28 YRS	15.38	14.93	17.84	17.68	16.20	16.95	16.06	18.10
29 YRS	15.62	15.17	18.27	18.07	16.56	17.26	16.32	18.48
30 YRS	15.86	15.42	18.70	18.46	16.92	17.56	16.58	18.86

Table 10.2. Age 69 – Female.

EDUCATION	BUSCHFR1	BRETRIE	REYA1	REYA2	REYA3	REYA4	REYA5	REYTOT	REYB1	REYA6
0 YRS	10.02	10.15	9.06	8.80	7.83	7.74	6.76	9.21	8.31	7.52
1 YRS	10.08	10.26	9.19	8.92	8.07	7.97	7.06	9.35	8.53	7.77
2 YRS	10.14	10.37	9.31	9.04	8.30	8.20	7.37	9.49	8.75	8.03
3 YRS	10.21	10.48	9.44	9.16	8.53	8.43	7.68	9.63	8.97	8.28
4 YRS	10.27	10.59	9.56	9.28	8.77	8.65	7.98	9.77	9.19	8.54
5 YRS	10.33	10.70	9.69	9.40	9.00	8.88	8.29	9.90	9.41	8.79
6 YRS	10.40	10.81	9.81	9.52	9.23	9.11	8.60	10.04	9.63	9.04
7 YRS	10.46	10.92	9.94	9.64	9.47	9.33	8.90	10.18	9.86	9.30
8 YRS	10.52	11.03	10.07	9.76	9.70	9.56	9.21	10.32	10.08	9.55
9 YRS	10.59	11.14	10.19	9.88	9.93	9.79	9.52	10.46	10.30	9.81
10 YRS	10.65	11.25	10.32	10.00	10.17	10.01	9.82	10.59	10.52	10.06
11 YRS	10.71	11.36	10.44	10.12	10.40	10.24	10.13	10.73	10.74	10.31
12 YRS	10.78	11.47	10.57	10.24	10.63	10.47	10.44	10.87	10.96	10.57
13 YRS	10.84	11.58	10.69	10.36	10.87	10.70	10.74	11.01	11.18	10.82
14 YRS	10.90	11.69	10.82	10.48	11.10	10.92	11.05	11.15	11.40	11.08
15 YRS	10.97	11.80	10.94	10.60	11.33	11.15	11.36	11.29	11.62	11.33
16 YRS	11.03	11.91	11.07	10.72	11.57	11.38	11.66	11.42	11.84	11.58
17 YRS	11.09	12.02	11.19	10.84	11.80	11.60	11.97	11.56	12.06	11.84
18 YRS	11.16	12.13	11.32	10.96	12.03	11.83	12.28	11.70	12.29	12.09
19 YRS	11.22	12.24	11.45	11.09	12.26	12.06	12.58	11.84	12.51	12.35
20 YRS	11.28	12.35	11.57	11.21	12.50	12.29	12.89	11.98	12.73	12.60
21 YRS	11.35	12.46	11.70	11.33	12.73	12.51	13.20	12.12	12.95	12.85
22 YRS	11.41	12.57	11.82	11.45	12.96	12.74	13.51	12.25	13.17	13.11
23 YRS	11.47	12.68	11.95	11.57	13.20	12.97	13.81	12.39	13.39	13.36
24 YRS	11.54	12.79	12.07	11.69	13.43	13.19	14.12	12.53	13.61	13.61
25 YRS	11.60	12.90	12.20	11.81	13.66	13.42	14.43	12.67	13.83	13.87
26 YRS	11.66	13.00	12.32	11.93	13.90	13.65	14.73	12.81	14.05	14.12
27 YRS	11.72	13.11	12.45	12.05	14.13	13.87	15.04	12.94	14.27	14.38
28 YRS	11.79	13.22	12.58	12.17	14.36	14.10	15.35	13.08	14.50	14.63
29 YRS	11.85	13.33	12.70	12.29	14.60	14.33	15.65	13.22	14.72	14.88
30 YRS	11.91	13.44	12.83	12.41	14.83	14.56	15.96	13.36	14.94	15.14

EDUCATION	CORRECT	DIGITSPA	WAISIMIL	WAISJUDG	VERBAL	ANIMAL	WAISBLOC	DIGIT
0 YRS	8.69	7.99	5.76	6.68	6.11	8.47	8.79	7.51
1 YRS	8.93	8.23	6.19	7.08	6.47	8.77	9.05	7.89
2 YRS	9.16	8.48	6.62	7.47	6.83	9.07	9.31	8.27
3 YRS	9.40	8.73	7.05	7.86	7.19	9.38	9.57	8.64
4 YRS	9.64	8.98	7.48	8.26	7.55	9.68	9.83	9.02
5 YRS	9.88	9.22	7.91	8.65	7.91	9.98	10.09	9.40
6 YRS	10.12	9.47	8.35	9.04	8.27	10.29	10.35	9.78
7 YRS	10.36	9.72	8.78	9.43	8.63	10.59	10.61	10.16
8 YRS	10.60	9.97	9.21	9.83	8.99	10.89	10.86	10.54
9 YRS	10.84	10.22	9.64	10.22	9.35	11.20	11.12	10.91
10 YRS	11.08	10.46	10.07	10.61	9.71	11.50	11.38	11.29
11 YRS	11.32	10.71	10.50	11.00	10.07	11.80	11.64	11.67
12 YRS	11.56	10.96	10.93	11.40	10.43	12.11	11.90	12.05
13 YRS	11.80	11.21	11.37	11.79	10.79	12.41	12.16	12.43
14 YRS	12.04	11.46	11.80	12.18	11.15	12.71	12.42	12.81
15 YRS	12.27	11.70	12.23	12.57	11.52	13.01	12.68	13.18
16 YRS	12.51	11.95	12.66	12.97	11.88	13.32	12.94	13.56
17 YRS	12.75	12.20	13.09	13.36	12.24	13.62	13.20	13.94
18 YRS	12.99	12.45	13.52	13.75	12.60	13.92	13.46	14.32
19 YRS	13.23	12.69	13.96	14.15	12.96	14.23	13.72	14.70
20 YRS	13.47	12.94	14.39	14.54	13.32	14.53	13.98	15.08
21 YRS	13.71	13.19	14.82	14.93	13.68	14.83	14.24	15.45
22 YRS	13.95	13.44	15.25	15.32	14.04	15.14	14.50	15.83
23 YRS	14.19	13.69	15.68	15.72	14.40	15.44	14.76	16.21
24 YRS	14.43	13.93	16.11	16.11	14.76	15.74	15.02	16.59
25 YRS	14.67	14.18	16.54	16.50	15.12	16.05	15.28	16.97
26 YRS	14.91	14.43	16.98	16.89	15.48	16.35	15.54	17.35
27 YRS	15.15	14.68	17.41	17.29	15.84	16.65	15.80	17.72
28 YRS	15.38	14.93	17.84	17.68	16.20	16.95	16.06	18.10
29 YRS	15.62	15.17	18.27	18.07	16.56	17.26	16.32	18.48
30 YRS	15.86	15.42	18.70	18.46	16.92	17.56	16.58	18.86

Table 11.1. Age 70 – Male.

EDUCATION	BUSCHFR1	BRETRIE	REYA1	REYA2	REYA3	REYA4	REYA5	REYTOT	REYB1	REYA6
0 YRS	9.90	9.99	8.96	8.69	7.68	7.60	6.61	9.06	8.15	7.36
1 YRS	9.96	10.10	9.09	8.81	7.92	7.82	6.92	9.20	8.37	7.61
2 YRS	10.03	10.21	9.22	8.93	8.15	8.05	7.22	9.34	8.59	7.87
3 YRS	10.09	10.32	9.34	9.05	8.38	8.28	7.53	9.48	8.81	8.12
4 YRS	10.15	10.42	9.47	9.17	8.62	8.50	7.84	9.62	9.03	8.38
5 YRS	10.22	10.53	9.59	9.30	8.85	8.73	8.14	9.75	9.25	8.63
6 YRS	10.28	10.64	9.72	9.42	9.08	8.96	8.45	9.89	9.47	8.88
7 YRS	10.34	10.75	9.84	9.54	9.32	9.19	8.76	10.03	9.69	9.14
8 YRS	10.40	10.86	9.97	9.66	9.55	9.41	9.06	10.17	9.91	9.39
9 YRS	10.47	10.97	10.09	9.78	9.78	9.64	9.37	10.31	10.13	9.65
10 YRS	10.53	11.08	10.22	9.90	10.02	9.87	9.68	10.45	10.36	9.90
11 YRS	10.59	11.19	10.34	10.02	10.25	10.09	9.98	10.58	10.58	10.15
12 YRS	10.66	11.30	10.47	10.14	10.48	10.32	10.29	10.72	10.80	10.41
13 YRS	10.72	11.41	10.60	10.26	10.72	10.55	10.60	10.86	11.02	10.66
14 YRS	10.78	11.52	10.72	10.38	10.95	10.77	10.90	11.00	11.24	10.92
15 YRS	10.85	11.63	10.85	10.50	11.18	11.00	11.21	11.14	11.46	11.17
16 YRS	10.91	11.74	10.97	10.62	11.41	11.23	11.52	11.27	11.68	11.42
17 YRS	10.97	11.85	11.10	10.74	11.65	11.46	11.82	11.41	11.90	11.68
18 YRS	11.04	11.96	11.22	10.86	11.88	11.68	12.13	11.55	12.12	11.93
19 YRS	11.10	12.07	11.35	10.98	12.11	11.91	12.44	11.69	12.34	12.19
20 YRS	11.16	12.18	11.47	11.10	12.35	12.14	12.74	11.83	12.57	12.44
21 YRS	11.23	12.29	11.60	11.22	12.58	12.36	13.05	11.97	12.79	12.69
22 YRS	11.29	12.40	11.73	11.34	12.81	12.59	13.36	12.10	13.01	12.95
23 YRS	11.35	12.51	11.85	11.46	13.05	12.82	13.67	12.24	13.23	13.20
24 YRS	11.42	12.62	11.98	11.58	13.28	13.04	13.97	12.38	13.45	13.45
25 YRS	11.48	12.73	12.10	11.70	13.51	13.27	14.28	12.52	13.67	13.71
26 YRS	11.54	12.84	12.23	11.82	13.75	13.50	14.59	12.66	13.89	13.96
27 YRS	11.61	12.95	12.35	11.94	13.98	13.73	14.89	12.79	14.11	14.22
28 YRS	11.67	13.06	12.48	12.06	14.21	13.95	15.20	12.93	14.33	14.47
29 YRS	11.73	13.17	12.60	12.18	14.45	14.18	15.51	13.07	14.55	14.72
30 YRS	11.80	13.28	12.73	12.30	14.68	14.41	15.81	13.21	14.77	14.98

EDUCATION	CORRECT	DIGITSPA	WAISIMIL	WAISJUDG	VERBAL	ANIMAL	WAISBLOC	DIGIT
0 YRS	8.53	7.92	5.66	6.62	6.05	8.35	8.67	7.29
1 YRS	8.77	8.17	6.09	7.01	6.41	8.65	8.93	7.67
2 YRS	9.01	8.42	6.52	7.41	6.77	8.96	9.19	8.05
3 YRS	9.25	8.66	6.96	7.80	7.13	9.26	9.45	8.42
4 YRS	9.49	8.91	7.39	8.19	7.49	9.56	9.71	8.80
5 YRS	9.73	9.16	7.82	8.58	7.85	9.87	9.97	9.18
6 YRS	9.97	9.41	8.25	8.98	8.22	10.17	10.23	9.56
7 YRS	10.21	9.65	8.68	9.37	8.58	10.47	10.49	9.94
8 YRS	10.45	9.90	9.11	9.76	8.94	10.78	10.75	10.32
9 YRS	10.69	10.15	9.54	10.15	9.30	11.08	11.01	10.69
10 YRS	10.92	10.40	9.98	10.55	9.66	11.38	11.27	11.07
11 YRS	11.16	10.65	10.41	10.94	10.02	11.69	11.53	11.45
12 YRS	11.40	10.89	10.84	11.33	10.38	11.99	11.79	11.83
13 YRS	11.64	11.14	11.27	11.73	10.74	12.29	12.05	12.21
14 YRS	11.88	11.39	11.70	12.12	11.10	12.59	12.31	12.59
15 YRS	12.12	11.64	12.13	12.51	11.46	12.90	12.57	12.96
16 YRS	12.36	11.89	12.57	12.90	11.82	13.20	12.83	13.34
17 YRS	12.60	12.13	13.00	13.30	12.18	13.50	13.09	13.72
18 YRS	12.84	12.38	13.43	13.69	12.54	13.81	13.35	14.10
19 YRS	13.08	12.63	13.86	14.08	12.90	14.11	13.61	14.48
20 YRS	13.32	12.88	14.29	14.47	13.26	14.41	13.87	14.86
21 YRS	13.56	13.12	14.72	14.87	13.62	14.72	14.12	15.23
22 YRS	13.80	13.37	15.15	15.26	13.98	15.02	14.38	15.61
23 YRS	14.03	13.62	15.59	15.65	14.34	15.32	14.64	15.99
24 YRS	14.27	13.87	16.02	16.04	14.70	15.63	14.90	16.37
25 YRS	14.51	14.12	16.45	16.44	15.06	15.93	15.16	16.75
26 YRS	14.75	14.36	16.88	16.83	15.42	16.23	15.42	17.13
27 YRS	14.99	14.61	17.31	17.22	15.78	16.53	15.68	17.50
28 YRS	15.23	14.86	17.74	17.61	16.14	16.84	15.94	17.88
29 YRS	15.47	15.11	18.18	18.01	16.50	17.14	16.20	18.26
30 YRS	15.71	15.36	18.61	18.40	16.86	17.44	16.46	18.64

Table 11.2. Age 70 – Female.

EDUCATION	BUSCHFR1	BRETRIE	REYA1	REYA2	REYA3	REYA4	REYA5	REYTOT	REYB1	REYA6
0 YRS	9.90	9.99	8.96	8.69	7.68	7.60	6.61	9.06	8.15	7.36
1 YRS	9.96	10.10	9.09	8.81	7.92	7.82	6.92	9.20	8.37	7.61
2 YRS	10.03	10.21	9.22	8.93	8.15	8.05	7.22	9.34	8.59	7.87
3 YRS	10.09	10.32	9.34	9.05	8.38	8.28	7.53	9.48	8.81	8.12
4 YRS	10.15	10.42	9.47	9.17	8.62	8.50	7.84	9.62	9.03	8.38
5 YRS	10.22	10.53	9.59	9.30	8.85	8.73	8.14	9.75	9.25	8.63
6 YRS	10.28	10.64	9.72	9.42	9.08	8.96	8.45	9.89	9.47	8.88
7 YRS	10.34	10.75	9.84	9.54	9.32	9.19	8.76	10.03	9.69	9.14
8 YRS	10.40	10.86	9.97	9.66	9.55	9.41	9.06	10.17	9.91	9.39
9 YRS	10.47	10.97	10.09	9.78	9.78	9.64	9.37	10.31	10.13	9.65
10 YRS	10.53	11.08	10.22	9.90	10.02	9.87	9.68	10.45	10.36	9.90
11 YRS	10.59	11.19	10.34	10.02	10.25	10.09	9.98	10.58	10.58	10.15
12 YRS	10.66	11.30	10.47	10.14	10.48	10.32	10.29	10.72	10.80	10.41
13 YRS	10.72	11.41	10.60	10.26	10.72	10.55	10.60	10.86	11.02	10.66
14 YRS	10.78	11.52	10.72	10.38	10.95	10.77	10.90	11.00	11.24	10.92
15 YRS	10.85	11.63	10.85	10.50	11.18	11.00	11.21	11.14	11.46	11.17
16 YRS	10.91	11.74	10.97	10.62	11.41	11.23	11.52	11.27	11.68	11.42
17 YRS	10.97	11.85	11.10	10.74	11.65	11.46	11.82	11.41	11.90	11.68
18 YRS	11.04	11.96	11.22	10.86	11.88	11.68	12.13	11.55	12.12	11.93
19 YRS	11.10	12.07	11.35	10.98	12.11	11.91	12.44	11.69	12.34	12.19
20 YRS	11.16	12.18	11.47	11.10	12.35	12.14	12.74	11.83	12.57	12.44
21 YRS	11.23	12.29	11.60	11.22	12.58	12.36	13.05	11.97	12.79	12.69
22 YRS	11.29	12.40	11.73	11.34	12.81	12.59	13.36	12.10	13.01	12.95
23 YRS	11.35	12.51	11.85	11.46	13.05	12.82	13.67	12.24	13.23	13.20
24 YRS	11.42	12.62	11.98	11.58	13.28	13.04	13.97	12.38	13.45	13.45
25 YRS	11.48	12.73	12.10	11.70	13.51	13.27	14.28	12.52	13.67	13.71
26 YRS	11.54	12.84	12.23	11.82	13.75	13.50	14.59	12.66	13.89	13.96
27 YRS	11.61	12.95	12.35	11.94	13.98	13.73	14.89	12.79	14.11	14.22
28 YRS	11.67	13.06	12.48	12.06	14.21	13.95	15.20	12.93	14.33	14.47
29 YRS	11.73	13.17	12.60	12.18	14.45	14.18	15.51	13.07	14.55	14.72
30 YRS	11.80	13.28	12.73	12.30	14.68	14.41	15.81	13.21	14.77	14.98

EDUCATION	CORRECT	DIGITSPA	WAISIMIL	WAISJUDG	VERBAL	ANIMAL	WAISBLOC	DIGIT
0 YRS	8.53	7.92	5.66	6.62	6.05	8.35	8.67	7.29
1 YRS	8.77	8.17	6.09	7.01	6.41	8.65	8.93	7.67
2 YRS	9.01	8.42	6.52	7.41	6.77	8.96	9.19	8.05
3 YRS	9.25	8.66	6.96	7.80	7.13	9.26	9.45	8.42
4 YRS	9.49	8.91	7.39	8.19	7.49	9.56	9.71	8.80
5 YRS	9.73	9.16	7.82	8.58	7.85	9.87	9.97	9.18
6 YRS	9.97	9.41	8.25	8.98	8.22	10.17	10.23	9.56
7 YRS	10.21	9.65	8.68	9.37	8.58	10.47	10.49	9.94
8 YRS	10.45	9.90	9.11	9.76	8.94	10.78	10.75	10.32
9 YRS	10.69	10.15	9.54	10.15	9.30	11.08	11.01	10.69
10 YRS	10.92	10.40	9.98	10.55	9.66	11.38	11.27	11.07
11 YRS	11.16	10.65	10.41	10.94	10.02	11.69	11.53	11.45
12 YRS	11.40	10.89	10.84	11.33	10.38	11.99	11.79	11.83
13 YRS	11.64	11.14	11.27	11.73	10.74	12.29	12.05	12.21
14 YRS	11.88	11.39	11.70	12.12	11.10	12.59	12.31	12.59
15 YRS	12.12	11.64	12.13	12.51	11.46	12.90	12.57	12.96
16 YRS	12.36	11.89	12.57	12.90	11.82	13.20	12.83	13.34
17 YRS	12.60	12.13	13.00	13.30	12.18	13.50	13.09	13.72
18 YRS	12.84	12.38	13.43	13.69	12.54	13.81	13.35	14.10
19 YRS	13.08	12.63	13.86	14.08	12.90	14.11	13.61	14.48
20 YRS	13.32	12.88	14.29	14.47	13.26	14.41	13.87	14.86
21 YRS	13.56	13.12	14.72	14.87	13.62	14.72	14.12	15.23
22 YRS	13.80	13.37	15.15	15.26	13.98	15.02	14.38	15.61
23 YRS	14.03	13.62	15.59	15.65	14.34	15.32	14.64	15.99
24 YRS	14.27	13.87	16.02	16.04	14.70	15.63	14.90	16.37
25 YRS	14.51	14.12	16.45	16.44	15.06	15.93	15.16	16.75
26 YRS	14.75	14.36	16.88	16.83	15.42	16.23	15.42	17.13
27 YRS	14.99	14.61	17.31	17.22	15.78	16.53	15.68	17.50
28 YRS	15.23	14.86	17.74	17.61	16.14	16.84	15.94	17.88
29 YRS	15.47	15.11	18.18	18.01	16.50	17.14	16.20	18.26
30 YRS	15.71	15.36	18.61	18.40	16.86	17.44	16.46	18.64

Table 12.1. Age 71 – Male.

EDUCATION	BUSCHFR1	BRETRIE	REYA1	REYA2	REYA3	REYA4	REYA5	REYTOT	REYB1	REYA6
0 YRS	9.78	9.82	8.87	8.59	7.53	7.45	6.46	8.91	7.98	7.20
1 YRS	9.84	9.93	8.99	8.71	7.77	7.67	6.77	9.05	8.20	7.45
2 YRS	9.91	10.04	9.12	8.83	8.00	7.90	7.08	9.19	8.43	7.71
3 YRS	9.97	10.15	9.24	8.95	8.23	8.13	7.38	9.33	8.65	7.96
4 YRS	10.03	10.26	9.37	9.07	8.47	8.36	7.69	9.47	8.87	8.22
5 YRS	10.10	10.37	9.49	9.19	8.70	8.58	8.00	9.60	9.09	8.47
6 YRS	10.16	10.48	9.62	9.31	8.93	8.81	8.30	9.74	9.31	8.72
7 YRS	10.22	10.59	9.75	9.43	9.17	9.04	8.61	9.88	9.53	8.98
8 YRS	10.29	10.70	9.87	9.55	9.40	9.26	8.92	10.02	9.75	9.23
9 YRS	10.35	10.81	10.00	9.67	9.63	9.49	9.22	10.16	9.97	9.49
10 YRS	10.41	10.92	10.12	9.79	9.87	9.72	9.53	10.30	10.19	9.74
11 YRS	10.48	11.03	10.25	9.91	10.10	9.94	9.84	10.43	10.41	9.99
12 YRS	10.54	11.14	10.37	10.03	10.33	10.17	10.14	10.57	10.63	10.25
13 YRS	10.60	11.25	10.50	10.15	10.56	10.40	10.45	10.71	10.86	10.50
14 YRS	10.67	11.36	10.62	10.27	10.80	10.63	10.76	10.85	11.08	10.76
15 YRS	10.73	11.47	10.75	10.39	11.03	10.85	11.06	10.99	11.30	11.01
16 YRS	10.79	11.58	10.88	10.51	11.26	11.08	11.37	11.12	11.52	11.26
17 YRS	10.86	11.69	11.00	10.63	11.50	11.31	11.68	11.26	11.74	11.52
18 YRS	10.92	11.80	11.13	10.76	11.73	11.53	11.98	11.40	11.96	11.77
19 YRS	10.98	11.91	11.25	10.88	11.96	11.76	12.29	11.54	12.18	12.03
20 YRS	11.05	12.02	11.38	11.00	12.20	11.99	12.60	11.68	12.40	12.28
21 YRS	11.11	12.13	11.50	11.12	12.43	12.22	12.90	11.82	12.62	12.53
22 YRS	11.17	12.24	11.63	11.24	12.66	12.44	13.21	11.95	12.84	12.79
23 YRS	11.24	12.35	11.75	11.36	12.90	12.67	13.52	12.09	13.07	13.04
24 YRS	11.30	12.46	11.88	11.48	13.13	12.90	13.82	12.23	13.29	13.29
25 YRS	11.36	12.57	12.01	11.60	13.36	13.12	14.13	12.37	13.51	13.55
26 YRS	11.43	12.68	12.13	11.72	13.60	13.35	14.44	12.51	13.73	13.80
27 YRS	11.49	12.79	12.26	11.84	13.83	13.58	14.75	12.64	13.95	14.06
28 YRS	11.55	12.90	12.38	11.96	14.06	13.80	15.05	12.78	14.17	14.31
29 YRS	11.62	13.01	12.51	12.08	14.30	14.03	15.36	12.92	14.39	14.56
30 YRS	11.68	13.12	12.63	12.20	14.53	14.26	15.67	13.06	14.61	14.82

EDUCATION	CORRECT	DIGITSPA	WAISIMIL	WAISJUDG	VERBAL	ANIMAL	WAISBLOC	DIGIT
0 YRS	8.38	7.85	5.57	6.56	6.00	8.23	8.56	7.07
1 YRS	8.62	8.10	6.00	6.95	6.36	8.54	8.82	7.45
2 YRS	8.86	8.35	6.43	7.34	6.72	8.84	9.08	7.83
3 YRS	9.10	8.60	6.86	7.73	7.08	9.14	9.34	8.20
4 YRS	9.34	8.85	7.29	8.13	7.44	9.45	9.60	8.58
5 YRS	9.57	9.09	7.72	8.52	7.80	9.75	9.86	8.96
6 YRS	9.81	9.34	8.15	8.91	8.16	10.05	10.12	9.34
7 YRS	10.05	9.59	8.59	9.31	8.52	10.36	10.37	9.72
8 YRS	10.29	9.84	9.02	9.70	8.88	10.66	10.63	10.10
9 YRS	10.53	10.08	9.45	10.09	9.24	10.96	10.89	10.47
10 YRS	10.77	10.33	9.88	10.48	9.60	11.27	11.15	10.85
11 YRS	11.01	10.58	10.31	10.88	9.96	11.57	11.41	11.23
12 YRS	11.25	10.83	10.74	11.27	10.32	11.87	11.67	11.61
13 YRS	11.49	11.08	11.18	11.66	10.68	12.17	11.93	11.99
14 YRS	11.73	11.32	11.61	12.05	11.04	12.48	12.19	12.37
15 YRS	11.97	11.57	12.04	12.45	11.40	12.78	12.45	12.74
16 YRS	12.21	11.82	12.47	12.84	11.76	13.08	12.71	13.12
17 YRS	12.44	12.07	12.90	13.23	12.12	13.39	12.97	13.50
18 YRS	12.68	12.32	13.33	13.62	12.48	13.69	13.23	13.88
19 YRS	12.92	12.56	13.76	14.02	12.84	13.99	13.49	14.26
20 YRS	13.16	12.81	14.20	14.41	13.20	14.30	13.75	14.63
21 YRS	13.40	13.06	14.63	14.80	13.56	14.60	14.01	15.01
22 YRS	13.64	13.31	15.06	15.20	13.92	14.90	14.27	15.39
23 YRS	13.88	13.55	15.49	15.59	14.29	15.21	14.53	15.77
24 YRS	14.12	13.80	15.92	15.98	14.65	15.51	14.79	16.15
25 YRS	14.36	14.05	16.35	16.37	15.01	15.81	15.05	16.53
26 YRS	14.60	14.30	16.79	16.77	15.37	16.11	15.31	16.90
27 YRS	14.84	14.55	17.22	17.16	15.73	16.42	15.57	17.28
28 YRS	15.08	14.79	17.65	17.55	16.09	16.72	15.83	17.66
29 YRS	15.32	15.04	18.08	17.94	16.45	17.02	16.09	18.04
30 YRS	15.55	15.29	18.51	18.34	16.81	17.33	16.35	18.42

Table 12.2. Age 71 – Female.

EDUCATION	BUSCHFR1	BRETRIE	REYA1	REYA2	REYA3	REYA4	REYA5	REYTOT	REYB1	REYA6
0 YRS	9.78	9.82	8.87	8.59	7.53	7.45	6.46	8.91	7.98	7.20
1 YRS	9.84	9.93	8.99	8.71	7.77	7.67	6.77	9.05	8.20	7.45
2 YRS	9.91	10.04	9.12	8.83	8.00	7.90	7.08	9.19	8.43	7.71
3 YRS	9.97	10.15	9.24	8.95	8.23	8.13	7.38	9.33	8.65	7.96
4 YRS	10.03	10.26	9.37	9.07	8.47	8.36	7.69	9.47	8.87	8.22
5 YRS	10.10	10.37	9.49	9.19	8.70	8.58	8.00	9.60	9.09	8.47
6 YRS	10.16	10.48	9.62	9.31	8.93	8.81	8.30	9.74	9.31	8.72
7 YRS	10.22	10.59	9.75	9.43	9.17	9.04	8.61	9.88	9.53	8.98
8 YRS	10.29	10.70	9.87	9.55	9.40	9.26	8.92	10.02	9.75	9.23
9 YRS	10.35	10.81	10.00	9.67	9.63	9.49	9.22	10.16	9.97	9.49
10 YRS	10.41	10.92	10.12	9.79	9.87	9.72	9.53	10.30	10.19	9.74
11 YRS	10.48	11.03	10.25	9.91	10.10	9.94	9.84	10.43	10.41	9.99
12 YRS	10.54	11.14	10.37	10.03	10.33	10.17	10.14	10.57	10.63	10.25
13 YRS	10.60	11.25	10.50	10.15	10.56	10.40	10.45	10.71	10.86	10.50
14 YRS	10.67	11.36	10.62	10.27	10.80	10.63	10.76	10.85	11.08	10.76
15 YRS	10.73	11.47	10.75	10.39	11.03	10.85	11.06	10.99	11.30	11.01
16 YRS	10.79	11.58	10.88	10.51	11.26	11.08	11.37	11.12	11.52	11.26
17 YRS	10.86	11.69	11.00	10.63	11.50	11.31	11.68	11.26	11.74	11.52
18 YRS	10.92	11.80	11.13	10.76	11.73	11.53	11.98	11.40	11.96	11.77
19 YRS	10.98	11.91	11.25	10.88	11.96	11.76	12.29	11.54	12.18	12.03
20 YRS	11.05	12.02	11.38	11.00	12.20	11.99	12.60	11.68	12.40	12.28
21 YRS	11.11	12.13	11.50	11.12	12.43	12.22	12.90	11.82	12.62	12.53
22 YRS	11.17	12.24	11.63	11.24	12.66	12.44	13.21	11.95	12.84	12.79
23 YRS	11.24	12.35	11.75	11.36	12.90	12.67	13.52	12.09	13.07	13.04
24 YRS	11.30	12.46	11.88	11.48	13.13	12.90	13.82	12.23	13.29	13.29
25 YRS	11.36	12.57	12.01	11.60	13.36	13.12	14.13	12.37	13.51	13.55
26 YRS	11.43	12.68	12.13	11.72	13.60	13.35	14.44	12.51	13.73	13.80
27 YRS	11.49	12.79	12.26	11.84	13.83	13.58	14.75	12.64	13.95	14.06
28 YRS	11.55	12.90	12.38	11.96	14.06	13.80	15.05	12.78	14.17	14.31
29 YRS	11.62	13.01	12.51	12.08	14.30	14.03	15.36	12.92	14.39	14.56
30 YRS	11.68	13.12	12.63	12.20	14.53	14.26	15.67	13.06	14.61	14.82

EDUCATION	CORRECT	DIGITSPA	WAISIMIL	WAISJUDG	VERBAL	ANIMAL	WAISBLOC	DIGIT
0 YRS	8.38	7.85	5.57	6.56	6.00	8.23	8.56	7.07
1 YRS	8.62	8.10	6.00	6.95	6.36	8.54	8.82	7.45
2 YRS	8.86	8.35	6.43	7.34	6.72	8.84	9.08	7.83
3 YRS	9.10	8.60	6.86	7.73	7.08	9.14	9.34	8.20
4 YRS	9.34	8.85	7.29	8.13	7.44	9.45	9.60	8.58
5 YRS	9.57	9.09	7.72	8.52	7.80	9.75	9.86	8.96
6 YRS	9.81	9.34	8.15	8.91	8.16	10.05	10.12	9.34
7 YRS	10.05	9.59	8.59	9.31	8.52	10.36	10.37	9.72
8 YRS	10.29	9.84	9.02	9.70	8.88	10.66	10.63	10.10
9 YRS	10.53	10.08	9.45	10.09	9.24	10.96	10.89	10.47
10 YRS	10.77	10.33	9.88	10.48	9.60	11.27	11.15	10.85
11 YRS	11.01	10.58	10.31	10.88	9.96	11.57	11.41	11.23
12 YRS	11.25	10.83	10.74	11.27	10.32	11.87	11.67	11.61
13 YRS	11.49	11.08	11.18	11.66	10.68	12.17	11.93	11.99
14 YRS	11.73	11.32	11.61	12.05	11.04	12.48	12.19	12.37
15 YRS	11.97	11.57	12.04	12.45	11.40	12.78	12.45	12.74
16 YRS	12.21	11.82	12.47	12.84	11.76	13.08	12.71	13.12
17 YRS	12.44	12.07	12.90	13.23	12.12	13.39	12.97	13.50
18 YRS	12.68	12.32	13.33	13.62	12.48	13.69	13.23	13.88
19 YRS	12.92	12.56	13.76	14.02	12.84	13.99	13.49	14.26
20 YRS	13.16	12.81	14.20	14.41	13.20	14.30	13.75	14.63
21 YRS	13.40	13.06	14.63	14.80	13.56	14.60	14.01	15.01
22 YRS	13.64	13.31	15.06	15.20	13.92	14.90	14.27	15.39
23 YRS	13.88	13.55	15.49	15.59	14.29	15.21	14.53	15.77
24 YRS	14.12	13.80	15.92	15.98	14.65	15.51	14.79	16.15
25 YRS	14.36	14.05	16.35	16.37	15.01	15.81	15.05	16.53
26 YRS	14.60	14.30	16.79	16.77	15.37	16.11	15.31	16.90
27 YRS	14.84	14.55	17.22	17.16	15.73	16.42	15.57	17.28
28 YRS	15.08	14.79	17.65	17.55	16.09	16.72	15.83	17.66
29 YRS	15.32	15.04	18.08	17.94	16.45	17.02	16.09	18.04
30 YRS	15.55	15.29	18.51	18.34	16.81	17.33	16.35	18.42

Table 13.1. Age 72 – Male.

EDUCATION	BUSCHFR1	BRETRIE	REYA1	REYA2	REYA3	REYA4	REYA5	REYTOT	REYB1	REYA6
0 YRS	9.66	9.66	8.77	8.48	7.38	7.30	6.31	8.76	7.82	7.04
1 YRS	9.73	9.77	8.90	8.60	7.62	7.53	6.62	8.90	8.04	7.29
2 YRS	9.79	9.88	9.02	8.72	7.85	7.75	6.93	9.04	8.26	7.55
3 YRS	9.85	9.99	9.15	8.84	8.08	7.98	7.24	9.18	8.48	7.80
4 YRS	9.92	10.10	9.27	8.97	8.32	8.21	7.54	9.32	8.70	8.06
5 YRS	9.98	10.21	9.40	9.09	8.55	8.43	7.85	9.45	8.93	8.31
6 YRS	10.04	10.32	9.52	9.21	8.78	8.66	8.16	9.59	9.15	8.56
7 YRS	10.11	10.43	9.65	9.33	9.01	8.89	8.46	9.73	9.37	8.82
8 YRS	10.17	10.54	9.77	9.45	9.25	9.12	8.77	9.87	9.59	9.07
9 YRS	10.23	10.65	9.90	9.57	9.48	9.34	9.08	10.01	9.81	9.33
10 YRS	10.30	10.76	10.03	9.69	9.71	9.57	9.38	10.15	10.03	9.58
11 YRS	10.36	10.87	10.15	9.81	9.95	9.80	9.69	10.28	10.25	9.83
12 YRS	10.42	10.98	10.28	9.93	10.18	10.02	10.00	10.42	10.47	10.09
13 YRS	10.49	11.09	10.40	10.05	10.41	10.25	10.30	10.56	10.69	10.34
14 YRS	10.55	11.20	10.53	10.17	10.65	10.48	10.61	10.70	10.91	10.60
15 YRS	10.61	11.31	10.65	10.29	10.88	10.70	10.92	10.84	11.13	10.85
16 YRS	10.68	11.42	10.78	10.41	11.11	10.93	11.22	10.97	11.36	11.10
17 YRS	10.74	11.53	10.90	10.53	11.35	11.16	11.53	11.11	11.58	11.36
18 YRS	10.80	11.64	11.03	10.65	11.58	11.39	11.84	11.25	11.80	11.61
19 YRS	10.86	11.75	11.16	10.77	11.81	11.61	12.14	11.39	12.02	11.87
20 YRS	10.93	11.86	11.28	10.89	12.05	11.84	12.45	11.53	12.24	12.12
21 YRS	10.99	11.97	11.41	11.01	12.28	12.07	12.76	11.67	12.46	12.37
22 YRS	11.05	12.08	11.53	11.13	12.51	12.29	13.06	11.80	12.68	12.63
23 YRS	11.12	12.19	11.66	11.25	12.75	12.52	13.37	11.94	12.90	12.88
24 YRS	11.18	12.30	11.78	11.37	12.98	12.75	13.68	12.08	13.12	13.13
25 YRS	11.24	12.41	11.91	11.49	13.21	12.97	13.98	12.22	13.34	13.39
26 YRS	11.31	12.52	12.03	11.61	13.44	13.20	14.29	12.36	13.57	13.64
27 YRS	11.37	12.63	12.16	11.73	13.68	13.43	14.60	12.49	13.79	13.90
28 YRS	11.43	12.74	12.28	11.85	13.91	13.66	14.90	12.63	14.01	14.15
29 YRS	11.50	12.85	12.41	11.97	14.14	13.88	15.21	12.77	14.23	14.40
30 YRS	11.56	12.96	12.54	12.10	14.38	14.11	15.52	12.91	14.45	14.66

EDUCATION	CORRECT	DIGITSPA	WAISIMIL	WAISJUDG	VERBAL	ANIMAL	WAISBLOC	DIGIT
0 YRS	8.22	7.79	5.47	6.49	5.94	8.12	8.44	6.85
1 YRS	8.46	8.04	5.90	6.89	6.30	8.42	8.70	7.23
2 YRS	8.70	8.28	6.33	7.28	6.66	8.72	8.96	7.61
3 YRS	8.94	8.53	6.76	7.67	7.02	9.03	9.22	7.98
4 YRS	9.18	8.78	7.20	8.06	7.38	9.33	9.48	8.36
5 YRS	9.42	9.03	7.63	8.46	7.74	9.63	9.74	8.74
6 YRS	9.66	9.28	8.06	8.85	8.10	9.94	10.00	9.12
7 YRS	9.90	9.52	8.49	9.24	8.46	10.24	10.26	9.50
8 YRS	10.14	9.77	8.92	9.63	8.82	10.54	10.52	9.87
9 YRS	10.38	10.02	9.35	10.03	9.18	10.85	10.78	10.25
10 YRS	10.62	10.27	9.79	10.42	9.54	11.15	11.04	10.63
11 YRS	10.86	10.51	10.22	10.81	9.90	11.45	11.30	11.01
12 YRS	11.09	10.76	10.65	11.20	10.26	11.75	11.56	11.39
13 YRS	11.33	11.01	11.08	11.60	10.62	12.06	11.82	11.77
14 YRS	11.57	11.26	11.51	11.99	10.99	12.36	12.08	12.14
15 YRS	11.81	11.51	11.94	12.38	11.35	12.66	12.34	12.52
16 YRS	12.05	11.75	12.37	12.78	11.71	12.97	12.60	12.90
17 YRS	12.29	12.00	12.81	13.17	12.07	13.27	12.86	13.28
18 YRS	12.53	12.25	13.24	13.56	12.43	13.57	13.12	13.66
19 YRS	12.77	12.50	13.67	13.95	12.79	13.88	13.38	14.04
20 YRS	13.01	12.75	14.10	14.35	13.15	14.18	13.63	14.41
21 YRS	13.25	12.99	14.53	14.74	13.51	14.48	13.89	14.79
22 YRS	13.49	13.24	14.96	15.13	13.87	14.79	14.15	15.17
23 YRS	13.73	13.49	15.40	15.52	14.23	15.09	14.41	15.55
24 YRS	13.97	13.74	15.83	15.92	14.59	15.39	14.67	15.93
25 YRS	14.20	13.98	16.26	16.31	14.95	15.69	14.93	16.31
26 YRS	14.44	14.23	16.69	16.70	15.31	16.00	15.19	16.68
27 YRS	14.68	14.48	17.12	17.09	15.67	16.30	15.45	17.06
28 YRS	14.92	14.73	17.55	17.49	16.03	16.60	15.71	17.44
29 YRS	15.16	14.98	17.99	17.88	16.39	16.91	15.97	17.82
30 YRS	15.40	15.22	18.42	18.27	16.75	17.21	16.23	18.20

Table 13.2. Age 72 – Female.

EDUCATION	BUSCHFR1	BRETRIE	REYA1	REYA2	REYA3	REYA4	REYA5	REYTOT	REYB1	REYA6
0 YRS	9.66	9.66	8.77	8.48	7.38	7.30	6.31	8.76	7.82	7.04
1 YRS	9.73	9.77	8.90	8.60	7.62	7.53	6.62	8.90	8.04	7.29
2 YRS	9.79	9.88	9.02	8.72	7.85	7.75	6.93	9.04	8.26	7.55
3 YRS	9.85	9.99	9.15	8.84	8.08	7.98	7.24	9.18	8.48	7.80
4 YRS	9.92	10.10	9.27	8.97	8.32	8.21	7.54	9.32	8.70	8.06
5 YRS	9.98	10.21	9.40	9.09	8.55	8.43	7.85	9.45	8.93	8.31
6 YRS	10.04	10.32	9.52	9.21	8.78	8.66	8.16	9.59	9.15	8.56
7 YRS	10.11	10.43	9.65	9.33	9.01	8.89	8.46	9.73	9.37	8.82
8 YRS	10.17	10.54	9.77	9.45	9.25	9.12	8.77	9.87	9.59	9.07
9 YRS	10.23	10.65	9.90	9.57	9.48	9.34	9.08	10.01	9.81	9.33
10 YRS	10.30	10.76	10.03	9.69	9.71	9.57	9.38	10.15	10.03	9.58
11 YRS	10.36	10.87	10.15	9.81	9.95	9.80	9.69	10.28	10.25	9.83
12 YRS	10.42	10.98	10.28	9.93	10.18	10.02	10.00	10.42	10.47	10.09
13 YRS	10.49	11.09	10.40	10.05	10.41	10.25	10.30	10.56	10.69	10.34
14 YRS	10.55	11.20	10.53	10.17	10.65	10.48	10.61	10.70	10.91	10.60
15 YRS	10.61	11.31	10.65	10.29	10.88	10.70	10.92	10.84	11.13	10.85
16 YRS	10.68	11.42	10.78	10.41	11.11	10.93	11.22	10.97	11.36	11.10
17 YRS	10.74	11.53	10.90	10.53	11.35	11.16	11.53	11.11	11.58	11.36
18 YRS	10.80	11.64	11.03	10.65	11.58	11.39	11.84	11.25	11.80	11.61
19 YRS	10.86	11.75	11.16	10.77	11.81	11.61	12.14	11.39	12.02	11.87
20 YRS	10.93	11.86	11.28	10.89	12.05	11.84	12.45	11.53	12.24	12.12
21 YRS	10.99	11.97	11.41	11.01	12.28	12.07	12.76	11.67	12.46	12.37
22 YRS	11.05	12.08	11.53	11.13	12.51	12.29	13.06	11.80	12.68	12.63
23 YRS	11.12	12.19	11.66	11.25	12.75	12.52	13.37	11.94	12.90	12.88
24 YRS	11.18	12.30	11.78	11.37	12.98	12.75	13.68	12.08	13.12	13.13
25 YRS	11.24	12.41	11.91	11.49	13.21	12.97	13.98	12.22	13.34	13.39
26 YRS	11.31	12.52	12.03	11.61	13.44	13.20	14.29	12.36	13.57	13.64
27 YRS	11.37	12.63	12.16	11.73	13.68	13.43	14.60	12.49	13.79	13.90
28 YRS	11.43	12.74	12.28	11.85	13.91	13.66	14.90	12.63	14.01	14.15
29 YRS	11.50	12.85	12.41	11.97	14.14	13.88	15.21	12.77	14.23	14.40
30 YRS	11.56	12.96	12.54	12.10	14.38	14.11	15.52	12.91	14.45	14.66

EDUCATION	CORRECT	DIGITSPA	WAISIMIL	WAISJUDG	VERBAL	ANIMAL	WAISBLOC	DIGIT
0 YRS	8.22	7.79	5.47	6.49	5.94	8.12	8.44	6.85
1 YRS	8.46	8.04	5.90	6.89	6.30	8.42	8.70	7.23
2 YRS	8.70	8.28	6.33	7.28	6.66	8.72	8.96	7.61
3 YRS	8.94	8.53	6.76	7.67	7.02	9.03	9.22	7.98
4 YRS	9.18	8.78	7.20	8.06	7.38	9.33	9.48	8.36
5 YRS	9.42	9.03	7.63	8.46	7.74	9.63	9.74	8.74
6 YRS	9.66	9.28	8.06	8.85	8.10	9.94	10.00	9.12
7 YRS	9.90	9.52	8.49	9.24	8.46	10.24	10.26	9.50
8 YRS	10.14	9.77	8.92	9.63	8.82	10.54	10.52	9.87
9 YRS	10.38	10.02	9.35	10.03	9.18	10.85	10.78	10.25
10 YRS	10.62	10.27	9.79	10.42	9.54	11.15	11.04	10.63
11 YRS	10.86	10.51	10.22	10.81	9.90	11.45	11.30	11.01
12 YRS	11.09	10.76	10.65	11.20	10.26	11.75	11.56	11.39
13 YRS	11.33	11.01	11.08	11.60	10.62	12.06	11.82	11.77
14 YRS	11.57	11.26	11.51	11.99	10.99	12.36	12.08	12.14
15 YRS	11.81	11.51	11.94	12.38	11.35	12.66	12.34	12.52
16 YRS	12.05	11.75	12.37	12.78	11.71	12.97	12.60	12.90
17 YRS	12.29	12.00	12.81	13.17	12.07	13.27	12.86	13.28
18 YRS	12.53	12.25	13.24	13.56	12.43	13.57	13.12	13.66
19 YRS	12.77	12.50	13.67	13.95	12.79	13.88	13.38	14.04
20 YRS	13.01	12.75	14.10	14.35	13.15	14.18	13.63	14.41
21 YRS	13.25	12.99	14.53	14.74	13.51	14.48	13.89	14.79
22 YRS	13.49	13.24	14.96	15.13	13.87	14.79	14.15	15.17
23 YRS	13.73	13.49	15.40	15.52	14.23	15.09	14.41	15.55
24 YRS	13.97	13.74	15.83	15.92	14.59	15.39	14.67	15.93
25 YRS	14.20	13.98	16.26	16.31	14.95	15.69	14.93	16.31
26 YRS	14.44	14.23	16.69	16.70	15.31	16.00	15.19	16.68
27 YRS	14.68	14.48	17.12	17.09	15.67	16.30	15.45	17.06
28 YRS	14.92	14.73	17.55	17.49	16.03	16.60	15.71	17.44
29 YRS	15.16	14.98	17.99	17.88	16.39	16.91	15.97	17.82
30 YRS	15.40	15.22	18.42	18.27	16.75	17.21	16.23	18.20

Table 14.1. Age 73 – Male.

EDUCATION	BUSCHFR1	BRETRIE	REYA1	REYA2	REYA3	REYA4	REYA5	REYTOT	REYB1	REYA6
0 YRS	9.54	9.50	8.67	8.38	7.23	7.15	6.17	8.61	7.66	6.88
1 YRS	9.61	9.61	8.80	8.50	7.47	7.38	6.47	8.75	7.88	7.13
2 YRS	9.67	9.72	8.92	8.62	7.70	7.60	6.78	8.89	8.10	7.39
3 YRS	9.73	9.83	9.05	8.74	7.93	7.83	7.09	9.03	8.32	7.64
4 YRS	9.80	9.94	9.18	8.86	8.16	8.06	7.40	9.17	8.54	7.90
5 YRS	9.86	10.05	9.30	8.98	8.40	8.29	7.70	9.30	8.76	8.15
6 YRS	9.92	10.16	9.43	9.10	8.63	8.51	8.01	9.44	8.98	8.40
7 YRS	9.99	10.27	9.55	9.22	8.86	8.74	8.32	9.58	9.20	8.66
8 YRS	10.05	10.37	9.68	9.34	9.10	8.97	8.62	9.72	9.43	8.91
9 YRS	10.11	10.48	9.80	9.46	9.33	9.19	8.93	9.86	9.65	9.17
10 YRS	10.18	10.59	9.93	9.58	9.56	9.42	9.24	10.00	9.87	9.42
11 YRS	10.24	10.70	10.05	9.70	9.80	9.65	9.54	10.13	10.09	9.67
12 YRS	10.30	10.81	10.18	9.82	10.03	9.87	9.85	10.27	10.31	9.93
13 YRS	10.37	10.92	10.31	9.94	10.26	10.10	10.16	10.41	10.53	10.18
14 YRS	10.43	11.03	10.43	10.06	10.50	10.33	10.46	10.55	10.75	10.44
15 YRS	10.49	11.14	10.56	10.18	10.73	10.56	10.77	10.69	10.97	10.69
16 YRS	10.56	11.25	10.68	10.30	10.96	10.78	11.08	10.82	11.19	10.94
17 YRS	10.62	11.36	10.81	10.43	11.20	11.01	11.38	10.96	11.41	11.20
18 YRS	10.68	11.47	10.93	10.55	11.43	11.24	11.69	11.10	11.64	11.45
19 YRS	10.75	11.58	11.06	10.67	11.66	11.46	12.00	11.24	11.86	11.71
20 YRS	10.81	11.69	11.18	10.79	11.90	11.69	12.30	11.38	12.08	11.96
21 YRS	10.87	11.80	11.31	10.91	12.13	11.92	12.61	11.52	12.30	12.21
22 YRS	10.94	11.91	11.43	11.03	12.36	12.15	12.92	11.65	12.52	12.47
23 YRS	11.00	12.02	11.56	11.15	12.59	12.37	13.22	11.79	12.74	12.72
24 YRS	11.06	12.13	11.69	11.27	12.83	12.60	13.53	11.93	12.96	12.97
25 YRS	11.13	12.24	11.81	11.39	13.06	12.83	13.84	12.07	13.18	13.23
26 YRS	11.19	12.35	11.94	11.51	13.29	13.05	14.14	12.21	13.40	13.48
27 YRS	11.25	12.46	12.06	11.63	13.53	13.28	14.45	12.34	13.62	13.74
28 YRS	11.32	12.57	12.19	11.75	13.76	13.51	14.76	12.48	13.84	13.99
29 YRS	11.38	12.68	12.31	11.87	13.99	13.73	15.06	12.62	14.07	14.24
30 YRS	11.44	12.79	12.44	11.99	14.23	13.96	15.37	12.76	14.29	14.50

EDUCATION	CORRECT	DIGITSPA	WAISIMIL	WAISJUDG	VERBAL	ANIMAL	WAISBLOC	DIGIT
0 YRS	8.07	7.72	5.37	6.43	5.88	8.00	8.33	6.63
1 YRS	8.31	7.97	5.81	6.82	6.24	8.30	8.59	7.01
2 YRS	8.55	8.22	6.24	7.21	6.60	8.61	8.85	7.38
3 YRS	8.79	8.47	6.67	7.61	6.96	8.91	9.11	7.76
4 YRS	9.03	8.71	7.10	8.00	7.32	9.21	9.37	8.14
5 YRS	9.27	8.96	7.53	8.39	7.69	9.52	9.63	8.52
6 YRS	9.51	9.21	7.96	8.78	8.05	9.82	9.88	8.90
7 YRS	9.74	9.46	8.40	9.18	8.41	10.12	10.14	9.28
8 YRS	9.98	9.71	8.83	9.57	8.77	10.43	10.40	9.65
9 YRS	10.22	9.95	9.26	9.96	9.13	10.73	10.66	10.03
10 YRS	10.46	10.20	9.69	10.36	9.49	11.03	10.92	10.41
11 YRS	10.70	10.45	10.12	10.75	9.85	11.33	11.18	10.79
12 YRS	10.94	10.70	10.55	11.14	10.21	11.64	11.44	11.17
13 YRS	11.18	10.94	10.98	11.53	10.57	11.94	11.70	11.55
14 YRS	11.42	11.19	11.42	11.93	10.93	12.24	11.96	11.92
15 YRS	11.66	11.44	11.85	12.32	11.29	12.55	12.22	12.30
16 YRS	11.90	11.69	12.28	12.71	11.65	12.85	12.48	12.68
17 YRS	12.14	11.94	12.71	13.10	12.01	13.15	12.74	13.06
18 YRS	12.38	12.18	13.14	13.50	12.37	13.46	13.00	13.44
19 YRS	12.62	12.43	13.57	13.89	12.73	13.76	13.26	13.82
20 YRS	12.85	12.68	14.01	14.28	13.09	14.06	13.52	14.19
21 YRS	13.09	12.93	14.44	14.67	13.45	14.37	13.78	14.57
22 YRS	13.33	13.18	14.87	15.07	13.81	14.67	14.04	14.95
23 YRS	13.57	13.42	15.30	15.46	14.17	14.97	14.30	15.33
24 YRS	13.81	13.67	15.73	15.85	14.53	15.27	14.56	15.71
25 YRS	14.05	13.92	16.16	16.25	14.89	15.58	14.82	16.09
26 YRS	14.29	14.17	16.60	16.64	15.25	15.88	15.08	16.46
27 YRS	14.53	14.41	17.03	17.03	15.61	16.18	15.34	16.84
28 YRS	14.77	14.66	17.46	17.42	15.97	16.49	15.60	17.22
29 YRS	15.01	14.91	17.89	17.82	16.33	16.79	15.86	17.60
30 YRS	15.25	15.16	18.32	18.21	16.69	17.09	16.12	17.98

Table 14.2. Age 73 – Female.

EDUCATION	BUSCHFR1	BRETRIE	REYA1	REYA2	REYA3	REYA4	REYA5	REYTOT	REYB1	REYA6
0 YRS	9.54	9.50	8.67	8.38	7.23	7.15	6.17	8.61	7.66	6.88
1 YRS	9.61	9.61	8.80	8.50	7.47	7.38	6.47	8.75	7.88	7.13
2 YRS	9.67	9.72	8.92	8.62	7.70	7.60	6.78	8.89	8.10	7.39
3 YRS	9.73	9.83	9.05	8.74	7.93	7.83	7.09	9.03	8.32	7.64
4 YRS	9.80	9.94	9.18	8.86	8.16	8.06	7.40	9.17	8.54	7.90
5 YRS	9.86	10.05	9.30	8.98	8.40	8.29	7.70	9.30	8.76	8.15
6 YRS	9.92	10.16	9.43	9.10	8.63	8.51	8.01	9.44	8.98	8.40
7 YRS	9.99	10.27	9.55	9.22	8.86	8.74	8.32	9.58	9.20	8.66
8 YRS	10.05	10.37	9.68	9.34	9.10	8.97	8.62	9.72	9.43	8.91
9 YRS	10.11	10.48	9.80	9.46	9.33	9.19	8.93	9.86	9.65	9.17
10 YRS	10.18	10.59	9.93	9.58	9.56	9.42	9.24	10.00	9.87	9.42
11 YRS	10.24	10.70	10.05	9.70	9.80	9.65	9.54	10.13	10.09	9.67
12 YRS	10.30	10.81	10.18	9.82	10.03	9.87	9.85	10.27	10.31	9.93
13 YRS	10.37	10.92	10.31	9.94	10.26	10.10	10.16	10.41	10.53	10.18
14 YRS	10.43	11.03	10.43	10.06	10.50	10.33	10.46	10.55	10.75	10.44
15 YRS	10.49	11.14	10.56	10.18	10.73	10.56	10.77	10.69	10.97	10.69
16 YRS	10.56	11.25	10.68	10.30	10.96	10.78	11.08	10.82	11.19	10.94
17 YRS	10.62	11.36	10.81	10.43	11.20	11.01	11.38	10.96	11.41	11.20
18 YRS	10.68	11.47	10.93	10.55	11.43	11.24	11.69	11.10	11.64	11.45
19 YRS	10.75	11.58	11.06	10.67	11.66	11.46	12.00	11.24	11.86	11.71
20 YRS	10.81	11.69	11.18	10.79	11.90	11.69	12.30	11.38	12.08	11.96
21 YRS	10.87	11.80	11.31	10.91	12.13	11.92	12.61	11.52	12.30	12.21
22 YRS	10.94	11.91	11.43	11.03	12.36	12.15	12.92	11.65	12.52	12.47
23 YRS	11.00	12.02	11.56	11.15	12.59	12.37	13.22	11.79	12.74	12.72
24 YRS	11.06	12.13	11.69	11.27	12.83	12.60	13.53	11.93	12.96	12.97
25 YRS	11.13	12.24	11.81	11.39	13.06	12.83	13.84	12.07	13.18	13.23
26 YRS	11.19	12.35	11.94	11.51	13.29	13.05	14.14	12.21	13.40	13.48
27 YRS	11.25	12.46	12.06	11.63	13.53	13.28	14.45	12.34	13.62	13.74
28 YRS	11.32	12.57	12.19	11.75	13.76	13.51	14.76	12.48	13.84	13.99
29 YRS	11.38	12.68	12.31	11.87	13.99	13.73	15.06	12.62	14.07	14.24
30 YRS	11.44	12.79	12.44	11.99	14.23	13.96	15.37	12.76	14.29	14.50

EDUCATION	CORRECT	DIGITSPA	WAISIMIL	WAISJUDG	VERBAL	ANIMAL	WAISBLOC	DIGIT
0 YRS	8.07	7.72	5.37	6.43	5.88	8.00	8.33	6.63
1 YRS	8.31	7.97	5.81	6.82	6.24	8.30	8.59	7.01
2 YRS	8.55	8.22	6.24	7.21	6.60	8.61	8.85	7.38
3 YRS	8.79	8.47	6.67	7.61	6.96	8.91	9.11	7.76
4 YRS	9.03	8.71	7.10	8.00	7.32	9.21	9.37	8.14
5 YRS	9.27	8.96	7.53	8.39	7.69	9.52	9.63	8.52
6 YRS	9.51	9.21	7.96	8.78	8.05	9.82	9.88	8.90
7 YRS	9.74	9.46	8.40	9.18	8.41	10.12	10.14	9.28
8 YRS	9.98	9.71	8.83	9.57	8.77	10.43	10.40	9.65
9 YRS	10.22	9.95	9.26	9.96	9.13	10.73	10.66	10.03
10 YRS	10.46	10.20	9.69	10.36	9.49	11.03	10.92	10.41
11 YRS	10.70	10.45	10.12	10.75	9.85	11.33	11.18	10.79
12 YRS	10.94	10.70	10.55	11.14	10.21	11.64	11.44	11.17
13 YRS	11.18	10.94	10.98	11.53	10.57	11.94	11.70	11.55
14 YRS	11.42	11.19	11.42	11.93	10.93	12.24	11.96	11.92
15 YRS	11.66	11.44	11.85	12.32	11.29	12.55	12.22	12.30
16 YRS	11.90	11.69	12.28	12.71	11.65	12.85	12.48	12.68
17 YRS	12.14	11.94	12.71	13.10	12.01	13.15	12.74	13.06
18 YRS	12.38	12.18	13.14	13.50	12.37	13.46	13.00	13.44
19 YRS	12.62	12.43	13.57	13.89	12.73	13.76	13.26	13.82
20 YRS	12.85	12.68	14.01	14.28	13.09	14.06	13.52	14.19
21 YRS	13.09	12.93	14.44	14.67	13.45	14.37	13.78	14.57
22 YRS	13.33	13.18	14.87	15.07	13.81	14.67	14.04	14.95
23 YRS	13.57	13.42	15.30	15.46	14.17	14.97	14.30	15.33
24 YRS	13.81	13.67	15.73	15.85	14.53	15.27	14.56	15.71
25 YRS	14.05	13.92	16.16	16.25	14.89	15.58	14.82	16.09
26 YRS	14.29	14.17	16.60	16.64	15.25	15.88	15.08	16.46
27 YRS	14.53	14.41	17.03	17.03	15.61	16.18	15.34	16.84
28 YRS	14.77	14.66	17.46	17.42	15.97	16.49	15.60	17.22
29 YRS	15.01	14.91	17.89	17.82	16.33	16.79	15.86	17.60
30 YRS	15.25	15.16	18.32	18.21	16.69	17.09	16.12	17.98

Table 15.1. Age 74 – Male.

EDUCATION	BUSCHFR1	BRETRIE	REYA1	REYA2	REYA3	REYA4	REYA5	REYTOT	REYB1	REYA6
0 YRS	9.43	9.33	8.58	8.27	7.08	7.00	6.02	8.46	7.50	6.72
1 YRS	9.49	9.44	8.70	8.39	7.31	7.23	6.33	8.60	7.72	6.97
2 YRS	9.55	9.55	8.83	8.51	7.55	7.46	6.63	8.74	7.94	7.23
3 YRS	9.62	9.66	8.95	8.64	7.78	7.68	6.94	8.88	8.16	7.48
4 YRS	9.68	9.77	9.08	8.76	8.01	7.91	7.25	9.02	8.38	7.74
5 YRS	9.74	9.88	9.20	8.88	8.25	8.14	7.55	9.15	8.60	7.99
6 YRS	9.81	9.99	9.33	9.00	8.48	8.36	7.86	9.29	8.82	8.24
7 YRS	9.87	10.10	9.45	9.12	8.71	8.59	8.17	9.43	9.04	8.50
8 YRS	9.93	10.21	9.58	9.24	8.95	8.82	8.48	9.57	9.26	8.75
9 YRS	10.00	10.32	9.71	9.36	9.18	9.05	8.78	9.71	9.48	9.01
10 YRS	10.06	10.43	9.83	9.48	9.41	9.27	9.09	9.85	9.70	9.26
11 YRS	10.12	10.54	9.96	9.60	9.65	9.50	9.40	9.98	9.93	9.51
12 YRS	10.19	10.65	10.08	9.72	9.88	9.73	9.70	10.12	10.15	9.77
13 YRS	10.25	10.76	10.21	9.84	10.11	9.95	10.01	10.26	10.37	10.02
14 YRS	10.31	10.87	10.33	9.96	10.35	10.18	10.32	10.40	10.59	10.28
15 YRS	10.38	10.98	10.46	10.08	10.58	10.41	10.62	10.54	10.81	10.53
16 YRS	10.44	11.09	10.58	10.20	10.81	10.63	10.93	10.67	11.03	10.78
17 YRS	10.50	11.20	10.71	10.32	11.05	10.86	11.24	10.81	11.25	11.04
18 YRS	10.57	11.31	10.84	10.44	11.28	11.09	11.54	10.95	11.47	11.29
19 YRS	10.63	11.42	10.96	10.56	11.51	11.32	11.85	11.09	11.69	11.55
20 YRS	10.69	11.53	11.09	10.68	11.74	11.54	12.16	11.23	11.91	11.80
21 YRS	10.76	11.64	11.21	10.80	11.98	11.77	12.46	11.37	12.14	12.05
22 YRS	10.82	11.75	11.34	10.92	12.21	12.00	12.77	11.50	12.36	12.31
23 YRS	10.88	11.86	11.46	11.04	12.44	12.22	13.08	11.64	12.58	12.56
24 YRS	10.95	11.97	11.59	11.16	12.68	12.45	13.38	11.78	12.80	12.81
25 YRS	11.01	12.08	11.71	11.28	12.91	12.68	13.69	11.92	13.02	13.07
26 YRS	11.07	12.19	11.84	11.40	13.14	12.90	14.00	12.06	13.24	13.32
27 YRS	11.14	12.30	11.97	11.52	13.38	13.13	14.30	12.19	13.46	13.58
28 YRS	11.20	12.41	12.09	11.64	13.61	13.36	14.61	12.33	13.68	13.83
29 YRS	11.26	12.52	12.22	11.77	13.84	13.59	14.92	12.47	13.90	14.08
30 YRS	11.32	12.63	12.34	11.89	14.08	13.81	15.22	12.61	14.12	14.34

EDUCATION	CORRECT	DIGITSPA	WAISIMIL	WAISJUDG	VERBAL	ANIMAL	WAISBLOC	DIGIT
0 YRS	7.92	7.66	5.28	6.36	5.83	7.88	8.21	6.41
1 YRS	8.16	7.90	5.71	6.76	6.19	8.19	8.47	6.79
2 YRS	8.39	8.15	6.14	7.15	6.55	8.49	8.73	7.16
3 YRS	8.63	8.40	6.57	7.54	6.91	8.79	8.99	7.54
4 YRS	8.87	8.65	7.01	7.94	7.27	9.10	9.25	7.92
5 YRS	9.11	8.90	7.44	8.33	7.63	9.40	9.51	8.30
6 YRS	9.35	9.14	7.87	8.72	7.99	9.70	9.77	8.68
7 YRS	9.59	9.39	8.30	9.11	8.35	10.01	10.03	9.06
8 YRS	9.83	9.64	8.73	9.51	8.71	10.31	10.29	9.43
9 YRS	10.07	9.89	9.16	9.90	9.07	10.61	10.55	9.81
10 YRS	10.31	10.14	9.59	10.29	9.43	10.91	10.81	10.19
11 YRS	10.55	10.38	10.03	10.68	9.79	11.22	11.07	10.57
12 YRS	10.79	10.63	10.46	11.08	10.15	11.52	11.33	10.95
13 YRS	11.03	10.88	10.89	11.47	10.51	11.82	11.59	11.33
14 YRS	11.26	11.13	11.32	11.86	10.87	12.13	11.85	11.70
15 YRS	11.50	11.37	11.75	12.25	11.23	12.43	12.11	12.08
16 YRS	11.74	11.62	12.18	12.65	11.59	12.73	12.37	12.46
17 YRS	11.98	11.87	12.62	13.04	11.95	13.04	12.63	12.84
18 YRS	12.22	12.12	13.05	13.43	12.31	13.34	12.89	13.22
19 YRS	12.46	12.37	13.48	13.83	12.67	13.64	13.14	13.60
20 YRS	12.70	12.61	13.91	14.22	13.03	13.95	13.40	13.97
21 YRS	12.94	12.86	14.34	14.61	13.39	14.25	13.66	14.35
22 YRS	13.18	13.11	14.77	15.00	13.76	14.55	13.92	14.73
23 YRS	13.42	13.36	15.21	15.40	14.12	14.85	14.18	15.11
24 YRS	13.66	13.61	15.64	15.79	14.48	15.16	14.44	15.49
25 YRS	13.90	13.85	16.07	16.18	14.84	15.46	14.70	15.87
26 YRS	14.14	14.10	16.50	16.57	15.20	15.76	14.96	16.24
27 YRS	14.37	14.35	16.93	16.97	15.56	16.07	15.22	16.62
28 YRS	14.61	14.60	17.36	17.36	15.92	16.37	15.48	17.00
29 YRS	14.85	14.84	17.79	17.75	16.28	16.67	15.74	17.38
30 YRS	15.09	15.09	18.23	18.14	16.64	16.98	16.00	17.76

Table 15.2. Age 74 – Female.

EDUCATION	BUSCHFR1	BRETRIE	REYA1	REYA2	REYA3	REYA4	REYA5	REYTOT	REYB1	REYA6
0 YRS	9.88	8.58	8.51	7.88	7.08	6.83	6.30	8.18	7.44	6.67
1 YRS	9.89	8.71	8.64	8.03	7.30	7.06	6.57	8.33	7.68	6.92
2 YRS	9.91	8.84	8.77	8.18	7.53	7.29	6.84	8.48	7.91	7.17
3 YRS	9.92	8.97	8.90	8.34	7.76	7.53	7.10	8.63	8.14	7.42
4 YRS	9.93	9.10	9.04	8.49	7.99	7.76	7.37	8.78	8.38	7.67
5 YRS	9.95	9.23	9.17	8.64	8.22	7.99	7.64	8.92	8.61	7.92
6 YRS	9.96	9.37	9.30	8.79	8.45	8.22	7.91	9.07	8.85	8.17
7 YRS	9.97	9.50	9.43	8.95	8.67	8.45	8.18	9.22	9.08	8.42
8 YRS	9.99	9.63	9.57	9.10	8.90	8.68	8.45	9.37	9.31	8.67
9 YRS	10.00	9.76	9.70	9.25	9.13	8.91	8.72	9.51	9.55	8.92
10 YRS	10.01	9.89	9.83	9.41	9.36	9.14	8.99	9.66	9.78	9.17
11 YRS	10.03	10.02	9.97	9.56	9.59	9.37	9.26	9.81	10.02	9.43
12 YRS	10.04	10.15	10.10	9.71	9.82	9.61	9.53	9.96	10.25	9.68
13 YRS	10.05	10.28	10.23	9.86	10.04	9.84	9.80	10.10	10.48	9.93
14 YRS	10.07	10.41	10.36	10.02	10.27	10.07	10.07	10.25	10.72	10.18
15 YRS	10.08	10.54	10.50	10.17	10.50	10.30	10.34	10.40	10.95	10.43
16 YRS	10.09	10.68	10.63	10.32	10.73	10.53	10.61	10.55	11.19	10.68
17 YRS	10.10	10.81	10.76	10.47	10.96	10.76	10.88	10.69	11.42	10.93
18 YRS	10.12	10.94	10.89	10.63	11.18	10.99	11.15	10.84	11.66	11.18
19 YRS	10.13	11.07	11.03	10.78	11.41	11.22	11.42	10.99	11.89	11.43
20 YRS	10.14	11.20	11.16	10.93	11.64	11.46	11.68	11.14	12.12	11.68
21 YRS	10.16	11.33	11.29	11.09	11.87	11.69	11.95	11.28	12.36	11.93
22 YRS	10.17	11.46	11.42	11.24	12.10	11.92	12.22	11.43	12.59	12.18
23 YRS	10.18	11.59	11.56	11.39	12.33	12.15	12.49	11.58	12.83	12.43
24 YRS	10.20	11.72	11.69	11.54	12.55	12.38	12.76	11.73	13.06	12.68
25 YRS	10.21	11.85	11.82	11.70	12.78	12.61	13.03	11.87	13.29	12.93
26 YRS	10.22	11.99	11.95	11.85	13.01	12.84	13.30	12.02	13.53	13.18
27 YRS	10.24	12.12	12.09	12.00	13.24	13.07	13.57	12.17	13.76	13.43
28 YRS	10.25	12.25	12.22	12.16	13.47	13.30	13.84	12.32	14.00	13.68
29 YRS	10.26	12.38	12.35	12.31	13.70	13.54	14.11	12.46	14.23	13.93
30 YRS	10.28	12.51	12.49	12.46	13.92	13.77	14.38	12.61	14.46	14.18

EDUCATION	TRUEPOSI	TRUENEGA	CORRECT	DIGITSPA	WAISIMIL	WAISJUDG	VERBAL	ANIMAL	WAISBLOC	DIGIT
0 YRS	8.07	8.87	7.83	8.03	6.08	7.13	6.23	7.98	8.40	6.58
1 YRS	8.21	8.98	8.07	8.24	6.43	7.45	6.55	8.26	8.64	6.94
2 YRS	8.34	9.09	8.30	8.45	6.79	7.76	6.86	8.54	8.88	7.29
3 YRS	8.48	9.19	8.53	8.67	7.14	8.08	7.18	8.83	9.13	7.65
4 YRS	8.61	9.30	8.76	8.88	7.50	8.40	7.49	9.11	9.37	8.01
5 YRS	8.75	9.41	8.99	9.09	7.85	8.72	7.81	9.39	9.61	8.36
6 YRS	8.88	9.52	9.22	9.31	8.21	9.04	8.13	9.68	9.85	8.72
7 YRS	9.02	9.63	9.46	9.52	8.56	9.36	8.44	9.96	10.09	9.08
8 YRS	9.15	9.74	9.69	9.73	8.92	9.67	8.76	10.24	10.33	9.43
9 YRS	9.29	9.85	9.92	9.94	9.27	9.99	9.07	10.52	10.58	9.79
10 YRS	9.42	9.95	10.15	10.16	9.63	10.31	9.39	10.81	10.82	10.15
11 YRS	9.56	10.06	10.38	10.37	9.99	10.63	9.71	11.09	11.06	10.50
12 YRS	9.69	10.17	10.61	10.58	10.34	10.95	10.02	11.37	11.30	10.86
13 YRS	9.83	10.28	10.84	10.80	10.70	11.27	10.34	11.66	11.54	11.21
14 YRS	9.97	10.39	11.08	11.01	11.05	11.59	10.65	11.94	11.79	11.57
15 YRS	10.10	10.50	11.31	11.22	11.41	11.90	10.97	12.22	12.03	11.93
16 YRS	10.24	10.61	11.54	11.44	11.76	12.22	11.28	12.50	12.27	12.28
17 YRS	10.37	10.71	11.77	11.65	12.12	12.54	11.60	12.79	12.51	12.64
18 YRS	10.51	10.82	12.00	11.86	12.47	12.86	11.92	13.07	12.75	13.00
19 YRS	10.64	10.93	12.23	12.07	12.83	13.18	12.23	13.35	12.99	13.35
20 YRS	10.78	11.04	12.47	12.29	13.18	13.50	12.55	13.64	13.24	13.71
21 YRS	10.91	11.15	12.70	12.50	13.54	13.82	12.86	13.92	13.48	14.06
22 YRS	11.05	11.26	12.93	12.71	13.89	14.13	13.18	14.20	13.72	14.42
23 YRS	11.18	11.37	13.16	12.93	14.25	14.45	13.50	14.48	13.96	14.78
24 YRS	11.32	11.48	13.39	13.14	14.60	14.77	13.81	14.77	14.20	15.13
25 YRS	11.45	11.58	13.62	13.35	14.96	15.09	14.13	15.05	14.45	15.49
26 YRS	11.59	11.69	13.85	13.57	15.31	15.41	14.44	15.33	14.69	15.85
27 YRS	11.72	11.80	14.09	13.78	15.67	15.73	14.76	15.62	14.93	16.20
28 YRS	11.86	11.91	14.32	13.99	16.02	16.04	15.07	15.90	15.17	16.56
29 YRS	11.99	12.02	14.55	14.21	16.38	16.36	15.39	16.18	15.41	16.92
30 YRS	12.13	12.13	14.78	14.42	16.73	16.68	15.71	16.47	15.66	17.27

Table 16.1. Age 75 – Male.

EDUCATION	BUSCHFR1	BRETRIE	REYA1	REYA2	REYA3	REYA4	REYA5	REYTOT	REYB1	REYA6
0 YRS	9.31	9.17	8.48	8.17	6.93	6.85	5.87	8.31	7.33	6.56
1 YRS	9.37	9.28	8.60	8.29	7.16	7.08	6.18	8.45	7.55	6.81
2 YRS	9.44	9.39	8.73	8.41	7.40	7.31	6.49	8.59	7.77	7.07
3 YRS	9.50	9.50	8.86	8.53	7.63	7.53	6.79	8.73	8.00	7.32
4 YRS	9.56	9.61	8.98	8.65	7.86	7.76	7.10	8.87	8.22	7.58
5 YRS	9.63	9.72	9.11	8.77	8.10	7.99	7.41	9.00	8.44	7.83
6 YRS	9.69	9.83	9.23	8.89	8.33	8.22	7.71	9.14	8.66	8.08
7 YRS	9.75	9.94	9.36	9.01	8.56	8.44	8.02	9.28	8.88	8.34
8 YRS	9.82	10.05	9.48	9.13	8.80	8.67	8.33	9.42	9.10	8.59
9 YRS	9.88	10.16	9.61	9.25	9.03	8.90	8.63	9.56	9.32	8.85
10 YRS	9.94	10.27	9.73	9.37	9.26	9.12	8.94	9.70	9.54	9.10
11 YRS	10.00	10.38	9.86	9.49	9.50	9.35	9.25	9.83	9.76	9.35
12 YRS	10.07	10.49	9.99	9.61	9.73	9.58	9.56	9.97	9.98	9.61
13 YRS	10.13	10.60	10.11	9.73	9.96	9.80	9.86	10.11	10.21	9.86
14 YRS	10.19	10.71	10.24	9.85	10.19	10.03	10.17	10.25	10.43	10.12
15 YRS	10.26	10.82	10.36	9.97	10.43	10.26	10.48	10.39	10.65	10.37
16 YRS	10.32	10.93	10.49	10.10	10.66	10.49	10.78	10.52	10.87	10.62
17 YRS	10.38	11.04	10.61	10.22	10.89	10.71	11.09	10.66	11.09	10.88
18 YRS	10.45	11.15	10.74	10.34	11.13	10.94	11.40	10.80	11.31	11.13
19 YRS	10.51	11.26	10.86	10.46	11.36	11.17	11.70	10.94	11.53	11.39
20 YRS	10.57	11.37	10.99	10.58	11.59	11.39	12.01	11.08	11.75	11.64
21 YRS	10.64	11.48	11.12	10.70	11.83	11.62	12.32	11.22	11.97	11.89
22 YRS	10.70	11.59	11.24	10.82	12.06	11.85	12.62	11.35	12.19	12.15
23 YRS	10.76	11.70	11.37	10.94	12.29	12.08	12.93	11.49	12.41	12.40
24 YRS	10.83	11.81	11.49	11.06	12.53	12.30	13.24	11.63	12.64	12.65
25 YRS	10.89	11.92	11.62	11.18	12.76	12.53	13.54	11.77	12.86	12.91
26 YRS	10.95	12.03	11.74	11.30	12.99	12.76	13.85	11.91	13.08	13.16
27 YRS	11.02	12.14	11.87	11.42	13.23	12.98	14.16	12.04	13.30	13.42
28 YRS	11.08	12.25	11.99	11.54	13.46	13.21	14.46	12.18	13.52	13.67
29 YRS	11.14	12.36	12.12	11.66	13.69	13.44	14.77	12.32	13.74	13.92
30 YRS	11.21	12.47	12.25	11.78	13.93	13.66	15.08	12.46	13.96	14.18

EDUCATION	CORRECT	DIGITSPA	WAISMIL	WAISJUDG	VERBAL	ANIMAL	WAISBLOC	DIGIT
0 YRS	7.76	7.59	5.18	6.30	5.77	7.77	8.10	6.19
1 YRS	8.00	7.84	5.62	6.69	6.13	8.07	8.36	6.57
2 YRS	8.24	8.09	6.05	7.09	6.49	8.37	8.62	6.94
3 YRS	8.48	8.33	6.48	7.48	6.85	8.68	8.88	7.32
4 YRS	8.72	8.58	6.91	7.87	7.21	8.98	9.13	7.70
5 YRS	8.96	8.83	7.34	8.26	7.57	9.28	9.39	8.08
6 YRS	9.20	9.08	7.77	8.66	7.93	9.58	9.65	8.46
7 YRS	9.44	9.33	8.20	9.05	8.29	9.89	9.91	8.84
8 YRS	9.68	9.57	8.64	9.44	8.65	10.19	10.17	9.21
9 YRS	9.91	9.82	9.07	9.83	9.01	10.49	10.43	9.59
10 YRS	10.15	10.07	9.50	10.23	9.37	10.80	10.69	9.97
11 YRS	10.39	10.32	9.93	10.62	9.73	11.10	10.95	10.35
12 YRS	10.63	10.57	10.36	11.01	10.09	11.40	11.21	10.73
13 YRS	10.87	10.81	10.79	11.41	10.46	11.71	11.47	11.11
14 YRS	11.11	11.06	11.23	11.80	10.82	12.01	11.73	11.48
15 YRS	11.35	11.31	11.66	12.19	11.18	12.31	11.99	11.86
16 YRS	11.59	11.56	12.09	12.58	11.54	12.62	12.25	12.24
17 YRS	11.83	11.80	12.52	12.98	11.90	12.92	12.51	12.62
18 YRS	12.07	12.05	12.95	13.37	12.26	13.22	12.77	13.00
19 YRS	12.31	12.30	13.38	13.76	12.62	13.53	13.03	13.38
20 YRS	12.55	12.55	13.82	14.15	12.98	13.83	13.29	13.75
21 YRS	12.79	12.80	14.25	14.55	13.34	14.13	13.55	14.13
22 YRS	13.02	13.04	14.68	14.94	13.70	14.43	13.81	14.51
23 YRS	13.26	13.29	15.11	15.33	14.06	14.74	14.07	14.89
24 YRS	13.50	13.54	15.54	15.72	14.42	15.04	14.33	15.27
25 YRS	13.74	13.79	15.97	16.12	14.78	15.34	14.59	15.65
26 YRS	13.98	14.04	16.40	16.51	15.14	15.65	14.85	16.02
27 YRS	14.22	14.28	16.84	16.90	15.50	15.95	15.11	16.40
28 YRS	14.46	14.53	17.27	17.30	15.86	16.25	15.37	16.78
29 YRS	14.70	14.78	17.70	17.69	16.22	16.56	15.63	17.16
30 YRS	14.94	15.03	18.13	18.08	16.58	16.86	15.89	17.54

Table 16.2. Age 75 – Female.

EDUCATION	BUSCHFR1	BRETRIE	REYA1	REYA2	REYA3	REYA4	REYA5	REYTOT	REYB1	REYA6
0 YRS	9.31	9.17	8.48	8.17	6.93	6.85	5.87	8.31	7.33	6.56
1 YRS	9.37	9.28	8.60	8.29	7.16	7.08	6.18	8.45	7.55	6.81
2 YRS	9.44	9.39	8.73	8.41	7.40	7.31	6.49	8.59	7.77	7.07
3 YRS	9.50	9.50	8.86	8.53	7.63	7.53	6.79	8.73	8.00	7.32
4 YRS	9.56	9.61	8.98	8.65	7.86	7.76	7.10	8.87	8.22	7.58
5 YRS	9.63	9.72	9.11	8.77	8.10	7.99	7.41	9.00	8.44	7.83
6 YRS	9.69	9.83	9.23	8.89	8.33	8.22	7.71	9.14	8.66	8.08
7 YRS	9.75	9.94	9.36	9.01	8.56	8.44	8.02	9.28	8.88	8.34
8 YRS	9.82	10.05	9.48	9.13	8.80	8.67	8.33	9.42	9.10	8.59
9 YRS	9.88	10.16	9.61	9.25	9.03	8.90	8.63	9.56	9.32	8.85
10 YRS	9.94	10.27	9.73	9.37	9.26	9.12	8.94	9.70	9.54	9.10
11 YRS	10.00	10.38	9.86	9.49	9.50	9.35	9.25	9.83	9.76	9.35
12 YRS	10.07	10.49	9.99	9.61	9.73	9.58	9.56	9.97	9.98	9.61
13 YRS	10.13	10.60	10.11	9.73	9.96	9.80	9.86	10.11	10.21	9.86
14 YRS	10.19	10.71	10.24	9.85	10.19	10.03	10.17	10.25	10.43	10.12
15 YRS	10.26	10.82	10.36	9.97	10.43	10.26	10.48	10.39	10.65	10.37
16 YRS	10.32	10.93	10.49	10.10	10.66	10.49	10.78	10.52	10.87	10.62
17 YRS	10.38	11.04	10.61	10.22	10.89	10.71	11.09	10.66	11.09	10.88
18 YRS	10.45	11.15	10.74	10.34	11.13	10.94	11.40	10.80	11.31	11.13
19 YRS	10.51	11.26	10.86	10.46	11.36	11.17	11.70	10.94	11.53	11.39
20 YRS	10.57	11.37	10.99	10.58	11.59	11.39	12.01	11.08	11.75	11.64
21 YRS	10.64	11.48	11.12	10.70	11.83	11.62	12.32	11.22	11.97	11.89
22 YRS	10.70	11.59	11.24	10.82	12.06	11.85	12.62	11.35	12.19	12.15
23 YRS	10.76	11.70	11.37	10.94	12.29	12.08	12.93	11.49	12.41	12.40
24 YRS	10.83	11.81	11.49	11.06	12.53	12.30	13.24	11.63	12.64	12.65
25 YRS	10.89	11.92	11.62	11.18	12.76	12.53	13.54	11.77	12.86	12.91
26 YRS	10.95	12.03	11.74	11.30	12.99	12.76	13.85	11.91	13.08	13.16
27 YRS	11.02	12.14	11.87	11.42	13.23	12.98	14.16	12.04	13.30	13.42
28 YRS	11.08	12.25	11.99	11.54	13.46	13.21	14.46	12.18	13.52	13.67
29 YRS	11.14	12.36	12.12	11.66	13.69	13.44	14.77	12.32	13.74	13.92
30 YRS	11.21	12.47	12.25	11.78	13.93	13.66	15.08	12.46	13.96	14.18

EDUCATION	CORRECT	DIGITSPA	WAISIMIL	WAISJUDG	VERBAL	ANIMAL	WAISBLOC	DIGIT
0 YRS	7.76	7.59	5.18	6.30	5.77	7.77	8.10	6.19
1 YRS	8.00	7.84	5.62	6.69	6.13	8.07	8.36	6.57
2 YRS	8.24	8.09	6.05	7.09	6.49	8.37	8.62	6.94
3 YRS	8.48	8.33	6.48	7.48	6.85	8.68	8.88	7.32
4 YRS	8.72	8.58	6.91	7.87	7.21	8.98	9.13	7.70
5 YRS	8.96	8.83	7.34	8.26	7.57	9.28	9.39	8.08
6 YRS	9.20	9.08	7.77	8.66	7.93	9.58	9.65	8.46
7 YRS	9.44	9.33	8.20	9.05	8.29	9.89	9.91	8.84
8 YRS	9.68	9.57	8.64	9.44	8.65	10.19	10.17	9.21
9 YRS	9.91	9.82	9.07	9.83	9.01	10.49	10.43	9.59
10 YRS	10.15	10.07	9.50	10.23	9.37	10.80	10.69	9.97
11 YRS	10.39	10.32	9.93	10.62	9.73	11.10	10.95	10.35
12 YRS	10.63	10.57	10.36	11.01	10.09	11.40	11.21	10.73
13 YRS	10.87	10.81	10.79	11.41	10.46	11.71	11.47	11.11
14 YRS	11.11	11.06	11.23	11.80	10.82	12.01	11.73	11.48
15 YRS	11.35	11.31	11.66	12.19	11.18	12.31	11.99	11.86
16 YRS	11.59	11.56	12.09	12.58	11.54	12.62	12.25	12.24
17 YRS	11.83	11.80	12.52	12.98	11.90	12.92	12.51	12.62
18 YRS	12.07	12.05	12.95	13.37	12.26	13.22	12.77	13.00
19 YRS	12.31	12.30	13.38	13.76	12.62	13.53	13.03	13.38
20 YRS	12.55	12.55	13.82	14.15	12.98	13.83	13.29	13.75
21 YRS	12.79	12.80	14.25	14.55	13.34	14.13	13.55	14.13
22 YRS	13.02	13.04	14.68	14.94	13.70	14.43	13.81	14.51
23 YRS	13.26	13.29	15.11	15.33	14.06	14.74	14.07	14.89
24 YRS	13.50	13.54	15.54	15.72	14.42	15.04	14.33	15.27
25 YRS	13.74	13.79	15.97	16.12	14.78	15.34	14.59	15.65
26 YRS	13.98	14.04	16.40	16.51	15.14	15.65	14.85	16.02
27 YRS	14.22	14.28	16.84	16.90	15.50	15.95	15.11	16.40
28 YRS	14.46	14.53	17.27	17.30	15.86	16.25	15.37	16.78
29 YRS	14.70	14.78	17.70	17.69	16.22	16.56	15.63	17.16
30 YRS	14.94	15.03	18.13	18.08	16.58	16.86	15.89	17.54

Table 17.1. Age 76 – Male.

EDUCATION	BUSCHFR1	BRETRIE	REYA1	REYA2	REYA3	REYA4	REYA5	REYTOT	REYB1	REYA6
0 YRS	9.19	9.01	8.38	8.06	6.78	6.71	5.73	8.16	7.17	6.40
1 YRS	9.25	9.12	8.51	8.18	7.01	6.93	6.03	8.30	7.39	6.65
2 YRS	9.32	9.23	8.63	8.31	7.25	7.16	6.34	8.44	7.61	6.91
3 YRS	9.38	9.34	8.76	8.43	7.48	7.39	6.65	8.58	7.83	7.16
4 YRS	9.44	9.45	8.88	8.55	7.71	7.61	6.95	8.72	8.05	7.42
5 YRS	9.51	9.56	9.01	8.67	7.95	7.84	7.26	8.85	8.27	7.67
6 YRS	9.57	9.67	9.14	8.79	8.18	8.07	7.57	8.99	8.50	7.92
7 YRS	9.63	9.78	9.26	8.91	8.41	8.29	7.87	9.13	8.72	8.18
8 YRS	9.70	9.89	9.39	9.03	8.65	8.52	8.18	9.27	8.94	8.43
9 YRS	9.76	10.00	9.51	9.15	8.88	8.75	8.49	9.41	9.16	8.69
10 YRS	9.82	10.11	9.64	9.27	9.11	8.98	8.79	9.55	9.38	8.94
11 YRS	9.89	10.22	9.76	9.39	9.34	9.20	9.10	9.68	9.60	9.19
12 YRS	9.95	10.33	9.89	9.51	9.58	9.43	9.41	9.82	9.82	9.45
13 YRS	10.01	10.43	10.01	9.63	9.81	9.66	9.71	9.96	10.04	9.70
14 YRS	10.08	10.54	10.14	9.75	10.04	9.88	10.02	10.10	10.26	9.96
15 YRS	10.14	10.65	10.27	9.87	10.28	10.11	10.33	10.24	10.48	10.21
16 YRS	10.20	10.76	10.39	9.99	10.51	10.34	10.64	10.37	10.71	10.46
17 YRS	10.27	10.87	10.52	10.11	10.74	10.56	10.94	10.51	10.93	10.72
18 YRS	10.33	10.98	10.64	10.23	10.98	10.79	11.25	10.65	11.15	10.97
19 YRS	10.39	11.09	10.77	10.35	11.21	11.02	11.56	10.79	11.37	11.23
20 YRS	10.46	11.20	10.89	10.47	11.44	11.25	11.86	10.93	11.59	11.48
21 YRS	10.52	11.31	11.02	10.59	11.68	11.47	12.17	11.07	11.81	11.73
22 YRS	10.58	11.42	11.14	10.71	11.91	11.70	12.48	11.20	12.03	11.99
23 YRS	10.65	11.53	11.27	10.83	12.14	11.93	12.78	11.34	12.25	12.24
24 YRS	10.71	11.64	11.40	10.95	12.38	12.15	13.09	11.48	12.47	12.49
25 YRS	10.77	11.75	11.52	11.07	12.61	12.38	13.40	11.62	12.69	12.75
26 YRS	10.84	11.86	11.65	11.19	12.84	12.61	13.70	11.76	12.91	13.00
27 YRS	10.90	11.97	11.77	11.31	13.08	12.83	14.01	11.89	13.14	13.26
28 YRS	10.96	12.08	11.90	11.44	13.31	13.06	14.32	12.03	13.36	13.51
29 YRS	11.03	12.19	12.02	11.56	13.54	13.29	14.62	12.17	13.58	13.76
30 YRS	11.09	12.30	12.15	11.68	13.77	13.52	14.93	12.31	13.80	14.02

EDUCATION	CORRECT	DIGITSPA	WAISIMIL	WAISJUDG	VERBAL	ANIMAL	WAISBLOC	DIGIT
0 YRS	7.61	7.53	5.09	6.24	5.71	7.65	7.98	5.97
1 YRS	7.85	7.77	5.52	6.63	6.07	7.95	8.24	6.35
2 YRS	8.09	8.02	5.95	7.02	6.43	8.26	8.50	6.72
3 YRS	8.33	8.27	6.38	7.41	6.79	8.56	8.76	7.10
4 YRS	8.56	8.52	6.81	7.81	7.16	8.86	9.02	7.48
5 YRS	8.80	8.76	7.25	8.20	7.52	9.16	9.28	7.86
6 YRS	9.04	9.01	7.68	8.59	7.88	9.47	9.54	8.24
7 YRS	9.28	9.26	8.11	8.99	8.24	9.77	9.80	8.62
8 YRS	9.52	9.51	8.54	9.38	8.60	10.07	10.06	8.99
9 YRS	9.76	9.76	8.97	9.77	8.96	10.38	10.32	9.37
10 YRS	10.00	10.00	9.40	10.16	9.32	10.68	10.58	9.75
11 YRS	10.24	10.25	9.84	10.56	9.68	10.98	10.84	10.13
12 YRS	10.48	10.50	10.27	10.95	10.04	11.29	11.10	10.51
13 YRS	10.72	10.75	10.70	11.34	10.40	11.59	11.36	10.88
14 YRS	10.96	11.00	11.13	11.73	10.76	11.89	11.62	11.26
15 YRS	11.20	11.24	11.56	12.13	11.12	12.20	11.88	11.64
16 YRS	11.44	11.49	11.99	12.52	11.48	12.50	12.14	12.02
17 YRS	11.67	11.74	12.43	12.91	11.84	12.80	12.39	12.40
18 YRS	11.91	11.99	12.86	13.30	12.20	13.11	12.65	12.78
19 YRS	12.15	12.23	13.29	13.70	12.56	13.41	12.91	13.15
20 YRS	12.39	12.48	13.72	14.09	12.92	13.71	13.17	13.53
21 YRS	12.63	12.73	14.15	14.48	13.28	14.01	13.43	13.91
22 YRS	12.87	12.98	14.58	14.88	13.64	14.32	13.69	14.29
23 YRS	13.11	13.23	15.01	15.27	14.00	14.62	13.95	14.67
24 YRS	13.35	13.47	15.45	15.66	14.36	14.92	14.21	15.05
25 YRS	13.59	13.72	15.88	16.05	14.72	15.23	14.47	15.42
26 YRS	13.83	13.97	16.31	16.45	15.08	15.53	14.73	15.80
27 YRS	14.07	14.22	16.74	16.84	15.44	15.83	14.99	16.18
28 YRS	14.31	14.47	17.17	17.23	15.80	16.14	15.25	16.56
29 YRS	14.54	14.71	17.60	17.62	16.16	16.44	15.51	16.94
30 YRS	14.78	14.96	18.04	18.02	16.53	16.74	15.77	17.32

Table 17.2. Age 76 – Female.

EDUCATION	BUSCHFR1	BRETRIE	REYA1	REYA2	REYA3	REYA4	REYA5	REYTOT	REYB1	REYA6
0 YRS	9.19	9.01	8.38	8.06	6.78	6.71	5.73	8.16	7.17	6.40
1 YRS	9.25	9.12	8.51	8.18	7.01	6.93	6.03	8.30	7.39	6.65
2 YRS	9.32	9.23	8.63	8.31	7.25	7.16	6.34	8.44	7.61	6.91
3 YRS	9.38	9.34	8.76	8.43	7.48	7.39	6.65	8.58	7.83	7.16
4 YRS	9.44	9.45	8.88	8.55	7.71	7.61	6.95	8.72	8.05	7.42
5 YRS	9.51	9.56	9.01	8.67	7.95	7.84	7.26	8.85	8.27	7.67
6 YRS	9.57	9.67	9.14	8.79	8.18	8.07	7.57	8.99	8.50	7.92
7 YRS	9.63	9.78	9.26	8.91	8.41	8.29	7.87	9.13	8.72	8.18
8 YRS	9.70	9.89	9.39	9.03	8.65	8.52	8.18	9.27	8.94	8.43
9 YRS	9.76	10.00	9.51	9.15	8.88	8.75	8.49	9.41	9.16	8.69
10 YRS	9.82	10.11	9.64	9.27	9.11	8.98	8.79	9.55	9.38	8.94
11 YRS	9.89	10.22	9.76	9.39	9.34	9.20	9.10	9.68	9.60	9.19
12 YRS	9.95	10.33	9.89	9.51	9.58	9.43	9.41	9.82	9.82	9.45
13 YRS	10.01	10.43	10.01	9.63	9.81	9.66	9.71	9.96	10.04	9.70
14 YRS	10.08	10.54	10.14	9.75	10.04	9.88	10.02	10.10	10.26	9.96
15 YRS	10.14	10.65	10.27	9.87	10.28	10.11	10.33	10.24	10.48	10.21
16 YRS	10.20	10.76	10.39	9.99	10.51	10.34	10.64	10.37	10.71	10.46
17 YRS	10.27	10.87	10.52	10.11	10.74	10.56	10.94	10.51	10.93	10.72
18 YRS	10.33	10.98	10.64	10.23	10.98	10.79	11.25	10.65	11.15	10.97
19 YRS	10.39	11.09	10.77	10.35	11.21	11.02	11.56	10.79	11.37	11.23
20 YRS	10.46	11.20	10.89	10.47	11.44	11.25	11.86	10.93	11.59	11.48
21 YRS	10.52	11.31	11.02	10.59	11.68	11.47	12.17	11.07	11.81	11.73
22 YRS	10.58	11.42	11.14	10.71	11.91	11.70	12.48	11.20	12.03	11.99
23 YRS	10.65	11.53	11.27	10.83	12.14	11.93	12.78	11.34	12.25	12.24
24 YRS	10.71	11.64	11.40	10.95	12.38	12.15	13.09	11.48	12.47	12.49
25 YRS	10.77	11.75	11.52	11.07	12.61	12.38	13.40	11.62	12.69	12.75
26 YRS	10.84	11.86	11.65	11.19	12.84	12.61	13.70	11.76	12.91	13.00
27 YRS	10.90	11.97	11.77	11.31	13.08	12.83	14.01	11.89	13.14	13.26
28 YRS	10.96	12.08	11.90	11.44	13.31	13.06	14.32	12.03	13.36	13.51
29 YRS	11.03	12.19	12.02	11.56	13.54	13.29	14.62	12.17	13.58	13.76
30 YRS	11.09	12.30	12.15	11.68	13.77	13.52	14.93	12.31	13.80	14.02

EDUCATION	CORRECT	DIGITSPA	WAISIMIL	WAISJUDG	VERBAL	ANIMAL	WAISBLOC	DIGIT
0 YRS	7.61	7.53	5.09	6.24	5.71	7.65	7.98	5.97
1 YRS	7.85	7.77	5.52	6.63	6.07	7.95	8.24	6.35
2 YRS	8.09	8.02	5.95	7.02	6.43	8.26	8.50	6.72
3 YRS	8.33	8.27	6.38	7.41	6.79	8.56	8.76	7.10
4 YRS	8.56	8.52	6.81	7.81	7.16	8.86	9.02	7.48
5 YRS	8.80	8.76	7.25	8.20	7.52	9.16	9.28	7.86
6 YRS	9.04	9.01	7.68	8.59	7.88	9.47	9.54	8.24
7 YRS	9.28	9.26	8.11	8.99	8.24	9.77	9.80	8.62
8 YRS	9.52	9.51	8.54	9.38	8.60	10.07	10.06	8.99
9 YRS	9.76	9.76	8.97	9.77	8.96	10.38	10.32	9.37
10 YRS	10.00	10.00	9.40	10.16	9.32	10.68	10.58	9.75
11 YRS	10.24	10.25	9.84	10.56	9.68	10.98	10.84	10.13
12 YRS	10.48	10.50	10.27	10.95	10.04	11.29	11.10	10.51
13 YRS	10.72	10.75	10.70	11.34	10.40	11.59	11.36	10.88
14 YRS	10.96	11.00	11.13	11.73	10.76	11.89	11.62	11.26
15 YRS	11.20	11.24	11.56	12.13	11.12	12.20	11.88	11.64
16 YRS	11.44	11.49	11.99	12.52	11.48	12.50	12.14	12.02
17 YRS	11.67	11.74	12.43	12.91	11.84	12.80	12.39	12.40
18 YRS	11.91	11.99	12.86	13.30	12.20	13.11	12.65	12.78
19 YRS	12.15	12.23	13.29	13.70	12.56	13.41	12.91	13.15
20 YRS	12.39	12.48	13.72	14.09	12.92	13.71	13.17	13.53
21 YRS	12.63	12.73	14.15	14.48	13.28	14.01	13.43	13.91
22 YRS	12.87	12.98	14.58	14.88	13.64	14.32	13.69	14.29
23 YRS	13.11	13.23	15.01	15.27	14.00	14.62	13.95	14.67
24 YRS	13.35	13.47	15.45	15.66	14.36	14.92	14.21	15.05
25 YRS	13.59	13.72	15.88	16.05	14.72	15.23	14.47	15.42
26 YRS	13.83	13.97	16.31	16.45	15.08	15.53	14.73	15.80
27 YRS	14.07	14.22	16.74	16.84	15.44	15.83	14.99	16.18
28 YRS	14.31	14.47	17.17	17.23	15.80	16.14	15.25	16.56
29 YRS	14.54	14.71	17.60	17.62	16.16	16.44	15.51	16.94
30 YRS	14.78	14.96	18.04	18.02	16.53	16.74	15.77	17.32

Table 18.1. Age 77 – Male.

EDUCATION	BUSCHFR1	BRETRIE	REYA1	REYA2	REYA3	REYA4	REYA5	REYTOT	REYB1	REYA6
0 YRS	9.07	8.84	8.29	7.96	6.63	6.56	5.58	8.01	7.01	6.24
1 YRS	9.14	8.95	8.41	8.08	6.86	6.78	5.89	8.15	7.23	6.49
2 YRS	9.20	9.06	8.54	8.20	7.10	7.01	6.19	8.29	7.45	6.75
3 YRS	9.26	9.17	8.66	8.32	7.33	7.24	6.50	8.43	7.67	7.00
4 YRS	9.33	9.28	8.79	8.44	7.56	7.46	6.81	8.57	7.89	7.26
5 YRS	9.39	9.39	8.91	8.56	7.80	7.69	7.11	8.70	8.11	7.51
6 YRS	9.45	9.50	9.04	8.68	8.03	7.92	7.42	8.84	8.33	7.76
7 YRS	9.52	9.61	9.16	8.80	8.26	8.15	7.73	8.98	8.55	8.02
8 YRS	9.58	9.72	9.29	8.92	8.49	8.37	8.03	9.12	8.77	8.27
9 YRS	9.64	9.83	9.42	9.04	8.73	8.60	8.34	9.26	9.00	8.53
10 YRS	9.71	9.94	9.54	9.16	8.96	8.83	8.65	9.40	9.22	8.78
11 YRS	9.77	10.05	9.67	9.28	9.19	9.05	8.95	9.53	9.44	9.03
12 YRS	9.83	10.16	9.79	9.40	9.43	9.28	9.26	9.67	9.66	9.29
13 YRS	9.90	10.27	9.92	9.52	9.66	9.51	9.57	9.81	9.88	9.54
14 YRS	9.96	10.38	10.04	9.65	9.89	9.74	9.87	9.95	10.10	9.80
15 YRS	10.02	10.49	10.17	9.77	10.13	9.96	10.18	10.09	10.32	10.05
16 YRS	10.09	10.60	10.29	9.89	10.36	10.19	10.49	10.22	10.54	10.30
17 YRS	10.15	10.71	10.42	10.01	10.59	10.42	10.80	10.36	10.76	10.56
18 YRS	10.21	10.82	10.54	10.13	10.83	10.64	11.10	10.50	10.98	10.81
19 YRS	10.28	10.93	10.67	10.25	11.06	10.87	11.41	10.64	11.21	11.07
20 YRS	10.34	11.04	10.80	10.37	11.29	11.10	11.72	10.78	11.43	11.32
21 YRS	10.40	11.15	10.92	10.49	11.53	11.32	12.02	10.92	11.65	11.57
22 YRS	10.46	11.26	11.05	10.61	11.76	11.55	12.33	11.05	11.87	11.83
23 YRS	10.53	11.37	11.17	10.73	11.99	11.78	12.64	11.19	12.09	12.08
24 YRS	10.59	11.48	11.30	10.85	12.23	12.01	12.94	11.33	12.31	12.33
25 YRS	10.65	11.59	11.42	10.97	12.46	12.23	13.25	11.47	12.53	12.59
26 YRS	10.72	11.70	11.55	11.09	12.69	12.46	13.56	11.61	12.75	12.84
27 YRS	10.78	11.81	11.67	11.21	12.92	12.69	13.86	11.74	12.97	13.10
28 YRS	10.84	11.92	11.80	11.33	13.16	12.91	14.17	11.88	13.19	13.35
29 YRS	10.91	12.03	11.93	11.45	13.39	13.14	14.48	12.02	13.42	13.60
30 YRS	10.97	12.14	12.05	11.57	13.62	13.37	14.78	12.16	13.64	13.86

EDUCATION	CORRECT	DIGITSPA	WAISIMIL	WAISJUDG	VERBAL	ANIMAL	WAISBLOC	DIGIT
0 YRS	7.45	7.46	4.99	6.17	5.66	7.53	7.87	5.75
1 YRS	7.69	7.71	5.42	6.57	6.02	7.84	8.13	6.12
2 YRS	7.93	7.96	5.86	6.96	6.38	8.14	8.39	6.50
3 YRS	8.17	8.20	6.29	7.35	6.74	8.44	8.64	6.88
4 YRS	8.41	8.45	6.72	7.74	7.10	8.74	8.90	7.26
5 YRS	8.65	8.70	7.15	8.14	7.46	9.05	9.16	7.64
6 YRS	8.89	8.95	7.58	8.53	7.82	9.35	9.42	8.02
7 YRS	9.13	9.19	8.01	8.92	8.18	9.65	9.68	8.39
8 YRS	9.37	9.44	8.45	9.31	8.54	9.96	9.94	8.77
9 YRS	9.61	9.69	8.88	9.71	8.90	10.26	10.20	9.15
10 YRS	9.85	9.94	9.31	10.10	9.26	10.56	10.46	9.53
11 YRS	10.08	10.19	9.74	10.49	9.62	10.87	10.72	9.91
12 YRS	10.32	10.43	10.17	10.88	9.98	11.17	10.98	10.29
13 YRS	10.56	10.68	10.60	11.28	10.34	11.47	11.24	10.66
14 YRS	10.80	10.93	11.03	11.67	10.70	11.78	11.50	11.04
15 YRS	11.04	11.18	11.47	12.06	11.06	12.08	11.76	11.42
16 YRS	11.28	11.43	11.90	12.46	11.42	12.38	12.02	11.80
17 YRS	11.52	11.67	12.33	12.85	11.78	12.69	12.28	12.18
18 YRS	11.76	11.92	12.76	13.24	12.14	12.99	12.54	12.56
19 YRS	12.00	12.17	13.19	13.63	12.50	13.29	12.80	12.93
20 YRS	12.24	12.42	13.62	14.03	12.86	13.59	13.06	13.31
21 YRS	12.48	12.66	14.06	14.42	13.23	13.90	13.32	13.69
22 YRS	12.72	12.91	14.49	14.81	13.59	14.20	13.58	14.07
23 YRS	12.96	13.16	14.92	15.20	13.95	14.50	13.84	14.45
24 YRS	13.19	13.41	15.35	15.60	14.31	14.81	14.10	14.83
25 YRS	13.43	13.66	15.78	15.99	14.67	15.11	14.36	15.20
26 YRS	13.67	13.90	16.21	16.38	15.03	15.41	14.62	15.58
27 YRS	13.91	14.15	16.65	16.77	15.39	15.72	14.88	15.96
28 YRS	14.15	14.40	17.08	17.17	15.75	16.02	15.14	16.34
29 YRS	14.39	14.65	17.51	17.56	16.11	16.32	15.40	16.72
30 YRS	14.63	14.90	17.94	17.95	16.47	16.63	15.65	17.10

Table 18.2. Age 77 – Female.

EDUCATION	BUSCHFR1	BRETRIE	REYA1	REYA2	REYA3	REYA4	REYA5	REYTOT	REYB1	REYA6
0 YRS	9.07	8.84	8.29	7.96	6.63	6.56	5.58	8.01	7.01	6.24
1 YRS	9.14	8.95	8.41	8.08	6.86	6.78	5.89	8.15	7.23	6.49
2 YRS	9.20	9.06	8.54	8.20	7.10	7.01	6.19	8.29	7.45	6.75
3 YRS	9.26	9.17	8.66	8.32	7.33	7.24	6.50	8.43	7.67	7.00
4 YRS	9.33	9.28	8.79	8.44	7.56	7.46	6.81	8.57	7.89	7.26
5 YRS	9.39	9.39	8.91	8.56	7.80	7.69	7.11	8.70	8.11	7.51
6 YRS	9.45	9.50	9.04	8.68	8.03	7.92	7.42	8.84	8.33	7.76
7 YRS	9.52	9.61	9.16	8.80	8.26	8.15	7.73	8.98	8.55	8.02
8 YRS	9.58	9.72	9.29	8.92	8.49	8.37	8.03	9.12	8.77	8.27
9 YRS	9.64	9.83	9.42	9.04	8.73	8.60	8.34	9.26	9.00	8.53
10 YRS	9.71	9.94	9.54	9.16	8.96	8.83	8.65	9.40	9.22	8.78
11 YRS	9.77	10.05	9.67	9.28	9.19	9.05	8.95	9.53	9.44	9.03
12 YRS	9.83	10.16	9.79	9.40	9.43	9.28	9.26	9.67	9.66	9.29
13 YRS	9.90	10.27	9.92	9.52	9.66	9.51	9.57	9.81	9.88	9.54
14 YRS	9.96	10.38	10.04	9.65	9.89	9.74	9.87	9.95	10.10	9.80
15 YRS	10.02	10.49	10.17	9.77	10.13	9.96	10.18	10.09	10.32	10.05
16 YRS	10.09	10.60	10.29	9.89	10.36	10.19	10.49	10.22	10.54	10.30
17 YRS	10.15	10.71	10.42	10.01	10.59	10.42	10.80	10.36	10.76	10.56
18 YRS	10.21	10.82	10.54	10.13	10.83	10.64	11.10	10.50	10.98	10.81
19 YRS	10.28	10.93	10.67	10.25	11.06	10.87	11.41	10.64	11.21	11.07
20 YRS	10.34	11.04	10.80	10.37	11.29	11.10	11.72	10.78	11.43	11.32
21 YRS	10.40	11.15	10.92	10.49	11.53	11.32	12.02	10.92	11.65	11.57
22 YRS	10.46	11.26	11.05	10.61	11.76	11.55	12.33	11.05	11.87	11.83
23 YRS	10.53	11.37	11.17	10.73	11.99	11.78	12.64	11.19	12.09	12.08
24 YRS	10.59	11.48	11.30	10.85	12.23	12.01	12.94	11.33	12.31	12.33
25 YRS	10.65	11.59	11.42	10.97	12.46	12.23	13.25	11.47	12.53	12.59
26 YRS	10.72	11.70	11.55	11.09	12.69	12.46	13.56	11.61	12.75	12.84
27 YRS	10.78	11.81	11.67	11.21	12.92	12.69	13.86	11.74	12.97	13.10
28 YRS	10.84	11.92	11.80	11.33	13.16	12.91	14.17	11.88	13.19	13.35
29 YRS	10.91	12.03	11.93	11.45	13.39	13.14	14.48	12.02	13.42	13.60
30 YRS	10.97	12.14	12.05	11.57	13.62	13.37	14.78	12.16	13.64	13.86

EDUCATION	CORRECT	DIGITSPA	WAISIMIL	WAISJUDG	VERBAL	ANIMAL	WAISBLOC	DIGIT
0 YRS	7.45	7.46	4.99	6.17	5.66	7.53	7.87	5.75
1 YRS	7.69	7.71	5.42	6.57	6.02	7.84	8.13	6.12
2 YRS	7.93	7.96	5.86	6.96	6.38	8.14	8.39	6.50
3 YRS	8.17	8.20	6.29	7.35	6.74	8.44	8.64	6.88
4 YRS	8.41	8.45	6.72	7.74	7.10	8.74	8.90	7.26
5 YRS	8.65	8.70	7.15	8.14	7.46	9.05	9.16	7.64
6 YRS	8.89	8.95	7.58	8.53	7.82	9.35	9.42	8.02
7 YRS	9.13	9.19	8.01	8.92	8.18	9.65	9.68	8.39
8 YRS	9.37	9.44	8.45	9.31	8.54	9.96	9.94	8.77
9 YRS	9.61	9.69	8.88	9.71	8.90	10.26	10.20	9.15
10 YRS	9.85	9.94	9.31	10.10	9.26	10.56	10.46	9.53
11 YRS	10.08	10.19	9.74	10.49	9.62	10.87	10.72	9.91
12 YRS	10.32	10.43	10.17	10.88	9.98	11.17	10.98	10.29
13 YRS	10.56	10.68	10.60	11.28	10.34	11.47	11.24	10.66
14 YRS	10.80	10.93	11.03	11.67	10.70	11.78	11.50	11.04
15 YRS	11.04	11.18	11.47	12.06	11.06	12.08	11.76	11.42
16 YRS	11.28	11.43	11.90	12.46	11.42	12.38	12.02	11.80
17 YRS	11.52	11.67	12.33	12.85	11.78	12.69	12.28	12.18
18 YRS	11.76	11.92	12.76	13.24	12.14	12.99	12.54	12.56
19 YRS	12.00	12.17	13.19	13.63	12.50	13.29	12.80	12.93
20 YRS	12.24	12.42	13.62	14.03	12.86	13.59	13.06	13.31
21 YRS	12.48	12.66	14.06	14.42	13.23	13.90	13.32	13.69
22 YRS	12.72	12.91	14.49	14.81	13.59	14.20	13.58	14.07
23 YRS	12.96	13.16	14.92	15.20	13.95	14.50	13.84	14.45
24 YRS	13.19	13.41	15.35	15.60	14.31	14.81	14.10	14.83
25 YRS	13.43	13.66	15.78	15.99	14.67	15.11	14.36	15.20
26 YRS	13.67	13.90	16.21	16.38	15.03	15.41	14.62	15.58
27 YRS	13.91	14.15	16.65	16.77	15.39	15.72	14.88	15.96
28 YRS	14.15	14.40	17.08	17.17	15.75	16.02	15.14	16.34
29 YRS	14.39	14.65	17.51	17.56	16.11	16.32	15.40	16.72
30 YRS	14.63	14.90	17.94	17.95	16.47	16.63	15.65	17.10

Table 19.1. Age 78 – Male.

EDUCATION	BUSCHFR1	BRETRIE	REYA1	REYA2	REYA3	REYA4	REYA5	REYTOT	REYB1	REYA6
0 YRS	8.95	8.68	8.19	7.85	6.48	6.41	5.43	7.86	6.84	6.08
1 YRS	9.02	8.79	8.31	7.98	6.71	6.64	5.74	8.00	7.07	6.33
2 YRS	9.08	8.90	8.44	8.10	6.94	6.86	6.05	8.14	7.29	6.59
3 YRS	9.14	9.01	8.57	8.22	7.18	7.09	6.35	8.28	7.51	6.84
4 YRS	9.21	9.12	8.69	8.34	7.41	7.32	6.66	8.42	7.73	7.10
5 YRS	9.27	9.23	8.82	8.46	7.64	7.54	6.97	8.55	7.95	7.35
6 YRS	9.33	9.34	8.94	8.58	7.88	7.77	7.27	8.69	8.17	7.60
7 YRS	9.40	9.45	9.07	8.70	8.11	8.00	7.58	8.83	8.39	7.86
8 YRS	9.46	9.56	9.19	8.82	8.34	8.22	7.89	8.97	8.61	8.11
9 YRS	9.52	9.67	9.32	8.94	8.58	8.45	8.19	9.11	8.83	8.37
10 YRS	9.59	9.78	9.44	9.06	8.81	8.68	8.50	9.25	9.05	8.62
11 YRS	9.65	9.89	9.57	9.18	9.04	8.91	8.81	9.38	9.28	8.87
12 YRS	9.71	10.00	9.69	9.30	9.28	9.13	9.11	9.52	9.50	9.13
13 YRS	9.78	10.11	9.82	9.42	9.51	9.36	9.42	9.66	9.72	9.38
14 YRS	9.84	10.22	9.95	9.54	9.74	9.59	9.73	9.80	9.94	9.64
15 YRS	9.90	10.33	10.07	9.66	9.98	9.81	10.03	9.94	10.16	9.89
16 YRS	9.97	10.44	10.20	9.78	10.21	10.04	10.34	10.07	10.38	10.14
17 YRS	10.03	10.55	10.32	9.90	10.44	10.27	10.65	10.21	10.60	10.40
18 YRS	10.09	10.66	10.45	10.02	10.68	10.49	10.95	10.35	10.82	10.65
19 YRS	10.16	10.77	10.57	10.14	10.91	10.72	11.26	10.49	11.04	10.91
20 YRS	10.22	10.88	10.70	10.26	11.14	10.95	11.57	10.63	11.26	11.16
21 YRS	10.28	10.99	10.82	10.38	11.37	11.18	11.88	10.77	11.48	11.41
22 YRS	10.35	11.10	10.95	10.50	11.61	11.40	12.18	10.90	11.71	11.67
23 YRS	10.41	11.21	11.08	10.62	11.84	11.63	12.49	11.04	11.93	11.92
24 YRS	10.47	11.32	11.20	10.74	12.07	11.86	12.80	11.18	12.15	12.17
25 YRS	10.54	11.43	11.33	10.86	12.31	12.08	13.10	11.32	12.37	12.43
26 YRS	10.60	11.54	11.45	10.98	12.54	12.31	13.41	11.46	12.59	12.68
27 YRS	10.66	11.65	11.58	11.11	12.77	12.54	13.72	11.59	12.81	12.94
28 YRS	10.73	11.76	11.70	11.23	13.01	12.76	14.02	11.73	13.03	13.19
29 YRS	10.79	11.87	11.83	11.35	13.24	12.99	14.33	11.87	13.25	13.44
30 YRS	10.85	11.98	11.95	11.47	13.47	13.22	14.64	12.01	13.47	13.70

EDUCATION	CORRECT	DIGITSPA	WAISIMIL	WAISJUDG	VERBAL	ANIMAL	WAISBLOC	DIGIT
0 YRS	7.30	7.39	4.90	6.11	5.60	7.42	7.75	5.53
1 YRS	7.54	7.64	5.33	6.50	5.96	7.72	8.01	5.90
2 YRS	7.78	7.89	5.76	6.89	6.32	8.02	8.27	6.28
3 YRS	8.02	8.14	6.19	7.29	6.68	8.32	8.53	6.66
4 YRS	8.26	8.39	6.62	7.68	7.04	8.63	8.79	7.04
5 YRS	8.50	8.63	7.06	8.07	7.40	8.93	9.05	7.42
6 YRS	8.73	8.88	7.49	8.46	7.76	9.23	9.31	7.80
7 YRS	8.97	9.13	7.92	8.86	8.12	9.54	9.57	8.17
8 YRS	9.21	9.38	8.35	9.25	8.48	9.84	9.83	8.55
9 YRS	9.45	9.62	8.78	9.64	8.84	10.14	10.09	8.93
10 YRS	9.69	9.87	9.21	10.04	9.20	10.45	10.35	9.31
11 YRS	9.93	10.12	9.64	10.43	9.56	10.75	10.61	9.69
12 YRS	10.17	10.37	10.08	10.82	9.92	11.05	10.87	10.07
13 YRS	10.41	10.62	10.51	11.21	10.29	11.36	11.13	10.44
14 YRS	10.65	10.86	10.94	11.61	10.65	11.66	11.39	10.82
15 YRS	10.89	11.11	11.37	12.00	11.01	11.96	11.65	11.20
16 YRS	11.13	11.36	11.80	12.39	11.37	12.27	11.90	11.58
17 YRS	11.37	11.61	12.23	12.78	11.73	12.57	12.16	11.96
18 YRS	11.61	11.86	12.67	13.18	12.09	12.87	12.42	12.34
19 YRS	11.84	12.10	13.10	13.57	12.45	13.17	12.68	12.71
20 YRS	12.08	12.35	13.53	13.96	12.81	13.48	12.94	13.09
21 YRS	12.32	12.60	13.96	14.35	13.17	13.78	13.20	13.47
22 YRS	12.56	12.85	14.39	14.75	13.53	14.08	13.46	13.85
23 YRS	12.80	13.09	14.82	15.14	13.89	14.39	13.72	14.23
24 YRS	13.04	13.34	15.26	15.53	14.25	14.69	13.98	14.61
25 YRS	13.28	13.59	15.69	15.93	14.61	14.99	14.24	14.98
26 YRS	13.52	13.84	16.12	16.32	14.97	15.30	14.50	15.36
27 YRS	13.76	14.09	16.55	16.71	15.33	15.60	14.76	15.74
28 YRS	14.00	14.33	16.98	17.10	15.69	15.90	15.02	16.12
29 YRS	14.24	14.58	17.41	17.50	16.05	16.21	15.28	16.50
30 YRS	14.48	14.83	17.84	17.89	16.41	16.51	15.54	16.88

Table 19.2. Age 78 – Female.

EDUCATION	BUSCHFR1	BRETRIE	REYA1	REYA2	REYA3	REYA4	REYA5	REYTOT	REYB1	REYA6
0 YRS	8.95	8.68	8.19	7.85	6.48	6.41	5.43	7.86	6.84	6.08
1 YRS	9.02	8.79	8.31	7.98	6.71	6.64	5.74	8.00	7.07	6.33
2 YRS	9.08	8.90	8.44	8.10	6.94	6.86	6.05	8.14	7.29	6.59
3 YRS	9.14	9.01	8.57	8.22	7.18	7.09	6.35	8.28	7.51	6.84
4 YRS	9.21	9.12	8.69	8.34	7.41	7.32	6.66	8.42	7.73	7.10
5 YRS	9.27	9.23	8.82	8.46	7.64	7.54	6.97	8.55	7.95	7.35
6 YRS	9.33	9.34	8.94	8.58	7.88	7.77	7.27	8.69	8.17	7.60
7 YRS	9.40	9.45	9.07	8.70	8.11	8.00	7.58	8.83	8.39	7.86
8 YRS	9.46	9.56	9.19	8.82	8.34	8.22	7.89	8.97	8.61	8.11
9 YRS	9.52	9.67	9.32	8.94	8.58	8.45	8.19	9.11	8.83	8.37
10 YRS	9.59	9.78	9.44	9.06	8.81	8.68	8.50	9.25	9.05	8.62
11 YRS	9.65	9.89	9.57	9.18	9.04	8.91	8.81	9.38	9.28	8.87
12 YRS	9.71	10.00	9.69	9.30	9.28	9.13	9.11	9.52	9.50	9.13
13 YRS	9.78	10.11	9.82	9.42	9.51	9.36	9.42	9.66	9.72	9.38
14 YRS	9.84	10.22	9.95	9.54	9.74	9.59	9.73	9.80	9.94	9.64
15 YRS	9.90	10.33	10.07	9.66	9.98	9.81	10.03	9.94	10.16	9.89
16 YRS	9.97	10.44	10.20	9.78	10.21	10.04	10.34	10.07	10.38	10.14
17 YRS	10.03	10.55	10.32	9.90	10.44	10.27	10.65	10.21	10.60	10.40
18 YRS	10.09	10.66	10.45	10.02	10.68	10.49	10.95	10.35	10.82	10.65
19 YRS	10.16	10.77	10.57	10.14	10.91	10.72	11.26	10.49	11.04	10.91
20 YRS	10.22	10.88	10.70	10.26	11.14	10.95	11.57	10.63	11.26	11.16
21 YRS	10.28	10.99	10.82	10.38	11.37	11.18	11.88	10.77	11.48	11.41
22 YRS	10.35	11.10	10.95	10.50	11.61	11.40	12.18	10.90	11.71	11.67
23 YRS	10.41	11.21	11.08	10.62	11.84	11.63	12.49	11.04	11.93	11.92
24 YRS	10.47	11.32	11.20	10.74	12.07	11.86	12.80	11.18	12.15	12.17
25 YRS	10.54	11.43	11.33	10.86	12.31	12.08	13.10	11.32	12.37	12.43
26 YRS	10.60	11.54	11.45	10.98	12.54	12.31	13.41	11.46	12.59	12.68
27 YRS	10.66	11.65	11.58	11.11	12.77	12.54	13.72	11.59	12.81	12.94
28 YRS	10.73	11.76	11.70	11.23	13.01	12.76	14.02	11.73	13.03	13.19
29 YRS	10.79	11.87	11.83	11.35	13.24	12.99	14.33	11.87	13.25	13.44
30 YRS	10.85	11.98	11.95	11.47	13.47	13.22	14.64	12.01	13.47	13.70

EDUCATION	CORRECT	DIGITSPA	WAISIMIL	WAISJUDG	VERBAL	ANIMAL	WAISBLOC	DIGIT
0 YRS	7.30	7.39	4.90	6.11	5.60	7.42	7.75	5.53
1 YRS	7.54	7.64	5.33	6.50	5.96	7.72	8.01	5.90
2 YRS	7.78	7.89	5.76	6.89	6.32	8.02	8.27	6.28
3 YRS	8.02	8.14	6.19	7.29	6.68	8.32	8.53	6.66
4 YRS	8.26	8.39	6.62	7.68	7.04	8.63	8.79	7.04
5 YRS	8.50	8.63	7.06	8.07	7.40	8.93	9.05	7.42
6 YRS	8.73	8.88	7.49	8.46	7.76	9.23	9.31	7.80
7 YRS	8.97	9.13	7.92	8.86	8.12	9.54	9.57	8.17
8 YRS	9.21	9.38	8.35	9.25	8.48	9.84	9.83	8.55
9 YRS	9.45	9.62	8.78	9.64	8.84	10.14	10.09	8.93
10 YRS	9.69	9.87	9.21	10.04	9.20	10.45	10.35	9.31
11 YRS	9.93	10.12	9.64	10.43	9.56	10.75	10.61	9.69
12 YRS	10.17	10.37	10.08	10.82	9.92	11.05	10.87	10.07
13 YRS	10.41	10.62	10.51	11.21	10.29	11.36	11.13	10.44
14 YRS	10.65	10.86	10.94	11.61	10.65	11.66	11.39	10.82
15 YRS	10.89	11.11	11.37	12.00	11.01	11.96	11.65	11.20
16 YRS	11.13	11.36	11.80	12.39	11.37	12.27	11.90	11.58
17 YRS	11.37	11.61	12.23	12.78	11.73	12.57	12.16	11.96
18 YRS	11.61	11.86	12.67	13.18	12.09	12.87	12.42	12.34
19 YRS	11.84	12.10	13.10	13.57	12.45	13.17	12.68	12.71
20 YRS	12.08	12.35	13.53	13.96	12.81	13.48	12.94	13.09
21 YRS	12.32	12.60	13.96	14.35	13.17	13.78	13.20	13.47
22 YRS	12.56	12.85	14.39	14.75	13.53	14.08	13.46	13.85
23 YRS	12.80	13.09	14.82	15.14	13.89	14.39	13.72	14.23
24 YRS	13.04	13.34	15.26	15.53	14.25	14.69	13.98	14.61
25 YRS	13.28	13.59	15.69	15.93	14.61	14.99	14.24	14.98
26 YRS	13.52	13.84	16.12	16.32	14.97	15.30	14.50	15.36
27 YRS	13.76	14.09	16.55	16.71	15.33	15.60	14.76	15.74
28 YRS	14.00	14.33	16.98	17.10	15.69	15.90	15.02	16.12
29 YRS	14.24	14.58	17.41	17.50	16.05	16.21	15.28	16.50
30 YRS	14.48	14.83	17.84	17.89	16.41	16.51	15.54	16.88

Table 20.1. Age 79 – Male.

EDUCATION	BUSCHFR1	BRETRIE	REYA1	REYA2	REYA3	REYA4	REYA5	REYTOT	REYB1	REYA6
0 YRS	8.84	8.52	8.09	7.75	6.33	6.26	5.29	7.71	6.68	5.92
1 YRS	8.90	8.63	8.22	7.87	6.56	6.49	5.59	7.85	6.90	6.17
2 YRS	8.96	8.74	8.34	7.99	6.79	6.71	5.90	7.99	7.12	6.43
3 YRS	9.03	8.85	8.47	8.11	7.03	6.94	6.21	8.13	7.34	6.68
4 YRS	9.09	8.96	8.59	8.23	7.26	7.17	6.51	8.27	7.57	6.94
5 YRS	9.15	9.07	8.72	8.35	7.49	7.39	6.82	8.40	7.79	7.19
6 YRS	9.22	9.18	8.84	8.47	7.73	7.62	7.13	8.54	8.01	7.44
7 YRS	9.28	9.29	8.97	8.59	7.96	7.85	7.43	8.68	8.23	7.70
8 YRS	9.34	9.40	9.10	8.71	8.19	8.08	7.74	8.82	8.45	7.95
9 YRS	9.41	9.51	9.22	8.83	8.43	8.30	8.05	8.96	8.67	8.21
10 YRS	9.47	9.62	9.35	8.95	8.66	8.53	8.35	9.10	8.89	8.46
11 YRS	9.53	9.73	9.47	9.07	8.89	8.76	8.66	9.23	9.11	8.71
12 YRS	9.60	9.84	9.60	9.19	9.13	8.98	8.97	9.37	9.33	8.97
13 YRS	9.66	9.95	9.72	9.32	9.36	9.21	9.27	9.51	9.55	9.22
14 YRS	9.72	10.06	9.85	9.44	9.59	9.44	9.58	9.65	9.78	9.48
15 YRS	9.79	10.17	9.97	9.56	9.83	9.67	9.89	9.79	10.00	9.73
16 YRS	9.85	10.28	10.10	9.68	10.06	9.89	10.19	9.92	10.22	9.98
17 YRS	9.91	10.39	10.23	9.80	10.29	10.12	10.50	10.06	10.44	10.24
18 YRS	9.98	10.49	10.35	9.92	10.52	10.35	10.81	10.20	10.66	10.49
19 YRS	10.04	10.60	10.48	10.04	10.76	10.57	11.11	10.34	10.88	10.75
20 YRS	10.10	10.71	10.60	10.16	10.99	10.80	11.42	10.48	11.10	11.00
21 YRS	10.17	10.82	10.73	10.28	11.22	11.03	11.73	10.62	11.32	11.25
22 YRS	10.23	10.93	10.85	10.40	11.46	11.25	12.03	10.75	11.54	11.51
23 YRS	10.29	11.04	10.98	10.52	11.69	11.48	12.34	10.89	11.76	11.76
24 YRS	10.36	11.15	11.10	10.64	11.92	11.71	12.65	11.03	11.98	12.01
25 YRS	10.42	11.26	11.23	10.76	12.16	11.94	12.96	11.17	12.21	12.27
26 YRS	10.48	11.37	11.36	10.88	12.39	12.16	13.26	11.31	12.43	12.52
27 YRS	10.55	11.48	11.48	11.00	12.62	12.39	13.57	11.44	12.65	12.78
28 YRS	10.61	11.59	11.61	11.12	12.86	12.62	13.88	11.58	12.87	13.03
29 YRS	10.67	11.70	11.73	11.24	13.09	12.84	14.18	11.72	13.09	13.28
30 YRS	10.74	11.81	11.86	11.36	13.32	13.07	14.49	11.86	13.31	13.54

EDUCATION	CORRECT	DIGITSPA	WAISIMIL	WAISJUDG	VERBAL	ANIMAL	WAISBLOC	DIGIT
0 YRS	7.15	7.33	4.80	6.05	5.54	7.30	7.64	5.31
1 YRS	7.38	7.58	5.23	6.44	5.90	7.60	7.89	5.68
2 YRS	7.62	7.82	5.67	6.83	6.26	7.90	8.15	6.06
3 YRS	7.86	8.07	6.10	7.22	6.62	8.21	8.41	6.44
4 YRS	8.10	8.32	6.53	7.62	6.99	8.51	8.67	6.82
5 YRS	8.34	8.57	6.96	8.01	7.35	8.81	8.93	7.20
6 YRS	8.58	8.82	7.39	8.40	7.71	9.12	9.19	7.58
7 YRS	8.82	9.06	7.82	8.79	8.07	9.42	9.45	7.95
8 YRS	9.06	9.31	8.25	9.19	8.43	9.72	9.71	8.33
9 YRS	9.30	9.56	8.69	9.58	8.79	10.03	9.97	8.71
10 YRS	9.54	9.81	9.12	9.97	9.15	10.33	10.23	9.09
11 YRS	9.78	10.05	9.55	10.36	9.51	10.63	10.49	9.47
12 YRS	10.02	10.30	9.98	10.76	9.87	10.94	10.75	9.85
13 YRS	10.26	10.55	10.41	11.15	10.23	11.24	11.01	10.22
14 YRS	10.49	10.80	10.84	11.54	10.59	11.54	11.27	10.60
15 YRS	10.73	11.05	11.28	11.93	10.95	11.85	11.53	10.98
16 YRS	10.97	11.29	11.71	12.33	11.31	12.15	11.79	11.36
17 YRS	11.21	11.54	12.14	12.72	11.67	12.45	12.05	11.74
18 YRS	11.45	11.79	12.57	13.11	12.03	12.75	12.31	12.12
19 YRS	11.69	12.04	13.00	13.51	12.39	13.06	12.57	12.49
20 YRS	11.93	12.29	13.43	13.90	12.75	13.36	12.83	12.87
21 YRS	12.17	12.53	13.87	14.29	13.11	13.66	13.09	13.25
22 YRS	12.41	12.78	14.30	14.68	13.47	13.97	13.35	13.63
23 YRS	12.65	13.03	14.73	15.08	13.83	14.27	13.61	14.01
24 YRS	12.89	13.28	15.16	15.47	14.19	14.57	13.87	14.39
25 YRS	13.13	13.52	15.59	15.86	14.55	14.88	14.13	14.76
26 YRS	13.36	13.77	16.02	16.25	14.91	15.18	14.39	15.14
27 YRS	13.60	14.02	16.45	16.65	15.27	15.48	14.65	15.52
28 YRS	13.84	14.27	16.89	17.04	15.63	15.79	14.91	15.90
29 YRS	14.08	14.52	17.32	17.43	16.00	16.09	15.16	16.28
30 YRS	14.32	14.76	17.75	17.82	16.36	16.39	15.42	16.66

Table 20.2. Age 79 – Female.

EDUCATION	BUSCHFR1	BRETRIE	REYA1	REYA2	REYA3	REYA4	REYA5	REYTOT	REYB1	REYA6
0 YRS	8.84	8.52	8.09	7.75	6.33	6.26	5.29	7.71	6.68	5.92
1 YRS	8.90	8.63	8.22	7.87	6.56	6.49	5.59	7.85	6.90	6.17
2 YRS	8.96	8.74	8.34	7.99	6.79	6.71	5.90	7.99	7.12	6.43
3 YRS	9.03	8.85	8.47	8.11	7.03	6.94	6.21	8.13	7.34	6.68
4 YRS	9.09	8.96	8.59	8.23	7.26	7.17	6.51	8.27	7.57	6.94
5 YRS	9.15	9.07	8.72	8.35	7.49	7.39	6.82	8.40	7.79	7.19
6 YRS	9.22	9.18	8.84	8.47	7.73	7.62	7.13	8.54	8.01	7.44
7 YRS	9.28	9.29	8.97	8.59	7.96	7.85	7.43	8.68	8.23	7.70
8 YRS	9.34	9.40	9.10	8.71	8.19	8.08	7.74	8.82	8.45	7.95
9 YRS	9.41	9.51	9.22	8.83	8.43	8.30	8.05	8.96	8.67	8.21
10 YRS	9.47	9.62	9.35	8.95	8.66	8.53	8.35	9.10	8.89	8.46
11 YRS	9.53	9.73	9.47	9.07	8.89	8.76	8.66	9.23	9.11	8.71
12 YRS	9.60	9.84	9.60	9.19	9.13	8.98	8.97	9.37	9.33	8.97
13 YRS	9.66	9.95	9.72	9.32	9.36	9.21	9.27	9.51	9.55	9.22
14 YRS	9.72	10.06	9.85	9.44	9.59	9.44	9.58	9.65	9.78	9.48
15 YRS	9.79	10.17	9.97	9.56	9.83	9.67	9.89	9.79	10.00	9.73
16 YRS	9.85	10.28	10.10	9.68	10.06	9.89	10.19	9.92	10.22	9.98
17 YRS	9.91	10.39	10.23	9.80	10.29	10.12	10.50	10.06	10.44	10.24
18 YRS	9.98	10.49	10.35	9.92	10.52	10.35	10.81	10.20	10.66	10.49
19 YRS	10.04	10.60	10.48	10.04	10.76	10.57	11.11	10.34	10.88	10.75
20 YRS	10.10	10.71	10.60	10.16	10.99	10.80	11.42	10.48	11.10	11.00
21 YRS	10.17	10.82	10.73	10.28	11.22	11.03	11.73	10.62	11.32	11.25
22 YRS	10.23	10.93	10.85	10.40	11.46	11.25	12.03	10.75	11.54	11.51
23 YRS	10.29	11.04	10.98	10.52	11.69	11.48	12.34	10.89	11.76	11.76
24 YRS	10.36	11.15	11.10	10.64	11.92	11.71	12.65	11.03	11.98	12.01
25 YRS	10.42	11.26	11.23	10.76	12.16	11.94	12.96	11.17	12.21	12.27
26 YRS	10.48	11.37	11.36	10.88	12.39	12.16	13.26	11.31	12.43	12.52
27 YRS	10.55	11.48	11.48	11.00	12.62	12.39	13.57	11.44	12.65	12.78
28 YRS	10.61	11.59	11.61	11.12	12.86	12.62	13.88	11.58	12.87	13.03
29 YRS	10.67	11.70	11.73	11.24	13.09	12.84	14.18	11.72	13.09	13.28
30 YRS	10.74	11.81	11.86	11.36	13.32	13.07	14.49	11.86	13.31	13.54

EDUCATION	CORRECT	DIGITSPA	WAISIMIL	WAISJUDG	VERBAL	ANIMAL	WAISBLOC	DIGIT
0 YRS	7.15	7.33	4.80	6.05	5.54	7.30	7.64	5.31
1 YRS	7.38	7.58	5.23	6.44	5.90	7.60	7.89	5.68
2 YRS	7.62	7.82	5.67	6.83	6.26	7.90	8.15	6.06
3 YRS	7.86	8.07	6.10	7.22	6.62	8.21	8.41	6.44
4 YRS	8.10	8.32	6.53	7.62	6.99	8.51	8.67	6.82
5 YRS	8.34	8.57	6.96	8.01	7.35	8.81	8.93	7.20
6 YRS	8.58	8.82	7.39	8.40	7.71	9.12	9.19	7.58
7 YRS	8.82	9.06	7.82	8.79	8.07	9.42	9.45	7.95
8 YRS	9.06	9.31	8.25	9.19	8.43	9.72	9.71	8.33
9 YRS	9.30	9.56	8.69	9.58	8.79	10.03	9.97	8.71
10 YRS	9.54	9.81	9.12	9.97	9.15	10.33	10.23	9.09
11 YRS	9.78	10.05	9.55	10.36	9.51	10.63	10.49	9.47
12 YRS	10.02	10.30	9.98	10.76	9.87	10.94	10.75	9.85
13 YRS	10.26	10.55	10.41	11.15	10.23	11.24	11.01	10.22
14 YRS	10.49	10.80	10.84	11.54	10.59	11.54	11.27	10.60
15 YRS	10.73	11.05	11.28	11.93	10.95	11.85	11.53	10.98
16 YRS	10.97	11.29	11.71	12.33	11.31	12.15	11.79	11.36
17 YRS	11.21	11.54	12.14	12.72	11.67	12.45	12.05	11.74
18 YRS	11.45	11.79	12.57	13.11	12.03	12.75	12.31	12.12
19 YRS	11.69	12.04	13.00	13.51	12.39	13.06	12.57	12.49
20 YRS	11.93	12.29	13.43	13.90	12.75	13.36	12.83	12.87
21 YRS	12.17	12.53	13.87	14.29	13.11	13.66	13.09	13.25
22 YRS	12.41	12.78	14.30	14.68	13.47	13.97	13.35	13.63
23 YRS	12.65	13.03	14.73	15.08	13.83	14.27	13.61	14.01
24 YRS	12.89	13.28	15.16	15.47	14.19	14.57	13.87	14.39
25 YRS	13.13	13.52	15.59	15.86	14.55	14.88	14.13	14.76
26 YRS	13.36	13.77	16.02	16.25	14.91	15.18	14.39	15.14
27 YRS	13.60	14.02	16.45	16.65	15.27	15.48	14.65	15.52
28 YRS	13.84	14.27	16.89	17.04	15.63	15.79	14.91	15.90
29 YRS	14.08	14.52	17.32	17.43	16.00	16.09	15.16	16.28
30 YRS	14.32	14.76	17.75	17.82	16.36	16.39	15.42	16.66

Table 21.1. Age 80 – Male.

EDUCATION	BUSCHFR1	BRETRIE	REYA1	REYA2	REYA3	REYA4	REYA5	REYTOT	REYB1	REYA6
0 YRS	8.72	8.35	7.99	7.65	6.18	6.11	5.14	7.56	6.52	5.76
1 YRS	8.78	8.46	8.12	7.77	6.41	6.34	5.45	7.70	6.74	6.01
2 YRS	8.85	8.57	8.25	7.89	6.64	6.57	5.75	7.84	6.96	6.27
3 YRS	8.91	8.68	8.37	8.01	6.88	6.79	6.06	7.98	7.18	6.52
4 YRS	8.97	8.79	8.50	8.13	7.11	7.02	6.37	8.12	7.40	6.78
5 YRS	9.04	8.90	8.62	8.25	7.34	7.25	6.67	8.25	7.62	7.03
6 YRS	9.10	9.01	8.75	8.37	7.58	7.47	6.98	8.39	7.85	7.28
7 YRS	9.16	9.12	8.87	8.49	7.81	7.70	7.29	8.53	8.07	7.54
8 YRS	9.23	9.23	9.00	8.61	8.04	7.93	7.59	8.67	8.29	7.79
9 YRS	9.29	9.34	9.12	8.73	8.28	8.15	7.90	8.81	8.51	8.05
10 YRS	9.35	9.45	9.25	8.85	8.51	8.38	8.21	8.95	8.73	8.30
11 YRS	9.42	9.56	9.38	8.97	8.74	8.61	8.51	9.08	8.95	8.55
12 YRS	9.48	9.67	9.50	9.09	8.98	8.84	8.82	9.22	9.17	8.81
13 YRS	9.54	9.78	9.63	9.21	9.21	9.06	9.13	9.36	9.39	9.06
14 YRS	9.60	9.89	9.75	9.33	9.44	9.29	9.43	9.50	9.61	9.32
15 YRS	9.67	10.00	9.88	9.45	9.67	9.52	9.74	9.64	9.83	9.57
16 YRS	9.73	10.11	10.00	9.57	9.91	9.74	10.05	9.77	10.05	9.82
17 YRS	9.79	10.22	10.13	9.69	10.14	9.97	10.35	9.91	10.28	10.08
18 YRS	9.86	10.33	10.25	9.81	10.37	10.20	10.66	10.05	10.50	10.33
19 YRS	9.92	10.44	10.38	9.93	10.61	10.42	10.97	10.19	10.72	10.59
20 YRS	9.98	10.55	10.51	10.05	10.84	10.65	11.27	10.33	10.94	10.84
21 YRS	10.05	10.66	10.63	10.17	11.07	10.88	11.58	10.47	11.16	11.09
22 YRS	10.11	10.77	10.76	10.29	11.31	11.11	11.89	10.60	11.38	11.35
23 YRS	10.17	10.88	10.88	10.41	11.54	11.33	12.19	10.74	11.60	11.60
24 YRS	10.24	10.99	11.01	10.53	11.77	11.56	12.50	10.88	11.82	11.85
25 YRS	10.30	11.10	11.13	10.65	12.01	11.79	12.81	11.02	12.04	12.11
26 YRS	10.36	11.21	11.26	10.78	12.24	12.01	13.12	11.16	12.26	12.36
27 YRS	10.43	11.32	11.38	10.90	12.47	12.24	13.42	11.29	12.49	12.62
28 YRS	10.49	11.43	11.51	11.02	12.71	12.47	13.73	11.43	12.71	12.87
29 YRS	10.55	11.54	11.63	11.14	12.94	12.69	14.04	11.57	12.93	13.12
30 YRS	10.62	11.65	11.76	11.26	13.17	12.92	14.34	11.71	13.15	13.38

EDUCATION	CORRECT	DIGITSPA	WAISIMIL	WAISJUDG	VERBAL	ANIMAL	WAISBLOC	DIGIT
0 YRS	6.99	7.26	4.71	5.98	5.49	7.18	7.52	5.09
1 YRS	7.23	7.51	5.14	6.37	5.85	7.48	7.78	5.46
2 YRS	7.47	7.76	5.57	6.77	6.21	7.79	8.04	5.84
3 YRS	7.71	8.01	6.00	7.16	6.57	8.09	8.30	6.22
4 YRS	7.95	8.25	6.43	7.55	6.93	8.39	8.56	6.60
5 YRS	8.19	8.50	6.86	7.94	7.29	8.70	8.82	6.98
6 YRS	8.43	8.75	7.30	8.34	7.65	9.00	9.08	7.36
7 YRS	8.67	9.00	7.73	8.73	8.01	9.30	9.34	7.73
8 YRS	8.90	9.25	8.16	9.12	8.37	9.61	9.60	8.11
9 YRS	9.14	9.49	8.59	9.51	8.73	9.91	9.86	8.49
10 YRS	9.38	9.74	9.02	9.91	9.09	10.21	10.12	8.87
11 YRS	9.62	9.99	9.45	10.30	9.45	10.52	10.38	9.25
12 YRS	9.86	10.24	9.89	10.69	9.81	10.82	10.64	9.63
13 YRS	10.10	10.48	10.32	11.09	10.17	11.12	10.90	10.00
14 YRS	10.34	10.73	10.75	11.48	10.53	11.42	11.16	10.38
15 YRS	10.58	10.98	11.18	11.87	10.89	11.73	11.41	10.76
16 YRS	10.82	11.23	11.61	12.26	11.25	12.03	11.67	11.14
17 YRS	11.06	11.48	12.04	12.66	11.61	12.33	11.93	11.52
18 YRS	11.30	11.72	12.48	13.05	11.97	12.64	12.19	11.89
19 YRS	11.54	11.97	12.91	13.44	12.33	12.94	12.45	12.27
20 YRS	11.78	12.22	13.34	13.83	12.69	13.24	12.71	12.65
21 YRS	12.01	12.47	13.77	14.23	13.06	13.55	12.97	13.03
22 YRS	12.25	12.72	14.20	14.62	13.42	13.85	13.23	13.41
23 YRS	12.49	12.96	14.63	15.01	13.78	14.15	13.49	13.79
24 YRS	12.73	13.21	15.06	15.40	14.14	14.46	13.75	14.16
25 YRS	12.97	13.46	15.50	15.80	14.50	14.76	14.01	14.54
26 YRS	13.21	13.71	15.93	16.19	14.86	15.06	14.27	14.92
27 YRS	13.45	13.95	16.36	16.58	15.22	15.37	14.53	15.30
28 YRS	13.69	14.20	16.79	16.98	15.58	15.67	14.79	15.68
29 YRS	13.93	14.45	17.22	17.37	15.94	15.97	15.05	16.06
30 YRS	14.17	14.70	17.65	17.76	16.30	16.27	15.31	16.43

Table 21.2. Age 80 – Female.

EDUCATION	BUSCHFR1	REYA1	REYA2	REYA3	REYA4	REYA5	REYTOT	REYB1	REYA6
0 YRS	8.72	7.99	7.65	6.18	6.11	5.14	7.56	6.52	5.76
1 YRS	8.78	8.12	7.77	6.41	6.34	5.45	7.70	6.74	6.01
2 YRS	8.85	8.25	7.89	6.64	6.57	5.75	7.84	6.96	6.27
3 YRS	8.91	8.37	8.01	6.88	6.79	6.06	7.98	7.18	6.52
4 YRS	8.97	8.50	8.13	7.11	7.02	6.37	8.12	7.40	6.78
5 YRS	9.04	8.62	8.25	7.34	7.25	6.67	8.25	7.62	7.03
6 YRS	9.10	8.75	8.37	7.58	7.47	6.98	8.39	7.85	7.28
7 YRS	9.16	8.87	8.49	7.81	7.70	7.29	8.53	8.07	7.54
8 YRS	9.23	9.00	8.61	8.04	7.93	7.59	8.67	8.29	7.79
9 YRS	9.29	9.12	8.73	8.28	8.15	7.90	8.81	8.51	8.05
10 YRS	9.35	9.25	8.85	8.51	8.38	8.21	8.95	8.73	8.30
11 YRS	9.42	9.38	8.97	8.74	8.61	8.51	9.08	8.95	8.55
12 YRS	9.48	9.50	9.09	8.98	8.84	8.82	9.22	9.17	8.81
13 YRS	9.54	9.63	9.21	9.21	9.06	9.13	9.36	9.39	9.06
14 YRS	9.60	9.75	9.33	9.44	9.29	9.43	9.50	9.61	9.32
15 YRS	9.67	9.88	9.45	9.67	9.52	9.74	9.64	9.83	9.57
16 YRS	9.73	10.00	9.57	9.91	9.74	10.05	9.77	10.05	9.82
17 YRS	9.79	10.13	9.69	10.14	9.97	10.35	9.91	10.28	10.08
18 YRS	9.86	10.25	9.81	10.37	10.20	10.66	10.05	10.50	10.33
19 YRS	9.92	10.38	9.93	10.61	10.42	10.97	10.19	10.72	10.59
20 YRS	9.98	10.51	10.05	10.84	10.65	11.27	10.33	10.94	10.84
21 YRS	10.05	10.63	10.17	11.07	10.88	11.58	10.47	11.16	11.09
22 YRS	10.11	10.76	10.29	11.31	11.11	11.89	10.60	11.38	11.35
23 YRS	10.17	10.88	10.41	11.54	11.33	12.19	10.74	11.60	11.60
24 YRS	10.24	11.01	10.53	11.77	11.56	12.50	10.88	11.82	11.85
25 YRS	10.30	11.13	10.65	12.01	11.79	12.81	11.02	12.04	12.11
26 YRS	10.36	11.26	10.78	12.24	12.01	13.12	11.16	12.26	12.36
27 YRS	10.43	11.38	10.90	12.47	12.24	13.42	11.29	12.49	12.62
28 YRS	10.49	11.51	11.02	12.71	12.47	13.73	11.43	12.71	12.87
29 YRS	10.55	11.63	11.14	12.94	12.69	14.04	11.57	12.93	13.12
30 YRS	10.62	11.76	11.26	13.17	12.92	14.34	11.71	13.15	13.38

EDUCATION	CORRECT	DIGITSPA	WAISIMIL	WAISJUDG	VERBAL	ANIMAL	WAISBLOC	DIGIT
0 YRS	6.99	7.26	4.71	5.98	5.49	7.18	7.52	5.09
1 YRS	7.23	7.51	5.14	6.37	5.85	7.48	7.78	5.46
2 YRS	7.47	7.76	5.57	6.77	6.21	7.79	8.04	5.84
3 YRS	7.71	8.01	6.00	7.16	6.57	8.09	8.30	6.22
4 YRS	7.95	8.25	6.43	7.55	6.93	8.39	8.56	6.60
5 YRS	8.19	8.50	6.86	7.94	7.29	8.70	8.82	6.98
6 YRS	8.43	8.75	7.30	8.34	7.65	9.00	9.08	7.36
7 YRS	8.67	9.00	7.73	8.73	8.01	9.30	9.34	7.73
8 YRS	8.90	9.25	8.16	9.12	8.37	9.61	9.60	8.11
9 YRS	9.14	9.49	8.59	9.51	8.73	9.91	9.86	8.49
10 YRS	9.38	9.74	9.02	9.91	9.09	10.21	10.12	8.87
11 YRS	9.62	9.99	9.45	10.30	9.45	10.52	10.38	9.25
12 YRS	9.86	10.24	9.89	10.69	9.81	10.82	10.64	9.63
13 YRS	10.10	10.48	10.32	11.09	10.17	11.12	10.90	10.00
14 YRS	10.34	10.73	10.75	11.48	10.53	11.42	11.16	10.38
15 YRS	10.58	10.98	11.18	11.87	10.89	11.73	11.41	10.76
16 YRS	10.82	11.23	11.61	12.26	11.25	12.03	11.67	11.14
17 YRS	11.06	11.48	12.04	12.66	11.61	12.33	11.93	11.52
18 YRS	11.30	11.72	12.48	13.05	11.97	12.64	12.19	11.89
19 YRS	11.54	11.97	12.91	13.44	12.33	12.94	12.45	12.27
20 YRS	11.78	12.22	13.34	13.83	12.69	13.24	12.71	12.65
21 YRS	12.01	12.47	13.77	14.23	13.06	13.55	12.97	13.03
22 YRS	12.25	12.72	14.20	14.62	13.42	13.85	13.23	13.41
23 YRS	12.49	12.96	14.63	15.01	13.78	14.15	13.49	13.79
24 YRS	12.73	13.21	15.06	15.40	14.14	14.46	13.75	14.16
25 YRS	12.97	13.46	15.50	15.80	14.50	14.76	14.01	14.54
26 YRS	13.21	13.71	15.93	16.19	14.86	15.06	14.27	14.92
27 YRS	13.45	13.95	16.36	16.58	15.22	15.37	14.53	15.30
28 YRS	13.69	14.20	16.79	16.98	15.58	15.67	14.79	15.68
29 YRS	13.93	14.45	17.22	17.37	15.94	15.97	15.05	16.06
30 YRS	14.17	14.70	17.65	17.76	16.30	16.27	15.31	16.43

Table 22.1. Age 81 – Male.

EDUCATION	BUSCHFR1	BRETRIE	REYA1	REYA2	REYA3	REYA4	REYA5	REYTOT	REYB1	REYA6
0 YRS	8.60	8.19	7.90	7.54	6.03	5.96	4.99	7.41	6.36	5.60
1 YRS	8.66	8.30	8.02	7.66	6.26	6.19	5.30	7.55	6.58	5.85
2 YRS	8.73	8.41	8.15	7.78	6.49	6.42	5.61	7.69	6.80	6.11
3 YRS	8.79	8.52	8.27	7.90	6.73	6.64	5.91	7.83	7.02	6.36
4 YRS	8.85	8.63	8.40	8.02	6.96	6.87	6.22	7.97	7.24	6.62
5 YRS	8.92	8.74	8.53	8.14	7.19	7.10	6.53	8.10	7.46	6.87
6 YRS	8.98	8.85	8.65	8.26	7.43	7.32	6.83	8.24	7.68	7.12
7 YRS	9.04	8.96	8.78	8.38	7.66	7.55	7.14	8.38	7.90	7.38
8 YRS	9.11	9.07	8.90	8.50	7.89	7.78	7.45	8.52	8.12	7.63
9 YRS	9.17	9.18	9.03	8.62	8.12	8.01	7.75	8.66	8.35	7.89
10 YRS	9.23	9.29	9.15	8.74	8.36	8.23	8.06	8.80	8.57	8.14
11 YRS	9.30	9.40	9.28	8.86	8.59	8.46	8.37	8.93	8.79	8.39
12 YRS	9.36	9.51	9.40	8.99	8.82	8.69	8.67	9.07	9.01	8.65
13 YRS	9.42	9.62	9.53	9.11	9.06	8.91	8.98	9.21	9.23	8.90
14 YRS	9.49	9.73	9.66	9.23	9.29	9.14	9.29	9.35	9.45	9.16
15 YRS	9.55	9.84	9.78	9.35	9.52	9.37	9.59	9.49	9.67	9.41
16 YRS	9.61	9.95	9.91	9.47	9.76	9.60	9.90	9.62	9.89	9.66
17 YRS	9.68	10.06	10.03	9.59	9.99	9.82	10.21	9.76	10.11	9.92
18 YRS	9.74	10.17	10.16	9.71	10.22	10.05	10.51	9.90	10.33	10.17
19 YRS	9.80	10.28	10.28	9.83	10.46	10.28	10.82	10.04	10.55	10.43
20 YRS	9.87	10.39	10.41	9.95	10.69	10.50	11.13	10.18	10.78	10.68
21 YRS	9.93	10.50	10.53	10.07	10.92	10.73	11.43	10.32	11.00	10.93
22 YRS	9.99	10.61	10.66	10.19	11.16	10.96	11.74	10.45	11.22	11.19
23 YRS	10.06	10.72	10.78	10.31	11.39	11.18	12.05	10.59	11.44	11.44
24 YRS	10.12	10.83	10.91	10.43	11.62	11.41	12.35	10.73	11.66	11.69
25 YRS	10.18	10.94	11.04	10.55	11.86	11.64	12.66	10.87	11.88	11.95
26 YRS	10.25	11.05	11.16	10.67	12.09	11.87	12.97	11.01	12.10	12.20
27 YRS	10.31	11.16	11.29	10.79	12.32	12.09	13.27	11.14	12.32	12.46
28 YRS	10.37	11.27	11.41	10.91	12.55	12.32	13.58	11.28	12.54	12.71
29 YRS	10.44	11.38	11.54	11.03	12.79	12.55	13.89	11.42	12.76	12.96
30 YRS	10.50	11.49	11.66	11.15	13.02	12.77	14.20	11.56	12.99	13.22

EDUCATION	CORRECT	DIGITSPA	WAISIMIL	WAISJUDG	VERBAL	ANIMAL	WAISBLOC	DIGIT
0 YRS	6.84	7.20	4.61	5.92	5.43	7.06	7.40	4.86
1 YRS	7.08	7.44	5.04	6.31	5.79	7.37	7.66	5.24
2 YRS	7.32	7.69	5.47	6.70	6.15	7.67	7.92	5.62
3 YRS	7.55	7.94	5.91	7.10	6.51	7.97	8.18	6.00
4 YRS	7.79	8.19	6.34	7.49	6.87	8.28	8.44	6.38
5 YRS	8.03	8.44	6.77	7.88	7.23	8.58	8.70	6.76
6 YRS	8.27	8.68	7.20	8.27	7.59	8.88	8.96	7.13
7 YRS	8.51	8.93	7.63	8.67	7.95	9.19	9.22	7.51
8 YRS	8.75	9.18	8.06	9.06	8.31	9.49	9.48	7.89
9 YRS	8.99	9.43	8.50	9.45	8.67	9.79	9.74	8.27
10 YRS	9.23	9.68	8.93	9.84	9.03	10.10	10.00	8.65
11 YRS	9.47	9.92	9.36	10.24	9.39	10.40	10.26	9.03
12 YRS	9.71	10.17	9.79	10.63	9.76	10.70	10.52	9.40
13 YRS	9.95	10.42	10.22	11.02	10.12	11.00	10.78	9.78
14 YRS	10.19	10.67	10.65	11.41	10.48	11.31	11.04	10.16
15 YRS	10.43	10.91	11.09	11.81	10.84	11.61	11.30	10.54
16 YRS	10.66	11.16	11.52	12.20	11.20	11.91	11.56	10.92
17 YRS	10.90	11.41	11.95	12.59	11.56	12.22	11.82	11.30
18 YRS	11.14	11.66	12.38	12.98	11.92	12.52	12.08	11.67
19 YRS	11.38	11.91	12.81	13.38	12.28	12.82	12.34	12.05
20 YRS	11.62	12.15	13.24	13.77	12.64	13.13	12.60	12.43
21 YRS	11.86	12.40	13.67	14.16	13.00	13.43	12.86	12.81
22 YRS	12.10	12.65	14.11	14.56	13.36	13.73	13.12	13.19
23 YRS	12.34	12.90	14.54	14.95	13.72	14.04	13.38	13.57
24 YRS	12.58	13.15	14.97	15.34	14.08	14.34	13.64	13.94
25 YRS	12.82	13.39	15.40	15.73	14.44	14.64	13.90	14.32
26 YRS	13.06	13.64	15.83	16.13	14.80	14.95	14.16	14.70
27 YRS	13.30	13.89	16.26	16.52	15.16	15.25	14.42	15.08
28 YRS	13.54	14.14	16.70	16.91	15.52	15.55	14.67	15.46
29 YRS	13.77	14.38	17.13	17.30	15.88	15.85	14.93	15.84
30 YRS	14.01	14.63	17.56	17.70	16.24	16.16	15.19	16.21

Table 22.2. Age 81 – Female.

EDUCATION	BUSCHFR1	BRETRIE	REYA1	REYA2	REYA3	REYA4	REYA5	REYTOT	REYB1	REYA6
0 YRS	8.60	8.19	7.90	7.54	6.03	5.96	4.99	7.41	6.36	5.60
1 YRS	8.66	8.30	8.02	7.66	6.26	6.19	5.30	7.55	6.58	5.85
2 YRS	8.73	8.41	8.15	7.78	6.49	6.42	5.61	7.69	6.80	6.11
3 YRS	8.79	8.52	8.27	7.90	6.73	6.64	5.91	7.83	7.02	6.36
4 YRS	8.85	8.63	8.40	8.02	6.96	6.87	6.22	7.97	7.24	6.62
5 YRS	8.92	8.74	8.53	8.14	7.19	7.10	6.53	8.10	7.46	6.87
6 YRS	8.98	8.85	8.65	8.26	7.43	7.32	6.83	8.24	7.68	7.12
7 YRS	9.04	8.96	8.78	8.38	7.66	7.55	7.14	8.38	7.90	7.38
8 YRS	9.11	9.07	8.90	8.50	7.89	7.78	7.45	8.52	8.12	7.63
9 YRS	9.17	9.18	9.03	8.62	8.12	8.01	7.75	8.66	8.35	7.89
10 YRS	9.23	9.29	9.15	8.74	8.36	8.23	8.06	8.80	8.57	8.14
11 YRS	9.30	9.40	9.28	8.86	8.59	8.46	8.37	8.93	8.79	8.39
12 YRS	9.36	9.51	9.40	8.99	8.82	8.69	8.67	9.07	9.01	8.65
13 YRS	9.42	9.62	9.53	9.11	9.06	8.91	8.98	9.21	9.23	8.90
14 YRS	9.49	9.73	9.66	9.23	9.29	9.14	9.29	9.35	9.45	9.16
15 YRS	9.55	9.84	9.78	9.35	9.52	9.37	9.59	9.49	9.67	9.41
16 YRS	9.61	9.95	9.91	9.47	9.76	9.60	9.90	9.62	9.89	9.66
17 YRS	9.68	10.06	10.03	9.59	9.99	9.82	10.21	9.76	10.11	9.92
18 YRS	9.74	10.17	10.16	9.71	10.22	10.05	10.51	9.90	10.33	10.17
19 YRS	9.80	10.28	10.28	9.83	10.46	10.28	10.82	10.04	10.55	10.43
20 YRS	9.87	10.39	10.41	9.95	10.69	10.50	11.13	10.18	10.78	10.68
21 YRS	9.93	10.50	10.53	10.07	10.92	10.73	11.43	10.32	11.00	10.93
22 YRS	9.99	10.61	10.66	10.19	11.16	10.96	11.74	10.45	11.22	11.19
23 YRS	10.06	10.72	10.78	10.31	11.39	11.18	12.05	10.59	11.44	11.44
24 YRS	10.12	10.83	10.91	10.43	11.62	11.41	12.35	10.73	11.66	11.69
25 YRS	10.18	10.94	11.04	10.55	11.86	11.64	12.66	10.87	11.88	11.95
26 YRS	10.25	11.05	11.16	10.67	12.09	11.87	12.97	11.01	12.10	12.20
27 YRS	10.31	11.16	11.29	10.79	12.32	12.09	13.27	11.14	12.32	12.46
28 YRS	10.37	11.27	11.41	10.91	12.55	12.32	13.58	11.28	12.54	12.71
29 YRS	10.44	11.38	11.54	11.03	12.79	12.55	13.89	11.42	12.76	12.96
30 YRS	10.50	11.49	11.66	11.15	13.02	12.77	14.20	11.56	12.99	13.22

EDUCATION	CORRECT	DIGITSPA	WAISIMIL	WAISJUDG	VERBAL	ANIMAL	WAISBLOC	DIGIT
0 YRS	6.84	7.20	4.61	5.92	5.43	7.06	7.40	4.86
1 YRS	7.08	7.44	5.04	6.31	5.79	7.37	7.66	5.24
2 YRS	7.32	7.69	5.47	6.70	6.15	7.67	7.92	5.62
3 YRS	7.55	7.94	5.91	7.10	6.51	7.97	8.18	6.00
4 YRS	7.79	8.19	6.34	7.49	6.87	8.28	8.44	6.38
5 YRS	8.03	8.44	6.77	7.88	7.23	8.58	8.70	6.76
6 YRS	8.27	8.68	7.20	8.27	7.59	8.88	8.96	7.13
7 YRS	8.51	8.93	7.63	8.67	7.95	9.19	9.22	7.51
8 YRS	8.75	9.18	8.06	9.06	8.31	9.49	9.48	7.89
9 YRS	8.99	9.43	8.50	9.45	8.67	9.79	9.74	8.27
10 YRS	9.23	9.68	8.93	9.84	9.03	10.10	10.00	8.65
11 YRS	9.47	9.92	9.36	10.24	9.39	10.40	10.26	9.03
12 YRS	9.71	10.17	9.79	10.63	9.76	10.70	10.52	9.40
13 YRS	9.95	10.42	10.22	11.02	10.12	11.00	10.78	9.78
14 YRS	10.19	10.67	10.65	11.41	10.48	11.31	11.04	10.16
15 YRS	10.43	10.91	11.09	11.81	10.84	11.61	11.30	10.54
16 YRS	10.66	11.16	11.52	12.20	11.20	11.91	11.56	10.92
17 YRS	10.90	11.41	11.95	12.59	11.56	12.22	11.82	11.30
18 YRS	11.14	11.66	12.38	12.98	11.92	12.52	12.08	11.67
19 YRS	11.38	11.91	12.81	13.38	12.28	12.82	12.34	12.05
20 YRS	11.62	12.15	13.24	13.77	12.64	13.13	12.60	12.43
21 YRS	11.86	12.40	13.67	14.16	13.00	13.43	12.86	12.81
22 YRS	12.10	12.65	14.11	14.56	13.36	13.73	13.12	13.19
23 YRS	12.34	12.90	14.54	14.95	13.72	14.04	13.38	13.57
24 YRS	12.58	13.15	14.97	15.34	14.08	14.34	13.64	13.94
25 YRS	12.82	13.39	15.40	15.73	14.44	14.64	13.90	14.32
26 YRS	13.06	13.64	15.83	16.13	14.80	14.95	14.16	14.70
27 YRS	13.30	13.89	16.26	16.52	15.16	15.25	14.42	15.08
28 YRS	13.54	14.14	16.70	16.91	15.52	15.55	14.67	15.46
29 YRS	13.77	14.38	17.13	17.30	15.88	15.85	14.93	15.84
30 YRS	14.01	14.63	17.56	17.70	16.24	16.16	15.19	16.21

Table 23.1. Age 82 – Male.

EDUCATION	BUSCHFR1	BRETRIE	REYA1	REYA2	REYA3	REYA4	REYA5	REYTOT	REYB1	REYA6
0 YRS	8.48	8.03	7.80	7.44	5.88	5.81	4.84	7.26	6.19	5.44
1 YRS	8.55	8.14	7.93	7.56	6.11	6.04	5.15	7.40	6.41	5.69
2 YRS	8.61	8.25	8.05	7.68	6.34	6.27	5.46	7.54	6.64	5.95
3 YRS	8.67	8.36	8.18	7.80	6.58	6.50	5.76	7.68	6.86	6.20
4 YRS	8.74	8.47	8.30	7.92	6.81	6.72	6.07	7.82	7.08	6.46
5 YRS	8.80	8.58	8.43	8.04	7.04	6.95	6.38	7.95	7.30	6.71
6 YRS	8.86	8.69	8.55	8.16	7.27	7.18	6.69	8.09	7.52	6.96
7 YRS	8.93	8.80	8.68	8.28	7.51	7.40	6.99	8.23	7.74	7.22
8 YRS	8.99	8.91	8.80	8.40	7.74	7.63	7.30	8.37	7.96	7.47
9 YRS	9.05	9.02	8.93	8.52	7.97	7.86	7.61	8.51	8.18	7.73
10 YRS	9.12	9.13	9.06	8.64	8.21	8.08	7.91	8.65	8.40	7.98
11 YRS	9.18	9.24	9.18	8.76	8.44	8.31	8.22	8.78	8.62	8.23
12 YRS	9.24	9.35	9.31	8.88	8.67	8.54	8.53	8.92	8.85	8.49
13 YRS	9.31	9.46	9.43	9.00	8.91	8.77	8.83	9.06	9.07	8.74
14 YRS	9.37	9.57	9.56	9.12	9.14	8.99	9.14	9.20	9.29	9.00
15 YRS	9.43	9.68	9.68	9.24	9.37	9.22	9.45	9.34	9.51	9.25
16 YRS	9.50	9.79	9.81	9.36	9.61	9.45	9.75	9.47	9.73	9.50
17 YRS	9.56	9.90	9.93	9.48	9.84	9.67	10.06	9.61	9.95	9.76
18 YRS	9.62	10.01	10.06	9.60	10.07	9.90	10.37	9.75	10.17	10.01
19 YRS	9.69	10.12	10.19	9.72	10.31	10.13	10.67	9.89	10.39	10.27
20 YRS	9.75	10.23	10.31	9.84	10.54	10.35	10.98	10.03	10.61	10.52
21 YRS	9.81	10.34	10.44	9.96	10.77	10.58	11.29	10.17	10.83	10.77
22 YRS	9.88	10.44	10.56	10.08	11.01	10.81	11.59	10.30	11.06	11.03
23 YRS	9.94	10.55	10.69	10.20	11.24	11.04	11.90	10.44	11.28	11.28
24 YRS	10.00	10.66	10.81	10.32	11.47	11.26	12.21	10.58	11.50	11.53
25 YRS	10.06	10.77	10.94	10.45	11.70	11.49	12.51	10.72	11.72	11.79
26 YRS	10.13	10.88	11.06	10.57	11.94	11.72	12.82	10.86	11.94	12.04
27 YRS	10.19	10.99	11.19	10.69	12.17	11.94	13.13	10.99	12.16	12.30
28 YRS	10.25	11.10	11.32	10.81	12.40	12.17	13.43	11.13	12.38	12.55
29 YRS	10.32	11.21	11.44	10.93	12.64	12.40	13.74	11.27	12.60	12.80
30 YRS	10.38	11.32	11.57	11.05	12.87	12.62	14.05	11.41	12.82	13.06

EDUCATION	CORRECT	DIGITSPA	WAISIMIL	WAISJUDG	VERBAL	ANIMAL	WAISBLOC	DIGIT
0 YRS	6.68	7.13	4.52	5.85	5.37	6.95	7.29	4.64
1 YRS	6.92	7.38	4.95	6.25	5.73	7.25	7.55	5.02
2 YRS	7.16	7.63	5.38	6.64	6.09	7.55	7.81	5.40
3 YRS	7.40	7.87	5.81	7.03	6.46	7.86	8.07	5.78
4 YRS	7.64	8.12	6.24	7.42	6.82	8.16	8.33	6.16
5 YRS	7.88	8.37	6.67	7.82	7.18	8.46	8.59	6.54
6 YRS	8.12	8.62	7.11	8.21	7.54	8.77	8.85	6.91
7 YRS	8.36	8.87	7.54	8.60	7.90	9.07	9.11	7.29
8 YRS	8.60	9.11	7.97	8.99	8.26	9.37	9.37	7.67
9 YRS	8.84	9.36	8.40	9.39	8.62	9.68	9.63	8.05
10 YRS	9.08	9.61	8.83	9.78	8.98	9.98	9.89	8.43
11 YRS	9.31	9.86	9.26	10.17	9.34	10.28	10.15	8.81
12 YRS	9.55	10.11	9.70	10.56	9.70	10.58	10.41	9.18
13 YRS	9.79	10.35	10.13	10.96	10.06	10.89	10.66	9.56
14 YRS	10.03	10.60	10.56	11.35	10.42	11.19	10.92	9.94
15 YRS	10.27	10.85	10.99	11.74	10.78	11.49	11.18	10.32
16 YRS	10.51	11.10	11.42	12.14	11.14	11.80	11.44	10.70
17 YRS	10.75	11.34	11.85	12.53	11.50	12.10	11.70	11.08
18 YRS	10.99	11.59	12.28	12.92	11.86	12.40	11.96	11.45
19 YRS	11.23	11.84	12.72	13.31	12.22	12.71	12.22	11.83
20 YRS	11.47	12.09	13.15	13.71	12.58	13.01	12.48	12.21
21 YRS	11.71	12.34	13.58	14.10	12.94	13.31	12.74	12.59
22 YRS	11.95	12.58	14.01	14.49	13.30	13.62	13.00	12.97
23 YRS	12.18	12.83	14.44	14.88	13.66	13.92	13.26	13.35
24 YRS	12.42	13.08	14.87	15.28	14.02	14.22	13.52	13.72
25 YRS	12.66	13.33	15.31	15.67	14.38	14.53	13.78	14.10
26 YRS	12.90	13.58	15.74	16.06	14.74	14.83	14.04	14.48
27 YRS	13.14	13.82	16.17	16.45	15.10	15.13	14.30	14.86
28 YRS	13.38	14.07	16.60	16.85	15.46	15.43	14.56	15.24
29 YRS	13.62	14.32	17.03	17.24	15.83	15.74	14.82	15.62
30 YRS	13.86	14.57	17.46	17.63	16.19	16.04	15.08	15.99

Table 23.2. Age 82 – Female.

EDUCATION	BUSCHFR1	BRETRIE	REYA1	REYA2	REYA3	REYA4	REYA5	REYTOT	REYB1	REYA6
0 YRS	8.48	8.03	7.80	7.44	5.88	5.81	4.84	7.26	6.19	5.44
1 YRS	8.55	8.14	7.93	7.56	6.11	6.04	5.15	7.40	6.41	5.69
2 YRS	8.61	8.25	8.05	7.68	6.34	6.27	5.46	7.54	6.64	5.95
3 YRS	8.67	8.36	8.18	7.80	6.58	6.50	5.76	7.68	6.86	6.20
4 YRS	8.74	8.47	8.30	7.92	6.81	6.72	6.07	7.82	7.08	6.46
5 YRS	8.80	8.58	8.43	8.04	7.04	6.95	6.38	7.95	7.30	6.71
6 YRS	8.86	8.69	8.55	8.16	7.27	7.18	6.69	8.09	7.52	6.96
7 YRS	8.93	8.80	8.68	8.28	7.51	7.40	6.99	8.23	7.74	7.22
8 YRS	8.99	8.91	8.80	8.40	7.74	7.63	7.30	8.37	7.96	7.47
9 YRS	9.05	9.02	8.93	8.52	7.97	7.86	7.61	8.51	8.18	7.73
10 YRS	9.12	9.13	9.06	8.64	8.21	8.08	7.91	8.65	8.40	7.98
11 YRS	9.18	9.24	9.18	8.76	8.44	8.31	8.22	8.78	8.62	8.23
12 YRS	9.24	9.35	9.31	8.88	8.67	8.54	8.53	8.92	8.85	8.49
13 YRS	9.31	9.46	9.43	9.00	8.91	8.77	8.83	9.06	9.07	8.74
14 YRS	9.37	9.57	9.56	9.12	9.14	8.99	9.14	9.20	9.29	9.00
15 YRS	9.43	9.68	9.68	9.24	9.37	9.22	9.45	9.34	9.51	9.25
16 YRS	9.50	9.79	9.81	9.36	9.61	9.45	9.75	9.47	9.73	9.50
17 YRS	9.56	9.90	9.93	9.48	9.84	9.67	10.06	9.61	9.95	9.76
18 YRS	9.62	10.01	10.06	9.60	10.07	9.90	10.37	9.75	10.17	10.01
19 YRS	9.69	10.12	10.19	9.72	10.31	10.13	10.67	9.89	10.39	10.27
20 YRS	9.75	10.23	10.31	9.84	10.54	10.35	10.98	10.03	10.61	10.52
21 YRS	9.81	10.34	10.44	9.96	10.77	10.58	11.29	10.17	10.83	10.77
22 YRS	9.88	10.44	10.56	10.08	11.01	10.81	11.59	10.30	11.06	11.03
23 YRS	9.94	10.55	10.69	10.20	11.24	11.04	11.90	10.44	11.28	11.28
24 YRS	10.00	10.66	10.81	10.32	11.47	11.26	12.21	10.58	11.50	11.53
25 YRS	10.06	10.77	10.94	10.45	11.70	11.49	12.51	10.72	11.72	11.79
26 YRS	10.13	10.88	11.06	10.57	11.94	11.72	12.82	10.86	11.94	12.04
27 YRS	10.19	10.99	11.19	10.69	12.17	11.94	13.13	10.99	12.16	12.30
28 YRS	10.25	11.10	11.32	10.81	12.40	12.17	13.43	11.13	12.38	12.55
29 YRS	10.32	11.21	11.44	10.93	12.64	12.40	13.74	11.27	12.60	12.80
30 YRS	10.38	11.32	11.57	11.05	12.87	12.62	14.05	11.41	12.82	13.06

EDUCATION	CORRECT	DIGITSPA	WAISIMIL	WAISJUDG	VERBAL	ANIMAL	WAISBLOC	DIGIT
0 YRS	6.68	7.13	4.52	5.85	5.37	6.95	7.29	4.64
1 YRS	6.92	7.38	4.95	6.25	5.73	7.25	7.55	5.02
2 YRS	7.16	7.63	5.38	6.64	6.09	7.55	7.81	5.40
3 YRS	7.40	7.87	5.81	7.03	6.46	7.86	8.07	5.78
4 YRS	7.64	8.12	6.24	7.42	6.82	8.16	8.33	6.16
5 YRS	7.88	8.37	6.67	7.82	7.18	8.46	8.59	6.54
6 YRS	8.12	8.62	7.11	8.21	7.54	8.77	8.85	6.91
7 YRS	8.36	8.87	7.54	8.60	7.90	9.07	9.11	7.29
8 YRS	8.60	9.11	7.97	8.99	8.26	9.37	9.37	7.67
9 YRS	8.84	9.36	8.40	9.39	8.62	9.68	9.63	8.05
10 YRS	9.08	9.61	8.83	9.78	8.98	9.98	9.89	8.43
11 YRS	9.31	9.86	9.26	10.17	9.34	10.28	10.15	8.81
12 YRS	9.55	10.11	9.70	10.56	9.70	10.58	10.41	9.18
13 YRS	9.79	10.35	10.13	10.96	10.06	10.89	10.66	9.56
14 YRS	10.03	10.60	10.56	11.35	10.42	11.19	10.92	9.94
15 YRS	10.27	10.85	10.99	11.74	10.78	11.49	11.18	10.32
16 YRS	10.51	11.10	11.42	12.14	11.14	11.80	11.44	10.70
17 YRS	10.75	11.34	11.85	12.53	11.50	12.10	11.70	11.08
18 YRS	10.99	11.59	12.28	12.92	11.86	12.40	11.96	11.45
19 YRS	11.23	11.84	12.72	13.31	12.22	12.71	12.22	11.83
20 YRS	11.47	12.09	13.15	13.71	12.58	13.01	12.48	12.21
21 YRS	11.71	12.34	13.58	14.10	12.94	13.31	12.74	12.59
22 YRS	11.95	12.58	14.01	14.49	13.30	13.62	13.00	12.97
23 YRS	12.18	12.83	14.44	14.88	13.66	13.92	13.26	13.35
24 YRS	12.42	13.08	14.87	15.28	14.02	14.22	13.52	13.72
25 YRS	12.66	13.33	15.31	15.67	14.38	14.53	13.78	14.10
26 YRS	12.90	13.58	15.74	16.06	14.74	14.83	14.04	14.48
27 YRS	13.14	13.82	16.17	16.45	15.10	15.13	14.30	14.86
28 YRS	13.38	14.07	16.60	16.85	15.46	15.43	14.56	15.24
29 YRS	13.62	14.32	17.03	17.24	15.83	15.74	14.82	15.62
30 YRS	13.86	14.57	17.46	17.63	16.19	16.04	15.08	15.99

Table 24.1. Age 83 – Male.

EDUCATION	BUSCHFR1	BRETRIE	REYA1	REYA2	REYA3	REYA4	REYA5	REYTOT	REYB1	REYA6
0 YRS	8.37	7.86	7.70	7.33	5.73	5.67	4.70	7.11	6.03	5.28
1 YRS	8.43	7.97	7.83	7.45	5.96	5.89	5.00	7.25	6.25	5.53
2 YRS	8.49	8.08	7.95	7.57	6.19	6.12	5.31	7.39	6.47	5.79
3 YRS	8.55	8.19	8.08	7.69	6.42	6.35	5.62	7.53	6.69	6.04
4 YRS	8.62	8.30	8.21	7.81	6.66	6.57	5.92	7.67	6.92	6.30
5 YRS	8.68	8.41	8.33	7.93	6.89	6.80	6.23	7.80	7.14	6.55
6 YRS	8.74	8.52	8.46	8.05	7.12	7.03	6.54	7.94	7.36	6.80
7 YRS	8.81	8.63	8.58	8.17	7.36	7.25	6.85	8.08	7.58	7.06
8 YRS	8.87	8.74	8.71	8.29	7.59	7.48	7.15	8.22	7.80	7.31
9 YRS	8.93	8.85	8.83	8.41	7.82	7.71	7.46	8.36	8.02	7.57
10 YRS	9.00	8.96	8.96	8.53	8.06	7.94	7.77	8.50	8.24	7.82
11 YRS	9.06	9.07	9.08	8.66	8.29	8.16	8.07	8.63	8.46	8.07
12 YRS	9.12	9.18	9.21	8.78	8.52	8.39	8.38	8.77	8.68	8.33
13 YRS	9.19	9.29	9.34	8.90	8.76	8.62	8.69	8.91	8.90	8.58
14 YRS	9.25	9.40	9.46	9.02	8.99	8.84	8.99	9.05	9.12	8.84
15 YRS	9.31	9.51	9.59	9.14	9.22	9.07	9.30	9.19	9.35	9.09
16 YRS	9.38	9.62	9.71	9.26	9.46	9.30	9.61	9.32	9.57	9.34
17 YRS	9.44	9.73	9.84	9.38	9.69	9.53	9.91	9.46	9.79	9.60
18 YRS	9.50	9.84	9.96	9.50	9.92	9.75	10.22	9.60	10.01	9.85
19 YRS	9.57	9.95	10.09	9.62	10.16	9.98	10.53	9.74	10.23	10.11
20 YRS	9.63	10.06	10.21	9.74	10.39	10.21	10.83	9.88	10.45	10.36
21 YRS	9.69	10.17	10.34	9.86	10.62	10.43	11.14	10.02	10.67	10.61
22 YRS	9.76	10.28	10.47	9.98	10.85	10.66	11.45	10.15	10.89	10.87
23 YRS	9.82	10.39	10.59	10.10	11.09	10.89	11.75	10.29	11.11	11.12
24 YRS	9.88	10.50	10.72	10.22	11.32	11.11	12.06	10.43	11.33	11.37
25 YRS	9.95	10.61	10.84	10.34	11.55	11.34	12.37	10.57	11.56	11.63
26 YRS	10.01	10.72	10.97	10.46	11.79	11.57	12.67	10.71	11.78	11.88
27 YRS	10.07	10.83	11.09	10.58	12.02	11.80	12.98	10.84	12.00	12.14
28 YRS	10.14	10.94	11.22	10.70	12.25	12.02	13.29	10.98	12.22	12.39
29 YRS	10.20	11.05	11.34	10.82	12.49	12.25	13.59	11.12	12.44	12.64
30 YRS	10.26	11.16	11.47	10.94	12.72	12.48	13.90	11.26	12.66	12.90

EDUCATION	CORRECT	DIGITSPA	WAISIMIL	WAISJUDG	VERBAL	ANIMAL	WAISBLOC	DIGIT
0 YRS	6.53	7.07	4.42	5.79	5.32	6.83	7.17	4.42
1 YRS	6.77	7.31	4.85	6.18	5.68	7.13	7.43	4.80
2 YRS	7.01	7.56	5.28	6.57	6.04	7.44	7.69	5.18
3 YRS	7.25	7.81	5.72	6.97	6.40	7.74	7.95	5.56
4 YRS	7.49	8.06	6.15	7.36	6.76	8.04	8.21	5.94
5 YRS	7.72	8.30	6.58	7.75	7.12	8.35	8.47	6.32
6 YRS	7.96	8.55	7.01	8.15	7.48	8.65	8.73	6.69
7 YRS	8.20	8.80	7.44	8.54	7.84	8.95	8.99	7.07
8 YRS	8.44	9.05	7.87	8.93	8.20	9.26	9.25	7.45
9 YRS	8.68	9.30	8.31	9.32	8.56	9.56	9.51	7.83
10 YRS	8.92	9.54	8.74	9.72	8.92	9.86	9.77	8.21
11 YRS	9.16	9.79	9.17	10.11	9.28	10.16	10.03	8.59
12 YRS	9.40	10.04	9.60	10.50	9.64	10.47	10.29	8.96
13 YRS	9.64	10.29	10.03	10.89	10.00	10.77	10.55	9.34
14 YRS	9.88	10.54	10.46	11.29	10.36	11.07	10.81	9.72
15 YRS	10.12	10.78	10.89	11.68	10.72	11.38	11.07	10.10
16 YRS	10.36	11.03	11.33	12.07	11.08	11.68	11.33	10.48
17 YRS	10.60	11.28	11.76	12.46	11.44	11.98	11.59	10.86
18 YRS	10.83	11.53	12.19	12.86	11.80	12.29	11.85	11.23
19 YRS	11.07	11.77	12.62	13.25	12.16	12.59	12.11	11.61
20 YRS	11.31	12.02	13.05	13.64	12.53	12.89	12.37	11.99
21 YRS	11.55	12.27	13.48	14.03	12.89	13.20	12.63	12.37
22 YRS	11.79	12.52	13.92	14.43	13.25	13.50	12.89	12.75
23 YRS	12.03	12.77	14.35	14.82	13.61	13.80	13.15	13.13
24 YRS	12.27	13.01	14.78	15.21	13.97	14.11	13.41	13.50
25 YRS	12.51	13.26	15.21	15.61	14.33	14.41	13.67	13.88
26 YRS	12.75	13.51	15.64	16.00	14.69	14.71	13.92	14.26
27 YRS	12.99	13.76	16.07	16.39	15.05	15.01	14.18	14.64
28 YRS	13.23	14.01	16.50	16.78	15.41	15.32	14.44	15.02
29 YRS	13.47	14.25	16.94	17.18	15.77	15.62	14.70	15.40
30 YRS	13.71	14.50	17.37	17.57	16.13	15.92	14.96	15.77

Table 24.2. Age 83 – Female.

EDUCATION	BUSCHFR1	BRETRIE	REYA1	REYA2	REYA3	REYA4	REYA5	REYTOT	REYB1	REYA6
0 YRS	8.37	7.86	7.70	7.33	5.73	5.67	4.70	7.11	6.03	5.28
1 YRS	8.43	7.97	7.83	7.45	5.96	5.89	5.00	7.25	6.25	5.53
2 YRS	8.49	8.08	7.95	7.57	6.19	6.12	5.31	7.39	6.47	5.79
3 YRS	8.55	8.19	8.08	7.69	6.42	6.35	5.62	7.53	6.69	6.04
4 YRS	8.62	8.30	8.21	7.81	6.66	6.57	5.92	7.67	6.92	6.30
5 YRS	8.68	8.41	8.33	7.93	6.89	6.80	6.23	7.80	7.14	6.55
6 YRS	8.74	8.52	8.46	8.05	7.12	7.03	6.54	7.94	7.36	6.80
7 YRS	8.81	8.63	8.58	8.17	7.36	7.25	6.85	8.08	7.58	7.06
8 YRS	8.87	8.74	8.71	8.29	7.59	7.48	7.15	8.22	7.80	7.31
9 YRS	8.93	8.85	8.83	8.41	7.82	7.71	7.46	8.36	8.02	7.57
10 YRS	9.00	8.96	8.96	8.53	8.06	7.94	7.77	8.50	8.24	7.82
11 YRS	9.06	9.07	9.08	8.66	8.29	8.16	8.07	8.63	8.46	8.07
12 YRS	9.12	9.18	9.21	8.78	8.52	8.39	8.38	8.77	8.68	8.33
13 YRS	9.19	9.29	9.34	8.90	8.76	8.62	8.69	8.91	8.90	8.58
14 YRS	9.25	9.40	9.46	9.02	8.99	8.84	8.99	9.05	9.12	8.84
15 YRS	9.31	9.51	9.59	9.14	9.22	9.07	9.30	9.19	9.35	9.09
16 YRS	9.38	9.62	9.71	9.26	9.46	9.30	9.61	9.32	9.57	9.34
17 YRS	9.44	9.73	9.84	9.38	9.69	9.53	9.91	9.46	9.79	9.60
18 YRS	9.50	9.84	9.96	9.50	9.92	9.75	10.22	9.60	10.01	9.85
19 YRS	9.57	9.95	10.09	9.62	10.16	9.98	10.53	9.74	10.23	10.11
20 YRS	9.63	10.06	10.21	9.74	10.39	10.21	10.83	9.88	10.45	10.36
21 YRS	9.69	10.17	10.34	9.86	10.62	10.43	11.14	10.02	10.67	10.61
22 YRS	9.76	10.28	10.47	9.98	10.85	10.66	11.45	10.15	10.89	10.87
23 YRS	9.82	10.39	10.59	10.10	11.09	10.89	11.75	10.29	11.11	11.12
24 YRS	9.88	10.50	10.72	10.22	11.32	11.11	12.06	10.43	11.33	11.37
25 YRS	9.95	10.61	10.84	10.34	11.55	11.34	12.37	10.57	11.56	11.63
26 YRS	10.01	10.72	10.97	10.46	11.79	11.57	12.67	10.71	11.78	11.88
27 YRS	10.07	10.83	11.09	10.58	12.02	11.80	12.98	10.84	12.00	12.14
28 YRS	10.14	10.94	11.22	10.70	12.25	12.02	13.29	10.98	12.22	12.39
29 YRS	10.20	11.05	11.34	10.82	12.49	12.25	13.59	11.12	12.44	12.64
30 YRS	10.26	11.16	11.47	10.94	12.72	12.48	13.90	11.26	12.66	12.90

EDUCATION	CORRECT	DIGITSPA	WAISIMIL	WAISJUDG	VERBAL	ANIMAL	WAISBLOC	DIGIT
0 YRS	6.53	7.07	4.42	5.79	5.32	6.83	7.17	4.42
1 YRS	6.77	7.31	4.85	6.18	5.68	7.13	7.43	4.80
2 YRS	7.01	7.56	5.28	6.57	6.04	7.44	7.69	5.18
3 YRS	7.25	7.81	5.72	6.97	6.40	7.74	7.95	5.56
4 YRS	7.49	8.06	6.15	7.36	6.76	8.04	8.21	5.94
5 YRS	7.72	8.30	6.58	7.75	7.12	8.35	8.47	6.32
6 YRS	7.96	8.55	7.01	8.15	7.48	8.65	8.73	6.69
7 YRS	8.20	8.80	7.44	8.54	7.84	8.95	8.99	7.07
8 YRS	8.44	9.05	7.87	8.93	8.20	9.26	9.25	7.45
9 YRS	8.68	9.30	8.31	9.32	8.56	9.56	9.51	7.83
10 YRS	8.92	9.54	8.74	9.72	8.92	9.86	9.77	8.21
11 YRS	9.16	9.79	9.17	10.11	9.28	10.16	10.03	8.59
12 YRS	9.40	10.04	9.60	10.50	9.64	10.47	10.29	8.96
13 YRS	9.64	10.29	10.03	10.89	10.00	10.77	10.55	9.34
14 YRS	9.88	10.54	10.46	11.29	10.36	11.07	10.81	9.72
15 YRS	10.12	10.78	10.89	11.68	10.72	11.38	11.07	10.10
16 YRS	10.36	11.03	11.33	12.07	11.08	11.68	11.33	10.48
17 YRS	10.60	11.28	11.76	12.46	11.44	11.98	11.59	10.86
18 YRS	10.83	11.53	12.19	12.86	11.80	12.29	11.85	11.23
19 YRS	11.07	11.77	12.62	13.25	12.16	12.59	12.11	11.61
20 YRS	11.31	12.02	13.05	13.64	12.53	12.89	12.37	11.99
21 YRS	11.55	12.27	13.48	14.03	12.89	13.20	12.63	12.37
22 YRS	11.79	12.52	13.92	14.43	13.25	13.50	12.89	12.75
23 YRS	12.03	12.77	14.35	14.82	13.61	13.80	13.15	13.13
24 YRS	12.27	13.01	14.78	15.21	13.97	14.11	13.41	13.50
25 YRS	12.51	13.26	15.21	15.61	14.33	14.41	13.67	13.88
26 YRS	12.75	13.51	15.64	16.00	14.69	14.71	13.92	14.26
27 YRS	12.99	13.76	16.07	16.39	15.05	15.01	14.18	14.64
28 YRS	13.23	14.01	16.50	16.78	15.41	15.32	14.44	15.02
29 YRS	13.47	14.25	16.94	17.18	15.77	15.62	14.70	15.40
30 YRS	13.71	14.50	17.37	17.57	16.13	15.92	14.96	15.77

Table 25.1. Age 84 – Male.

EDUCATION	BUSCHFR1	BRETRIE	REYA1	REYA2	REYA3	REYA4	REYA5	REYTOT	REYB1	REYA6
0 YRS	8.25	7.70	7.61	7.23	5.57	5.52	4.55	6.96	5.87	5.12
1 YRS	8.31	7.81	7.73	7.35	5.81	5.74	4.86	7.10	6.09	5.37
2 YRS	8.37	7.92	7.86	7.47	6.04	5.97	5.16	7.24	6.31	5.63
3 YRS	8.44	8.03	7.98	7.59	6.27	6.20	5.47	7.38	6.53	5.88
4 YRS	8.50	8.14	8.11	7.71	6.51	6.43	5.78	7.52	6.75	6.14
5 YRS	8.56	8.25	8.23	7.83	6.74	6.65	6.08	7.65	6.97	6.39
6 YRS	8.63	8.36	8.36	7.95	6.97	6.88	6.39	7.79	7.19	6.64
7 YRS	8.69	8.47	8.49	8.07	7.21	7.11	6.70	7.93	7.42	6.90
8 YRS	8.75	8.58	8.61	8.19	7.44	7.33	7.00	8.07	7.64	7.15
9 YRS	8.82	8.69	8.74	8.31	7.67	7.56	7.31	8.21	7.86	7.41
10 YRS	8.88	8.80	8.86	8.43	7.91	7.79	7.62	8.35	8.08	7.66
11 YRS	8.94	8.91	8.99	8.55	8.14	8.01	7.93	8.48	8.30	7.91
12 YRS	9.01	9.02	9.11	8.67	8.37	8.24	8.23	8.62	8.52	8.17
13 YRS	9.07	9.13	9.24	8.79	8.61	8.47	8.54	8.76	8.74	8.42
14 YRS	9.13	9.24	9.36	8.91	8.84	8.70	8.85	8.90	8.96	8.68
15 YRS	9.20	9.35	9.49	9.03	9.07	8.92	9.15	9.04	9.18	8.93
16 YRS	9.26	9.46	9.62	9.15	9.30	9.15	9.46	9.17	9.40	9.18
17 YRS	9.32	9.57	9.74	9.27	9.54	9.38	9.77	9.31	9.62	9.44
18 YRS	9.39	9.68	9.87	9.39	9.77	9.60	10.07	9.45	9.85	9.69
19 YRS	9.45	9.79	9.99	9.51	10.00	9.83	10.38	9.59	10.07	9.95
20 YRS	9.51	9.90	10.12	9.63	10.24	10.06	10.69	9.73	10.29	10.20
21 YRS	9.58	10.01	10.24	9.75	10.47	10.28	10.99	9.87	10.51	10.45
22 YRS	9.64	10.12	10.37	9.87	10.70	10.51	11.30	10.00	10.73	10.71
23 YRS	9.70	10.23	10.49	10.00	10.94	10.74	11.61	10.14	10.95	10.96
24 YRS	9.77	10.34	10.62	10.12	11.17	10.97	11.91	10.28	11.17	11.21
25 YRS	9.83	10.45	10.75	10.24	11.40	11.19	12.22	10.42	11.39	11.47
26 YRS	9.89	10.56	10.87	10.36	11.64	11.42	12.53	10.56	11.61	11.72
27 YRS	9.96	10.67	11.00	10.48	11.87	11.65	12.83	10.69	11.83	11.98
28 YRS	10.02	10.78	11.12	10.60	12.10	11.87	13.14	10.83	12.06	12.23
29 YRS	10.08	10.89	11.25	10.72	12.34	12.10	13.45	10.97	12.28	12.48
30 YRS	10.15	11.00	11.37	10.84	12.57	12.33	13.75	11.11	12.50	12.74

EDUCATION	CORRECT	DIGITSPA	WAISIMIL	WAISJUDG	VERBAL	ANIMAL	WAISBLOC	DIGIT
0 YRS	6.37	7.00	4.33	5.73	5.26	6.71	7.06	4.20
1 YRS	6.61	7.25	4.76	6.12	5.62	7.02	7.32	4.58
2 YRS	6.85	7.50	5.19	6.51	5.98	7.32	7.58	4.96
3 YRS	7.09	7.74	5.62	6.90	6.34	7.62	7.84	5.34
4 YRS	7.33	7.99	6.05	7.30	6.70	7.93	8.10	5.72
5 YRS	7.57	8.24	6.48	7.69	7.06	8.23	8.36	6.10
6 YRS	7.81	8.49	6.92	8.08	7.42	8.53	8.62	6.47
7 YRS	8.05	8.73	7.35	8.47	7.78	8.84	8.88	6.85
8 YRS	8.29	8.98	7.78	8.87	8.14	9.14	9.14	7.23
9 YRS	8.53	9.23	8.21	9.26	8.50	9.44	9.40	7.61
10 YRS	8.77	9.48	8.64	9.65	8.86	9.74	9.66	7.99
11 YRS	9.01	9.73	9.07	10.04	9.23	10.05	9.92	8.37
12 YRS	9.25	9.97	9.50	10.44	9.59	10.35	10.17	8.74
13 YRS	9.48	10.22	9.94	10.83	9.95	10.65	10.43	9.12
14 YRS	9.72	10.47	10.37	11.22	10.31	10.96	10.69	9.50
15 YRS	9.96	10.72	10.80	11.62	10.67	11.26	10.95	9.88
16 YRS	10.20	10.97	11.23	12.01	11.03	11.56	11.21	10.26
17 YRS	10.44	11.21	11.66	12.40	11.39	11.87	11.47	10.64
18 YRS	10.68	11.46	12.09	12.79	11.75	12.17	11.73	11.01
19 YRS	10.92	11.71	12.53	13.19	12.11	12.47	11.99	11.39
20 YRS	11.16	11.96	12.96	13.58	12.47	12.78	12.25	11.77
21 YRS	11.40	12.20	13.39	13.97	12.83	13.08	12.51	12.15
22 YRS	11.64	12.45	13.82	14.36	13.19	13.38	12.77	12.53
23 YRS	11.88	12.70	14.25	14.76	13.55	13.69	13.03	12.90
24 YRS	12.12	12.95	14.68	15.15	13.91	13.99	13.29	13.28
25 YRS	12.36	13.20	15.11	15.54	14.27	14.29	13.55	13.66
26 YRS	12.59	13.44	15.55	15.93	14.63	14.59	13.81	14.04
27 YRS	12.83	13.69	15.98	16.33	14.99	14.90	14.07	14.42
28 YRS	13.07	13.94	16.41	16.72	15.35	15.20	14.33	14.80
29 YRS	13.31	14.19	16.84	17.11	15.71	15.50	14.59	15.17
30 YRS	13.55	14.44	17.27	17.50	16.07	15.81	14.85	15.55

Table 25.2. Age 84 – Female.

EDUCATION	BUSCHFR1	BRETRIE	REYA1	REYA2	REYA3	REYA4	REYA5	REYTOT	REYB1	REYA6
0 YRS	8.25	7.70	7.61	7.23	5.57	5.52	4.55	6.96	5.87	5.12
1 YRS	8.31	7.81	7.73	7.35	5.81	5.74	4.86	7.10	6.09	5.37
2 YRS	8.37	7.92	7.86	7.47	6.04	5.97	5.16	7.24	6.31	5.63
3 YRS	8.44	8.03	7.98	7.59	6.27	6.20	5.47	7.38	6.53	5.88
4 YRS	8.50	8.14	8.11	7.71	6.51	6.43	5.78	7.52	6.75	6.14
5 YRS	8.56	8.25	8.23	7.83	6.74	6.65	6.08	7.65	6.97	6.39
6 YRS	8.63	8.36	8.36	7.95	6.97	6.88	6.39	7.79	7.19	6.64
7 YRS	8.69	8.47	8.49	8.07	7.21	7.11	6.70	7.93	7.42	6.90
8 YRS	8.75	8.58	8.61	8.19	7.44	7.33	7.00	8.07	7.64	7.15
9 YRS	8.82	8.69	8.74	8.31	7.67	7.56	7.31	8.21	7.86	7.41
10 YRS	8.88	8.80	8.86	8.43	7.91	7.79	7.62	8.35	8.08	7.66
11 YRS	8.94	8.91	8.99	8.55	8.14	8.01	7.93	8.48	8.30	7.91
12 YRS	9.01	9.02	9.11	8.67	8.37	8.24	8.23	8.62	8.52	8.17
13 YRS	9.07	9.13	9.24	8.79	8.61	8.47	8.54	8.76	8.74	8.42
14 YRS	9.13	9.24	9.36	8.91	8.84	8.70	8.85	8.90	8.96	8.68
15 YRS	9.20	9.35	9.49	9.03	9.07	8.92	9.15	9.04	9.18	8.93
16 YRS	9.26	9.46	9.62	9.15	9.30	9.15	9.46	9.17	9.40	9.18
17 YRS	9.32	9.57	9.74	9.27	9.54	9.38	9.77	9.31	9.62	9.44
18 YRS	9.39	9.68	9.87	9.39	9.77	9.60	10.07	9.45	9.85	9.69
19 YRS	9.45	9.79	9.99	9.51	10.00	9.83	10.38	9.59	10.07	9.95
20 YRS	9.51	9.90	10.12	9.63	10.24	10.06	10.69	9.73	10.29	10.20
21 YRS	9.58	10.01	10.24	9.75	10.47	10.28	10.99	9.87	10.51	10.45
22 YRS	9.64	10.12	10.37	9.87	10.70	10.51	11.30	10.00	10.73	10.71
23 YRS	9.70	10.23	10.49	10.00	10.94	10.74	11.61	10.14	10.95	10.96
24 YRS	9.77	10.34	10.62	10.12	11.17	10.97	11.91	10.28	11.17	11.21
25 YRS	9.83	10.45	10.75	10.24	11.40	11.19	12.22	10.42	11.39	11.47
26 YRS	9.89	10.56	10.87	10.36	11.64	11.42	12.53	10.56	11.61	11.72
27 YRS	9.96	10.67	11.00	10.48	11.87	11.65	12.83	10.69	11.83	11.98
28 YRS	10.02	10.78	11.12	10.60	12.10	11.87	13.14	10.83	12.06	12.23
29 YRS	10.08	10.89	11.25	10.72	12.34	12.10	13.45	10.97	12.28	12.48
30 YRS	10.15	11.00	11.37	10.84	12.57	12.33	13.75	11.11	12.50	12.74

EDUCATION	CORRECT	DIGITSPA	WAISIMIL	WAISJUDG	VERBAL	ANIMAL	WAISBLOC	DIGIT
0 YRS	6.37	7.00	4.33	5.73	5.26	6.71	7.06	4.20
1 YRS	6.61	7.25	4.76	6.12	5.62	7.02	7.32	4.58
2 YRS	6.85	7.50	5.19	6.51	5.98	7.32	7.58	4.96
3 YRS	7.09	7.74	5.62	6.90	6.34	7.62	7.84	5.34
4 YRS	7.33	7.99	6.05	7.30	6.70	7.93	8.10	5.72
5 YRS	7.57	8.24	6.48	7.69	7.06	8.23	8.36	6.10
6 YRS	7.81	8.49	6.92	8.08	7.42	8.53	8.62	6.47
7 YRS	8.05	8.73	7.35	8.47	7.78	8.84	8.88	6.85
8 YRS	8.29	8.98	7.78	8.87	8.14	9.14	9.14	7.23
9 YRS	8.53	9.23	8.21	9.26	8.50	9.44	9.40	7.61
10 YRS	8.77	9.48	8.64	9.65	8.86	9.74	9.66	7.99
11 YRS	9.01	9.73	9.07	10.04	9.23	10.05	9.92	8.37
12 YRS	9.25	9.97	9.50	10.44	9.59	10.35	10.17	8.74
13 YRS	9.48	10.22	9.94	10.83	9.95	10.65	10.43	9.12
14 YRS	9.72	10.47	10.37	11.22	10.31	10.96	10.69	9.50
15 YRS	9.96	10.72	10.80	11.62	10.67	11.26	10.95	9.88
16 YRS	10.20	10.97	11.23	12.01	11.03	11.56	11.21	10.26
17 YRS	10.44	11.21	11.66	12.40	11.39	11.87	11.47	10.64
18 YRS	10.68	11.46	12.09	12.79	11.75	12.17	11.73	11.01
19 YRS	10.92	11.71	12.53	13.19	12.11	12.47	11.99	11.39
20 YRS	11.16	11.96	12.96	13.58	12.47	12.78	12.25	11.77
21 YRS	11.40	12.20	13.39	13.97	12.83	13.08	12.51	12.15
22 YRS	11.64	12.45	13.82	14.36	13.19	13.38	12.77	12.53
23 YRS	11.88	12.70	14.25	14.76	13.55	13.69	13.03	12.90
24 YRS	12.12	12.95	14.68	15.15	13.91	13.99	13.29	13.28
25 YRS	12.36	13.20	15.11	15.54	14.27	14.29	13.55	13.66
26 YRS	12.59	13.44	15.55	15.93	14.63	14.59	13.81	14.04
27 YRS	12.83	13.69	15.98	16.33	14.99	14.90	14.07	14.42
28 YRS	13.07	13.94	16.41	16.72	15.35	15.20	14.33	14.80
29 YRS	13.31	14.19	16.84	17.11	15.71	15.50	14.59	15.17
30 YRS	13.55	14.44	17.27	17.50	16.07	15.81	14.85	15.55

Table 26.1. Age 85 – Male.

EDUCATION	BUSCHFR1	BRETRIE	REYA1	REYA2	REYA3	REYA4	REYA5	REYTOT	REYB1	REYA6
0 YRS	8.13	7.54	7.51	7.12	5.42	5.37	4.40	6.81	5.71	4.96
1 YRS	8.19	7.65	7.64	7.24	5.66	5.60	4.71	6.95	5.93	5.21
2 YRS	8.26	7.76	7.76	7.36	5.89	5.82	5.02	7.09	6.15	5.47
3 YRS	8.32	7.87	7.89	7.48	6.12	6.05	5.32	7.23	6.37	5.72
4 YRS	8.38	7.98	8.01	7.60	6.36	6.28	5.63	7.37	6.59	5.98
5 YRS	8.45	8.09	8.14	7.72	6.59	6.50	5.94	7.50	6.81	6.23
6 YRS	8.51	8.20	8.26	7.84	6.82	6.73	6.24	7.64	7.03	6.48
7 YRS	8.57	8.31	8.39	7.96	7.06	6.96	6.55	7.78	7.25	6.74
8 YRS	8.64	8.42	8.51	8.08	7.29	7.18	6.86	7.92	7.47	6.99
9 YRS	8.70	8.53	8.64	8.20	7.52	7.41	7.16	8.06	7.69	7.25
10 YRS	8.76	8.64	8.77	8.33	7.76	7.64	7.47	8.20	7.92	7.50
11 YRS	8.83	8.75	8.89	8.45	7.99	7.87	7.78	8.33	8.14	7.75
12 YRS	8.89	8.86	9.02	8.57	8.22	8.09	8.08	8.47	8.36	8.01
13 YRS	8.95	8.97	9.14	8.69	8.45	8.32	8.39	8.61	8.58	8.26
14 YRS	9.02	9.08	9.27	8.81	8.69	8.55	8.70	8.75	8.80	8.52
15 YRS	9.08	9.19	9.39	8.93	8.92	8.77	9.01	8.89	9.02	8.77
16 YRS	9.14	9.30	9.52	9.05	9.15	9.00	9.31	9.02	9.24	9.02
17 YRS	9.20	9.41	9.64	9.17	9.39	9.23	9.62	9.16	9.46	9.28
18 YRS	9.27	9.52	9.77	9.29	9.62	9.46	9.93	9.30	9.68	9.53
19 YRS	9.33	9.63	9.89	9.41	9.85	9.68	10.23	9.44	9.90	9.79
20 YRS	9.39	9.74	10.02	9.53	10.09	9.91	10.54	9.58	10.13	10.04
21 YRS	9.46	9.85	10.15	9.65	10.32	10.14	10.85	9.72	10.35	10.29
22 YRS	9.52	9.96	10.27	9.77	10.55	10.36	11.15	9.85	10.57	10.55
23 YRS	9.58	10.07	10.40	9.89	10.79	10.59	11.46	9.99	10.79	10.80
24 YRS	9.65	10.18	10.52	10.01	11.02	10.82	11.77	10.13	11.01	11.05
25 YRS	9.71	10.29	10.65	10.13	11.25	11.04	12.07	10.27	11.23	11.31
26 YRS	9.77	10.40	10.77	10.25	11.49	11.27	12.38	10.41	11.45	11.56
27 YRS	9.84	10.50	10.90	10.37	11.72	11.50	12.69	10.54	11.67	11.82
28 YRS	9.90	10.61	11.02	10.49	11.95	11.73	12.99	10.68	11.89	12.07
29 YRS	9.96	10.72	11.15	10.61	12.19	11.95	13.30	10.82	12.11	12.32
30 YRS	10.03	10.83	11.28	10.73	12.42	12.18	13.61	10.96	12.33	12.58

EDUCATION	CORRECT	DIGITSPA	WAISIMIL	WAISJUDG	VERBAL	ANIMAL	WAISBLOC	DIGIT
0 YRS	6.22	6.93	4.23	5.66	5.20	6.60	6.94	3.98
1 YRS	6.46	7.18	4.66	6.05	5.56	6.90	7.20	4.36
2 YRS	6.70	7.43	5.09	6.45	5.93	7.20	7.46	4.74
3 YRS	6.94	7.68	5.53	6.84	6.29	7.51	7.72	5.12
4 YRS	7.18	7.93	5.96	7.23	6.65	7.81	7.98	5.50
5 YRS	7.42	8.17	6.39	7.62	7.01	8.11	8.24	5.88
6 YRS	7.66	8.42	6.82	8.02	7.37	8.42	8.50	6.25
7 YRS	7.90	8.67	7.25	8.41	7.73	8.72	8.76	6.63
8 YRS	8.13	8.92	7.68	8.80	8.09	9.02	9.02	7.01
9 YRS	8.37	9.16	8.11	9.20	8.45	9.32	9.28	7.39
10 YRS	8.61	9.41	8.55	9.59	8.81	9.63	9.54	7.77
11 YRS	8.85	9.66	8.98	9.98	9.17	9.93	9.80	8.14
12 YRS	9.09	9.91	9.41	10.37	9.53	10.23	10.06	8.52
13 YRS	9.33	10.16	9.84	10.77	9.89	10.54	10.32	8.90
14 YRS	9.57	10.40	10.27	11.16	10.25	10.84	10.58	9.28
15 YRS	9.81	10.65	10.70	11.55	10.61	11.14	10.84	9.66
16 YRS	10.05	10.90	11.14	11.94	10.97	11.45	11.10	10.04
17 YRS	10.29	11.15	11.57	12.34	11.33	11.75	11.36	10.41
18 YRS	10.53	11.40	12.00	12.73	11.69	12.05	11.62	10.79
19 YRS	10.77	11.64	12.43	13.12	12.05	12.36	11.88	11.17
20 YRS	11.00	11.89	12.86	13.51	12.41	12.66	12.14	11.55
21 YRS	11.24	12.14	13.29	13.91	12.77	12.96	12.40	11.93
22 YRS	11.48	12.39	13.72	14.30	13.13	13.26	12.66	12.31
23 YRS	11.72	12.63	14.16	14.69	13.49	13.57	12.92	12.68
24 YRS	11.96	12.88	14.59	15.08	13.85	13.87	13.18	13.06
25 YRS	12.20	13.13	15.02	15.48	14.21	14.17	13.43	13.44
26 YRS	12.44	13.38	15.45	15.87	14.57	14.48	13.69	13.82
27 YRS	12.68	13.63	15.88	16.26	14.93	14.78	13.95	14.20
28 YRS	12.92	13.87	16.31	16.66	15.30	15.08	14.21	14.58
29 YRS	13.16	14.12	16.75	17.05	15.66	15.39	14.47	14.95
30 YRS	13.40	14.37	17.18	17.44	16.02	15.69	14.73	15.33

Table 26.2. Age 85 – Female.

EDUCATION	BUSCHFR1	BRETRIE	REYA1	REYA2	REYA3	REYA4	REYA5	REYTOT	REYB1	REYA6
0 YRS	8.13	7.54	7.51	7.12	5.42	5.37	4.40	6.81	5.71	4.96
1 YRS	8.19	7.65	7.64	7.24	5.66	5.60	4.71	6.95	5.93	5.21
2 YRS	8.26	7.76	7.76	7.36	5.89	5.82	5.02	7.09	6.15	5.47
3 YRS	8.32	7.87	7.89	7.48	6.12	6.05	5.32	7.23	6.37	5.72
4 YRS	8.38	7.98	8.01	7.60	6.36	6.28	5.63	7.37	6.59	5.98
5 YRS	8.45	8.09	8.14	7.72	6.59	6.50	5.94	7.50	6.81	6.23
6 YRS	8.51	8.20	8.26	7.84	6.82	6.73	6.24	7.64	7.03	6.48
7 YRS	8.57	8.31	8.39	7.96	7.06	6.96	6.55	7.78	7.25	6.74
8 YRS	8.64	8.42	8.51	8.08	7.29	7.18	6.86	7.92	7.47	6.99
9 YRS	8.70	8.53	8.64	8.20	7.52	7.41	7.16	8.06	7.69	7.25
10 YRS	8.76	8.64	8.77	8.33	7.76	7.64	7.47	8.20	7.92	7.50
11 YRS	8.83	8.75	8.89	8.45	7.99	7.87	7.78	8.33	8.14	7.75
12 YRS	8.89	8.86	9.02	8.57	8.22	8.09	8.08	8.47	8.36	8.01
13 YRS	8.95	8.97	9.14	8.69	8.45	8.32	8.39	8.61	8.58	8.26
14 YRS	9.02	9.08	9.27	8.81	8.69	8.55	8.70	8.75	8.80	8.52
15 YRS	9.08	9.19	9.39	8.93	8.92	8.77	9.01	8.89	9.02	8.77
16 YRS	9.14	9.30	9.52	9.05	9.15	9.00	9.31	9.02	9.24	9.02
17 YRS	9.20	9.41	9.64	9.17	9.39	9.23	9.62	9.16	9.46	9.28
18 YRS	9.27	9.52	9.77	9.29	9.62	9.46	9.93	9.30	9.68	9.53
19 YRS	9.33	9.63	9.89	9.41	9.85	9.68	10.23	9.44	9.90	9.79
20 YRS	9.39	9.74	10.02	9.53	10.09	9.91	10.54	9.58	10.13	10.04
21 YRS	9.46	9.85	10.15	9.65	10.32	10.14	10.85	9.72	10.35	10.29
22 YRS	9.52	9.96	10.27	9.77	10.55	10.36	11.15	9.85	10.57	10.55
23 YRS	9.58	10.07	10.40	9.89	10.79	10.59	11.46	9.99	10.79	10.80
24 YRS	9.65	10.18	10.52	10.01	11.02	10.82	11.77	10.13	11.01	11.05
25 YRS	9.71	10.29	10.65	10.13	11.25	11.04	12.07	10.27	11.23	11.31
26 YRS	9.77	10.40	10.77	10.25	11.49	11.27	12.38	10.41	11.45	11.56
27 YRS	9.84	10.50	10.90	10.37	11.72	11.50	12.69	10.54	11.67	11.82
28 YRS	9.90	10.61	11.02	10.49	11.95	11.73	12.99	10.68	11.89	12.07
29 YRS	9.96	10.72	11.15	10.61	12.19	11.95	13.30	10.82	12.11	12.32
30 YRS	10.03	10.83	11.28	10.73	12.42	12.18	13.61	10.96	12.33	12.58

EDUCATION	CORRECT	DIGITSPA	WAISIMIL	WAISJUDG	VERBAL	ANIMAL	WAISBLOC	DIGIT
0 YRS	6.22	6.93	4.23	5.66	5.20	6.60	6.94	3.98
1 YRS	6.46	7.18	4.66	6.05	5.56	6.90	7.20	4.36
2 YRS	6.70	7.43	5.09	6.45	5.93	7.20	7.46	4.74
3 YRS	6.94	7.68	5.53	6.84	6.29	7.51	7.72	5.12
4 YRS	7.18	7.93	5.96	7.23	6.65	7.81	7.98	5.50
5 YRS	7.42	8.17	6.39	7.62	7.01	8.11	8.24	5.88
6 YRS	7.66	8.42	6.82	8.02	7.37	8.42	8.50	6.25
7 YRS	7.90	8.67	7.25	8.41	7.73	8.72	8.76	6.63
8 YRS	8.13	8.92	7.68	8.80	8.09	9.02	9.02	7.01
9 YRS	8.37	9.16	8.11	9.20	8.45	9.32	9.28	7.39
10 YRS	8.61	9.41	8.55	9.59	8.81	9.63	9.54	7.77
11 YRS	8.85	9.66	8.98	9.98	9.17	9.93	9.80	8.14
12 YRS	9.09	9.91	9.41	10.37	9.53	10.23	10.06	8.52
13 YRS	9.33	10.16	9.84	10.77	9.89	10.54	10.32	8.90
14 YRS	9.57	10.40	10.27	11.16	10.25	10.84	10.58	9.28
15 YRS	9.81	10.65	10.70	11.55	10.61	11.14	10.84	9.66
16 YRS	10.05	10.90	11.14	11.94	10.97	11.45	11.10	10.04
17 YRS	10.29	11.15	11.57	12.34	11.33	11.75	11.36	10.41
18 YRS	10.53	11.40	12.00	12.73	11.69	12.05	11.62	10.79
19 YRS	10.77	11.64	12.43	13.12	12.05	12.36	11.88	11.17
20 YRS	11.00	11.89	12.86	13.51	12.41	12.66	12.14	11.55
21 YRS	11.24	12.14	13.29	13.91	12.77	12.96	12.40	11.93
22 YRS	11.48	12.39	13.72	14.30	13.13	13.26	12.66	12.31
23 YRS	11.72	12.63	14.16	14.69	13.49	13.57	12.92	12.68
24 YRS	11.96	12.88	14.59	15.08	13.85	13.87	13.18	13.06
25 YRS	12.20	13.13	15.02	15.48	14.21	14.17	13.43	13.44
26 YRS	12.44	13.38	15.45	15.87	14.57	14.48	13.69	13.82
27 YRS	12.68	13.63	15.88	16.26	14.93	14.78	13.95	14.20
28 YRS	12.92	13.87	16.31	16.66	15.30	15.08	14.21	14.58
29 YRS	13.16	14.12	16.75	17.05	15.66	15.39	14.47	14.95
30 YRS	13.40	14.37	17.18	17.44	16.02	15.69	14.73	15.33

Table 27.1. Age 86 – Male.

EDUCATION	BUSCHFR1	BRETRIE	REYA1	REYA2	REYA3	REYA4	REYA5	REYTOT	REYB1	REYA6
0 YRS	8.01	7.38	7.41	7.02	5.27	5.22	4.26	6.66	5.54	4.80
1 YRS	8.07	7.49	7.54	7.14	5.51	5.45	4.56	6.80	5.76	5.05
2 YRS	8.14	7.60	7.66	7.26	5.74	5.67	4.87	6.94	5.99	5.31
3 YRS	8.20	7.71	7.79	7.38	5.97	5.90	5.18	7.08	6.21	5.56
4 YRS	8.26	7.82	7.92	7.50	6.21	6.13	5.48	7.22	6.43	5.82
5 YRS	8.33	7.92	8.04	7.62	6.44	6.36	5.79	7.35	6.65	6.07
6 YRS	8.39	8.03	8.17	7.74	6.67	6.58	6.10	7.49	6.87	6.32
7 YRS	8.45	8.14	8.29	7.86	6.91	6.81	6.40	7.63	7.09	6.58
8 YRS	8.52	8.25	8.42	7.98	7.14	7.04	6.71	7.77	7.31	6.83
9 YRS	8.58	8.36	8.54	8.10	7.37	7.26	7.02	7.91	7.53	7.09
10 YRS	8.64	8.47	8.67	8.22	7.60	7.49	7.32	8.05	7.75	7.34
11 YRS	8.71	8.58	8.79	8.34	7.84	7.72	7.63	8.18	7.97	7.59
12 YRS	8.77	8.69	8.92	8.46	8.07	7.94	7.94	8.32	8.19	7.85
13 YRS	8.83	8.80	9.04	8.58	8.30	8.17	8.24	8.46	8.42	8.10
14 YRS	8.90	8.91	9.17	8.70	8.54	8.40	8.55	8.60	8.64	8.36
15 YRS	8.96	9.02	9.30	8.82	8.77	8.63	8.86	8.74	8.86	8.61
16 YRS	9.02	9.13	9.42	8.94	9.00	8.85	9.16	8.87	9.08	8.86
17 YRS	9.09	9.24	9.55	9.06	9.24	9.08	9.47	9.01	9.30	9.12
18 YRS	9.15	9.35	9.67	9.18	9.47	9.31	9.78	9.15	9.52	9.37
19 YRS	9.21	9.46	9.80	9.30	9.70	9.53	10.09	9.29	9.74	9.63
20 YRS	9.28	9.57	9.92	9.42	9.94	9.76	10.39	9.43	9.96	9.88
21 YRS	9.34	9.68	10.05	9.54	10.17	9.99	10.70	9.57	10.18	10.13
22 YRS	9.40	9.79	10.17	9.67	10.40	10.21	11.01	9.70	10.40	10.39
23 YRS	9.47	9.90	10.30	9.79	10.64	10.44	11.31	9.84	10.63	10.64
24 YRS	9.53	10.01	10.43	9.91	10.87	10.67	11.62	9.98	10.85	10.89
25 YRS	9.59	10.12	10.55	10.03	11.10	10.90	11.93	10.12	11.07	11.15
26 YRS	9.66	10.23	10.68	10.15	11.33	11.12	12.23	10.26	11.29	11.40
27 YRS	9.72	10.34	10.80	10.27	11.57	11.35	12.54	10.39	11.51	11.66
28 YRS	9.78	10.45	10.93	10.39	11.80	11.58	12.85	10.53	11.73	11.91
29 YRS	9.85	10.56	11.05	10.51	12.03	11.80	13.15	10.67	11.95	12.16
30 YRS	9.91	10.67	11.18	10.63	12.27	12.03	13.46	10.81	12.17	12.42

EDUCATION	CORRECT	DIGITSPA	WAISIMIL	WAISJUDG	VERBAL	ANIMAL	WAISBLOC	DIGIT
0 YRS	6.07	6.87	4.13	5.60	5.15	6.48	6.83	3.76
1 YRS	6.31	7.12	4.57	5.99	5.51	6.78	7.09	4.14
2 YRS	6.54	7.36	5.00	6.38	5.87	7.09	7.35	4.52
3 YRS	6.78	7.61	5.43	6.78	6.23	7.39	7.61	4.90
4 YRS	7.02	7.86	5.86	7.17	6.59	7.69	7.87	5.28
5 YRS	7.26	8.11	6.29	7.56	6.95	8.00	8.13	5.65
6 YRS	7.50	8.36	6.72	7.95	7.31	8.30	8.39	6.03
7 YRS	7.74	8.60	7.16	8.35	7.67	8.60	8.65	6.41
8 YRS	7.98	8.85	7.59	8.74	8.03	8.90	8.91	6.79
9 YRS	8.22	9.10	8.02	9.13	8.39	9.21	9.17	7.17
10 YRS	8.46	9.35	8.45	9.52	8.75	9.51	9.43	7.55
11 YRS	8.70	9.59	8.88	9.92	9.11	9.81	9.68	7.92
12 YRS	8.94	9.84	9.31	10.31	9.47	10.12	9.94	8.30
13 YRS	9.18	10.09	9.75	10.70	9.83	10.42	10.20	8.68
14 YRS	9.42	10.34	10.18	11.09	10.19	10.72	10.46	9.06
15 YRS	9.65	10.59	10.61	11.49	10.55	11.03	10.72	9.44
16 YRS	9.89	10.83	11.04	11.88	10.91	11.33	10.98	9.82
17 YRS	10.13	11.08	11.47	12.27	11.27	11.63	11.24	10.19
18 YRS	10.37	11.33	11.90	12.67	11.63	11.94	11.50	10.57
19 YRS	10.61	11.58	12.33	13.06	12.00	12.24	11.76	10.95
20 YRS	10.85	11.83	12.77	13.45	12.36	12.54	12.02	11.33
21 YRS	11.09	12.07	13.20	13.84	12.72	12.84	12.28	11.71
22 YRS	11.33	12.32	13.63	14.24	13.08	13.15	12.54	12.09
23 YRS	11.57	12.57	14.06	14.63	13.44	13.45	12.80	12.46
24 YRS	11.81	12.82	14.49	15.02	13.80	13.75	13.06	12.84
25 YRS	12.05	13.06	14.92	15.41	14.16	14.06	13.32	13.22
26 YRS	12.29	13.31	15.36	15.81	14.52	14.36	13.58	13.60
27 YRS	12.53	13.56	15.79	16.20	14.88	14.66	13.84	13.98
28 YRS	12.76	13.81	16.22	16.59	15.24	14.97	14.10	14.36
29 YRS	13.00	14.06	16.65	16.98	15.60	15.27	14.36	14.73
30 YRS	13.24	14.30	17.08	17.38	15.96	15.57	14.62	15.11

Table 27.2. Age 86 – Female.

EDUCATION	BUSCHFR1	BRETRIE	REYA1	REYA2	REYA3	REYA4	REYA5	REYTOT	REYB1	REYA6
0 YRS	8.01	7.38	7.41	7.02	5.27	5.22	4.26	6.66	5.54	4.80
1 YRS	8.07	7.49	7.54	7.14	5.51	5.45	4.56	6.80	5.76	5.05
2 YRS	8.14	7.60	7.66	7.26	5.74	5.67	4.87	6.94	5.99	5.31
3 YRS	8.20	7.71	7.79	7.38	5.97	5.90	5.18	7.08	6.21	5.56
4 YRS	8.26	7.82	7.92	7.50	6.21	6.13	5.48	7.22	6.43	5.82
5 YRS	8.33	7.92	8.04	7.62	6.44	6.36	5.79	7.35	6.65	6.07
6 YRS	8.39	8.03	8.17	7.74	6.67	6.58	6.10	7.49	6.87	6.32
7 YRS	8.45	8.14	8.29	7.86	6.91	6.81	6.40	7.63	7.09	6.58
8 YRS	8.52	8.25	8.42	7.98	7.14	7.04	6.71	7.77	7.31	6.83
9 YRS	8.58	8.36	8.54	8.10	7.37	7.26	7.02	7.91	7.53	7.09
10 YRS	8.64	8.47	8.67	8.22	7.60	7.49	7.32	8.05	7.75	7.34
11 YRS	8.71	8.58	8.79	8.34	7.84	7.72	7.63	8.18	7.97	7.59
12 YRS	8.77	8.69	8.92	8.46	8.07	7.94	7.94	8.32	8.19	7.85
13 YRS	8.83	8.80	9.04	8.58	8.30	8.17	8.24	8.46	8.42	8.10
14 YRS	8.90	8.91	9.17	8.70	8.54	8.40	8.55	8.60	8.64	8.36
15 YRS	8.96	9.02	9.30	8.82	8.77	8.63	8.86	8.74	8.86	8.61
16 YRS	9.02	9.13	9.42	8.94	9.00	8.85	9.16	8.87	9.08	8.86
17 YRS	9.09	9.24	9.55	9.06	9.24	9.08	9.47	9.01	9.30	9.12
18 YRS	9.15	9.35	9.67	9.18	9.47	9.31	9.78	9.15	9.52	9.37
19 YRS	9.21	9.46	9.80	9.30	9.70	9.53	10.09	9.29	9.74	9.63
20 YRS	9.28	9.57	9.92	9.42	9.94	9.76	10.39	9.43	9.96	9.88
21 YRS	9.34	9.68	10.05	9.54	10.17	9.99	10.70	9.57	10.18	10.13
22 YRS	9.40	9.79	10.17	9.67	10.40	10.21	11.01	9.70	10.40	10.39
23 YRS	9.47	9.90	10.30	9.79	10.64	10.44	11.31	9.84	10.63	10.64
24 YRS	9.53	10.01	10.43	9.91	10.87	10.67	11.62	9.98	10.85	10.89
25 YRS	9.59	10.12	10.55	10.03	11.10	10.90	11.93	10.12	11.07	11.15
26 YRS	9.66	10.23	10.68	10.15	11.33	11.12	12.23	10.26	11.29	11.40
27 YRS	9.72	10.34	10.80	10.27	11.57	11.35	12.54	10.39	11.51	11.66
28 YRS	9.78	10.45	10.93	10.39	11.80	11.58	12.85	10.53	11.73	11.91
29 YRS	9.85	10.56	11.05	10.51	12.03	11.80	13.15	10.67	11.95	12.16
30 YRS	9.91	10.67	11.18	10.63	12.27	12.03	13.46	10.81	12.17	12.42

EDUCATION	CORRECT	DIGITSPA	WAISMIL	WAISJUDG	VERBAL	ANIMAL	WAISBLOC	DIGIT
0 YRS	6.07	6.87	4.13	5.60	5.15	6.48	6.83	3.76
1 YRS	6.31	7.12	4.57	5.99	5.51	6.78	7.09	4.14
2 YRS	6.54	7.36	5.00	6.38	5.87	7.09	7.35	4.52
3 YRS	6.78	7.61	5.43	6.78	6.23	7.39	7.61	4.90
4 YRS	7.02	7.86	5.86	7.17	6.59	7.69	7.87	5.28
5 YRS	7.26	8.11	6.29	7.56	6.95	8.00	8.13	5.65
6 YRS	7.50	8.36	6.72	7.95	7.31	8.30	8.39	6.03
7 YRS	7.74	8.60	7.16	8.35	7.67	8.60	8.65	6.41
8 YRS	7.98	8.85	7.59	8.74	8.03	8.90	8.91	6.79
9 YRS	8.22	9.10	8.02	9.13	8.39	9.21	9.17	7.17
10 YRS	8.46	9.35	8.45	9.52	8.75	9.51	9.43	7.55
11 YRS	8.70	9.59	8.88	9.92	9.11	9.81	9.68	7.92
12 YRS	8.94	9.84	9.31	10.31	9.47	10.12	9.94	8.30
13 YRS	9.18	10.09	9.75	10.70	9.83	10.42	10.20	8.68
14 YRS	9.42	10.34	10.18	11.09	10.19	10.72	10.46	9.06
15 YRS	9.65	10.59	10.61	11.49	10.55	11.03	10.72	9.44
16 YRS	9.89	10.83	11.04	11.88	10.91	11.33	10.98	9.82
17 YRS	10.13	11.08	11.47	12.27	11.27	11.63	11.24	10.19
18 YRS	10.37	11.33	11.90	12.67	11.63	11.94	11.50	10.57
19 YRS	10.61	11.58	12.33	13.06	12.00	12.24	11.76	10.95
20 YRS	10.85	11.83	12.77	13.45	12.36	12.54	12.02	11.33
21 YRS	11.09	12.07	13.20	13.84	12.72	12.84	12.28	11.71
22 YRS	11.33	12.32	13.63	14.24	13.08	13.15	12.54	12.09
23 YRS	11.57	12.57	14.06	14.63	13.44	13.45	12.80	12.46
24 YRS	11.81	12.82	14.49	15.02	13.80	13.75	13.06	12.84
25 YRS	12.05	13.06	14.92	15.41	14.16	14.06	13.32	13.22
26 YRS	12.29	13.31	15.36	15.81	14.52	14.36	13.58	13.60
27 YRS	12.53	13.56	15.79	16.20	14.88	14.66	13.84	13.98
28 YRS	12.76	13.81	16.22	16.59	15.24	14.97	14.10	14.36
29 YRS	13.00	14.06	16.65	16.98	15.60	15.27	14.36	14.73
30 YRS	13.24	14.30	17.08	17.38	15.96	15.57	14.62	15.11

Table 28.1. Age 87 – Male.

EDUCATION	BUSCHFR1	BRETRIE	REYA1	REYA2	REYA3	REYA4	REYA5	REYTOT	REYB1	REYA6
0 YRS	7.89	7.21	7.32	6.91	5.12	5.07	4.11	6.51	5.38	4.64
1 YRS	7.96	7.32	7.44	7.03	5.36	5.30	4.42	6.65	5.60	4.89
2 YRS	8.02	7.43	7.57	7.15	5.59	5.53	4.72	6.79	5.82	5.15
3 YRS	8.08	7.54	7.69	7.27	5.82	5.75	5.03	6.93	6.04	5.40
4 YRS	8.15	7.65	7.82	7.39	6.05	5.98	5.34	7.07	6.26	5.66
5 YRS	8.21	7.76	7.94	7.51	6.29	6.21	5.64	7.20	6.49	5.91
6 YRS	8.27	7.87	8.07	7.63	6.52	6.43	5.95	7.34	6.71	6.16
7 YRS	8.34	7.98	8.19	7.75	6.75	6.66	6.26	7.48	6.93	6.42
8 YRS	8.40	8.09	8.32	7.87	6.99	6.89	6.56	7.62	7.15	6.67
9 YRS	8.46	8.20	8.45	8.00	7.22	7.11	6.87	7.76	7.37	6.93
10 YRS	8.53	8.31	8.57	8.12	7.45	7.34	7.18	7.90	7.59	7.18
11 YRS	8.59	8.42	8.70	8.24	7.69	7.57	7.48	8.03	7.81	7.43
12 YRS	8.65	8.53	8.82	8.36	7.92	7.80	7.79	8.17	8.03	7.69
13 YRS	8.72	8.64	8.95	8.48	8.15	8.02	8.10	8.31	8.25	7.94
14 YRS	8.78	8.75	9.07	8.60	8.39	8.25	8.40	8.45	8.47	8.20
15 YRS	8.84	8.86	9.20	8.72	8.62	8.48	8.71	8.59	8.70	8.45
16 YRS	8.91	8.97	9.32	8.84	8.85	8.70	9.02	8.72	8.92	8.70
17 YRS	8.97	9.08	9.45	8.96	9.09	8.93	9.32	8.86	9.14	8.96
18 YRS	9.03	9.19	9.58	9.08	9.32	9.16	9.63	9.00	9.36	9.21
19 YRS	9.10	9.30	9.70	9.20	9.55	9.39	9.94	9.14	9.58	9.47
20 YRS	9.16	9.41	9.83	9.32	9.79	9.61	10.25	9.28	9.80	9.72
21 YRS	9.22	9.52	9.95	9.44	10.02	9.84	10.55	9.42	10.02	9.97
22 YRS	9.29	9.63	10.08	9.56	10.25	10.07	10.86	9.55	10.24	10.23
23 YRS	9.35	9.74	10.20	9.68	10.48	10.29	11.17	9.69	10.46	10.48
24 YRS	9.41	9.85	10.33	9.80	10.72	10.52	11.47	9.83	10.68	10.73
25 YRS	9.48	9.96	10.45	9.92	10.95	10.75	11.78	9.97	10.90	10.99
26 YRS	9.54	10.07	10.58	10.04	11.18	10.97	12.09	10.11	11.13	11.24
27 YRS	9.60	10.18	10.71	10.16	11.42	11.20	12.39	10.24	11.35	11.50
28 YRS	9.66	10.29	10.83	10.28	11.65	11.43	12.70	10.38	11.57	11.75
29 YRS	9.73	10.40	10.96	10.40	11.88	11.66	13.01	10.52	11.79	12.00
30 YRS	9.79	10.51	11.08	10.52	12.12	11.88	13.31	10.66	12.01	12.26

EDUCATION	CORRECT	DIGITSPA	WAISIMIL	WAISJUDG	VERBAL	ANIMAL	WAISBLOC	DIGIT
0 YRS	5.91	6.80	4.04	5.53	5.09	6.36	6.71	3.54
1 YRS	6.15	7.05	4.47	5.93	5.45	6.67	6.97	3.92
2 YRS	6.39	7.30	4.90	6.32	5.81	6.97	7.23	4.30
3 YRS	6.63	7.55	5.33	6.71	6.17	7.27	7.49	4.68
4 YRS	6.87	7.79	5.77	7.10	6.53	7.58	7.75	5.06
5 YRS	7.11	8.04	6.20	7.50	6.89	7.88	8.01	5.43
6 YRS	7.35	8.29	6.63	7.89	7.25	8.18	8.27	5.81
7 YRS	7.59	8.54	7.06	8.28	7.61	8.48	8.53	6.19
8 YRS	7.83	8.79	7.49	8.67	7.97	8.79	8.79	6.57
9 YRS	8.07	9.03	7.92	9.07	8.33	9.09	9.05	6.95
10 YRS	8.30	9.28	8.36	9.46	8.70	9.39	9.31	7.33
11 YRS	8.54	9.53	8.79	9.85	9.06	9.70	9.57	7.70
12 YRS	8.78	9.78	9.22	10.25	9.42	10.00	9.83	8.08
13 YRS	9.02	10.02	9.65	10.64	9.78	10.30	10.09	8.46
14 YRS	9.26	10.27	10.08	11.03	10.14	10.61	10.35	8.84
15 YRS	9.50	10.52	10.51	11.42	10.50	10.91	10.61	9.22
16 YRS	9.74	10.77	10.94	11.82	10.86	11.21	10.87	9.60
17 YRS	9.98	11.02	11.38	12.21	11.22	11.52	11.13	9.97
18 YRS	10.22	11.26	11.81	12.60	11.58	11.82	11.39	10.35
19 YRS	10.46	11.51	12.24	12.99	11.94	12.12	11.65	10.73
20 YRS	10.70	11.76	12.67	13.39	12.30	12.42	11.91	11.11
21 YRS	10.94	12.01	13.10	13.78	12.66	12.73	12.17	11.49
22 YRS	11.18	12.26	13.53	14.17	13.02	13.03	12.43	11.87
23 YRS	11.41	12.50	13.97	14.56	13.38	13.33	12.69	12.24
24 YRS	11.65	12.75	14.40	14.96	13.74	13.64	12.94	12.62
25 YRS	11.89	13.00	14.83	15.35	14.10	13.94	13.20	13.00
26 YRS	12.13	13.25	15.26	15.74	14.46	14.24	13.46	13.38
27 YRS	12.37	13.49	15.69	16.14	14.82	14.55	13.72	13.76
28 YRS	12.61	13.74	16.12	16.53	15.18	14.85	13.98	14.14
29 YRS	12.85	13.99	16.56	16.92	15.54	15.15	14.24	14.51
30 YRS	13.09	14.24	16.99	17.31	15.90	15.46	14.50	14.89

Table 28.2. Age 87 – Female.

EDUCATION	BUSCHFR1	BRETRIE	REYA1	REYA2	REYA3	REYA4	REYA5	REYTOT	REYB1	REYA6
0 YRS	7.89	7.21	7.32	6.91	5.12	5.07	4.11	6.51	5.38	4.64
1 YRS	7.96	7.32	7.44	7.03	5.36	5.30	4.42	6.65	5.60	4.89
2 YRS	8.02	7.43	7.57	7.15	5.59	5.53	4.72	6.79	5.82	5.15
3 YRS	8.08	7.54	7.69	7.27	5.82	5.75	5.03	6.93	6.04	5.40
4 YRS	8.15	7.65	7.82	7.39	6.05	5.98	5.34	7.07	6.26	5.66
5 YRS	8.21	7.76	7.94	7.51	6.29	6.21	5.64	7.20	6.49	5.91
6 YRS	8.27	7.87	8.07	7.63	6.52	6.43	5.95	7.34	6.71	6.16
7 YRS	8.34	7.98	8.19	7.75	6.75	6.66	6.26	7.48	6.93	6.42
8 YRS	8.40	8.09	8.32	7.87	6.99	6.89	6.56	7.62	7.15	6.67
9 YRS	8.46	8.20	8.45	8.00	7.22	7.11	6.87	7.76	7.37	6.93
10 YRS	8.53	8.31	8.57	8.12	7.45	7.34	7.18	7.90	7.59	7.18
11 YRS	8.59	8.42	8.70	8.24	7.69	7.57	7.48	8.03	7.81	7.43
12 YRS	8.65	8.53	8.82	8.36	7.92	7.80	7.79	8.17	8.03	7.69
13 YRS	8.72	8.64	8.95	8.48	8.15	8.02	8.10	8.31	8.25	7.94
14 YRS	8.78	8.75	9.07	8.60	8.39	8.25	8.40	8.45	8.47	8.20
15 YRS	8.84	8.86	9.20	8.72	8.62	8.48	8.71	8.59	8.70	8.45
16 YRS	8.91	8.97	9.32	8.84	8.85	8.70	9.02	8.72	8.92	8.70
17 YRS	8.97	9.08	9.45	8.96	9.09	8.93	9.32	8.86	9.14	8.96
18 YRS	9.03	9.19	9.58	9.08	9.32	9.16	9.63	9.00	9.36	9.21
19 YRS	9.10	9.30	9.70	9.20	9.55	9.39	9.94	9.14	9.58	9.47
20 YRS	9.16	9.41	9.83	9.32	9.79	9.61	10.25	9.28	9.80	9.72
21 YRS	9.22	9.52	9.95	9.44	10.02	9.84	10.55	9.42	10.02	9.97
22 YRS	9.29	9.63	10.08	9.56	10.25	10.07	10.86	9.55	10.24	10.23
23 YRS	9.35	9.74	10.20	9.68	10.48	10.29	11.17	9.69	10.46	10.48
24 YRS	9.41	9.85	10.33	9.80	10.72	10.52	11.47	9.83	10.68	10.73
25 YRS	9.48	9.96	10.45	9.92	10.95	10.75	11.78	9.97	10.90	10.99
26 YRS	9.54	10.07	10.58	10.04	11.18	10.97	12.09	10.11	11.13	11.24
27 YRS	9.60	10.18	10.71	10.16	11.42	11.20	12.39	10.24	11.35	11.50
28 YRS	9.66	10.29	10.83	10.28	11.65	11.43	12.70	10.38	11.57	11.75
29 YRS	9.73	10.40	10.96	10.40	11.88	11.66	13.01	10.52	11.79	12.00
30 YRS	9.79	10.51	11.08	10.52	12.12	11.88	13.31	10.66	12.01	12.26

EDUCATION	CORRECT	DIGITSPA	WAISIMIL	WAISJUDG	VERBAL	ANIMAL	WAISBLOC	DIGIT
0 YRS	5.91	6.80	4.04	5.53	5.09	6.36	6.71	3.54
1 YRS	6.15	7.05	4.47	5.93	5.45	6.67	6.97	3.92
2 YRS	6.39	7.30	4.90	6.32	5.81	6.97	7.23	4.30
3 YRS	6.63	7.55	5.33	6.71	6.17	7.27	7.49	4.68
4 YRS	6.87	7.79	5.77	7.10	6.53	7.58	7.75	5.06
5 YRS	7.11	8.04	6.20	7.50	6.89	7.88	8.01	5.43
6 YRS	7.35	8.29	6.63	7.89	7.25	8.18	8.27	5.81
7 YRS	7.59	8.54	7.06	8.28	7.61	8.48	8.53	6.19
8 YRS	7.83	8.79	7.49	8.67	7.97	8.79	8.79	6.57
9 YRS	8.07	9.03	7.92	9.07	8.33	9.09	9.05	6.95
10 YRS	8.30	9.28	8.36	9.46	8.70	9.39	9.31	7.33
11 YRS	8.54	9.53	8.79	9.85	9.06	9.70	9.57	7.70
12 YRS	8.78	9.78	9.22	10.25	9.42	10.00	9.83	8.08
13 YRS	9.02	10.02	9.65	10.64	9.78	10.30	10.09	8.46
14 YRS	9.26	10.27	10.08	11.03	10.14	10.61	10.35	8.84
15 YRS	9.50	10.52	10.51	11.42	10.50	10.91	10.61	9.22
16 YRS	9.74	10.77	10.94	11.82	10.86	11.21	10.87	9.60
17 YRS	9.98	11.02	11.38	12.21	11.22	11.52	11.13	9.97
18 YRS	10.22	11.26	11.81	12.60	11.58	11.82	11.39	10.35
19 YRS	10.46	11.51	12.24	12.99	11.94	12.12	11.65	10.73
20 YRS	10.70	11.76	12.67	13.39	12.30	12.42	11.91	11.11
21 YRS	10.94	12.01	13.10	13.78	12.66	12.73	12.17	11.49
22 YRS	11.18	12.26	13.53	14.17	13.02	13.03	12.43	11.87
23 YRS	11.41	12.50	13.97	14.56	13.38	13.33	12.69	12.24
24 YRS	11.65	12.75	14.40	14.96	13.74	13.64	12.94	12.62
25 YRS	11.89	13.00	14.83	15.35	14.10	13.94	13.20	13.00
26 YRS	12.13	13.25	15.26	15.74	14.46	14.24	13.46	13.38
27 YRS	12.37	13.49	15.69	16.14	14.82	14.55	13.72	13.76
28 YRS	12.61	13.74	16.12	16.53	15.18	14.85	13.98	14.14
29 YRS	12.85	13.99	16.56	16.92	15.54	15.15	14.24	14.51
30 YRS	13.09	14.24	16.99	17.31	15.90	15.46	14.50	14.89

Table 29.1. Age 88 – Male.

EDUCATION	BUSCHFR1	BRETRIE	REYA1	REYA2	REYA3	REYA4	REYA5	REYTOT	REYB1	REYA6
0 YRS	7.78	7.05	7.22	6.81	4.97	4.92	3.96	6.36	5.22	4.48
1 YRS	7.84	7.16	7.34	6.93	5.20	5.15	4.27	6.50	5.44	4.73
2 YRS	7.90	7.27	7.47	7.05	5.44	5.38	4.58	6.64	5.66	4.99
3 YRS	7.97	7.38	7.60	7.17	5.67	5.60	4.88	6.78	5.88	5.24
4 YRS	8.03	7.49	7.72	7.29	5.90	5.83	5.19	6.92	6.10	5.50
5 YRS	8.09	7.60	7.85	7.41	6.14	6.06	5.50	7.05	6.32	5.75
6 YRS	8.15	7.71	7.97	7.53	6.37	6.29	5.80	7.19	6.54	6.00
7 YRS	8.22	7.82	8.10	7.65	6.60	6.51	6.11	7.33	6.76	6.26
8 YRS	8.28	7.93	8.22	7.77	6.84	6.74	6.42	7.47	6.99	6.51
9 YRS	8.34	8.04	8.35	7.89	7.07	6.97	6.72	7.61	7.21	6.77
10 YRS	8.41	8.15	8.47	8.01	7.30	7.19	7.03	7.75	7.43	7.02
11 YRS	8.47	8.26	8.60	8.13	7.54	7.42	7.34	7.88	7.65	7.27
12 YRS	8.53	8.37	8.73	8.25	7.77	7.65	7.64	8.02	7.87	7.53
13 YRS	8.60	8.48	8.85	8.37	8.00	7.87	7.95	8.16	8.09	7.78
14 YRS	8.66	8.59	8.98	8.49	8.24	8.10	8.26	8.30	8.31	8.04
15 YRS	8.72	8.70	9.10	8.61	8.47	8.33	8.56	8.44	8.53	8.29
16 YRS	8.79	8.81	9.23	8.73	8.70	8.56	8.87	8.57	8.75	8.54
17 YRS	8.85	8.92	9.35	8.85	8.94	8.78	9.18	8.71	8.97	8.80
18 YRS	8.91	9.03	9.48	8.97	9.17	9.01	9.48	8.85	9.20	9.05
19 YRS	8.98	9.14	9.60	9.09	9.40	9.24	9.79	8.99	9.42	9.31
20 YRS	9.04	9.25	9.73	9.21	9.63	9.46	10.10	9.13	9.64	9.56
21 YRS	9.10	9.36	9.86	9.34	9.87	9.69	10.40	9.27	9.86	9.81
22 YRS	9.17	9.47	9.98	9.46	10.10	9.92	10.71	9.40	10.08	10.07
23 YRS	9.23	9.58	10.11	9.58	10.33	10.14	11.02	9.54	10.30	10.32
24 YRS	9.29	9.69	10.23	9.70	10.57	10.37	11.33	9.68	10.52	10.57
25 YRS	9.36	9.80	10.36	9.82	10.80	10.60	11.63	9.82	10.74	10.83
26 YRS	9.42	9.91	10.48	9.94	11.03	10.83	11.94	9.96	10.96	11.08
27 YRS	9.48	10.02	10.61	10.06	11.27	11.05	12.25	10.09	11.18	11.34
28 YRS	9.55	10.13	10.73	10.18	11.50	11.28	12.55	10.23	11.40	11.59
29 YRS	9.61	10.24	10.86	10.30	11.73	11.51	12.86	10.37	11.63	11.84
30 YRS	9.67	10.35	10.98	10.42	11.97	11.73	13.17	10.51	11.85	12.10

EDUCATION	CORRECT	DIGITSPA	WAISIMIL	WAISJUDG	VERBAL	ANIMAL	WAISBLOC	DIGIT
0 YRS	5.76	6.74	3.94	5.47	5.03	6.25	6.60	3.32
1 YRS	6.00	6.98	4.38	5.86	5.40	6.55	6.86	3.70
2 YRS	6.24	7.23	4.81	6.25	5.76	6.85	7.12	4.08
3 YRS	6.48	7.48	5.24	6.65	6.12	7.16	7.38	4.46
4 YRS	6.72	7.73	5.67	7.04	6.48	7.46	7.64	4.84
5 YRS	6.95	7.98	6.10	7.43	6.84	7.76	7.90	5.21
6 YRS	7.19	8.22	6.53	7.83	7.20	8.06	8.16	5.59
7 YRS	7.43	8.47	6.97	8.22	7.56	8.37	8.42	5.97
8 YRS	7.67	8.72	7.40	8.61	7.92	8.67	8.68	6.35
9 YRS	7.91	8.97	7.83	9.00	8.28	8.97	8.93	6.73
10 YRS	8.15	9.22	8.26	9.40	8.64	9.28	9.19	7.11
11 YRS	8.39	9.46	8.69	9.79	9.00	9.58	9.45	7.48
12 YRS	8.63	9.71	9.12	10.18	9.36	9.88	9.71	7.86
13 YRS	8.87	9.96	9.55	10.57	9.72	10.19	9.97	8.24
14 YRS	9.11	10.21	9.99	10.97	10.08	10.49	10.23	8.62
15 YRS	9.35	10.45	10.42	11.36	10.44	10.79	10.49	9.00
16 YRS	9.59	10.70	10.85	11.75	10.80	11.10	10.75	9.38
17 YRS	9.82	10.95	11.28	12.14	11.16	11.40	11.01	9.75
18 YRS	10.06	11.20	11.71	12.54	11.52	11.70	11.27	10.13
19 YRS	10.30	11.45	12.14	12.93	11.88	12.00	11.53	10.51
20 YRS	10.54	11.69	12.58	13.32	12.24	12.31	11.79	10.89
21 YRS	10.78	11.94	13.01	13.72	12.60	12.61	12.05	11.27
22 YRS	11.02	12.19	13.44	14.11	12.96	12.91	12.31	11.65
23 YRS	11.26	12.44	13.87	14.50	13.32	13.22	12.57	12.02
24 YRS	11.50	12.69	14.30	14.89	13.68	13.52	12.83	12.40
25 YRS	11.74	12.93	14.73	15.29	14.04	13.82	13.09	12.78
26 YRS	11.98	13.18	15.17	15.68	14.40	14.13	13.35	13.16
27 YRS	12.22	13.43	15.60	16.07	14.77	14.43	13.61	13.54
28 YRS	12.46	13.68	16.03	16.46	15.13	14.73	13.87	13.91
29 YRS	12.70	13.92	16.46	16.86	15.49	15.04	14.13	14.29
30 YRS	12.93	14.17	16.89	17.25	15.85	15.34	14.39	14.67

Table 29.2. Age 88 – Female.

EDUCATION	BUSCHFR1	BRETRIE	REYA1	REYA2	REYA3	REYA4	REYA5	REYTOT	REYB1	REYA6
0 YRS	7.78	7.05	7.22	6.81	4.97	4.92	3.96	6.36	5.22	4.48
1 YRS	7.84	7.16	7.34	6.93	5.20	5.15	4.27	6.50	5.44	4.73
2 YRS	7.90	7.27	7.47	7.05	5.44	5.38	4.58	6.64	5.66	4.99
3 YRS	7.97	7.38	7.60	7.17	5.67	5.60	4.88	6.78	5.88	5.24
4 YRS	8.03	7.49	7.72	7.29	5.90	5.83	5.19	6.92	6.10	5.50
5 YRS	8.09	7.60	7.85	7.41	6.14	6.06	5.50	7.05	6.32	5.75
6 YRS	8.15	7.71	7.97	7.53	6.37	6.29	5.80	7.19	6.54	6.00
7 YRS	8.22	7.82	8.10	7.65	6.60	6.51	6.11	7.33	6.76	6.26
8 YRS	8.28	7.93	8.22	7.77	6.84	6.74	6.42	7.47	6.99	6.51
9 YRS	8.34	8.04	8.35	7.89	7.07	6.97	6.72	7.61	7.21	6.77
10 YRS	8.41	8.15	8.47	8.01	7.30	7.19	7.03	7.75	7.43	7.02
11 YRS	8.47	8.26	8.60	8.13	7.54	7.42	7.34	7.88	7.65	7.27
12 YRS	8.53	8.37	8.73	8.25	7.77	7.65	7.64	8.02	7.87	7.53
13 YRS	8.60	8.48	8.85	8.37	8.00	7.87	7.95	8.16	8.09	7.78
14 YRS	8.66	8.59	8.98	8.49	8.24	8.10	8.26	8.30	8.31	8.04
15 YRS	8.72	8.70	9.10	8.61	8.47	8.33	8.56	8.44	8.53	8.29
16 YRS	8.79	8.81	9.23	8.73	8.70	8.56	8.87	8.57	8.75	8.54
17 YRS	8.85	8.92	9.35	8.85	8.94	8.78	9.18	8.71	8.97	8.80
18 YRS	8.91	9.03	9.48	8.97	9.17	9.01	9.48	8.85	9.20	9.05
19 YRS	8.98	9.14	9.60	9.09	9.40	9.24	9.79	8.99	9.42	9.31
20 YRS	9.04	9.25	9.73	9.21	9.63	9.46	10.10	9.13	9.64	9.56
21 YRS	9.10	9.36	9.86	9.34	9.87	9.69	10.40	9.27	9.86	9.81
22 YRS	9.17	9.47	9.98	9.46	10.10	9.92	10.71	9.40	10.08	10.07
23 YRS	9.23	9.58	10.11	9.58	10.33	10.14	11.02	9.54	10.30	10.32
24 YRS	9.29	9.69	10.23	9.70	10.57	10.37	11.33	9.68	10.52	10.57
25 YRS	9.36	9.80	10.36	9.82	10.80	10.60	11.63	9.82	10.74	10.83
26 YRS	9.42	9.91	10.48	9.94	11.03	10.83	11.94	9.96	10.96	11.08
27 YRS	9.48	10.02	10.61	10.06	11.27	11.05	12.25	10.09	11.18	11.34
28 YRS	9.55	10.13	10.73	10.18	11.50	11.28	12.55	10.23	11.40	11.59
29 YRS	9.61	10.24	10.86	10.30	11.73	11.51	12.86	10.37	11.63	11.84
30 YRS	9.67	10.35	10.98	10.42	11.97	11.73	13.17	10.51	11.85	12.10

EDUCATION	CORRECT	DIGITSPA	WAISIMIL	WAISJUDG	VERBAL	ANIMAL	WAISBLOC	DIGIT
0 YRS	5.76	6.74	3.94	5.47	5.03	6.25	6.60	3.32
1 YRS	6.00	6.98	4.38	5.86	5.40	6.55	6.86	3.70
2 YRS	6.24	7.23	4.81	6.25	5.76	6.85	7.12	4.08
3 YRS	6.48	7.48	5.24	6.65	6.12	7.16	7.38	4.46
4 YRS	6.72	7.73	5.67	7.04	6.48	7.46	7.64	4.84
5 YRS	6.95	7.98	6.10	7.43	6.84	7.76	7.90	5.21
6 YRS	7.19	8.22	6.53	7.83	7.20	8.06	8.16	5.59
7 YRS	7.43	8.47	6.97	8.22	7.56	8.37	8.42	5.97
8 YRS	7.67	8.72	7.40	8.61	7.92	8.67	8.68	6.35
9 YRS	7.91	8.97	7.83	9.00	8.28	8.97	8.93	6.73
10 YRS	8.15	9.22	8.26	9.40	8.64	9.28	9.19	7.11
11 YRS	8.39	9.46	8.69	9.79	9.00	9.58	9.45	7.48
12 YRS	8.63	9.71	9.12	10.18	9.36	9.88	9.71	7.86
13 YRS	8.87	9.96	9.55	10.57	9.72	10.19	9.97	8.24
14 YRS	9.11	10.21	9.99	10.97	10.08	10.49	10.23	8.62
15 YRS	9.35	10.45	10.42	11.36	10.44	10.79	10.49	9.00
16 YRS	9.59	10.70	10.85	11.75	10.80	11.10	10.75	9.38
17 YRS	9.82	10.95	11.28	12.14	11.16	11.40	11.01	9.75
18 YRS	10.06	11.20	11.71	12.54	11.52	11.70	11.27	10.13
19 YRS	10.30	11.45	12.14	12.93	11.88	12.00	11.53	10.51
20 YRS	10.54	11.69	12.58	13.32	12.24	12.31	11.79	10.89
21 YRS	10.78	11.94	13.01	13.72	12.60	12.61	12.05	11.27
22 YRS	11.02	12.19	13.44	14.11	12.96	12.91	12.31	11.65
23 YRS	11.26	12.44	13.87	14.50	13.32	13.22	12.57	12.02
24 YRS	11.50	12.69	14.30	14.89	13.68	13.52	12.83	12.40
25 YRS	11.74	12.93	14.73	15.29	14.04	13.82	13.09	12.78
26 YRS	11.98	13.18	15.17	15.68	14.40	14.13	13.35	13.16
27 YRS	12.22	13.43	15.60	16.07	14.77	14.43	13.61	13.54
28 YRS	12.46	13.68	16.03	16.46	15.13	14.73	13.87	13.91
29 YRS	12.70	13.92	16.46	16.86	15.49	15.04	14.13	14.29
30 YRS	12.93	14.17	16.89	17.25	15.85	15.34	14.39	14.67

Table 30.1. Age 89 – Male.

EDUCATION	BUSCHFR1	BRETRIE	REYA1	REYA2	REYA3	REYA4	REYA5	REYTOT	REYB1	REYA6
0 YRS	7.66	6.89	7.12	6.70	4.82	4.77	3.82	6.21	5.06	4.32
1 YRS	7.72	7.00	7.25	6.82	5.05	5.00	4.12	6.35	5.28	4.57
2 YRS	7.78	7.11	7.37	6.94	5.29	5.23	4.43	6.49	5.50	4.83
3 YRS	7.85	7.22	7.50	7.06	5.52	5.46	4.74	6.63	5.72	5.08
4 YRS	7.91	7.33	7.62	7.18	5.75	5.68	5.04	6.77	5.94	5.34
5 YRS	7.97	7.44	7.75	7.30	5.99	5.91	5.35	6.90	6.16	5.59
6 YRS	8.04	7.55	7.88	7.42	6.22	6.14	5.66	7.04	6.38	5.84
7 YRS	8.10	7.66	8.00	7.54	6.45	6.36	5.96	7.18	6.60	6.10
8 YRS	8.16	7.77	8.13	7.67	6.69	6.59	6.27	7.32	6.82	6.35
9 YRS	8.23	7.87	8.25	7.79	6.92	6.82	6.58	7.46	7.04	6.61
10 YRS	8.29	7.98	8.38	7.91	7.15	7.05	6.88	7.60	7.26	6.86
11 YRS	8.35	8.09	8.50	8.03	7.39	7.27	7.19	7.73	7.49	7.11
12 YRS	8.42	8.20	8.63	8.15	7.62	7.50	7.50	7.87	7.71	7.37
13 YRS	8.48	8.31	8.75	8.27	7.85	7.73	7.80	8.01	7.93	7.62
14 YRS	8.54	8.42	8.88	8.39	8.08	7.95	8.11	8.15	8.15	7.88
15 YRS	8.61	8.53	9.01	8.51	8.32	8.18	8.42	8.29	8.37	8.13
16 YRS	8.67	8.64	9.13	8.63	8.55	8.41	8.72	8.42	8.59	8.38
17 YRS	8.73	8.75	9.26	8.75	8.78	8.63	9.03	8.56	8.81	8.64
18 YRS	8.80	8.86	9.38	8.87	9.02	8.86	9.34	8.70	9.03	8.89
19 YRS	8.86	8.97	9.51	8.99	9.25	9.09	9.64	8.84	9.25	9.15
20 YRS	8.92	9.08	9.63	9.11	9.48	9.32	9.95	8.98	9.47	9.40
21 YRS	8.99	9.19	9.76	9.23	9.72	9.54	10.26	9.12	9.70	9.65
22 YRS	9.05	9.30	9.88	9.35	9.95	9.77	10.56	9.25	9.92	9.91
23 YRS	9.11	9.41	10.01	9.47	10.18	10.00	10.87	9.39	10.14	10.16
24 YRS	9.18	9.52	10.13	9.59	10.42	10.22	11.18	9.53	10.36	10.41
25 YRS	9.24	9.63	10.26	9.71	10.65	10.45	11.48	9.67	10.58	10.67
26 YRS	9.30	9.74	10.39	9.83	10.88	10.68	11.79	9.81	10.80	10.92
27 YRS	9.37	9.85	10.51	9.95	11.12	10.90	12.10	9.95	11.02	11.18
28 YRS	9.43	9.96	10.64	10.07	11.35	11.13	12.41	10.08	11.24	11.43
29 YRS	9.49	10.07	10.76	10.19	11.58	11.36	12.71	10.22	11.46	11.68
30 YRS	9.56	10.18	10.89	10.31	11.82	11.59	13.02	10.36	11.68	11.94

EDUCATION	CORRECT	DIGITSPA	WAISIMIL	WAISJUDG	VERBAL	ANIMAL	WAISBLOC	DIGIT
0 YRS	5.60	6.67	3.85	5.41	4.98	6.13	6.48	3.10
1 YRS	5.84	6.92	4.28	5.80	5.34	6.43	6.74	3.48
2 YRS	6.08	7.17	4.71	6.19	5.70	6.74	7.00	3.86
3 YRS	6.32	7.41	5.14	6.58	6.06	7.04	7.26	4.24
4 YRS	6.56	7.66	5.58	6.98	6.42	7.34	7.52	4.62
5 YRS	6.80	7.91	6.01	7.37	6.78	7.64	7.78	4.99
6 YRS	7.04	8.16	6.44	7.76	7.14	7.95	8.04	5.37
7 YRS	7.28	8.41	6.87	8.15	7.50	8.25	8.30	5.75
8 YRS	7.52	8.65	7.30	8.55	7.86	8.55	8.56	6.13
9 YRS	7.76	8.90	7.73	8.94	8.22	8.86	8.82	6.51
10 YRS	8.00	9.15	8.16	9.33	8.58	9.16	9.08	6.89
11 YRS	8.24	9.40	8.60	9.72	8.94	9.46	9.34	7.26
12 YRS	8.47	9.65	9.03	10.12	9.30	9.77	9.60	7.64
13 YRS	8.71	9.89	9.46	10.51	9.66	10.07	9.86	8.02
14 YRS	8.95	10.14	9.89	10.90	10.02	10.37	10.12	8.40
15 YRS	9.19	10.39	10.32	11.30	10.38	10.68	10.38	8.78
16 YRS	9.43	10.64	10.75	11.69	10.74	10.98	10.64	9.15
17 YRS	9.67	10.88	11.19	12.08	11.10	11.28	10.90	9.53
18 YRS	9.91	11.13	11.62	12.47	11.47	11.58	11.16	9.91
19 YRS	10.15	11.38	12.05	12.87	11.83	11.89	11.42	10.29
20 YRS	10.39	11.63	12.48	13.26	12.19	12.19	11.68	10.67
21 YRS	10.63	11.88	12.91	13.65	12.55	12.49	11.94	11.05
22 YRS	10.87	12.12	13.34	14.04	12.91	12.80	12.19	11.42
23 YRS	11.11	12.37	13.78	14.44	13.27	13.10	12.45	11.80
24 YRS	11.35	12.62	14.21	14.83	13.63	13.40	12.71	12.18
25 YRS	11.58	12.87	14.64	15.22	13.99	13.71	12.97	12.56
26 YRS	11.82	13.12	15.07	15.61	14.35	14.01	13.23	12.94
27 YRS	12.06	13.36	15.50	16.01	14.71	14.31	13.49	13.32
28 YRS	12.30	13.61	15.93	16.40	15.07	14.62	13.75	13.69
29 YRS	12.54	13.86	16.36	16.79	15.43	14.92	14.01	14.07
30 YRS	12.78	14.11	16.80	17.19	15.79	15.22	14.27	14.45

Table 30.2. Age 89 – Female.

EDUCATION	BUSCHFR1	BRETRIE	REYA1	REYA2	REYA3	REYA4	REYA5	REYTOT	REYB1	REYA6
0 YRS	7.66	6.89	7.12	6.70	4.82	4.77	3.82	6.21	5.06	4.32
1 YRS	7.72	7.00	7.25	6.82	5.05	5.00	4.12	6.35	5.28	4.57
2 YRS	7.78	7.11	7.37	6.94	5.29	5.23	4.43	6.49	5.50	4.83
3 YRS	7.85	7.22	7.50	7.06	5.52	5.46	4.74	6.63	5.72	5.08
4 YRS	7.91	7.33	7.62	7.18	5.75	5.68	5.04	6.77	5.94	5.34
5 YRS	7.97	7.44	7.75	7.30	5.99	5.91	5.35	6.90	6.16	5.59
6 YRS	8.04	7.55	7.88	7.42	6.22	6.14	5.66	7.04	6.38	5.84
7 YRS	8.10	7.66	8.00	7.54	6.45	6.36	5.96	7.18	6.60	6.10
8 YRS	8.16	7.77	8.13	7.67	6.69	6.59	6.27	7.32	6.82	6.35
9 YRS	8.23	7.87	8.25	7.79	6.92	6.82	6.58	7.46	7.04	6.61
10 YRS	8.29	7.98	8.38	7.91	7.15	7.05	6.88	7.60	7.26	6.86
11 YRS	8.35	8.09	8.50	8.03	7.39	7.27	7.19	7.73	7.49	7.11
12 YRS	8.42	8.20	8.63	8.15	7.62	7.50	7.50	7.87	7.71	7.37
13 YRS	8.48	8.31	8.75	8.27	7.85	7.73	7.80	8.01	7.93	7.62
14 YRS	8.54	8.42	8.88	8.39	8.08	7.95	8.11	8.15	8.15	7.88
15 YRS	8.61	8.53	9.01	8.51	8.32	8.18	8.42	8.29	8.37	8.13
16 YRS	8.67	8.64	9.13	8.63	8.55	8.41	8.72	8.42	8.59	8.38
17 YRS	8.73	8.75	9.26	8.75	8.78	8.63	9.03	8.56	8.81	8.64
18 YRS	8.80	8.86	9.38	8.87	9.02	8.86	9.34	8.70	9.03	8.89
19 YRS	8.86	8.97	9.51	8.99	9.25	9.09	9.64	8.84	9.25	9.15
20 YRS	8.92	9.08	9.63	9.11	9.48	9.32	9.95	8.98	9.47	9.40
21 YRS	8.99	9.19	9.76	9.23	9.72	9.54	10.26	9.12	9.70	9.65
22 YRS	9.05	9.30	9.88	9.35	9.95	9.77	10.56	9.25	9.92	9.91
23 YRS	9.11	9.41	10.01	9.47	10.18	10.00	10.87	9.39	10.14	10.16
24 YRS	9.18	9.52	10.13	9.59	10.42	10.22	11.18	9.53	10.36	10.41
25 YRS	9.24	9.63	10.26	9.71	10.65	10.45	11.48	9.67	10.58	10.67
26 YRS	9.30	9.74	10.39	9.83	10.88	10.68	11.79	9.81	10.80	10.92
27 YRS	9.37	9.85	10.51	9.95	11.12	10.90	12.10	9.95	11.02	11.18
28 YRS	9.43	9.96	10.64	10.07	11.35	11.13	12.41	10.08	11.24	11.43
29 YRS	9.49	10.07	10.76	10.19	11.58	11.36	12.71	10.22	11.46	11.68
30 YRS	9.56	10.18	10.89	10.31	11.82	11.59	13.02	10.36	11.68	11.94

EDUCATION	CORRECT	DIGITSPA	WAISIMIL	WAISJUDG	VERBAL	ANIMAL	WAISBLOC	DIGIT
0 YRS	5.60	6.67	3.85	5.41	4.98	6.13	6.48	3.10
1 YRS	5.84	6.92	4.28	5.80	5.34	6.43	6.74	3.48
2 YRS	6.08	7.17	4.71	6.19	5.70	6.74	7.00	3.86
3 YRS	6.32	7.41	5.14	6.58	6.06	7.04	7.26	4.24
4 YRS	6.56	7.66	5.58	6.98	6.42	7.34	7.52	4.62
5 YRS	6.80	7.91	6.01	7.37	6.78	7.64	7.78	4.99
6 YRS	7.04	8.16	6.44	7.76	7.14	7.95	8.04	5.37
7 YRS	7.28	8.41	6.87	8.15	7.50	8.25	8.30	5.75
8 YRS	7.52	8.65	7.30	8.55	7.86	8.55	8.56	6.13
9 YRS	7.76	8.90	7.73	8.94	8.22	8.86	8.82	6.51
10 YRS	8.00	9.15	8.16	9.33	8.58	9.16	9.08	6.89
11 YRS	8.24	9.40	8.60	9.72	8.94	9.46	9.34	7.26
12 YRS	8.47	9.65	9.03	10.12	9.30	9.77	9.60	7.64
13 YRS	8.71	9.89	9.46	10.51	9.66	10.07	9.86	8.02
14 YRS	8.95	10.14	9.89	10.90	10.02	10.37	10.12	8.40
15 YRS	9.19	10.39	10.32	11.30	10.38	10.68	10.38	8.78
16 YRS	9.43	10.64	10.75	11.69	10.74	10.98	10.64	9.15
17 YRS	9.67	10.88	11.19	12.08	11.10	11.28	10.90	9.53
18 YRS	9.91	11.13	11.62	12.47	11.47	11.58	11.16	9.91
19 YRS	10.15	11.38	12.05	12.87	11.83	11.89	11.42	10.29
20 YRS	10.39	11.63	12.48	13.26	12.19	12.19	11.68	10.67
21 YRS	10.63	11.88	12.91	13.65	12.55	12.49	11.94	11.05
22 YRS	10.87	12.12	13.34	14.04	12.91	12.80	12.19	11.42
23 YRS	11.11	12.37	13.78	14.44	13.27	13.10	12.45	11.80
24 YRS	11.35	12.62	14.21	14.83	13.63	13.40	12.71	12.18
25 YRS	11.58	12.87	14.64	15.22	13.99	13.71	12.97	12.56
26 YRS	11.82	13.12	15.07	15.61	14.35	14.01	13.23	12.94
27 YRS	12.06	13.36	15.50	16.01	14.71	14.31	13.49	13.32
28 YRS	12.30	13.61	15.93	16.40	15.07	14.62	13.75	13.69
29 YRS	12.54	13.86	16.36	16.79	15.43	14.92	14.01	14.07
30 YRS	12.78	14.11	16.80	17.19	15.79	15.22	14.27	14.45

Table 31.1. Age 90 – Male.

EDUCATION	BUSCHFR1	BRETRIE	REYA1	REYA2	REYA3	REYA4	REYA5	REYTOT	REYB1	REYA6
0 YRS	7.54	6.72	7.03	6.60	4.67	4.63	3.67	6.06	4.89	4.16
1 YRS	7.60	6.83	7.15	6.72	4.90	4.85	3.98	6.20	5.11	4.41
2 YRS	7.67	6.94	7.28	6.84	5.14	5.08	4.28	6.34	5.33	4.67
3 YRS	7.73	7.05	7.40	6.96	5.37	5.31	4.59	6.48	5.56	4.92
4 YRS	7.79	7.16	7.53	7.08	5.60	5.53	4.90	6.62	5.78	5.18
5 YRS	7.86	7.27	7.65	7.20	5.84	5.76	5.20	6.75	6.00	5.43
6 YRS	7.92	7.38	7.78	7.32	6.07	5.99	5.51	6.89	6.22	5.68
7 YRS	7.98	7.49	7.90	7.44	6.30	6.22	5.82	7.03	6.44	5.94
8 YRS	8.05	7.60	8.03	7.56	6.54	6.44	6.12	7.17	6.66	6.19
9 YRS	8.11	7.71	8.15	7.68	6.77	6.67	6.43	7.31	6.88	6.45
10 YRS	8.17	7.82	8.28	7.80	7.00	6.90	6.74	7.45	7.10	6.70
11 YRS	8.24	7.93	8.41	7.92	7.23	7.12	7.04	7.58	7.32	6.95
12 YRS	8.30	8.04	8.53	8.04	7.47	7.35	7.35	7.72	7.54	7.21
13 YRS	8.36	8.15	8.66	8.16	7.70	7.58	7.66	7.86	7.77	7.46
14 YRS	8.43	8.26	8.78	8.28	7.93	7.80	7.96	8.00	7.99	7.72
15 YRS	8.49	8.37	8.91	8.40	8.17	8.03	8.27	8.14	8.21	7.97
16 YRS	8.55	8.48	9.03	8.52	8.40	8.26	8.58	8.27	8.43	8.22
17 YRS	8.62	8.59	9.16	8.64	8.63	8.49	8.88	8.41	8.65	8.48
18 YRS	8.68	8.70	9.28	8.76	8.87	8.71	9.19	8.55	8.87	8.73
19 YRS	8.74	8.81	9.41	8.88	9.10	8.94	9.50	8.69	9.09	8.99
20 YRS	8.80	8.92	9.54	9.01	9.33	9.17	9.80	8.83	9.31	9.24
21 YRS	8.87	9.03	9.66	9.13	9.57	9.39	10.11	8.97	9.53	9.49
22 YRS	8.93	9.14	9.79	9.25	9.80	9.62	10.42	9.10	9.75	9.75
23 YRS	8.99	9.25	9.91	9.37	10.03	9.85	10.72	9.24	9.97	10.00
24 YRS	9.06	9.36	10.04	9.49	10.27	10.07	11.03	9.38	10.20	10.25
25 YRS	9.12	9.47	10.16	9.61	10.50	10.30	11.34	9.52	10.42	10.51
26 YRS	9.18	9.58	10.29	9.73	10.73	10.53	11.64	9.66	10.64	10.76
27 YRS	9.25	9.69	10.41	9.85	10.97	10.76	11.95	9.80	10.86	11.02
28 YRS	9.31	9.80	10.54	9.97	11.20	10.98	12.26	9.93	11.08	11.27
29 YRS	9.37	9.91	10.67	10.09	11.43	11.21	12.57	10.07	11.30	11.52
30 YRS	9.44	10.02	10.79	10.21	11.66	11.44	12.87	10.21	11.52	11.78

EDUCATION	CORRECT	DIGITSPA	WAISIMIL	WAISJUDG	VERBAL	ANIMAL	WAISBLOC	DIGIT
0 YRS	5.45	6.61	3.75	5.34	4.92	6.01	6.37	2.88
1 YRS	5.69	6.85	4.19	5.73	5.28	6.32	6.63	3.26
2 YRS	5.93	7.10	4.62	6.13	5.64	6.62	6.89	3.64
3 YRS	6.17	7.35	5.05	6.52	6.00	6.92	7.15	4.02
4 YRS	6.41	7.60	5.48	6.91	6.36	7.22	7.41	4.39
5 YRS	6.65	7.84	5.91	7.30	6.72	7.53	7.67	4.77
6 YRS	6.89	8.09	6.34	7.70	7.08	7.83	7.93	5.15
7 YRS	7.12	8.34	6.77	8.09	7.44	8.13	8.19	5.53
8 YRS	7.36	8.59	7.21	8.48	7.80	8.44	8.44	5.91
9 YRS	7.60	8.84	7.64	8.88	8.16	8.74	8.70	6.29
10 YRS	7.84	9.08	8.07	9.27	8.53	9.04	8.96	6.66
11 YRS	8.08	9.33	8.50	9.66	8.89	9.35	9.22	7.04
12 YRS	8.32	9.58	8.93	10.05	9.25	9.65	9.48	7.42
13 YRS	8.56	9.83	9.36	10.45	9.61	9.95	9.74	7.80
14 YRS	8.80	10.08	9.80	10.84	9.97	10.26	10.00	8.18
15 YRS	9.04	10.32	10.23	11.23	10.33	10.56	10.26	8.56
16 YRS	9.28	10.57	10.66	11.62	10.69	10.86	10.52	8.93
17 YRS	9.52	10.82	11.09	12.02	11.05	11.16	10.78	9.31
18 YRS	9.76	11.07	11.52	12.41	11.41	11.47	11.04	9.69
19 YRS	10.00	11.32	11.95	12.80	11.77	11.77	11.30	10.07
20 YRS	10.23	11.56	12.39	13.19	12.13	12.07	11.56	10.45
21 YRS	10.47	11.81	12.82	13.59	12.49	12.38	11.82	10.83
22 YRS	10.71	12.06	13.25	13.98	12.85	12.68	12.08	11.20
23 YRS	10.95	12.31	13.68	14.37	13.21	12.98	12.34	11.58
24 YRS	11.19	12.55	14.11	14.77	13.57	13.29	12.60	11.96
25 YRS	11.43	12.80	14.54	15.16	13.93	13.59	12.86	12.34
26 YRS	11.67	13.05	14.97	15.55	14.29	13.89	13.12	12.72
27 YRS	11.91	13.30	15.41	15.94	14.65	14.20	13.38	13.10
28 YRS	12.15	13.55	15.84	16.34	15.01	14.50	13.64	13.47
29 YRS	12.39	13.79	16.27	16.73	15.37	14.80	13.90	13.85
30 YRS	12.63	14.04	16.70	17.12	15.73	15.10	14.16	14.23

Table 31.2. Age 90 – Female.

EDUCATION	BUSCHFR1	BRETRIE	REYA1	REYA2	REYA3	REYA4	REYA5	REYTOT	REYB1	REYA6
0 YRS	7.54	6.72	7.03	6.60	4.67	4.63	3.67	6.06	4.89	4.16
1 YRS	7.60	6.83	7.15	6.72	4.90	4.85	3.98	6.20	5.11	4.41
2 YRS	7.67	6.94	7.28	6.84	5.14	5.08	4.28	6.34	5.33	4.67
3 YRS	7.73	7.05	7.40	6.96	5.37	5.31	4.59	6.48	5.56	4.92
4 YRS	7.79	7.16	7.53	7.08	5.60	5.53	4.90	6.62	5.78	5.18
5 YRS	7.86	7.27	7.65	7.20	5.84	5.76	5.20	6.75	6.00	5.43
6 YRS	7.92	7.38	7.78	7.32	6.07	5.99	5.51	6.89	6.22	5.68
7 YRS	7.98	7.49	7.90	7.44	6.30	6.22	5.82	7.03	6.44	5.94
8 YRS	8.05	7.60	8.03	7.56	6.54	6.44	6.12	7.17	6.66	6.19
9 YRS	8.11	7.71	8.15	7.68	6.77	6.67	6.43	7.31	6.88	6.45
10 YRS	8.17	7.82	8.28	7.80	7.00	6.90	6.74	7.45	7.10	6.70
11 YRS	8.24	7.93	8.41	7.92	7.23	7.12	7.04	7.58	7.32	6.95
12 YRS	8.30	8.04	8.53	8.04	7.47	7.35	7.35	7.72	7.54	7.21
13 YRS	8.36	8.15	8.66	8.16	7.70	7.58	7.66	7.86	7.77	7.46
14 YRS	8.43	8.26	8.78	8.28	7.93	7.80	7.96	8.00	7.99	7.72
15 YRS	8.49	8.37	8.91	8.40	8.17	8.03	8.27	8.14	8.21	7.97
16 YRS	8.55	8.48	9.03	8.52	8.40	8.26	8.58	8.27	8.43	8.22
17 YRS	8.62	8.59	9.16	8.64	8.63	8.49	8.88	8.41	8.65	8.48
18 YRS	8.68	8.70	9.28	8.76	8.87	8.71	9.19	8.55	8.87	8.73
19 YRS	8.74	8.81	9.41	8.88	9.10	8.94	9.50	8.69	9.09	8.99
20 YRS	8.80	8.92	9.54	9.01	9.33	9.17	9.80	8.83	9.31	9.24
21 YRS	8.87	9.03	9.66	9.13	9.57	9.39	10.11	8.97	9.53	9.49
22 YRS	8.93	9.14	9.79	9.25	9.80	9.62	10.42	9.10	9.75	9.75
23 YRS	8.99	9.25	9.91	9.37	10.03	9.85	10.72	9.24	9.97	10.00
24 YRS	9.06	9.36	10.04	9.49	10.27	10.07	11.03	9.38	10.20	10.25
25 YRS	9.12	9.47	10.16	9.61	10.50	10.30	11.34	9.52	10.42	10.51
26 YRS	9.18	9.58	10.29	9.73	10.73	10.53	11.64	9.66	10.64	10.76
27 YRS	9.25	9.69	10.41	9.85	10.97	10.76	11.95	9.80	10.86	11.02
28 YRS	9.31	9.80	10.54	9.97	11.20	10.98	12.26	9.93	11.08	11.27
29 YRS	9.37	9.91	10.67	10.09	11.43	11.21	12.57	10.07	11.30	11.52
30 YRS	9.44	10.02	10.79	10.21	11.66	11.44	12.87	10.21	11.52	11.78

EDUCATION	CORRECT	DIGITSPA	WAISIMIL	WAISJUDG	VERBAL	ANIMAL	WAISBLOC	DIGIT
0 YRS	5.45	6.61	3.75	5.34	4.92	6.01	6.37	2.88
1 YRS	5.69	6.85	4.19	5.73	5.28	6.32	6.63	3.26
2 YRS	5.93	7.10	4.62	6.13	5.64	6.62	6.89	3.64
3 YRS	6.17	7.35	5.05	6.52	6.00	6.92	7.15	4.02
4 YRS	6.41	7.60	5.48	6.91	6.36	7.22	7.41	4.39
5 YRS	6.65	7.84	5.91	7.30	6.72	7.53	7.67	4.77
6 YRS	6.89	8.09	6.34	7.70	7.08	7.83	7.93	5.15
7 YRS	7.12	8.34	6.77	8.09	7.44	8.13	8.19	5.53
8 YRS	7.36	8.59	7.21	8.48	7.80	8.44	8.44	5.91
9 YRS	7.60	8.84	7.64	8.88	8.16	8.74	8.70	6.29
10 YRS	7.84	9.08	8.07	9.27	8.53	9.04	8.96	6.66
11 YRS	8.08	9.33	8.50	9.66	8.89	9.35	9.22	7.04
12 YRS	8.32	9.58	8.93	10.05	9.25	9.65	9.48	7.42
13 YRS	8.56	9.83	9.36	10.45	9.61	9.95	9.74	7.80
14 YRS	8.80	10.08	9.80	10.84	9.97	10.26	10.00	8.18
15 YRS	9.04	10.32	10.23	11.23	10.33	10.56	10.26	8.56
16 YRS	9.28	10.57	10.66	11.62	10.69	10.86	10.52	8.93
17 YRS	9.52	10.82	11.09	12.02	11.05	11.16	10.78	9.31
18 YRS	9.76	11.07	11.52	12.41	11.41	11.47	11.04	9.69
19 YRS	10.00	11.32	11.95	12.80	11.77	11.77	11.30	10.07
20 YRS	10.23	11.56	12.39	13.19	12.13	12.07	11.56	10.45
21 YRS	10.47	11.81	12.82	13.59	12.49	12.38	11.82	10.83
22 YRS	10.71	12.06	13.25	13.98	12.85	12.68	12.08	11.20
23 YRS	10.95	12.31	13.68	14.37	13.21	12.98	12.34	11.58
24 YRS	11.19	12.55	14.11	14.77	13.57	13.29	12.60	11.96
25 YRS	11.43	12.80	14.54	15.16	13.93	13.59	12.86	12.34
26 YRS	11.67	13.05	14.97	15.55	14.29	13.89	13.12	12.72
27 YRS	11.91	13.30	15.41	15.94	14.65	14.20	13.38	13.10
28 YRS	12.15	13.55	15.84	16.34	15.01	14.50	13.64	13.47
29 YRS	12.39	13.79	16.27	16.73	15.37	14.80	13.90	13.85
30 YRS	12.63	14.04	16.70	17.12	15.73	15.10	14.16	14.23

Table 32. *T* Score Means and Standard Deviations for Subject Samples.

Test Measure	Base Sample	Validation Sample
BUSCHFR1		
Mean	50.03	49.22
SD	9.96	10.61
BRETRIE		
Mean	50.02	49.48
SD	9.99	10.67
WAISBLOC		
Mean	50.01	50.52
SD	9.99	10.67
WAISIMIL		
Mean	50.00	50.40
SD	9.99	11.65
DIGITSPA		
Mean	50.01	51.88
SD	9.98	10.88
DIGIT		
Mean	49.99	52.26
SD	9.99	10.42
WAISJUDG		
Mean	49.98	50.30
SD	10.02	12.64
REYA1		
Mean	50.02	51.80
SD	9.99	10.12
REYA2		
Mean	49.96	49.70
SD	10.00	9.59
REYA3		
Mean	49.99	48.84
SD	10.02	10.94
REYA4		
Mean	50.00	47.14
SD	10.00	10.14
REYA5		
Mean	49.99	48.90
SD	10.02	11.92
REYA6		
Mean	49.97	49.66
SD	10.02	10.49
REYB1		
Mean	50.01	52.78
SD	10.00	10.78
REYTOT		
Mean	49.99	48.98
SD	10.00	10.65
VERBAL		
Mean	49.97	50.40
SD	9.95	9.51
CORRECT		
Mean	50.01	47.64
SD	9.98	9.84
ANIMAL		
Mean	50.02	49.42
SD	9.99	11.71

Table 33. Predicted and Actual Percentage of Subjects in the Base and Validation Normal Samples Scoring within Seven T Score Ranges.

T Score Range	0–24	25–34	35–44	45–54	55–64	65–74	75+
Predicted From Normal Distribution	0.5	5.5	22.9	38.2	25.4	6.7	0.7
Test Measure							
BUSCHFR1	1%	4%	28%	34%	26%	8%	0%
BRETRIE	2%	5%	23%	34%	30%	6%	0%
REYA1	0%	5%	22%	38%	26%	8%	1%
REYA2	0%	5%	24%	40%	25%	6%	1%
REYA3	0%	6%	22%	40%	24%	8%	0%
REYA4	1%	7%	24%	34%	26%	8%	0%
REYA5	0%	6%	27%	31%	27%	9%	0%
REYTOT	0%	6%	22%	38%	26%	8%	0%
REYB1	0%	4%	23%	41%	22%	9%	1%
REYA6	0%	6%	24%	37%	26%	7%	1%
CORRECT	1%	8%	19%	38%	29%	5%	0%
DIGITSPA	0%	4%	31%	32%	25%	8%	0%
WAISIMIL	0%	10%	20%	28%	38%	5%	0%
WAISJUDG	1%	8%	20%	38%	26%	6%	2%
VERBAL	0%	5%	24%	42%	20%	8%	1%
ANIMAL	0%	5%	24%	44%	19%	6%	2%
WAISBLOC	0%	5%	26%	38%	22%	10%	0%
DIGIT	0%	6%	20%	42%	24%	6%	2%

Table 34. Optimal Cutoff Scores for Each Measure.

Test Measure	T Score
BUSCHFR1	36
BRETRIE	34
REYA1	46
REYA2	42
REYA3	41
REYA4	37
REYA5	35
REYTOT	38
REYB1	45
REYA6	38
CORRECT	45
DIGITSPA	49
WAISIMIL	43
WAISJUDG	47
VERBAL	40
ANIMAL	40
WAISBLOC	45
DIGIT	39

Table 35. Range of Sensitivity (Proportion of True Positives) from Optimal T Score Cutoffs for Each Test Variable.

Test Measure	Optimal T Score -2	Optimal T Score -1	Optimal T Score	Optimal T Score 1	Optimal T Score 2
BUSCHFR1	.71	.75	.77	.78	.78
BRETRIE	.81	.82	.83	.84	.85
REYA1	.60	.66	.70	.75	.82
REYA2	.70	.74	.76	.80	.82
REYA3	.75	.76	.78	.83	.85
REYA4	.68	.71	.75	.77	.78
REYA5	.73	.74	.78	.80	.81
REYTOT	.80	.81	.82	.86	.87
REYB1	.48	.55	.57	.62	.64
REYA6	.75	.80	.83	.88	.89
CORRECT	.82	.84	.86	.88	.89
DIGITSPA	.51	.57	.59	.63	.64
WAISIMIL	.71	.73	.74	.77	.79
WAISJUDG	.67	.68	.72	.75	.79
VERBAL	.51	.58	.62	.66	.68
ANIMAL	.63	.66	.68	.74	.76
WAISBLOC	.70	.72	.75	.80	.82
DIGIT	.65	.67	.70	.75	.76

Table 36. Range of Specificity (Proportion of True Negatives) from Optimal T Score Cutoffs for Each Test Variable.

Test Measure	Optimal T Score -2	Optimal T Score -1	Optimal T Score	Optimal T Score 1	Optimal T Score 2
BUSCHFR1	.95	.95	.93	.93	.92
BRETRIE	.96	.94	.94	.94	.93
REYA1	.74	.71	.66	.64	.60
REYA2	.86	.82	.81	.80	.75
REYA3	.87	.84	.81	.80	.77
REYA4	.95	.93	.91	.91	.89
REYA5	.97	.95	.94	.93	.90
REYTOT	.93	.91	.90	.87	.84
REYB1	.80	.73	.71	.67	.64
REYA6	.93	.89	.87	.87	.84
CORRECT	.77	.75	.73	.72	.68
DIGITSPA	.60	.58	.56	.55	.49
WAISIMIL	.79	.78	.75	.74	.71
WAISJUDG	.72	.71	.68	.65	.60
VERBAL	.91	.88	.86	.85	.81
ANIMAL	.92	.89	.87	.83	.78
WAISBLOC	.76	.73	.70	.70	.67
DIGIT	.88	.87	.87	.85	.82

Table 37. Frequency of Occurrence of Each Subcategory Within the CIND Diagnosis from CSHA-1.

Category	Percent in Community Sample
Delirium	0.8
Drug and Alcohol Abuse	8.8
Psychiatric	9.4
Age Associated Memory Impairment	28.7
Mental Retardation	1.0
Other	29.9
Cerebral and General Vascular	14.8
Other Neurological – Parkinson's Epilepsy	1.2
Socio-cultural/Isolation	3.2
Sensory Loss	2.2

Table 38. Percentage of Subjects in the Normal Validation Sample, Cognitively Impaired Not Dementia (CIND) and Dementia Groups Scoring Below Optimal Cutoff Point for Identifying Dementia.

Group	Normal	CIND	Dementia
Test Measure			
BUSCHFR1	8%	38%	77%
BRETRIE	10%	45%	83%
REYA1	22%	58%	70%
REYA2	18%	47%	76%
REYA3	22%	54%	78%
REYA4	18%	43%	75%
REYA5	12%	44%	78%
REYTOT	12%	51%	82%
REYB1	18%	44%	57%
REYA6	12%	53%	83%
CORRECT	34%	69%	86%
DIGITSPA	42%	60%	59%
WAISIMIL	24%	55%	74%
WAISJUDG	34%	64%	72%
VERBAL	12%	51%	62%
ANIMAL	18%	44%	68%
WAISBLOC	32%	62%	75%
DIGIT	2%	44%	70%

Table 39. Percentage of Subjects in the Normal Validation Sample, Cognitively Impaired Not Dementia (CIND) and Dementia Groups Scoring Below a *T* Score of 40.

Group	Normal	CIND	Dementia
Test Measure			
BUSCHFR1	24%	53%	83%
BRETRIE	16%	58%	88%
REYA1	12%	33%	49%
REYA2	16%	40%	70%
REYA3	18%	51%	76%
REYA4	20%	57%	80%
REYA5	22%	59%	86%
REYTOT	16%	59%	87%
REYB1	8%	23%	38%
REYA6	16%	60%	89%
CORRECT	20%	54%	75%
DIGITSPA	12%	25%	24%
WAISIMIL	18%	47%	61%
WAISJUDG	18%	43%	53%
VERBAL	12%	51%	62%
ANIMAL	18%	43%	68%
WAISBLOC	16%	42%	59%
DIGIT	6%	49%	75%

Table 40. Percent of Cases Falling below Optimal Cut-off Points for Identifying Normal Versus Dementia.

Number of Measures Falling below Optimal Cut-Off	Normal	CIND	Dementia
Memory Measures*			
0	57.4	10.7	1.6
1	32.1	25.6	4.8
2	7.9	18.7	8.6
3	1.5	25.6	27.8
4	1.1	19.5	57.2
Abstract Thinking (WAIS – R Similarities)			
0	75.5	45.3	26.2
1	24.5	54.7	73.8
Judgment (WAIS – R Comprehension)			
0	67.5	35.7	28.3
1	32.5	64.3	71.7
Language Measures+			
0	75.5	34.4	18.2
1	20.8	36.8	33.2
2	3.8	28.8	48.7
Construction (WAIS – R Block Design)			
0	69.4	38.4	24.6
1	30.6	61.6	75.4
Other (WAIS – R Digit Symbol)			
0	88.7	56	30.5
1	11.3	44	69.5

Note. * Buschke Retrieval, Rey Auditory Verbal Learning Test Total, Rey Auditory Verbal Learning Test List A6, Benton Visual Retention Test – Multiple Choice Correct.
+ Word Fluency, Animal Fluency.

Table 41. Percentage of Subjects in the CIND Group Scoring within Seven *T* Score Ranges.

T Score Range Predicted From	0–24	25–34	35–44	45–54	55–64	65–74	75+
Normal Distribution	0.5	5.5	22.9	38.2	25.4	6.7	0.7
Test Measure							
BUSCHFR1	15%	21%	30%	23%	9%	2%	1%
BRETRIE	25%	23%	22%	21%	7%	1%	0%
REYA1	2%	10%	40%	35%	10%	2%	0%
REYA2	3%	19%	40%	30%	7%	1%	0%
REYA3	6%	23%	37%	26%	6%	1%	0%
REYA4	10%	26%	38%	19%	6%	2%	0%
REYA5	17%	27%	29%	19%	6%	3%	0%
REYTOT	9%	34%	32%	19%	5%	2%	0%
REYB1	1%	10%	33%	32%	22%	2%	1%
REYA6	11%	32%	31%	20%	5%	1%	0%
CORRECT	17%	25%	27%	19%	11%	1%	0%
DIGITSPA	2%	14%	31%	31%	14%	6%	1%
WAISIMIL	3%	25%	35%	27%	8%	2%	0%
WAISJUDG	5%	22%	32%	26%	13%	2%	0%
VERBAL	3%	26%	38%	24%	7%	2%	0%
ANIMAL	5%	19%	37%	28%	10%	2%	0%
WAISBLOC	3%	21%	38%	26%	10%	2%	0%
DIGIT	9%	23%	36%	24%	7%	1%	0%

Table 42. Percentage of Subjects in the Demented Group within Seven *T* Score Ranges.

T Score Range Predicted From	0–24	25–34	35–44	45–54	55–64	65–74	75+
Normal Distribution	0.5	5.5	22.9	38.2	25.4	6.7	0.7
Test Measure							
BUSCHFR1	55%	20%	13%	9%	3%	0%	0%
BRETRIE	74%	11%	7%	5%	2%	1%	0%
REYA1	3%	29%	34%	29%	4%	0%	0%
REYA2	10%	30%	45%	14%	1%	0%	0%
REYA3	20%	41%	28%	9%	2%	0%	0%
REYA4	25%	43%	22%	7%	1%	1%	0%
REYA5	41%	37%	16%	6%	1%	0%	0%
REYTOT	19%	54%	21%	5%	1%	0%	0%
REYB1	3%	13%	41%	32%	10%	1%	1%
REYA6	34%	41%	17%	7%	1%	0%	0%
CORRECT	39%	25%	22%	10%	5%	0%	0%
DIGITSPA	4%	11%	27%	38%	17%	4%	0%
WAISIMIL	4%	33%	42%	16%	5%	1%	0%
WAISJUDG	12%	22%	33%	24%	7%	2%	1%
VERBAL	5%	34%	33%	20%	6%	1%	0%
ANIMAL	18%	29%	36%	13%	3%	1%	0%
WAISBLOC	7%	36%	32%	17%	6%	1%	1%
DIGIT	22%	35%	28%	11%	4%	0%	0%

Table 43. Probability of Dementia Based on Classification from Logistic Regression Analyses.

Probability of Dementia	Normal Base Sample (n = 224)	Normal Validation Sample	CIND	Dementia
< .10	80.5	74.0	17.9	1.6
.11–.19	6.5	12.0	6.7	2.7
.20–.29	5.1	4.0	5.1	3.2
.30–.39	1.9	4.0	7.5	0.5
.40–.49	1.9	0.0	4.0	2.1
.50–.59	0.9	0.0	5.1	1.6
.60–.69	1.9	0.0	5.6	3.2
.70–.79	0.5	4.0	4.8	2.1
.80–.89	0.5	2.0	7.5	5.9
.90–.99	0.5	0.0	36.0	77.0

Table A1. Correlations with Age, Education.

Test Measure	Age	Education
Wechsler Memory Scale – Information subtest	−0.19 $p = .006$	0.20 $p = .003$
Buschke Acquisition	0.13 $p = .05$	0.15 $p = .02$
Buschke Retention	0.03 $p = .61$	0.21 $p = .002$
Rey AVLT* True Positives	−0.11 $p = .10$	0.12 $p = .08$
Rey AVLT* True Negatives	−0.04 $p = .60$	0.14 $p = .04$
Token Test	−0.21 $p = .002$	0.29 $p = .000$

Note. *Auditory Verbal Learning Test Recognition.

Table A2. Identified Cut-Off Scores not Affected by Age and Education.

Test Measure	Percent of Base Sample	
	<16	>16
Wechsler Memory Scale – Information subtest	0–4	5–6
Buschke Retention	0–11	12
Rey AVLT* True Positives	0–12	13–15
Rey AVLT* True Negatives	0–13	14–15

Note. *Auditory Verbal Learning Test Recognition.

Table A3. Identified Cut-Off Scores for Buschke Acquisition by Age.

Age	Percent of Base Sample	
	<16	>16
65–84	0–35	36
85+	0–34	35–36

Table A4. Identified Cut-Off Scores for Token Test by Age and Education.

Age	Percent of Base Sample	
	<16	>16
65–74	0–36	37–44
75–84	0–34	35–44
85+	0–30	31–44
Years of Education		
<12	0–32	33–44
>12	0–38	39–44

Table A5. Mann-Whitney U Comparisons of the Combined Normal Samples ($n = 265$) and the Dementia Sample ($n = 187$).

Test Measure	Z	P
Wechsler Memory Scale – Information subtest	−15.21	.000
Buschke Acquisition	−13.89	.000
Buschke Retention	−15.35	.000
Rey AVLT* True Positives	−8.25	.000
Rey AVLT* True Negatives	−14.07	.000
Token Test	−9.33	.000

Note. *Auditory Verbal Learning Test Recognition.

T Score Conversions.

Test Name	Raw Score	Scaled Score	Predicted Score	Education	Sex
					T Score
Buschke's Cued Recall FR1	_____	_____	− _____ / 2.89	= ___ × 10 = ___ + 50 = _____	
Bretrie	_____	_____	− _____ / 2.80	= ___ × 10 = ___ + 50 = _____	
Rey Auditory Verbal Learning A1	_____	_____	− _____ / 2.90	= ___ × 10 = ___ + 50 = _____	

Table continues.

T Score Conversions (continued).

Test Name	Raw Score	Scaled Score	Predicted Score	Education	Sex
					T Score
Rey Auditory Verbal Learning A2	_____	_____	$-$ _____ / 2.85 = ___ × 10 = ___ + 50 = _____		
Rey Auditory Verbal Learning A3	_____	_____	$-$ _____ / 2.67 = ___ × 10 = ___ + 50 = _____		
Rey Auditory Verbal Learning A4	_____	_____	$-$ _____ / 2.65 = ___ × 10 = ___ + 50 = _____		
Rey Auditory Verbal Learning A5	_____	_____	$-$ _____ / 2.54 = ___ × 10 = ___ + 50 = _____		
Rey Auditory Verbal Total	_____	_____	$-$ _____ / 2.60 = ___ × 10 = ___ + 50 = _____		
Rey Auditory Verbal Learning B1	_____	_____	$-$ _____ / 2.69 = ___ × 10 = ___ + 50 = _____		
Rey Auditory Verbal Learning A6	_____	_____	$-$ _____ / 2.79 = ___ × 10 = ___ + 50 = _____		
Correct	_____	_____	$-$ _____ / 2.72 = ___ × 10 = ___ + 50 = _____		
Digitspa	_____	_____	$-$ _____ / 2.83 = ___ × 10 = ___ + 50 = _____		
WAIS – R Similarities	_____	_____	$-$ _____ / 2.51 = ___ × 10 = ___ + 50 = _____		
WAIS – R Comprehension	_____	_____	$-$ _____ / 2.58 = ___ × 10 = ___ + 50 = _____		
Verbal Fluency	_____	_____	$-$ _____ / 2.68 = ___ × 10 = ___ + 50 = _____		
Animal Fluency	_____	_____	$-$ _____ / 2.61 = ___ × 10 = ___ + 50 = _____		
WAIS – R Block	_____	_____	$-$ _____ / 2.70 = ___ × 10 = ___ + 50 = _____		
Digit	_____	_____	$-$ _____ / 2.33 = ___ × 10 = ___ + 50 = _____		

Profile Grid

X = Optimal Cut Off

Test Name	T Scores						
	< 20	30	40	50	60	70	80 >
Buschke's Cued Recall FR1			X				
Bretrie			X				
Rey Auditory Verbal Learning A1				X			
Rey Auditory Verbal Learning A2			X				
Rey Auditory Verbal Learning A3			X				
Rey Auditory Verbal Learning A4			X				
Rey Auditory Verbal Learning A5			X				
Rey Auditory Verbal Total		X					
Rey Auditory Verbal Learning B1				X			
Rey Auditory Verbal Learning A6			X				
Correct			X				
Digitspa				X			
WAIS-R Similarities				X			
WAIS-R Comprehension				X			
Verbal Fluency			X				
Animal Fluency			X				
WAIS-R Block				X			
Digit				X			

APPENDIX A

Information on the Measures Removed from the Regression Analyses Due to Non-normality of Regression Residual.

As noted in the section describing the development of the demographic correction system, the following variables were dropped at this point due to non-normality of regression residuals: Wechsler Memory Scale – Information subtest; Buschke Acquisition; Buschke Retention; Rey Auditory Verbal Learning Test – Recognition: True Positives and True Negatives; and the Token Test. For these tests, the vast majority of respondents in the base sample made very few errors, resulting in negatively skewed regression residuals. Table 5 summarizes the raw score results of the Base sample on each of the 24 measures in the battery.

As age and education correlated significantly with some of the variables (see Table A1), the frequency distributions of the scores for each measure was examined by age (i.e., 65–74, 75–84, 85+) and education (i.e., less than or equal to 12 years of education, greater than 12 tears of (education) groups. Given the skewed nature of the distributions of scores on these measures, normative data were categorized as falling at or below the 16th percentile and scores falling above the 16th percentile. No clinically meaningful differences in identified cutoff scores were apparent by age for four of the six measures. No clinically meaningful differences in cutoff scores were identified by education for any measure except the Token Test. The identified cutoff scores for each measure are shown in Table A2–A4.

When the identified cutoff scores from the Base sample ($n = 215$), determined above, were applied to the Validation sample ($n = 50$), typically less than 16% of the Validation sample fell below the score. The only exceptions were for the Token Test. For persons aged 85 and older, 23% performed at or below the identified cutoff of 30 and 42.9% performed at or below the identified cutoff of 38 for persons with greater than 12 years of education.

When the Base and Validation samples were combined ($n = 265$), and compared to the Dementia ($n = 187$) sample (see Subject Samples), p. 2) using Mann-Whitney U tests, differences were apparent for all six variables (see Table A5).

APPENDIX B

Possible Contamination and Estimating the Probability of Dementia

It has been noted that the neuropsychological test data was included in formulating the diagnosis (i.e., diagnosis derived from a multidisciplinary case conference) for the cases described in this document. It could be argued that the diagnosis is thus contaminated by the inclusion of the neuropsychological data. In the CSHA, both the physician and the neuropsychologist made independent preliminary diagnoses with all available information being combined to formulate the final diagnosis. The extent to which the present normative sample differed from a sample diagnosed without inclusion of the neuropsychological information was examined. Only 2/274 cases were diagnosed differently (i.e., as dementia) at the physician's preliminary diagnosis. With inclusion of the neuropsychological data, the diagnoses for these 2 people were changed to indicate no cognitive loss. Thus, the diagnoses for the present sample shows little evidence of contamination and can be viewed as equivalent to the independently diagnosed sample.

As mentioned above, a stepwise logistic regression was used to determine the combination of tests that optimally discriminate between individuals with no cognitive loss and dementia for the CSHA neuropsychological battery. These derived logistic regression weights may be applied to an individual patient's test scores to yield probability estimates for the presence of dementia. Initially, the individual's T scores are multiplied by the logistic regression weights (and the constant added) as specified by the following equation (Hosmer & Lemeshow, 1989):

$$g = 19.309 + (-.0917 \times \text{BRetriev}) + (-.0713 \times \text{ReyA1 score}) + (-.1212 \times \text{ReyA6 score}) + (-.0469 \times \text{BVRT Correct score}) + (-.0689 \times \text{Verbal score}) + (-.0769 \times \text{Digit Symbol score}).$$

The value **g** is then entered into the formula:

$$\text{Probability of Dementia: } e^g/(1 + e^g),$$

where e is the exponential.*

* – the value of e^g can be determined using most calculators with function keys. Enter the value for **g**, and press the key marked e^x.

Journal of Clinical and Experimental Neuropsychology
1997, Vol. 19, No. 6, pp. 889–896

Use of the Odds Ratio to Translate Neuropsychological Test Scores into Real-World Outcomes: From Statistical Significance to Clinical Significance*

Linas A. Bieliauskas[1,2], Philip S. Fastenau[3], Maureen A. Lacy[2], and Brad L. Roper[5]

[1]Psychology Service (116B), VA Medical Center, Ann Arbor, MI, [2]Division of Neuropsychology, Department of Psychiatry, University of Michigan Medical Center, Ann Arbor, MI, [3]Indiana University Purdue University, Indianapolis, IN, and [4]Psychology Service (116B), VA Medical Center, Memphis, TN

ABSTRACT

Standard parametric tests generate p values and effect sizes, but often these are difficult to translate into real-world outcomes. In this study, the odds ratio was applied to neuropsychological testing and was compared to parametric approaches. Participants were 26 community-dwelling adults with possible or probable Alzheimer's disease and 25 matched healthy community-dwelling volunteers. Odds ratios were computed to estimate the probability of concurrent diagnosis given neuropsychological performance level. Odds ratios discriminated the groups at magnitudes that could not be discerned from t-test significance tables. These values were compared to sensitivity, specificity, and overall accuracy. Clinical and research applications and implications were addressed.

A major focus of research in neuropsychology is to identify the degree and nature of cognitive change associated with CNS trauma or disease, such as dementia. Various empirical paradigms are employed to demonstrate the sensitivity and specificity of neuropsychological measures in the assessment of dementia. Most studies that employ standard parametric analyses readily demonstrate significant differences between demented and nondemented individuals on almost any cognitive task. Unfortunately, those results give little information as to the discriminative power of such differences.

Epidemiological studies routinely assess risk. For example, it has long been established through prospective longitudinal cohort studies that hypercholesteremia, alcohol intake, and smoking increase the risk of coronary heart disease (Inter-Society Commission for Heart Disease Resources, 1970). One major tool that is often used in such studies is the odds ratio, a measure of association between the incidence of disease in a given situation versus the incidence of disease without that situation. Thus, the odds ratio represents the ratio of the 'probability that (an) event occurs to the probability that it does not' (Wickens, 1989).

It also indicates the direction and strength of the association; 'odds ratios close to 1 indicate only weak associations, whereas ratios over about 3 for positive associations, or near zero for negative associations indicate strong associations' (Sandercock, 1989, p. 818). Use of odds ratio analysis for clinical prediction, even in case-control

*This research was undertaken through the University of Michigan Alzheimer Disease Research Center, the Department of Neurology and the Neuropsychology Division, Department of Psychiatry, and supported by Grant #P50-AG08671 from the NIH/NIA. This manuscript is an elaboration of a paper presented at the Annual Meeting of the International Neuropsychological Society in Orlando, FL, February. 1997.
Address correspondence to: L.A. Bieliauskas, Division of Neuropsychology, Box 0840. Department of Psychiatry, University of Michigan Medical Center, Ann Arbor, MI 48109-0840, USA.
Accepted for publication: June 9, 1997.

studies, has been supported in neuroscience research (Sandercock).

It has been suggested that when highly significant differences on cognitive test performance between impaired and unimpaired elderly patients are subjected to risk analysis, prediction of cognitive decline is often less than impressive (Bieliauskas, 1993). This is particularly important in clinical practice if one is predicting a terminal course of cognitive decline for these patients.

It was the purpose of this study to evaluate the application of the odds ratio to performance on standard clinical neuropsychological tasks, comparing the odds ratio to standard parametric approaches. Comparisons between patients diagnosed with Alzheimer's disease and matched controls were used to exemplify the use of the odds ratio in clinical neuropsychology.

METHOD

Participants and Measures

Control Group
The normal control sample consisted of 25 currently healthy community-dwelling adults, aged 51 to 83 years, who volunteered to complete a neuropsychological battery. All participants in the study met the following criteria: (1) no expressed concerns of cognitive compromise; (2) no active central nervous system or psychiatric conditions; (3) no active or residual cognitive deficits from injury or disease; and (4) no level of medication use that could result in cognitive compromise.

Patient Sample
The patient sample consisted of 26 community-dwelling adults, aged 57–86, who were evaluated at an outpatient geriatric clinic as part of a dementia work-up. All patients met NINCDS/ADRDA criteria (McKhann, Drachman, Katzman, Price, & Stradlan, 1984) for possible or probable Alzheimer's disease; diagnoses were determined by comprehensive neurological work-up and, therefore, were largely independent of individual scores on neuropsychological tests. Patients were *not* classified into the dementia group on the basis of the neuropsychological cutoff scores used here. Demographics for both samples are shown in Table 1.

Patients and controls were matched on education, $t(48) = 0.22$, $p > .10$; gender, $\chi^2 = 0.04$, $p > .10$; and handedness, $\chi^2 = 4.47$, $p > .10$. The two groups differed on age, $t(48) = -6.34$, $p < .001$, but all individuals'

Table 1. Comparisons between Patients and Controls on Demographic Data and on Selected Wechsler Memory Scale Scores.

Variable	Controls ($n = 25$) M	(SD)	Patients ($n = 26$) M	(SD)	t	p	o'	Clo'	Sens	Spec	Accur
Age	61.1	(10.1)	77.0	(7.6)	-6.34	<.001					
Education	16.2	(2.8)	16.0	(2.6)	0.22	.82					
% Female	32.0	(34.6)	0.04	.84[a]							
% Right-Handed	76.0	(96.2)	4.47	.11[a]							
LM % Retained	77.5	(15.0)	13.3	(21.1)	12.21	<.0005	100.3	13.6–742.5	96	88	91.8
VR % Retained	91.0	(21.9)	29.5	(25.8)	9.09	<.0005	44.9	8.6–233.5	92	84	88.0
Paired Associates	15.8	(3.4)	7.1	(2.4)	10.38	<.0005	27.7	1.5–506.9	35	100	66.7
Mental Control	7.8	(1.3)	4.8	(2.3)	5.69	<.0005	19.6	1.1–366.1	77	83	80.0
Digit Span	11.8	(2.2)	9.4	(1.8)	4.20	<.0005	4.2	0.6–27.8	58	83	70.0

Note. LM = Logical Memory; VR = Visual Reproductions; p = level of significance associated with a t test comparing the two groups; o' = corrected odds ratio; CLo' = 95% confidence interval around o; Sens = Sensitivity; Spec = Specificity; Accur = Overall Accuracy; Demographic significance tests were two-tailed; cognitive significance tests were one-tailed.
[a] Chi – square.

scores were corrected for age using published, age-appropriate norms. The measures administered included the Russell revision of the Wechsler Memory Scale (WMS; Russell, 1975; Wechsler, 1945). Dependent variables from the WMS were Logical Memory (LM) Percent Retained (after a 30-min delay), Visual Reproductions (VR) Percent Retained, Paired Associate Learning, Mental Control, and Digit Span.

Design and Analyses

This study followed a comparative retrospective (or case-control) design. Several potential biases to this design have been described at length in many classic papers (e.g., Cornfield, 1951; Cornfield & Haenszel, 1960; White & Bailar, 1956) and are recapitulated in more recent reviews and commentaries (e.g., Feinstein, 1979; Sackett, 1979). Although the retrospective design is susceptible to misapplication and over-interpretation, it is nonetheless a powerful statistical tool (Ibrahim & Spitzer, 1979). Compared to cross-sectional and prospective designs, the case-control procedure maximizes precision and power and minimizes the confidence interval in analyses of 2 × 2 contingency tables (Fleiss, 1981). It was argued to be the 'method of choice' by Mantel and Haenszel (1959).

The odds ratio is considered the optimal statistic for analyzing 2 × 2 contingency tables because it 'is suggested by a mathematical model, ... remains valid under alternative models, ... can serve as the basis of a test of a hypothesis, and ... is invariant under different methods of studying association' (Fleiss, 1981, p. 92). In our study, the odds ratio was computed using the correction proposed by Fleiss, which is designated o'. This correction adds 0.5 to the raw frequency of each cell in the 2 × 2 table, so that empty cells will not produce an undefined entity (i.e., a zero in the denominator of the odds ratio formula).

The confidence interval (CI) was derived using the natural logarithm of the corrected odds ratio, or ln (o'), and the standard error of ln (o'). The logarithm of o' adds the property of an absolute zero, which the standard o' lacks. The CI was converted back to standard values by taking the antilog of the lower and upper bounds (Fleiss, 1981). A step-by-step procedure for computing the odds ratio and confidence interval is described in the Appendix.

Neuropsychological scores were dichotomized into negative and positive risk factors using a cut-off of one standard deviation beyond the age-appropriate normative mean (using published norms), in the direction of impaired performance. Specifically, for a given score, if the participant scored at or below $-1.0\ SD$ (or $\geq +1.0$, where positive scores indicate greater impairment, such is the case with error scores), that person was classified as 'at risk' on the neuropsychological dimension.

RESULTS

The descriptives for the two samples are presented in Table 1; also reported in the table are the t values comparing the two groups by conventional methods of analysis of case-control data in neuropsychology, the alpha (p) associated with that t test, the o' measure of association, and the CI on o'. Sensitivity, specificity, and overall accuracy (sum of accurately classified cases divided by the total number of cases) are also tabulated. Classification rates by cell (true positive, false positive, true negative, and false negative) are presented for each dependent variable in Table 2. It is apparent from these data that all of the neuropsychological measures discriminated the two groups at levels that resulted in very small and indistinguishable p values using a standard parametric test, even after correcting for age by using age-appropriate norms for each individual. The most exact p value provided by either computer program (SPSS, 1994) or by statistics textbook was $p < .0005$; this applies to any t value exceeding 3.55 for a sample this size, a criterion exceeded by all of the neuropsychological tests in this study.

By contrast to the measurable p values, the odds ratios varied considerably in their magnitude. Retention of new verbal information (Logical Memory) indicated a concurrent diagnosis of Alzheimer's disease far better than did retention of new visual information (Visual Reproductions). The three other variables (Digit Span, Mental Control, and Paired Associates) were much less indicative. In fact, the odds ratio CI for each of those three scores approached or included the value 1.0. An odds ratio of 1.0 indicates an equal probability of being diagnosed with the disorder regardless of whether or not people score beyond the neuropsychological cutoff.

Table 2. Classification of Participants by Neuro-psychological Test Variables.

	Positive		Negative	
	True	False	True	False
LM % Retained	24	3	21	1
VR % Retained	23	4	21	2
Paired Associates	9	0	25	17
Mental Control	20	4	20	6
Digit Span	15	4	20	11

At least two of these ratios (Digit Span and Mental Control) would be considered clinically non-significant even though they reached statistical significance by conventional parametric hypothesis testing ($p \leq .0005$). Thus, the odds ratio data yielded considerably more information that is not reflected in the parametric data.

DISCUSSION

In this study, patients with Alzheimer's disease were compared to a control group in order to exemplify and evaluate the application of the odds ratio in clinical neuropsychology. Using standard parametric tests, all five neuropsychological measures that were examined distinguished patients from controls at very discriminating levels, as depicted by the magnitude of the t values. But beyond its use in ranking the variables within this study, how does one interpret individual t values? One way to assign further meaning is to determine the associated p value, but there are several limits to this approach. First, for any $t > 3.55$ (such as all is in this study), t tables generate the same significance level, $p < .0005$. Beyond this point, effect sizes are virtually indistinguishable.

There is a second limitation of using p as an index of effect size: These values vary with sample size and are not comparable between samples. As a final limitation, even if we can ascertain the exact values and make comparisons solely within a single study, how do we compare $p = .00005$ to $p = .0001$ with regard to the real-world impact of the diagnostic test? One index of effect size for group comparisons is the point-biserial correlation. This can be a fairly useful index for social scientists, who use and interpret correlation coefficients on a frequent basis. Other consumers of clinical neuropsychological test data, on the other hand, may be less versed in the meaning of correlation coefficients. Furthermore, even sophisticated social scientists would have a difficult time translating a point-biserial correlation into classification rates and probabilities.

These limitations of parametric values can be contrasted to the odds ratio to exemplify the advantages of the latter. First, odds ratios showed considerable differences in magnitude that could not be discerned from standard parametric p values. For example, at least two of the ratios examined in this study (Digit Span and Mental Control) would be considered clinically non-significant by the confidence interval on the odds ratio, even though they resulted in the smallest p value listed in a conventional parametric table ($p < .0005$). As a further advantage over the p values, these odds ratios can be compared to odds ratios generated from other studies, even if the sample sizes are different. Finally, the o' values have an inherent and clinically interpretable meaning: For individuals who score beyond the cutoff score on a neuropsychological test, the probability that they will be diagnosed with dementia by a neurologist *concurrently* (by the present design) is o' times greater than that for people scoring in the unimpaired range on that same test. A scientifically responsible statement of such results in a clinical report might use the lower bound as a means of controlling for error of estimate. For example, 'We can be 97.5% (one-tailed) confident that people this patient's age who retain less than xx% (the -1.0 SD cutoff) of new verbal information are at least 13 times more likely to have diagnosable dementia than are those who retain more on that same test.'

Other common diagnostic statistics are sensitivity and specificity. Sensitivity is the proportion of diseased individuals who are correctly identified by a diagnostic test. Specificity is the proportion of healthy individuals who are correctly identified as such by a diagnostic test. These can be combined into a summary index using 'overall accuracy', which is the sum of accurately classified cases (true positive + true negative) divided by the total number of cases. Because these statistics also derive from 2×2 contingency tables, they are related to the odds ratio. This is evident in Table 1, where the two tests with the highest odds ratios also carry the best combination of sensitivity and specificity values and the highest overall accuracy values. Both the odds ratio and the sensitivity-specificity values offer unique advantages: used together, therefore, they yield even more information.

It should be emphasized that the research design in the present study is not a true retrospective/case-control design but more of what we would call a 'concurrent/case-control design.'

Whereas a retrospective study would compare current diagnosis to a past predictor (exposure), our study compares current diagnosis with a *current* indicator (neuropsychological performance). The odds ratio generated from this design can be interpreted as the probability that people who are 'positive' by neuropsychological evaluation would be diagnosed by a neurologist as having dementia *at or near that same point* in time. This application of neuropsychological testing is typical of diagnostic settings, in which neuropsychologists are often asked to confirm or clarify a patient's present diagnosis. In contrast to true retrospective designs, this 'concurrent' design does not permit interpretations of future prediction. Prediction from the odds ratio can be inferred only if a retrospective or prospective design is used.

There is another caveat to the use of the odds ratio in neuropsychology, computation of an odds ratio requires the classification of neuropsychological scores into 'impaired' versus 'unimpaired.' Forcing continuous variables into discrete variables results in a loss of precision (Ragland, 1992; Zhao & Kolonel, 1992). However, such a dichotomy can facilitate communication in medical settings where decision making occurs under time constraints.

Sample size and power estimation also warrant special considerations in using odds ratios. Unlike many commonly used statistics. CIs around o' are only loosely related to sample size. Rather, they are more related to the distribution of scores within the 2 × 2 contingency table. For example, if 100 people were distributed with perfect classification (50 scoring beyond the cutoff all being diagnosed as positive; 50 scoring within normal limits being diagnosed as negative), the o' would be over 10,000 (95% CI: 198 < o' < 524,058). If those same 100 people were distributed with poor classification (equally across the four cells), o' would be 1.00 (95% CI: 0.46 < o' < 2.17). Multiplying that sample by 10 in the perfect classification scenario would escalate the o' and the CI range ($o' = 1$ million; 95% CI: 19.536 < o' < 49.721,975); in the poor classification scenario this distribution would maintain the o' but tighten the CI ($o' = 1.00$; 95% CI: 0.78 < o' < 1.28). Nonetheless, there are considerations for planning the sample size in a proposed study. For more information, the reader might consult

Fleiss and Levin (1988); Mendell, Thode, and Finch (1991); and Smith, Connett, and McHugh (1985). Statistical power for odds ratios is also estimable (Hirji, Tang, Vollset, & Elashoff, 1994).

In conclusion, this index can be useful to clinical neuropsychology. Clinically, it adapts neuropsychological test data to everyday decision-making models. It yields a statement, based on appropriate analysis, that can be easily incorporated into a clinical report and that can be easily understood by many different groups of referring professionals. In research, also, this statistic can provide an interpretable index on which to compare different measures, different patient groups, and different studies, from a probability perspective. Although this tool should not replace the more precise parametric statistics for continuous variables, it can certainly be a valuable complement to them. We recommend the reporting of *both* parametric statistics and odds ratios in designs that lend themselves to such analyses.

REFERENCES

Bieliauskas, L.A., (1993). Risk ratios and prediction of cognitive decline in dementing illness [Abstract]. *Journal of Clinical and Experimental Neuropsychology, 15*, 391.

Cornfield, J. (1951). A method of estimating comparative rates from clinical data: Applications to cancer of the lung, breast, and cervix. *Journal of the National Cancer Institute, 11*, 1269–1275.

Cornfield, J., & Haenszel, W. (1960). Some aspects of retrospective studies. *Journal of Chronic Disease, 11*, 523–534.

Feinstein, A.R. (1979). Methodologic problems and standards in case-control research. *Journal of Chronic Disease, 32*, 35–41.

Fleiss, J.L. (1979). Confidence intervals for the odds ratio in case-control studies: The state of the art. *Journal of Chronic Disease, 32*, 69–77.

Fleiss, J.L. (1981). *Statistical methods for rates and proportions* (2nd ed.). New York: Wiley & Sons.

Fleiss, J.L., & Levin, B. (1988). Sample size determination in studies with matched pairs. *Journal of Clinical Epidemiology, 41*, 727–730.

Hirji, K.F., Tang, M.L., Vollset, S.E., & Elashoff, R.M. (1994). Efficient power computation for exact and mid-P tests for the common odds ratio in several 2 × 2 tables. *Statistics in Medicine, 13*, 1539–1549.

Ibrahim, M.A., & Spitzer, W.O. (1979). The case-control study: The problem and the prospect. *Journal of Chronic Disease, 32*, 139–144.

Inter-Society Commission for heart disease resources (1970). Primary prevention of the atherosclerotic diseases. *Circulation, 42*, A55.

Mantel, N., & Haenszel, W. (1959). Statistical aspects of the analysis of data from retrospective studies of disease. *Journal of the National Cancer Institute, 22*, 719–748.

McKhann, G., Drachman, D., Folstein, M., Katzman, R., Price, D., & Stadlan, E.M. (1984). Clinical diagnosis of Alzheimer's Disease: Report of the NINCDS-ADRDA work group under the auspices of the Department of Health and Human Services task force on Alzheimer's disease. *Neurology, 34*, 939–944.

Mendell, N.R., Thode, H.C. Jr., & Finch, S.J. (1991). The likelihood ratio test for the two-component normal mixture problem: Power and sample size analysis. *Biometrics, 47*, 1143–1148.

Ragland, D.R. (1992). Dichotomizing continuous outcome variables: Dependence of the magnitude of association and statistical power on the cutpoint. *Epidemiology, 3*, 434–440.

Russell, E.W. (1975). A multiple scoring method for the assessment of complex memory functions. *Journal of Consulting and Clinical Psychology, 43*, 800–809.

Sackett, D.L. (1979). Bias in analytic research. *Journal of Chronic Disease, 32*, 51–63.

Sandercock, P. (1989). The odds ratio: A useful tool in neurosciences. *Journal of Neurology, Neurosurgery, and Psychiatry, 52*, 817–820.

Smith, J., Connett, J., & McHugh, R. (1985). Planning the size of a matched case-control study for estimation of the odds ratio. *American Journal of Epidemiology, 122*, 345–347.

SPSS (1994). *SPSS 6.1 for Windows* [Computer software].Chicago, IL: Author.

Wechsler, D. (1945). A standardized memory scale for clinical use. *Journal of Psychology, 19*, 87–95.

White, C., & Bailar, J.C. (1956). Retrospective and prospective methods of studying association in medicine. *American Journal of Public Health, 46*, 35–44.

Wickens. T.D. (1989). *Multiway contingency tables analysis for the social sciences.* Hillsdale, NJ: Lawrence Erlbaum.

Zhao, L.P., & Kolonel, L.N. (1992). Efficiency loss from categorizing quantitative exposures into qualitative exposures in case-control studies. *American Journal of Epidemiology, 136*, 464–474.

Child Neuropsychology
1995, Vol. 1, No. 1, pp. 26–37

Diagnosing Autism Using ICD-10 Criteria: A Comparison of Neural Networks and Standard Multivariate Procedures*

Domenic V. Cicchetti[1,2], Fred Volkmar[3], Ami Klin[3], and Donald Showalter[4]

[1]West Haven VAMC and [2]Yale University, [3]Yale University Child Study Center and [4]West Haven VAMC

ABSTRACT

In a sample of 976 consecutive cases derived from the recent world-wide Field Trial of Autism and other Pervasive Developmental Disorders, we tested the accuracy of the 15 ICD-10 criteria for the diagnosis of Autism, by comparing neural network models (NN) to more conventional multivariate competitors, namely, linear and quadratic discriminant function analyses and logistic regression. NNs were less accurate than competitors, both in terms of cross-validation results as well as in levels of shrinkage from training to test conditions. The clinical research implications of these results are discussed.

The purpose of this research investigation was to examine critically the extent to which various multivariate procedures, including neural networks (NN), compare to each other as appropriate candidates for assessing the accuracy of the clinical diagnosis of autism, on the basis of an ICD-10 classification system. The major focus is on data deriving from a recent world-wide Field Trial of Autism and other Pervasive Developmental Disorders.

In a recent article, Cohen, Sudhalter, Landon-Jiminez, and Keogh (1993) compared an NN approach to linear discriminant function analysis (LDFA) in the classification of Autism. While the authors report that NN was superior to LDFA for both *training* (92% vs. 85%) and *test* cases (92% vs. 82%), they were careful to note the need for replication studies necessitated by study sample limitations. A major methodologic deficiency of this investigation is that the subject-to-variable ratio of only 5:1 is not sufficient to produce valid results (see especially, Astion & Wilding, 1992a).

In order to overcome this problem and to produce more comprehensive and generalizable findings,

we designed our study to: (1) include a substantially larger number of Autistic (+) and Non-Autistic (−) cases relative to input parameters; (2) use a broader comparison group, comprised of non-autistic cases with or without pervasive developmental disorder (PDD), mental retardation, or other developmental disorder; (3) broaden the multivariate approaches against which to compare the diagnostic accuracy of NN, to include not only LDFA but also Quadratic Discriminant Function Analysis (QDFA) and Logistic Regression (LOGREG).

REVIEW OF RELEVANT LITERATURE

A brief but critically important computer simulation literature has begun to develop, over the past decade and a half, that focuses upon the critical relationship between the number of subjects (S) per input variable (V), or S/V ratio, and the accuracy of classification, for: LDFA (Fletcher, Rice, & Ray, 1978); QDFA (Rawlings, Rae, Graubard, Eckardt, & Ryback, 1982); and, most recently, NN (Astion & Wilding, 1992a).

* Address correspondence to: Domenic V. Cicchetti, Ph.D., Senior Research Psychologist and Biostatistician, West Haven VA Medical Center & Yale University, 950 Campbell Avenue, West Haven, CT, O65 16, USA.
Accepted for publication: October 20, 1994.

In each of these studies, recommendations were based upon equal sample sizes in the disordered (diseased) and nondisordered (control or normal) group. The work of Fletcher et al. (1978) indicates that, for accurate results to be obtained when applying LDFA, the S/V needs to be at least 5:1 to produce shrinkage levels at about 10%. The later work of Rawlings et al. (1982) suggests that a corresponding S/V ratio of about 10:1 is required for QDFA.

As noted recently by one of the authors (Cicchetti, 1992), the importance of the size of the S/V ratio has not been recognized as a critical variable in designing NN studies. As a result, NN studies in both medicine (see Astion & Wilding, 1992b and, most recently, Wu, Giger, Doi, Vyborny, Schmidt, & Metz, 1993) and the behavioral sciences (e.g., Cohen et al., 1993) have used S/V ratios of 5:1 or less. Nonetheless, the computer simulation studies just cited for NN, LDFA, and QDFA indicate clearly that there is a strong inverse linear relationship between the size of S/V and the level of accuracy of classification. More specifically, the lower the S/V, the higher the inaccuracy rate. This is another way of documenting the extent of shrinkage that can be expected to occur from training set accuracy to test or cross-validation set accuracy, whenever one applies a given multivariate technique to test the accuracy of diagnosis.

Using random numbers and varying the S/V so that the expected level of accuracy of classification into one of two outcome groups could be defined as 50%, Fletcher et al. (1978) were able to show, in their pioneering study, that neither the sample size (S) alone nor the number of variables (V) alone was responsible for differences in shrinkage levels. Rather, it was the S/V ratio itself that made the difference. Specifically, Fletcher et al. (1978), as summarized by Cicchetti (1992), demonstrated the following:

When the ratio is 1:1, whether the number of subjects in the two groups is 10, 25, or 50, the expected shrinkage estimates vary within the narrow band of 34% to 36%. For a ratio of 2:1, group sizes of 20, 50, and 100 produced shrinkage estimates ranging between 21% and 23%; for a 3:1 ratio and corresponding samples of 30, 75, and 150, the shrinkage estimates were all 17%; for 4:1, and group sizes 40, 100,

and 200, the shrinkage estimates were between 13% and 15%; and, finally, for ratios of 5:1 and sample sizes of 50, 125, and 250, the shrinkages were between 9% and 12%. (p. 9)

Using the previous work of Fletcher et al. (1978), as a model, Astion and Wilding (1992a) were able to show that shrinkage rates for NN are a joint function of both the S/V ratio and the number of hidden neurons. Specifically, these authors examined S/V ratios of 1:1, 3:1, 5:1, 10:1, 20:1, 25:1, and 30:1. For each S/V, the number of hidden neurons was set at 1, 3, or 10. Results indicated the following: For a *single* hidden neuron, the respective shrinkages, as S/V increased from 1:1 to 30:1, were 42%, 21%, 12%, 10%, 8%, 5%, and 1%. For *three* hidden neurons, the corresponding shrinkages were 50%, 37%, 28%, 12%, 12%, 7%, and 5%. Finally, for 10 hidden neurons, shrinkage rates were, respectively, 50%, 50%, 47%, 33%, 21%, 20%, and 17%. The upshot of this is that, when the number of hidden neurons is restricted to only one, the work of Astion and Wilding (1992a) indicates a ratio of 20:1 in order to keep shrinkage at about 10%. However, at the same S/V of 20:1, shrinkage increases to 12% for 3 and 21% for 10 hidden neurons (i.e., Astion & Wilding, 1992a, Table 1, p. 998). It is quite informative that, on a purely mathematical/statistical basis, the conjoint role of S/V and the number of hidden neurons in a given feed-forward, back-propagation NN is quite consistent with both approximation and estimation theory (e.g., see, most recently, Barron, 1994).

As we shall see, the data deriving from the rather definitive computer simulation work on LDFA, QDFA, and NN render it possible to formulate some specific hypotheses for comparing critically the accuracy of a given multivariate technique for diagnosing or differentiating autistic from nonautistic disorders. These hypotheses will be articulated in the next section of the exposition.

METHOD

Subjects
Subjects were 977 consecutive patients, deriving from 20 field sites in the U.S. (11 sites), as well as sites in Canada, England, France, Holland, Israel, Japan, Korea, New Zealand, and Spain. Varying numbers of patients

were obtained from these multiple sites, with the minimum number seldom fewer than 20 cases. The 125 examiners rated, on average, about 8 cases each. The intent in the design of the Autism Field Trial was to include a broad sample of autistic individuals representative of the range of syndrome expression of the disorder, namely, from preschool age to adulthood, and with intellectual levels ranging from profound mental retardation

Table 1. Demographic Characteristics of Patients and Evaluators in Autism Field Trial.

	Autistic	Non-Autistic	Total sample
N	454	523	977
Sex ratio	4.49:1	2.94:1	
(Male/female)			
% Mute	54%	34%	
Mean age	8.99	9.70	
Mean IQ	58.1	71.6	
Race ethnicity			
White			67.4%
Black			11.9%
Hispanic			7.4%
Asian			8.9%
Other			4.6%
Placement			
Regular school			11.6%
Special classes			20.5%
Special school			38.5%
Not in school			
or NA			29.4%
Living situation			
Home			79.7%
Residential			13.0%
Other			7.3%

to normal or average IQ. The age range for children was between 3 and 20 years (98% of the total sample). Adults, between 21 and 60 years of age, comprised the remaining 2% of the sample. Control or comparison cases were defined to include individuals with disorders that would be anticipated to enter into a differential diagnosis of Autism. This would reasonably include mental retardation and developmental language disorders but probably would not include conduct disorders. Cases were also recruited to fill potential gaps in coverage that would be expected to occur as a result of our consecutive sample design. These cases included higher functioning autistic females, and those with Rett's Syndrome, Childhood Disintegrative Disorder, or Asperger's Syndrome. For such cases, evaluations were based less frequently on currently examination than on past contact with the patients.

The demographic characteristics of the patient and evaluator samples are provided in Tables 1, 2, and 3.

Procedure

Study Design Procedure

A standard protocol was used at each site. On the basis of both interviews and other sources of information provided in clinical records, patients were always given an initial overall clinical diagnosis. Each examiner then rated the patient on each of the DSM-III, DSM-III-R, DSM-IV, or ICD-10 criteria. These four classification systems were presented in randomized order.

For 118 cases, two independent examiners provided reliability data on the overall diagnosis of Autism. This resulted in a kappa value of .81, a level of chance-corrected agreement that is considered excellent by the clinical criteria of Cicchetti and Sparrow (1981), Fleiss (1981), and almost perfect (.80–1.00) by Landis and Koch (1977). (See footnotes 1–4)

Table 2. Primary Clinical Diagnoses of Non-Autistic Cases.

Other PDD ($n = 240$) (Not Autistic)		Non-PDD ($n = 283$) Disorders	
Rett Syndrome	13 Cases	Mental retardation	132 Cases
Heller Syndrome	16 Cases	Developmental language	88 Cases
Asperger Syndrome	48 Cases	Childhood schizophrenia	9 Cases
PDD-NO	116 Cases	Other	54 Cases
Atypical Autism	47 Cases		

[1] Independent clinical diagnoses produced a level of 92% agreement for Autistic cases, 89% for Non-Autistic cases, 91% for positive and negative diagnoses combined, and the resulting kappa of .81.

[2] This same sample of 118 patients was rated independently by two examiners producing the following levels of agreement: 81% for Autistic cases, 82% for Non-Autistic cases, 81% for Autistic and Non-Autistic cases combined, and a kappa of .63 (in the "GOOD" range, i.e., the criteria of Cicchetti & Sparrow, 1981).

As in all research of this genre, the focus is in identifying those methods (usually multivariate) that best predict the extent to which a number of input variables $(X_1, X_2, \ldots, X_n)$ distinguish between the presence or absence of a given disorder or disease process, usually designated as (Y). In our research, Y, a dichotomous dependent variable, would represent the overall clinician diagnosis, defined as **presence** $(+)$ or **absence** $(-)$ of Autism and the input variables $X_1, X_2, \ldots, X_{15}$ would represent the 15 ICD-10 criteria (each also scored as **present** $(+)$ or **absent** $(-)$), as they are classified under the relevant diagnostic parameters pertaining to the following defining features of Autism, namely: Onset; Qualitative impairments in reciprocal social interaction; Qualitative impairments in communication; and

Restricted, repetitive and stereotyped patterns of behavior, interests and activities. This information is presented in Table 4.

Before considering data analytic strategies, one additional critical issue needs to be addressed, namely, the extent to which each of the 15 predictor variables (in this case ICD-10 criteria) is correlated, one with the other. From a clinical point of view, we are concerned with avoiding redundancy of information provided by the individual ICD-10 criteria as prognostic indices of an overall best clinical diagnosis of Autism. Viewed in terms of biostatistical soundness, we are concerned with the issue of multicollinearity (e.g., Cohen & Cohen, 1983) or the extent to which highly correlated input variables can invalidate the results of a multivariate predictive model.

In our research investigation, the 15 ICD-10 predictor variables produced an intercorrelation matrix comprised of $R(R - 1)$ or $(15 \times 14)/2 = 105$ Rs, or Phi coefficients. Of these, 95 (or 90.5%) ranged between .07 and .49. The remaining 10 (or 9.5%) were between .50 and .59, with a median Phi value of .34. In terms of how each ICD-10 criterion correlated with a best clinical diagnosis of Autism: 8 produced Phis ranging between .24 and .39; 4 were between .43 and .47; and the remaining 3 were between .50 and .55. Given these results, none of the 15 ICD-10 criteria needed to be deleted as predictor variables. Setting beyond .60 as a minimal criterion for redundancy of information is consistent with that set in other research investigations (e.g., McCarthy et al., 1982; and J. Fletcher, personal communication).

Data Analytic Strategies

The overall strategy involved dividing the total group of 977 patients into a training and test set (cross-validation set). Since there were 523 patients in the Non-Autistic group and 454 in the Autistic group, one case was randomly deleted from the Non-Autistic group in order to produce an equal number of 488 patients in both the *training* and *test* sets. In order to insure further that there would be an equal number of Autistic and Non-Autistic subjects in both the *training* and *test* groups, we used the technique of pairing and stratified random assignment, as delineated in Fleiss (1981, p. 53). This produced 227 Autistic $(+)$ and 261 Non-Autistic $(-)$ patients in both the *training* and *test* sets.

Table 3. Characteristics of 125 Evaluators.[a]

A. *Profession*	n
Psychiatrist	54
Resident	18
Psychologist	23
Psychology trainee	9
Speech therapist	3
Nurse	4
Social worker	1
Educator	7
Other	6
Total	125
B. *Degree*	
MD	76
PhD/PsyD	23
MS/MA	14
BS/BA	15
Total	128
C. *Age*	
20–29	23
30–39	67
40–49	25
50–59	5
60+	5
Total	125

Note. [a] The n for highest degree obtained exceeds 125 because of 3 evaluators with more than one professional degree, e.g., MD/PhD.

---

[3] Whether independent clinical examiners were used to compare an ICD-10 diagnosis with the clinical diagnosis or the same clinical examiner made both assessments, the results were very similar.

Specifically, examiner 1's level of ICD-10 accuracy with the clinical diagnosis was 85% when the two evaluations were made independently and 86% when made by the same examiner. Corresponding accuracies for the

second examiner were 80% (independent diagnoses) and 79% (non-independent assessments).

[4] In the DSM-IV trials, the clinical diagnoses were made independently by each examiner, followed by application of the ICD criteria. The ICD-10 diagnosis was made by the investigators in the later scoring of each patient protocol. The rule used was not available to field trial participants.

Table 4. ICD-10 Criteria for Diagnosis of Autism.

Onset

Presence of abnormal/impaired development from before the age of 3 years.

Usually there is no prior period of unequivocally normal development but, when present the period of normality does not extent BEYOND AGE 3 YEARS. Delay and/or abnormal patterns of functioning before 3 years (whether or not recognized as such at the time) in at least one out of the following areas is required: (**Rate A1–A3**)

A1. Receptive and/or expressive language as used in social communication
A2. The development of selective social attachments and/or of reciprocal social interaction
A3. Functional and/or symbolic play.

Qualitative impairments in reciprocal social interaction

B1. Failure adequately to use eye-to-eye gaze, facial expression, body posture, and gesture to regulate social interaction
B2. Failure to develop (in a manner appropriate to mental age and despite ample opportunities) peer relationships that involve a mutual sharing of interests, activities, and emotions
B4. Lack of shared enjoyment in terms of vicarious pleasure in other people's happiness and/or a spontaneous seeking to share their own enjoyment through joint involvement with others
B5. A lack of social-emotional reciprocity as shown by an impaired or deviant response to other people's emotions, and/or lack of modulation of behavior according to social context, and/or a weak integration of social, emotional, and communicative behaviors.

Qualitative impairments in communication

C1. A delay in, or total lack of development of spoken language that is *not* accompanied by an attempt to compensate through the use of gesture or mime as alternative modes of communication (often preceded by a lack of communicative babbling)
C2. Relative failure to initiate or sustain conversational interchange (at whatever level of language skills are present) in which there is no reciprocal to and from responsiveness to the communications of the other person
C3. Stereotyped and repetitive use of language and/or idiosyncratic use of words or phrases
C4. A lack of varied spontaneous make-believe play or (when young) in social imitative play.

Restricted, repetitive, and stereotyped patterns of behavior, interests, and activities

D1. An encompassing preoccupation with stereotyped and restricted patterns of interest
D3. Apparently compulsive adherence to specific, nonfunctional, routines or rituals
D4. Stereotyped and repetitive motor mannerisms that involve either hand/finger flapping or twisting, or complex whole body movements
D5. Preoccupations with part-objects or nonfunctional elements of play materials (such as their odor, the feel of their surface, or the noise/vibration that they generate).

The resulting subject to variable ratios (S/V) then became 227/15 or 15:1 for the *Autistic* (+) and 261/15 or 17:1 for the *Non-Autistic* (−) patients.

Hypotheses

Given that our S/V was 15:1 for Autistic (+) cases and 17:1 for Non-Autistic (−) cases, we hypothesized that shrinkage levels for LDFA, QDFA, and LOGREG would be consistently below 10%, for overall diagnostic accuracy as well as for sensitivity (Se), specificity (Sp), predicted positive accuracy (PPA), and predicted negative accuracy (PNA). This derives from the aforementioned work of Fletcher et al. (1978) (for LDFA) and Rawlings et al. (1982) (for QDFA).

LOGREG would be expected to produce very similar levels of accuracy to LDFA, when the sample size of each of the two outcome groups is the same or similar (e.g., see Fleiss, Williams, & Dubro, 1986, p. 195). This led logically to the prediction that LOGREG would produce results at levels similar to those produced by LDFA. Since we also reasoned that the relationship between number of positive ICD-10 signs and the probability of an overall clinical diagnosis of Autism is primarily, though not exclusively, a linear phenomenon, this reinforced the prediction of essentially no clinically meaningful difference in the level of diagnostic accuracy produced by the various multivariate techniques LDFA, QDFA, and LOGREG.

Our prediction for the accuracy of NN was based upon the following reasoning. Given S/V ratios of only 15:1 and 17:1, with 8 or 9 hidden neurons, we hypothesized, on the basis of the comprehensive computer simulation of Astion and Wilding (1992a), that shrinkage rates for NN would be far in excess of 10%, in fact, approaching the 20% level.

Neural Networks

As in the Cohen et al. research, we employed a feed-forward NN with back-propagation training. We utilized Brainmaker (1992, 6th ed.) for NN software. Hardware consisted of a Hyundai 286E, with 640 K. Training was accomplished by "setting" the connection weights among the simulated neurons at a random level. We also applied the "generalized delta rule" (see Astion & Wilding, 1992b, p. 36) to minimize the error or maximize the probability of correct classification of each training case. After each iteration, the resulting errors – which tend, on average, to consistently decrease – were back-propagated to both the input and hidden layers. The result is a point at which the classification of the training cases is at a maximum (or asymptote).

As for any NN model, we needed to define the following parameters: the number of hidden layers, the number of hidden neurons, the tolerance for defining the outcome diagnosis (Autism-Yes/No), and the optimal number of computer runs to define asymptote or optimal training criterion. Ours occurred consistently at approximately 500 iterations of the training set.

Although the remaining parameters were varied over a large range of hidden neurons and error tolerance levels, the best results (lowest shrinkage levels) are our focus for NN comparison with its competitors, namely, LDFA, QDFA, and LOGREG. Specifically, each of our back-propagation NNs used an error tolerance of .5 to define presence of Autism. This meant that an output value, based upon a summation of weights between .5 and 1.0, signified presence of a clinical diagnosis of Autism, while values below .5 defined a negative or Non-Autistic diagnosis. This selection makes biostatistical sense in that a 50% criterion is analogous to the threshold used for classification in LDFA, QDFA, and LOGREG.

In order to define an appropriate number of hidden layers and hidden neurons, we applied two typical rules of thumb used in NN analysis, as given, for example, in Lawrence (1991). Each of these rules advises starting with a single hidden layer. In deciding upon the number of hidden neurons within the hidden layer, one rule specifies the *smaller* of the number of input (in our case 15) or output (in our case 2) neurons. The second rule of thumb defines the number of hidden neurons on the basis of approximately one half the combined number of input (15) and output (2) neurons. In our case $(.5)(15 + 2) = 8.5$, or between 8 and 9 hidden neurons. These criteria were used for both the training and test (cross-validation) cases.

Finally, we addressed, for the first time, an issue that is specific to the determination of optimal classification by NN's competitors, namely, LDFA, QDFA, and LOGREG.

This is the variation in classification accuracy that can occur as a function of how cross-validation accuracy is measured. There are three commonly used methods. The typical data analytic procedure is for an investigator to choose one of them only, depending upon either sample size limitations (the usual determinant) or ready availability or awareness of other classificatory strategies. The various available techniques are described briefly, as follows.

The usual technique is to apply the classificatory "rule" (mathematical equation) derived from the training sample to the test sample. Specifically, the LDFA, QDFA, or LOGREG discriminant function used to classify the training set is then applied to classify subjects in the test set. This technique was, for example, utilized by Astion and Wilding (1992b) to cross-validate the accuracy of age and nine laboratory tests, based on blood plasma or serum specimens, to distinguish benign from malignant breast lesions.

Another technique is to treat the training and test sets as if they were two independent, but similarly designed, studies performed in two different research settings. In this case, the discriminant rule derived from each independent sample is applied to that sample only.

A third technique is chosen primarily because of sample size limitations, and, therefore, most likely inadequate or borderline S/V ratios. This technique is known as jackknifing, or the leaving one out, or $(N - 1)$ classificatory method (Lachenbruch & Mickey, 1968). In this case, one performs a discriminant function for *each* subject in the training group by basing his classification in the ersatz test group on the discriminant rule based upon all the $(N - 1)$ remaining subjects. This technique has been utilized for the following: distinguishing Autism from mental retardation (Cohen et al., 1993); differentiating among three types of liver disease (Reibnegger, Weiss, Werner-Felmayer, Judmaier, & Wachter, 1991); and to diagnose malignancies of the breast (Wu et al., 1993).

RESULTS

General

1. As hypothesized, NN consistently performed poorer than any of its competitors (highest training level accuracy but correspondingly highest level of shrinkage).

2. Also as hypothesized, the 2 hidden neuron NN performed consistently better (demonstrated higher levels of diagnostic accuracy) than did either the 8 or 9 hidden neuron networks.

3. Finally, and again as hypothesized, NN's alternatives, LDFA, QDFA, and LOGREG were

consistently more accurate, produced much lower levels of shrinkage from training to test sets, and were very similar one to the other as classificatory methods.

Specific

Specific results rank NN and its alternatives on the basis of a sensitivity-specificity model (e.g., Cicchetti, in press; Feinstein, 1987). The specific components of the model, briefly reviewed, are, as follows:

1. *Overall Accuracy* (OA): The percentage of total cases (ICD-10 (+) and ICD-10 (−)) that agree with the overall clinical diagnosis of either Autism or Non-Autism.
2. *Sensitivity* (Se): The percentage of Autistic cases that are correctly identified by ICD-10 criteria.
3. *Specificity* (Sp): The percentage of Non-Autistic cases that are correctly identified by ICD-10 criteria.
4. *Positive Predictive Accuracy* (PPA): The percentage of ICD-10 (+) cases that are *confirmed positive* by the overall clinical diagnosis of Autism.
5. *Negative Predictive Accuracy* (NPA): The percentage of ICD-10 (−) cases that are *confirmed negative* by the overall clinical diagnosis of Non-Autism.

In an earlier publication, two of the authors and colleagues defined 70% as a minimal criterion of diagnostic reliability to be considered clinically useful (Volkmar et al., 1988). In generalizing and applying this criterion to the accuracy of the diagnosis of the *presence* or *absence* of Autism, on the basis of ICD-10 criteria, we shall utilize the following set of clinical guidelines:

Level of Diagnostic Accuracy

OA, Se, Sp, PPA, PNA	Clinical significance
Below 70%	POOR
70%–79%	FAIR
80%–89%	GOOD
90%–100%	EXCELLENT

The results of overall diagnostic accuracy of ID-10 criteria are spread in Table 5 and illustrate the following:

1. NN produces the highest levels of training accuracy, or from 90% (for 2 hidden neurons

(2H)) to 96% (for 8H), but much higher levels of shrinkage than do its *competitors* (10% for 2H to 17% for both 8H and 9H).
2. NN's *competitors* (LDFA, QDFA, and LOGREG) consistently produce *training* levels of accuracy that fall into the GOOD range (84%–87%), and shrinkage levels are almost always under 10%. This narrow band of variability indicates that NN's *competitors* are indistinguishable from each other as diagnostic statistical tools for distinguishing Autistic from Non-Autistic disorders.

Very similar results occur for Se, Sp, PPA, and PNA. These are shown in Tables 6 through 9, respectively.

DISCUSSION

The results support our hypotheses and indicate that NN's *competitors* consistently produce levels

Table 5. Overall Accuracy of ICD-10 Criteria for Clinical Diagnosis of Autism.[a]

Classificatory training	Training set	Test set	Shrinkage (−) or gain (+)
NN (8H)	96%	79%	−17%
NN (9H)	95%	78%	−17%
NN (2H)	90%	80%	−10%
LDFA	84%	83%	−1%
LOGREG	84%	81%	−3%
QDFA	87%	82%	−5%

Note. [a] NN refers to neural networks; H designates the number of artificial neurons in the hidden layer; LDFA designates linear discriminant function analysis; LOGREG refers to logistic regression; and QDFA designates quadratic discriminant function analysis.

Table 6. Sensitivity of ICD-10 Criteria for Clinical Diagnosis of Autism.

Classificatory training	Training set	Test set	Shrinkage (−) or gain (+)
NN (9H)	97%	80%	−17%
NN (8)	96%	81%	−15%
LOGREG	85%	86%	+1%
NN (2H)	93%	88%	−5%
LDFA	90%	86%	−4%
QDFA	88%	77%	−11%

of accuracy of the ICD-10 diagnosis of Autism that can be characterized as more stable in the specific sense of being subject to much lower levels of cross-validation shrinkage. Also, it is not just a matter of the amount of shrinkage: The best *competitor* **test** set is consistently more accurate than is the best NN **test** set. This can be illustrated as follows:

1. For overall accuracy (OA) of the ICD-10 diagnosis of Autism (Table 5), the best NN test set performance (NN 2H) is 80%, with a shrinkage of 10%. In contrast, the best *competitor* test set accuracy occurs for LDFA with 83% and a shrinkage rate of only 1%.

Table 7. Specificity of ICD-10 Criteria for Clinical Diagnosis of Autism.

Classificatory training	Training set	Test set	Shrinkage (−) or gain (+)
NN (8H)	95%	78%	−17%
NN (2H)	88%	73%	−15%
NN (9H)	94%	80%	−14%
LOGREG	83%	77%	−6%
LDFA	80%	80%	0%
QDFA	86%	86%	0%

Table 8. Predictive Positive Accuracy of ICD-10 Criteria for Clinical Diagnosis of Autism.

Classificatory training	Training set	Test set	Shrinkage (−) or gain (+)
NN (8H)	95%	76%	−19%
NN (9H)	93%	74%	−19%
NN (2H)	87%	74%	−13%
LOGREG	82%	76%	−6%
LDFA	79%	79%	0%
QDFA	84%	83%	−1%

Table 9. Predictive Negative Accuracy of ICD-10 Criteria for Clinical Diagnosis of Autism.

Classificatory training	Training set	Test set	Shrinkage (−) or gain (+)
NN (8H)	97%	81%	−16%
NN (9H)	97%	83%	−14%
NN (2H)	93%	87%	−6%
LDFA	90%	87%	−3%
LOGREG	87%	86%	−1%
QDFA	89%	81%	−8%

2. For Se (Table 6), the best NN test set (NN 2H) performs at an accuracy level of 88%, with a shrinkage of 5%. Here the best test set for competitors is LOGREG with 86% and essentially the same as the training set accuracy of 85%.
3. For Sp (Table 7), the best NN test set (here, NN 9H) is at 80%, with a shrinkage level of 14%. This compares to QDFA with a test set performance accuracy of 86% and no shrinkage.
4. For PPA (Table 8), NN 8H performs best with a test set accuracy level of 76% and a shrinkage level of 19%, as compared to a QDFA test set performance level of 83%, and a shrinkage level of only 1%.
5. Finally, for PNA (Table 9), the best NN test set accuracy is at 2H with a level of 87% and 6% shrinkage. The best competitor is LOGREG with a test set accuracy of 86% and, again, a shrinkage level of only 1%.
6. The fact that the test set accuracies are consistently lower for NN than for competitors, tends to vitiate any argument that the NNs were overtrained. For a discussion of this issue, see Astion and Wilding (1991a).

On the basis of these data we would conclude the following: Under rather stringent conditions (S/V ratios between 15:1 and 17:1), and commonly recommended general rules of thumb, NN, in terms of a feed-forward back-propagation model, appears to have little to offer, as compared to more traditional methods. That said, it is also the case that our study is one in which the outcome variable is dichotomous and the phenomenon appears to be essentially a linear one. Whether other NN models, with differently scaled outcome and input parameters, will fare better is a matter to be decided by appropriately designed future research investigations in the specific area of the nosology of Autism as well as more generally.

Most past NN research has: (a) utilized S/V ratios of 5:1 or less (usually the latter); (b) usually not handled the issue of highly intercorrelated input variables; and (c) almost never utilized more than one NN competitor. Our conclusion is that results stand in the context of the most well-designed, comprehensive NN feed-forward, back-propagation diagnostic studies accomplished to date.

As we noted earlier, we also designed this investigation in order to be able to compare various methods of assessing shrinkage in the test cases for NN's multivariate competitors (LDFA, QDFA, and LOGREG). These methods were as follows: (1) applying the classificatory or discriminant function derived from the training set to the test set; (2) treating the training and test sets as two independent samples; and (3) applying the Lachenbruch and Mickey (1968) (N − 1) or leaving one out jackknifing method. We can conclude from these analyses that the levels of accuracy and shrinkage were very similar across each of the three methods and emphasize that, as long as the S/V ratios are adequate (in our case 15:1 or 17:1), cross-validation methods will probably produce similar results.

As one example, the data just discussed were based upon applying the discriminant rule from the **training** to the test sample. The corresponding overall accuracy (OA) levels for LDFA, QDFA, and LOGREG, were 83%, 82%, and 81%, respectively. Similarly, when the **training** and **test** sets were treated as two **independent samples**, overall accuracy (OA) levels for LOGREG, LDFA, and QDFA were 79%, 80%, and 84%, respectively. As one might expect, similar results were obtained when the two methods were compared for Se, Sp, PPA, and PNA. In short, regardless of the three methods used, the levels ranged between the high 70s and high 80s with the great majority in the low to middle 80s. By the criteria we specified earlier, the levels of accuracy pro-duced by traditional multivariate techniques were almost always in the good range (80–89% accuracy).

However, one caveat needs to be inserted here. In our research, and in the Cohen et al. (1993) research, as well as in the LDFA, QDFA, and NN computer simulation research, the numbers of subjects in each of the two outcome groups were equal or similar in size. One would predict that, when outcome groups are unequal in sample size, the effect upon shrinkage levels will also be linear. Specifically, the greater the subject to variable (S/V) ratio **difference** between the two outcome groups, the greater the resulting shrinkage upon cross-validation or test cases. Our program of research is investigating this phenomenon through appropriately designed computer simulation studies as recently delineated in Astion and Wilding (1992a) and Cicchetti (1992).

Other important caveats are specific to NN as a multivariate classification technique. It is important to emphasize the following: (a) the full responsibility for designing any given NN falls directly upon a given research investigator; (b) the specific choices that are made for given parameters affect **strongly** both NN training and test classification accuracies (Ahmad & Tesauro, 1989; Kolen & Pollack, 1991); and (c) new NN architectures are being reported at a prolific rate (e.g., the work of Denoeux & Lengellé, 1993; Rumelhart & McClelland, 1986; and most recently, Bremner, Gotts, & Denham, 1994). Again, these new models affect greatly the resulting NN training and outcome accuracies. The situation is such that a myriad of techniques is available to NN afficionados that enables them to be essentially at liberty to attempt a large number of NN approaches on a given data set and then rationalize why the one that was reported (which just happened to produce the best results) was clearly the method of choice. Because of this phenomenon, we relied on available rules of thumb and available computer simulation studies to design our NN research and to derive our specific hypotheses.

As a final note, it should be stated that there is evidence to suggest that NN models rest on a rather unstable theoretical foundation. The major impetus behind the early development of NNs derived specifically from the neuropsychological theorizing of Donald Hebb (1949), concerning how human neurons function. The rationale underlying the training of NNs is based upon the *Hebb rule* or Hebbian *learning*, specifically, "the assumption that the simultaneous excitation of two neurons strengthens the link between them" (Lisboa, 1992, p. 270). As noted by Rumelhart and McClelland (1986), the Hebb rule "has some serious limitations, and, to our knowledge, no theorists continue to use it in this simple form" (p. 37). This has resulted in the use of other rules, notably among them the generalized Delta rule, for the back-propagation of error information from the output layer. This information is then utilized for changing the NNs connection weights (e.g., Astion & Wilding, 1992a, p. 997).

It is further informative that the concept of back-propagation NNs (or "back-prop nets") itself seems to bear little relationship to how neural connections are made and strengthened in the human brain. In commenting about this relationship, Crick (1989) notes the following:

But is this what the brain actually does? Alas, the back-drop nets are unrealistic in almost every respect, as indeed some of their inventors have admitted. They usually violate the rule that the outputs of a single neuron, at least in the neocortex, are either excitatory synapses or inhibitory ones, but not both. It is also extremely difficult to see how neurons would implement the back-prop algorithm. Taken at its face value this seems to require the rapid transmission of information backwards along the axon, that is, antidromically from each of its synapses. It seems highly unlikely that this actually happens in the brain. Attempts to make more realistic nets to do this, though ingenious, seem to me to be very forced. (p. 130)

Neural network models have also been described, quite understandably, as black-boxes with known inputs and outputs but internal workings that remain obscure (Hart & Wyatt, 1990).

Given the very large ($\geq$25:1) subject-to-variable ratios required for the valid application of NN methodology (Astion & Wilding, 1992a), and the many theoretical and empirical controversies that surround the technology, it would be prudent for the clinical research investigator with an interest in this area of inquiry to proceed with extreme caution.

REFERENCES

Ahmad, S., & Tesauro, G. (1989). Scaling and generalization in neural networks: A case study. In S.D. Touretzky (Ed.), Advances in neural information processing systems (Vol. 1, pp. 160–168). San Mateo, CA: Morgan Kauffman.

American Psychiatric Association (1980). Diagnostic and statistical manual of mental disorders–DSM-III (3rd ed.). Washington, DC: Author.

American Psychiatric Association (1987). Diagnostic and statistical manual of mental disorders–DSM-III-R (3rd ed. rev.). Washington, DC: Author.

American Psychiatric Association (1994). Diagnostic and statistical manual of mental disorders–DSM-IV (4th ed.). Washington, DC: Author.

Astion, M.L., & Wilding, P. (1992a). The application of backpropagation neural networks to problems in pathology and laboratory medicine. Archives of Pathology and Laboratory Medicine, 116, 995–1001.

Astion, M.L., & Wilding, P. (1992b). Application of neural networks to the interpretation of laboratory data in cancer diagnosis. Clinical Chemistry, 38, 34–38.

Barron, A.R. (1994). Approximation and estimation bounds for artificial neural networks. Machine Learning, 14, 115–133.

Bremner, F.J., Gotts, S.J., & Denham, D.L. (1994). Hinton diagrams: Viewing connection strengths in neural networks. Behavioral Research Methods, Instruments, & Computers, 26, 215–218.

California Scientific Software (1992). BrainMaker: User's guide and reference manual (6th ed.). Nevada City, CA: Author.

Cicchetti, D.V. (1992). Neural networks and diagnosis in the clinical laboratory: State of the art. Clinical Chemistry, 38, 9–10.

Cicchetti, D.V. (in press). Guidelines, criteria and rules of thumb for evaluating normed and standardized assessment instruments in psychology. Psychological Assessment.

Cicchetti, D.V., & Sparrow, S.S. (1981). Developing criteria for establishing interrater reliability of specific items: Applications to assessment of adaptive behavior. American Journal of Mental Deficiency, 86, 127–137.

Cohen, J., & Cohen, P. (1983). Applied multiple regression/correlation analysis for the behavioral sciences (2nd ed.). Hillsdale, NJ: Lawrence Erlbaum.

Cohen, I.L., Sudhalter, V., Landon-Jimenez, D., & Keogh, M. (1993). A neural network approach to the classification of autism. Journal of Autism and Developmental Disorders, 23, 443–466.

Crick, F. (1989). The recent excitement about neural networks. Nature, 337, 129–132.

Denoeux, T., & Lengellé, R. (1993). Initializing back propagation networks with prototypes. Neural Networks, 6, 351–363.

Feinstein, A.R. (1987). Clinimetrics. New Haven: Yale University Press.

Fleiss, J.L. (1981). Statistical methods for rates and proportions (2nd ed.). New York: Wiley.

Fleiss, J.L., Williams, J.B.W., & Dubro, A.R. (1986). The logistic regression analysis of psychiatric data. Journal of Psychiatric Research, 20, 195–209.

Fletcher, J.M., Rice, W.J., & Ray, R.M. (1978). Linear discriminant function analysis in neuropsychological research: Some uses and abuses. Cortex, 14, 564–577.

Hart, A., & Wyatt, J. (1990). Evaluating black-boxes as medical decision aids: Issues arising from a study of neural networks. Medical Informatics, 15, 229–236.

Hebb, D.O. (1949). The organization of behavior. New York: Wiley.

Kolen, J.F., & Pollack, J.B. (1991). Back propagation is sensitive to initial conditions. In J.E. Moody &

D.S. Touretzky (Eds.), *Advances in neural information processing systems* (Vol. 3, pp. 860–867). San Mateo, CA: Morgan Kauffman.

Lachenbruch, P.A., & Mickey, M.R. (1968). Estimation of error rates in discriminant analysis. *Technometrics, 10*, 1–10.

Landis, J.R., & Koch, G.G. (1977). The measurement of observer agreement of categorical data. *Biometrics, 33*, 259–274.

Lisboa, P.G.J. (1992). *Neural networks: Current applications.* New York: Chapman & Hall.

Lawrence, J. (1991). *Introduction to neural networks.* Grass Valley, CA: California Scientific Software.

McCarthy, P., Sharpe, M.R., Spiesel, S.Z., Dolan, T.F., Forsyth, B.W., DeWitt, T.G., Fink, H.D., Baron, M.A., & Cicchetti, D.V. (1982). Observation scales to identify serious illness in febrile children. *Pediatrics, 70*, 802–809.

Rawlings, R.R., Rae, D.S., Graubard, B.I., Eckardt, M.J., & Ryback, R.S. (1982). A methodology for construction of a multivariate diagnostic instrument: An application to alcohol abuse screening. *Computers and Biomedical Research, 15*, 228–239.

Reibnegger, G., Weiss, G., Werner-Felmayer, G., Judmaier, G., & Wachter, H. (1991). Neural networks as a tool for utilizing laboratory information: Comparison with linear discriminant analysis and with classification and regression trees. *Proceedings of the National Academy of Science, USA, 88*, 11426–11430.

Rumelhart, D.E., & Mc Clelland, J.L. (1986). *Parallel distributed processing: Explorations in the microstructure of cognition.* (Vol. 1, p. 34: *Foundations*). Cambridge, MA: MIT Press.

Volkmar, F.R., Cicchetti, D.V., Dykens, E., Sparrow, S.S., Lechman, J.F., & Cohen, D.J. (1988). An evaluation of the Autism Behavior Checklist. *Journal of Autism and Developmental Disorders, 18*, 81–97.

World Health Organization (1990). *International classification of diseases, 10th revision, Chapter V.: Mental and behavioral disorders (including disorders of psychological development) diagnostic criteria for research* (May 1990 draft for field trials). Geneva, Switzerland: WHO (unpublished).

Wu, Y., Giger, M.L., Doi, K., Vyborny, C.J., Schmidt, R.A., & Metz, C.E. (1993). Artificial neural networks in mammography: Application to decision making in the diagnosis of breast cancer. *Radiology, 187*, 81–87.

The Clinical Neuropsychologist
1999, Vol. 13, No. 1, pp. 54–65

VIII-B

Construct Validity of the Continuous Recognition Memory Test*

Kathleen L. Fuchs[1], H. Julia Hannay[1], Wendy M. Huckeba[2], and Kimberley Andrews Espy[3]

[1]The University of Houston, Houston, TX, [2]Psychological Corporation, San Antonio, TX, and [3]Department of Behavioral & Social Sciences, School of Medicine, Southern Illinois University, Carbondale, IL

ABSTRACT

A principal factor analysis was performed on variables derived from a neuropsychological battery administered to 100 healthy young adults in order to investigate the construct validity of the Continuous Recognition Memory test (CRM). It was hypothesized that CRM "hits" and "false alarms" would load on different factors. The factors that emerged in the analysis were labeled "Verbal Ability", "Divided Attention", "Attention to Visual Detail", "Visuomotor Integration and Planning", and "Learning and Memory". As expected, CRM hits had a significant loading on the Learning and Memory factor. However, CRM false alarms did not have a significant loading on the Divided Attention factor as expected and, instead, loaded significantly on the Attention to Visual Detail factor. A second analysis was performed using variables from the delayed condition of the memory measures. In this analysis, the CRM delayed recognition variable had significant loadings on both a "Nonverbal Memory" factor and a "Verbal Memory" factor. These analyses support the construct validity of CRM hits as a measure of learning and memory and suggest that false alarms provide a measure of attention to visual detail.

The Continuous Recognition Memory test (CRM) was designed to assess memory deficits in patients with closed-head injuries (Hannay & Levin, 1988a). Unlike many memory measures that call for a written or multiword verbal response, the CRM makes minimal response demands on the subject thus making it possible to assess memory in individuals with motor and/or speech output deficits. Performance on the CRM has been shown to be related to severity of injury but not to age, sex, or educational level in adolescents and adults (Hannay & Levin, 1988b, Hannay, Levin, & Grossman, 1979).

The CRM consists of 120 stimulus cards with a black and white line drawing of a familiar, living object on each. After presentation of the first block of 20 stimulus drawings, 8 of the stimulus drawings are repeated in each of the subsequent five blocks interspersed with drawings that are semantically and/or perceptually similar as well as with drawings that are dissimilar. The subject's task is to respond with the word "old" every time a drawing is presented that is identical to one previously presented and "new" each time a drawing is presented for the first time. In this way, the CRM was designed as an analogue to a signal detection task; a subject can correctly identify a previously seen target item (a hit), incorrectly reject a previously seen item (a miss), incorrectly identify a new item (a false alarm), or correctly reject a new item (a correct

* We would like to acknowledge the assistance of the following individuals for data collection and scoring: Michelle Davis, Ronetta Fairchild, Emily Ford, Helena Grant-Huckabee, Kurt Krider, Paul Laurienti, Josette LeDoux, Stephen McCauley, Beth Neitman, Holly Rickert, and Carole Smith. Portions of this study were presented at the International Neuropsychological Society Twenty Sixth Annual Meeting, February, 1998.
Address correspondence to: H. Julia Hannay, Ph.D., Department of Psychology, The University of Houston, Houston, TX 77204-5341, USA.
Accepted for publication: October 23, 1998.

rejection). As in the case of a signal detection task, there are two types of trials: a "signal plus noise" trial in which the target is presented and the subject's response will either be scored as a hit or a miss; and a "noise only" trial in which a correct rejection or false alarm is scored. The total correct score for the CRM consists of the number of hits plus the number of correct rejections (which equals hits plus 60 minus the number of false alarms).

Because the stimulus drawings are of familiar living things, Hannay and Levin (1988b) point out that the test may be less confusing to impaired subjects than other memory tests which utilize geometric or nonsense designs. Even though the items are presented visually and not named by the examiner, they lend themselves to verbal description and thus could be encoded verbally and/or nonverbally. In this way the task was designed not to be lateralizing, and studies with head-injured subjects have supported this premise (Hannay et al., 1979, Hannay & Levin, 1988b). Because poor performance on the CRM could be due to impaired visual-perceptual abilities rather than memory deficits, a discrimination post-test is given to subjects to investigate this possibility. The discrimination test consists of eight pages each with one of the target stimulus drawings at the top and six drawings below – one identical to the target and five perceptually similar drawings from the same semantic category. If a subject has difficulty discriminating the target drawing from the distracters, failure on the CRM may be attributable to impaired visual-perceptual processing (Hannay & Levin, 1988a).

The CRM has been shown to be sensitive to the diffuse effects of head injury in that it is not lateralizing and can discriminate between levels of severity of injury (Hannay et al., 1979). However, as Loring and Papanicolaou (1987) point out, our constructs of cognitive operations should not be based solely on tests sensitive to brain damage. In other words, although the CRM renders discriminating data, we are not yet certain if it measures memory, attention, visual perception, a combination of these, or other cognitive operations. For instance, Walker (1991) found that performance on the CRM during recovery from head injury was a good overall predictor of subsequent vocational performance, but was not related to subsequent on-the-job memory ratings. Kaufmann,

Fletcher, Levin, Miner, and Ewing-Cobbs (1993) found that CRM hit and false alarm scores did not correlate with each other in a sample of adolescents post head injury and proposed that the two scores measure different and perhaps independent abilities. They also suggested that disinhibition and impulsivity accounted for much of the variance in the CRM total score.

In an exploratory factor analysis using data from neurologically intact young adults, Drake, Hannay, and Burkhart (1993) obtained a four-factor solution in which the CRM hits loaded highly on a "General Learning and Memory" factor, but not on a "Visual/Perceptual/Motor" factor. The General Learning and Memory factor included measures of both verbal and nonverbal memory and thus did not support a dissociation of these memory abilities. This lack of dissociation is a common finding in factor analytic studies (Larrabee & Curtiss, 1995). In the Drake et al. study, the CRM false alarm score loaded significantly on an "Attention/ Concentration" factor that was distinct from an "Impulsivity/Disinhibition" factor. Thus, in contrast to the report of Kaufmann et al., Drake et al. concluded that CRM scores do not relate to disinhibition in cognitively intact adults. Additionally, because they loaded on different factors, CRM hit and false alarm scores appear to be indices of different abilities, and important clinical information about test performance would be obscured by combining hits and false alarms into a total correct score.

Drake et al. also included a separate analysis involving delayed memory measures. The CRM delayed recognition test is given 30 min after completion of the CRM and prior to the discrimination post-test. It utilizes the eight-page discrimination post-test booklet but with the target drawing at the top of each page covered. The subject is asked to pick out the drawing that was presented many times during the test (the one that was "old") from a group of drawings that includes the "old" target stimulus and the perceptually similar drawings that were used as distracters during the test. Although the subject has been previously exposed to all the drawings, only the target drawing was presented a total of six times during the initial test. In the analysis using delayed memory variables, Drake et al. obtained a three-factor solution similar to that obtained for the immediate condition. The CRM delayed recognition memory variable loaded with other delayed memory variables on a single factor distinct from a Visual/Perceptual/Motor factor and a Disinhibition/Impulsivity factor. CRM false alarms were not included in the delayed condition analysis as they are part of the immediate, input condition. Thus the second analysis resulted in only a three-factor solution with no factor reflecting an attention/concentration construct.

In a recent factor analytic study investigating the construct validity of verbal and visual memory tests, Larrabee and Curtiss (1995) utilized data from neuropsychological test batteries given to a variety of individuals seen as outpatients in a neuropsychological private practice. The sample was heterogeneous in term of age (16 to 70), education (7 to 18 years), and diagnosis (i.e., individuals with neurological findings were included with those who had received psychiatric diagnoses only). Separate analyses were performed utilizing variables for immediate and delayed conditions of the memory measures. For the immediate condition, the CRM total correct score loaded with the Continuous Visual Memory Test (CVMT) total correct score, the number of words consistently recalled in Verbal Selective Reminding (CLTR score), the Serial Digits (a supraspan digit sequence learning test) score, and a score for a modified version of the Wechsler Memory Scale (WMS) paired associates test on a factor the authors called "General (Visual and Verbal) Memory". Other factors that emerged in the analysis included a "Visual-Spatial Intelligence/Ability" factor with high loadings from WAIS-R Block Design, Object Assembly, Trail Making Part B, and Visual Reproduction from the WMS; an "Attention/ Immediate Memory and Information Processing" factor consisting of loadings from the Paced Auditory Serial Addition Test, Digit Span, Serial Digits, and WMS Mental Control; and a "Verbal Intelligence/Ability" factor consisting of loadings from WAIS-R Information and Vocabulary subtests. It should be noted that CRM hits and false alarms were not considered separately in the analysis. Although the results of the study indicated that the CRM is a measure of general memory, more fine-grained information regarding the processes involved in test performance may have been obfuscated by the failure to separate the total score into its hit and false alarm components, as was done in the Drake et al. study.

Larrabee and Curtiss (1995) obtained similar results for a factor analysis using delayed recall and recognition measures. In that analysis, the CRM delayed recognition score, CVMT delayed recognition score, Verbal Selective Reminding delayed recall score, modified paired associate delayed recall score, Serial Digits score, and WMS delayed Visual Reproduction score all loaded on a "General Memory" factor. The other three factors that emerged in the second analysis were defined in the same manner as in the first analysis. Because the WMS Visual Reproduction score loaded on the General Memory factor in the delayed condition only, the authors suggested that the CRM and CVMT may be considered "purer" measures of memory. A possible reason for this might be that WMS Visual Reproduction acquisition is confounded with visuoconstructive ability whereas CRM and CVMT acquisition are not. An important finding in this study was the lack of a specific, visual memory factor. Instead, measures that employed visual presentation of stimuli loaded on the General Memory factor along with measures that utilized orally presented stimuli. Likewise, measures using verbal material loaded together with measures utilizing pictorial material.

Despite the data that have accumulated thus far on the utility and factor structure of the CRM, further exploration of the construct validity of the CRM in both healthy and neurologically impaired populations remains to be done. The present study used exploratory factor analysis to examine performance by healthy young adults on a large battery of tests to determine if factors tapped by specific tests correlated with variables derived from the CRM such that the underlying factor structure of the CRM could be elucidated. Although this type of work was initiated by Drake et al. (1993), the number and range of variables selected for analysis in that study were not really sufficient. Cattell (1988) advocates for the use of a minimum of two "marker variables" for each factor expected to emerge from the factor analysis. These variables should be selected on the basis of their strong and distinct loadings in previous studies. Cattell also suggests that a factor analysis should include "background markers" – variables that will contrast with the variables of interest. Together, the markers and background markers help to define the factors and thus the constructs under investigation.

Drake et al. did not include variables from measures of verbal ability in their analysis and thus the contribution of verbal abilities to CRM performance may not have been captured. Also, it is perhaps not surprising that they found no dissociation between verbal and nonverbal memory abilities because too few verbal and nonverbal memory measures were used to define separate factors according to guidelines suggested by Cattell (1988), Gorsuch (1988), and Streiner (1994). Likewise, measures of divided and focused attention were inadequately represented. It also appears that the criterion for determining a significant factor loading was applied inconsistently, such that at least one factor (Attention/Concentration) may have been mislabeled. The present study also differs from that by Larrabee and Curtiss (1995) in variable selection, the separation of the CRM total score into its hit and false alarm components, and in subject demographics. The subjects in this study were neurologically intact college students so that data analysis would be relatively uncontaminated by variance resulting from differences in age, education, and clinical diagnosis. At least in that regard, the present study was more similar to the Drake et al. study.

We expected that in our analysis of variables from a neuropsychological test battery, the CRM hit score would load with marker variables for memory abilities on a factor that was distinct from factors defined by measures of language ability, visuoconstructional ability, divided attention, and impulsivity. We also expected that the CRM false alarm score would help define a factor for divided attention. Although Drake et al. (1993) found that the CRM false alarm score loaded on a factor which they called "Attention/Concentration", the processes involved in remembering previously presented target items while rejecting perceptually similar stimuli presented in "noise only" trials seems to better represent the definition of a divided attention task (Lezak, 1995; Van Zomeren & Brouwer, 1994). Additionally, we expected that the CRM false alarm score would not load on

a factor defined by measures of impulsivity, if indeed it is a measure of primary attentional abilities and not a measure of impulsivity or disinhibition as suggested by Kaufmann et al. (1993). When delayed condition variables were used in a factor analysis, we expected that the CRM recognition memory score would load on a factor with other measures of memory and that the overall factor structure would be similar to that obtained in the first analysis.

METHOD

Subjects were solicited for participation from undergraduate psychology classes at a large university that draws its students from a racially and economically diverse urban community. Individuals were deemed ineligible for the study if they had a history of closed-head injury, neurological disorder, psychiatric disorder, substance abuse, or learning disability. Of the 122 individuals who consented to participate in the study, 100 subjects produced complete, valid data for analysis (60 females, 35 males, 5 whose sex was not recorded). The median age of the subjects was 19 years (range = 17 to 41 years) whereas the mean age was 21.3 years (SD = 5.1 years).

The subjects completed a comprehensive neuropsychological battery over two testing sessions. The tests selected from this battery for analysis were expected to assess the areas of verbal ability (WAIS-R Vocabulary, WAIS-R Information, Controlled Oral Word Association), visuoperception and visuoconstruction (WAIS-R Block Design, WAIS-R Picture Completion, Rey-Osterreith Complex Figure copy, Judgment of Line Orientation), divided attention (Paced Auditory Serial Addition Test total score, Digit Span backward, Trail Making Test, Part B, CVMT false alarms), focused attention (WAIS-R Arithmetic, Digit Span forward, Trail Making Test, Part A), immediate verbal and nonverbal memory (CVMT hits, WMS-R Logical Memory immediate recall, Consistent Long-Term Retrieval from the Verbal Selective Reminding Test), delayed verbal and nonverbal memory (CVMT delayed recognition, Logical Memory delayed recall, Verbal Selective Reminding Test delayed recall, Rey-Osterreith Complex Figure delayed reproduction) and impulsivity (MMPI-2 scale 4, Porteus Mazes qualitative error score, Kagan's Matching Familiar Figures error score). Descriptions of these tests and scoring criteria can be found in Lezak (1995). All delay periods were 30 min, and strict scoring rules were used for the Rey-Osterreith Complex Figure and the Porteus Mazes. Additionally, the variables of interest from the CRM – hits, false alarms, and delayed recognition – were included. Test protocols were scored according to standard scoring procedures given in test manuals.

Raw scores for the variables of interest for all subjects with complete data were entered into two SAS data sets – one in which variables for memory tests were from the immediate condition, and one in which variables for memory tests were from the delayed condition. Raw scores were used rather than scaled or standardized scores to better capture the variability in test performance across subjects in this fairly homogeneous sample. Also, because the tests used in the battery have been normed on different populations, converting the raw scores we obtained to z scores or T scores might introduce error into the analyses as a result of differences in the normative populations rather than actual variability within our sample.

RESULTS

Initial univariate analysis of the variables indicated that the score distributions for Judgment of Line Orientation and Kagan's Matching Familiar Figures were skewed to the extent that they did not approximate a normal distribution even with mathematical transformation. Examination of the squared multiple correlation of each variable, where it serves as a dependent variable with all other variables in the analysis as independent variables, indicated that the variable derived from the MMPI-2 was not sufficiently related to the other variables in the set. These three variables were thus not included in further analyses.

The variables that remained were subjected to principal factor analysis using the SAS system according to the steps outlined by Tabachnick and Fidell (1989) and by Hatcher (1994). The number of factors to be retained for rotation after initial extraction was determined by a combination of examination of the Scree plot, the amount of variance accounted for by each factor, and the number of variables with significant loadings on each factor.

For the analysis using variables from the immediate condition of the memory measures, a five-factor solution satisfied the criteria recommended by Hatcher as the final factor retained accounted for 10% of the variance in the set of variables, appeared before a drop in the Scree plot, and had significant loadings (>.35) from at least three variables. The five factors were submitted to

oblique rotation using Promax, which first produces an orthogonal rotation through Varimax. As the obliquely and orthogonally rotated solutions did not differ substantially, the orthogonal rotation was retained for ease of interpretation.

The process was repeated substituting the delay condition variables for the immediate condition variables of the memory measures. A four-factor solution emerged that satisfied the above criteria and, again, as the orthogonal and oblique rotations did not produce substantially different factor patterns and loadings, the orthogonal rotation solution was retained for interpretation.

Immediate Condition

Means and standard deviations for the variables used in the analysis are given in Table 1. Principal factor analysis produced a five-factor solution using the squared multiple correlation for each variable as its prior communality estimate. Significant factor loadings after orthogonal rotation ($\geqslant.35$) are given in Table 2 along with the final communality estimate (h^2) for each variable, the proportion of variance accounted for by each factor, and the proportion of covariance accounted for by each factor.

The first factor to emerge in the analysis accounted for 10% of the total variance in the variable set and 24% of the common variance. It contained significant variable loadings from WAIS-R Vocabulary, WAIS-R Information, WMS-R Logical Memory (immediate recall), and WAIS-R Arithmetic and was labeled "Verbal Ability". The magnitude of the factor loadings for Vocabulary and Information were much larger than those for Logical Memory and Arithmetic. Inspection of the final communality estimates also indicated that much of the variance in Logical Memory and Arithmetic was not accounted for in this analysis. However, these variables shared a significant amount of variance with Vocabulary and Information. It is likely that the underlying ability responsible for this covariance was verbal ability in that responses appear to require access to a semantic store and manipulation of verbal information.

The second factor to emerge also contained a significant loading from WAIS-R Arithmetic, as well as significant loadings from PASAT, Digit Span backwards, Controlled Oral Word Association

Table 1. Simple Statistics for the Variables Used in the Analyses (Raw Scores).

	Mean	Standard Deviation
CRM Hits	38.6	1.55
CRM False Alarms	7.9	5.92
CRM Delay	7.3	0.93
WAIS-R Vocabulary	49.3	10.17
WAIS-R Information	19.3	4.12
WAIS-R Arithmetic	13.3	2.52
WAIS-R Block Design	36.4	8.69
WAIS-R Picture Completion	16.3	1.68
WAIS-R Digits Backward	8.1	2.21
WAIS-R Digits Forward	9.2	1.93
PASAT	152.2	24.43
Trail Making Test, Part A	25.4	7.96
Trail Making Test, Part B	49.7	16.01
Controlled Oral Word Association	40.6	9.22
Verbal Selective Reminding Test – CLTR	105.8	26.12
Verbal Selective Reminding Test – Delay	11.3	1.13
Logical Memory – Immediate Recall	31.2	5.93
Logical Memory – Delayed Recall	28.5	6.19
CVMT Hits	37.0	3.34
CVMT False Alarms	8.2	6.31
CVMT Delay	5.6	1.4
Rey-Osterreith Complex Figure Copy	30.8	2.90
Rey-Osterreith Complex Figure Delay	22.9	4.81
Porteus Mazes – Error score	16.0	12.58

Table 2. Orthogonally Rotated Factor Pattern – Immediate Condition.

	1	2	3	4	5	h^2
Vocabulary	**.80**	.05	−.17	−.05	.12	.68
Information	**.72**	.14	−.14	−.03	.26	.62
Logical Memory	**.39**	.23	−.17	.15	.02	.25
Arithmetic	**.39**	**.40**	−.20	.10	−.00	.36
Digits Forward	.33	.21	−.08	−.32	−.04	.27
PASAT	.22	**.74**	−.03	−.05	.11	.62
Digits Backward	.20	**.54**	−.18	−.18	.13	.42
COWA	.03	**.45**	−.09	−.03	−.09	.22
CVMT false alarms	−.08	−.11	**.74**	.15	−.13	.61
CRM false alarms	−.11	−.05	**.72**	.09	.10	.55
Picture Completion	.15	.08	**−.37**	.19	.07	.21
Block Design	.25	.20	**−.43**	.07	.29	.38
Rey Complex Figure Copy	.18	.07	**−.43**	.33	.08	.33
Trail Making Test, Part A	.11	−.20	.08	**.63**	−.08	.47
Trail Making Test, Part B	−.07	**−.44**	−.05	**.50**	−.22	.49
Porteus Mazes	.08	−.29	.13	**−.45**	−.15	.34
CRM hits	.08	−.01	−.04	−.10	**.61**	.39
SRT CLTR	.28	−.07	−.16	.09	**.50**	.37
CVMT hits	−.03	**.38**	.03	.04	**.47**	.37
Proportion of Variance	10%	9.8%	9.5%	6.5%	6.2%	Total Variance = 42%
Proportion of Covariance	24%	23%	22%	16%	15%	Total Covariance = 100%

Note. Loadings ≥.35 were deemed significant.

(COWA), and CVMT hits. The Trail Making Test, Part B also showed a significant negative loading on this factor. The negative loading was expected as a high score on this variable is indicative of poor performance (time to complete the task) whereas a high score on the other measures is related to good performance on those tasks. Three of these variables – PASAT, Digit Span backwards, and Trail Making, Part B – were selected for this analysis as marker variables for divided attention, and thus this factor was labeled "Divided Attention." Although COWA is often thought of as a test of verbal ability, it did not have a significant loading on the Verbal Ability factor. The final communality estimate for the COWA variable indicated that most of the variance was not accounted for in this analysis, and it is possible that only the attentional component of the task was captured on this factor. The Divided Attention factor accounted for nearly 10% of the total variance and 23% of the common variance in the variable set.

Marker variables for focused attention also were included in the analysis – WAIS-R Arithmetic, Digit Span forward, and the Trail Making Test, Part A. These variables did not load together to form a distinct factor as Arithmetic loaded significantly on the Verbal Ability and Divided Attention factors, Digit Span forward had loadings that approached but did not reach significance on the first and fourth factor, and Trail Making, Part A loaded significantly on the fourth factor only.

The third factor to emerge in the analysis accounted for 9.5% of the total variance and 22% of the common variance. This factor was defined by significant loadings from the false alarm variables from the CRM and CVMT, WAIS-R Picture Completion, WAIS-R Block Design, and the Rey-Osterreith Complex Figure copy. It was expected that the sign of the loadings from the false alarm variables would be opposite of that from the other variables, as a high false alarm score is indicative of poor performance. The variables for Picture Completion, Block Design, and the Rey-Osterreith Complex Figure were selected for analysis as marker variables to define a "Visuoperception and Visuoconstruction" factor, but this factor might be better labeled "Attention to Visual Detail". The high loadings from the CRM and CVMT false alarm variables on this factor indicate that the false

alarm scores were more related to attention to visual detail than other abilities, such as divided attention.

The fourth factor was labeled "Visuomotor Integration and Planning" as it was defined by variables that involved manipulating a pencil under a time pressure to plan and execute a route from one point to another. This factor accounted for 6.5% of the total variance and 16% of the common variance and was defined by significant loadings from Trail Making, Part A, Trail Making, Part B, and the qualitative error score from Porteus Mazes. Whereas the variables for Trail Making Parts A and B are reflective of speed of performance and had positive loadings on this factor, the variable from Porteus Mazes is related to accuracy of execution regardless of speed and had a negative loading. Thus, a high score on the Trail Making Test and a low error score for Porteus Mazes might indicate a planned, careful response to a visuomotor task.

The final factor to emerge in the analysis accounted for 6.2% of the total variance and 16% of the common variance. This factor was labeled "Learning and Memory" as it contained significant loadings from CRM hits, CVMT hits, and Consistent Long-Term Retrieval (CLTR) from the Verbal Selective Reminding Test. This variable was not simply labeled "memory" as the three measures rely on learning repeated stimuli unlike other variables with immediate recall conditions such as WMS-R Logical Memory and Digit Span forward.

Delay Condition

Principal factor analysis was repeated using delay rather than immediate condition variables for the memory measures. There were fewer variables in this analysis because hits and false alarms from the CRM and CVMT were replaced by the delayed recognition memory measures from each of these tests. Significant factor loadings after orthogonal rotation are given in Table 3 along with the final communality estimate (h^2) for each variable, the proportion of variance accounted for by each factor, and the proportion of covariance accounted for by each factor.

The first factor to emerge in the analysis accounted for 10% of the total variance in the variable set and 23% of the common variance. Similar to the immediate condition analysis, it

Table 3. Orthogonally Rotated Factor Pattern – Delayed Condition.

	1	2	3	4	5	h^2
Vocabulary	**.78**	.10	.02	.24	−.01	.67
Information	**.72**	.15	.20	.23	−.00	.64
Digits Forward	**.38**	.20	.03	−.01	−.25	.25
Arithmetic	**.37**	**.42**	.19	.11	.13	.38
PASAT	.18	**.75**	.11	.02	−.12	.63
Digits Backward	.21	**.54**	.14	.07	−.19	.40
COWA	.03	**.43**	.10	−.07	−.07	.20
Picture Completion	.19	.08	.33	−.10	.07	.17
Block Design	.30	.16	**.67**	.01	.00	.57
Rey Complex Figure Delay	−.18	.14	**.61**	.32	.19	.56
CVMT Delay Recognition	−.00	.17	**.59**	.26	−.17	.47
CRM Delay Recognition	.08	−.05	**.43**	**.57**	−.04	.52
SRT Delay Recall	.14	−.08	.04	**.60**	−.10	.40
Logical Memory Delay	.26	.19	.04	**.54**	.18	.43
Trail Making Test, Part A	.03	−.15	−.05	.02	**.70**	.52
Trail Making Test, Part B	−.07	**−.40**	.08	−.17	**.60**	.56
Porteus Mazes	.16	−.31	−.23	−.15	**−.37**	.34
Proportion of Variance	10%	10%	9.7%	7.9%	7.3%	Total Variance = 45%
Proportion of Covariance	23%	22%	21%	17%	16%	Total Covariance = 100%

Note. Loadings ≥.35 were deemed significant.

contained significant variable loadings from WAIS-R Vocabulary, WAIS-R Information, and WAIS-R Arithmetic. In this analysis, the loading from Digit Span forward reached the significance criterion (≥.35). As in the immediate condition analysis, this factor was labeled "Verbal Ability".

The second factor to emerge accounted for 10% of the total variance in the set and 22% of the common variance. This factor was nearly identical in variable composition and magnitude of loadings to the second factor in the immediate condition and was likewise labeled "Divided Attention".

The third factor accounted for 9.7% of the total variance and 21% of the common variance in the variable set. Like the third factor from the immediate condition analysis, this factor contained significant loadings from the WAIS-R Block Design variable, as well as the delayed memory variables from the Rey Complex Figure, the CRM, and the CVMT. Notably, WAIS-R Picture Completion failed to produce a significant loading in this analysis and its final communality estimate (.17) indicates that it did not share a great deal of variance with the other variables in this analysis. Although the Rey Complex Figure, CRM, and CVMT variables were all from delayed memory

conditions, WAIS-R Block Design was not. It is not entirely clear why Block Design loaded on this factor (perhaps because all the measures involve visual perception), but the factor was deemed a "Nonverbal Memory" factor.

The fourth factor accounted for 7.9% of the total variance and 17% of the common variance in the delay condition analysis. This factor was defined by significant loadings from CRM delayed recognition, Verbal Selective Reminding delayed recall, and WMS-R Logical Memory delayed recall. The latter two variables are clearly based on verbal material and, as it appears that the nonverbal aspects of the CRM recognition variable were captured on the third factor, it is likely that the significant loading from the CRM recognition variable on this factor represented the verbal encoding aspect of the CRM stimuli. Thus, this factor was labeled "Verbal Memory".

The final factor to emerge accounted for 7.3% of the total variance and 16% of the common variance in the variable set. This factor was identical in variable loadings with similar loading magnitudes to the fourth factor in the immediate condition analysis and was thus labeled "Visuomotor Integration and Planning".

DISCUSSION

The present analyses support the construct validity of the CRM as a measure of learning and memory. Importantly, the two components of the CRM total score – hits and false alarms – loaded on separate factors indicating that these variables are indices of different abilities within the same test. CRM hits loaded with other variables that defined a Learning and Memory factor whereas CRM false alarms loaded significantly on a factor defined by measures requiring attention to visual detail. The other factors that emerged in the analysis of the immediate condition variables were labeled Verbal Ability, Divided Attention, and Visuomotor Integration and Planning. Further, the analysis using delayed memory measures again supports the proposition that the CRM stimuli can be encoded verbally or nonverbally, as the CRM delay variable showed significant loadings on both the verbal and nonverbal memory factors.

We expected that CRM hits and false alarms would load on separate factors in this analysis. It may not be intuitively obvious that hits and false alarms would depend on different cognitive abilities; however, as the CRM was constructed as an analogue to a signal detection task, hits and false alarms occur under two different test conditions. False alarms occur in "noise only" trials where the stimuli have not been previously presented. Good performance is thus dependent upon attention to visual detail. If attention is not paid to the details of the stimuli, differences between targets and distracters may not be readily apparent and a subject may endorse a distracter item as one that had been previously seen because it is perceptually or semantically "close" to a previously seen target. Prior to our analysis, the process that occurs in noise only trials appeared to us to meet the definitions for divided attention provided by Lezak (1995) and Van Zomeren and Brouwer (1994). One class of information (previously seen items) must be remembered while an operation (attention to visual detail) is performed on a task-related item and a match/no match decision is made. However, our analysis suggests that it is not divided attention but attention to visual detail that is measured by the CRM false alarm score. Hits occur in "signal plus noise" trials in which all

stimuli have been previously seen and thus the task is one of recognition memory – all items thus should "match" the memory trace of the item even if the subject is unsure of the details of the drawing. Additionally, the target items are presented several times in the course of the test. This should strengthen the memory trace (i.e., learning) of the target and make it easier to recognize as the test progresses. CRM hits did indeed load on the Learning and Memory factor. Though the false alarm variable from the CVMT differs from that of the CRM in that the CVMT utilizes abstract line drawings rather than drawings of recognizable living things, they both showed significant loadings on the same factor indicating that the cognitive process that supports test performance is similar regardless of the type of stimuli used.

Following the recommendation of Cattell (1988), some of the variables used in the analyses were selected as "marker variables" for certain abilities to help define and label the factors that emerged. As expected, WAIS-R Information and Vocabulary loaded together to help define the Verbal Ability factor, PASAT and Digit Span backward defined the Divided Attention factor, Block Design, Picture Completion, and copy of the Rey-Osterreith Complex Figure defined what we initially were inclined to call a Visuoperception/Visuoconstruction factor but is most likely an Attention to Visual Detail factor, and the CVMT hits and Consistent Long-Term Retrieval from the Verbal Selective Reminding Test helped define the Learning and Memory factor. However, some of the variables selected for the analyses did not "behave" as expected. Notably, variables for the MMPI-2 (Scale 4) and Kagan's Matching Familiar Figures Test were dropped from the analyses due to poor correlation with other variables and extremely skewed score distributions. These variables were expected to load together to define a factor for disinhibition/impulsivity, and without these variables in the analysis, no such factor emerged. It may be that a clinical population would produce greater variability in scores on these measures such that these variables could be included in an analysis.

Also, it was expected that the variables from WAIS-R Arithmetic, Digit Span forward, and Trail Making, Part A would define a factor for focused attention. This factor did not emerge as Digit Span forward failed to load significantly on any factor in the immediate condition analysis, and Arithmetic loaded on both the Verbal Ability and Divided Attention factors. The variance from Trail Making, Part A was captured on a factor that seemed best labeled Visuomotor Integration and Planning as that factor also included significant loadings from Trail Making, Part B and the qualitative error score from Porteus Mazes.

Another unexpected finding was that the variable from the Controlled Oral Word Association did not load on the Verbal Ability factor whereas the immediate recall variable from the WMS-R Logical Memory did. This finding is striking, as COWA is often considered a test of verbal fluency, and it has been shown to correlate highly with vocabulary (desRosiers & Kavanagh, 1987). However, Ruff, Light, Parker, and Levin (1997) have shown that COWA correlates as well with Digit Span (.45) as with Vocabulary (.41) in a large sample of healthy adults. They propose that the abilities tapped by COWA are word knowledge, as well as attention and concentration in order to avoid breaking the rules under a speeded condition.

Factor analytic studies of neuropsychological test variables with mixed populations (neurologic and psychiatric patients) have shown that Logical Memory I consistently loads highly on a visual/verbal memory factor and also produces a smaller but significant loading on a verbal ability/verbal expression factor (Larrabee, Kane, Schuck, & Francis, 1985; Ryan, Rosenberg, & Mittenber, 1984). The low final communality estimates (h^2) for COWA (.22) and Logical Memory (.25) in the immediate condition analysis indicates that much of the variance in these measures was not accounted for in the analysis. Thus, it may be the secondary features – divided attention for COWA and verbal ability for Logical Memory – that were captured in the present study. In the delay condition analysis, the final communality estimate for Logical Memory was much higher (.43), and this variable loaded, as expected, with measures of verbal memory.

In contrast to other factor analytic studies (Drake, Hannay, & Burkhart, 1993; Larrabee & Curtiss, 1995; Larrabee et al., 1985), the analysis using delay condition variables from the memory measures supported a dissociation between mem-

ory for verbal material and nonverbal material. Although CRM and CVMT hits loaded together in the immediate condition analysis, and delayed recognition from these tests loaded together on the Nonverbal Memory factor, only the CRM delayed recognition also showed a significant loading on the Verbal Memory factor along with the Verbal Selective Reminding delayed recall and the Logical Memory delayed recall. It appears that in the immediate condition, the learning aspect of the CRM, CVMT, and Verbal Selective Reminding predominates as these three tests utilize repeated stimuli whereas Logical Memory does not utilize repeated stimuli and, in fact, did not load with these other variables in the immediate condition. However, recall and recognition after a delay may rely more on the manner in which the material was encoded and thus the verbal and nonverbal aspects of memory are more separable. If this be the case, the results from this study support the contention of Hannay and Levin (1988b) that the CRM is a nonlateralizing test of memory function as performance on the CRM delayed recognition appears to draw from both verbal and nonverbal memory abilities.

In contrast to the Drake et al. (1993) factor analytic study of the CRM, this study included a wider range and number of variables to help define the factors, as well as clearer decision rules as to the designation of significant factor loadings. This study also differed from that of Larrabee and Curtiss (1995) in variable selection and in the use of a neurologically intact population. Although the current study represents a further definition of the constructs that underlie performance on the CRM, there are some limitations that should be pointed out. Whereas the subject to variable ratio remained above that commonly recommended (Streiner, 1994; Tabachnick & Fidell, 1989), the sample size just meets the minimum requirements given for performing a factor analysis. With a minimum sample size, it may be that the factor structure that emerged is unstable and would not be obtained in a similar sample of 100 or more subjects. Additionally, the individuals who participated in the study were young adults with some college education. Thus, the results from this study might not generalize to other populations, such as older individuals or individuals with neurological disorders. However, the results of the current study provide a useful contrast to other studies which utilize the CRM.

REFERENCES

Cattell, R.B. (1988). The meaning and strategic use of factor analysis. In J. R. Nesselroade & R. B. Cattell (Eds.), *Handbook of multivariate experimental psychology*. (pp. 131–203). New York: Plenum Press.

desRosiers, G., & Kavanagh, D. (1987). Cognitive assessment in closed-head injury: Stability, validity, and parallel forms for two neuropsychological measures of recovery. *International Journal of Clinical Neuropsychology*, *9*, 162–173.

Drake, A.I., Hannay, H.J., & Burkhart, B. (1993, February). *The construct validity of the Continuous Recognition Memory Test.* Poster session presented at the 21st annual meeting of the International Neuropsychological Society, Galveston, Texas.

Gorsuch, R.L. (1988). Exploratory factor analysis. In J. R. Nesselroade & R. B. Cattell (Eds.), *Handbook of multivariate experimental psychology* (pp. 231–258). New York: Plenum Press.

Hannay, H.J., & Levin, H.S. (1988a). *The Continuous Recognition Memory Test: A Manual.* [Available from the first author].

Hannay, H.J., & Levin, H.S. (1988b). Visual continuous recognition memory in normal and closed head-injured adolescents. *Journal of Clinical and Experimental Neuropsychology*, *4*, 444–460.

Hannay, H.J., Levin, H.S., & Grossman, R.G. (1979). Impaired recognition memory after head injury. *Cortex*, *15*, 269–283.

Hatcher, L. (1994). *A step-by-step approach to using the SAS system for factor analysis and structural equation modeling.* Cary, NC: SAS Institute Inc.

Kaufmann, P.M., Fletcher, J.M., Levin, H.S., Miner, M., & Ewing-Cobbs, L. (1993). Attentional disturbance following closed-head injury. *Journal of Child Neurology*, *8*, 348–353.

Larrabee, G.J., & Curtiss, G. (1995). Construct validity of various verbal and visual memory tests. *Journal of Clinical and Experimental Neuropsychology*, *17*, 536–547.

Larrabee, G.J., Kane, R.L., Schuck, J.R., & Francis, D.J. (1985). Construct validity of various memory testing procedures. *Journal of Clinical and Experimental Neuropsychology*, *7*, 239–250.

Lezak, M.D. (1995). *Neuropsychological assessment* (3rd ed.). New York: Oxford University Press.

Loring, D.W., & Papanicolaou, A.C. (1987). Memory assessment in neuropsychology: Theoretical considerations and practical utility. *Journal of Clinical and Experimental Neuropsychology*, *9*, 340–358.

Ruff, R.M., Light, R.H., Parker, S.B., & Levin, H.S. (1997). The psychological construct of word fluency. *Brain and Language 57*, 394–405.

Ryan, J.J., Rosenberg, S.J., & Mittenberg, W. (1984). Factor analysis of the Rey Auditory-Verbal Learning Test. *International Journal of Clinical Neuropsychology*, *6*, 239–241.

Streiner, D.L. (1994). Figuring out factors: The use and misuse of factor analysis. *Canadian Journal of Psychiatry*, *39*, 135–140.

Tabachnick, B.G., & Fidell, L.S. (1989). *Using multivariate statistics* (2nd ed.). New York: Harper Collins Publishers.

Van Zomeren, A.M., & Brouwer, W.H. (1994). *Clinical neuropsychology of attention.* New York: Oxford University Press.

Walker, M.L. (1991). *Utility of the continuous recognition memory test in the prediction of outcome after closed head injury.* Unpublished doctoral dissertation, University of Houston.

Child Neuropsychology
1996, Vol. 2, No. 1, pp. 39–47

A Structural Equation Analysis of the Wide Range Assessment of Memory and Learning in the Standardization Sample*

Donald Bradley Burton[1], Jacques Donders[2], and Wiley Mittenberg[3]

[1]University of Mississippi Medical Center, [2]Mary Free Bed Hospital, and [3]Nova University

ABSTRACT

A maximum likelihood confirmatory factor analysis was performed by applying LISREL VII to the Wide Range Assessment of Memory and Learning standardization sample ($N = 2363$). Analyses were designed to determine which of nine hypothesized oblique factor solutions could best explain memory as measured by the WRAML. Competing latent variable models were identified in previous studies and monographs on memory. Models were tested separately in two samples of children used in the standardization of the scale, providing a cross-validation of results. Findings supported a three-factor model including Verbal Memory, Visual Memory, and Attention/Concentration factors. Our results are consistent with previous characterizations of attention as an important component of memory as measured by the WRAML. A distinct Learning Index was not empirically supported in the current analysis.

The ability to learn and recall new information is known to be affected adversely by cerebral injury in children, including congenital conditions such as hydrocephalus (Cull & Wyke, 1984; Tromp & Van Den Burg, 1982) as well as acquired conditions such as traumatic brain injury (Dalby & Obrzut, 1991; Donders, 1993). Until recently, there were no comprehensive, standardized, and age-normed instruments available for the assessment of children's memory.

The Wide Range Assessment of Memory and Learning (WRAML) was specifically constructed to be a comprehensive measure of memory and normative data were provided for 2363 children in 21 age groups ranging from 5 to 17 years (Sheslow & Adams, 1990). Additionally, the normative sample was stratified by race, sex, residence, and region based on 1980 U.S. Census figures. The WRAML is composed of nine subtests (Picture Memory, Design Memory, Verbal Learning, Story Memory, Finger Windows, Sound Symbol, Sentence Memory, Visual Learning, and Number/Letter Memory) that are thought to measure both common and unique aspects of memory. Four summary indexes can be calculated that are hypothesized to provide measures of General Memory, Verbal Memory, Visual Memory, and Learning. The Verbal, Visual, and Learning Indexes are composed of linear combinations of three subtests each and reflect the test authors' hypotheses about the latent dimensions of memory that underlie children's performance on the WRAML. The results of previous research have called into question the validity of the Learning Memory Index and have suggested that an attention/concentration dimension may exist.

Gioia (1991) performed an exploratory factor analysis of the standardization sample and compared his results to the principal-components analysis (PCA) presented by the test authors. Gioia (1991) reported results that differed from those provided by the test authors and interpreted his findings

---

* Address correspondence to: D.B. Burton, Ph.D., University of Mississippi Medical Center, School of Medicine, Dept. of Psychiatry and Human Behavior, 2500 North State Street, Jackson, MS 39216-4505, USA.
Accepted for publication: November 17, 1995.

as calling into question the validity of making a distinction between the learning and memory indexes.

In a subsequent investigation with a mixed clinical sample, Aylward, Gioia, Verhulst, and Bell (1994) employed a principal-factors analysis to assess the viability of two-, three-, and four-factor solutions, none of which corresponded to the three-scale configuration suggested by Sheslow and Adams (1990). They found that a three-factor model accounted for the most variance among the subtests. This model included a "verbal content" factor, a "visual content" factor, and a "verbal short-term content" factor. On this basis, Aylward et al. (1994) argued that the indexes provided by the test authors should not be used for purposes of clinical interpretation.

Haut, Haut, and Franzen (1992) compared the individual WRAML subtests to commonly used measures of attention and what they termed "cognitive processing" measures. They found that the Number/Letter and Finger Windows subtests were more strongly correlated with measures of attention (Knox Cube and Digit Span) than they were with "cognitive processing" measures and other WRAML subtests. Sentence Memory, although correlated with attentional measures, was more strongly correlated with Story Memory, and the authors interpreted this finding as indicating that Sentence Memory was more related to "verbal processing" than to attention. They interpreted their results as providing evidence that the WRAML contains a strong attention/concentration component.

Haut, Haut, Callahan, and Franzen (1992) factor-analyzed data from a clinical sample of 103 children referred for neuropsychological examination. In two separate analyses of the WRAML subtests alone and in combination with common measures of attention/concentration, a distinct learning factor failed to emerge. On the basis of their results, these authors suggested that the verbal and visual memory distinction may have some validity but that attention/concentration also had a strong impact on WRAML subtest performance.

The WRAML manual presents the results of a PCA of the standardization sample data as supporting the validity of the proposed Learning and Memory Indexes. The test authors reported a three-factor model (Verbal Memory, Visual Memory, and Learning) that, they argued, corresponded to the

WRAML summary indexes. Inspection of the factor pattern matrix presented in the WRAML manual (Sheslow & Adams, 1990) suggests that the verbal and visual memory dichotomy is an empirically valid subdivision of the WRAML subtests. Whether a Learning Factor is supported by the authors' factor analysis is, perhaps, open to debate. The Verbal Factor that Sheslow and Adams (1990) presented, composed of the Sentence Memory and Number/ Letter subtests, might also be characterized as an attentional factor, consistent with the findings of other researchers (Aylward et al., 1994; Haut, Haut, Callahan, & Franzen, 1992; Haut, Haut, & Franzen, 1992). The Learning Factor, which included the Verbal Learning, Story Memory, and Sound Sym-bol subtests, could also be characterized as a Verbal Memory Factor. As such, the factor analysis presented by the test authors could be interpreted as supporting a three-factor model composed of Verbal Memory, Visual Memory, and Attention/ Concentration Factors rather than a model consistent with the published WRAML Indexes.

The current study examined the construct validity of the WRAML summary indexes using structural equation analysis. Nine latent variable models were evaluated for goodness of fit across the two major subdivisions of the WRAML standardization sample (age 8 years and younger; 9 years and older). Structural models were chosen in order to provide a comprehensive test of the proposed latent dimensions that underlie performance on the WRAML.

Model I was a one-factor model hypothesizing a General Memory Factor. Models II and III were two-factor models hypothesizing subdivisions between general memory and learning (consistent with Sheslow & Adams, 1990) and general memory and attention (Haut, Haut, Callahan, & Franzen, 1992). Model IV was a two-factor model that tested the hypothesis that WRAML subtest variability could be accounted for by a verbal/nonverbal dichotomy (Haut, Haut, Callahan, & Franzen, 1992). Model V was a three-factor model hypothesizing the existence of an attentional component in addition to the verbal and nonverbal memory factors, consistent with the findings of Haut, Haut, and Franzen, (1992) and Aylward et al., (1994). Model VI was a three-factor model that corresponded to the summary indexes constructed by the WRAML authors (Sheslow & Adams, 1990). Models VII, VIII, and IX evaluated the viability of different orderings of the Sentence Memory, Number/Letter, and Finger Windows subtests in order to empirically derive an Attention/concentration factor. These last three models were included to test the fit of various subtests that have been proposed to constitute the Attention/Concentration factor (e.g., Aylward et al., 1994; Haut, Haut, & Franzen, 1992).

The nine models can be summarized as follows:

Model I: General Memory

Model II: General Memory and Learning

Model III: General Memory and Attention

Model IV: Verbal Memory and Nonverbal Memory

Model V: Verbal Memory, Nonverbal Memory, and Attention (composed of Sentence Memory, Finger Windows, and Number/Letter)

Model VI: Verbal Memory, Nonverbal Memory, and Learning

Model VII: Verbal Memory, Nonverbal Memory, and Attention (composed of Sentence Memory and Number/Letter)

Model VIII: Verbal Memory, Nonverbal Memory, and Attention (composed of Sentence Memory and Finger Windows)

Model IX: Verbal Memory, Nonverbal Memory, and Attention (composed of Number/Letter and Finger Windows)

METHOD

The two Pearson product-moment intercorrelation matrices (for ages 8 and younger, $n = 903$ and 9 or older, $n = 1460$) of the nine WRAML subtests used to derive the maximum likelihood estimates were obtained from the WRAML manual (Sheslow & Adams, 1990). Data were collected as part of the standardization of the scale and full probability sampling was employed by the test authors, such that the sample was stratified by age, race, sex, region, and urban versus rural residence.

The confirmatory factor analysis was performed by using the LISREL VII software (Joreskog & Sorbom, 1989) and the SAS CALIS procedure (SAS, 1993). The correlations obtained for each pair of WRAML subtests in the two samples were subjected to confirmatory factor analysis by calculating a set of simultaneous structural equations for each of the nine hypothetical models using the Linear Structural Relationship Model. Structural

coefficients were estimated from the structural equations using the "Maximum Likelihood Fit Function" (Hayduk, 1988; Joreskog & Sorbom, 1989). A multivariate probability density formula was used to determine the likelihood that a given set of structural estimates resulted in a difference between the estimated correlation matrix and the actual correlation matrix that was entirely due to chance fluctuation (Hayduk, 1988).

The Chi-Square statistic divided by its Degrees of Freedom (df) and the Adjusted Goodness of Fit Index (AGFI) were used to assess model fit. Lower values of the Chi-Square/df ratio were assumed to represent a greater fit between the hypothesized correlation matrix and the actual correlation matrix. Additionally, higher AGFI values were associated with better fitting models. Three additional goodness of fit indexes were also selected for use in assessing model viability: Akaike's Information Criterion (Akaike, 1987), the Comparative Fit Index (Bentler, 1989), and the Parsimonious Normed Fit Index (Netemeyer, Johnston, & Burton, 1990). Smaller values of Akaike's Information Criterion were interpreted as indicating better model fit (Akaike, 1987), while higher values ($>.90$) of the Comparative Fit Index were viewed as consistent with better model fit (Bentler, 1989). Parsimonious Normed Fit Indexes greater than .60 were interpreted as indicating that an increase in the number of freed model parameters resulted in a significant increase in the predictive validity of the model over more parsimonious orderings of subtests (Netemeyer et al., 1990). Finally, Chi-Squares of difference were computed between selected nested models in order to determine whether freeing additional model parameters significantly increased model fit over simpler models.

RESULTS

The goodness of fit indexes for each of the nine models tested in the younger age group (8 years and below) are contained in Table 1. Model VII displayed the lowest Chi-Square/df ratio (2.98) and the highest AGFI (.967). Additionally, Model VII displayed the lowest Akaike's Information Criterion Index (23.51), the highest Comparative Fit Index (0.966), and a Parsimonious Normed Fit Index above .60 (.633). Model VII contained Visual Memory, Verbal Memory, and Attention/Concentration factors, with Attention/Concentration composed of Sentence Memory and Number/Letter. A distinct Learning factor composed of Verbal Learning, Visual Learning, and Sound Symbol failed to be supported in the younger age group (Models II and VI).

A modification of Model VII was tested post hoc in order to determine if the Finger Windows subtest measured both Visual and Attention/Concentration factors or loaded on the Visual Memory factor alone. This modification (Model X) was performed because the Finger Windows subtest was found by some researchers to contain a primary attentional component (e.g., Haut, Haut, & Franzen, 1992), whereas other authors found it to primarily measure visual memory (Aylward et al., 1994). Model X empirically assessed whether Finger Windows was unifactorial or multifactorial in nature. Review of Table 1 does support Model X as representing a significant improvement in model fit over the other models tested in our analysis including Model VII (i.e., lower Chi-Square/df ratio = 56.92, higher AGFI = .972, lowest Akaike's Information

Criteria = 10.92, highest Comparative Fit Index = .975, and a Parsimonious Normed Fit Index above .60. Table 2 contains the standardized structural coefficients (factor loadings) for Model X.

Table 3 contains the Chi-Square difference tests for selected nested comparisons. Review of these results revealed that adding the Learning (Model II) or Attention/Concentration (Model III) factors significantly improved model fit when compared to the one-factor General Memory Model. Model IV, which hypothesized separate Verbal and Nonverbal Memory factors, also resulted in significantly improved model fit when compared to the one-factor Model I. The addition of the verbal/nonverbal component reflected in Models V and VI resulted in significantly improved fit as compared to the two-factor models not containing the verbal/nonverbal dichotomy (Models II and III). A nested

Table 1. Summary of Goodness of Fit Statistics for Models Measured in the 8 and Younger Age Group (n = 903).

Model	Chi-Sq.	df	p	Chi-Sq./df	AGFI	AIC	CFI	PNFI
I	296.05	27	.00	10.96	.879	342.06	.805	.593
II	276.35	26	.00	10.63	.876	224.36	.819	.581
III	130.11	26	.00	5.00	.945	78.12	.925	.656
IV	234.20	26	.00	9.01	.890	182.21	.849	.603
V	107.14	24	.00	4.46	.952	59.14	.940	.616
VI	166.47	24	.00	6.94	.925	118.47	.897	.588
VII	71.51	24	.00	2.98	.967	23.51	.966	.633
VIII	219.74	24	.00	9.16	.895	171.74	.858	.563
IX	247.76	24	.00	10.32	.882	199.77	.838	.550
X*	56.92	23	.00	2.47	.972	10.92	.975	.613

Note. Chi-Sq. = Chi-Square; df = degrees of freedom; AGFI = adjusted goodness of fit index; AIC = Akaike's information criterion; CFI = comparative fit index; PNFI = parsimonious normed fit index; p = probability value; * = best fitting model.

Table 2. Standardized Oblique Structural Coefficients for Model X in the 8 and Younger Age Group (n = 903).

Variable	Factor		
	Nonverbal	Verbal	Attention
Number/Letter	.000	.000	**.614**
Sentence Memory	.000	.000	**.963**
Story Memory	.000	**.624**	.000
Finger Windows	**.346**	.000	**.158**
Design Memory	**.628**	.000	.000
Picture Memory	**.446**	.000	.000
Verbal Learning	.000	**.570**	.000
Visual Learning	**.512**	.000	.000
Sound Symbol	.000	**.432**	.000

Table 3. Nested Comparisons for selected Models Tested in the 8 and Younger Age Group.

Comparison	Chi-Sq. diff.	df diff.	p
I vs. II	19.70	1	.001
I vs. III	165.94	1	.001
I vs. IV	61.85	1	.001
III vs. V	22.97	2	.001
II vs. VI	109.88	2	.001
IV vs. V	127.06	2	.001
IV vs. VI	67.73	2	.001
VII vs. X	14.59	1	.001

Note. Chi-Sq. diff. = Chi-Square difference; df = degrees of freedom; p = probability value.

comparison of Model IV versus Model V revealed that the addition of the Attention/Concentration factor significantly improved model fit. Also, Model VI fit significantly better than Model IV, thus supporting the addition of a third factor. Finally, Model X represented a significant improvement in model fit as compared to Model VII where the Finger Windows subtest was allowed to load only on the Nonverbal Memory factor.

Results in the older age group (9 years and above) mirror those found in the younger group, supporting Model X as the best fit among the set of models evaluated in our analysis. Examination of Table 4 reveals that Model X obtained the lowest Chi-Square/*df* ratio (4.43), the highest AGFI (.970), the lowest Akaike's Information Criteria (55.95), the highest Comparative Fit Index (.973), and a Parsimonious Normed Fit Index greater

than .60 (.617) as compared to the other models tested in our analysis. Table 5 contains the standardized structural coefficients for Model X.

Nested comparisons of selected models, the results of which are contained in Table 6, were also consistent with findings in the younger portion of the standardization sample. Adding the Learning (Model II) and Attention/Concentration (Model II) and Attention/Concentration (Model III) factors and dividing the General Memory Factor into a verbal/nonverbal dichotomy (Model IV) significantly improved model fit in all instances as compared to Model I. Additionally, including the verbal/nonverbal dichotomy (Models V and VI) improved model fit as compared to the two-factor models not containing this dichotomy (Models II and III). The addition of a third factor (Models V and VI) resulted in improved model fit as

Table 4. Summary of Goodness of Fit Statistics for Models Measured in the 9 and Older Age Group (*n* = 1460).

Model	Chi-Sq.	df	p	Chi-Sq./df	AGFI	AIC	CFI	PNFI
I	612.27	27	.00	22.68	.852	558.27	.799	.594
II	596.91	26	.00	22.96	.845	544.92	.803	.576
III	295.12	26	.00	11.35	.922	243.12	.908	.650
IV	486.58	26	.00	18.71	.870	434.58	.842	.603
V	188.51	24	.00	7.85	.948	140.51	.944	.624
VI	368.33	24	.00	15.35	.900	320.33	.882	.583
VII	150.55	24	.00	6.27	.958	102.55	.957	.633
VIII	392.64	24	.00	16.36	.888	344.64	.873	.578
IX	450.29	24	.00	18.76	.877	402.29	.854	.565
*X	101.95	23	.00	4.43	.970	55.95	.973	.617

Note. Chi-Sq. = Chi-Square; df = degrees of freedom; AGFI = adjusted goodness of fit index; AIC = Akaike's information criterion; CFI = comparative fit index; PNFI = parsimonious normed fit index; p = probability value; * = best fitting model.

Table 5. Standardized Oblique Structural Coefficients for Model X in the 9 and Older Age Group (*n* = 1460).

Variable	Factor		
	Nonverbal	Verbal	Attention
Number/Letter	.000	.000	**.662**
Sentence Memory	.000	.000	**.914**
Story Memory	.000	**.642**	.000
Finger Windows	**.317**	.000	**.218**
Design Memory	**.643**	.000	.000
Picture Memory	**.536**	.000	.000
Verbal Learning	.000	**.541**	.000
Visual Learning	**.644**	.000	.000
Sound Symbol	.000	**.597**	.000

Table 6. Nested Comparisons for Selected Models Tested in the 9 and Older Age Group.

Comparison	Chi-Sq. diff.	df diff.	P
I vs. II	15.36	1	.001
I vs. III	317.15	1	.001
I vs. IV	125.69	1	.001
III vs. V	106.61	2	.001
II vs. VI	228.58	2	.001
IV vs. V	298.07	2	.001
IV vs. VI	118.25	2	.001
VII vs. X	48.60	1	.001

Note. Chi-Sq. diff. = Chi-Square difference; df = degrees of freedom; p = probability value.

compared to Model IV which contained the Verbal/Nonverbal factors only. Model X was found to represent a significant improvement in model fit over the more parsimonious Model VII that allowed the Finger Windows subtest to load only on the Nonverbal Memory factor.

DISCUSSION

The results of the current investigation support a three-factor model including Visual Memory, Verbal Memory, and Attention/Concentration as the most predictive of WRAML subtest variability in the group of models that we tested. This finding calls into question the validity of the published WRAML Indexes. The three-factor model presented by the WRAML authors (Verbal Memory, Nonverbal Memory, and Learning) was substantially less predictive of subtest co-variability than were other models tested in this analysis. The Learning factor did not emerge as a strong predictor of subtest covariability. Instead, the Verbal Learning and Sound Symbol subtests appeared to be mea-sures of verbal memory rather than measures of learning per se. Likewise, the Visual Learning subtest appeared to be primarily a measure of visual memory function and did not emerge as a specific index of learning function.

Our results support the conclusions of Gioia (1991) who found the WRAML Learning Index to have questionable construct validity. Moreover, the current results are consistent with the findings of Aylward et al. (1994), who questioned the viability of the indexes provided by the test authors and reported a three-factor model that was very similar to the model we found to be the best fit. Their model contained verbal and nonverbal memory factors, but also contained a dimension that they termed "verbal short-term content" that was similar to the current attention/concentration factor. The "verbal short-term content" factor consisted of Number/Letter and Sentence Memory.

In constructing the Learning Index, it appears that the WRAML authors hoped to provide a measure of a child's capacity to assimilate new information strategically over repeated presentations. In the WRAML manual, the test authors defined learning as "the acquisition of new information over trials"

(Sheslow & Adams, 1990, p. 10). They interpreted the Learning Index as a "procedure to allow the evaluation of a child's memory strategies" (p. 7).

On the basis of our results, it appears that the WRAML does a poor job of empirically differen-tiating between strategic memory processes and declarative memory processes in the standardiza-tion sample. The subtests that make up the WRAML Learning Index do present information redundantly and provide a measure of the amount of information retained over trials. However, only the Verbal Learning subtest presents children with a set of unstructured information that apparently requires them to organize that material strategically in a conceptually meaningful manner.

This strategic component appears to be lacking in the Sound Symbol and Visual Learning sub-tests. These two subtests present information redundantly, but the stimuli to be remembered are not presented as a set. For these two subtests the child is not required to organize the entire set of material in a meaningful manner and then freely recall the entire set. These two subtests present what may be termed "paired associates" and thus appear to be a measure of verbal and nonverbal cued retrieval rather than a measure of learning (or strategic memory). The apparent absence of the necessity to exert strategic organization over the material contained in the Sound Symbol and Visual Learning subtests may be the factor that renders these subtests more declarative and less strategic in nature. Had this strategic/organiza-tional component been included, a Learning factor might have been empirically supported.

In the present analysis, our Attention/ Concentration factor emerged consistently as a strong predictor of WRAML subtest variability. This Attention/Concentration factor was com-posed of the Number/Letter, Sentence Memory, and Finger Windows subtests. Because of the "digit span" quality of these subtests, they were interpreted as involving the application of imme-diate memory span and attention/concentration functions. In each of these subtests, children are presented with increasingly complex sequences of stimuli that require them to sustain their attention throughout the presentation, retain the sequence in short-term memory, and then immediately retrieve the material.

Our results are consistent with those of Haut, Haut, and Franzen (1992) who found the Number/ Letter, Finger Windows, and, to a lesser extent, Sentence Memory subtests to be highly correlated with commonly accepted measures of attention. Similarly, Haut, Haut, Callahan, and Franzen (1992) performed an exploratory factor analysis of the WRAML subtests in conjunction with measures of attention and immediate memory span. They derived what they termed a "combined memory" factor and an attentional factor that included the Number/Letter, Sentence Memory, and Finger Windows subtests.

We allowed the Finger Windows subtest to load on both the Attention/Concentration and Visual Memory factors because it appeared to have a significant visual component and also because there seemed to be conflicting findings in the literature. Aylward et al., (1994) found Finger Windows to load exclusively on a nonverbal memory factor, while Haut, Haut, and Franzen (1992) found Finger Windows to be more highly correlated with measures of attention than with either verbal or nonverbal memory measures. In a related study, Haut, Haut, Callahan, and Franzen (1992) derived an attentional factor that included the Finger Windows subtest. Our analysis suggests that both authors were correct because our results strongly imply that the Finger Windows subtest contains both attentional and visuo-perceptual components. As such, clinical interpretations of this subtest should include a consideration of both sources of variability.

Additional factor analyses should be conducted in order to further substantiate the current findings. Results of our analysis in the standardization sample should be compared to patterns of latent variability found in various clinical groups. It may be that the pattern of latent variability will be different in diagnostically distinct clinical samples. WRAML factor structure should also be examined across different developmental periods. Experience with other measures, such as the Wechsler Adult Intelligence Scale – Revised, suggests that patterns of latent variability can differ between separate age groups (Leckliter, Matarazzo, & Silverstein, 1986).

By examining changes in the patterns of relationships among WRAML subtests across developmental periods, substantial knowledge could be gained about the development of memory processes in children and adolescents. Groups differing on other meaningful demographic and neuropsychological variables should also be compared in terms of WRAML latent variability. For example, the dimensions underlying standardized psychometric instruments have been demonstrated to vary by gender (Burton, Ryan, Paolo, & Mittenberg, 1994). The latent variability of the WRAML should be evaluated for gender differences as well in order to determine whether males and females approach the WRAML memory tasks differently.

Other tests should be assessed in combination with the WRAML to determine if a strategic memory factor can be demonstrated. For example, the California Verbal Learning Test for children (CVLT-C) was designed to provide a measure of children's learning and mnemonic organizational abilities (Delis, Kramer, Kaplan, & Ober, 1994). Analysis of a combined WRAML/CVLT-C memory battery may provide results supporting a strategic memory/learning factor. It may be that the WRAML Learning Memory subtest is a measure of strategic memory function and that a structural equation analysis of the WRAML in combination with the CVLT-C will reveal a factor structure including Attention/Concentration, Verbal and Visual Memory, and Strategic Memory/Learning.

Overall, the WRAML is an adequately normed and potentially useful memory battery for children and adolescents. However, on the basis of the current results, it would appear that clinicians should be cautious when using the published WRAML Indexes. A potentially more useful and possibly more valid way of scoring the WRAML may be to combine the subtests into linear combinations of Verbal, Visual, and Attention/Concentration indexes as suggested in the current analysis. A scaled and normed measure of attention/concentration appears to be a potentially important addition to the WRAML.

In our clinical practice, referrals for psychometric evaluation frequently involve questions about an individual child's capacity to focus and maintain attention during the learning process. Reorganizing the WRAML subtests on the basis of our analysis of the standardization sample in order to provide Verbal Memory, Visual Memory, and Attention/ Concentration indexes might increase the clinical utility of the scale. Such an Attention/

Concentration Index would allow the clinician to assess the extent to which the memory performance of children is being effected by impaired ability to focus their cognitive resources on the task.

REFERENCES

Akaike, H. (1987). Factor analysis and AIC. *Psychometrika, 52,* 317–332.

Aylward, G.P., Gioia, G.A., Verhulst, S.J., & Bell, S. (1994). *Factor structure of the WRAML in a clinical population.* Paper presented at the meeting of the International Neuropsychological Society, Cincinnati, OH.

Bentler, P.M. (1989). *EQS structural equations program.* Los Angeles: BMDP statistical software.

Burton, D.B., Ryan, J.J., Paolo, A.M., & Mittenberg, W. (1994). Structural equation analysis of the Wechsler Adult Intelligence Scale – Revised in a normal elderly sample. *Psychological Assessment, 6,* 380–387.

Cull, C., & Wyke, M.A. (1984). Memory function of children with spina bifida and shunted hydrocephalus. *Developmental Medicine and Child Neurology. 26,* 177–183.

Dalby, P.R., & Obrzut, H.E. (1991). Epidemiologic characteristics of closed head-injured children and adolescents: A review. *Developmental Neuropsychology, 7,* 35–68.

Delis, D.C., Kramer, J.H., Kaplan, E., & Ober, B.A., (1994). *California Verbal Learning Test: Children's version.* San Antonio, TX: The Psychological Corporation.

Donders, J. (1993). Memory functioning after traumatic brain injury in children. *Brain Injury, 7,* 431–437.

Gioia, G.A. (1991). *Re-analysis of the factor structure of the Wide Range Assessment of Memory and Learning: Implications for clinical interpretation.* Paper presented at the meeting of the International Neuropsychological Society, San Antonio, TX.

Haut, J.S., Haut, M.W., Callahan, T.S., & Franzen, M.D. (1992). *Factor analysis of the Wide Range Assessment of Memory and Learning (WRAML) scores in a clinical sample.* Paper presented at the Meeting of the National Academy of Neuropsychology, Pittsburgh, PA.

Haut, J.S., Haut, M.W., & Franzen, M.D. (1992). *Assessment of an attentional component of Wide Range Assessment of Memory and Learning (WRAML) subtests.* Paper presented at the meeting of the International Neuropsychological Society, San Diego, CA.

Hayduk, L.A. (1988). *Structural equation modeling with LISREL.* Baltimore: John Hopkins University Press.

Joreskog, K.G., & Sorbom, D. (1989). LISREL VII, *user's reference guide.* Scientific Software.

Leckliter, I.N., Matarazzo, J.D., & Silverstein, A.B. (1986). A literature review of the factor analytic studies of the WAIS-R. *Journal of Clinical Psychology, 42,* 332–342.

Netemeyer, R.G., Johnston, M.W., & Burton, S. (1990). Analysis of role conflict and role ambiguity in a structural equations framework. *Journal of Applied Psychology, 75,* 148–157.

SAS (1993). *SAS/STAT User's guide, version 6* (8th ed., volume 1). Cary, NC: SAS Institute.

Sheslow, D., & Adams, W. (1990). *Wide Range Assessment of Memory and Learning Administration Manual.* Delaware: Jastak Associates.

Tromp, C.N., & Van Den Burg, W. (1982). Verbal memory impairment in treated hydrocephalic children. *Zeitschrift fur Kinderchirurgie, 37,* 175–178.

Journal of Clinical and Experimental Neuropsychology
1992, Vol. 14, No. 4, pp. 625–637

A Five-Factor Model for Motor, Psychomotor, and Visual-Spatial Tests Used in the Neuropsychological Assessment of Children*

David J. Francis[1], Jack M. Fletcher[2], Byron P. Rourke[3], and Mary J. York[4]

[1]University of Houston, [2]Department of Pediatrics, Univ. of Texas Medical School-Houston,
[3]University of Windsor, and [4]University of Houston

ABSTRACT

Previous confirmatory factor analysis has supported a distinction between simple and complex motor skill tests in a modified and expanded Halstead Reitan test battery (HRB). The present study used a sample of 722 right-handed boys and girls, aged 9 through 12, and expanded the sample of motor, psychomotor, and visual-spatial tests to further clarify this distinction. Restricted maximum-likelihood factor analysis resulted in correlated factors of Simple Motor Skill, Complex Visual-Spatial Relations, Simple Spatial Motor Operations, Motor Steadiness, and Speeded Motor Sequencing. These results provide additional evidence for the discriminant validity of this particular battery of tests, and explicate further the skills and abilities measured in neuropsychological assessments of children referred for evaluation.

In recent years, the psychometric properties of neuropsychological tests for children have come under increased scrutiny. Although studies of the validity of such tests for assessing various childhood learning and behavioral disorders certainly exist, the reliability and construct dimensions of these tests have not been extensively studied. Systematic analysis of child-neuropsychological tests is needed to delineate more precisely the measurement characteristics of these frequently employed procedures.

Attempts to study the measurement dimensions of neuropsychological tests with exploratory factoring methods have been hampered by the inclusion of tests measuring motor skills with both the left and right hand. In an earlier study (Francis, Fletcher, & Rourke, 1988), we used confirmatory factor analysis to assess the discriminant validity

of several motor tests, viz., Finger Tapping, Grip Strength, Grooved Pegboard, and the Maze Test from the Halstead Reitan and Kløve motor batteries (Reitan & Davison, 1974; Kløve, 1963). This study revealed no evidence for discriminant validity of right- and left-hand versions of the same test, but supported the discriminant validity of the different types of motor test. Although results suggested the presence of at least two motoric factors (Simple and Complex), the study lacked a sufficient variety of tests to describe adequately the nature of these different motor skills factors.

The present study reports the results of some additional confirmatory factor analyses of the motor tests included in Francis et al. (1988) and other measures used in the neuropsychological assessment of children (Rourke, Fisk, & Strang, 1986).

*Preparation of this article was supported in part by National Institutes of Health Grant CA33097-08, "The Neuropsychological Assessment of Children with Cancer," and National Institute of Child Health and Human Development Grants HD21888, "Psycholinguistic and Biological Mechanisms in Dyslexia" and P50 HD25802, "Center for Learning and Attention Disorders."

Address reprint requests to David J. Francis, Ph.D., Department of Psychology, University of Houston, Houston TX 77204-5341, USA.

Accepted for publication: November 10, 1991.

These analyses were designed specifically to describe more precisely the differences among the motor skill and other nonlanguage tests of the modified HRB under consideration. Confirmatory factor analysis (CFA) was used instead of exploratory factor analysis because CFA permits estimation and statistical evaluation of restricted measurement models, that is, models with some factor loadings constrained to be zero. Also, in assessing model fit, CFA approaches permit evaluation of statistical assumptions underlying the common factor model (e.g., that all intervariable associations are via the common factors).

METHOD

Subjects

Subjects for the study were 722 right-handed boys and girls who were 9 ($n = 229$), 10 ($n = 190$), 11 ($n = 158$), or 12 ($n = 145$) years of age, and who had been tested at the Neuropsychology Service of a children's service in Windsor, Ontario from June, 1967 to March, 1981. The sample was approximately 80% male in each age cohort. Inclusion was based on recorded diagnosis, which was made at the time of the neuropsychological report. The majority of children (72.6% overall, ranging from 71.1% to 73.8% in the four age groups) had received a diagnosis of "learning disability." The diagnosis of learning disability required that the child have a Full Scale IQ above 84, at least one centile score <30 on the Wide Range Achievement Test (WRAT), and clear evidence of an information-processing deficiency. A small sample of children ($n = 29, 29, 31,$ and 23 in ages 9 through 12, respectively) were included in the study who had Full Scale IQs between 70 and 84. Also included was a somewhat smaller sample of children ($n = 33, 26, 12,$ and 15 in ages 9 through 12, respectively) who had Full Scale IQs above 84, but who did not meet all of the criteria for diagnosis of learning disability. Children who showed evidence of (a) mental retardation (Full Scale IQ less than 70), (b) neurological disorder, (c) emotional disturbance, or (d) environmental deprivation were excluded.

Measures

Twelve neuropsychological tests thought to measure motor, psychomotor, and visual spatial skills and abilities were included in the study. Sample means and standard deviations for these 12 tests and for the WISC IQ (Wechsler, 1949) scales and the WRAT (Jastak & Jastak, 1965) are given in Table 1. These tests have been widely employed in child clinical neuropsychological assessment

over the last three decades (Reitan, 1971; Rourke, Bakker, Fisk, & Strang, 1983). Details for test administration and scoring are provided in Rourke et al. (1986) with the following modification: scores for Finger Tapping, Grip Strength, Grooved Pegboard, Mazes, and Holes represent the sum of left- and right-hand performances. The decision to combine left- and right-hand scores into a single index for these tests was based on our previous research which found no evidence for discriminant validity of left- and right-hand versions of these tests (Francis et al., 1988).

Tests of visual-spatial ability (e.g., WISC Block Design, Object Assembly) were included in the study with the motor and psychomotor tests for two reasons. First, the Grooved Pegboard and Maze tests, considered measures of complex motor skill from the previous study (Francis et al., 1988), have a potential visual-spatial component. Secondly, some of the measures of visual-spatial ability have possible motor components due to their response format (e.g., WISC Block Design and Object Assembly). To assess these potential relations, it was essential that both types of tests be included in the analysis.

Two variable transformations were also employed in the factor analysis. Interpretation of factor loadings and correlations is complicated when some measures are scored positively and others are scored negatively (i.e., higher scores indicate poorer performance, such as with time and error measures). Thus, in order to facilitate interpretation of the factors, all time scores were reflected in the factor analysis so that higher scores indicate better performance on all measures. This transformation applies only to tables of factor loadings and variable/factor correlations, where positive factor loadings and positive variable/factor correlations indicate that higher scores on the factor are associated with *better* test performance.

A second transformation was also applied to the time measures to make the data more consistent with the factor analytic assumption of linear relations between measures and factors. Specifically, because time data tend to be positively skewed, with some extreme, high observations, confirmatory factor-analyses of time data often produce poorly fitting models with evidence for correlated errors of measurement. To reduce the effects of extreme observations, and to reduce the amount of skew in variable distributions, all time measures were first submitted to logarithmic transformation. After logarithmic transformation of the original observations, time scores were reflected for the reasons described above.

Procedures

Prior to assessing the factor structure of the 12 measures, evidence for age-related differences in correlations was examined using LISREL VII (Jöreskog & Sörbom, 1989). This test indicated that the hypothesis

Table 1. Means and Standard Deviations for Neuropsychological and Achievement Tests.

Test	Age Group							
	9		10		11		12	
	(n = 229)		(n = 190)		(n = 158)		(n = 145)	
	M	SD	M	SD	M	SD	M	SD
Finger Tapping[a] (# taps)	60.4	9.0	65.3	9.5	69.6	9.7	75.1	11.2
Grip Strength[a]	25.4	7.2	28.5	7.2	33.6	9.1	38.0	9.2
Trail Making Test, Part A, (Time)	29.7	17.6	23.7	9.6	21.9	8.9	20.0	7.1
WISC Object Assembly	10.4	3.2	10.5	3.3	10.3	3.2	10.5	3.2
WISC Block Design	10.4	2.8	10.3	3.0	9.9	3.0	10.4	3.0
WISC Picture Completion	10.6	3.2	10.6	2.9	10.2	3.2	10.5	2.9
Grooved Pegboard (Time)[a]	182.9	39.9	170.0	39.8	156.5	29.7	147.4	27.4
Target Test (# Correct)	14.3	3.2	15.4	3.2	16.2	2.9	16.7	2.6
Holes (Contact Time)[a]	66.7	24.9	56.3	22.8	55.6	24.5	45.1	20.9
Mazes (Contact Time)[a]	16.5	9.4	12.7	8.6	10.5	6.8	8.6	6.9
TPT (Total Time)	10.1	5.0	9.5	5.1	7.9	3.6	6.8	3.0
WISC Coding	9.6	2.7	9.5	3.1	9.6	3.3	9.4	2.8
WISC VIQ[b]	95.3	11.0	93.4	11.2	92.0	9.9	91.8	11.9
WISC PIQ[b]	101.7	13.8	101.0	14.9	99.7	14.4	100.6	14.1
WISC FSIQ[b]	98.2	11.8	96.8	11.9	95.2	11.8	95.6	12.2
WRAT Reading %ile[b]	27.5	26.5	28.1	26.0	22.6	24.2	23.6	25.5
WRAT Spelling %ile[b]	21.1	21.3	19.4	21.0	15.1	16.8	14.6	18.6
WRAT Arithmetic %ile[b]	26.0	16.1	20.2	14.2	16.7	11.5	14.4	14.5

Note. All times are given in seconds, except for TPT, which is in minutes. All WISC subtests are reported as scaled scores.
[a] Sum of left- and right-hand scores
[b] Test not included in factor analysis

of equal correlation matrices in different age groups could not be rejected ($\chi^2 = 200.21$, df = 198, $p = .443$). Consequently, factor analysis was performed on the maximum likelihood estimate of the common correlation matrix. The matrix of estimated correlations is provided in Appendix A.

To clarify the nature of the motor, psychomotor, and visual-spatial tests included in the battery, five nested factor models were compared using the computer program LISREL VII (Jöreskog & Sörbom, 1989). These models were named according to the number of factors in the model, viz., 1, 3, 4, 5, and 5A. Factors were considered correlated in all multi-factor models, and none of the models allowed for correlated errors among tests (i.e., all intervariable relations were explained only by the common factors).

Model Description

Model 1 was included to serve as a null model and specified that the tests were one-dimensional. Models 3, 4, and 5 were saturated models, and may be conceptualized as tests of the number of underlying factors, viz., 3, 4, and 5 factors, respectively. The results of

Francis et al. (1988) suggested that at least three factors would be necessary. For this reason, the substantive models considered in this study began with three factors instead of two.

Multi-factor models were specified to yield specific factors by selecting an index variable for each factor and allowing all other factor loadings and factor correlations to be estimated. Index variables load on only a single factor and, thereby, define the factor pattern. Model 3 specified the following: a Simple Motor Factor indexed by Grip Strength; a Motor Steadiness Factor indexed by the Holes test; and a Complex Visual-Spatial Relations factor indexed by WISC Block Design. Model 4 added a Speeded Motor-Sequencing factor using WISC Coding as the index variable. Finally, Model 5 separated the Motor Steadiness Factor of Models 3 and 4 into two factors: Simple Spatial-Motor indexed by the Target Test, and Motor Steadiness indexed by the Holes test.

Selecting different index variables in Models 3, 4 or 5 would alter the factor loadings and possibly the factor interpretation if a non-pure index variable were chosen, or if the number of factors were inadequately specified.

However, indices of model fit (χ^2 and residual statistics) are unaffected by the choice of index variable in these models because the models are saturated. Most important, no restricted model with the same number of factors can yield a better fit than the saturated model without relaxing the restriction of uncorrelated errors. Thus, the chi-square tests for Models 1, 3, 4 and 5 are best conceptualized as testing the number of factors needed to reproduce the data, although it should be kept in mind that specific factors were expected as reflected in the choice of index variables.

Model 5A represents a restricted version of Model 5 that was obtained by restricting to zero all factor loadings in Model 5 with t values less than 1.7 in absolute value. In addition, Model 5A allowed the Finger Tapping measure to load on the Motor Steadiness factor for reasons described below. Thus, Model 5A can be considered a test of the interpretive structure of Model 5. Ultimately, one would like to be able to propose Model 5A a priori on the basis of theory. However, when theory development with respect to measurement in a given area does not allow for articulation of specific models for investigation, it is still possible to employ restricted factor models in a tentative hypothesis-testing framework, which is the strategy adopted in these analyses.

RESULTS

Factor models were compared using the chi-square difference test and incremental fit ratios (Sobel & Bohrnstedt, 1985). These results are presented in Table 2. It is apparent from the information in Table 2 that a five-factor model fits the data quite

well in a global sense. The statistics in Table 2 also indicate that a saturated model with fewer factors is inadequate to explain the relationships among the variables. These conclusions are borne out by the nonsignificant overall chi-square for Model 5, the significant χ^2 for Models 1, 3 and 4, and the significant χ^2 difference between models 4 and 5. The χ^2 difference reflects the improvement of adding a fifth factor to a model with four factors.

Nonstatistical determination of the number of factors, using the eigenvalue >1 criterion, and the scree test indicated only three factors. These criteria were examined because χ^2 is known to be sensitive to sample size and multivariate non-normality, which tends to inflate chi-square (Anderson & Gerbing, 1984; Bearden, Sharma, & Teal, 1982; Boomsma, 1982).

Examination of the three- and four-factor models indicated that these solutions were problematic. The three-factor model produced many large residual correlations, including one residual of .214 for the correlation between Trail Making Test, Part A, and WISC Coding subtest. In all, 22 standardized residual correlations exceeded 2.0 in absolute value, indicating that they were statistically different from zero. The three-factor model also produced many significant modification indices corresponding to correlated errors of measurement. Specifically, with only three common factors, 20 of the 66 pairs of measures showed significant evidence of association not related to the factors.

Table 2. Comparison of Models 1, 3, 4, 5 and 5A.

Model	χ^2	df	p<	Difference with preceding model[a]			NFI[b]
				χ^2	df	p<	
1	584.27	54	.001				
3	186.39	33	.001	397.88	21	.001	.681
4	53.02	24	.001	133.37	9	.001	.909
5	14.69	16	.547	38.33	8	.001	.975
5A	33.35	35	.548	18.66	19	.479	.943

Note. Models 3 and 4 cannot be directly compared with Model 5A.
[a] In the case of Models 3, 4, and 5, this difference χ^2 tests the improvement over Model 1, 3, and 4, respectively. For Model 5A, the difference χ^2 tests the lack of fit introduced by restrictions in Model 5A over Model 5.
[b] Normed Fit Index (Bentler & Bonnett, 1980). All fit ratios are expressed as improvements over Model 1, with Model 1 also serving as the null Model.

The four-factor model was similarly problematic. First, this model produced a negative residual variance estimate of .336 for the Maze test. Although this negative estimate could indicate a true residual variance of zero, it may also result from extracting an incorrect number of factors, or from non-normality in the distribution of Maze scores. In addition to the problematic variance estimate, the four-factor model produced 12 standardized residuals larger than 2.0 in absolute value, and another 12 between 1.5 and 2.0.

In contrast to the three- and four-factor models, the five-factor model produced no improper estimates, and yielded only two standardized residuals as large as 2.0 in absolute value, and another two residuals between 1.5 and 2.0. The incremental fit ratios in Table 2 show that the three- and four-factor models explain 68.1% and 90.9% of the information left unexplained by the one-factor model, as compared to 97.5% for the five-factor model. Moreover, the five-factor model explains 72.3% of the information left unexplained by the four-factor model. In short, Model 5 fits the data well, and provides substantial improvements over Model 4 and Model 3.

Of the 35 free factor loadings in Model 5, 20 were associated with t statistics less than 1.65 in absolute value, which corresponds to the critical t for a one-sided p value of .05. When these 20 factor loadings were simultaneously restricted to zero, the loading for Finger Tapping on the Motor Steadiness factor was associated with a significant modification index of 11.24, indicating that the model fit would be significantly improved if this factor loading were not fixed at zero. Consequently, we re-estimated the restricted five-factor model without this loading constrained to be zero. This model is reported as Model 5A.

The overall chi-square difference between models 5 and 5A suggests that no lack of fit has been introduced by fixing these 19 factor loadings at zero. This finding is not fully expected because the 19 t values that led to the choice of constraints are not independent, such that fixing some loadings at zero may cause others to become important. Thus, it is entirely possible that a comparison of models 5 and 5A would have yielded a significant chi-square difference indicating a lack of fit introduced by the constraints of Model 5A.

Table 3. Additional Fit Statistics for Model 5A.

$\chi^2/d.f.$	= .953
Goodness of Fit Index	= .992
Adjusted Goodness of Fit Index	= .983
Root Mean Square Residual	= .017
Residuals $\geq$ .05	1 (.054)
Normalized Residuals $\geq$ 2.0 in absolute value	3

It is important to point out that Models 3, 4, and 5A are not directly comparable because they are not nested. These models can only be indirectly compared through comparison with Models 1 and 5. Such a comparison shows that Model 5A accounts for 94.3% of the information left unexplained by Model 1. It should also be pointed out that, whereas Model 5A has more factors than Models 3 and 4, Model 5A is more parsimonious than these models because it involves fewer free parameters. Additional fit information for Model 5A is provided in Table 3, and indicates that the restricted five-factor model fits the data extremely well.

Factor loadings, squared multiple correlations, and factor intercorrelations are presented for Model 5A in Table 4. Squared multiple correlations represent the proportion of variance in each variable explained by the set of factors. It can be seen from the squared multiple correlations that some variables are poorly explained by the set of factors, specifically the Finger Tapping, Trail A, Picture Completion, Holes, and Tactual Performance Tests. However, the squared multiple correlations predicting each measure from the 11 remaining measures are generally low (less than .25, except for the Holes Test which was .33) for these five measures. Thus, these low squared multiple Rs for predicting the measures from the factors result more from the low intercorrelations for these variables in this data matrix than from inadequacy in the factor solution. It is likely that additional factors may underlie performance on measures with small squared multiple correlations, but that the data matrix does not contain a sufficient number of indicators of these factors for them to be uncovered. Alternatively some such measures may have poor reliability in this population, although recent analysis of the test-retest reliability of these measures in a larger sample of these children (Brown, Rourke, & Cicchetti, 1989) does not support that proposition.

Table 4. Results of Maximum Likelihood Confirmatory Factor Analysis for Model 5A ($N = 722$).

Measure	Factor Loadings and Variance Explained					
	Factor					
	I	II	III	IV	V	R^2
Finger Tapping	.493			.208		.326
Grip Strength	.689					.475
Trail Making Test, Part A			.137		.494	.343
WISC Object Assembly		1.209	−.693		.361	.727
WISC Block Design		.756				.572
WISC Picture Completion		.525				.276
Grooved Pegboard Test		.401		.351	.136	.449
Target Test			.728			.530
Holes Test				.632		.399
Mazes Test			.469	1.016	−.550	.909
Tactual Performance Test		.408			.177	.246
WISC Coding					.721	.519

Note. Metrics for all tests are as given in Table 1.

Factor Correlations	I	II	III	IV
I Simple Motor				
II Complex Visual-Spatial Relations	.423			
III Simple Spatial-Motor Operations	.419	.799		
IV Motor Steadiness	.197	.192	.333	
V Speeded Motor Sequencing	.201	.333	.595	.586

Note. Blank factor loadings indicate loadings constrained to 0. All scores have been reflected so that higher scores indicate better performance.

The intercorrelations among the factors in Model 5A are all positive, and range from small to moderate in size except for the correlation between Simple Spatial-Motor and Complex Visual-Spatial Relations, which is large. All of the unconstrained factor loadings in Table 4 are statistically significant at $p < .01$. In addition, none of the parameter estimates for Model 5A were inadmissible (e.g., negative error variances or correlations that exceeded 1.0). Factor loadings that exceed 1.0 are possible when the factors are correlated, hence the loading of 1.2 for Object Assembly on the Complex Visual-Spatial Relations factor is admissible. Although the factors are correlated, interpretation of the factors from the pattern of loadings is possible because each factor includes at least one indicator which loads on only that factor (Gorsuch, 1983).

It must also be kept in mind that the factor loading reflects the contribution of a factor to performance on a test after controlling for all other factors. Consequently, correlations among variables and

factors are presented in Table 5 to facilitate understanding of the variable/factor relations. The correlations indicate that all of the variable/factor relations are in the appropriate direction in that higher factor scores are associated with better performance on each test. For example, although the loading of Object Assembly on the Simple Spatial-Motor factor is −.693, the correlation of Object Assembly with this factor is +.489. Similarly, the factor loading of Mazes on Speeded Motor Sequencing is −.550, but the correlation of Mazes with this factor is +.325. With regard to the Mazes test, it must also be kept in mind that scores have been reflected so that higher scores reflect better performance.

DISCUSSION

In a previous study of the measurement characteristics of the Windsor version of the Halstead-Reitan

Table 5. Correlations between Neuropsychological Tests and Factors ($N = 722$).

Measure	Factor				
	I	II	III	IV	V
Finger Tapping	.534	.249	.276	.306	.221
Grip Strength	.688	.291	.289	.136	.139
Trail Making Test, Part A	.156	.274	.431	.336	.576
WISC Object Assembly	.294	.776	.489	.214	.353
WISC Block Design	.319	.756	.604	.146	.251
WISC Picture Completion	.221	.525	.420	.101	.175
Grooved Pegboard Test	.266	.513	.518	.508	.476
Target Test	.304	.600	.728	.242	.433
Holes Test	.124	.122	.210	.632	.371
Mazes Test	.286	.386	.481	.850	.325
Tactual Performance Test	.207	.467	.461	.182	.312
WISC Coding	.144	.239	.429	.423	.720

Note. Metrics for all tests are as given in Table 1. All scores have been scaled so that higher scores indicate better performance.

Neuropsychological Battery for children, we found evidence for the presence of multiple motor-related factors (Francis et al., 1988). The present study shows that this battery contains at least three primary motor factors. One factor is represented by tests of simple motor function, such as Finger Tapping and Grip Strength. The second factor includes more complex motor tasks, such as the Grooved Pegboard, Holes, and Mazes. Each of these latter tasks places demands on manual dexterity and the capacity to benefit from visual proprioceptive feedback. We interpret this factor to be Motor Steadiness because of the pure loading of the Holes test on this factor, and because of the contribution of this factor to two other complex psychomotor tasks that require steadiness, viz., the Pegs and Mazes tests. Although, with the exception of the Holes test, each of the tests loading on this factor loads on one or more other factors, it is certainly the case that performance on these measures is affected by motor steadiness. Whereas the pattern of zero loadings for the Holes test is partially constrained by design, there was no evidence for cross-loading of the Holes test in Model 5A.

We have interpreted a third factor to be primarily spatial in nature with minimal motor contributions, viz., Factor III, Simple Spatial-Motor. This factor had loadings from the Target Test, Trails A, and Mazes tests, with a negative loading for Object Assembly. We considered that this factor

might be described more aptly as Spatial-Motor except for the fact that four tests which loaded on the Complex Visual-Spatial Relations factor have an obvious component of spatial-motor operations (e.g., rotation of objects in two and three dimensions), viz., the Grooved Pegboard, Tactual Per-formance Test, Block Design Subtest, and Object Assembly Subtest. Consequently, we added the modifier "Simple" to Factor III reflecting the different nature of the spatial-motor operations involved in tests loading on this factor as compared to those involved in tests loading on the Complex Visual-Spatial Relations factor.

The clarity of the Motor Steadiness and Simple Motor factors emerged when additional tests measuring visual-spatial relations were added. The Complex Visual-Spatial Relations factor is represented by the WISC subtests of Block Design, Object Assembly, and Picture Completion, along with the Grooved Pegboard and Tactual Performance test (TPT). All of these tasks are visual in nature, except for the TPT. The latter task is administered blindfolded, but requires the use of visual imagery for correct block placement. All tasks have obvious, prominent requirements for spatial processing. This processing includes the spatial construction components of the Block Design and Object Assembly subtests, and the need to perform complex two- and three-dimensional manipultions of objects. These findings correspond with previous studies of the WISC which yielded a Perceptual Organization factor (Kaufman, 1979).

The inclusion of the Grooved Pegboard Test on this factor may reflect two characteristics of this test. First, the test requires proper orientation of pegs before they can be placed. Secondly, the test requires that the holes be filled from left to right, beginning with the first row and proceeding to the final row. It is conceivable that rotation and alignment of the pegs with the grooved holes, and the constraints on filling the holes in order increase the visual-spatial processing demands of the Grooved Pegboard Test. This hypothesis could be tested in a confirmatory factor study that included the Purdue Pegboard Test, which does not make such demands on the testee.

The fact that some tests load on more than one factor simply indicates that performance on some of these measures is multi-determined. Hence, a complex measure such as the Grooved Pegboard Test has visual-spatial and motor steadiness components, whereas spatial relations tests such as the Object Assembly subtest and the Tactual Performance Test are also affected by differences in motor sequencing skills.

One of the advantages of confirmatory factor analysis is its capacity to elucidate these types of relationships by placing restrictions on the factor pattern and assessing the lack of fit introduced by these restrictions. The emergence of the fifth factor, which we labeled Speeded Motor Sequencing, is of particular interest. We originally hypothesized that this factor simply involved motor learning. However, the shared relationship of the WISC Coding subtest with the Mazes Test, Tactual Performance Test, and Trails A suggests a broader interpretation of this factor to include some type of executive (sequencing or planning) function. Each of these tests requires motor output, but also requires the ability to form cognitive plans and learn from experience. Hence, this factor appears to involve higher level executive functions as well as motor output.

Examining the relations of this factor with other indices of executive functions (e.g., Category Test, Wisconsin Card Sorting Test) is an obvious direction for future research. In addition, measures of language and attentional skills could be included in an effort to elucidate further a measurement model for this modified version of the Halstead-Reitan tests for children. The results of this research should be more precise characterizations of performance patterns in children with various learning and behavioral disorders.

Clinical Implications

The results of this study carry some implications for the neuropsychological assessment of children within the 9- to 14-year age-group, as follows:

(1) With respect to coverage, the implication would seem to be that a test battery made up of Grip Strength, the WISC Object Assembly subtest, the Target Test, the Mazes Test, and the WISC Coding subtest would, to a significant and clinically relevant extent, tap the major dimensions assessed by the 12 tests analyzed in this study.

(2) A battery comprised of Grip Strength and the Grooved Pegboard Test, although sacrificing a significant amount with respect to coverage, would probably contribute significant clinical assessment information for children in this age group.

(3) A potentially important dimension of increasing complexity may be nascent within the five factors isolated: That is, there may be a clinically significant progression from (I) "simple motor" to (IV) "motor steadiness" to (III) "simple spatial-motor" operations to (II) "complex visual-spatial relations" to (V) "speeded motor sequencing." If this is, in fact, a hierarchically arranged set of motor/psychomotor/visual spatial/sequencing-planning skills and abilities, the clinician may be in a position to make a systematic analysis of the point in this hierarchy at which the child's performance breaks down. For example, a child who exhibits nonverbal learning disabilities (Rourke, 1989) may not be able to perform adequately beyond the simplest (Factor I) stage in this hierarchy. On the other hand, a child with a psycholinguistically based learning disability may be able to perform adequately on Factors I through IV, and do poorly only when the requirement for the guiding of behavior through symbolic/verbal means is added (Factor V). Further light should be shed upon these and related issues when we extend this analysis to a consideration of the verbal/linguistic aspects of the Windsor battery.

REFERENCES

Anderson, J.C., & Gerbing, D.W. (1984). The effect of sampling error on convergence, improper solutions, and goodness-of-fit indices for maximum-likelihood confirmatory factor analysis. *Psychometrika, 49,* 155–173.

Bearden, W.O., Sharma, S., & Teal, J.E. (1982). Sample size effects on chi-square and other statistics used in evaluating causal models. *Journal of Marketing Research, 19,* 425–430.

Bentler, P.M., & Bonnet, D.G. (1980). Significance tests and goodness-of-fit in the analysis of covariance structures. *Psychological Bulletin, 88,* 588–606.

Boomsma, A. (1982). The robustness of LISREL against small sample sizes in factor analysis models. In K. G. Jöreskog & H. Wold (Eds.), *Systems under indirect observation: Causality, structure, prediction. Part I* (pp. 149–173). Amsterdam: North Holland.

Brown, S.J., Rourke, B.P., & Cicchetti, D. (1989). Reliability of tests and measures used in the neuropsychological assessment of children. *The Clinical Neuropsychologist, 3,* 353–368.

Francis, D.J., Fletcher, J.M., & Rourke, B.P. (1988). Discriminant validity of lateral sensorimotor tests in children, *Journal of Clinical and Experimental Neuropsychology, 10,* 779–799.

Gorsuch, R.L. (1983). *Factor analysis* (2nd ed.). Hillsdale: Lawrence Erlbaum.

Jastak, J.F., & Jastak, S.R. (1965). *The Wide Range Achievement Test.* Wilmington, DE: Guidance Associates.

Jöreskog, K.G., & Sörbom, D. (1989). *LISREL VII: Analysis of linear structural relationships by the method of maximum-likelihood.* Chicago: National Educational Resources.

Kaufman, A. (1979). *Intelligent testing with the WISC-R.* New York: Academic Press.

Kløve, H. (1963). Clinical neuropsychology. In F. M. Forster (Ed.), *The medical clinics of North America* (pp. 1647–1658). New York: Saunders.

Reitan, R. M. (1971). Sensorimotor functions in brain-damaged and normal children of early school-age. *Perceptual and Motor Skills. 33,* 655–664.

Reitan, R.M., & Davison, L. (1974). *Clinical neuropsychology: Current status and applications.* New York: Winston/Wiley.

Rourke, B.P. (1989). *Nonverbal learning disabilities: The syndrome and the model.* New York: Guilford Press.

Rourke, B.P., Bakker, D.J., Fisk, J.L., & Strang, J.D. (1983). *Child neuropsychology: An introduction to theory, research, and clinical practice.* New York: Guilford Press.

Rourke, B.P., Fisk, J.L., & Strang, J.D. (1986). *Neuropsychological assessment of children: A treatment-oriented approach.* New York: Guilford Press.

Sobel, M.E., & Bohrnstedt, G.W. (1985). Use of null models in evaluating the fit of covariance structure models. In N. Tuma (Ed.), *Sociological methodology 1985* (pp. 152–178). San Francisco: Jossey-Bass.

Wechsler, D. (1949). *Wechsler Intelligence Scale for Children.* New York: Psychological Corporation.

APPENDIX A

Maximum-likelihood Estimate of Common Correlation in Children Aged 9–12 ($n = 722$).

Measure	Correlation with Measure Number										
	1	2	3	4	5	6	7	8	9	10	11
1. Finger Tapping											
2. Grip Strength	.368										
3. Trail Making Test, Part A	.118	.103									
4. WISC Object Assembly	.162	.193	.217								
5. WISC Block Design	.212	.236	.179	.592							
6. WISC Picture Completion	.128	.159	.121	.412	.396						
7. Target Test	.188	.186	.346	.360	.437	.311					
8. Grooved Pegboard Test	.276	.226	.287	.424	.365	.273	.388				
9. Holes Test	.198	.060	.184	.135	.105	.064	.144	.305			
10. Mazes Test	.315	.197	.194	.249	.313	.175	.348	.501	.535		
11. Tactual Performance Test	.165	.137	.224	.374	.351	.239	.302	.347	.100	.211	
12. WISC Coding	.171	.106	.416	.271	.204	.125	.295	.345	.290	.254	.209

Note. Metrics for measures are as reported in Table 1. Correlations are reported for transformed measures used in the factor analysis, not the original untransformed scores. Measure transformations are described in the Methods section.

Child Neuropsychology
2003, Vol. 9, No. 1, pp. 10–21

VIII-D

Cognitive Development of Lead Exposed Children from Ages 6 to 15 Years: An Application of Growth Curve Analysis

Juliet M. Coscia[1,2], M. Douglas Ris[1,2], Paul A. Succop[2], and Kim N. Dietrich[1,2]

[1]Children's Hospital Medical Center, and [2]University of Cincinnati College of Medicine, Cincinnati, OH, USA

ABSTRACT

The effect of lead exposure on cognitive growth patterns was assessed in a longitudinal study of 196 children. Performances on tests of verbal comprehension and perceptual organization (Vocabulary & Block Design, Wechsler Intelligence Scales for Children) were measured at ages 6.5, 11 and 15 years. Growth curve analyses revealed that the quadratic model best described the relationship between test scores and age. Children with higher lead levels, as measured at age 15 years, demonstrated lower verbal comprehension scores over time and greater decline in their rate of Vocabulary development at age 15 years, as compared to children with lower lead levels. Lead exposure was not significantly associated with growth in perceptual organization test scores. Socioeconomic status and maternal intelligence were statistically significantly associated with growth patterns for both test scores, independent of the effects of lead. The findings suggest that lead negatively impacts the developmental progression of specific cognitive skills from childhood through adolescence.

COGNITIVE DEVELOPMENT OF LEAD EXPOSED CHILDREN FROM AGES 6 TO 15 YEARS

Studies of the development of infants and children exposed to inorganic lead (Pb) have documented a negative relationship between Pb levels and cognitive performance in a number of domains including intelligence, visual spatial reasoning, visual-motor skills, motor speed, vocabulary, reading skills and language processing (e.g., Baghurst et al., 1992; Campbell, Needleman, Riess, & Tobin, 2000; Dietrich, Berger, & Succop, 1993; Dietrich, Berger, Succop, Hammond, & Bornschein, 1993; Needleman, Schell, Bellinger, Leviton, & Allred, 1990; Ris, Dietrich, Succop, Berger, & Bornschein, 2002; Wasserman et al., 2000). These cognitive deficits, when broadly categorized, fall into the domains of verbal and nonverbal reasoning

skills. There is also suggestion in the literature that specific skill areas may be especially vulnerable to Pb exposure at different stages of development. For example, Dietrich et al. (1993) found that postnatal blood Pb concentration was significantly associated with perceptual organization skills (Performance IQ) but not verbal comprehension skills (Verbal IQ) at age 6.5 years. In contrast, Needleman et al. (1990) found a significant association between tooth Pb concentration during childhood and measures of vocabulary, but not between Pb and measures of perceptual organization/complex constructional skills (e.g., Rey–Osterreith complex figure) during late adolescence. While these differing findings could be explained by the use of varying measurement tools across studies, they nonetheless indicate that Pb may be associated with the rate of growth in specific cognitive domains at different age points. Furthermore,

Address correspondence to: Juliet M. Coscia, Department of Psychology, Mary Free Bed Hospital & Rehabilitation Center, 235 Wealthy SE, Grand Rapids, MI 49503-5299, USA. Tel.: + 1-616-242-9201. E-mail: jcoscia@mfbrc.com
Accepted for publication: October 10, 2002.

only a few published reports document the developmental outcomes of Pb exposed children in adolescence and early adulthood. Needleman and colleagues' findings represent evidence of cognitive deficits in the oldest cohort of Pb exposed individuals published to date ($M = 18$ years). Collectively, these findings suggest that: (1) Pb influences multiple cognitive skills; (2) these skill areas may be differentially impacted by Pb at different developmental stages; and (3) Pb influences development into adolescence and early adulthood.

An outstanding question in the literature on Pb effects is how Pb exposure early in life impacts the developmental progression of cognitive skills across the lifespan. As summarized above, the literature to date has largely emphasized mean performance scores from cross-sectional data. Regression analyses have also been typically utilized to examine the relationship between Pb and environmental risk factors on cognitive outcome at any one point in time. Several studies have indirectly addressed the question of developmental change and correlates of change using longitudinal data from children undergoing chelation treatment (Rogan et al., 2001; Ruff, Bijur, Markowitz, Ma, & Rosen, 1993; Ruff, Markowitz, Bijur, & Rosen, 1996). However, these studies examined difference or change in developmental scores over narrow windows of time (e.g., 6 and 36 months) in children of varying ages. Thus, only very limited conclusions can be drawn about development across childhood on the basis of these studies. Two studies (Tong, Baghurst, Sawyer, Burns, & McMichael, 1998; Wasserman et al., 2000) represent the first attempts to directly examine the relationship between changes in blood Pb levels and changes in IQ scores in children studied longitudinally. Tong and colleagues followed 375 children from birth to between 11 and 13 years (Port Pirie Cohort Study), and Wasserman and colleagues followed 442 children from birth to age 7 years (Yugoslavia Prospective Lead Study). In the Port Pirie Study, analysis of variance was used to examine the relationship between difference in cognitive scores and change in blood lead concentrations across the interval between pairs of developmental assessments (e.g., between ages 2 and 11–13 years, 4 and 11–13 years, and 7 and 11–13 years). The disadvantages to using such difference scores

include the difficulty with their interpretation, including the assumption of change as linear when in fact it may not be (see Cronbach & Furby, 1970; Rogosa & Willett, 1985). Analyses using the entire growth curve would enhance our understanding of potential nonlinear change processes. Both the Port Pirie and Yugoslavia studies involved administration of three different standardized age-appropriate intellectual measures across the age span. The issue of instrument transitions is one of the most challenging in longitudinal analyses as the question inevitably arises as to whether the data reflect actual cognitive growth or changing measurement instruments (Lindsey, O'Donnell, & Brouwers, 2000). In sum, to our knowledge, no studies have examined change in cognitive development in Pb exposed children, or factors related to change, using appropriate longitudinal statistical techniques and using similar measurement tools across assessment points.

The availability of a longitudinal data set spanning childhood and adolescence, with similar cognitive assessment measures, offers the unique opportunity to apply growth curve analysis to the study of Pb exposed children. Growth curve analysis allows examination of impact of various factors on the rates of change for individual children of varying developmental skills (Francis, Fletcher, Stuebing, Davidson, & Thompson, 1991). Growth curve analysis examines both the rate (i.e., speed) and level (i.e., outcome at any specific point in time) of change occurring for each individual. When applied to longitudinal data with more than two time points, growth curve modeling offers the advantage of estimating nonlinear change processes (e.g., quadratic change). As such, it avoids the problems inherent with the use of incremental change or difference scores (Cronbach & Furby, 1970). Furthermore, the additional opportunity to examine correlates of change yields insight into the relation among multiple environmental factors and the rate and level of growth in cognitive skills. Growth curve modeling has been successfully applied to the study of development in children with other chronic health conditions. For example, growth curve modeling has been utilized to examine the cognitive recovery of children with traumatic brain injury (Francis et al., 1991) and to examine the effects of radiation therapy on IQ scores over time in children with medulloblastoma (Ris, Packer, Goldwein, Jones-Wallace, & Boyett, 2001).

The growth curve analytic strategy followed in this paper differs from the individual growth curve approach often applied to repeated measurements. A mixed model approach, which is a type of regression model applied to repeated observations, was utilized (Statistical Analysis System Institute, 1997). This allowed us to estimate the longitudinal effects of Pb in a model that correctly accounts for the within- and between-subject variation. This strategy was also preferred so as to utilize all available data in this longitudinal data set and to minimize biases that result from missing data points.

Growth curve modeling also offers the advantage of examination of correlates of developmental change. This is particularly relevant to the study of Pb exposed children because of evidence that both biological and contextual factors independently contribute to suboptimal development. Development is believed to be directly related to the effects of Pb on the developing central nervous system (for a review see Finkelstein, Markowitz, & Rosen, 1998) and adverse social effects (Dietrich, Ris, Succop, Berger, & Bornschein, 2001). With regards to the latter, Pb exposure is often associated with other environmental risk factors, such as poverty, undernutrition and suboptimal caregiving (Dietrich, 1995). Such factors account for unique variance in developmental scores in Pb exposed children (e.g., Baghurst et al., 1992). Finally, it is well accepted that sociohereditary variables that influence the home environment (e.g., maternal IQ, quality of caregiving, socioeconomic status) influence individual intellectual growth patterns in healthy, full-term children (Espy, Molfese, & DiLalla, 2001). In order to comprehensively assess factors that contribute to developmental growth in this at risk population, it is necessary to include these sociohereditary variables.

The present study advances the scientific knowledge of the impact of Pb exposure on cognitive development in several respects. This is the first study to utilize growth curve analysis to document the developmental progression of a large sample of Pb exposed individuals followed prenatally through adolescence. The study assesses differences in patterns of developmental growth as a function of the severity of Pb exposure. Outcome measures include verbal comprehension and perceptual organization skills to assess whether Pb has a differential impact on the development of these skills. Moreover, the present study includes analyses of sociohereditary variables (i.e., quality of the home environment, socioeconomic status, maternal IQ), those measures that typically predict performance on cognitive tests. It was hypothesized that blood Pb and measures of the sociohereditary environment would systematically influence developmental growth patterns in verbal comprehension and perceptual organization skills.

METHOD

Participants

The children and adolescents who participated in this study were part of the Cincinnati Lead Study (CLS). The CLS represents a birth cohort of approximately 300 subjects that have been followed since prenatal recruitment began in 1979 and concluded in early 1985 (Dietrich, Berger, Succop, Hammond et al., 1993; Dietrich et al., 1987; Dietrich, Succop, Berger, Hammond, & Bornschein, 1991). Women were recruited from obstetrical clinics located in the catchment area. Women were excluded from the study if they were known to be addicted to drugs, alcoholic, diabetic or had a neurologic disorder, psychosis or mental retardation. Infants were excluded if they were less than 35 weeks gestation or less than 1,500 g at birth or if they had a genetic syndrome or other disqualifying medical conditions at birth (Dietrich et al., 1987).

For this study, children who were tested longitudinally at approximately 6.5, 11 and 15 years were included in the analyses. Although most of the children participated in testing at each age ($n = 152$), some children missed assessments due to factors such as refusals, chronically missed appointments, inability to locate subjects' family, long-term incarceration, homicide, severe developmental disability, and scheduling problems. In order to take advantage of all of the data available and to minimize biases that result from missing data points, children with one ($n = 9$) or two ($n = 35$) missing data points were included in the analyses. Therefore, a total of 196 children (104 females; 92 males) were included in the sample. Table 1 contains the demographic characteristics of the children included in the study.

Measures

Blood Lead
The microanalytical laboratory at the University of Cincinnati Department of Environmental Health

Table 1. Descriptive Statistics for the Sample of Children ($n = 196$).

	M or %	SD	Minimum	Maximum
Age (years)				
1st assessment ($n = 175$)	6.55	0.12	6.44	7.23
2nd assessment ($n = 167$)	11.40	1.04	10.33	15.00
3rd assessment ($n = 193$)	15.50	0.85	12.60	17.83
Males	47%			
African-American	92%			
Birthweight (g)	3107.79	473.30	1814.00	4400.00
Gestational age (weeks)	39.42	1.76	35.00	43.00
OCS raw score	33.47	2.71	27.00	39.00
PCS raw score	9.38	1.10	3.00	10.00
SES (Age < 5 years)	18.10	4.38	11.00	36.25
SES (Age > 11 years)	24.26	9.21	6.00	58.00
Maternal IQ[a]	75.28	9.20	55.00	110.00
HOME[b]	−0.03	0.85	−2.85	1.71
Blood lead (ug/dl)				
PbBPre	8.53	3.90	0.90	26.80
MPB1	10.73	5.13	3.10	35.00
MPB2	17.03	8.13	5.70	49.30
MPB3	16.25	7.31	4.30	49.70
MPB4	14.30	7.03	3.90	45.20
MPB5	12.02	6.20	3.30	38.30
MPB6	9.78	5.18	3.20	32.40
MPBLife	13.46	5.87	4.70	37.20
PB78	8.27	4.67	1.80	33.90
PB15Y	2.80	1.29	1.00	11.30

Note. OCS = Obstetrical Complication Scale (Littman & Parmelee, 1978); PCS = Postnatal Complication Scale (Littman & Parmelee, 1978); SES = Socioeconomic Status (Hollingshead, 1985); HOME = Home Observation for Measurement of the Environment (Caldwell & Bradley, 1978); PbBPre = prenatal blood lead; MPB1 = mean blood lead for Year 1; MPB2 = mean blood lead for Year 2; MPB3 = mean blood lead level for Year 3; MPB4 = mean blood lead level for Year 4; MPB5 = mean blood lead level for Year 5; MPB6 = mean blood lead level for Year 6; MPBLife = mean blood lead for Years 1 through 6 plus at 66 and 72 months of age; PB78 = blood lead level at 78 months; PB15Y = blood lead level at 15 years.
[a] Maternal IQ estimated using the Vocabulary and Block Design subtests of the WAIS-R (Silverstein, 1982).
[b] HOME score represents the mean score for administrations at 6, 12, 24 and 36 months of age and is represented as a z score.

performed the measurements of Pb in whole blood (PbB). For a description of the procedures used to obtain and analyze blood samples, the reader is referred to earlier reports (Dietrich et al., 1987, 1991). Blood was collected prenatally from the mother near the end of the first trimester of pregnancy (PbBPre), approximately 10 days after birth, and at quarterly intervals to the age of 5 years. Blood was also sampled at 66, 72, and 78 months (PbB78) and at approximately 15 years (PbB15Y). Postnatal Pb exposures were expressed as the mean PbB concentrations of the 1st through 6th year of life (Mean PbB1–6). Average lifetime blood Pb level was defined as the mean of 20 quarterly PbB assessments and the PbBs at 66 and 72 months of age (MPbBLife).

Cognitive Assessment
Raw score performances on the Vocabulary and Block Design subtests from the Wechsler Intelligence Scale for Children-Revised (WISC-R; Wechsler, 1974) at ages 6.5 and 11 years and from the Wechsler Intelligence Scale for Children – 3rd Edition (WISC-III; Wechsler, 1991) at age 15 years were used in the growth curve analysis. The WISC-R was the primary intelligence measure for longitudinal analysis at ages 6.5 and 11 years. At the 15 year assessment, the Vocabulary and Block Design subtests from the WISC-III were chosen as estimates of intelligence because of their high correlations with global intelligence or g (Sattler, 1992). The Vocabulary and Block Design subtests are especially

suited for this growth curve analysis for several reasons. First, in studies examining the factor structure of intellectual and neuropsychological measures, these two subtests load on separate cognitive factors representing verbal reasoning and visual perception (Chittooran, D'Amato, Lassiter, & Dean, 1993; Livingston, Gray, Haak, & Jennings, 1997). Second, these subtests have strong reliability across both versions of the WISC (Wechsler, 1974, 1991). Third, in order to improve upon past studies where different cognitive measures were used at varying time points, we wanted to use the same cognitive measure, or measures that were as similar as possible, across the three assessment points. Although these subtests have been modified in the newer version of the WISC (WISC-III), there is still considerable overlap between the items across versions (Wechsler, 1991). Furthermore, correlations between these subtests across the two versions are high; 0.77 between Vocabulary subtests and 0.76 between Block Design subtests (Wechsler, 1991). In appreciation of the modifications to the WISC-III subtests and in keeping with the goal of using raw scores in the growth curve analysis, we adjusted for the slight differences in raw score ranges between the two versions of the WISC. This was accomplished by converting the raw score on the WISC-III to the appropriate scaled score, and then using the raw score on the WISC-R that corresponds with that same scaled score. This process of transforming scores onto a similar scale has been supported in the literature as an appropriate technique for handling test transitions in pediatric longitudinal studies and clinical trials (Lindsey et al., 2000). Only one experienced examiner (KD) administered the tests at ages 6.5 and 11 years. At age 15 years, two examiners administered the tests (KD and a trained assistant psychometrician).

Assessment of Covariates

A variety of covariates and potential confounders were assessed in this investigation, including measures of fetal distress and growth, perinatal complications, and maternal IQ. Both the average socioeconomic status score (Hollingshead, 1985) measured prior to age 5 years and that measured on a single occasion after age 11 years were investigated. In addition, the home observation for measurement of the environment (HOME) inventory (Caldwell & Bradley, 1978) was administered at ages 6, 12, 24 and 36 months to measure of the quality and quantity of social and physical stimulation available in the child's home. The procedures for the assessment of these cofactors are presented in previous articles (Dietrich et al., 1991; Dietrich, Succop, Berger, & Keith, 1992).

Statistical Methods

A mixed regression model (Statistical Analysis System PROC MIXED) was used to fit the quadratic regression curve to the unadjusted and covariate-adjusted Vocabulary and Block Design scores over three time points (Statistical Analysis System Institute, 1997). This technique is well suited for this data set because it makes use of all available data, including those children with less than three assessment points ($n = 44$). This technique also allows for the estimation of the population growth curve in a single-stage within- and between-subject analysis. The within-subject effects represent those variables that predict the changes in the Block Design and Vocabulary scores over the course of the study whereas the between-subject effects are main effects that modify the expected baseline or intercept of the regression curve. A separate covariate-adjusted regression model was fit for each of the 10 PbB levels. While keeping in mind the risks of inflating Type 1 error, these 10 PbB levels were chosen because they have been investigated in our previous research (e.g., Dietrich et al., 1992) and because they included PbB levels taken during adolescence in order to investigate the possibility that early lead exposure might lead to cognitive deficits that are not observable or recognized until adolescence. The effect of PbB and each of the covariates were tested for their effects on the linear and quadratic components of the growth curve by interacting each of these independent variables with child's age and age squared in the initial models. The main effects of PbB and each of the covariates were also included in the initial models to test for any baseline differences that might be related to these variables. For each of the covariate-adjusted models, insignificant main effects (i.e., PbB or a covariate) or interaction effects (e.g., covariate by age or PbB by age) were removed in a backward elimination process. A main effect was not a candidate for removal until both of its interactions with the linear (age) and quadratic components (age squared) were eliminated. An insignificant interaction with the quadratic component of age was removed before the interaction with the linear age component was tested for possible elimination from the model. Final models were derived that included only statistically significant interactions and statistically significant main effects. The main effects of PbB and the linear and quadratic age components were retained in all models regardless of their statistical significance. A two-tailed alpha level of 0.05 was used to judge statistical significance. The 0.05 level was chosen since the size of the Pb effects was expected to be relatively small, particularly after covariate control.

RESULTS

The means and standard deviations for the ages of assessment, PbB measures and covariates are depicted in Table 1. Table 2 shows the means and

Table 2. Mean Vocabulary and Block Design Scaled Scores as a Function of Age of Assessment ($n = 196$).

WISC scores	M	SD	Minimum			Maximum		
	Raw	Scaled	Raw	Scaled	Raw	Scaled	Raw	Scaled
Block design								
6.5 years ($n = 175$)	6.59	8.05	3.53	2.20	0	2.0	20.0	13.0
11 years ($n = 167$)	24.85	7.91	10.57	2.60	4.5	1.0	52.3	14.0
15 years* ($n = 193$)	37.51	6.05	13.27	3.24	6.0	1.0	64.0	13.0
Vocabulary								
6.5 years ($n = 175$)	12.07	8.18	3.49	2.42	3.8	3.0	21.6	15.0
11 years ($n = 167$)	25.82	7.37	6.16	2.76	11.3	1.0	42.2	13.0
15 years* ($n = 193$)	27.80	5.26	8.30	2.93	11.0	1.0	50.0	12.0

Note. Scaled scores are shown for ease of interpretability. Analyses were conducted using raw scores.
   * Vocabulary and Block Design scores for the 15 year assessment are adjusted raw scores.

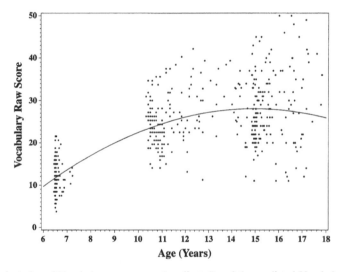

Fig. 1. Growth trajectories of Vocabulary raw scores (unadjusted) and the predicted Vocabulary raw scores as a function of age in years.

standard deviations for the raw and scaled scores from the cognitive measures at each assessment. In Figures 1 and 2 the respective Vocabulary and Block Design raw scores and predicted scores were plotted as a function of age for each of the 196 participants.

Unadjusted models: Examination of within subject change

Results for the unadjusted models are graphically represented in Figures 1 and 2. For both Vocabulary and Block Design scores, a quadratic regression model best fit the data. For the Vocabulary

scores, the quadratic term was negative and statistically significant (beta = -0.229, $t = -11.91$, $p < 0.0001$). Group Vocabulary performance visibly increased with age between 6.5 and 11 years, and then plateaued between the ages of 11–15 years, with evidence of declines in rate of growth occurring post 15 years of age (see Fig. 1). The term for a quadratic trend in the Block Design scores, although not as striking as for the Vocabulary scores, was also negative and statistically significant (beta = -0.094, $t = -2.75$, $p < 0.01$). As seen in Figure 2, Block Design scores showed the same pattern of increase between ages 6.5 and 11 years,

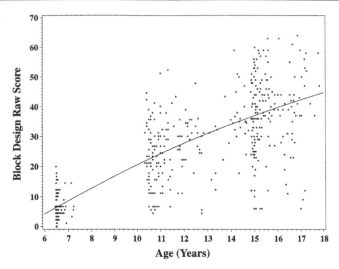

Fig. 2. Growth trajectories of Block Design raw scores (unadjusted) and the predicted Block Design raw scores as a function of age in years.

however, scores from age 11 on demonstrated a deceleration in growth rather than a decline.

Additional analyses to support the superiority of the quadratic term over the linear term for both cognitive scores were conducted. A model R-square was calculated to examine the increase in prediction by including the quadratic terms. The unadjusted models' R-squares increased from 0.503 to 0.554 ($p < 0.0001$) when including the quadratic term for the Vocabulary scores, and increased from 0.622 to 0.627 ($p < 0.01$) when including the quadratic term for the Block Design scores. Consistent with the findings above, this suggests a marked improvement in prediction for the Vocabulary scores and milder improvement for the Block Design scores.

Covariate-Adjusted Models: Correlates of Within Subject Parameters

The covariate by age and PbB by age interactions remaining in the final models after eliminating insignificant factors were very consistent for each of the models (see Table 3). For the Block Design scores, child's race and gender, family SES (>11 years), maternal IQ and scores on the obstetrical complications scale (OCS) all were statistically significantly related to scores both as main effects and as interaction effects with age. That is, as the children aged, whites, males, children whose families

had higher SES or mothers with higher IQs and those with higher OCS scores tended to have higher scores on the Block Design subscale. None of the ten PbB levels were statistically significantly related to the Block Design scores, either as main effects or as interactions with age.

For the Vocabulary scores, child's birthweight and family SES were statistically significantly related to test scores as interactions with age; the interactions between maternal IQ and both the linear and quadratic components of age were statistically significant; and the HOME score was statistically significantly associated with Vocabulary scores as a main effect. Greater birth-weight was more beneficial to the Vocabulary scores as the child aged, whereas SES (>11 years) and maternal IQ had their greatest effects on Vocabulary scores between 6.5 and 11 years, and the strength of this statistically significant association decreased after age 11 years. The HOME score was uniformly positive in its effect on Vocabulary scores throughout the growth curve. PbB measured at approximately 15 years of age was statistically significantly related to the Vocabulary scores, as an interaction with the quadratic age component (beta $= -0.046$; $t = -2.87$; $p < 0.01$), indicating that PbB burden is detrimental at some point during adolescence.

Table 3. Results of Backward Elimination Regression Analysis: Significant Betas ($n = 196$).

	Main effect	SE	Linear effect	SE	Quadratic effect	SE
Dependent variable: Block design scores						
Age	7.57*	16.07	−0.75	1.41	−0.09	0.03
Race	−7.43	4.58	0.84	0.34		
Sex	2.97	2.28	−0.43	0.18		
SES (>11 years)	−0.14	0.13	0.02	0.01		
Maternal IQ	−0.09	0.12	0.03	0.01		
OCS	−0.71	0.42	0.11	0.03		
Dependent variable: Vocabulary scores						
Age	−44.18*	17.82	11.07	3.34	−0.54	0.14
PbB15Y	−4.01	1.78	0.95	0.35	−0.05	0.02
Birthweight	−0.01	0.01	0.01	0.01		
SES (>11 years)	−0.01	0.07	0.01	0.01		
Maternal IQ	0.51	0.21	−0.11	0.04	0.01	0.01
HOME	0.89	0.45				

Note. Regression model for the Vocabulary and Block Design scores is for the 1st year PbB data; significant betas are shown for those variables with significant interactions and main effects; see Table 1 for references to specific variables; main effect = intercept and linear effects of covariates and Pb; linear effect = linear effects of age and the interaction of covariates with age; quadratic effect = quadratic effects of age and interaction of covariates with the quadratic age term.
* Main effects for age represent the intercept.

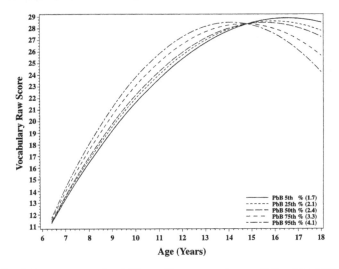

Fig. 3. Predicted Vocabulary raw scores for children with average values on birthweight, SES, maternal IQ and HOME scores and 15 year PbB at the 5th, 25th, 50th, 75th and 95th percentiles. Note that value in parentheses represents actual PbB level (ug/dl).

Figure 3 demonstrates the predicted course for Vocabulary scores for children with average values on each of the significant covariates (birthweight, SES, maternal IQ and HOME) and PbB at the 5th, 25th, 50th, 75th and 95th percentiles of the 15 year PbB distribution. This figure demonstrates that as PbB increases, the predicted decline in the rate of Vocabulary scores becomes steeper and begins at an earlier age. The effect sizes for PbB on the vocabulary scores can also be determined from Figure 3. The approximate difference in expected (predicted) Vocabulary values is 4 raw score points, reflecting an approximate deficit of 1–2 scaled scores.

DISCUSSION

This growth curve analysis is, to our knowledge, the first to examine the developmental trajectory of cognitive skills of Pb exposed children from childhood through adolescence. Several interesting findings emerge from these data. First, a quadratic term best described the relationship between age and measures of verbal comprehension and perceptual organization skills. Both verbal comprehension and perceptual organization scores increased between ages 6.5 and 11 years, but then showed slightly different patterns thereafter. Verbal comprehension scores plateaued between 11 and 15 years with evidence of declines in the rate of growth post 15 years. Perceptual organization scores from age 11 years on demonstrated a deceleration in growth. This study also confirmed the results of previous cross-sectional studies in demonstrating that Pb exposure is associated with cognitive test scores from childhood through adolescence. We found that Pb is differentially associated with cognitive skills; Pb was associated with growth in verbal comprehension and not perceptual organization skills. Perhaps global measures of development (vs. tests of neuropsychological domains) may not necessarily be more sensitive to Pb effects (Bellinger, 1995). The findings of a statistically significant negative association between the most recently measured Pb levels (i.e., at age 15 years) and Vocabulary scores across the growth curve were intriguing. The smaller variance of the 15-year-PbB levels could produce attenuated relationships with cognitive scores. Yet, this finding is consistent with several other studies in which the more recent measures of Pb are more strongly associated with cognitive outcomes (e.g., Baghurst et al., 1992; Dietrich et al., 1993; Factor-Litvak, Wasserman, Kline, & Graziano, 1999). Perhaps later measures of PbB are markers for some physiologically based genetic factors reflecting Pb metabolism and retention (e.g., Schwartz, Lee, et al., 2000; Schwartz, Stewart, et al., 2000).

Although the focus of this study was on Pb effects, these findings also support the importance of the sociohereditary environment in the growth of cognitive skills independent of the effects of Pb. The relationships between birthweight, socio-economic status, maternal IQ and HOME scores and verbal comprehension scores across the growth curve were statistically significant. Race, gender, SES, maternal IQ and obstetrical complication scores were statistically significantly associated with perceptual organization skills across the curve independent of the effects of Pb. Statistically significant associations between genetic factors, the home environment and cognitive outcomes are well documented among Pb exposed and healthy preschool and school age children (e.g., Bradley Leviton, Waternaux, Needleman, & Rabinowitz, 1989; Dietrich et al., 1985; Espy et al., 2001). However, less is known about these relationships for both at risk and healthy children during late childhood and adolescence. These findings suggest that such associations persist well into late adolescence for this at risk population. Although the focus of this study was on longitudinal analysis of cognitive outcome, future research will also be critical to understand the potential moderating role of genetics and the home environment on the relationship between Pb and cognitive outcomes. For example, recent animal studies that suggest that enriched environments help protect against neurotoxicity and neurobehavioral deficits related to Pb exposure (Schneider, 2001). Studies of Pb exposed children conducted by Bellinger and colleagues (e.g., Bellinger, Leviton, & Sloman, 1990; Bellinger et al., 1989) also support the moderating role of SES on the relationship between Pb and cognitive outcome. Future studies planned in our laboratory that incorporate structural equation modeling will address this important question.

These findings suggest that, in this socially disadvantaged population, early Pb exposure predicts cognitive growth patterns into adolescence. However, limitations of this study should be examined before final conclusions can be made. As with all longitudinal studies, this study was vulnerable to attrition. We attempted to minimize bias through the inclusion of those children who missed one or two of the three assessment points. When reviewing the data it became apparent that those adolescents whose evaluation was delayed until after age 15 years, when the declines in the rate of Vocabulary scores were most apparent, may differ from the rest of the cohort in terms of IQ or other sociodemographic factors. However, subjects who participated in the final analysis at age 15 years did not differ significantly from those lost to follow-up in terms of measures of Pb exposure, perinatal health, early school intelligence or socioeconomic status (Dietrich et al., 2001). Yet another factor to consider is the potential impact of changing measurement tools at age 15 years to the newest revision of the WISC. Although the method of transforming raw scores has been supported in the literature (Lindsey et al., 2000), we did rely on scaled scores for this transformation. When relying on scaled scores in this manner, it is assumed that the normative data between the WISC-R and WISC-III are stable when they may not be. This could potentially introduce additional error into the estimation of curvilinear function. Another issue to consider when transforming data is item overlap. The WISC-III Vocabulary and Block Design subscales do in fact share many items with the WISC-R subscales (i.e., there are 18 shared items across the two versions of the Vocabulary subscale and 10 shared items across the versions of the Block Design subscale) and the scaled scores are highly correlated across the two versions, lending additional confidence in this transformation approach.

While these results need to be replicated, they are also intriguing in that they may support one neuropsychological mediator pathway that has been proposed for the observed relationship between early Pb exposure and delinquent/antisocial behavior (Dietrich et al., 2001; Ris et al., 2002). More specifically, it has been proposed that early Pb exposure may contribute to weak verbal abilities leading to slow or impaired acquisition of reading skills. These interact with other liabilities to deflect such youth's development in an antisocial direction. The differential impact, reported here, on the downstream development of verbal comprehension skills (which tend to be more strongly correlated to both academic success and delinquency than perceptual organization skills) would lend partial support to such a formulation.

This study represents an initial step in applying advanced longitudinal methodology to the

investigation of Pb effects throughout development. Studies that incorporate the assessment of other neuropsychological domains, such as attention, executive functioning and learning and memory, will enhance our understanding of other specific cognitive Pb effects across the developmental lifespan. Such information will be critical for the creation of models that elucidate the complex genetic and neuropathophysiological underpinnings of Pb related neurobehavioral effects. Advances in our knowledge of etiological mechanisms may lead to enhanced prevention and pharmacological treatments.

AUTHOR NOTE

Juliet M. Coscia and M. Douglas Ris, Division of Psychology, Children's Hospital Medical Center, Cincinnati, OH and Department of Pediatrics, University of Cincinnati College of Medicine.

Paul A. Succop, Department of Environmental Health, Division of Epidemiology and Biostatistics, University of Cincinnati College of Medicine.

Kim N. Dietrich, Departments of Pediatrics and Environmental Health, University of Cincinnati College of Medicine.

Juliet M. Coscia is now at Department of Psychology, Mary Free Bed Hospital & Rehabilitation Center, Grand Rapids, MI.

REFERENCES

Baghurst, P.A., McMichael, A.J., Wigg, N.R., Vimpani, G.V., Robertson, E.F., Roberts, R.J., & Tong, S. (1992). Environmental exposure to lead and children's intelligence at the age of seven years: The Port Pirie Cohort Study. *New England Journal of Medicine*, *327*, 1279–1284.

Bellinger, D. (1995). Interpreting the literature on lead and child development: The neglected role of the "experimental system." *Neurotoxicology and Teratology*, *17*, 201–212.

Bellinger, D., Leviton, A., & Sloman, J. (1990). Antecedents and correlates of improved cognitive performance in children exposed in utero to low levels of lead. *Environmental Health Perspectives*, *89*, 5–11.

Bellinger, D., Leviton, A., Waternaux, C., Needleman, H., & Rabinowitz, M. (1989). Low-level lead exposure, social class, and infant development. *Neurotoxicology and Teratology*, *10*, 497–503.

Bradley, R.H., Caldwell, B.M., Rock, S.L., Barnard, K.E., Gray, C., Hammond, M.A., Mitchell, S., Siegel, L.,

Ramey, C.T., Gottfried, A.W., & Johnson, D.L. (1989). Home environment and cognitive development in the first three years of life: A collaborative study involving six sites and three ethnic groups in North America. *Developmental Psychology, 25*, 217–235.

Caldwell, B.M., & Bradley, R.H. (1978). *Administration manual: Home observation for measurement of the environment.* Little Rock: University of Arkansas.

Campbell, T.F., Needleman, H.L., Riess, J.A., & Tobin, M.J. (2000). Bone lead levels and language processing performance. *Developmental Neuropsychology, 18*, 171–186.

Chittooran, M.M., D'Amato, R.C., Lassiter, K.S., & Dean, R.S. (1993). Factor structure of psychoeducational and neuropsychological measures of learning-disabled children. *Psychology in the Schools, 30*, 109–118.

Cronbach, L.J., & Furby, L. (1970). How we should measure "change": Or should we? *Psychological Bulletin, 74*, 68–80.

Dietrich, K.N. (1995). A higher level of analysis: Bellinger's interpreting the literature on lead and child development. *Neurotoxicology and Teratology, 17*, 223–225.

Dietrich, K.N., Berger, O.G., & Succop, P.A. (1993). Lead exposure and the motor developmental status of urban six-year-old children in the Cincinnati Prospective Study. *Pediatrics, 91*, 301–307.

Dietrich, K.N., Berger, O.G., Succop, P.A., Hammond, P.B., & Bornschein, R.L. (1993). The developmental consequences of low to moderate prenatal and postnatal lead exposure: Intellectual attainment in the Cincinnati Lead Study Cohort following school entry. *Neurotoxicology and Teratology, 15*, 37–44.

Dietrich, K.N., Krafft, K.M., Bornschein, R.L., Hammond, P.B., Berger, O., Succop, P.A., & Bier, M. (1987). Low-level fetal lead exposure effect on neurobehavioral development in early infancy. *Pediatrics, 80*, 721–730.

Dietrich, K.N., Krafft, K.M., Pearson, D.T., Harris, L.C., Bornschein, R.L., Hammond, P.B., & Succop, P. (1985). Contribution of social and developmental factors to lead exposure during the first year of life. *Pediatrics, 75*, 1114–1119.

Dietrich, K.N., Ris, M.D., Succop, P.A., Berger, O.G., & Bronschein, R.L. (2001). Early exposure to lead and juvenile delinquency. *Neurotoxicology and Teratology, 23*, 511–518.

Dietrich, K.N., Succop, P.A., Berger, O.G., Hammond, P.B., & Bornschein, R.L. (1991). Lead exposure and the cognitive development of urban preschool children: The Cincinnati Lead Study cohort at age 4 years. *Neurotoxicology and Teratology, 13*, 203–211.

Dietrich, K.N., Succop, P.A., Berger, O.G., & Keith, R.W. (1992). Lead exposure and the central auditory processing abilities and cognitive development of urban children: The Cincinnati Lead Study cohort at age 5 years. *Neurotoxicology and Teratology, 14*, 51–56.

Espy, K.A., Molfese, V.J., & DiLalla, L.F. (2001). Effects of environmental measures on intelligence in young children: Growth curve modeling of longitudinal data. *Merrill-Palmer Quarterly, 47*, 42–73.

Factor-Litvak, P., Wasserman, G., Kline, J.K., & Graziano, J. (1999). The Yugoslavia prospective study of environmental lead exposure. *Environmental Health Perspectives, 107*, 9–15.

Finkelstein, Y., Markowitz, M.E., & Rosen, J.F. (1998). Low-level lead-induced neurotoxicity in children: An update on central nervous system effects. *Brain Research Review, 27*, 168–176.

Francis, D.J., Fletcher, J.M., Stuebing, K.K., Davidson, K.C., & Thompson, N.M. (1991). Analysis of change: Modeling individual growth. *Journal of Consulting and Clinical Psychology, 59*, 27–37.

Hollingshead, A.B. (1985). *Four factor index of social status* (Unpublished manual). New Haven: Yale University.

Lindsey, J.C., O'Donnell, K., & Brouwers, P. (2000). Methodological issues in analyzing psychological test scores in pediatric clinical trials. *Developmental and Behavioral Pediatrics, 21*, 141–151.

Littman, B., & Parmelee, A.H. (1978). Medical correlates of infant development. *Pediatrics, 61*, 470–474.

Livingston, R.B., Gray, R.M., Haak, R.A., & Jennings, E. (1997). Factor structure of the Halstead–Reitan Neuropsychological Test Battery for older children. *Child Neuropsychology, 3*, 176–191.

Needleman, H.L., Schell, A., Bellinger, D., Leviton, A., & Allred, E.N. (1990). The long-term effects of exposure to low doses of lead in childhood. An 11-year follow-up report. *New England Journal of Medicine, 322*, 83–88.

Ris, M.D., Dietrich, K.N., Succop, P.A., Berger, O., & Bornschein, R.L. (2003). *Early exposure to lead and neuropsychological outcome in adolescence.* Manuscript submitted for publication.

Ris, M.D., Packer, R., Goldwein, J., Jones-Wallace, D., & Boyett, J.M. (2001). Intellectual outcome after reduced-dose radiation therapy plus adjuvant chemotherapy for medulloblastoma: A Children's Cancer Group study. *Journal of Clinical Oncology, 19*, 3470–3476.

Rogan, W.J., Dietrich, K.N., Ware, J.H., Dockery, D.W., Salganik, M., Radcliffe, J., Jones, R.L., Ragan, N.B., Chisolm, J.J., & Rhoads, G.G. (2001). The effect of chelation therapy with succimer on neuropsychological development in children exposed to lead. *New England Journal of Medicine,* *344*, 1421–1426.

Rogosa, D.R., & Willett, J.B. (1985). Understanding correlates of change by modeling individual differences in growth. *Psychometrika, 50,* 203–228.

Ruff, H.A., Bijur, P.E., Markowitz, M., Ma, Y., & Rosen, J. (1993). Declining blood lead levels and cognitive changes in moderately lead-poisoned children. *Journal of the American Medical Association, 269,* 1641–1646.

Ruff, H.A., Markowitz, M.E., Bijur, P.E., & Rosen, J.F. (1996). Relationships among blood lead levels, iron deficiency, and cognitive development in two-year-old children. *Environmental Health Perspectives, 104,* 180–185.

Sattler, J.M. (1992). *Assessment of children: WISC-III and WPPSI-R supplement.* San Diego: Author.

Schneider, J.S. (2001). Enriched environment during development is protective against lead-induced neurotoxicity. *Brain Research, 896,* 48–55.

Schwartz, B.S., Lee, B.K., Lee, G.S., Stewart, W.F., Simon, D., Kelsey, K., & Todd, A.C. (2000). Associations of blood lead, dimercaptosuccinic acid-chelatable lead, and tibia lead with polymorphisms in the vitamin D receptor and [delta]-aminolevulinic acid dehydratase genes. *Environmental Health Perspectives, 108,* 949–954.

Schwartz, B.S., Stewart, W.F., Kelsey, K.T., Simon, D., Park, S., Links, J.M., & Todd, A.C. (2000). Associations of tibia lead levels with Bsml polymorphisms in the vitamin D receptor in former organolead manufacturing workers. *Environmental Health Perspectives, 108,* 199–203.

Silverstein, A.B. (1982). Two- and four-subtest short forms of the Wechsler Adult Intelligence Scale – Revised. *Journal of Consulting and Clinical Psychology, 50,* 415–418.

Statistical Analysis System Institute. (1997). *SAS/STAT software: Changes and enhancements through release 6.12.* Cary, NC: Author.

Tong, S., Baghurst, P.A., Sawyer, M.G., Burns, J., & McMichael, A.J. (1998). Declining blood lead levels and changes in cognitive function during childhood: The Port Pirie Cohort Study. *Journal of the American Medical Association, 280,* 1915–1919.

Wasserman, G.A., Liu, X., Popovac, D., Factor-Litvak, P., Kline, J., Waternaux, C., LoIacono, N., & Graziano, J.H. (2000). The Yugoslavia Prospective Lead Study: Contributions of prenatal and postnatal lead exposure to early intelligence. *Neurotoxicology and Teratology, 22,* 811–818.

Wasserman, G.A., Musabegovic, A., Liu, X., Kline, J., Factor-Litvak, P., & Graziano, J.H. (2000). Lead exposure and motor functioning in 4 1/2 year old children: The Yugoslavia Prospective Study. *Journal of Pediatrics, 137,* 555–561.

Wechsler, D. (1974). *Manual for the Wechsler Intelligence Scale for Children – Revised.* San Antonio: The Psychological Corporation.

Wechsler, D. (1991). *Manual for the Wechsler Intelligence Scale for Children – Third Edition.* San Antonio: The Psychological Corporation.

Child Neuropsychology
1997, Vol. 3, No. 2, pp. 98–133

A Typology of Psychosocial Functioning in Pediatric Closed-Head Injury*

Katy Butler[1], Byron P. Rourke[1,2], Darren R. Fuerst[3], and John L. Fisk[4*]

[1]University of Windsor, [2]Yale University, [3]Wayne State University School of Medicine, and [4]Henry Ford Hospital

ABSTRACT

A typology of psychosocial functioning following pediatric closed-head injury (CHI) was derived by subjecting Personality Inventory for Children – Revised (PIC-R) profiles to cluster analyses. Participants ($N = 128$) aged 6 to 16 years were classified into mild, moderate, and severe injury groups based on loss of consciousness (LOC), Glasgow Coma Scale (GCS), and so forth. On average, subjects were injured at 8.78 years of age and were assessed 2.12 years following their injury. Using four hierarchical-agglomerative clustering techniques, a seven-subtype typology was derived that overlapped, in part, with typologies previously reported for children with learning disabilities (LD). Based on clinical scale elevations of the mean PIC-R profiles, the subtypes were labeled Normal, Cognitive Deficit, Somatic Concern, Mild Anxiety, Internalized Psychopathology, Antisocial, and Social Isolation. Statistically significant relationships were found between psychosocial subtype membership and (a) injury severity, and (b) age at injury. Children assigned to the Social Isolation subtype were more likely to have severe CHI, and to have been injured at younger ages. Children tested after longer intervals since sustaining their CHI also tended to be assigned to the Social Isolation subtype. This subtype had elevations on the PIC-R cognitive triad and Psychosis scales, and may represent a persistent pattern of psychosocial disturbance following childhood CHI.

It is generally contended that children who sustain head injuries, particularly severe head injuries, tend to manifest psychosocial and behavioral problems as a result of those injuries. Interestingly, relatively few studies have addressed this issue in any detail, and comparisons among the existing investigations are difficult due to variations in methodology. Among the most common differences are the operational definition of head injury severity, the presence and rigor of an assessment of premorbid behavior, the manner in which cases are selected, and the range of outcome measures employed (Asarnow, Satz, Light, Lewis, & Neumann, 1991).

Although certain outcome measures are used more commonly than others, variability in the instruments used contributes to poor generalizability across studies. Although brief, open-ended interviews may elicit more detailed information from the caregiver, they tend to have poor or absent criteria for determining behavior problems and cannot be compared to normative standards. Standardized measures for which age-and gender-stratified normative data have been collected are generally preferred for this purpose, in part because many of the sequelae of head injury occur with some frequency in the general population (Asarnow et al., 1991).

---

* This study is based on a dissertation submitted by the first author to the University of Windsor in partial fulfillment of the requirements for the degree of Doctor of Philosophy. Aspects of this study were presented at the Annual Meeting of the International Neuropsychological Society, Chicago, 1996. John L. Fisk is now at Foote Memorial Hospital.

Address correspondence to: Katy Butler, University of Medicine and Dentistry of New Jersey, Robert Wood Johnson Medical School (UMDNJ-RWJMS), Division of Child and Adolescent Psychiatry, 675 Hoes Lane, Piscataway, NJ 08854, USA.

Accepted for publication: February 14, 1996.

The Child Behavior Checklist (CBCL; Achenbach & Edelbrock, 1983), Teacher's Report Form (TRF; Achenbach & Edelbrock, 1986), and the Vineland Adaptive Behavior Scales (Vineland; Sparrow, Balla, & Cicchetti, 1984) are the most commonly used instruments of this nature. The Conners' Behavior Scales (Conners, 1973), including both the Conners' Parent Questionnaire (CPQ) and the Conners' Teacher Questionnaire (CTQ), have also been used to assess the degree of behavior disorders in head-injured children. Although these measures survey a broad range of psychosocial and behavioral problems, they may provide only partial coverage of the problems inherent to head injury.

There is also considerable controversy over the use of appropriate control groups. Some authors (e.g., Brown, Chadwick, Shaffer, Rutter, & Traub, 1981) have elected to include a control group of children who sustained orthopedic injuries as an attempt to control for the nonspecific stresses related to trauma and hospitalization. However, the possibility of minor head injury, as well as the effects of pain and analgesics, may contaminate the comparison (Levin, Ewing-Cobbs, & Fletcher, 1989). Others have recruited normal classmates as control subjects (e.g., Shaffer, Chadwick, & Rutter, 1975). Further difficulties in the use of a control group arise with serial assessments, particularly with normal controls. Uninjured children may be expected to benefit more from repeated exposure to test materials than would head-injured children. In addition, normal children make significant improvements in test performance due to maturation, even over the course of a 6-month test-retest interval (Levin et al., 1989). For these reasons, many investigators have argued that the use of a comparison group is problematic and have opted to use standardized measures with age- and gender-stratified normative data (e.g., Fletcher, Ewing-Cobbs, Miner, Levin, & Eisenberg, 1990). This method may provide a more objective means of determining the rate of target disorders in the experimental group in comparison to population-based norms.

Research

Rutter, Chadwick, and colleagues have conducted a thorough prospective study of groups of children with mild and severe head injuries, as well as orthopedic controls matched on several social and demographic variables (Brown et al., 1981; Chadwick, Rutter, Schaffer, & Shrout, 1981; Rutter, 1981; Rutter, Chadwick, Shaffer, & Brown, 1980). Brown et al. (1981) investigated the rate of acquisition of new behavior disorders following head injury in children aged 5 to 14 years. Parents were interviewed immediately following the accident to ascertain the child's behavior, emotions, and family relationships, as well as medical, developmental, and school history prior to the injury. In addition, the CPQ administered to parents and teachers completed the Rutter's teacher scale. Follow-up evaluations were conducted at 4 months, 1 year, and approximately 2 years postinjury. At the final assessment, the teacher most familiar with each severely head-injured child was also interviewed, and a thorough neurological examination was conducted. The results revealed that children who had sustained mild head injuries demonstrated greater behavioral disturbance preinjury, based on the CPQ and teacher questionnaires, than did either severely head-injured children or matched orthopedic controls. At 4 months postinjury, the children in the severe head-injury group manifested greater behavioral disturbance than did the controls, and this rate continued to rise during the 2-year follow-up period. Onehalf of the severely head-injured children were found to develop new behavior disorders postinjury. The authors concluded that the increases in new psychiatric disorders following severe, but not mild, head injury suggest that severe head injury results in psychiatric problems as a result of brain damage. Disorders attributable to the head injury alone were characterized by a pattern of marked social disinhibition.

Fletcher et al. (1990) report longitudinal assessments of behavioral adjustment following head injury in children aged 3 to 15 years at the time of injury. Severe head injury was found to be associated with declines in adaptive behavior assessed with the Vineland, but not with problem behaviors identified on the CBCL. These results are different from those obtained by Brown et al. (1981) in that the mild and moderate groups in Fletcher et al.'s study did not demonstrate increased behavior problems at the time of the injury. However, this sample was carefully screened for premorbid psychosocial difficulties: Fletcher et al. excluded cases with premorbid history of learning disability (LD), attention deficit disorder (ADD), mental retardation (MR), or other developmental disabilities, which may have decreased the likelihood of premorbid behavioral differences between the groups. However, they also used a small sample, limiting the power of their analyses. Brown et al. (1981) did not screen for premorbid behavior problems; however, the inclusion of these cases did permit the demonstration of the relationship between mild head injury and behavior problems that antedate it.

The studies also differed in the criteria used to classify the severity of the injuries. In the Fletcher et al. (1990) study, many of the children in the moderate group, based on length of loss of consciousness (LOC), would have been classified as mild by Brown et al. (1981) using the unstandardized criterion of duration of PTA. In the Brown study, posttraumatic amnesia (PTA) of less than 7 days defined mild closed-head injury (CHI), while PTA greater than or equal to 7 days was defined as severe CHI. However, this difference alone does not account for the disparate results, as Fletcher et al. (1990) found no differences between the mild and moderate groups on either the Vineland or the CBCL. Taken together, the results of these two studies suggest that behavioral problems following mild head injury in children may be due to preexisting problems. Brown et al. (1981) found that among unscreened cases, the mild group had significantly more premorbid behavior problems than did either orthopedic controls or severely head-injured children. Fletcher et al. (1990) found no significant differences between premorbid behavior problems in carefully screened mild, moderate, and severe head-injury groups.

Asarnow et al. (1991) directly addressed the controversy over whether children who sustain mild head injuries have premorbid psychosocial problems, versus the hypothesis that mild injuries result directly in psychosocial morbidity. They attempted to overcome what they saw as three major methodological limitations of previous studies: (1) To reduce the likelihood that psychosocial problems identified in the study were merely premorbid, they excluded children with a history of central nervous system (CNS) damage, significant developmental delay, or behavior problems; (2) Children were evaluated at least 1 year postinjury to exclude transient reactions to the stress of the injury; and (3) Standardized measures with age- and gender-based normative data were used to determine deviance, rather than small control groups that may not be comparable to the experimental sample.

These investigators found that mildly and severely head-injured children obtained elevated scores on the Internalizing and Externalizing scales of the CBCL 1 year following the resolution of PTA. Although the mild injury group demonstrated no decline in adaptive functioning based on the Vineland, severely injured children were impaired on this measure. These results were consistent with previous findings of increased psychosocial morbidity following severe head injury. Conversely, mild CHI was not associated with increased impairment of adaptive functioning, which is congruent with other studies that have controlled for premorbid adaptive behavior problems or developmental delay (e.g., Fletcher et al., 1990). However, mildly head-injured children did demonstrate a level of behavior problems on the CBCL that was greater than that exhibited by the standardization sample, as well as similar to the proportion of children in the severe group manifesting behavior problems (Asarnow et al., 1991). In contrast to Asarnow et al., Fletcher et al. (1990) found that mild CHI did not result in elevations on the CBCL. The findings of behavior problems following mild head injury was unlikely to be due to premorbid dysfunction because the subjects were screened for premorbid psychopathology. Thus, there is evidence to suggest that there is at least a subgroup of children with mild CHI who manifest behavior problems that did not exist prior to their injury.

Donders (1992) investigated 85 children with recent traumatic brain injury (TBI) secondary to head trauma who were selected from consecutive admissions to a pediatric rehabilitation unit. The subjects were aged 6 to 16 years at the time of injury. He found that a greater proportion of children sustaining mild or moderate, versus severe, head injuries were involved in high risk activities when the trauma occurred. However, all children, regardless of injury severity, obtained normal scores on the CBCL and TRF assessing preinjury behavior. These findings suggest that the rate of premorbid behavioral and adjustment problems among children who sustain traumatic brain injuries (11%) is very similar to that expected in the general population of nonreferred children at any one time (10%; Achenbach & Edelbrock, 1983). These findings are in disagreement with those of Brown et al. (1981), who used semi-structured interviews with parents to measure premorbid behavior, versus the more objective age-normed and standardized behavior rating scales used by Donders. In addition, Brown et al. used unstandardized PTA estimates to assess injury severity, whereas Donders used Glasgow Coma Scale (GCS) scores and computed tomography (CT) findings. Fletcher et al. (1990), who also used standardized instruments to measure behavior, similarly found no differences inpremorbid behavior among groups of varying severity of head injury. Donders (1992) points out that his results cannot be generalized to the acute care setting, because the rehabilitation population is biased toward the prevalence of severe injuries. Children with mild injuries may be discharged without referral to an inpatient rehabilitation facility.

Knights et al. (1991) conducted a prospective investigation of 76 children between the ages of 5 to 17 years admitted to a large children's hospital for treatment of head trauma. The authors found that severely head-injured children studied at intake, 3, and 9 months postinjury were more impaired than were mild and moderate injury groups only on the Conners' scales of hyperactivity and learning problems. In addition, a behavior problem checklist administered 1 year postinjury to the parents of the severely injured children revealed them to have significantly more problems than did children in the other groups. The majority of the Conners' scales revealed no differences between the severe versus the mild and moderate injury groups. This is a common problem when statistical analyses are based on groups, masking the characteristics of individual subjects (Knights & Stoddart, 1981). Knights et al. (1991) also propose that the impact of an injury to a child on the psychosocial functioning of the family makes the assessment of psychosocial functioning in the child difficult. In addition, parents of severely injured children may be more tolerant of behavioral and other problems.

Summary

In the foregoing review of the literature, there is a paucity of research investigating psychosocial and behavioral sequelae of head injuries sustained during childhood. Moreover, comparisons among these studies and the extent to which the findings can be generalized are often limited by vast differences in methodology and small sample sizes. In general, the majority of the investigators to date have concluded that severe head injury, when compared with mild or moderate injury groups, normal or orthopedic controls, or population-based norms, results in the manifestation of behavior, psychiatric, and/or adaptive behavior disturbances (Asarnow et al., 1991; Brown et al., 1981; Fletcher et al., 1990; Knights et al., 1991). Considerable controversy exists regarding the behavioral sequelae of mild head injury, however. Although one investigation reported that behavioral disturbance following mild head injury antedated the injury (Brown et al., 1981), others have not found elevated rates of pre-injury behavior disturbance in mildly head-injured children (Donders, 1992; Fletcher et al., 1990).

Considerable variability is also apparent in the choice of measures used to assess behavioral outcome. It is interesting to note that, to our knowledge, the Personality Inventory for Children – Revised (PIC-R) has not been used to study behavioral and psychiatric sequelae in head-injured children. Whereas some investigators have argued that open-ended or semi-structured interviews elicit more relevant data, others have opted for standardized measures with age- and gender-stratified normative data available for comparison. Often the latter procedure has been used in lieu of a control group, although still others have opted to use normal or orthopedic controls. Although many investigators have obtained data from both parents and teachers in an attempt to reduce possible biases introduced by surveying the parents alone, in all cases the results of the teacher's questionnaires were comparable, though less robust, than were those of the parent questionnaires.

In summary: (1) Many indices of injury severity have been used to assign subjects to groups, but the overriding factor determining outcome appears to be severity, regardless of the way in which it is measured; (2) The use of various normal and orthopedic control groups is often problematic and controversial. An acceptable alternative seems to be the use of population-based, age- and gender-stratified normed measures; (3) Given the limitations of the behavior problem checklists commonly employed in this area of research, the use of a psychosocial and behavioral measure with a broader and increased depth of focus, such as the PIC-R, may prove useful; (4) Furthermore, a profile analysis approach may elucidate differences that are masked in the contrasting-groups comparisons used to date; and (5) The addition of teacher questionnaires to the data pool has not been shown to provide additional or disparate information to that obtained from the parents.

Principal Conclusions

Based on the foregoing review of the literature, the following general conclusions can be drawn regarding the effects of head injury on psychosocial functioning in children: (1) Although few investigators have pursued the issue, it is generally contended that children who sustain head injuries, particularly severe head injuries, manifest a range of behavior, psychiatric, and/or adaptive behavior disturbances as a result of those injuries; (2) Investigators who have studied psychosocial functioning following pediatric head injury frequently criticize the measures that they employ. Open-ended interviews provide more information, but are limited because they are not standardized and tend to be subjective. Brief rating scales have the advantage of age- and gender-stratified normative data, but limit the scope of the data obtained. Regardless, no investigation to date has employed a more comprehensive, standardized measure such as the PIC-R; (3) The use of a comparison group with this population is often problematic and an acceptable alternative seems to be the use of standardized measures with population-based normative data.

Hypotheses

The present investigation sought to examine the psychosocial sequelae of pediatric closed-head injury using the PIC-R. PIC-R profiles of head-injured children were subjected to cluster analyses. Given that this instrument has not previously been used with this population, this study was, by necessity, somewhat exploratory. However, some general predictions were made and, in this light, the following hypotheses (with their associated rationales) were generated:

1. The major focus of the present investigation was to develop a PIC-R-based psychosocial

typology of children with CHI. The best known empirical PIC-R psychosocial typology, with demonstrated internal and external validity, is that of Rourke and Fuerst (1991). However, that typology was developed for children with LD, and the generalizability of that typology to other populations is currently unknown. Therefore, two issues were of major interest as follows: (a) Considering the range of subtypes found in the Rourke and Fuerst (1991) typology, it was expected that at least some of the subtypes in the LD-typology would also be recovered from children with CHI. However, additional subtypes which differ from those previously identified were expected in the CHI-derived typology, and (b) if a similar typology, or at least a subset of similar subtypes were to be found, it was expected that children with CHI, overall, would be more likely to be found in frankly pathological subtypes than would children with LD, because psychosocial disturbance is frequently associated with CHI.

2. In many studies of psychosocial functioning following CHI, severity of injury, no matter how defined, has been found to be associated with greater psychosocial disturbance. Thus, it was expected that (a) the proportions of mild/moderate versus severe CHI cases within each subtype would differ, with the severe CHI cases tending to fall within the most pathological PIC subtypes. In addition, it was hypothesized that (b) the children with severe CHI would also show the greatest PIC-R profile elevation within subtypes.

3. The relationship between age at injury and psychosocial outcome was also investigated. Although previous studies have not found an association between age at injury and psychosocial outcome, worse neuropsychological outcome has been found in children severely injured at younger ages. It was hypothesized that the use of a more comprehensive measure of psychosocial functioning would permit a more sensitive test of this hypothesis. Given the residual neuropsychological deficits found in children injured at younger ages, it was expected that these children would also show worse psychosocial outcomes.

4. Also of interest was whether time since injury influenced psychosocial outcome. On one hand,

some improvement in psychosocial functioning might be expected to occur with recovery, so that children tested soon after injury may show worse functioning than children tested later. On the other hand, Rourke (1989) has argued that particular patterns of chronic cognitive deficits may eventuate in disordered psychosocial functioning over time. Therefore, at least some children tested at longer periods since injury were expected to show greater psychopathology than would children tested soon after injury.

METHOD

Subjects

Prospective participants were ascertained from two large urban clinics and one large urban private practice, all of which accept referrals for neuropsychological assessment because of difficulties suspected to be related to cerebral dysfunction. All cases had been administered a comprehensive neuropsychological test battery in the manner recommended by Rourke, Fisk, and Strang (1986). Two hundred and six (206) consecutive referrals for CHI between the ages of 6 and 16 years were reviewed for inclusion in the present investigation. Exclusion criteria consisted of the following: (1) parental report of a head injury, but no consultation with medical services (to exclude very mild injuries that may not have resulted in brain injury); (2) history of prior head injury; (3) any history of CNS damage or disease prior to the head injury (e.g., epilepsy, brain tumor); (4) evidence of learning disabilities, attention-deficit hyperactivity disorder, mental retardation, or other significant developmental disorder; (5) a history of premorbid behavioral or psychosocial problems; (6) evidence of educational or cultural deprivation; (7) evidence of child abuse; and (8) incomplete or invalid PIC-R profiles. One hundred and twenty-eight cases (77 males and 51 females) met the criteria for inclusion in the study. The mean age at which subjects sustained the CHI, chronological age at the time of the neuropsychological assessment, and the interval between the injury and the assessment are summarized in Table 1 across levels of injury severity.

Cases were divided into mild, moderate, and severe injury groups using information available regarding injury severity. There is a precedent in the literature for using this method in retrospective investigations of pediatric head injury (Winogron, Knights, & Bawden, 1984). To ensure that the children in the mild group had sustained a brain injury, mild CHI was operationally defined as loss of consciousness (LOC) less than 20 min with no evidence of mass lesion, brain swelling, or skull

fracture; Glasgow Coma Scale (GCS) score at admission of 13 to 15; and no deterioration of level of consciousness. Children who experienced no coma following the injury, but had a history of concussive symptoms and a short PTA after the injury also qualified for the mild injury group. Moderate CHI was defined as an admission GCS score of 9 to 12, or GCS of 13 to 15 with skull fracture, mass lesion, or other indication of specific brain injury; or LOC greater than 20 min. Severe CHI was defined as an initial GCS score of 3 to 8; intracranial hematoma; depressed skull fracture with neurological deficit, bruising, contusion, or loss of brain tissue; subarachnoid hemorrhage; CT scan findings, such as edema; or LOC greater than 48 hr. These criteria were in accordance with those used most often in the literature reviewed.

Measures

The Personality Inventory for Children – Revised (PIC-R; Lachar, 1982) is based on the comprehensive, empirically derived Personality Inventory for Children (Wirt, Lachar, Klinedinst, & Seat, 1977). Four hundred and twenty descriptive statements are responded to as true or false by the child's primary caretaker, usually the biological mother. Although up to 33 separate scales can be constructed from the results of the PIC-R, only 16 of these are typically used: 3 validity scales (Lie, F, and Defensiveness), 1 general measure of psychosocial adjustment (Adjustment), and 12 clinical scales (Achievement, Intellectual Screening, Development, Somatic Concern, Depression, Family Relations, Delinquency, Withdrawal, Anxiety, Psychosis, Hyperactivity, and Social Skills). PIC-R scale scores are expressed as T scores, with elevations above the mean indicating an increased likelihood of significant psychopathology.

Table 1. Mean Age at Injury (Years), Age at Test (Years), and Time Since Injury (Years) Across Levels of Injury Severity.

Injury severity	Age at injury	Age at Test 1	Time since injury
Mild	8.71 (3.36)	10.79 (2.80) $n = 36$	2.07 (1.84)
Moderate	9.12 (4.63)	11.35 (3.23) $n = 55$	2.25 (3.60)
Severe	8.36 (4.03)	10.33 (3.24) $n = 37$	1.96 (2.03)
Overall	8.78 (4.15)	10.90 (3.13) $N = 128$	2.12 (2.76)

Note. Means (Standard Deviations).

Analyses

Study 1
Subtype generation by cluster analysis   All 12 of the
PIC-R clinical scale scores were included in the cluster
analysis. In this study, as in previous research in our
laboratories, we were interested in grouping subjects on
the basis of similarity of PIC profile shape. Thus, for
each subject, the elements of profile elevation and dispersion were eliminated by standardizing each subject's
12 PIC-R scale scores across that subject's profile. This
was necessary because SAS clustering software limits
similarity measures to Euclidean distance. To do this,
each subject's 12 PIC-R scale scores were standardized
across that subject's profile using the transformation
$z = X - M/SD$ (X = a subject's raw scale score; M =
mean of that subject's profile; SD = standard deviation of
that subject's profile. M and SD are calculated across the
12 scales; z = resulting standard score; Lorr, 1983).

Whenever multivariate subtyping techniques are
applied in an exploratory fashion to data with relatively
unknown statistical properties, reliability of the resulting
typology is of particular concern. Even when applied to
random data, multivariate subtyping techniques, such as
cluster analysis, will always produce groups of subjects.
Moreover, different statistical subtyping techniques often
can, and do, generate different solutions from the same
data set. Therefore, replicating subtypes across either
different samples from the same population, or across
different subtyping techniques, is an important step in
determining the validity of subtypes generated with cluster
analysis (Fletcher, 1985; Fuerst, Fisk, & Rourke, 1989).

Numerous cluster analysis techniques exist, with
little evidence suggesting that any particular method
is superior, in part because of differences and interactions
between methods, measures, and samples (Aldenderfer &
Blashfield, 1984; Lorr, 1983). Four widely used and
relatively well understood hierarchical agglomerative
clustering methods were applied in the present investigation: Ward's Minimum-Variance method (Ward,
1963); the complete linkage method (Sorensen, 1948);
the weighted pair-group method using arithmetic averages (WPGMA; Sokal & Michener, 1958); and the
unweighted pair-group method using arithmetic averages (UPGMA; Sokal & Michener, 1958). In addition,
one relatively new technique, the equal-variance maximum likelihood method (EML; Sarle, 1985) was utilized. The SAS Version 6 implementation of these
algorithms was used (Sarle, 1985).

The primary method of assessing agreement between
various solutions involved three external criteria measures: Rand's statistic (Rand, 1971) and the two adjustments to Rand's statistic suggested by Morey and Agresti
(1984) and Hubert and Arabie (1985). Rand's statistic
measures the agreement between two different cluster
solutions by assessing the degree to which pairs of

subjects are clustered together or apart. Simply put, for
different solutions to agree, pairs of subjects clustered
together in one solution must also be clustered together
in the other solution and, similarly, pairs not clustered
together should be so in both solutions. The adjustments
to Rand's statistic (Morey & Agresti, 1984; Hubert &
Arabie, 1985) include corrections for chance agreement
between solutions (Milligan & Cooper, 1986). As a second method for assessing agreement, correlations were
calculated between the mean PIC-R profiles of the subtypes generated with the hierarchical method chosen as
the standard and those derived by the other four hierarchical techniques. These correlations provided a measure of the degree of similarity of mean PIC-R profile
shape among the various hierarchical subtypes.

Relationship to known subtypes   It was hypothesized
that at least some of the subtypes derived from children
with CHI would bear some relationship to those found
previously in LD samples. Therefore, the subtypes
derived from the cluster analysis in this study were
compared to those reported in previous research (Porter
& Rourke, 1985; Fuerst et al., 1989; Fuerst, Fisk, &
Rourke, 1990; Fuerst & Rourke, 1993). Rourke and
Fuerst (1991) reviewed the results of these studies and
used correlation coefficients to match corresponding
subtypes across studies, resulting in the identification of
seven distinct subtypes (Normal, Mild Hyperactive,
Mild Anxiety, Somatic Concern, Conduct Disorder, Internalized Psychopathology, and Externalized Psychopathology). "Prototypical" mean PIC profiles were
generated for each of the seven subtypes by averaging
the PIC scores of corresponding subtypes across studies.

Two methods were used to assess the relationship
between the seven Rourke and Fuerst (1991) LD subtypes and subtypes generated in this study for head-
injured children. First, correlations between the subtypes,
using the mean PIC-R scores on all 16 scales, were calculated and compared. This method assessed the degree
of similarity of mean PIC profile shape between the subtypes and prototypes (Hypothesis 1a). Second, the subtypes generated in the present study were compared to the
prototypes based on the proportion of subjects assigned
to each of the subtypes (Hypothesis 1b) using exact probability tests. This allowed for a comparison of the relative
frequency of each of the subtypes in head-injured children and children with LD (proportions taken from the
psychosocial typology of Rourke and Fuerst, 1991).

*Relationship of injury severity with psychosocial
functioning*   To determine if severity of injury was related
to psychosocial functioning (Hypothesis 2a), a cross-
tabulation of severity of injury classification (mild, moderate, and severe) with psychosocial subtype was carried
out. This table was visually inspected to determine if
severely injured children make up a disproportionate ratio
of the most severely disordered psychosocial subtypes.
This table was also subjected to a Chi-Square test of
independence of the cross-tabulation, and to Chi-Square

goodness-of-fit tests comparing the proportions of subjects in each injury severity group within each subtype.

To explore further the relationship between injury severity and psychosocial outcome (Hypothesis 2b), a one-way ANOVA with injury severity classification as the independent variable and mean profile elevation on the 12 PIC-R clinical scales as the dependent variable, was also performed. This analysis was done both across the entire sample and within each PIC-R subtype.

To determine if age at injury was related to psychosocial outcome (Hypothesis 3), a one-way ANOVA with age as the dependent variable and PIC-R subtype membership as the independent variable was performed. To determine if time since injury was related to psychosocial outcome (Hypothesis 4), a one-way ANOVA with time since injury as the dependent variable and PIC-R subtype membership as the independent variable was performed.

Study 2

Changes in psychosocial functioning with time: Test-retest analyses To determine if children who have sustained CHI show any change in their psychosocial functioning over time, the psychosocial subtype to which a child was assigned at the first assessment was compared with the subtype to which they were assigned at the second assessment (Hypothesis 4). This was evaluated in two ways. First, whether or not children change subtype over time was examined, with the initial subtype membership determined by the results of the cluster analysis. Given that fewer cases could be entered into this analysis, a second cluster analysis of subtype membership could not be performed on the PIC-R profiles obtained at retest. Therefore, the profile matching algorithm of Fuerst (1991) was used to assign subjects to subtypes within the typology developed in the initial cluster analysis.

The extent to which subjects move from or remain in their initial subtype was assessed using the adjusted value of Rand's statistic comparing initial and retest subtype membership. If subjects tend to remain in their initial subtype, the adjusted value of Rand's statistic for the two solutions was expected to be relatively high (.7 or better). A repeated measures ANOVA with mean elevation on the 12 PIC-R clinical scales as the dependent measure and test or retest as the independent measure was carried out to determine if level of psychosocial adjustment changes from initial assessment to retest.

RESULTS

Study 1

Subtype Derivation
Because the cluster analysis methods used in this study are known to be sensitive to the presence

of outliers, the initial sample was screened using the technique described by Fuerst and Rourke (1995), and 10% (13 subjects) of the subjects were judged to be outliers and were deleted from the sample. The most reliable (replicable) solution of the hierarchical methods, EML, was chosen as the standard. Examination of the R^2 and pseudo-F values for 2 to 30 cluster solutions suggested the presence of seven subtypes. For clarity of exposition, descriptive labels (Normal, Cognitive Deficit, Somatic Concern, Mild Anxiety, Internalized Psychopathology, Antisocial, and Social Isolation) summarizing the major features of the PIC-R profile (as outlined in Wirt, Lachar, Klinedinst, & Seat, 1984), were assigned to each subtype. For each of the seven subtypes, mean PIC-R scores on all 16 scales were calculated to obtain the profiles presented in Figures 1 through 7.

All versions of Rand's statistic were greater than 0.65, demonstrating that these seven subtypes were replicated with good accuracy by Ward's method, the Complete Linkage, and the WPGMA clustering techniques. although difficult to interpret, an adjusted value of 0.0 for Rand's statistic theoretically indicates purely chance agreement, and 1.0 indicates complete agreement. Empirical studies have demonstrated that adjusted values of Rand's statistic greater than 0.2 indicate agreement between solutions that is better than chance (Milligan & Cooper, 1986). Adjusted values of Rand's statistic greater than 0.65 suggest good agreement between cluster solutions.

As a further comparison of the agreement between the different cluster solutions, the mean PIC-R profiles of the clusters derived from Ward's method, Complete Linkage, and WPGMA cluster analysis were also derived and compared to the mean PIC-R profiles of the EML subtypes. Correlations between the mean PIC-R profiles of the EML subtypes and each of the replicated subtypes were calculated. All subtypes derived using the three replication methods correlated better than .64 with their corresponding EML subtypes, and most subtypes showed correlations at or above .94. That is, Ward's method, WPGMA, and Complete Linkage produced subtypes with PIC-R profiles that were very similar in shape to their corresponding EML subtypes.

Relationship to Known Subtypes

Visual inspection of Figures 1 through 7 suggested that four CHI subtypes appeared very similar to four of the seven prototypical PIC subtypes obtained in previous research of children with LD.

Subsequent to visual matching, correlations were calculated between the mean PIC-R profiles of the subtypes derived in this study and the mean PIC profiles of the prototypes. The CHI Cognitive Deficit subtype replicated with excellent accuracy

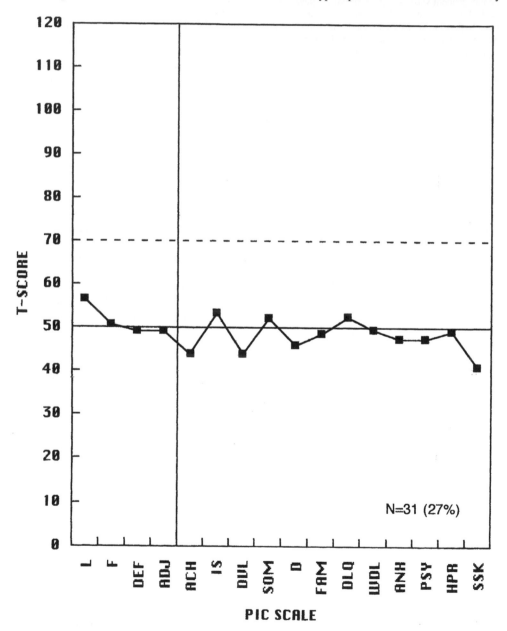

Fig. 1. Mean PIC-R profile for the Normal subtype.

the prototypical LD Normal subtype ($r = .91$). The mean PIC profiles for these two subtypes are presented in Figure 8. The prototypical LD Internalized Psychopathology subtype was replicated with excellent accuracy in the CHI sample ($r = .91$), although the elevation was more extreme in the CHI subtype. The mean PIC profiles for these two subtypes are presented in Figure 9.

The prototypical LD Somatic Concern subtype was replicated in the CHI with good accuracy

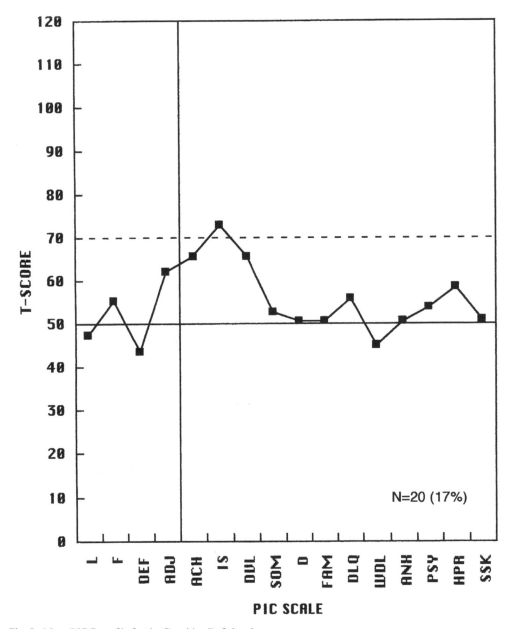

Fig. 2. Mean PIC-R profile for the Cognitive Deficit subtype.

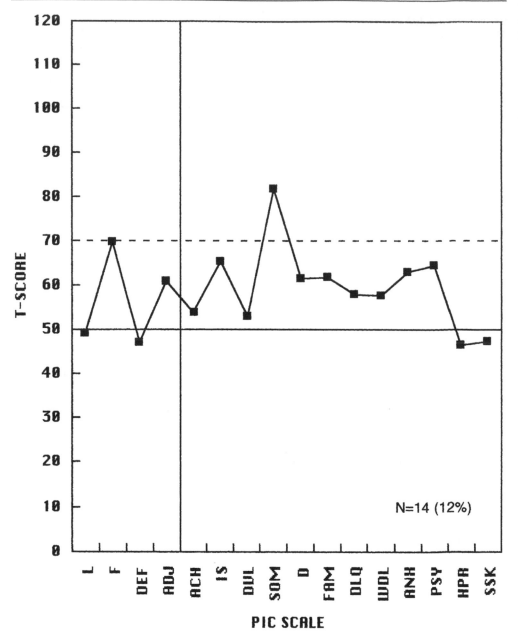

Fig. 3. Mean PIC-R profile for the Somatic Concern subtype.

($r = .79$). The mean PIC profiles for these two subtypes are presented in Figure 10. In addition, a subtype clearly resembling the LD Mild Anxiety prototype was recovered from the CHI cluster analysis ($r = .71$). The mean PIC profiles for these two subtypes are presented in Figure 11.

The subtypes recovered from the CHI sample were also compared to the prototypes in terms of

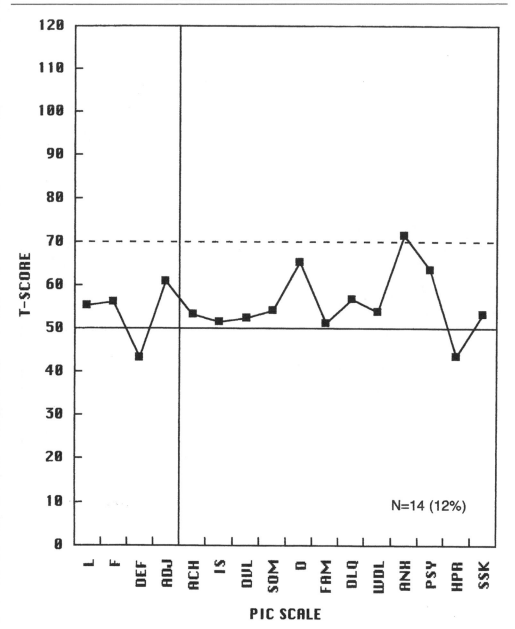

Fig. 4. Mean PIC-R profile for the Mild Anxiety subtype.

the percentages of subjects assigned to each of the subtypes (see Table 2). Inspection of Table 2 reveals that the percentage of CHI and LD subjects falling into the Mild Anxiety and Somatic Concern subtypes were very similar. However, relatively fewer CHI subjects were assigned to the Cognitive Deficit/LD Normal and Internalized Psychopathology subtypes than were LD subjects.

Exact probability tests of the percentages of assigned subjects within prototypical subtypes

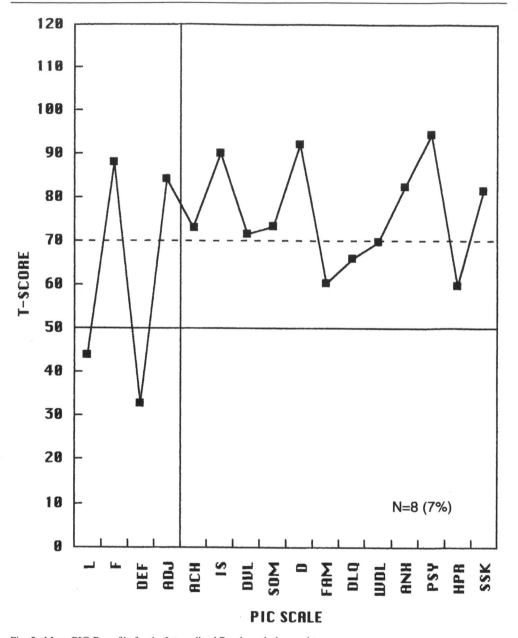

Fig. 5. Mean PIC-R profile for the Internalized Psychopathology subtype.

(LD) and subtypes derived by cluster analysis (CHI) revealed no significant differences for the Mild Anxiety and Somatic Concern subtypes. However, exact probability tests demonstrated that the deviation from expected values (proportions in prototypes) was significant for the proportion of CHI subjects assigned to the Cognitive Deficit (LD Normal; $p = .0075$) and Internalized Psychopathology ($p = .004$) subtypes. Therefore, a difference between the two populations was evident

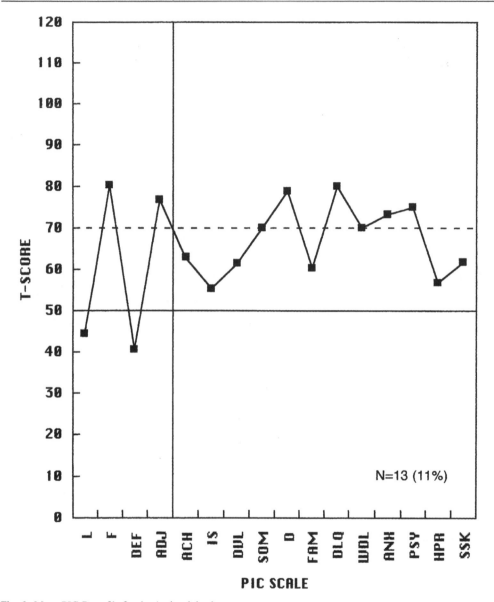

Fig. 6. Mean PIC-R profile for the Antisocial subtype.

in terms of the relative size of the Cognitive Deficit and Internalized Psychopathology subtypes.

Relationship of Injury Severity with Psychosocial Functioning

A cross-tabulation of severity of injury classification (mild, moderate, and severe) with psychosocial subtype was constructed. The percentages of mild, moderate, and severe injury participants is presented in Figure 12. Visual inspection of Figure 12 revealed that, in general, children sustaining severe head injuries were not assigned disproportionately to the most severely disturbed psychosocial subtypes. Based on the number of scales

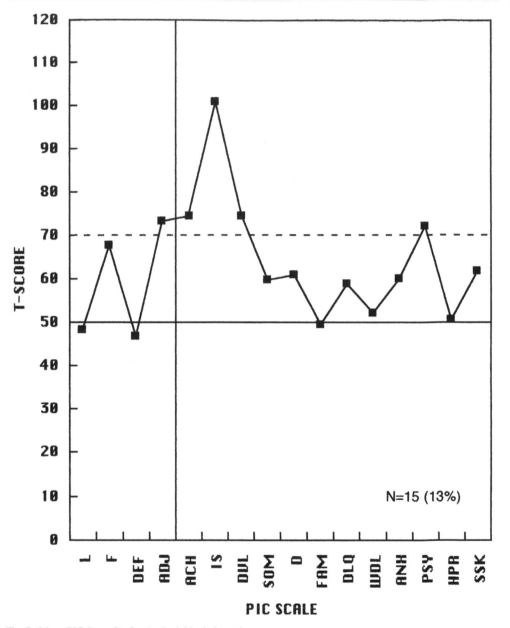

Fig. 7. Mean PIC-R profile for the Social Isolation subtype.

elevated and the degree of elevation, the Internalized Psychopathology and Antisocial subtypes
were the most severely disturbed. However, a
clear preponderance of severely injured subjects
was evident only in the Social Isolation subtype.

It was also apparent from Figure 12 that the
Cognitive Deficit subtype contained a majority of
mild and moderately injured subjects, whereas the
Normal and Antisocial subtypes contained relatively greater proportions of moderately injured

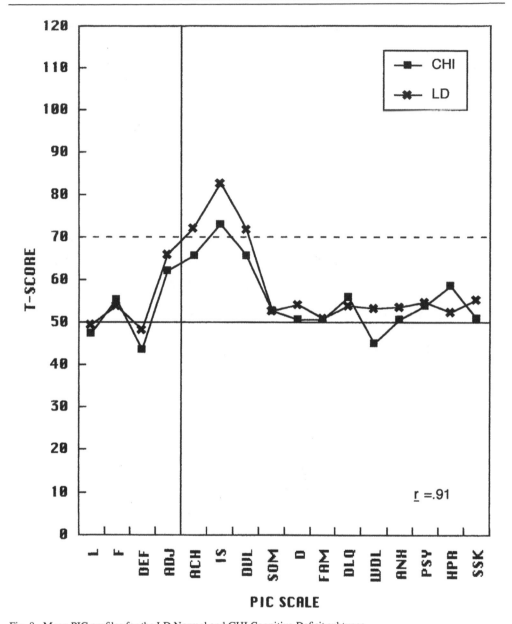

Fig. 8. Mean PIC profiles for the LD Normal and CHI Cognitive Deficit subtypes.

children. A slight preponderance of moderately and severely injured subjects was evident in the Somatic Concern subtype. Finally, the Mild Anxiety and Internalized Psychopathology subtypes were made up of relatively equal numbers of mild, moderate, and severe injury children.

A Chi-Square test of independence of the cross-tabulation demonstrated that there was a significant association between severity of injury and the psychosocial subtype to which subjects were assigned ($\chi^2(12) = 21.44$, $p < .05$). Chi-Square goodness-of-fit tests of the proportion of subjects

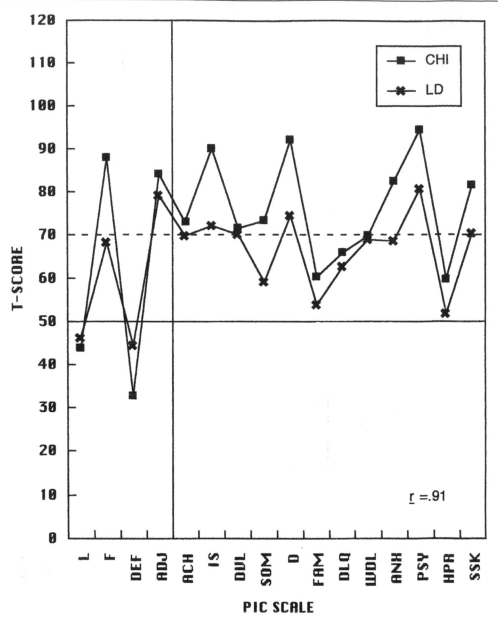

Fig. 9. Mean PIC profiles for the LD and CHI Internalized Psychopathology subtypes.

in each injury severity group for each subtype taken separately revealed a significant difference only for the Social Isolation subtype ($\chi^2(2) =$ 11.20, $p < .01$). An examination of the relative frequencies suggested that a disproportionate

number of severely injured children were assigned to this subtype.

A one-way ANOVA with injury severity classification as the independent variable and mean PIC-R profile elevation on the 12 clinical scales as

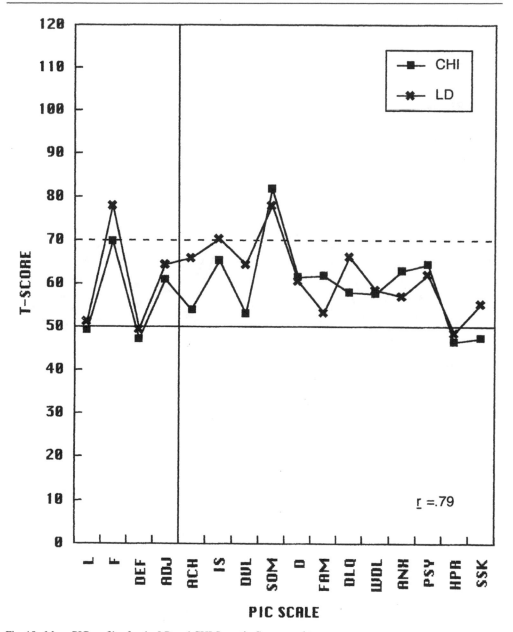

Fig. 10. Mean PIC profiles for the LD and CHI Somatic Concern subtypes.

the dependent variable for all subtypes combined revealed no significant difference in profile elevation across levels of injury severity ($p = .87$).

A one-way ANOVA with injury severity classification as the independent variable and mean PIC-R profile elevation on the 12 clinical scales as the dependent variable was repeated within each PIC-R subtype. This analysis revealed that mean PIC-R profile elevation was significantly different across levels of severity within the Antisocial

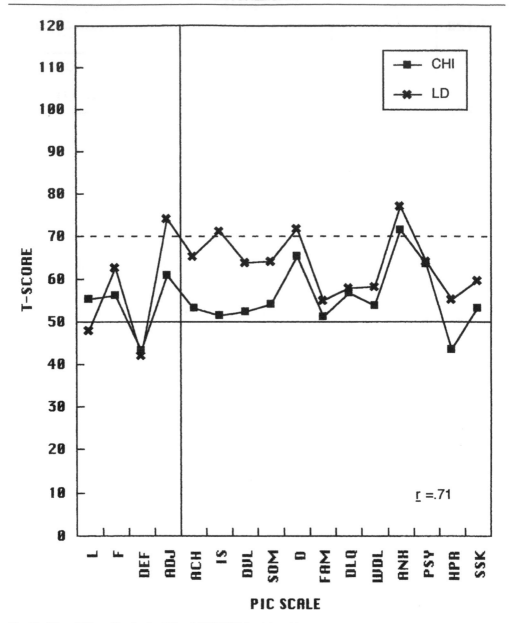

Fig. 11. Mean PIC profiles for the LD and CHI Mild Anxiety subtypes.

subtype $(F(2,10) = 9.14, \quad p < .05)$. Post-hoc comparisons using Tukey's HSD revealed that children in the mild injury group obtained significantly lower profile elevations than did children in either the moderate or severe injury group. Mean

PIC-R profile elevation was also significantly different across levels of severity within the Mild Anxiety subtype $(F(2,11) = 5.83, p < .05)$. Post-hoc comparisons using Tukey's HSD revealed that children in the mild injury group obtained

Table 2. Percentages of Subjects Assigned to Prototypical Subtypes (LD) and Subtypes Derived from the CHI Sample.

	Subtype						
	Cog. Def. (LD Normal)	Mild Anxiety	Somatic	Internal	Antisoc	Soc. Isol.	Normal
Prototype	28	11	11	16			
CHI	17	12	12	7	11	13	27

Note. Subjects in the prototype studies were also assigned to three additional subtypes (Externalized Psychopathology, Mild Hyperactivity, and Conduct Disorder) not represented in the CHI group. Cog. Def. = Cognitive Deficit; Somatic = Somatic Concern; Antisoc = Antisocial; Soc. Isol. = Social Isolation.

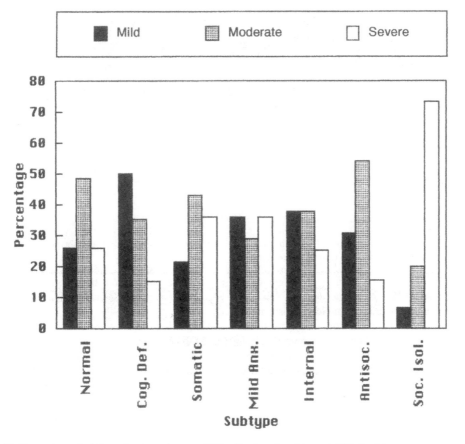

Fig. 12. Percentage of mild, moderate, and severe CHI subjects assigned to each PIC-R subtype.

significantly higher profile elevations than did children in the moderate injury group, with profile elevation for the severe group falling between these two.

Differences in mean PIC-R profile elevation across levels of severity within the Cognitive Deficit subtype approached statistical significance ($F(2, 17) = 2.82$, $p = .09$). (Although the results

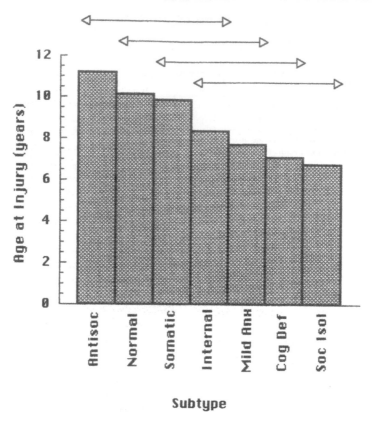

Fig. 13. Mean age at injury across PIC-R subtype. (*Note.* The arrows represent groups of subtypes which do not
differ significantly with respect to age at injury.)

of post-hoc tests in the absence of a significant
omnibus ANOVA are of questionable validity,
they are reported here in the interest of discerning
trends present in this exploratory study.) Post-hoc
comparisons using Tukey's HSD revealed that
children in the moderate injury group obtained
significantly higher profile elevations than did
children in the severe injury group, with profile
elevations for the mild group falling between
these two values.

Differences in mean PIC-R profile elevation
across levels of severity within the Normal subtype
also approached statistical significance ($F(2, 28) =$
2.62, $p = .09$). Post-hoc comparisons using
Tukey's HSD revealed no significant differences
in mean profile elevation across the three levels
of injury severity. Differences in mean PIC-R
profile elevation across levels of severity were

nonsignificant for the Somatic Concern, Internalized
Psychopathology, and Social Isolation subtypes.

*Relationship of Age at Injury with
Psychosocial Functioning*

A one-way ANOVA, with age at injury as the
dependent variable and PIC-R subtype membership as the independent variable, yielded a significant effect of age at injury ($F(6, 108) = 2.97$,
$p < .05$). Post-hoc pair-wise comparisons using
Tukey's HSD method failed to demonstrate significant differences between the group means,
despite the significant overall F statistic. For this
reason, differences between group means were
examined using Fisher's least significant difference method (LSD) with an alpha level of .05.
Mean age at injury across psychosocial subtype
membership and the results of LSD tests are

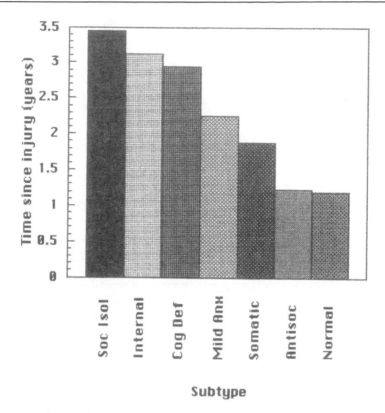

Subtype

Fig. 14. Group means for time since injury (years) as a function of psychosocial subtype.

presented in Figure 13. As can be seen, age at injury for the Antisocial subtype was significantly greater than age at injury for the Mild Anxiety, Cognitive Deficit, and Social Isolation subtypes. In addition, age at injury for the Normal subtype was significantly greater than age at injury for the Cognitive Deficit, and Social Isolation subtypes. Finally, age at injury for the Somatic Concern subtype was significantly greater than age at injury for the Social Isolation subtype. Put simply, children injured at younger ages were significantly more likely to be assigned to the Social Isolation, Cognitive Deficit, and Mild Anxiety subtypes.

Relationship of Time Since Injury With Psychosocial Functioning
A one-way ANOVA with time since injury as the dependent variable and PIC-R subtype membership as the independent variable approached statistical

significance ($F(6, 108) = 2.07, p = .06$). Post-hoc pair-wise comparisons using Tukey's HSD method did not demonstrate significant differences between the group means. Differences between group means (see Figure 14) were examined using Fisher's LSD method with an alpha of .05. These comparisons demonstrated that subjects assigned to the Social Isolation subtype exhibited significantly longer time since injury than did the Antisocial and Normal subtypes.

Study 2

Changes in Psychosocial Functioning With Time: Test-Retest Analyses
The profile matching algorithm of Fuerst (1991) was used to assign subjects, based on their PIC-R profiles, to subtypes within the typology developed in the initial cluster analysis. Of the 36 subjects

KATY BUTLER ET AL.

Table 3. Psychosocial Subtype Membership at Test 1 and Test 2.

Test 1	Test 2							
	Normal	Cog. Def.	Somatic	Mild Anx	Internal	Antisoc	Soc. Isol.	Total
Normal	4	0	1	1	0	0	1	7
Cog. Def.	0	4	0	0	1	0	1	6
Somatic	0	1	0	0	0	0	2	3
Mild Anx	0	0	0	3	0	0	1	4
Internal	0	0	0	0	0	0	0	0
Antisoc	0	0	0	1	1	2	0	4
Soc. Isol.	0	0	0	0	1	0	3	4
Total	4	5	1	5	3	2	8	28

Note. Cog. Def. = Cognitive Deficit; Somatic = Somatic Concern; Mild Anx = Mild Anxiety; Internal = Internalized Psychopathology; Antisoc = Antisocial; Soc. Isol. = Social Isolation.

receiving a second assessment, 28 could be assigned to one of the seven subtypes. The adjusted value of Rand's statistic comparing initial and retest subtype membership (.80) suggested relatively close agreement between the two solutions. In other words, the psychosocial subtypes to which subjects were assigned on the basis of their PIC-R profiles at Test 1 tended to remain the same at Test 2.

A repeated measures ANOVA with mean elevation on the 12 PIC-R clinical scales as the dependent measure and test or retest as the independent measure revealed no significant differences in level of psychosocial adjustment from initial assessment to retest. These results were supported by a Chi-Square test of independence of the cross-tabulation of subtype membership at Test 1 and Test 2 (presented in Table 3) which demonstrated that there was a statistically significant association between subtype membership at Test 1 and subtype membership at Test 2 ($\chi^2(30) = 58.322, p < .01$).

DISCUSSION

The major goal of this investigation was the development of a typology of psychosocial functioning in children who had sustained closed-head injuries, based on cluster analysis of the PIC-R. The psychosocial subtypes derived were examined in relation to the following: (1) subtypes derived previously in samples of children with LD; (2) the severity of the CHI (mild, moderate, or severe); (3) the age at which the CHI was sustained; (4) the duration of the interval between sustaining the

CHI and the assessment; and (5) changes over time in a within-subjects (test-retest) design.

The results of the cluster analysis suggested the presence of seven distinct psychosocial subtypes. Four of these subtypes were very similar to subtypes that have been derived previously in samples of children with LD, whereas three subtypes were unique to this sample of children with CHI. Relationships were found between the subtype to which children were assigned and injury severity, age at injury, and the length of time between the injury and the assessment. In an analysis of test-retest data, it appeared that children tended to remain in the subtypes to which they were originally assigned. These conclusions are discussed in greater detail below in relation to the hypotheses posed and issues related to them.

Hypothesis 1

Description of the Typology
In the interest of clarity when discussing the subtypes derived in this study, descriptive labels were assigned to each subtype based on the character-istics of the clinical scales that were elevated above 70 T (i.e., to a clinically significant level in the direction of psychopathology). When a subtype's mean PIC-R profile closely resembled one that had been obtained in previous research, the same label was assigned (with the exception of the LD Normal or CHI Cognitive Deficit subtype). It must be born in mind that the PIC-R is completed by the child's primary caretakers (usually the biological mother) and, thus, reflects their

concerns regarding the child. This is not necessarilyreflective of the child's actual behavior. In the following section, each subtype is discussed in terms of the expected behavioral characteristics of children assigned to that subtype in light of the pattern of scale elevations.

The mean PIC-R profiles of two of the subtypes were characteristic of normal psychosocial functioning. The profile for the Normal subtype did not contain any clinically significant elevations, resulting in a very flat profile across both the cognitive triad (Achievement, Intellectual Screening, and Development scales) and clinical scales. The caretakers of children in this subtype were not expressing undue concern about their child's cognitive, academic, or psychosocial functioning. This subtype was the largest, accounting for 27% of the sample.

The Cognitive Deficit subtype had a mean PIC-R profile that also suggested relatively normal psychosocial functioning, with the exception of a single elevation above $70\,T$ on the Intellectual Screening scale. Although they did not reach the level of strict clinical significance, high scores on the Achievement and Development scales suggested a profile very similar to those characterized by elevation of the cognitive triad. (The shape of the profile is important, even if the elevation of some scales is somewhat less than $70\,T$, because the profile representative of each subtype is an *average* of all children in that subtype.) This subtype was very similar to the Normal subtype identified in children with LD. (Of course, the "normal" subtype in an LD population is normal only with respect to the "clinical" scales; it is expected to exhibit elevations on the cognitive triad.)

Elevations on the cognitive triad scales in the absence of clinical scale elevations are considered "normal" in a sample of children with known learning problems. However, this profile is not considered to be strictly normal in the CHI population, particularly in light of the completely "normal" profile described above. For this reason, the profile labeled as "Normal" in the LD typology was labeled "Cognitive Deficit" in this study. Parents of children assigned to the Cognitive Deficit subtype were most concerned about their child's cognitive skills, age-appropriate development, and/or academic performance, but did not express concerns

regarding psychosocial functioning. This subtype was the second largest, containing approximately 17% of the children.

Two of the subtypes had mean PIC-R profiles that suggested mild degrees of psychosocial dysfunction (i.e., profiles with a single clinically significant elevation). The Somatic Concern subtype consisted of a relatively flat PIC-R profile witha single significant elevation (above $70\,T$) on the Somatic Concern scale. Children with similar PIC-R profiles are described as having health-related complaints such as frequent fatigue, headaches, or aches and pains. Further evaluation of such children would be necessary to determine if these complaints are maladaptive (e.g., employed to avoid responsibilities or withdraw from uncomfortable situations) versus "organic" in nature and requiring medical attention. The possibility of an organic basis for somatic complaints is particularly germane in the context of a CHI sample, because these children, by definition, have suffered at least one significant physical injury. This subtype comprised 12% of the sample.

The Mild Anxiety subtype was also characterized by a relatively normal PIC-R profile, with the exception of a single significant elevation on the Anxiety scale. Caretakers' descriptions of the behavior of children in this subtype may reflect fearfulness and worry, with specific complaints including multiple fears, difficulties with sleep, and distrust of others. This subtype also accounted for 12% of the sample.

The PIC-R profiles of the remaining three subtypes were indicative of greater degrees of psychosocial disturbance. The Internalized Psychopathology subtype had a mean PIC-R profile with rather high elevations (greater than $80\,T$) on the Intellectual Screening, Depression, Anxiety, Psychosis, and Social Skills scales. Secondary, significant elevations (above $70\,T$) were present on the Achievement, Development, Somatic Concern, and Withdrawal scales. Children in this subtype are likely to suffer from relatively severe, internalized psychopathology, including problems with depression, anxiety, emotional lability, inappropriate affect, reality testing, and social isolation. This was the smallest of subtypes, accounting for only 7% of the sample.

The Antisocial subtype had a mean PIC-R profile with significant elevations above $70\,T$ on the

Somatic Concern, Depression, Withdrawal, Anxiety, and Psychosis scale, with the highest elevation on the Delinquency scale. The behavioral characteristics of children in this subtype are similar to those in the Internalized Psychopathology subtype, with the addition of those reflected by elevations of the Delinquency scale. The Delinquency scale is elevated in children who resist authority and may be irresponsible, impulsive, hostile, argumentative, and poorly socialized. This subtype included 11% of the sample.

The final subtype, Social Isolation, was characterized by significant PIC-R profile elevations on the Achievement, Intellectual Screening, and Development scales (i.e., the cognitive triad), and Psychosis scale. Caretakers of children in this subtype were concerned about their child's cognitive development and academic performance, in addition to their social adaptation. Elevations on the Psychosis scale may reflect behaviors characteristic of social isolation and emotional lability. Thirteen percent of the sample was assigned to this subtype.

Internal Validity (Reliability) of the Typology
The demonstration of internal validity is crucial whenever multivariate subtyping techniques are applied in an exploratory fashion to a data set with unknown or poorly understood structure, as was the case in this study. Replication of the subtypes in a different sample from the same population or replication using different subtyping techniques are two commonly used methods of demonstrating reliability. In this study, reliability was demonstrated by replicating the obtained cluster solution using three additional clustering techniques. Good agreement between the four clustering methods suggested that the seven cluster typology described herein is reliable.

Relationship to known Subtypes
A second method of assessing the reliability of the subtypes generated in this study was to examine their relationship to subtypes generated in previous investigations (i.e., replication across samples and, in this case, populations). The best known empirical PIC-R psychosocial typology, with demonstrated reliability and external validity, is that of Rourke and Fuerst (1991) that was developed for children with LD.

Hypothesis 1a Considering the range of subtypes found in the Rourke and Fuerst (1991) typology, it was expected that at least some of the subtypes in the LD typology would also be recovered from children with CHI. However, additional subtypes differing from those previously identified were also expected in the CHI-derived typology. Support for this hypothesis was found, based on the observation that four of the CHI subtypes were very similar to four of the prototypical LD subtypes (LD Normal/CHI Cognitive Deficit, Internalized Psychopathology, Somatic Concern, and Mild Anxiety). Finding these four subtypes in a second population supports the reliability of these subtypes. They have now been identified across numerous samples of children with LD as well as in this sample of children with CHI. The three remaining subtypes (CHI Normal, Antisocial, and Social Isolation) appear to be unique to the CHI sample or, at the very least, have not been identified previously in an LD sample. Replication of these subtypes using several clustering techniques provides support for their reliability; however, replication in a second CHI sample is needed.

Hypothesis 1b It was expected that, overall, children with CHI would be more likely to be found in frankly pathological subtypes than would children with LD because psychosocial disturbance is thought to be frequently associated with CHI. Support for this hypothesis was not found, based on the relatively equal proportions of LD and CHI children falling into the Mild Anxiety and Somatic Concern subtypes (both with mild levels of psychosocial disturbance) and the greater proportion of children with LD versus CHI falling into the Internalized Psychopathology subtype. Although the proportion of LD in the LD Normal/Cognitive Deficit subtype was significantly larger than in the CHI sample, a large percentage of the CHI sample was assigned to the Normal subtype in the CHI typology.

The relative percentages of children with CHI and LD assigned to the subtypes found in each typology are spread in Table 4. Overall, 44% of the children with CHI were assigned to the Normal and Cognitive Deficit subtypes, whereas only 28% of children with LD were assigned to the Normal subtype (i.e., subtypes with no psychopathology). Conversely, 24% of children with CHI were

Table 4. Percentages of Children with CHI and LD (From Rourke & Fuerst, 1991) Assigned to Psychosocial Subtypes with Normal and Mildly or Severely Disturbed Levels of Psychosocial Functioning.

Degree of Pathology	CHI			LD		
	Subtype	%	Combined	Subtype	%	Combined
Normal	Normal	27	44	Normal	28	28
	Cog. Def.	17				
Mild	Somatic	12	24	Mild Hyp	11	41
	Mild Anx	12		Cond Dis	8	
				Somatic	11	
				Mild Anx	11	
Severe	Internal	7	31	Internal	16	32
	Antisoc	11		External	16	
	Soc. Isol.	13				

Note. Cog. Def. = Cognitive Deficit; Somatic = Somatic Concern; Mild Anx = Mild Anxiety; Internal = Internalized Psychopathology; Antisoc = Antisocial; Soc. Isol. = Social Isolation; Mild Hyp = Mild Hyperactivity; Cond Dis = Conduct Disorder; External = Externalized Psychopathology.

assigned to subtypes with a mild level of psychosocial disturbance, versus 41% of children with LD (Mild Hyperactive, Conduct Disorder, Somatic Concern, and Mild Anxiety subtypes). Relatively equal proportions of children with CHI and LD (31% and 32%, respectively) were assigned to subtypes with severely disturbed psychosocial functioning. Therefore, there is no evidence suggesting that children sustaining CHIs are more likely to fall into the more pathological psychosocial subtypes than are children with LD. However, there is little a priori reason to expect either similarities or differences in terms of subtype assignment between these two populations, given that they have not previously been compared in terms of psychosocial functioning.

Relationship to a psychiatric sample   Further support of the reliability of the typology derived in this study is provided by its considerable overlap with a PIC typology derived using a psychiatric sample (Gdowski, Lachar, & Kline, 1985; LaCombe, Kline, Lachar, Butkus, & Hillman, 1991). The CHI Normal subtype closely resembles the Type 1 (Within Normal Limits; WNL) profile identified by Gdowski et al. Type 2 profiles in the Gdowski et al. typology contain a single elevation, as do the Mild Anxiety and Somatic Concern subtypes derived in the present study. The CHI Social Isolation subtype is very similar to the Type 5 profile, which also shows elevations on only the cognitive triad and Psychosis scales.

LaCombe et al. describe Type 6 as a "pure" cognitive dysfunction group, closely resembling the CHI Cognitive Deficit subtype. Type 7 is described as exhibiting both internalized and externalized psychopathology (LaCombe et al., 1991), with a PIC profile that is very similar to that of the CHI Antisocial subtype. Finally, LaCombe et al. describe their Type 9 profile as "pure internalization", a pattern similar to that seen in the Internalized Psychopathology group identified herein. Thus, all 7 subtypes derived in this investigation bear close resemblance to 6 of the 12 patterns identified in children referred to a psychiatric facility.

External Validity of the Typology
When multivariate subtyping techniques are applied to any data set, a subtype structure will be imposed upon it and, therefore, the demonstration of internal validity is important. However, equally important is the demonstration of external validity. Although a statistically elegant cluster solution may be discovered, it is only as useful as its utility in guiding theory, research, and clinical practice.

All of the subtypes derived in the present investigation were readily interpretable within the framework recommended in the PIC-R manual (Wirt et al., 1984), thus supporting their clinical interpretability. These subtypes were also in accordance with patterns of behavior observed in clinical settings, as well as patterns of behavior identified in previous studies of children who have sustained CHI. None of the investigations reviewed has used a measure as comprehensive as the PIC-R, or a sample as large as the one employed in this study. Not surprisingly then, no single study has reported all of the psychosocial sequelae represented in the typology derived in this investigation. However, the combined results of several previous investigations overlap considerably with those of the present study.

For example, Brown et al. (1981) found that the most common postinjury behavioral deficit attributable to brain injury alone (i.e., in the absence of any indication of premorbid behavioral disturbance) was a "disinhibited state" characterized by marked socially disinhibited behavior, such as being over talkative and outspoken, inappropriate personal remarks, or a disregard for social conventions. Asarnow et al. (1991) found that mild and severely head-injured children obtained elevated scores on the Internalizing and Externalizing scales of the CBCL one year following the resolution of PTA. In addition, severely injured children were impaired on the communication, socialization, and daily living skills domains of the Vineland and on its adaptive behavior composite. Fletcher et al. (1990) also found that the Vineland composite and domain scores declined over the course of follow-up assessments at 6 and 12 months in the severe injury group. The psychosocial characteristics of the subjects in these studies are very similar to the behavioral characteristics of children assigned to the Internalized Psychopathology, Social Isolation, and Antisocial subtypes derived in this investigation.

Knights et al. (1991) found that severely head-injured children studied at intake, 3, and 9 months postinjury were more impaired than were mild and moderate injury groups only on the CPQ scales of hyperactivity and learning problems. In addition, a behavior problem checklist administered 1 year postinjury to the parents of the severely injured children revealed that these children had significantly more behavior problems (e.g., irritable mood, distractibility, peer problems, memory and motor coordination problems, and learning problems) than did children in the other groups. Similarly, the present investigation identified learning problems, as evidenced by elevations on the cognitive triad scales, in a number of the subtypes (Cognitive Deficit, Internalized Psychopathology, and Social Isolation).

Whereas Knights et al. (1991) found evidence of hyperactivity following CHI, Brown et al. (1981) found that overall restlessness and increased activity were less frequent in disorders attributable to brain injury. In accord with Brown's findings, the results of this investigation did not include, for example, Mild Hyperactive or Externalized Psychopathology subtypes found in previous psychosocial subtyping studies of children with LD. In the Knights et al. (1991) study, the majority of the CPQ scales revealed no differences between the severe versus the mild and moderate injury groups. This is a common problem when statistical analyses are based on groups, masking the characteristics of individual subjects (Knights & Stoddart, 1981). The present investigation overcame this obstacle by using a profile analysis approach.

Hypothesis 2

Relationship of Injury Severity and Psychosocial Functioning

In many studies of psychosocial functioning following CHI, severity of injury, no matter how defined, has been found to be associated with greater psychosocial disturbance. One way of examining the severity of the psychosocial disturbance of various subtypes obtained in this study would be to evaluate the severity of each subtype individually on the basis of the number and degree of clinical scale elevations. This can be done quantitatively by summing the T scores of the 12 clinical scales within each subtype. This results in the following rank-order of the subtypes from greatest to least psychopathology: Internalized Psychopathology, Antisocial, Social Isolation, Somatic Concern, Mild Anxiety, Cognitive Deficit, and Normal. This ranking of the subtypes in terms of degree of psychosocial disturbance has face validity in a clinical sense, and was used in subsequent comparisons.

Hypothesis 2a It was expected that the proportions of mild and moderate versus severe CHI would differ within each subtype, with the severe CHI cases tending to be assigned to the most pathological PIC subtypes. In general, this hypothesis was not supported. Although there was a significant association between severity of injury and psychosocial subtype membership, subjects sustaining severe head injuries were not assigned disproportionately to the most severely disturbed psychosocial subtypes. In fact, the Internalized Psychopathology and Antisocial subtypes, the most severely disturbed, contained proportionately fewer severely injured children. A clear preponderance of severely injured children was evident in only the Social Isolation subtype, which ranks third in the hierarchy of severity of psychosocial pathology. The Social Isolation subtype had higher elevations on the scales comprising the cognitive triad than did any of the other subtypes; this may be one important factor contributing to the preponderance of severely injured subjects in this subtype.

Hypothesis 2b One of the reasons for performing subtype analyses is to reveal differences between groups that may be masked by examining any given sample as a whole. Nevertheless, some general indices of psychosocial dysfunction can be examined across all subtypes combined. It was hypothesized that the children with severe CHI would show the greatest PIC-R profile elevation across subtypes. However, the results revealed no significant difference in profile elevation across levels of injury severity. This is not surprising, given the heterogeneity evident across the seven subtypes.

Mean PIC-R profile elevations were also examined within each subtype. Significant differences in mean PIC-R profile elevations across levels of injury severity were found for the Antisocial subtype, with the mild injury group obtaining significantly lower profile elevations than did subjects in either the moderate or severe injury group. Significant differences were also found in the Mild Anxiety subtype, with the mild injury group obtaining significantly *higher* profile elevations than did subjects in the moderate injury group. These results suggest that, within the Antisocial subtype (one of the more severely disturbed subtypes), severe CHIs result in a greater degree of psychosocial deficit. Conversely, within the Mild Anxiety subtype (a subtype with a mild level of disturbance), children sustaining mild, versus moderate or severe, head injuries are most likely to demonstrate the greatest overall psychosocial deficit (as indexed by mean profile elevation). The presence of these opposing patterns may have contributed to the nonsignificant overall comparison of PIC-R profile elevation with injury severity.

The pattern observed in the Mild Anxiety subtype is interesting and runs contrary to what might

be expected. It is possible that children in this subtype manifested symptoms resembling the post-concussion syndrome that has been reasonably well delineated in adults who have sustained mild head injuries (Dikmen, Temkin, & Armsden, 1989; Rutherford, 1989). The early symptoms of concussion – such as headache, dizziness, nausea, and vomiting – are reported by the patient as soon as consciousness is regained. However, the late symptoms of concussion are generally reported a few weeks postinjury, and/or up to several years later. In addition to headache and dizziness, late post-concussion symptoms include anxiety, irritability, and depression. Given that the children in this study were assessed, on average, 2 years postinjury, the items endorsed on the PIC-R could be considered as "late" symptoms. In this respect, children assigned to the Mild Anxiety psychosocial subtype show some similarities to adults manifesting the post-concussion syndrome, specifically in terms of anxiety.

The finding in this study that the mild CHI group obtained the highest PIC-R profile elevations within the Mild Anxiety subtype may suggest that a subset of children sustaining mild CHIs suffer from post-concussional complaints that are similar to those observed in some mildly head-injured adults. Although one previous investigation concluded that mildly head-injured children manifest relatively few post-concussion symptoms, the criteria employed for mild CHI excluded children who had suffered any loss of consciousness or had any neurological symptoms (Casey, Ludwig, & McCormick, 1986). These criteria are more stringent than those typically employed, and more stringent than the criteria used in this investigation. It is possible that the mild head injury group in the Casey et al. study did not sustain any brain injury. Furthermore, in contrast to the comprehensive behavioral measure employed in this investigation, Casey et al. evaluated the presence of the post-concussion syndrome by using a symptom checklist.

Hypothesis 3

Relationship of Age at Injury with Psychosocial Functioning
Although previous studies have not found an association between age at injury and psychosocial

outcome, worse neuropsychological outcome has been found in children severely injured at younger ages. It was hypothesized that the use of a more comprehensive measure of psychosocial functioning would permit a more sensitive test of this hypothesis. Given the residual neuropsychological deficits found previously in children injured at younger ages, it was not unreasonable to expect that these children would also show worse psychosocial outcomes. Although support for a relationship between age at injury and subtype membership was found, the results did not necessarily support the contention that children injured at younger ages demonstrate worse psychosocial outcome.

No significant relationship between age at injury and psychosocial functioning in terms of mean elevation on the clinical scales was found. However, as has been discussed previously, this is not surprising because of the heterogeneity of the sample in terms of psychosocial functioning. Further analyses revealed that age at injury for the Antisocial subtype was significantly higher than age at injury for the Mild Anxiety, Cognitive Deficit, and Social Isolation subtypes. In addition, age at injury for the Normal subtype was significantly higher than age at injury for the Cognitive Deficit and Social Isolation subtypes. Finally, age at injury for the Somatic Concern subtype was significantly higher than was age at injury for the Social Isolation subtype. Put simply, children injured at younger ages were significantly more likely to be assigned to the Social Isolation, Cognitive Deficit, and Mild Anxiety subtypes, whereas children injured at older ages were more likely to be assigned to the Antisocial, Normal, or Somatic Concern subtypes.

It is possible that children who sustain a CHI near puberty, a time associated with many changes in developmental demands, are more likely to act out, resist authority, and/or disrupt relationships within the family. In other words, children injured at this age may manifest exacerbations of the problems with which many adolescents struggle. On the other hand, children injured at younger ages may have most difficulty with the developmental challenges most germane in their lives at the time of the injury: namely, academic success and the fostering of interpersonal skills that

suddenly become necessary following immersion in the vast social network of school.

Hypothesis 4

Relationship of Time since Injury with Psychosocial Functioning

Of interest was whether the interval between the CHI and the assessment (time since injury) influenced psychosocial outcome. On one hand, some improvement in psychosocial functioning might be expected to occur with recovery, so children tested soon after injury may show worse functioning than children tested later. On the other hand, Rourke (1989) has argued that particular patterns of chronic cognitive deficits can eventuate in increasing levels and types of disordered psychosocial functioning over time. This possibility was evaluated in two ways. First, the time since injury was compared to psychosocial subtype membership in the original sample of 115 children. At least some children tested later were expected to actually show greater pathology than did children tested soon after injury. Second, a subset of children who had undergone serial assessments were evaluated in a test-retest analysis. These children were expected to demonstrate a pattern of either decline or recovery of psychosocial function at Test 2.

Time since injury The analyses of time since injury approached commonly accepted levels of statistical significance, with post-hoc comparisons (reported in the interest of discerning possible trends in the data) demonstrating that subjects assigned to the Social Isolation subtype had significantly longer time since injury than did the Antisocial and Normal subtypes. Overall, it does appear that children tested several years after sustaining their CHI tend to fall into two of the three more pathological subtypes (i.e., Social Isolation and Internalized Psychopathology). On the other hand, children tested soon after their injury tend to be assigned to the Normal or Antisocial subtypes, only one of which represents serious psychosocial maladjustment. Thus, there is support for the hypothesis that longer durations between injury and test are related to psychosocial outcome. However, the precise nature of this relationship is not entirely clear. It is possible that a referral bias is involved: Children who were not referred for neuropsychological assessment soon after their injury may only have been referred at a later date if they were experiencing significant problems.

Test-retest The assignment of children at their second assessment (using profile matching) to the subtypes derived through cluster analysis revealed that the psychosocial subtypes to which subjects were assigned on the basis of their PIC-R profiles at Test 1 tended to remain the same at Test 2. There was also a statistically significant association between subtype membership at Test 1 and subtype membership at Test 2. Further, no significant differences in level of psychosocial adjustment from initial assessment to retest were found. Thus, the results of the test-retest analysis do not suggest that the psychosocial sequelae of pediatric CHI, overall, change (statistically) over time. The weight of the evidence obtained herein is in favor of little change in psychosocial functioning over time, with a trend (though not statistically significant) for time since injury to determine subtype membership. In this connection, it is important to point out an essential difference between the CHI sample investigated in this study and the LD samples employed in previous subtyping studies of the PIC-R.

Whereas conditions such as LD may be thought of as chronic, a CHI is an acute event that may or may not result in some level of chronic cerebral dysfunction. Even if we assume that severe CHIs do eventuate in chronic dysfunction, the length of the interval between the head injury and the assessment (i.e., time since injury) could not possibly be equivalent with the duration of chronicity experienced by the child with LD. This may be an essential difference between these populations in terms of the long-term effects of their disabilities on psychosocial functioning. Therefore, Rourke's (1989) hypothesis regarding declines in psychosocial functioning in the context of chronic cerebral dysfunction may not apply to children who have sustained acute cerebral trauma. On the other hand, the results of this investigation do not suggest that the converse is true. No improvement in psychosocial functioning was seen over time. It is possible that if these children were to be studied across longer test-retest intervals, declines in psychosocial functioning may be evident as a result of the chronic cognitive deficits due to brain injury.

Summary

The following is a brief summary of the results of this investigation in terms of the hypotheses put forth.

1. The major goal of the present investigation, to develop a PIC-R-based psychosocial typology of children with CHI, was accomplished. Using cluster analysis, a seven-subtype typology was derived that overlapped, in part, with typologies previously reported for children with LD. This was expected, as was the finding of additional subtypes that appear to be unique to the CHI sample. However, no evidence was found to support the expectation that, overall, the CHI sample would fall disproportionately into the more severely disturbed subtypes when compared with the LD samples.

2. The results did not support the hypothesis that severe (vs mild or moderate) CHI would be associated with more severe psychosocial dysfunction, either in terms of assignment to the more disturbed subtypes or greater mean PIC-R profile elevation. However, a significant relationship between level of injury severity and psychosocial functioning was found in terms of the proportions of severely injured subjects assigned to each subtype.

3. No consistent support was found for the hypothesis that children injured at younger ages would demonstrate worse psychosocial outcome. However, a significant relationship between age at injury and subtype membership was found, demonstrating that younger age at injury tends to result in assignment to one particular psychosocial subtype (Social Isolation).

4. Contrary to expectations, the results of a test-retest analysis did not suggest that psychosocial functioning either improves or declines over time. However, children tested after longer intervals since sustaining their CHI tended to be assigned to one particular subtype (Social Isolation).

GENERAL CONCLUSIONS

One major contribution of this investigation was the demonstration that the psychosocial sequelae of pediatric CHI are heterogeneous. This may seem so simplistic and self-evident that it need not be stated at all. Although clinicians are well aware that this is most likely the case, researchers have continued to attempt to describe psychosocial deficits following head injury based on the results of single, generally narrow, measures that obscure differences between individuals. Therefore, the application of cluster analytic techniques to a pediatric CHI sample has contributed significantly to the existing body of literature. The results of this investigation led to the conclusion that the psychosocial sequelae of CHI during childhood cover a variety of patterns, ranging from normal to mildly disturbed in circumscribed areas (such as anxiety, intellectual and academic problems, or somatic complaints) to rather severe disturbances characterized by internalized psychopathology or antisocial behavior.

The proportions of children assigned to each subtype suggested that well over one half of the children sustaining even severe CHIs suffer no, or only minor, psychosocial difficulties. Indeed, a disproportionate number of severely injured children was evident in only one subtype (Social Isolation), characterized by cognitive, academic, and developmental problems in addition to social isolation, withdrawal, and emotional lability. Throughout the course of this investigation, the Social Isolation subtype appeared to be of key importance in terms of the relationships between psychosocial functioning and a host of other variables.

As mentioned above, the Social Isolation subtype contained a disproportionately high percentage of severely injured subjects. The mean PIC-R profile of the Social Isolation subtype also showed higher elevations on the cognitive triad than did any of the other subtypes. However, within the Social Isolation subtype, the cognitive triad was not significantly higher for the severe CHI subjects than for the mild or moderately injured subjects. This suggests that the tendency for children in the Social Isolation subtype to obtain the lowest scores on psychometric intelligence, academic, and some neuropsychological measures (Butler, Rourke, Fuerst, & Fisk, 1997) was not due solely to elevations on the cognitive triad. Rather, the combination of the elevated Psychosis and cognitive triad scales seems important in the robust pattern of neuropsychological deficits evident for children assigned to this psychosocial subtype.

The Social Isolation subtype was also comprised of children with the longest time since injury (the duration between sustaining their CHI and being assessed). Across all subtypes, children with the longest time since injury also obtained higher elevations on the cognitive triad and Social Skills scales. These findings may suggest that the constellation of psychosocial deficits represented in the Social Isolation subtype may be persistent sequelae of CHI in a subset of children. Children injured at younger ages also tended to be assigned to the Social Isolation subtype.

Taken together, these findings suggest that the pattern of deficits evident in the Social Isolation subtype are of particular relevance in pediatric CHI. It may be useful for clinicians to be aware of the potential risks for the development of psychosocial pathology when they assess children with some of the above characteristics: Children with severe, and likely persistent, deficits across a wide range of psychometric intelligence, academic, and neuropsychological measures are at risk for the development of psychosocial problems that may include social isolation, withdrawal, and emotional lability. It is also likely that these psychosocial problems will persist over a period of atleast several years, as demonstrated by the time since injury data presented herein. Children injured at younger ages are at greater risk for developing this pattern of psychosocial deficits. Conversely, children injured at older ages are more likely to present with a combined pattern of internalized psychopathology and antisocial behavior that may worsen over time, but is not as likely to persist over a period of several years following the head injury.

Finally, the results of this investigation provide sufficient evidence to conclude that the psychosocial sequelae of pediatric CHI are related, possibly in a causal fashion, to the brain injuries sustained during the head trauma. Support for this assertion is demonstrated by the significant relationships found between psychosocial functioning (subtype membership) and (a) CHI severity, and (b) many neuropsychological variables (Butler et al., 1997).

Limitations and Suggestions for Future Research
This was the first study to attempt the development of a psychosocial typology using the PIC-R in

closed-head-injured children. It is clear that future research could provide significant contributions to this field. First and foremost, the results of the current investigation provide a good basis for the inclusion of the PIC-R in a prospective study of the psychosocial sequelae of pediatric CHI. This would help to control for some of the drawbacks to conducting retrospective research, and would also provide the opportunity to replicate the results of this investigation in a different sample of children with CHI. Replication of the results obtained in this investigation would provide additional support for the reliability of the typology derived. In particular, the reliability of the three subtypes not previously identified (CHI Normal, Antisocial, and Social Isolation) needs to be evaluated.

The validity of the typology derived herein was demonstrated, in part, by its overlap with the PIC typology derived from a psychiatric sample by Gdowski et al. (1985). Visual inspection revealed that the 7 CHI psychosocial subtypes closely resembled 6 of Gdowski's 12 profile types. The overlap between the two typologies could be examined quantitatively by applying the classification rules proposed by LaCombe et al. (1991) to the CHI sample and calculating the concordance (with Rand's statistic, for example).

A future prospective study would remedy problems with sample bias that may have been present in this investigation. The sources of subjects for the present study were three neuropsychology clinics. Therefore, only children who had been referred for neuropsychological assessment were included. It is possible that only children experiencing significant problems following the CHI were referred for this type of assessment. Similarly, the children returning for reassessment may have been those who experienced continuing difficulties. The enrollment of subjects in a prospective fashion would eliminate this possible source of sample bias.

Although the results of this study indicated clearly a relationship between psychosocial functioning and injury severity, the precise nature of this relationship needs to be elucidated. Whereas the overall sample size was large for a study of this nature, the cell sizes of injury severity groups within each subtype were small. This may have contributed to the somewhat muddy nature of the findings regarding severity of injury and

psychosocial functioning. Future investigations with larger sample sizes (perhaps a large multi-center study) may help to clarify this relationship.

The finding that the mild CHI group obtained the highest mean PIC-R profile elevations within the Mild Anxiety subtype raises the possibility of the post-concussion syndrome in this group of children. No evidence for this has been reported previously, but children sustaining mild CHIs have not been the object of intense investigation. The results of this investigation support the need for research examining the psychosocial sequelae of mildly head-injured children in greater depth.

Whereas the results of this investigation supported a relationship between age at injury and psychosocial functioning, previous investigations have not. It was concluded that differences due to age at injury were obtained because of the comprehensive nature of the psychosocial measure used in this study versus those used in the past. However, given that this is an unprecedented finding, demonstration of its reliability through replication in future investigations is necessary.

Changes in psychosocial functioning over time can only be discerned through further investigation. The results of this investigation support the notion that increases in degree of psychopathology within certain subtypes may occur over time. There was also a trend toward membership in specific subtypes depending on the duration between the injury and the assessment. However, a larger sample of children receiving serial assessments is necessary in order to test these hypotheses in a more rigorous manner.

REFERENCES

Achenbach, T.M., & Edelbrock, C.S. (1983). *Manual for the Child Behavior Checklist and the Revised Behavior Profile*. Burlington, VA: Department of Psychiatry, University of Vermont.

Achenbach, T.M., & Edelbrock, C.S. (1986). *Teacher's Report Form*. Burlington, VT: Author.

Aldenderfer, M.S., & Blashfield, R.K. (1984). *Cluster analysis*. Beverly Hills, CA: Sage.

Asarnow, R.F., Satz, P., Light, R., Lewis, R., & Neumann, E. (1991). Behavior problems and adaptive functioning in children with mild and severe closed head injury. *Journal of Pediatric Psychology*, *16*, 543–555.

Brown, G., Chadwick, O., Shaffer, D., Rutter, M., & Traub, M. (1981). A prospective study of children with head injuries: III. Psychiatric sequelae. *Psychological Medicine, 11*, 63–78.

Butler, K., Rourke, B.P., Fuerst, D.R., & Fisk, J.L. (1997). *Neuropsychological sequelae of childhood closed head injury.* Manuscript in preparation.

Casey, R., Ludwig, S., & McCormick, M.C. (1986). Morbidity following minor head trauma in children. *Pediatrics, 78*, 497–502.

Chadwick, O., Rutter, M., Shaffer, D., & Shrout, P.E. (1981). A prospective study of children with head injuries: IV. Specific cognitive deficits. *Journal of Clinical Neuropsychology, 3*, 101–120.

Conners, C.K. (1973). Rating scales for use in drug studies with children. *Psychopharmacology Bulletin, 9*, 24–84.

Dikmen, S.S., Temkin, N., & Armsden, G. (1989). Neuropsychological recovery: Relationship to psychosocial functioning and postconcussional complaints. In H.S. Levin, H. M. Eisenberg, & A.L. Benton (Eds.), *Mild head injury.* (pp. 229–241). New York: Oxford University Press.

Donders, J. (1992). Premorbid behavior and psychosocial adjustment of children with traumatic brain injury. *Journal of Abnormal Child Psychology, 20*, 233–246.

Fletcher, J.M. (1985). External validation of learning disability typologies. In B.P. Rourke (Ed.), *Neuropsychology of learning disabilities: Essentials of subtype analysis.* (pp. 187–211). New York: Guilford Press.

Fletcher, J.M., Ewing-Cobbs, L., Miner, M.E., Levin, H.S., & Eisenberg, H.M. (1990). Behavioral changes after closed head injury in children. *Journal of Consulting and Clinical Psychology, 58*, 93–98.

Fuerst, D.R. (1991). *Psychosocial functioning of children with learning disabilities: The relations between psychosocial subtypes and neuropsychological functioning at three age levels.* Unpublished doctoral dissertation, University of Windsor, Ontario.

Fuerst, D.R., Fisk, J.L., & Rourke, B.P. (1989). Psychosocial functioning of learning-disabled children: Reliability of statistically derived subtypes. *Journal of Consulting and Clinical Psychology, 57*, 275–280.

Fuerst, D.R., Fisk, J.L., & Rourke, B.P. (1990). Psychosocial functioning of learning-disabled children: Relationships between WISC Verbal IQ – Performance IQ discrepancies and personality subtypes. *Journal of Consulting and Clinical Psychology, 58*, 657–660.

Fuerst, D.R., & Rourke, B.P. (1993). Psychosocial functioning of children: Relations between personality subtypes and academic achievement. *Journal of Abnormal Child Psychology, 21*, 597–607.

Fuerst, D.R., & Rourke, B.P. (1995). Psychosocial functioning of children with learning disabilities at three age levels. *Child Neuropsychology, 1*, 38–55.

Gdowski, C.L., Lachar, D., & Kline, R.B. (1985). A PIC profile typology of children and adolescents: I. An empirically derived alternative to traditional diagnosis. *Journal of Abnormal Psychology, 94*, 346–361.

Hubert, L., & Arabie, P. (1985). Comparing partitions. *Journal of Classification, 2*, 193–218.

Knights, R.M., Ivan, L.P., Ventureyra, E.C.G., Bentivoglio, C., Stoddart, C., Winogron, W., & Bawden, H.N. (1991). The effects of head injury in children on neuropsychological and behavioural functioning. *Brain Injury, 5*, 339–351.

Knights, R.M., & Stoddart, C. (1981). Profile approaches to neuropsychological diagnosis in children. In G.W. Hynd & J.E. Obrzut (Eds.), *Neuropsychological assessment and the school-age child.* (pp. 335–351). New York: Grune & Stratton.

Lachar, D. (1982). *Personality Inventory for Children (PIC): Revised format manual supplement.* Los Angeles: Western Psychological Services.

LaCombe, J.A., Kline, R.B., Lachar, D., Butkus, M., & Hillman, S.B. (1991). Case history correlates of a Personality Inventory for Children (PIC) profile typology. *Journal of Consulting and Clinical Psychology, 3*, 678–687.

Levin, H.S., Ewing-Cobbs, L., & Fletcher, J.M. (1989). Neurobehavioral outcome of mild head injury in children. In H.S. Levin, H.M. Eisenberg, & A.L. Benton (Eds.), *Mild head injury.* (pp. 189–213). New York: Oxford University Press.

Lorr, M. (1983). *Cluster analysis for social scientists.* San Francisco: Jossey-Bass.

Milligan, G.W., & Cooper, M.C. (1986). A study of the comparability of external criteria for hierarchical cluster analysis. *Multivariate Behavioral Research, 21*, 441–458.

Morey, L., & Agresti, A. (1984). The measurement of classification agreement: An adjustment to the Rand statistic for chance agreement. *Educational and Psychological Measurement, 44*, 33–37.

Porter, J., & Rourke, B.P. (1985). Socioemotional functioning of learning-disabled children: A subtypal analysis of personality patterns. In B.P. Rourke (Ed.), *Neuropsychology of learning disabilities: Essentials of subtype analysis.* (pp. 257–279). New York: Guilford Press.

Rand, W.M. (1971). Objective criteria for the evaluation of clustering methods. *Journal of the American Statistical Association, 66*, 846–850.

Rourke, B.P. (1989). *Nonverbal learning disabilities: The syndrome and the model.* New York: Guilford Press.

Rourke, B.P., Fisk, J.L., & Strang, J.D. (1986). *Neuropsychological assessment of children: A treatment-oriented approach.* New York: Guilford Press.

Rourke, B.P., & Fuerst, D.R. (1991). *Learning disabilities and psychosocial functioning: A neuropsychological perspective.* New York: Guilford Press.

Rutherford, W.H. (1989). Postconcussion symptoms: Relationship to acute neurological indices, individual differences, and circumstances of injury. In H.S. Levin, H.M. Eisenberg, & A.L. Benton (Eds.), *Mild head injury* (pp. 217–228). New York: Oxford University Press.

Rutter, M. (1981). Psychological sequelae of brain damage in children. *American Journal of Psychiatry, 138,* 1533–1544.

Rutter, M., Chadwick, O., Shaffer, D., & Brown, G. (1980). A prospective study of children with head injuries: I. Design and methods. *Psychological Medicine, 10,* 633–645.

Sarle, W.S. (1985). The CLUSTER procedure. In S.P. Joyner (Ed.), *SAS user's guide: Statistics, version 5 edition* (pp. 255–315). Cary, NC: SAS Institute.

Shaffer, D., Chadwick, O., & Rutter, M. (1975). Psychiatric outcome of localized head injury in children. *Outcome of severe damage to the CNS: Ciba Foundation Symposium, (new series),* 191–210.

Sokal, R., & Michener, C. (1958). A statistical method for evaluating systematic relationships. *University of Kansas Scientific Bulletin, 38,* 1409–1438.

Sorensen, T. (1948). A method of establishing groups of equal amplitude in plant sociology based on similarity of species content and its application to analyses of the vegetation on Danish commons. *Biologiske Skrifter, 5,* 1–34.

Sparrow, S., Balla, D., & Cicchetti, D. (1984). *Vineland Adaptive Behavior Scales.* Circle Pines, MN: American Guidance Service.

Ward, J. (1963). Hierarchical grouping to optimize an object function. *Journal of the American Statistical Association, 58,* 236–244.

Winogron, H.W., Knights, R.M., & Bawden, H.N. (1984). Neuropsychological deficits following head injury in children. *Journal of Clinical Neuropsychology, 6,* 269–286.

Wirt, R.D., Lachar, D., Klinedinst, J.K., & Seat, P.D. (1977). *Multidimensional description of child personality: A manual for the Personality Inventory for Children.* Los Angeles: Western Psychological Services.

Wirt, R.D., Lachar, D., Klinedinst, J.K., & Seat, P.D. (1984). *Multidimensional description of child personality: A manual for the Personality Inventory for Children Revised 1984.* Los Angeles: Western Psychological Services.

Journal of Clinical and Experimental Neuropsychology
1996, Vol. 18, No. 3, pp. 349–370

Neuropsychological Subgroups of Patients with Alzheimer's Disease*

Nancy J. Fisher[1], Byron P. Rourke[1,2], Linas Bieliauskas[3,4], Bruno Giordani[4], Stanley Berent[4], and Norman L. Foster[4]

[1]University of Windsor, [2]Yale University, and [3]VA Medical Center/[4]University of Michigan

ABSTRACT

Neuropsychological data from 134 patients diagnosed with *probable* Alzheimer's disease (AD) were studied retrospectively to investigate whether subgroups of patients with qualitatively distinct profiles could be identified. Three empirical classification approaches were undertaken in this regard: Q-type factor analysis, hierarchical agglomerative cluster analysis, and iterative partitioning. Three subgroups were consistently identified across the clustering methods. Subgroup 1, the largest of the groups, was marked by moderate to severe anomia and constructional dyspraxia. Individuals in subgroup 2 displayed relatively spared visual-perceptual/constructional functioning but severe anomia. Members of subgroup 3 exhibited intact naming and nonverbal reasoning and moderate difficulty in copying overlapping figures. The three subgroups did not differ with respect to age, age at disease onset, duration of illness, educational level, or Hamilton depression rating. Detailed description of the data analyses are provided as a tutorial outlining subtyping methodology. Results are discussed in terms of the *subgroup* and the *stage* model approaches to the conceptualization of AD.

Alzheimer's disease (AD) remains a devastatingly incurable process of neurodegeneration, which results in increasingly more widespread and severe neuropsychological disintegration with the passage of time. Although a treatment that may improve symptoms has recently become available, this drug (Tacrine) must be administered early in the course of AD in order to provide benefit (Farlow et al., 1992; Knapp et al., 1994; Swash et al., 1991). Thus, the clinical neuropsychologist, by providing early detection/diagnosis, makes an extremely important contribution in the battle against AD. However, despite the fundamental importance of diagnosis, research in this area has been largely inadequate with respect to AD. The diagnosis of AD remains one of exclusion, and a classificatory system accounting for clinical variability has yet to be developed.

Historically, neuropsychologists have attempted to distinguish AD from other, reversible forms of dementia. As such, initial research focused on the goal of identifying a signature profile of AD, often

* The research described herein was conducted as a Master's thesis by the first author, under the supervision of the second two authors, in partial fulfillment of the requirements of the Clinical Neuropsychology doctoral programme at the University of Windsor. This paper was presented at the 24th Annual Meeting of the International Neuropsychological Society. Chicago, IL, USA. February 15th, 1996. While preparing this article for publication, the first author was supported by a Doctoral Training Award from the Alzheimer Society of Canada. This research was undertaken through the University of Michigan Alzheimer's Disease Research Center, the Department of Neurology; the Neuropsychology Division, Department of Psychiatry; and supported by Grant # P50-AG08671 from the NIH/NIA. The project was reviewed and approved by the University of Michigan IRB and the Michigan Alzheimer's Disease Research Center.
Address correspondence to: Nancy J. Fisher at the University of Windsor, Department of Psychology, Windsor, Ontario, Canada, N9B 3P4.
Accepted for publication: January 3, 1996.

guided by underlying hypotheses regarding a neurochemical system thought to be central in the production of characteristic memory deficits (e.g., Fuld, 1984). Such largely unsuccessful research (see reviews by Goldman, Axelrod, Tandon, & Berent, 1993; Kaufman, 1990) involved comparing the average neuropsychological performance of suspected AD patients with those from groups of healthy controls and/or with patients diagnosed with other forms of dementia. As Martin (1988, 1990) points out, such group comparison research may have been misguided in its assumption that AD represents a homogeneous disease state; that is, averaging data across AD patients may obscure subgroups of patients with qualitatively distinct neuropsychological profiles. Indeed, in recent years, a substantial body of research spanning several fields has suggested that AD is not a unitary entity (Fisher, Rourke, & Bieliauskas, under review). Of particular interest in the present context are clinical observations of heterogeneous symptom presentation. Many clinical researchers agree that patients with early AD vary greatly in regard to their clinical presentation (Becker, Huff, Nebes, Holland, & Boller, 1988; Jagust, Davies, Tiller-Borcich, & Reed, 1990; Joanette, Ska, Poissant, & Beland, 1992; Martin, 1990; Martin, Cox, Brouwers, & Fedio, 1985; Neary et al., 1986; Price et al., 1993; Schwartz, 1987; Shuttleworth, 1984; Swash et al., 1991). This work points to the fact that, although memory deficits can almost always be shown to be present in AD if adequate neuropsychological testing is undertaken, considerable interindividual variability is apparent with respect to other areas of neuropsychological impairment and in psychiatric and strictly neurological symptomatology. There are two models of AD that attempt to explain the heterogeneity of symptom presentation among AD patients: the *subgroup*[1] and *stage* models. Each is described briefly as follows.

Proponents of the *subgroup model* of AD contend that patients vary with regard to their evolving pattern of neuropsychological/psychiatric/neurological impairment. In this way, it is proposed that individuals at comparable phases of the illness exhibit not only distinct patterns of spared and affected cognitive and functional abilities but also varying degrees of impairment of these capacities.

Furthermore, according to this view, not only do the neuropsychological functions affected differ among individuals in the early and middle period of AD, but the patterns by which the subcomponents of these functions break down also show inter-individual variability (Joanette et al., 1992; Jorm, 1985; Martin et al., 1986). The goal of research conducted by those adhering to this conceptual framework of AD is to identify subgroups of patients with similar patterns of degeneration. Such identification would allow for study of these individual "subgroups," which may have etiologic, prognostic, and/or therapeutic import.

In contrast to the view of individuals at comparable phases of AD as heterogeneous in symptom presentation, opponents argue that deficits incurred by AD victims are homogeneous or relatively equal across all domains. In this way, strict proponents of the classical *stage model* approach contend that differences between AD sufferers merely reflect the distinct stages of the disease and, hence, the severity and/or duration of the disorder (Constantinidis, 1978; Hom, 1992; Reisberg, Ferris, & Crook, 1982). Various stage models have been presented in the literature (e.g., Cummings & Benson, 1992), each assuming a more or less global, homogeneous deterioration of cognitive functioning that increases quantitatively as a function of disease progression. Qualitatively distinct symptoms among AD victims are recognized by proponents of these stage models, but are attributed to specific stages of disease progression (e.g., see Reisberg et al., 1982) that are thought to adhere to a strict timetable.

It must be emphasized that proponents of the subgroup approach recognize the progressive nature of AD, and generally agree that certain symptoms of AD appear to be developmental markers of

---

[1] The term "subgroup" is used throughout this paper to refer to homogeneous groups of patients according to some dimension, which may or may not be of etiologic significance (Jorm, 1985). The term "subtype" has been reserved for groups of patients with purportedly different etiologies (e.g., familial AD). The latter topic is not addressed directly in this article; the interested reader is referred to Chui (1987) and Boller, Forette, Khachaturian, Poncet, and Christen (1992) for epidemiological reviews. This terminological distinction between "subgroup" and "subtype" (as per Jorm, 1985) is observed here to prevent confusion.

disease progression (e.g., myoclonus). However, they believe that within this general framework, different patterns of progression exist, particularly with respect to neuropsychological functioning.

There are several limitations of the stage model approach to the conceptualization of AD. First, the fact that *several* different stage models are available in the literature, some of which clash markedly in terms of the temporal sequence in which certain symptoms are thought to first appear (e.g., personality disturbance; Martin et al., 1986), raises questions concerning the validity of this approach (Liston, 1979; Schwartz, 1987). Furthermore, there does not appear to be a consensus regarding the appropriate number of stages of the disease or the approximate duration of each of the different stages (see Schwartz [1987] for a review of stage models).

A second difficulty with the stage approach is that it does not account for autopsy-confirmed case examples in the literature that contradict the assumption of homogeneous dissolution of memory, visual-spatial, and language functions. For example, AD may initially present as an isolated memory impairment in the context of otherwise normal neuropsychological functioning (Berent et al., 1995; Haxby et al., 1988; Neary et al., 1986; Price et al., 1993). Furthermore, individuals have been identified who exhibit severe impairment on neuropsychological measures of visual construction while maintaining relatively normal levels of performance on tests of word generation and naming, and vice versa (e.g., Martin, 1990). Other contradictory autopsy-confirmed examples include AD initially presenting most prominently as a slowly progressive attentional deficit (Price et al., 1993), fluent aphasia (Pogacar & Williams, 1984), and parietal lobe syndrome (Crystal, Horoupian, Katzman, & Jotkowitz, 1982).

As a further limitation regarding the hypothesis of "homogeneous dissolution of function," not only do certain AD cases initially present with circumscribed impairment but, in general, the most prominent initial area of deficit remains salient during the course of the disease. Preserved areas remain relatively less affected until the terminal stages are reached, at which time all areas of neuropsychological functioning become disrupted profoundly (see Price et al. [1993] for several autopsy-confirmed examples).

A final major weakness of the stage approach is its adherence to a time schedule by which the appearance of certain qualitatively distinct symptoms are supposed to appear, as several autopsy-confirmed cases of AD do not follow such a sequence. For example, motor deficits may appear early in the course of AD (e.g., Funkenstein et al., 1993; Jagust et al., 1990), but most stage models do not schedule this type of impairment to occur until the final stages of the disease. Similarly, personality and/or affective disturbance may present as an initial symptom in some patients, while in others this does not occur until the later stages of AD (Adams & Victor, 1993).

As can be appreciated from the above critique of the stage model approach, the assertion that the deficits of AD progress in a parallel and/or predictable sequence is questionable on several grounds; strong contradictory evidence is readily available in the literature, and has been for at least the past decade. Some proponents of the stage approach dismiss as "atypical" the cases mentioned above that contradict their models. However, since these cases were autopsy-confirmed as AD, such a dismissal is difficult to justify. A subgroup model would appear to be much more adequate in terms of accounting for the case history literature to date. Extensive support for this approach is offered by Fisher, Rourke, and Bieliauskas (under review).

Despite these weaknesses, throughout the short history of neuropsychology, the stage model has dominated. The Geneva school held that AD manifested neuropsychologically as an "aphaso-agnoso-apractic syndrome," or as homogeneous impairment of language, perception, and gestural functioning (Joanette et al., 1992). It was not until the late 1960s that the first subgrouping study appeared in the published literature. McDonald (1969) recognized discrepancies regarding the features of senile dementia, and sought to subgroup patients on the basis of neuropsychological test performance. By examining data distributions for bimodality, he identified parietal function preserved and impaired subgroups, the latter of which was subsequently shown to have a considerably poorer prognosis.

Unfortunately, the study of McDonald (1969) did not appear to generate much interest at the time. Although some authors wrote about the apparent heterogeneity of AD (e.g., Liston, 1979), no further subgrouping studies were attempted (or at least published), and the majority of clinicians and researchers seemed to maintain the "homogeneous dissolution" conceptualization of the disease. Perhaps due to ageism, or the distorted view of AD as involving normal age-related loss of memory and intellectual faculties, this view of AD as a homogeneous neuropsychological entity persisted until quite recently, and is evident in the group comparison approach to the study of AD (e.g., Fuld, 1984; Hom, 1992). Although this view remains entrenched, the acknowledgement of the possibility of AD representing a heterogeneous neuropsychological disorder is becoming increasingly evident in the current approach to the study of individuals so afflicted (e.g., Delis et al., 1992; Freed, Corkin, Growdon, & Nissen, 1989). This changing conceptualization of AD within the field of neuropsychology is likely associated with the mounting evidence from several fields (e.g., epidemiology, neurochemistry, neuropathology, etc.) suggesting the heterogeneity of the disease (see Boller et al., 1992).

Martin and colleagues (1986) have conducted the landmark AD neuropsychological subgrouping research. These researchers studied a small group of AD patients ($N = 42$) at relatively equivalent periods of the disease (i.e., in terms of duration of illness), in search of qualitatively distinct profiles of impaired and spared abilities. After administering a wide range of neuropsychological measures to these patients, qualitative inspection of the data revealed that while a majority of patients exhibited deficits in all domains assessed, some demonstrated intact visual-spatial abilities coupled strikingly with impaired access to semantic knowledge, while another small group demonstrated the reverse pattern of performance.

In order to verify these observations quantitatively, Martin and colleagues subsequently subjected the results of the three measures of accessibility of semantic knowledge (i.e., Boston Naming Test, Verbal Fluency subtest of the Mattis Dementia Rating Scale, Associate Learning subtest of the Wechsler Memory Scale-easy items only) and the three measures of visual-spatial functioning (Block Design, Rey-Osterrieth Complex Figure-copy, Mosaic Comparison Test) to a factor analysis.

Varimax rotation of the principal components solution yielded two relatively independent factors, each with high loadings for one set of tests (i.e., either those assessing semantic knowledge or visual-spatial skill) and low loadings for the other. This two-factor solution accounted for 70.5% of the variance, suggesting the potential existence of subgroups of patients. (A stage model of AD would predict a single general factor on which all measures are highly loaded.) In order to test this hypothesis, the factor scores assigned to each subject were utilized in plotting the patients' data graphically in two-dimensional space. This revealed a tendency for patients to cluster into different groups. To verify these groupings statistically, cluster analysis (utilizing Ward's algorithm only) of the factor scores was undertaken, and revealed three qualitatively distinct subgroups: (1) those with relatively equal impairment of both semantic knowledge and visual-spatial skills ($n = 25$), (2) those with impaired semantic knowledge coupled with relatively spared visual-spatial functioning ($n = 9$), and (3) those with relatively intact access to semantic knowledge accompanied by visual-spatial impairment ($n = 8$). Linear discriminant analysis utilizing factor scores to predict subgroup membership successfully reassigned 41 of the 42 patients.

Following the above described statistical analysis, PET images of patients ($n = 19$) from each of the three subgroups were examined (Martin et al., 1986). Although the subgroups did not differ with respect to overall rate of cortical glucose metabolism, post-hoc comparisons indicated that metabolic differences were consistent with subgroup assignment: those with deficits in both cognitive domains (subgroup 1) displayed bilateral hypometabolism of the temporal and parietal lobes; those with impaired semantic knowledge accompanied by relatively spared visual-spatial abilities (subgroup 2) exhibited significantly greater hypometabolism in the left temporal region relative to other cortical regions; and those with the reverse cognitive pattern (subgroup 3) exhibited significantly greater hypometabolism in the right parietal region.[2] Thus,

---

[2] Many similar imaging studies have reported results consistent with those of Martin and colleagues (1986) (e.g., Foster et al., 1983; see Fisher, Rourke, & Bieliauskas, under review, for extensive review).

it appears that the PET analysis provided external validation of the cluster analytic results.

The patients involved in this original study (Martin et al., 1986) were followed and retested on the six measures of verbal and visual-spatial functioning at 1- to 2-year intervals following the initial assessment in 1986. Martin (1990) reports that results of the re-evaluations indicate distinct patterns of deterioration based on subgroup membership. Those in subgroup 1, who initially displayed equal impairment in both domains, continued with this general global decline in functioning. However, patients in subgroups 2 and 3 exhibited significantly greater deterioration in the area (i.e., either verbal or visual-spatial functioning) that was impaired at the initial evaluation. These results suggest that patterns of deterioration may be predicted through knowledge of initial subgroup membership. Moreover, AD may initially invade rather focal regions in some patients, and these regions of most marked pathology may show inter-patient variability, thus producing qualitatively distinct neuropsychological profiles (Martin et al., 1986).

If these findings are confirmed, they may have implications for models of AD progression (i.e., patterns of deterioration). In this way, unitary models of the course of AD (e.g., Zec, 1993) may need to be reconceptualized or broadened to account for subgroup differences. Each neuropsychological subgroup may correspond to distinct neuropathological routes of disease progression. Martin (1990) speculates on this issue and offers what he refers to as a "minimal model" of AD progression.

Becker and co-investigators (1988) have partially replicated the study of Martin et al. (1986) utilizing a larger sample of 86 patients. These patients underwent comprehensive neuropsychological evaluation. Subsequently, data obtained on measures of semantic knowledge and visual-spatial functioning, similar to those utilized by Martin et al. (1986), were submitted to the same type of factor analysis discussed above. The factors obtained were essentially the same as those reported by Martin et al. (1986). These researchers identified subgroups similar to the Martin et al. subgroups 2 and 3 by calculating composite scores for the two neuropsychological domains. However, they did not proceed with a cluster analysis.

The above described investigations strongly suggest a double dissociation between accessibility of semantic knowledge and visual-spatial constructional skill, implying the independence of corresponding neural systems. Subsequent AD subgrouping research has dealt mainly with patient heterogeneity *within* the domains of visual-spatial (Delis et al., 1992; Massman et al., 1993), attentional (Freed et al., 1988, 1989), semantic (Bandera, Della Sala, Laiacona, Luzzatti, & Spinnler, 1991) and amnestic (Becker, 1988) functioning. While these research efforts are contributory, the original studies of Martin et al. (1986) and Becker et al. (1988) have not been replicated in a manner that addresses their methodological limitations. For example, Martin et al. (1986) performed only one cluster analytic technique on their data (i.e., Ward's method). This represents a significant shortcoming, as lone cluster analytic solutions have been demonstrated to be unreliable (Blashfield & Aldenderfer, 1988; Everitt, 1974; Morris, Blashfield, & Satz, 1981). While a handful of other subgrouping studies have been conducted, such efforts have either failed to utilize the NINCDS-ADRDA criteria for subject selection (e.g., Naugle, Cullum, Bigler, & Massman, 1985), did not employ cluster analytic techniques (e.g., Rasmusson & Brandt, 1995), or did not replicate classificatory solutions across clustering approaches (e.g., Naugle et al., 1985). Thus, the purpose of the current research was to replicate the findings of Martin et al. (1986), employing a methodology that addresses these shortcomings.

Detailed description of the methodology utilized is provided throughout the remainder of this paper, intended as a tutorial for researchers interested in pursuing similar research. Given that one of the goals of this paper is to provide an illustrative methodological example, strict conformity to the customary methods and results section standards for inclusion are relaxed in order to facilitate an integrated understanding of the underlying procedure.

A final goal of the present research involved evaluation and extension of an earlier proposed neuropsychological model of AD accounting for variations in early clinical presentation (Martin, 1990). Martin (1990) theorized that heterogeneous AD patterns may suggest different underlying pathways of neuropathological progression, such that the brains of those with spared semantic knowledge or visual-spatial/constructional abilities are initially affected asymmetrically.

In the present study, we hypothesized that three neuropsychological "ideal types" (Morris & Fletcher, 1988) of AD would emerge, possibly reflecting distinct patterns of underlying neuropathological involvement: (1) Global AD (GAD), affecting the brain symmetrically in a manner progressing from posterior to anterior regions; (2) Left AD (LAD), initially involving more left hemisphere pathology; and (3) Right AD (RAD), initially involving relatively asymmetric right hemisphere degeneration. Those in subgroup 1 (GAD), representing about half of the sample, were predicted to display relatively equal impairments in (a) accessing semantic knowledge and (b) visual-spatial functioning. It was hypothesized, on the basis of past research (see Fisher, Rourke, & Bieliauskas, under review, for review), that the LAD and RAD subgroups would appear only in early AD, eventually giving way to global pathology and accompanying global decline in functioning. Thus, it was predicted that, in terms of overall functioning (i.e., Mini-Mental State Examination scores), the GAD group would be more severely impaired than the LAD and RAD subgroups. Similarly, since AD appears to originate posteriorly, advancing in an anterior direction, it was hypothesized that performance on motor tests would be most impaired in the GAD group (i.e., the more severely impaired group).

Based on past research (Martin et al., 1986), the other two subgroups (LAD and RAD) were predicted to account for approximately equal numbers of the remaining patients. Those of the LAD type were predicted to encounter difficulty accessing semantic knowledge while retaining relatively normal visual-spatial functioning. Individuals with the RAD pattern were expected to exhibit relatively intact access to semantic knowledge but impaired visual-spatial/constructional skills. Additionally, drawing on the Goldberg-Costa model of hemispheric specialization (Goldberg & Costa, 1981), patients with the RAD pattern were expected to evince lower PIQ as compared to VIQ, whereas those with the LAD pattern were expected to demonstrate the reverse pattern of performance on the Wechsler Adult Intelligence Scale-Revised (Wechsler, 1981) (i.e., IQ < PIQ).

(See Fisher, Rourke, & Bieliauskas, under review, for theoretical discussion.) It was further predicted that the LAD group would be less impaired on visual as compared to verbal memory tasks, and that the RAD group would display the reverse pattern (as per Becker, Lopez, & Wess, 1992; Martin et al., 1985).

METHOD

Subject Selection

Demographic and neuropsychological test data from patients meeting the NINCDS-ADRDA diagnostic criteria for *probable* AD (McKhann et al., 1984), housed in the University of Michigan's Alzheimer's Disease Research Center database, were utilized in the current investigation. These subjects were selected from a larger group of more than 3000 individuals who were referred to the University of Michigan Medical Center (Neuropsychology Division, Department of Psychiatry; Cognitive Disorders Clinic, Department of Neurology; and the various cores of the Michigan Alzheimer's Disease Research Center) or the Michigan Dementia Program for inpatient/outpatient consultation regarding suspected dementia. None had a history of any of the following: severe ongoing cardiac, hepatic, pulmonary, or renal disease (or other significant medical illness such as malignancy or HIV seropositivity); substance abuse; head injury with loss of consciousness exceeding 1 hr; anoxia or diffuse ischemia resulting in cognitive decline; psychiatric disorder unrelated to present illness; consistent non-compliance with medical treatment. Additionally, all subjects met the following inclusionary criteria: (1) adequate hearing and visual acuity, (2) persistent cognitive symptoms even when CNS drugs were with drawn, (3) if depressed, neuropsychological deficits had not been reversed with psychotherapy or antidepressants, (4) cognitive decline occurred over a period of at least 6 months and had resulted in impaired activities of daily living.

All patients received general medical and neurological examinations. The following laboratory screening studies were conducted on each subject, revealing no abnormalities: complete blood count (CBC); electrolyte, glucose, blood urea nitrogen (BUN), and creatinine level analysis; liver and thyroid function tests; B12 and folate level assessment; FTA-Abs test for syphilis; sedimentation rate; urinalysis. No patient displayed focal primary motor or sensory findings on neurological exam, and all had modified scores of less than four on the Hachinski Ischemic Scale (Hachinski et al., 1975). All patients underwent CT and MRI scanning which failed to reveal any significant focal abnormalities.

Aside from the above inclusionary/exclusionary criteria, all patients registered in the database were included in the current investigation if sufficient neuropsychological data were available (i.e., test data available from the measures described below). Demographic and test data were retrieved directly from the database and were double-checked manually via chart review. Best estimates of symptom duration were gleaned from reports of the referring physicians and file notes recorded by a neuropsychologist (or supervised trainee) during interviews conducted with family members/friends of the subjects. In the rare event that these two information sources differed, a mean estimated length of symptom duration, weighing each value equally, was calculated.

Neuropsychological Measu res

Psychometric evaluation included the following: Mini-Mental State Examination (MMSE) (Folstein, Folstein, & McHugh, 1975), Hamilton Rating Scale for Depression (Hamilton, 1967; Warren, 1994), Grip Strength Test (Reitan & Davison, 1974), Finger Tapping Test (Reitan & Davison, 1974), Blessed Dementia Rating Scale (Blessed, Tomlinson, & Roth, 1968), Wechsler Memory Scale (WMS) (Wechsler, 1945), Wechsler Adult Intelligence Scale – Revised (WAIS-R) (Wechsler, 1981), Boston Naming Test (BNT) (Kaplan, Goodglass, & Weintraub, 1983), Controlled Oral Word Association Test (COWAT) (Benton & Hamsher, 1989; Spreen & Benton, 1977), Animal Name Fluency Test (Isaacs & Kennie, 1973; Spreen & Strauss, 1991), Southern California Figure-Ground Visual Perception Test (Ayres, 1966). These tests were administered in the standard fashion (see respective manuals cited). For test descriptions, see individual sources cited.

Overview of Statistical Analyses

Because many different statistical procedures/strategies were employed in this research, a synopsis of the major paths taken, and the rationale behind each, is provided at this point. SPSS-X Version 4.0 (Norusis, 1990) implementations were utilized in all analyses.

The first major step of data analysis involved the conversion of raw patient scores on seven measures [BNT, COWAT, Animal Fluency, Easy Paired Associates (from WMS), Block Design, Figure-Ground, Pentagon Copy task (from MMSE)] to demographically corrected T scores for comparative purposes. Subsequently, the T scores were submitted to an R-type factor analysis. These tests were chosen for analysis due to their similarity to those utilized by Martin et al. (1986) and Becker et al. (1988). As expected, a two-factor solution emerged, with a high degree of intercorrelation between the verbal measures and between the spatial measures, but minimal relations across the two domains (i.e., suggesting the possibility of subgroups).

Following the R-analysis, a Q-type factor analysis was undertaken, in which product-moment correlations were calculated between all possible column pairs (i.e., between subject profiles). An initial Q-type factor analysis was thought beneficial in that this alternative "clustering" method has no bias against creating relatively small clusters; many cluster analysis techniques are biased toward creating clusters of equal size. Furthermore, Q-analysis controls for the presence of outliers because every case is not necessarily assigned to a cluster.

Because, as predicted, the Q-analysis identified qualitatively distinct subgroups of individuals (as evaluated via multivariate analysis of variance and profile analysis procedures), various cluster analyses were performed on the T score data in an attempt to generate similar subgroupings across multiple methods (i.e., to assess reliability or "internal validity"). Only those clusters emerging via the majority of methods were accepted as reliable. The product-moment correlation coefficient was chosen as the primary similarity measure (i.e., utilized in three of the four analyses) because the principal interest of this study involves qualitative pattern (i.e., shape) variability (Aldenderfer & Blashfield, 1984; Everitt, 1974; Morris, Blashfield, & Satz, 1981). Three hierarchical agglomerative methods (average linkage between groups, average linkage within groups, and Ward's method) were utilized first, followed by an iterative partitioning procedure (i.e., k-means) in which squared Euclidean distance served as the similarity measure. The appropriate number of clusters in the data were determined by inspection of the cluster fusion coefficients at each stage (i.e., for sudden drop) in addition to the corresponding icicle plots and dendrograms (Everitt & Dunn, 1991).

Following satisfactory evaluation of the emerging cluster solution (via misclassification analysis, qualitative comparison of subgroup profiles across clustering techniques, and examination of a multiprofile-multimethod matrix of intercorrelations), demographic and other neuropsychological data were provided for each of the subgroups which emerged. Comparisons were made between the subgroups to determine whether age, duration of illness, severity of the illness, and other such factors differed between the groups, in addition to whether the groups displayed distinct patterns of performance on verbal and nonverbal memory measures and on tests of motor functioning.

RESULTS

Sample Characteristics

A total of 134 patients (57 males, 77 females) met the criteria for inclusion. A descriptive chart comprising the demographic characteristics of the sample and their average level of performance on the WAIS-R, MMSE, Blessed Dementia Rating Scale, Hamilton Rating Scale for Depression, and the neuropsychological tests of interest is provided in Table 1. All subjects employed in this study were born between the years 1903 and 1941. The majority were right-handed (96.3%), and only 11% of the sample had significant extrapyramidal signs. As can be appreciated from Table 1, this sample is highly educated; 43% of the subjects had completed high school and some college ($M = 12.8$ years). However, this is a more representative mean educational level than that reported by Martin and colleagues (1986) (i.e., 14.5 years). The age range of the current sample (50–91) is also more representative than that of Martin and colleagues (1986) (i.e., 43–74 years), including representation of the "very-old" elderly. Forty-one percent of the subjects were 75 years old or older; 16% were ≥80 years of age. Eighty-three percent of the subjects were classified as "not depressed" by clinicians' ratings on the Hamilton Depression Scale.

Raw scores were converted to T scores ($M = 50$, $SD = 10$) demographically corrected for age (in addition to education and gender, when such normative information was available) using normative data presented by the following authors (tests in parentheses): Van Gorp, Satz, Kiersch, and Henry (1986) (BNT, age and educational level; if education ≥ 12 years); Ross, Lichtenberg, and Christensen (1994) (BNT, age and educational level; if education < 12 years); Bieliauskas, Newberry, and Gerstenberger (1988) (Figure-Ground, sex-corrected only); Read (1987) (COWAT, Animals; age and education); Wechsler (1945) (Easy Associates, MQ; age corrected only); Wechsler (1981) (Block Design, VIQ, PIQ; age corrected only). Because no norms were available for the copy task scoring system created for this project, a T score of 50 was considered the normal mean [corresponding to a perfect score of 5, because normal elderly have no difficulty copying the figures (Folstein et al., 1975)]. The scores of 4, 3, 2, and 1 were assigned T scores of 40, 30, 20, and 10, respectively.

The following T scores from each patient were averaged and expressed graphically (see Figure 1) to demonstrate the goodness of fit of this sample as compared to other AD samples: VIQ, PIQ, MQ, Semantic Memory (sum of T scores from COWAT, Animal Fluency, Boston Naming and Easy-Paired

Table 1. Characteristics of the Sample.

Demographic variable	M	SD	Range	
Age (years)	72.2	7.6	50–91	
Estimated Age of Onset	67.7	8.5	42–86	
Education (years)	12.8	3.1	5–20	
Duration of Illness (years)	4.5	3.3	1–19	
Psychological test	M	SD	Range	N
WAIS-R – VIQ	82.3	14.4	53–123	121
– PIQ	79.3	14.5	57–120	121
– FSIQ	80.5	13.9	50–123	133
WMS – MQ	75.3	13.5	50–117	133
– LM	2.5	2.4	0–20	133
– VR	3.0	1.9	0–9	133
HDR	5.5	4.2	0–20	128
MMSE (Total)	16.6	5.2	1–27	134
Blessed	6.8	3.9	0–19.5	134

Note. VIQ = Verbal Intelligence Quotient; PIQ = Performance Intelligence Quotient; FSIQ = Full Scale Intelligence Quotient; WMS = Wechsler Memory Scale; MQ = Memory Quotient; LM = Logical Memory; VR = Visual Reproduction; HDR = Hamilton Depression Rating; MMSE = Mini-Mental State Exam.

Associates divided by 4 for each individual), Visual- Perception (sum of *T* scores from Block Design, Figure-Ground and Copy task divided by 3). The typical pattern evinces depression of VIQ, PIQ, and MQ, with PIQ slightly lower than VIQ, MQ lower than PIQ, and relatively equal means for Semantic Memory and Visual-Perception. Figure 1 illustrates the pattern obtained in this sample as compared to that reported by Martin et al. (1986) for their group of patients.

As can be seen from this graph, when mean overall performance across all patients is considered, the current sample fits the above outlined pattern of performance normally observed amongst AD samples in general, in addition to that obtained by Martin et al. (1986) in terms of VIQ > PIQ > MQ. However, the present sample is a great deal less impaired than the group studied by Martin and colleagues. Furthermore, with respect to semantic and visual-perceptual/constructional functioning, the current sample exhibited the opposite pattern to that of the Martin et al. (1986) sample: Visual-perceptual-constructional abilities appear slightly more impaired than semantic knowledge. This may be due to the slightly different visual-perceptual tests utilized in the current research (e.g., Pentagon Copy Task, Figure-Ground Test). In addition, the method by which *T* scores were calculated for the Figure-Ground Test (due to lack of age-appropriate

normative data) probably over-estimated levels of impairment on this measure.

R-Factor Analysis

The *T* score data from the AD patients on the four measures of lexical/semantic access and three measures of visual-perceptual/constructional skill were subsequently submitted to a principal components analysis using Varimax orthogonal rotation of the principal components solution. The criterion for factor extraction was an eigenvalue of greater than 1 (i.e., Mineigen = 1; the latent root criterion) (Afifi & Clark, 1990; Hair, Anderson, Tatham, & Black, 1992; West, 1991). This criterion for selecting the appropriate number of factors was observed to correspond with that suggested by examination of the scree plot, in addition to the commonly utilized rule of thumb regarding selection of only those components that explain at least 100 ÷ N (N = the number of variables) percent of the total variance (100 ÷ 7, or at least 14.3% in this sample) (Afifi & Clark, 1990). A two-component solution emerged, accounting for 61.6% of the total variance, which is considered to be a satisfactory solution (Hair et al., 1992). The eigenvalues for the first and second components were 3.3 and 1.04, respectively. As expected, the variables loading highly on Factor I were as follows: BNT, COWAT, Animal Fluency, and Easy Paired Associates. Those with significant loadings on Factor II included the

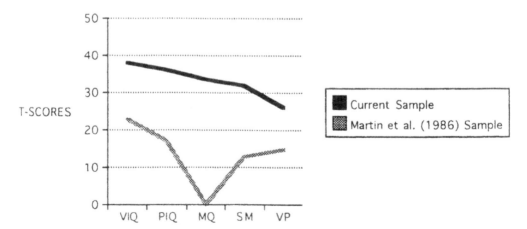

Fig. 1. *T* Scores comparing the present sample to that of Martin et al. (1986). VIQ = Verbal Intelligence Quotient; PIQ = Performance Intelligence Quotient; MQ = Memory Quotient; SM = Semantic Memory; VP = Visual-Perception/Construction.

following: Block Design, Figure-Ground, and the Copy task. Thus, the dissociation between accessibility of semantic knowledge and visual-perceptual/constructional functioning among AD patients reported by Martin and colleagues (1986) was replicated on this independent sample, that utilized similar neuropsychological test data and substantially less impaired patients. However, the factor loadings were not as high as those reported by Martin et al. (1986).

Q-Factor Analysis

Q-type factor analysis (McKeown & Thomas, 1988) was accomplished by creating a correlation matrix in which the individual respondents represented the rows and the test variables represented the columns. The resulting matrix was then transposed, and correlation (i.e., similarity) coefficients were calculated between the profiles of each pair of subjects in the sample, creating a 134×134 (i.e., $N \times N$) matrix of intercorrelations. Subsequently, this new matrix was submitted to a principal components factor analysis. Only those factors with eigenvalues $\geq$ the ratio of the number of subjects to the number of variables (i.e., $134 \div 7$, or 19.14) were retained (Del Dotto & Rourke, 1985). This criterion yielded three factors that accounted for 80% of the common variance. The three emerging factors were subjected to Varimax orthogonal rotation. Patients were assigned to

each subgroup on the basis of the factor for which they demonstrated a loading at or above .50. Subjects without at least one loading of .50 on a factor and those with significant loadings (i.e., $\geq .50$) on more than one factor were not considered in the determination of subgroups. This assignment procedure resulted in the subgrouping of 97 patients, or 72.39% of the sample. Thirty-four percent of these subjects were assigned to subgroup 1 (i.e., Factor I); subgroups II and III were comprised of 21.64% and 17.16% of the reduced sample, respectively.

Following this, T score means from the seven test variables used in the R- and Q-type analyses were computed for each subgroup and plotted graphically (Figure 2). Examination of these profiles revealed that all three subgroups performed similarly on some of the measures. For example, all three groups demonstrated similar levels of performance on the Figure-Ground Test, earning mean T scores of 19.98 (subgroup 1), 20.97 (subgroup 2), and 21.52 (subgroup 3). This suggests that these variables had little or no utility as discriminators between the groups.

Multivariate analysis of variance (MANOVA) was undertaken to determine whether the three groups differed significantly, utilizing the Q-defined subgroups as the independent variable and the seven neuropsychological measures as the dependent variables. Utilizing Wilks' Lambda as the criterion,

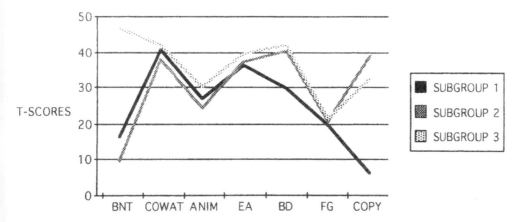

Fig. 2. Mean T Scores of the three subgroups derived by Q-factor analysis. BNT = Boston Naming Test; COWAT = Controlled Oral Word Association Test; ANIM = Animal Fluency; EA = Easy Associates; BD = Block Design; FG = Figure Ground; COPY = Pentagon Copy Task.

this analysis revealed that the groups were significantly different from each other on the combined dependent measures $F(14, 176) = 26.44, p < .001$. A commonly employed equation for calculating the proportion of variance accounted for by this significant subgroup effect ($h^2 = 1 - \lambda$) indicated that 89.6% of the variance in the best linear combination of test scores was accounted for by subgroup assignment (Tabachnick & Fidell, 1989). Subsequent univariate F tests revealed that the BNT [$F(2, 94) = 52.5$, $p < .001$], Block Design [$F(2, 94) = 26.04$, $p < .001$], and Copy Task [$F(2, 94) = 69.68$, $p < .001$] were significant contributors to these overall group differences. Due to the increased Type I error rate resulting from computation of multiple ANOVAs, more stringent α levels were set via a Bonferroni type adjustment. Conservative α values of .001 (.0014286, to be precise; i.e., $.01 \div 7$) were assigned for each of the seven variables, and the overall level considered necessary for a signifiant result for the set of dependent variables (i.e., .01) conformed to the following equaion: $\alpha = 1 - (1 - \alpha_1) - (1 - \alpha_2) \cdots (1 - \alpha_7)$ (Tabachnick & Fidell, 1989).

Because there were significant pooled within-group correlations among the test variables, a stepwise analysis was also performed, as suggested by Tabachnick and Fidell (1989). This involved an original univariate F test for the first variable (i.e., BNT), followed by analyses of covariance (i.e., a series of ANCOVAs) for each of the remaining variables, one at a time. Thus, the remaining six variables were evaluated as to the amount of new information (in terms of variance accounted for) that they added to the combination of dependent variables already tested. This was done within the context of controlling for the effects of all previously entered variables in a manner analogous to hierarchical stepwise analysis of the independent variables in multiple regression. Retaining the previous α adjusted for inflated Type I error rate, similar results emerged, with COWAT, Easy Associates, Animal Fluency and Figure-Ground F ratios not reaching statistical significance. Subsequent profile analyses indicated that the overall patterns of performance on the seven tests were significantly different between the three groups [(Wilks' U = .063) F (12, 162) = 40.15,

$p < .001$]. Indeed, eta square (i.e., the strength of the association; $\eta^2 = 1 -$ Wilks' Lambda) revealed that 94% of the variance about adjacent line segments of the profiles was accounted for by the varying shapes of the profiles.

Cluster Analyses

In order to evaluate the reliability of the Q-derived subgroups, four different clustering algorithms were applied to the same data in an attempt to replicate identification of the three Q-groups across various methods. As mentioned previously, such replication is required because cluster analysis often generates inconsistent results across different approaches, algorithms, and similarity measures (Afifi & Clark, 1990). If, indeed, subgroups exist, a design incorporating different approaches, algorithms, and similarity measures should produce consistent results. Only then can one be assured that results obtained are not simply an artifact of the particular methodology utilized (Campbell & Fiske, 1959).

Four widely used techniques were chosen on the basis of their availability and demonstrated utility in previous studies (see Blashfield & Aldenderfer, 1988; Everitt & Dunn, 1991): Ward's method (Ward, 1963), average linkage between groups (Sneath & Sokal, 1973), average linkage within groups (Sneath & Sokal, 1973), and k-means iterative partitioning (MacQueen, 1967). The correlation coefficient was selected as the similarity measure for the hierarchical analyses; squared Euclidean distance was employed in the k-means procedure.

Inspection of the amalgamation coefficients, icicle plots, and dendrograms generated by the three hierarchical methods suggested the presence of distinct homogeneous clusters of individuals. The average linkage (within groups) and Ward's algorithms clearly suggested a three-group solution. The other hierarchical technique, average linkage between groups, suggested either three- or four-group solutions as optimal. However, when a three-group solution was forced, each and every individual from the fourth group joined group one. Because no qualitative distinction could be made between the patterns of performance of group one and four, the three-cluster solution was considered to best explain the structure of the data.

The SPSS-X k-means procedure requires the researcher to select the number of clusters to be derived from the data. Because the Q-analysis and two of the three hierarchical procedures clearly suggested the presence of three groups, k was set at 3 for the iterative partitioning procedure. Initial cluster seeds were randomly selected by the program, in accordance with the one-stage k-means procedure outlined by DeLuca, Adams, and Rourke (1991). When the procedure was re-run utilizing the Q-derived means of the seven variables for the three subgroups as the initial cluster seeds (i.e., two-stage procedure; DeLuca et al., 1991), the results were nearly identical.

The results of the five analyses were evaluated in three ways, in a manner similar to that of previous systematic clustering studies (Del Dotto & Rourke, 1985; Fuerst, Fisk, & Rourke, 1989): (1) visual comparison of graphic profiles constructed by plotting the means of each subgroup on the seven measures (i.e., for each of the five methods), (2) misclassification analysis, and (3) construction of a multiprofile-multimethod matrix (Campbell & Fiske, 1959). Profile plotting and subsequent inspection of the patterns that each method generated for the three subgroups were qualitatively judged as highly similar (see Figures 3–5).

Misclassification analysis involved the use of the Q-defined groups as the criterion subgroups.

Counts were made of the number of subjects misclassified to the Q-factor groups by the other four clustering methods (see Table 2). As can be seen in Table 2, misclassifications were evident for each of the methods. However, the vast majority of subjects (81–93%) were correctly classified by each method. The average-linkage within groups and Ward's algorithms were most successful in correctly classifying the subjects. These two methods classified all of the Q-derived subgroup 1 subjects correctly. The k-means procedure performed the worst (although still quite well) of all the algorithms. This was probably a reflection of the use of a distance measure as the similarity measure with this algorithm: Distance measures are not as sensitive to profile shape as are correlation coefficients (Morris, Blashfield, & Satz, 1981).

As a third, and perhaps most powerful, means of assessing the similarity of the three subgroups generated by each of the five clustering approaches, a multiprofile-multimethod matrix of intercorrelations was constructed (see Table 3) in the tradition of Campbell and Fiske (1959). In order to demonstrate satisfactory internal validity of a subgroup, one is obligated to demonstrate high correlations between profiles of the same subgroup derived by different techniques. As well, one must also

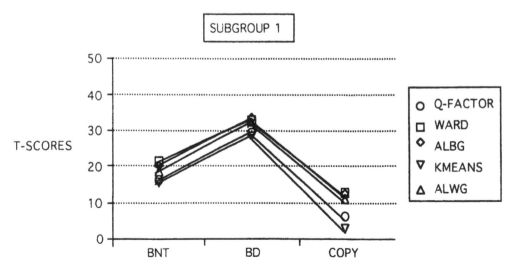

Fig. 3. Subgroup 1 (GAD) profiles by five clustering methods. ALBG = Average Linkage Between Groups; ALWG = Average Linkage Within Groups; BNT = Boston Naming Test; BD = Block Design; COPY = Pentagon Copy Task.

demonstrate that these coefficients are higher than those between distinct subgroup profiles derived by distinct methods, in addition to those between different subgroups generated by the same method. It should be noted that the correlations computed between the same subgroup profiles across different methods are extremely high, ranging from .79 to .99. Also, the majority of heteroprofile-heteromethod and heteroprofile-monomethod coefficients were substantially lower.

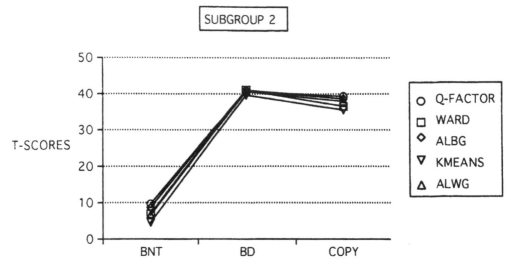

Fig. 4. Subgroup 2 (LAD) profiles by five clustering methods. ALBG = Average Linkage Between Groups; ALWG = Average Linkage Within Groups; BNT = Boston Naming Test; BD = Block Design; COPY = Pentagon Copy Task.

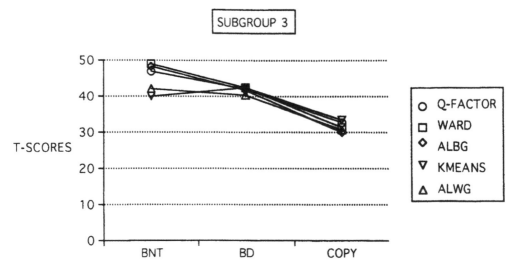

Fig. 5. Subgroup 3 (RAD) profiles by five clustering methods. ALBG = Average Linkage Between Groups; ALWG = Average Linkage Within Groups; BNT = Boston Naming Test; BD = Block Design; COPY = Pentagon Copy Task.

Table 2. Misclassification Analysis: Number of Patients Wrongfully Assigned to each Q-Factor Group by the Cluster Analytic Methods.

Clustering methods	Q-Derived subgroups			Total misclass. (n = 97)	% Correctly classified
	1 (n = 45)	2 (n = 29)	3 (n = 23)		
Ward's	0	4	6	10	90
ALBG	5	4	6	15	85
K-Means*	8	8	2	18	81
ALWG	0	4	3	7	93

Note. ALBG = average linkage between groups; ALWG = average linkage within groups; misclass. = misclassifications; * also known as nearest centroid sorting.

Table 3. Multiprofile-Multimethod Matrix.

	Q-Factor			Ward's			ALB			K-Means			ALW		
	Q1	Q2	Q3	W1	W2	W3	A1	A2	A3	K1	K2	K3	B1	B2	B3
Q1															
Q2	35														
Q3	0.32	0.08													
W1	**0.96**	0.43	0.54												
W2	0.41	**0.99**	0.03	0.47											
W3	0.27	0.08	**0.96**	0.46	−0.12										
A1	**0.96**	0.47	0.52	**0.99**	0.50	0.43									
A2	0.37	**0.99**	0.02	0.43	**0.99**	−0.14	0.47								
A3	0.30	−0.08	**0.96**	0.48	−0.12	**0.99**	0.45	−0.13							
K1	**0.98**	0.35	0.45	**0.98**	0.40	0.41	**0.98**	0.36	0.44						
K2	0.43	**0.99**	0.06	0.49	**0.99**	−0.10	0.52	**0.99**	−0.10	0.42					
K3	0.61	0.38	**0.90**	0.79	0.35	**0.79**	0.78	0.33	**0.81**	0.68	0.37				
B1	**0.98**	0.44	0.43	**0.99**	0.49	0.36	**0.99**	0.45	0.38	**0.98**	0.51	0.71			
B2	0.38	**0.99**	0.02	0.44	**0.99**	−0.14	0.47	**0.99**	−0.14	0.37	**0.99**	0.33	0.46		
B3	0.43	0.21	**0.97**	0.64	0.16	**0.91**	0.63	0.14	**0.92**	0.55	0.19	**0.93**	0.54	0.14	

Note. ALB = average-linkage between groups; ALW = average-linkage within groups. After Campbell & Fiske (1959).

The subgroups identified by the Q-analysis and replicated by the three hierarchical agglomerative algorithms and the iterative partitioning technique resemble the hypothetical subgroups global AD (GAD), left AD (LAD), and right AD (RAD). Those with the GAD pattern (subgroup 1) performed poorly on tests of naming, block construction, and copying of overlapping figures. This subgroup represented decline in the areas of both semantic knowledge and visual-perceptual functioning. The LAD patients' (subgroup 2) performance on the naming measure was severely impaired, whereas their visual-spatial constructions were relatively spared, falling within the borderline-low average range. The RAD patients

(subgroup 3) displayed the reverse trend, demonstrating preserved naming abilities, borderline block design performance, and mildly to moderately impaired ability to copy overlapping figures. In general, the RAD subgroup exhibited best performances of the three subgroups.

Because the three methods evaluating the reliability of the Q-factor analysis derived subgroups strongly supported the predicted existence of three qualitatively distinct subgroups, difference tests (i.e., ANOVAs) between the groups on measures not employed in their derivation were undertaken (Aldenderfer & Blashfield, 1984; Fletcher, 1985) (see Table 4). The groups did not differ significantly in terms of age, estimated age at disease onset,

Table 4. Means and Standard Deviations for the Three Q-Factor Analysis Derived Subgroups (S1, S2, S3).

Variable	S1		S2		S3		Paired Comparison (p < .05)[‡]
	M	(SD)	M	(SD)	M	(SD)	
AGE	71.16	(8.17)	69.72	(8.21)	73.87	(7.26)	None
EAO	67.42	(9.09)	65.68	(8.60)	69.00	(7.90)	None
LOI	3.73	(2.82)	4.00	(2.39)	4.91	(3.23)	None
EDUC	12.69	(3.12)	13.59	(2.31)	12.52	(3.33)	None
FSIQ	74.27	(11.94)	80.48	(9.23)	87.17	(13.5)[†]	1&2, 1&3
VIQ	78.66	(12.70)	79.46	(9.93)	90.53	(14.38)[*]	1&3, 2&3
PIQ	70.75	(11.38)	83.00	(12.06)	86.47	(11.4)[††]	1&2, 1&3
MMSE	14.82	(5.16)	18.03	(4.32)	18.83	(4.52)[*]	1&2, 1&3
Blessed	7.48	(3.67)	6.02	(3.67)	5.76	(3.11)	None
Hamilton	5.31	(4.30)	5.04	(4.12)	5.50	(4.01)	None
TVR	40.69	(4.56)	45.03	(5.89)	47.83	(6.56)[††]	1&2, 1&3
TLM	35.33	(10.72)	34.62	(4.79)	38.35	(9.81)	None
TTAPD	39.55	(13.37)	45.93	(14.01)	45.59	(10.77)	None
TTAPND	37.84	(15.02)	42.97	(12.90)	44.23	(10.27)	None
TGRIPD	38.89	(9.25)	38.38	(11.36)	40.09	(8.88)	None
TGRIPND	38.50	(10.70)	38.54	(13.52)	41.09	(9.47)	None

Note. EAO = estimated age at onset of AD; LOI = length since onset of illness (years); EDUC = Education (years); TVR = T score for Visual Reproduction; TLM = T score for Logical Memory; TTAPD = T score for finger tapping (dominant hand); TTAPND = T score for finger tapping (nondominant hand); TGRIPD = T score for grip strength (dominant hand); TGRIPND; T score for grip strength (nondominant hand).
[‡] Tukey's alternate procedure
[*] p < .002
[†] p < .0002
[‡‡] p < .00001

duration of illness, educational level, or Hamilton Depression Scale rating.

Univariate F tests were also conducted in order to test the a priori hypotheses that (1) the RAD subgroup would demonstrate relatively lower PIQ and visual memory performance as compared to the LAD subgroup, while (2) the LAD patients would show significantly more impairment on tests of verbal memory and crystallized verbal intelligence (i.e., VIQ). Due to the multitude of F tests conducted, the corrected alpha level required for significance became .0006 in order to maintain a conservative total alpha of .01. However, two measures demonstrated differences between the groups at the .002 level (equivalent to less than total p < .05), and are reported. To determine specifically which of the three groups differed from each other, multiple pairwise comparisons were conducted for the variables that yielded significant differences between the groups via the univariate F tests. Tukey's alternate procedure was selected as appropriate for the multiple comparisons (Jaccard, Becker, & Wood, 1984).

The GAD subgroup was significantly more impaired than the other two subgroups in terms of Mini-Mental State Exam scores (p < .002), FSIQ (p < .0002), PIQ (p < .05), and Visual Reproduction performance (p < .05). The RAD subgroup had a significantly higher VIQ than both the GAD and LAD subgroups (p < .05). Additionally, the RAD subgroup displayed the VIQ > PIQ pattern, while the LAD subgroup exhibited the reverse pattern on the WAIS-R (PIQ > VIQ).

There were no differences between the groups on the Logical Memory subtest of the WMS. No differences on the motor measures (i.e., grip strength and finger tapping) were apparent across the three groups. However, correlations computed between finger tapping performance and disease severity (as assessed by MMSE scores; higher MMSE scores indicate lower levels of impairment) were positive [dominant r = .45, p < .01; nondominant r = .33, p < .01]. Correlations between grip strength and level of symptom severity were not significant.

DISCUSSION

Summary of Results

In accord with previous research (e.g., Martin et al., 1986), three neuropsychological subgroups were identified. Overall, subgroup 3 (labelled RAD) appears as the highest functioning of the three groups. This subgroup demonstrated preserved naming abilities and Block Design performance, although some difficulty in copying simple overlapping figures was in evidence. Subgroup 2 (LAD) demonstrated severe anomia in the context of relatively spared visual-perceptual/constructional functioning. Subgroup 1 (GAD) was marked by moderate to severe anomia, mildly to moderately impaired Block Design performance, and a virtual inability to copy a simple drawing of two overlapping figures.

The results of this study demonstrated that reliable subgroups of patients diagnosed with mild to moderate *probable* AD, each displaying qualitatively distinct patterns of performance on neuropsychological measures, can be identified via Q-type factor analysis. These findings were replicated with three different hierarchical agglomerative cluster analysis algorithms, in addition to a non-hierarchical iterative partitioning technique. Such results stand in sharp contrast to "stage model" predictions regarding AD. The subgroups did not differ in terms of duration of illness, and the presence of simultaneous (i.e., non-AD) CNS processes accounting for the qualitative variation is unlikely, given the stringent exclusionary and inclusionary criteria for subject selection.

The subgroups identified in this study are not inconsistent with those reported by Martin and colleagues (1986). For example, their globally impaired group may correspond to subgroup 1 (i.e., GAD) of the current study. Furthermore, although clearly less impaired than the subjects studied by Martin et al. (1986), subgroup 2 (i.e., LAD) demonstrated a pattern that may be a precursor to the spared visual-perceptual functioning in the face of severe impairment of accessibility of semantic knowledge pattern identified by these researchers. In a similar fashion, subgroup 3 (i.e., RAD) may represent a precursor to the group identified by Martin and colleagues (1986) as exhibiting relatively intact access to semantic

knowledge in the face of impaired visual-perceptual/constructional abilities.

Outliers were not removed from the data prior to analysis. However, given that the same three groups were apparent across clustering approaches, algorithms, and similarity measures, it is unlikely that these data distorted the results in any significant way.

Evaluation of Hypotheses

It was predicted that three subgroups would be identified by the various clustering techniques employed. The largest subgroup was expected to be comprised of individuals displaying relatively equal neuropsychological impairment on measures tapping accessibility of semantic knowledge and those gauging visual-perceptual/constructional functioning. A second subgroup was predicted to comprise patients exhibiting relatively intact visual-perceptual functioning coupled with impaired semantic abilities; a third subgroup was predicted to display the opposite pattern. These second two subgroups were expected to account for approximately equal numbers of the remaining patients. Furthermore, based on the theoretical model of disease progression presented by Fisher and colleagues (under review), it was predicted that the first subgroup would contain subjects at all severity levels (i.e., mild, moderate, and severe), while the second two subgroups would only represent mild and moderate cases. It was expected that the asymmetrical patterns of impairment underlying these groups would eventually give way to global pathology, and corresponding diffuse neuropsychological dysfunction.

In general, this cluster of hypotheses was supported. The Q-type factor analysis and three hierarchical clustering approaches suggested the presence of three subgroups, and the groups were successfully replicated by the one- and two-stage k-means iterative partitioning procedures.

Subgroup 1 is analogous to the first group expected to emerge. This group represented the majority of patients, and was marked by moderate to severe anomia and moderate to severe compromise of constructional abilities. Support for the theoretical model of progression was also obtained, in that subgroup 1 (GAD) evinced significantly greater levels of impairment on the

MMSE and FSIQ as compared to the two remaining subgroups. Thus, individuals classified into this globally impaired group were more likely to evince greater overall impairment than were those assigned to the other two subgroups.

The correspondence of subgroups 2 and 3 to those predicted is less striking, yet present. In accordance with prediction, these two subgroups were comprised of relatively equal numbers of the remaining subjects. Subgroup 2 exhibited the expected impaired access to semantic knowledge, accompanied by relative sparing of visual-perceptual constructional abilities. This group displayed poor BNT performance (T score = 9.66), while scoring within borderline normal limits on the Block Design (T score = 40.55) and Copy (T score = 39.23) tasks.

Subgroup 3 resembles the group predicted to display sparing of semantic knowledge accessibility in the presence of visual-constructional impairment (i.e., BNT T score = 46.82; Copy T score = 36.61). However, the mean Block Design performance of this group fell just within normal limits (T =42.7), clouding the interpretation of this subgroup's constructional performance. This subgroup is the least well defined, and the discrepancy between the scores on the Block Design and Copy tasks is puzzling. It may be that this seeming contradiction can be accounted for in terms of the global-local demands of the two tasks. In this manner, while Block Design can be approached with both local (primarily left hemisphere?) and global (primarily right hemisphere?) strategies, it would appear that the pentagon copy task (drawing item from MMSE) is more dependent on preserved global processing capacities.

A further hypothesis predicted that subgroups 2 (LAD) and 3 (RAD) would demonstrate material-specific memory loss in the maximally impaired domain. Thus, it was predicted that subgroup 2 would evince higher levels of performance on the Visual Reproduction subtest of the WMS as compared to scores on Logical Memory, and that subgroup 3 would demonstrate the reverse pattern. This hypothesis was only partially supported: Whereas the performance of subgroup 2 on the Visual Reproduction test exceeded that on the Logical Mem-ory test, all three subgroups performed better on the Visual Reproduction test than on the Logical

Memory test, suggesting that this subtest may be somewhat easy for AD patients in general.

It was also predicted that correlations calculated between scores on the motor measures (i.e., finger tapping and grip strength) and decreasing severity of cognitive symptoms would be positive. This hypothesis originated from the disease progression model. It was theorized, on the basis of past research, that the frontal cortex (and, specifically, the motor areas) is spared of AD pathology until the advanced phase of the disease. Thus, it was reasoned that degree of impairment on these measures should be correlated with MMSE scores, and that the GAD group would perform worse on these tests. This hypothesis was partially supported with respect to finger tapping performance: as finger tapping performance declined, MMSE scores dropped, indicating greater degrees of disease severity. However, the correlation between grip strength performance and MMSE scores did not reach significance, and the GAD group performed no more poorly than did the LAD and RAD groups.

In accordance with the Goldberg and Costa model (1981) of hemispheric specialization, the final hypothesis predicted that those with the RAD pattern (i.e., impaired visual-constructional functioning in the context of relatively better preserved accessibility of semantic knowledge) would display a PIQ < VIQ pattern of performance, suggesting impaired fluid abilities as opposed to overlearned crystallized knowledge. Conversely, the LAD-like group was predicted to display the reverse WAIS-R pattern (i.e., PIQ > VIQ). This hypothesis was supported: Subgroup 2 (LAD-like subgroup) displayed superior PIQ compared to VIQ, whereas subgroup 3 (RAD-like subgroup) displayed the reverse pattern.

Limitations of the Present Study

Although the present study yielded some significant findings, several limitations must be noted. The reliability of the scoring criteria developed for the pentagon copy task is unknown. Each individual's drawings were scored by only one investigator, precluding the assessment of interrater reliability. Hence, these results must be interpreted cautiously. Similarly, given the lack of geriatric norms for the Figure-Ground Test and the observation that the three subgroups performed similarly on this measure, these results must also be viewed with caution. Because somewhat inappropriate age norms were utilized in calculating the T scores for this measure, it is quite possible that the suggested impairment across all subgroups represents a normal age-related decline.

Second, given that the current sample consisted mainly of highly educated, white, upper middle-class individuals, the generalizability of these results is limited to this population. As well, the sample is biased in terms of individuals willing to participate in research.

Another limitation of the present research involves the sample size. Although meeting the minimum number of subjects for powerful factor/cluster analytic research, utilization of a larger sample may have improved the stability of the results obtained.

As more of a conceptual limitation, neuropsychologically heterogeneous manifestations of AD may reflect inter-individual differences in brain organization (and, hence, distinct patterns of breakdown corresponding to these differences). Thus, differential changes in brain organization as a function of age, and/or the heterogeneity of the normal aging process itself, which leaves individuals differentially vulnerable to losses in certain areas (Joanette et al., 1992) is possible. It is also possible that cognitive decline associated with normal aging may not proceed in a homogeneous fashion. Thus, neuropsychologically identified subgroups of AD may, at least in part, reflect differences in premorbid levels of functioning (i.e., premorbid strengths and weaknesses). As such, distinct weak areas of neuropsychological functioning before AD strikes may become more pronounced when AD initially begins. If this were the case, heterogeneity would not be attributable to AD itself but to premorbid individual differences. Thus, the significance of neuropsychologically defined subgroups may represent regional neuropathological susceptibility rather than distinct evolutionary sequences related to different etiologies (Chui, 1987).

Some support, though minimal, for this potential confounding factor is provided by a cluster analytic study of neuropsychological data collected from healthy elderly individuals (Valdois, Joanette, Poissant, Ska, & Dehaut, 1990). This analysis yielded six subgroups, most of which represented quantitative differences, but two of which represented uninterpretable, though qualitatively distinct, profiles of neuropsychological functioning. Notably, these qualitatively distinct clusters were comprised only of the most severely impaired subjects and did not overlap with those determined by Martin et al. (1986), by Becker et al. (1988), or in the present study. Furthermore, the researchers did not elaborate the extent of their exclusionary screening process beyond simply stating that the subjects were "without obvious clinical signs of brain damage or psychiatric disorders" (p. 589). Given these difficult to evaluate inclusionarycriteria, it is quite possible that early AD patients with subtle signs were not screened out. In spite of these limitations, the Valdois et al. study is valuable as a caveat to overinterpretation of subgroup study results. More stringently designed studies (i.e., utilizing health screening criteria similar to those suggested by the NINCDS-ADRDA Work Group) of normal elderly individuals will surely resolve this issue.

Another limitation of this study, which could not be controlled, involves the source of the data. Due to the research criteria for the diagnosis of AD, which require deficits in at least two areas of neuropsychological functioning (one of which is memory), AD patients presenting atypically may have been excluded from the database utilized in this investigation (Becker et al., 1992; Martin, 1990). Identification of subgroups very early in their development represents a challenging task, and the results of the present study are limited in this regard.

Directions for Future Research

Future research should be directed toward improving upon the limitations of the current investigation. This research requires replication on a larger, independent, more representative (i.e., of minorities and low SES groups) sample. In addition, it would be beneficial to repeat the current analyses utilizing data collected from cognitively intact normal elderly controls (e.g., spouses of current subjects; non-neurological medical sample) in order to determine if the three subgroups do or do not exist among such individuals. As well, longitudinal research in which individuals from the three subgroups are followed and reevaluated yearly would be beneficial to delineate further patterns of progression. Such outcome research would be beneficial in determining prognostic differences. Future subgrouping studies should include patients with *possible* AD (yet low Hachinski scores), in order to prevent exclusion of atypical early presentations of AD. Neuroimaging studies on members of the individual subgroups would allow for external validation of the classification scheme suggested herein. Finally, research endeavours pertaining to neuropsychological functioning of AD patients should involve within-group comparisons rather than averaging patient data and comparing these to healthy controls. This should allow further differences between subgroups of AD patients to emerge.

REFERENCES

Adams, R.D., & Victor, M. (1993). *Principles of neurology* (5th ed.). New York: McGraw-Hill.

Afifi, A.A., & Clark, V. (1990). *Computer-aided multivariate analysis* (2nd ed.). Los Angeles: Van Nostrand Reinhold.

Aldenderfer, M.S., & Blashfield, R.K. (1984). *Cluster analysis*. Beverly Hills: Sage.

Ayres, A.J. (1966). *The Southern California Figure-Ground Visual Perception Test manual*. Los Angeles: Western Psychological Services.

Bandera, L., Della Sala, S., Laiacona, M., Luzzatti, C., & Spinnler, H. (1991). Generative associative naming in dementia of Alzheimer's type. *Neuropsychologia*, 29, 291–304.

Becker, J.T. (1988). Working memory and secondary memory deficits in Alzheimer's disease. *Journal of Clinical and Experimental Neuropsychology*, 10, 739–753.

Becker, J.T., Huff, J.F., Nebes, R.D., Holland, A., & Boller, F. (1988). Neuropsychological function in Alzheimer's disease: Pattern of impairment and rates of progression. *Archives of Neurology*, 45, 263–268.

Becker, J.T., Lopez, O.L., & Wess, J. (1992). Material-specific memory loss in probable Alzheimer's disease. *Journal of Neurology, Neurosurgery and Psychiatry*, 55, 1177–1181.

Benton, A.L., & Hamsher, K. (1989). *Multilingual Aphasia Examination: Manual of instructions* (2nd ed.). Iowa City: AJA.

Berent, S., Giordani, B., Minoshima, S., Foster, N.L., Koeppe, R.A., & Kuhl, D.E. (1995). Isolated memory impairment (IMI): Relationship to cognition, brain metabolism and Alzheimer's disease. *Journal of Cerebral Blood Flow and Metabolism*, 15, 102.

Bieliauskas, L.A., Newberry, B.H., & Gerstenberger, T.J. (1988). Young adult norms for the Southern California Figure-Ground Visual Perception Test. *The Clinical Neuropsychologist*, 2, 239–245.

Blashfield, R.K., & Aldenderfer, M.S. (1988). The methods and problems of cluster analysis. In J.R. Nesselroade & R.B. Cattell (Eds.), *Handbook of multivariate experimental psychology* (2nd ed.). (pp.447–473). New York: Plenum Press.

Blessed, G., Tomlinson, B.E., & Roth, M. (1968). The association between quantitative measures of dementia and of senile change in the cerebral grey matter of elderly subjects. *British Journal of Psychiatry*, 114, 797–811.

Boller, F., Forette, F., Khachaturian, Z., Poncet, M., & Christen, Y. (1992). *Heterogeneity of Alzheimer's disease*. (International Fondation Ipsen Symposium Proceedings, France Conference). Berlin: Springer-Verlag.

Campbell, D.T., & Fiske, D.W. (1959). Convergent and discriminant validation by the multitrait-multimethod matrix. *Psychological Bulletin*, 56, 81–105.

Chui, C.H. (1987). The significance of clinically defined subgroups of Alzheimer's disease. *Journal of Neural Transmission. (suppl.)*, 24, 57–68.

Constantinidis, J. (1978). Is Alzheimer's disease a major form of senile dementia? Clinical, anatomical, and genetic data. In R. Katzman, R.D. Terry, & K.L. Bick (Eds.), *Alzheimer's disease: Senile dementia and related disorders* (Aging, Vol.7, pp.15–25). New York: Raven Press.

Crystal, H.A., Horoupian, D.S., Katzman, R., & Jotkowitz, S. (1982). Biopsy-proved Alzheimer disease presenting as a right parietal lobe syndrome. *Annals of Neurology*, 12, 186–188.

Cummings, J.L., & Benson, F.D. (1992). *Dementia: A clinical approach*. Boston: Butterworth-Heinemann.

Del Dotto, J.E., & Rourke, B.P. (1985). Subtypes of left-handed learning-disabled children. In B.P. Rourke, *Neuropsychology of learning disabilities: Essentials of subtype analysis* (pp.89–130). New York: Guilford Press.

Delis, D.C., Massman, P.J., Butters, N., Salmon, D.P., Shear, P.K., Demadura, T., & Filoteo, J.V. (1992). Spatial cognition in Alzheimer's disease: Subtypes of global-local impairment. *Journal of Clinical and Experimental Neuropsychology*, 14, 463–477.

DeLuca, J.W., Adams, K.M., & Rourke, B.P. (1991). Methodological and statistical issues in cluster analysis. In B.P. Rourke (Ed.), *Neuropsychological validation of learning disability subtypes* (pp.45–54). New York: Guilford Press.

Everitt, B. (1974). *Cluster analysis*. London: Heinemann Educational Books.

Everitt, B.S., & Dunn, G. (1991). Cluster analysis.In B.S. Everitt & G. Dunn (Eds.), *Applied multivariate data analysis* (pp. 99–125). London: Edward Arnold.

Farlow, M., Gracon, S.I., Hershey, L.A., Lewis, K.W., Sadowsky, C.H., & Dolan-Ureno, J. (1992). A controlled trial of tacrine in Alzheimer's disease. The tacrine study group. *Journal of the American Medical Association, 268*, 2523–2529.

Fisher, N.J., Rourke, B.P., & Bieliauskas, L.A. Heterogeneity of Alzheimer's disease. (under review).

Fletcher, J. (1985). External validation of learning disability typologies. In B.P. Rourke, (Ed.), *Neuropsychology of learning disabilities: Essentials of subtype analysis* (pp. 187–211). New York: Guilford Press.

Folstein, M.F., Folstein, S.E., & McHugh, P.R. (1975). "Mini- Mental State": A practical method for grading the cognitive state of patients for the clinician. *Journal of Psychiatric Research, 12*, 189–198.

Foster, N.L., Chase, T.N., Fedio, P., Patronas, N.J., Brooks, R.A., & Di Chiro, G. (1983). Alzheimer's disease: Focal cortical changes shown by positron emission tomography. *Neurology, 33*, 961–965.

Freed, D.M., Corkin, S., Growdon, J.H., & Nissen, M.J. (1988). Selective attention in Alzheimer's disease: CSF correlates of behavioral impairments. *Neuropsychologia, 26*, 895–902.

Freed, D.M., Corkin, S., Growdon, J.H., & Nissen, M.J. (1989). Selective attention in Alzheimer's disease: Characterizing cognitive subgroups of patients. *Neuropsychologia, 27*, 325–339.

Fuerst, D.R., Fisk, J.L., & Rourke, B.P. (1989). Psychosocial functioning of learning-disabled children: Replicability of statistically derived subtypes. *Journal of Consulting and Clinical Psychology, 57*, 275–280.

Fuld, P.A. (1984). Test profile of cholinergic dysfunction and of Alzheimer-type dementia. *Journal of Clinical Neuropsychology, 6*, 380–392.

Funkenstein, H.H., Albert, M.S., Cook, N.R., West, C.G., Scherr, P.A., Chown, M.J., Pilgrim, D., & Evans, D.A. (1993). Extrapyramidal signs and other neurologic findings in clinically diagnosed Alzheimer's disease. A community-based study. *Archives of Neurology, 50*, 51–56.

Goldberg, E., & Costa, L.D. (1981). Hemisphere differences in the acquisition and use of descriptive systems. *Brain and Language, 14*, 144–173.

Goldman, R.S., Axelrod, B.N., Tandon, R., & Berent, S. (1993). Spurious WAIS-R cholinergic profiles in schizophrenia. *The Clinical Neuropsychologist, 7*, 171–178.

Hachinski, V.C., Iliff, L.D., Zilhka, E., Du Boulay, G.H., McAllister, V.L., Marshall, J., Russell, R.W., & Symon, L. (1975). Cerebral blood flow in dementia. *Archives of Neurology, 32*, 632–637.

Hair, J.F., Anderson, R.E., Tatham, R.L., & Black, W.C. (1992). *Multivariate data analysis* (3rd ed.). New York: Macmillan.

Hamilton, M. (1967). Development of a rating scale for primary depressive illness. *British Journal of Social and Clinical Psychology, 6*, 278–296.

Haxby, J.V., Grady, C.L., Koss, E., Horwitz, B., Schapiro, M., Friedland, R.P., & Rapoport, S.I. (1988). Heterogeneous anterior-posterior patterns in dementia of the Alzheimer type. *Neurology, 38*, 1853–1863.

Hom, J. (1992). General and specific cognitive dysfunctions in patients with Alzheimer's disease. *Archives of Clinical Neuropsychology, 7*, 121–133.

Isaacs, B., & Kennie, A.T. (1973). The set test as an aid to the detection of dementia in old people. *British Journal of Psychiatry, 123*, 467–470.

Jaccard, J., Becker, M.A., & Wood, G. (1984). Pairwise multiple comparison procedures: A review. *Psychological Bulletin, 96*, 589–596.

Jagust, W.J., Davies, P., Tiller-Borcich, J.K., & Reed, B.R. (1990). Focal Alzheimer's disease. *Neurology, 40*, 14–19.

Joanette, Y., Ska, B., Poissant, A., & Beland, R. (1992). Neuropsychological aspects of Alzheimer's disease: Evidence for inter- and intra-function heterogeneity. In F. Boller, F. Forette, Z. Khachaturian, M. Poncet, & Y. Christen (Eds.), *Heterogeneity of Alzheimer's disease* (pp. 33–42). Berlin: Springer-Verlag.

Jorm, A.F. (1985). Subtypes of Alzheimer's dementia: A conceptual analysis and critical review. *Psychological Medicine, 15*, 543–553.

Kaplan, E.F., Goodglass, H., & Weintraub, S. (1983). *The Boston Naming Test* (2nd ed.). Philadelphia: Lea & Febiger.

Kaufman, A.S. (1990). *Assessing adolescent and adult intelligence.* Boston: Allyn & Bacon.

Knapp, M.J., Knopman, D.S., Solomon, P.R., Pendlebury, W.W., Davis, C.S., & Gracon, S.I. (1994). The tacrine study group. A 30-week randomized controlled trial of high-dose tacrine in patients with Alzheimer's disease. *Journal of the American Medical Association, 271*, 985–991.

Liston, E.H. (1979). The clinical phenomenology of presenile dementia: A critical review of the literature. *Journal of Mental and Nervous Disease, 167*, 329–336.

MacQueen, J.B. (1967). Some methods for classification and analysis of multivariate observations. *Proceedings of the Fifth Berkeley Symposium on Mathematical Statistics and Probability, 1*, 281–297.

Martin, A. (1988). The search for the neuropsychological profile of a disease state: A mistaken enterprise? *Journal of Clinical and Experimental Neuropsychology, 10*, 22–23.

Martin, A. (1990). Neuropsychology of Alzheimer's disease: The case for subgroups. In M.F. Schwartz (Ed.), *Modular deficits in Alzheimer-type dementia* (pp.144–175). Cambridge, MA: MIT Press.

Martin, A., Brouwers, P., Lalonde, F., Cox, C., Teleska, P., Fedio, P., Foster, N.L., & Chase, T.N. (1986). Towards a behavioral typology of Alzheimer's patients. *Journal of Clinical and Experimental Neuropsychology*, 8, 594–610.

Martin, A., Cox, C., Brouwers, P., & Fedio, P. (1985). A note on different patterns of impaired and preserved cognitive abilities and their relation to episodic memory deficits in Alzheimer's patients. *Brain and Language*, 26, 181–185.

Massman, P.J., Delis, D.C., Filoteo, V.J., Butters, N., Salmon, D.P., & Demadura, T.L. (1993). Mechanisms of spatial impairment in Alzheimer's disease subgroups: Differential breakdown of directed attention to global-local stimuli. *Neuropsychology*, 7, 172–181.

McDonald, C. (1969). Clinical heterogeneity in senile dementia. *British Journal of Psychiatry*, 115, 267–271.

McKeown, B., & Thomas, D. (1988). *Q methodology.* Sage University Paper Series on quantitative applications in the social sciences, 07-066. Beverly Hills: Sage.

McKhann, G., Drachman, D., Folstein, M., Katzman, R., Price, D., & Stadlan, E.M. (1984). Clinical diagnosis of Alzheimer's disease: Report on the NINCDS-ADRDA work group under the auspices of department of health and human services task force on Alzheimer's disease. *Neurology*, 34, 939–944.

Morris, R., Blashfield, R., & Satz, P. (1981). Neuropsychology and cluster analysis: Potentials and problems. *Journal of Clinical Neuropsychology*, 3, 79–99.

Morris, R.D., & Fletcher, J.M. (1988). Classification in neuropsychology: A theoretical framework and research paradigm. *Journal of Clinical and Experimental Neuropschology*, 10, 640–658.

Naugle, R.I., Cullum, M.C., Bigler, E.D., & Massman, P.J. (1985). Neuropsychological and computerized axial tomography volume characteristics of empirically derived dementia subgroups. *Journal of Mental and Nervous Disease*, 173, 596–603.

Neary, D., Snowden, J.S., Bowen, D.M., Sims, N.R., Mann, D.M.A., Benton, J.S., Northen, B., Yates, P.O., & Davison, A.N. (1986). Neuropsychological syndromes in presenile dementia due to cerebral atrophy. *Journal of Neurology, Neurosurgery, and Psychiatry*, 49, 163–174.

Norusis, M.J. (1990). *SPSS advanced statistics student guide.* Chicago: SPSS.

Pogacar, S., & Williams, R.S. (1984). Alzheimer's disease presenting as slowly progressive aphasia. *Rhode Island Medical Journal*, 67, 181–185.

Price, B.H., Gurvit, H., Weintraub, S., Geula, C., Leimkuhler, E., & Mesulam, M. (1993). Neuropsychological patterns and language deficits in 20 consecutive cases of autopsy-confirmed Alzheimer's disease. *Archives of Neurology, 50*, 931–937.

Rasmusson, D.X., & Brandt, J. (1995). Instability of cognitive asymmetry in Alzheimer's disease. *Journal of Clinical and Experimental Neuropsychology, 17*, 449–458.

Read, D.E. (1987). *Neuropsychological assessment of memory in early dementia: Normative data for a new battery of memory tests.* Unpublished manuscript, University of Victoria, British Columbia.

Reisberg, B., Ferris, S.H., & Crook, T. (1982). Signs, symptoms, and course of age-associated cognitive decline. In S. Corkin, K.L. Davis, J.H. Growdon, & R.J. Wurthman (Eds.), *Alzheimer's Disease: A report of progress in research* (Aging, Vol. 19). (pp. 177–181). New York: Raven Press.

Reitan, R.M., & Davidson, L.A. (1974). *Clinical neuropsychology: Current status and implications.* Washington, DC: Winston & Sons.

Ross, T., Lichtenberg, P., & Christiansen, B. (1994). Age and education corrected norms for the Boston Naming Test. (In press).

Schwartz, M.F. (1987). Focal cognitive deficits in dementia of the Alzheimer type. *Neuropsychology, 1*, 27–35.

Shuttleworth, E.C. (1984). Atypical presentations of dementia of the Alzheimer type. *Journal of the American Geriatrics Society, 32*, 485–490.

Sneath, P., & Sokal, R. (1973). *Numerical taxonomy.* San Francisco: Freeman.

Spreen, O., & Benton, A.L. (1977). N*neurosensory Center Comprehensive Examination for Aphasia (NCCEA)* (rev. ed.). Victoria: University of Victoria.

Spreen, O., & Strauss, E. (1991). *A compendium of neuropsychological tests: Administration, norms, and commentary.* New York: Oxford University Press.

Swash, M., Brooks, D.N., Day, N.E., Frith, C.D., Levy, R., & Warlow, C.P. (1991). Clinical trials in Alzheimer's disease. *Journal of Neurology, Neurosurgery, and Psychiatry, 54*, 178–181.

Tabachnick, B.G., & Fidell, L.S. (1989). *Using multivariate statistics* (2nd ed.). New York: Harper-Collins.

Valdois, S., Joanette, Y., Poissant, A., Ska, B., & Dehaut, F. (1990). Heterogeneity in the cognitive profile of normal elderly. *Journal of Clinical and Experimental Neuropsychology, 12*, 578–596.

Van Gorp, W.G., Satz, P., Kiersch, M.E., & Henry, R. (1986). Normative data on the Boston Naming Test for a group of normal older adults. *Journal of Clinical and Experimental Neuropsychology, 8*, 702–705.

Ward, J.H. (1963). Hierarchical grouping to optimize on objective function. *Journal of the American Statistical Association, 58,* 236–244.

Warren, W.L. (1994). *Revised Hamilton Rating Scale for Depression manual.* Los Angeles: Western Psychological Services.

Wechsler, D. (1945). *Wechsler Memory Scale manual.* New York: The Psychological Corporation.

Wechsler, D. (1981). *Manual for the Wechsler Adult Intelligence Scale – Revised (WAIS-R).* San Antonio, TX: The Psychological Corporation.

West, R. (1991). *Computing for psychologists: Statistical analysis using SPSS and Minitab.* London: Harwood Academic.

Zec, R.F. (1993). Neuropsychological functioning in Alzheimer's disease. In R.W. Parks, R.F. Zec, & R.S. Wilson (Eds.), *Neuropsychology of Alzheimer's disease and other dementias* (pp. 3–80). New York: Oxford University Press.

Journal of Clinical and Experimental Neuropsychology
1999, Vol. 21, No. 4, pp. 488–518

Neuropsychological Subgroups of Patients with Alzheimer's Disease: An Examination of the First 10 Years of CERAD Data*

Nancy J. Fisher[1], Byron P. Rourke[1,2], and Linas A. Bieliauskas[3,4]

[1]University of Windsor, Ontario, Canada, [2]Yale University, New Haven, CT, [3]Ann Arbor VA Medical Center, MI, and [4]University of Michigan, Ann Arbor, MI

ABSTRACT

Neuropsychological CERAD data from 960 patients with Alzheimer's disease and 465 controls were subjected to separate yet identical classification procedures. Consistent with past research, three patient subgroups were reliably identified: Subgroup 1 (LAD; $n = 312$) was characterized by severe naming impairment yet borderline-normal figure-copying skills; Subgroup 2 (RAD; $n = 247$) displayed average naming ability but moderately-impaired copying performance; Subgroup 3 (GAD; $n = 161$) evinced profound anomia and constructional dyspraxia. LAD patients were older and less educated than those of the other subgroups. Control subgroups ($n = 2$) did not resemble the patient subgroups. Initial patterns of performance remained discernible across time for LAD and GAD, but were less consistent for RAD. Members from patient subgroups were present across disease stage.

Several studies have consistently reported three qualitatively distinct clinical subgroups of patients with Alzheimer's disease (AD) based on patterns of performance on semantic and visual-perceptual/constructional neuropsychological measures (Becker, Huff, Neves, Holland, & Boller, 1988; Fisher et al., 1996; Martin et al., 1986; Strite, Massman, Cooke, & Doody, 1997). This research has suggested that whereas many patients with AD undergo global decline in cognitive functioning, significant numbers of patients demonstrate relatively preserved functioning in one of these neuropsychological domains (either semantic or visual-perceptual/constructional functioning) during the early and middle periods of the disease. These studies served a valuable role in shifting the conceptualization of AD from one of a global unitary process to one acknowledging its heterogeneous neuropsychological manifestations.

Notwithstanding the value of the above studies, two central questions remain unanswered: (1) Do the initial subgroup patterns remain consistent with progression of the disease? and (2) Are these patterns simply mere reflections of premorbid

* The research described herein was conducted as a doctoral dissertation by the first author, under the supervision of the other authors, in partial fulfillment of the requirements of the Clinical Neuropsychology programme at the University of Windsor. Portions of this paper were presented at the 26th Annual Meeting of the International Neuropsychological Society, Honolulu, HI, USA, February, 1998.

The first author was supported by a Doctoral Training Award from the Alzheimer Society of Canada while conducting this research. This project was approved by the CERAD steering committee in October of 1995. The authors wish to acknowledge the 24 participating CERAD sites/investigators who contributed the data utilized in this investigation (see Appendix).

Address correspondence to: Nancy J. Fisher, Geriatric Research – A438, Sunnybrook and Women's College Health Sciences Centre, University of Toronto, 2075 Bayview Avenue, Toronto, Ontario, Canada, M4N 3M5. E-mail: nancy.fisher@swchsc.on.ca

Accepted for publication: January 4, 1999.

strengths and weaknesses? These questions are important because: (1) if the initial subgroup patterns do not remain consistent for a significant period, then aside from the inherent diagnostic value awareness of heterogeneous presentations brings, subgroup classification may have little (i.e., short-lived) practical value as a basis for making treatment recommendations; (2) if these patterns merely reflect premorbid strengths and weaknesses, then the theoretical notion of underlying initial symmetrical versus asymmetrical neuropathology as a function of variants of the disease (i.e., global vs. right- and left-hemisphere subtypes), would not hold. That is, the disease would then need to be conceptualized as global in all instances, with any apparent subgroups merely reflecting protective and/or exacerbatory effects of premorbid strengths and weaknesses. Studies to date have been limited in their ability to address these stability and premorbidity issues, due to the employment of case study (Fisher, Rourke, Bieliauskas, et al., 1997; Martin, 1990) or cross-sectional (Fisher et al., 1996; Martin et al., 1986; Strite et al., 1997) patient-only designs. Even in research involving the application of objective classificatory methodology (Fisher et al., 1996; Martin et al., 1986), one-time tested, patient-only samples were used.

In the current investigation, empirical classification techniques were utilized in a large scale examination of the neuropsychological profiles of patients with AD. This project was conducted with the goal of replicating the results of an earlier, much smaller study, in which three neuropsychological subgroups of patients with AD were reliably identified across objective classification methods (Fisher et al., 1996). The current study employed methodological improvements over the previous one, by inclusion of a demographically similar non-demented comparison group, utilization of a larger, multicenter sample, and incorporation of a longitudinal design. Employment of a longitudinal design and inclusion of a control group allowed exploration of the above-mentioned subgroup stability and premorbid pattern issues. The longitudinal nature of the data also allowed for evaluation and refinement of an earlier developed subgroup-specific neuropsychological model of AD (Fisher, Rourke, & Bieliauskas, 1997). This model incorporates both the Subgroup and Stage Models of the disease, by outlining progression patterns for each of three neuropsychological subgroups.

It was hypothesized (hypothesis 1) that three subgroups of patients with AD would be reliably identifiable when data from visual-constructional and semantic measures were analyzed via objective classification techniques. In accord with past research (Fisher et al., 1996; Martin et al., 1986), it was expected (hypothesis 2) that these subgroups would resemble the theoretical ideal types (Fisher, Rourke, & Bieliauskas, 1997) as follows: (a) GAD (global AD), those with global impairment (impaired access to semantic knowledge and impaired visual-constructional functioning); (b) RAD (right-hemisphere AD), those with relatively spared accessibility of semantic knowledge yet impaired visual-constructional functioning; and (c) LAD (left-hemisphere AD), those with impaired ability to access semantic knowledge, but relatively unimpaired visual-constructional functioning. It was further predicted (hypothesis 3) that similar subgroups would not emerge when identical analyses were performed on normal control data. That is, it was hypothesized that the three previously identified subgroups were specific to AD, and not mere reflections/pronouncements of premorbid patterns. Past research has demonstrated that when data from elderly samples are subjected to empirical classification techniques, significant interpretable subgroups resembling RAD and LAD do not emerge among the unimpaired subjects (Mitrushina, Uchiyama, & Satz, 1995; Valdois, Joanette, Poissant, Ska, & Dehaut, 1990). Clearly, it was expected that normal elderly persons may show different patterns of relative strengths and weaknesses (i.e., on memory measures; Mitrushina et al., 1995). However, it was expected that they would demonstrate consistent levels of performance in both the semantic and visual-constructional domains (i.e., like GAD patients, yet within the normal range of functioning) (Mitrushina et al., 1995).

In terms of subgroup stability, hypothesis 4 predictions were guided by an earlier proposed subgroup-progression model (Fisher, Rourke, & Bieliauskas, 1997). It was expected that the GAD profile would remain consistent throughout the course of the disease. That is, as the disease

progressed, it was predicted that levels of performance on the semantic and visual-constructional
measures would decrease, but remain relatively
equivalent to one another. RAD and LAD profiles
were predicted to remain detectable (i.e., stable)
over the early and middle course of the disease.
However, for these two subgroups, the discrepancy between the initially preserved and impaired
domains of functioning was expected to diminish
with disease progression. This fourth hypothesis
was based on past case study research which has
suggested that the initial neuropsychological patterns defining these subgroups (i.e., RAD & LAD)
remain detectable across time (Fisher, Rourke,
Bieliauskas, et al., 1997; Martin, 1990; Price et al.,
1993). It is known however that AD is progressive, and eventually results in widespread cognitive impairment (Price et al., 1993). As such, it was
predicted that the RAD and LAD subgroups would
eventually evince a GAD pattern.

METHOD

CERAD
The Consortium to Establish a Registry for Alzheimer's
Disease (CERAD) was established in 1986 as a united
effort to collect uniform longitudinal clinical, neuropsychological, and neuropathological data on a large sample of patients with AD. Patients are recruited from
dozens of university medical centers across the United
States (Consortium to Establish a Registry for
Alzheimer's Disease [CERAD], 1996). Data from normal
elderly individuals are also collected. Patients and controls are administered standardized evaluations yearly,
allowing for large-scale tracking of the natural progression of AD (CERAD, 1996). The data are pooled and
managed at a central location, and made available for
research use by CERAD and non-CERAD investigators.

Subject Selection
Clinical, demographic, and neuropsychological CERAD
data from patients with AD and non-demented controls
were utilized in this investigation. All subjects had
agreed to participate in the longitudinal data collection
process and had consented to the terms of the CERAD
study. Inclusionary criteria for both patients and controls
were as follows: (a) must be at least 50 years of age; (b)
must be free of major health problems, such as cancer,
cardiac or respiratory disease, hypertension, current
major depression or psychiatric illness, and/or recent
substance abuse; (c) must have normal consciousness

with no signs of delirium; (d) must be willing and cooperative research participants; (e) must be able to read and
comprehend the language on the neuropsychological
forms; and (f) must have an informant willing to provide
information (CERAD, 1996).
    All patients met the criteria for *probable* AD
(McKhann et al., 1984), between the years 1986 and
1996, after having been referred to a CERAD site for
consultation regarding suspected dementia. (A list of
participating CERAD sites is provided in the Appendix.)
In addition, as a criterion for inclusion, each patient had
suffered gradual progression of cognitive loss for at least
12 months, sufficient enough to have interfered with
daily activities. None of the patients had a history of
abrupt onset of dementia or evidence of other central
nervous system disorders or metabolic disturbances that
might account for the dementia.
    The comparison (i.e., control) group comprised
spouses or caregivers/friends of the patients; they were
selected so as to be similar to the patients in terms
of demographic characteristics (CERAD, 1996). All
controls met comparable exclusionary criteria as the
patients, and none had a history of cognitive impairment
(CERAD, 1996). Aside from the above inclusionary/
exclusionary criteria, all patients with *probable* AD and
non-demented controls registered in the CERAD database between the years 1986 and 1996 (Heyman, 1996)
were included in the current investigation if complete
neuropsychological data from at least the initial testing
were available.

The CERAD Assessment Battery
The CERAD standardized battery was established in
order to ensure that data collected at different research
centers are comparable; prior to its development, differing test protocols made across-research-center comparisons difficult to evaluate (Morris et al., 1989). There are
two parts to the CERAD assessment battery: (a) the clinical evaluation, and (b) the neuropsychological assessment. Both have been outlined in detail previously
(Morris et al., 1989). Measures from the clinical assessment utilized in the current investigation included the
Blessed Dementia Scale (Blessed, Tomlinson, & Roth,
1968), a measure of functional ability, and the Clinical
Dementia Rating Scale (CDR; Berg, 1984; Hughes,
Berg, Danziger, Coben, & Martin, 1982; Morris, 1993),
a staging measure.
    The following five measures comprise the CERAD
neuropsychological battery: Animal Category Verbal
Fluency (Isaacs & Kennie, 1973), Modified Boston
Naming Test (Kaplan, Good-glass, & Weintraub,
1978), Mini-Mental State Exam (Folstein, Folstein, &
McHugh, 1975), Word List Memory (Atkinson &
Shiffrin, 1971), and Constructional Praxis (i.e., copying
four geometric forms; Rosen, Mohs, & Davis, 1984).
These measures are well-known to clinicians and

described in detail elsewhere (Morris et al., 1989; Morris et al., 1993). In the current study, the Animal Category Verbal Fluency Test (VF) and the Modified Boston Naming Test (BNT) were utilized as measures of semantic knowledge accessibility; the Constructional Praxis (PRAX) test was used as a measure of visual-constructional functioning; and the Word List Memory test was used to measure immediate (IVBM), delayed (DVBM), and recognition (RECOG) verbal memory. The Mini-Mental State Exam (MMSE) was utilized as a measure of dementia severity.

Psychometric Properties of the CERAD Neuropsychological Battery

In a study of data from 16 CERAD sites, interrater scoring reliability was demonstrated to be high; intraclass correlation coefficients ranged from .92 to 1.0 (Morris et al., 1989). Test-retest reliability after one month was shown to be more than adequate for each of the neuropsychological measures (Morris et al., 1989). The battery has also been demonstrated to accurately distinguish demented from non-demented subjects (Morris et al., 1989; Welsh, Butters, Hughes, Mohs, & Heyman, 1992), and to be sensitive to increasing cognitive decline over time (Morris et al., 1989; Morris et al., 1993; Welsh et al., 1992). An initial factor analysis of the CERAD neuropsychological data from 354 patients with AD revealed three factors accounting for 73% of the total variance among the measures: (I) Memory; (II) Language; and (III) Constructional Praxis (Morris et al., 1989). In a more recent factor analytic study of CERAD data from 202 patients with AD, two factors (i.e., memory and nonmemory) were reported, accounting for 51% of the variance (Larrain & Cimino, 1998).

Overview of Statistical Analysis

The first step of data analysis involved conversion of raw patient scores on the measures of semantic accessibility, visual-construction, and memory (modified Boston Naming Test (BNT), Animal Fluency (VF), Constructional Praxis (PRAX), Word-List immediate free recall (IVBM), Word-List delayed recall (DVBM), Word-List recognition (RECOG)) to demographically corrected standard T scores for comparative purposes, utilizing normative data provided by Welsh et al. (1994). Subsequently, Q-type factor analysis was undertaken, in which product-moment correlations were calculated between subject profiles. An initial Q-type factor analysis was thought beneficial in that this alternative "clustering" method has no bias against creating relatively small clusters; many cluster analytic techniques are biased toward creating clusters of equal size (Aldenderfer & Blash-field, 1984; Edelbrock, 1979; Hair, Anderson, Tatham, & Black, 1992). Furthermore, Q-analysis controls for the presence of outliers, as every case is not necessarily required assignment to a cluster.

The Q-analysis identified significant qualitatively distinct subgroups of patients (as evaluated via multivariate analysis of variance and profile analysis procedures), and as such, various cluster analyses were performed on the T-score data, in an attempt to generate similar subgroupings across multiple methods. Only those clusters emerging via the majority of methods were accepted as reliable. Solutions derived by the cluster analytic techniques were subsequently compared to those generated by the Q-factor analysis to evaluate replicability. Demographic and psychometric data were provided for the Q-derived subgroups, and comparisons were made to determine whether the subgroups differed in terms of age, education, duration of illness, and/or severity of the illness. Following the patient data analyses, the same procedures outlined above were performed on the control sample data.

Longitudinal analyses aimed at evaluating stability of initial patient profiles were also conducted. In meeting this end, 5 subjects from each subgroup were randomly selected, and their patterns of discrepancy between semantic and visual-constructional functioning qualitatively examined across time. Following this, discrepancy scores (i.e., differences between BNT and PRAX performances) were calculated for the patients at each testing, and correlations between discrepancy scores and testing occasion were calculated. For subgroups LAD and RAD, diminishing discrepancy scores were expected across time, whereas for GAD, this was not expected to be the case. A between-subgroup ANOVA was also conducted with discrepancy score serving as the dependent variable. Due to restrictions with the data, separate ANOVAs were conducted on the data from each testing, with subgroup serving as the independent variable and mean discrepancy score, the dependent variable. (Note: The originally planned repeated measures ANOVA with the independent variables being (a) the assessment number, and (b) subgroup, and mean discrepancy score serving as the dependent variable, was not carried out. This repeated measures design could not be employed due to limitations in consistency of patients returning for follow-up visits, which resulted in empty cells and great variability in terms of inter-follow-up assessment intervals.)

In further investigating progression patterns, the patient sample was cross-sectionally divided into severity groupings (i.e., stage levels) on the basis of CDR ratings. Correlations between initial discrepancy scores and CDR ratings were calculated for the subgroups. Following this, mean discrepancy scores for each subgroup were compared across severity levels. With respect to GAD, no substantial differences across stage were expected. In regard to RAD and LAD however, it was expected that the differences between semantic and visual-constructive functioning would be greatest for the mildly impaired patients, become less prominent for

Table 1. Descriptive Statistics for Demographic and Neuropsychological Data.

Variable	AD				NC			
	N	M	(SD)	Range	N	M	(SD)	Range
Demographics (raw)								
Age (years)	960	72.07	(7.93)	50–97	465	68.38	(8.04)	50–93
Education (years)	960	12.30	(3.70)	0–26	465	13.67	(3.31)	2–25
Male	396				160			
Female	564			G	305			
White	784				429			
Black	158				34			
Hispanic	18				2			
General Impairment Ratings (raw)								
CDR	960	1.47	(.64)	0.5–5				
MMSE	926	17.40	(5.77)	1–29	461	28.73	(1.62)	17–30
Blessed	959	4.57	(2.48)	0–14				
Neuropsychological Tests (*T* scores)								
BNT	960	18.44	(20.59)	0–57	465	48.10	(12.37)	0–57
VF	960	28.34	(9.83)	9–60	465	49.47	(9.96)	28–85
PRAX	960	28.18	(19.41)	0–62	465	49.39	(10.83)	7–62
IVBM	960	2.36	(7.46)	0–71	465	48.85	(24.49)	0–117
DVBM	960	15.50	(8.34)	1–54	464	49.30	(10.63)	9–71
RECOG	960	7.03	(15.02)	0–62	465	51.39	(14.13)	0–62

Note. AD = Alzheimer's patients; NC = Normal Controls; CDR = Clinical Dementia Rating; MMSE = Mini-Mental State Exam; BNT = Boston Naming Test; VF = Verbal Fluency (Animal Category); PRAX = Constructional Praxis; IVBM = Immediate Verbal Recall; DVBM = Delayed Verbal Recall; RECOG = Recognition Memory.

the moderately impaired cases, and evince the least discrepancy in the severely demented groups.

RESULTS

Sample Characteristics

A total of 960 patients and 465 controls met the criteria for inclusion. The average duration of time since onset of first AD symptoms was 4.21 years ($SD = 2.64$). With respect to the staging of AD, the mean CDR score fell directly between the mildly and moderately demented stages ($M = 1.47$; $SD = .64$). Table 1 presents the demographic characteristics of the patient and control samples and their average levels of performance on neuropsychological measures. The control group was statistically younger ($p < .05$) and more educated ($p < .05$) than the patient sample, although the age and educational ranges and frequency distributions were similar, and the actual differences were quite small, as found in previous CERAD studies (e.g., Morris et al., 1993). Both groups were highly educated and predominantly Caucasian.

Q-Factor Analyses

Patients

Q-type factor analysis (McKeown & Thomas, 1988) was accomplished in the same manner outlined in the previous study (Fisher et al., 1996). This yielded three factors, accounting for 93.8% of the common variance. Patients were assigned to each subgroup on the basis of the factor for which they demonstrated a loading at or above .50. Subjects without at least one loading of .50 on a factor, in addition to those with significant loadings (i.e., $\geq.50$) on more than one factor, were not considered in the determination of subgroups. This assignment procedure resulted in the subgrouping of 720 patients, or 75% of the sample. Approximately 43% of these subjects were assigned to Subgroup I (i.e., Factor I); Subgroups II and III were comprised of 34.3% and 22.4% of the reduced sample, respectively.

Following this, T-score means from the six test variables used in the factor analysis were computed for each subgroup and plotted graphically (see Fig. 1). Examination of these profiles revealed that all three subgroups demonstrated a similar qualitative pattern of performance on the memory measures. In terms of levels of performance, the three groups were all severely impaired on these measures. Thus, with respect to both profile shape and levels of performance, it appeared that the memory variables had little or no utility as discriminators between the groups. Despite their similar memory performances, the three subgroups did demonstrate qualitatively distinct patterns on the remaining variables (i.e., BNT, PRAX, VF).

MANOVA revealed that the groups were significantly different from each other on the combined dependent measures [$F(12, 1424) = 380.32$, $p < .001$]. Subsequent univariate F tests (using Bonferroni adjustments for inflated Type I error rate) revealed that the BNT [$F(2, 717) = 2120.06$, $p < .001$], PRAX [$F(2, 717) = 401.40, p < .001$], VF [$F(2, 717) = 75.98$, $p < .001$], and DVBM [$F(2, 717) = 9.80$, $p < .001$] variables were significant contributors to these overall group differences.

Because there were significant pooled within-group correlations among the test variables, a stepwise analysis was also performed, as suggested by Tabachnick and Fidell (1989). This involved an original univariate F test for the first variable (i.e., BNT), followed by analyses of covariance (i.e., a series of ANCOVAs) for each of the remaining variables. Retaining the previous α adjusted for inflated Type I error rate (i.e., .002), the Fs for the DVBM ($p = .028$) and IVBM ($p = .048$) measures failed to reach significance, indicating that these variables were not significant in explaining additional variance. Subsequent profile analysis also indicated that the overall patterns of performance on the six tests were significantly different between the three groups [(Wilks' $\lambda = .066$) $F(10, 1426) = 411.88$, $p < .001$]. Eta square (i.e., the strength of the association; $\eta^2 = 1 - $ Wilks' λ) revealed that 93.4% of the variance about adjacent line segments of the profiles was accounted for by the varying shapes of the profiles.

Controls

A Q-factor analysis identical to that outlined above was next conducted on the control data. This yielded two factors, accounting for 76.8% of the common variance. Controls were assigned to

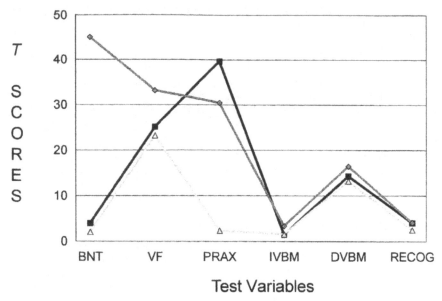

Test Variables

Fig. 1. Mean performance profiles of patient subgroups derived by Q-factor analysis. Q1 ■ = Q-group 1 (n = 312); Q2 ◆ = Q-Group 2 (n = 247); Q3 ▲ = Q-Group 3 (n = 161); BNT = Boston Naming Test; VF = Verbal Fluency; PRAX = Constructional Praxis; IVBM = Immediate Verbal Memory; DVBM = Delayed Verbal Memory; RECOG = Recognition Verbal Memory.

subgroups utilizing the same criteria outlined above for the patients. This assignment procedure resulted in the subgrouping of 207 control subjects, or 44.5% of the sample. Seventy-seven percent of these subjects were assigned to Subgroup I; Sub group II was comprised of 23% of the reduced sample.

Following this, T-score means from the six test variables were computed for each Q subgroup (Q1 and Q2) in addition to the remaining controls not assigned to a group by the Q analysis (i.e., designated as group Q0) and plotted graphically (see Fig. 2). Examination of these profiles revealed that the three groups generally performed within normal limits on the measures. However, Q1 demonstrated isolated impairment on IVBM.

MANOVA indicated that the two true Q groups (i.e., Q1 and Q2) were significantly different from each other on the combined dependent measures [$F(6, 200) = 54.05$, $p < .001$]. Subsequent univariate F tests using Bonferroni corrections revealed that all of the test variables were significant contributors to these overall group differences: IVBM [$F(1, 205) = 70.98$, $p < .001$], VF [$F(1, 205) = 24.93$, $p < .001$], DVBM [$F(1,$ 205) $= 23.20$, $p < .001$], RECOG [$F(1, 205) = 22.57$, $p < .001$], PRAX [$F(1, 205) = 18.11$, $p < .001$]. (Of note, BNT, the variable with the highest F for the patients, had the lowest F for the controls. Also, the variable with the highest F for the controls, IVBM, failed to reach univariate significance for the patients.) Due to significant pooled within-group correlations among the test variables, a stepwise analysis was also performed, retaining the previous α adjusted for inflated Type I error rate. Similar results emerged, with all variables reaching significance at the .001 level. Subsequent profile analysis indicated that the overall patterns of performance on the six tests were significantly different between the two groups [(Wilks' λ = .415) $F(5, 201) = 56.75$, $p < .001$]. Calculation of eta squared revealed that 58.5% of the variance about adjacent line segments of the profiles was accounted for by the varying shapes of the profiles.

When an additional Q-analysis of the control subjects' data was undertaken after eliminating those with MMSEs < 25, in an attempt to make the control sample more stringently normal, the

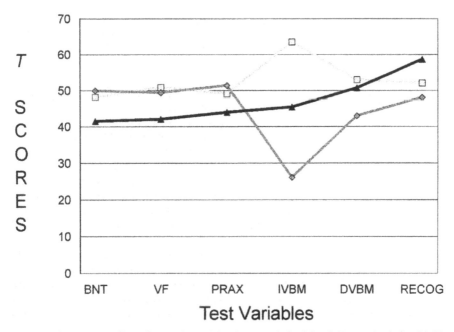

Fig. 2. Mean performance profiles of normal control subgroups derived by Q-Factor Analysis. Q0 ■ = non-classified controls (*n* = 258); Q1 ◆ = Q-group 1 (*n* = 160); Q2 ▲ = Q-group 2 (*n* = 47); BNT = Boston Naming Test; VF = Verbal Fluency; PRAX = Contructional Praxis; IVBM = Immediate Verbal Memory; DVBM = Delayed Verbal Memory; RECOG = Recognition Verbal Memory.

same results were obtained. That is, the Q-analysis again identified two subgroups, accounting for 77% of the variance. Subgroup I comprised 78% of the subjects. These subgroups highly resembled those derived on the entire control sample. As such, the full control sample was retained in the subsequent cluster analyses.

Cluster Analyses

To evaluate the reliability of the Q-derived subgroups, different clustering algorithms were utilized on the same data, in an attempt to replicate identification of the Q-groups across various methods. Such replication is required, because empirical classification techniques have been known to generate inconsistent results across different approaches (Afifi & Clark, 1990). Four widely used techniques were chosen, given their availability and success in previous studies (Blashfield & Aldenderfer, 1988; Everitt & Dunn, 1991): Ward's method (Ward, 1963), average linkage within groups (Sneath & Sokal, 1973), complete linkage

(Sokal & Michener, 1958), and K-Means iterative partitioning (MacQueen, 1967). The correlation coefficient was selected as the similarity measure for the hierarchical analyses, whereas squared Euclidean distance was employed in the K-Means procedure. Data from all 960 patients were used in the patient analyses, and those from all 465 controls were used in the control analyses (i.e., outliers were not removed; these analyses were not performed on the Q-reduced samples).

Patients

Inspection of the amalgamation coefficients and dendrograms generated by the hierarchical methods suggested the presence of three distinct homogeneous clusters of patients. As the Q-analysis and the hierarchical procedures clearly suggested the presence of three groups, *k* was set at 3 for the iterative partitioning procedure. The Q-derived means of the six variables for each of the three subgroups were utilized as the initial cluster seeds. When the procedure was re-run utilizing initial cluster seeds randomly selected by the program, the results were identical.

Controls

Inspection of the amalgamation coefficients and dendrograms generated by the Ward and average linkage hierarchical methods suggested the presence of two clusters of control subjects. The amalgamation coefficients and dendrogram for the complete linkage algorithm suggested either a two- or three-group solution. Because two of the three hierarchical methods and the Q-factor analysis had clearly indicated two clusters, k was set at 2 for the iterative partitioning procedure. The means of the six variables from the two Q-derived subgroups were utilized as the initial cluster seeds. When the procedure was rerun utilizing initial cluster seeds randomly selected by the program, the results were identical.

Evaluation of Clustering Results

For both the patient and control groups, the results of the five subgrouping analyses were evaluated three ways, in a manner similar to that of previous well-designed clustering studies (Del Dotto &

Rourke, 1985; Fuerst, Fisk, & Rourke, 1989; Fisher et al., 1996): (a) across-method visual comparison of graphic profiles constructed by plotting the means of each subgroup on the six measures, (b) misclassification analysis, and (c) construction of a multiprofile-multimethod matrix (Campbell & Fiske, 1959).

Patients

Inspection of the mean subgroup profiles generated by each clustering method revealed that the same three qualitative patterns were apparent across the methods. Misclassification analysis involved the use of the Q-defined groups as the criterion subgroups. Counts were made as to the number of subjects misclassified to the Q-factor groups by the other four clustering methods (see Table 2a). The vast majority of subjects (74–97%) were correctly classified by each method. Construction of a multiprofile-multimethod matrix of intercorrelation, revealed that correlations computed between the same subgroup profiles across different methods were generally high, with the majority (i.e., 25 out of 30) exceeding r values of .90 ($M_r = .90$).

Table 2. Misclassification Analysis.

(a) Patients

Clustering Method	Misclassifications			Total Misclassifications ($N = 720$)	% Correctly Classified
	Q1 ($n = 312$)	Q2 ($n = 247$)	Q3 ($n = 161$)		
ALWG	6	10	3	19	97.4
Ward	59	16	4	79	89.0
Complete	34	0	153	187	74.0
K-Means	45	32	3	80	88.9

(b) Controls

Clustering Method	Misclassifications		Total Misclassifications ($N = 207$)	% Correctly Classified
	Q1 ($n = 160$)	Q2 ($n = 47$)		
ALWG	1	25	26	87.4
Ward	2	11	13	93.7
Complete	12	31	43	79.2
K-Means	16	21	37	82.1

Note. ALWG = Average Linkage Within Groups; Q1 = Q-group 1; Q2 = Q-group 2; Q3 = Q-group 3.

In addition, the majority of heteroprofile-heteromethod and heteroprofile-homomethod coefficients were lower ($M_r = .38$).

Controls

The profiles for the control subgroups were also consistent across methods. Although misclassifications were evident for each of the methods, the majority of control subjects (79–94%) were correctly classified to the Q-criterion groups (see Table 2b). Correlations between the same subgroup profiles generated by the different methods averaged .81. The heteroprofile-heteromethod and heteroprofile-homomethod coefficients were substantially lower ($M_r = -.73$).

Inter-Subgroup Comparisons

Given that the findings from the three methods evaluating the reliability of the Q-factor analysis derived subgroups were satisfactory, difference tests (i.e., ANOVAs; adjusted $\alpha = .001$) were performed between the groups on measures not employed in their derivation (Aldenderfer & Blashfield, 1984; Fletcher, 1985) (see Table 3). Whereas the groups did not differ significantly in terms of duration of illness [$F(2, 707) = .801$, $p = .445$], significant between-subgroup differences were detected on the following variables: age [$F(2, 717) = 52.52$, $p < .001$], education [$F(2, 717) = 15.43, p < .001$], MMSE [$F(2, 693) = 81.58$, $p < .001$], CDR [$F(2, 717) = 42.08$, $p < .001$], Blessed [$F(2, 716) = 34.19, p < .001$]. Games-Howell multiple comparisons (Howell, 1992; Jaccard, Becker, &

Wood, 1984) indicated that members of Subgroup 1 were older and less educated than those in Sub groups 2 and 3. In terms of the dementia severity measures, those in Subgroup 3 were most impaired, followed next by those in Subgroup 1. The control subgroups (i.e., Q1 and Q2) did not differ in terms of age [$t(205) = -.628, p = .53$], education [$t(205) = 1.29, p = .20$], or MMSE scores [$t(205) = .08, p = .93$].

Longitudinal Findings

Stability of Profiles

In selecting patients from each Q-subgroup for longitudinal profile stability analysis, the initial Q-sample was reduced to include only those patients who had undergone three or more follow-up assessments. Five cases were randomly selected from each of the reduced subgroup samples, and the BNT and PRAX scores were plotted graphically for each testing session (see Figs. 3–5). (The BNT and PRAX scores were used in examining semantic accessibility vs. visual-constructional discrepancies in these and subsequent longitudinal analyses as they have been suggested by past research as the most sensitive to such domain-specific differences (Fisher et al., 1996; Fisher et al., 1997). In addition, these variables had the highest univariate Fs following the Q-MANOVA in the current investigation.) The longitudinal discrepancy profiles for Q1 were generally indicative of stability: four out of the five clearly suggested consistently superior

Table 3. Means and Standard Deviations for the Q-Factor Derived Patient Subgroups on Measures not Employed in their Derivation.

Variable	Subgroup 1		Subgroup 2		Subgroup 3		Significant ($p < .05$) Paired Comparisons[a]
	M	*(SD)*	*M*	*(SD)*	*M*	*(SD)*	
Age*	75.12	(6.68)	70.38	(7.51)	68.43	(8.42)	1 & 2; 1 & 3
DOI	4.25	(2.65)	4.22	(2.76)	4.54	(2.48)	–
Education*	11.48	(3.99)	12.85	(3.41)	13.14	(3.00)	1 & 2; 1 & 3
MMSE*	16.84	(5.67)	19.87	(4.28)	12.97	(5.81)	1 & 2; 1 & 3; 2 & 3
CDR*	1.52	(0.67)	1.24	(0.50)	1.81	(0.69)	1 & 2; 1 & 3; 2 & 3
Blessed*	4.70	(2.55)	3.80	(2.01)	5.81	(2.66)	1 & 2; 1 & 3; 2 & 3

Note. DOI = Duration since onset of illness; MMSE = Mini-Mental State Exam; CDR = Clinical Dementia Rating.
[a] Games-Howell test.
* $p < .001$ (ANOVA).

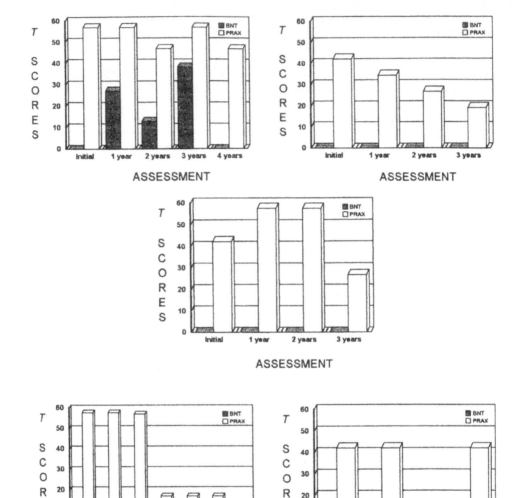

Fig. 3. Histograms depicting BNT/PRAX *T* Score discrepancies across time for 5 randomly selected Q1 patients. BNT = Boston Naming Test; PRAX = Contructional Praxis; Q1 = Q-Factor Derived Subgroup 1.

PRAX performance (i.e., normal range) as compared to BNT performance (impaired range), especially in the earlier years (see Fig. 3). The longitudinal profiles for the Q2 group were less stable, with only two out of the five cases showing stability of the initial profile across time (see Fig. 4). Profiles for the Q3 group were, in the main, stable, with both performances consistently impaired (see Fig. 5).

Discrepancy Score Changes with Time
In further investigating BNT/PRAX discrepancies across time, discrepancy scores were calculated for each of the Q-classified subjects. For Subgroup 1,

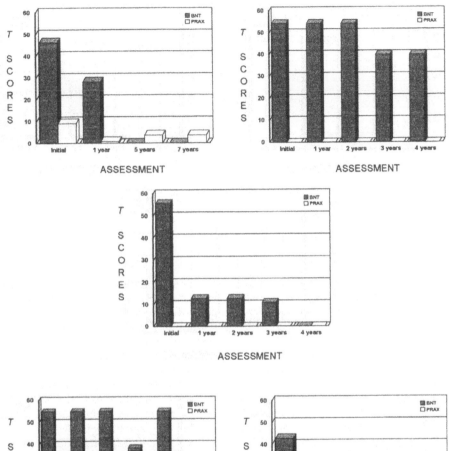

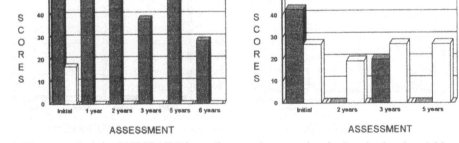

Fig. 4. Histograms depicting BNT PRAX T Score discrepancies across time for 5 randomly selected Q2 patients. BNT = Boston Naming Test; PRAX = Contructional Praxis; Q2 = Q-Factor derived Subgroup 2.

this score was calculated by subtracting the patient's BNT T score from their PRAX T score. For Subgroup 2, the discrepancy score was computed by subtracting the PRAX T score from the BNT T score. For the third subgroup, the discrepancy score was the absolute value of the BNT T score minus the PRAX T score. These scores were computed for every subject who appeared at each testing interval.

A Pearson product-moment correlation was calculated between discrepancy scores and testing number, revealing a significant negative correlation between these two variables for the patient sample as a whole [$r = -.31$, $p < .01$); $n = 1588$]. To detect between-subgroup differences, mean BNT/PRAX discrepancies at each assessment were calculated for each subgroup, and plotted graphically

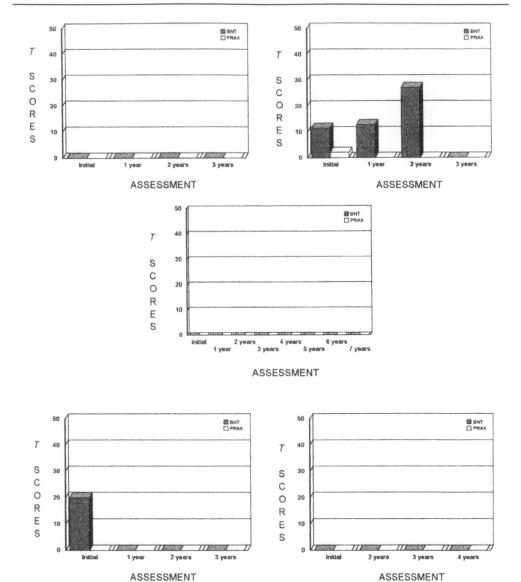

Fig. 5. Histograms depicting BNT PRAX T Score discrepancies across time for 5 randomly selected Q3 patients. BNT = Boston Naming Test; PRAX = Contructional Praxis; Q3 = Q-Factor derived Subgroup 3.

(see Fig. 6). As diminishing discrepancy scores across time were suggested by these plots, especially for Subgroups 1 and 2, separate Pearson correlations between testing number and discrepancy scores were calculated for each subgroup. These coefficients revealed significant negative correlations for Subgroup 1 [$r = -.36$, $p < .01$); $n = 647$] and Subgroup 2 [$r = -.34$, $p < .01$);

$n = 656$], and a nonsignificant correlation for Subgroup 3 [$r = .05, p = .43$); $n = 284$].

The findings of negative mean discrepancy scores for Subgroup 2 (from follow-up testings 4 through 7; see Fig. 6) suggested a reversal of the initial BNT > PRAX pattern with time. To investigate this further, mean BNT and PRAX scores were plotted by testing number for this subgroup, and for the

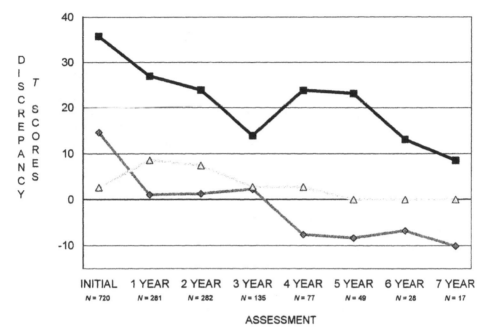

Fig. 6. BNT/PRAX Discrepancy *T* Scores for the patients across time. (Q1 = ■; Q2 = ◆; Q3 = ▲)

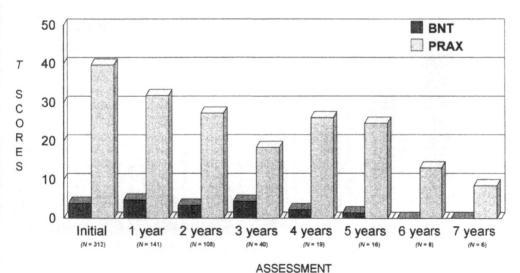

Fig. 7. Mean BNT and PRAX *T* Scores across testings for the Q1 group.

other subgroups for comparative purposes (see Figs. 7–9). Inspection of Figure 7 revealed the expected consistency of PRAX > BNT over time, even at the 7th year follow-up assessment, for the Q1 group.

Q3 (Fig. 8) showed little discrepancy in terms of BNT and PRAX performances across testings.

However, as suggested by the negative discrepancy scores obtained after follow-up testing

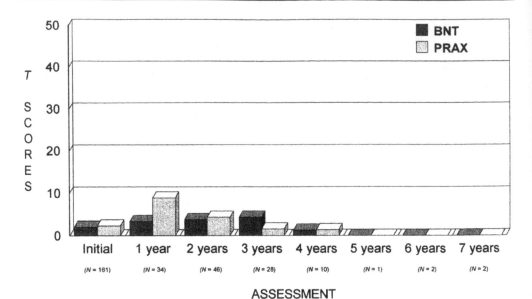

Fig. 8. Mean BNT and PRAX *T* Scores across testings for the Q3 group.

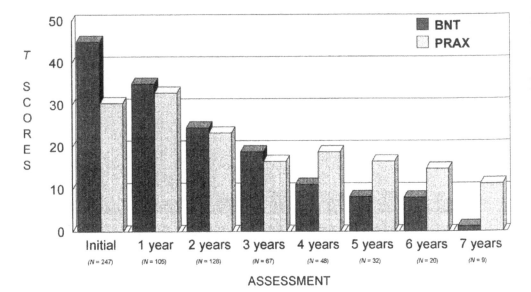

Fig. 9. Mean BNT and PRAX *T* Scores across testings for the Q2 group.

number 3, Q2 did evince little stability of the initial BNT > PRAX pattern (see Fig. 9). At follow-up assessment 1, this subgroup's mean performance on the two measures appeared to equalize until the 4th year follow-up assessment, at which time mean PRAX scores began to exceed mean BNT scores, although both performances were clearly within severely impaired limits. It should be noted that the number of subjects decreased markedly with each follow-up testing, and as such, these results should be interpreted cautiously.

Table 4. Mean BNT/PRAX Discrepancy T Scores across Assessments.

Assessment	Subgroup 1		Subgroup 2		Subgroup 3		Significant ($p < .05$) Paired Comparisons[a]
	M	(SD)	M	(SD)	M	(SD)	
Initial*	35.75	(12.19)	14.60	(17.82)	2.63	(4.21)	1 & 2, 1 & 3, 2 & 3
1 year*	26.94	(17.20)	2.10	(21.47)	8.57	(14.73)	1 & 2, 1 & 3
2 years*	23.85	(20.72)	1.24	(25.06)	7.41	(14.34)	1 & 2, 1 & 3
3 years*	13.92	(16.24)	2.26	(20.35)	2.77	(8.24)	1 & 2, 1 & 3
4 years*	23.77	(19.92)	−7.63	(20.21)	2.71	(5.72)	1 & 2, 1 & 3, 2 & 3
5 years*	23.12	(16.93)	−8.34	(20.52)	0	(0)	N.S.
6 years	13.10	(24.71)	−6.80	(17.89)	0	(0)	−
7 years	8.51	(20.84)	−10.11	(14.91)	0	(0)	−

Note. BNT = Boston Naming Test; PRAX = Constructional Praxis; N.S. = None Significant.
    *$p < .005$ (between-subgroup ANOVA difference).

A follow up 3×8 factorial ANOVA with sub-group and assessment number serving as the independent variables, and discrepancy score serving as the dependent variable revealed significant main effects for subgroup [$F(2, 1563) = 76.7$, $p < .001$] and assessment number [$F(7, 1563) = 13.05$, $p < .001$], in addition to a significant two-way interaction effect between the two independent variables [$F(14, 1563) = 5.4$, $p < .001$]. Although this analysis violated the ANOVA assumption of independent groups, the appropriate repeated measures ANOVA design could not be employed due to limitations with the data. Given these limitations, separate ANOVAs were conducted on the data from each testing, with subgroup serving as the independent variable and mean discrepancy score serving as the dependent variable. These analyses revealed significant between-group differences in discrepancy scores for the initial assessment [$F(2, 717) = 372.96$, $p < .001$], the 1st year follow-up [$F(2, 277) = 55.87$, $p < .001$], in addition to the 2nd [$F(2, 279) = 31.65$, $p < .001$], 3rd [$F(2, 132) = 6.25$, $p < .003$], 4th [$F(2, 74) = 18.66$, $p < .001$], and 5th year [$F(2, 46) = 14.0$, $p < .001$] follow-up assessments. However, between-subgroup differences in discrepancy scores from the 6th [$F(2, 25) = 2.51, p = .101$] and 7th [$F(2, 14) = 2.24, p = .144$] year follow-up assessments were not significant (see Table 4).

Post hoc multiple comparisons (i.e., Games-Howell) revealed that for the initial assessment, significant differences between all three subgroups were apparent, with Subgroup 1 showing the most discrepant scores, followed by Subgroup 2. At the first, second and third follow-up testings, significant differences were apparent between Subgroups 1 and 2, and Subgroups 1 and 3, but not between Subgroups 2 and 3. At the 4th year follow-up testing all the groups' discrepancy scores differed significantly from each other but the difference between Subgroups 2 and 3 was due to negative discrepancy scores for Subgroup 2. At this testing the discrepancy score of Subgroup 1 was significantly greater than that of Subgroups 2 or 3. Following this fourth follow-up testing, the groups did not differ with regard to their discrepancy scores (see Table 4).

Stage Findings
The patient sample was divided into severity groupings (i.e., stage levels) on the basis of CDR ratings. A Pearson product-moment correlation computed for the entire Q-sample ($N = 720$) between CDR stage and initial BNT/PRAX discrepancy scores (i.e., from the initial assessment), suggested no relationship between these two variables [$r = .06$, $p = .14$; $n = 720$]. Following this, separate Pearson correlations between CDR ratings and initial discrepancy scores were calculated for each subgroup. These coefficients revealed significant (yet modest) negative correlations for Subgroups 1 [$r = −.18$, $p < .01$; $n = 312$] and 3 [$r = −.24$, $p < .01$; $n = 161$], and a significant positive correlation for Subgroup 2 [$r = .23$, $p < .01$; $n = 247$], suggesting that with more severe dementia in terms of stage, discrepancy scores decline for Subgroups 1 and 3, but not Subgroup 2.

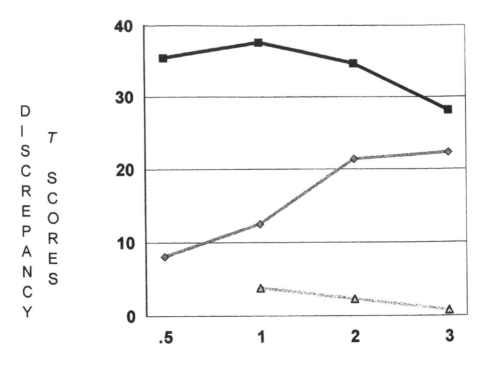

CLINICAL DEMENTIA RATING (CDR) SCORE

Fig. 10. Plots of initial BNT/PRAX mean discrepancy scores by CDR stage for each subgroup. BNT = Boston Naming Test; PRAX = Contructional Praxis; Q1 ■ = Subgroup 1; Q2 ♦ = Subgroup 2; Q3 ▲ = Subgroup 3. CDR 5 = questionable dementia; CDR 1 = mildly demented; CDR 2 = moderately demented; CDR 3 = severely demented.

Next, ANOVAs comparing mean discrepancy scores across severity levels (i.e., CDR stages) for each subgroup were conducted. The analysis was significant for the Q1 subgroup [$F(3, 307) = 4.11$, $p < .05$]. A graphical plot of mean discrepancy score by CDR stage suggested that this subgroup displays a trend for consistently decreasing discrepancy scores across stages 1 (mild dementia) through 3 (severe dementia) (see Fig. 10). However, post hoc comparisons revealed the decrease in discrepancy scores to be significant only between CDR stages 1 and 3 (i.e., not between stages 1 and 2 or 2 and 3). Significant Fs were also obtained for Q2 [$F(3, 243) = 4.81$, $p < .01$] and Q3 [$F(2, 156) = 4.23$, $p < .05$]. Examination of discrepancy by stage plots (Fig. 10) suggested that the discrepancy scores of Subgroup 2 increased with CDR

stages of dementia. Paired comparisons revealed that these increases were significant ($p < .05$) between stages .5 and 2, .5 and 3, 1 and 2, and 1 and 3. With respect to Subgroup 3, discrepancy scores decreased slightly with advancing CDR stage. Post hoc comparisons revealed that these declines were significant ($p < .05$) only between stages 1 and 3.

DISCUSSION

Summary of Results

The results of this study demonstrated that reliable subgroupings of patients with *probable* AD, each displaying qualitatively distinct patterns of performance on CERAD neuropsychological measures, can be identified via Q-type factor analysis. In accordance with previous research, three patient subgroups were identified, who did not differ from each other in terms of duration of illness. Whereas all three groups displayed a similar pattern of performance on a verbal list learning task, clinically meaningful distinctions on the semantic and visual-constructional measures were evident. These subgroups resembled the hypothetical groups RAD, LAD, and GAD. LAD and GAD profiles were consistently identifiable across time. The RAD profile demonstrated less stability across assessments, although some cases did demonstrate consistency of their initial pattern. Analyses of the control data revealed two subgroups, which did not resemble those of the patients. This suggests that the above three-subgroup classification is unique to AD, not merely attributable to patterns of strengths and weaknesses found among normal elderly individuals.

Evaluation of Hypotheses

The first hypothesis of this study predicted that the current sample of patients with *probable* AD could be reliably differentiated into three empirically derived neuropsychological subgroups. This hypothesis was fully supported: the Q-factor analysis and the hierarchical techniques all clearly indicated three subgroups of patients. Furthermore, when the K-Means procedure was run with k set at 3, the resulting subgroups resembled those produced by the Q-factor analysis and the hierarchical agglomerative techniques.

It was further hypothesized (hypothesis 2) that the three patient subgroups would be distinguishable on the basis of performance in two domains of neuropsychological functioning: visual-constructional ability and semantic knowledge accessibility. In this regard, it was expected that in accord with past research (Fisher et al., 1996; Martin et al., 1986), the three subgroups of AD patients would resemble the theoretical ideal types (Fisher, Rourke, Bieliauskas, et al., 1997) (a) GAD, those with global impairment (i.e., impaired access to semantic knowledge and impaired visual-constructional functioning); (b) LAD, those with impaired ability to access semantic knowledge, but relatively unimpaired visual-constructional functioning; and (c) RAD, those with relatively spared accessibility of semantic knowledge but impaired visual-constructional functioning.

This second hypothesis was also supported; the three subgroups did indeed resemble the hypothetical subtypes outlined above with respect to their performance patterns on visual-constructional and confrontational naming measures. Subgroup 1 resembled LAD. Patients in this group earned a mean naming T score of 4 (severely impaired) and a mean T score of 40 (borderline-normal) on the constructional praxis measure. Subgroup 2 earned mean T scores of 45 (average) and 30 (mildly-moderately impaired), on the naming and constructional measures respectively, displaying a pattern consistent with RAD. The third subgroup clearly resembled GAD, earning mean T scores of 2 on both measures, indicating severe impairment in both the naming and visual-constructional domains.

The RAD subgroup performed significantly better than the other subgroups on the Animal Verbal Fluency task, which is not inconsistent with hypothesis 2. However, all three subgroups displayed impairment on this measure. This finding of impairment across the subgroups on animal name generation accords with those of previous studies (e.g., Fisher et al., 1996). It appears that performance on this task becomes quickly impaired for members of all AD subgroups, perhaps for different neuropsychological reasons (see Fisher, Rourke, Bieliauskas, et al., 1997, for discussion).

Hypothesis 3 predicted that the non-demented comparison group employed in this investigation would not display neuropsychological patterns resembling those of the LAD and RAD patient subgroups. Whereas it was expected that normal elderly might show different patterns of relative strengths and weaknesses on memory measures (Mitrushina et al., 1995), it was predicted that their level of performance in the visual-constructional and semantic knowledge realms would remain within the same range of functioning. This hypothesis was generally supported. Unlike that with the patient sample, the Q-analysis of the control data was largely unsuccessful, classifying less than half the sample into two subgroups. These two subgroups did not resemble those derived from the patient data. With respect to the semantic and visual constructional measures, the control subgroups displayed patterns of flat lines, revealing equivalent (and normal) levels of performance in the two domains. The flat lines ran across all three non-memory measures (i.e., BNT, VF, PRAX), rendering the control profiles dissimilar even to the GAD profile. (The GAD profile had a peak on VF.)

The comparison group profiles on the memory measures were not flat, with both control subgroups performing best on recognition, then delayed recall, and least well on the immediate recall measure. This pattern is inconsistent with that observed for the three patient subgroups, in which delayed verbal recall was slightly better than immediate recall and recognition performance, although all three were severely impaired. It should be noted that control Subgroup 1 performed within the impaired range on the immediate recall measure, an unexpected finding. This subgroup appeared to perform relatively better on the visual constructional and semantic tasks as compared to their performance on the memory measures. Subgroup 2 was characterized by a relatively flat profile, with slightly better performance on the memory measures compared to the semantic and visual-constructional variables.

The final hypothesis (i.e., hypothesis 4) concerned the specific progression patterns of AD for each subgroup. It was predicted that, in the early and middle period of the disease, the initial impairment pattern of each subgroup would remain consistently identifiable. It was expected that those with the GAD pattern would continue to show impairment in both the semantic knowledge and visual-constructional realms of functioning, consistently exhibiting a pattern of relatively equivalent decline in the two domains.

Those with RAD were expected to continue to show sparing of semantic knowledge accessibility for a period of time, and though impairment in this domain was theorized to eventually occur, it was predicted to be relatively less severe than that of visual-constructional functioning, until late in the disease, when all functioning is profoundly disrupted. The prediction for patients with LAD was the opposite of that for the RAD group. Those classified with LAD were expected to initially display visual-constructional functioning within normal limits, in the face of difficulty in the area of semantic knowledge accessibility. Although with time and progression of the disease, visual-constructional functioning was expected to eventually decline into

the impaired range, it was predicted to continue to be relatively less severely affected than word finding ability, until the latest period of the disease. Indeed, it was expected that late in the disease course, all three subgroups would be rendered indistinguishably globally impaired as floor effects of the neuropsychological measures were reached.

Operationally, it was predicted that longitudinal analyses of performance discrepancies between semantic and visual-constructional functioning would reveal that such discrepancies diminish over time for the RAD and LAD groups only, but remain relatively consistent for the GAD group. Similarly, it was expected that cross-sectional analyses of discrepancies between the two domains for each CDR stratification would reveal stable discrepancies across stage for the GAD subgroup, and declining discrepancies for the RAD and LAD subgroups with successive stages.

This set of hypotheses was largely supported for the GAD and LAD groups. The performance of the GAD subgroup on the naming and visual-constructional measures remained consistent across testing sessions. This was apparent upon examination of the performances of randomly selected GAD patients across time, in addition to inspection of the mean naming and constructional performance patterns of this subgroup at each testing session. As well, correlations computed between discrepancy scores and assessment number were not significant for this subgroup, suggesting minimal change over time from the initial pattern. With respect to the cross-sectional analysis of discrepancy scores across CDR stage, the GAD subgroup showed a significant yet slight decrease in discrepancy scores with advanced stage. Post hoc inspection of these data suggests that this finding was contributed to by floor effects.

The discrepancy findings for the LAD subgroup were in accord with those predicted. Examination of the individual profiles from the randomly selected subgroup members revealed consistent PRAX > BNT patterns across assessment intervals. The mean performance patterns of this subgroup at each testing session also displayed consistent patterns of relatively superior constructional as opposed to semantic functioning. Correlations computed between assessment number and discrepancy scores were significantly negative for this subgroup, suggesting declining discrepancies with progression of the disease. With respect to the cross-sectional analysis of discrepancy scores across CDR stage, the LAD subgroup showed a significant yet slight decrease in discrepancy scores with advanced stage.

The longitudinal and cross-sectional discrepancy findings for the RAD group were generally inconsistent with those predicted. Examination of the individual profiles from the 5 randomly selected subgroup members revealed consistent BNT > PRAX patterns across assessment intervals for 2 of the subjects; only 2 of the 5 subjects retained their initially normal level of naming performance at the 1st year follow-up assessment. This finding is in distinct contrast to that of the LAD subgroup; 80% of the randomly selected LAD cases retained their PRAX performance within normal limits for at least one year following the initial assessment.

Examination of the mean performances of the RAD subgroup at each follow-up testing session revealed only minimally superior semantic as opposed to constructional functioning up until follow-up assessment 4. After the fourth assessment, the scores of this subgroup demonstrated a reversal effect, with PRAX performance becoming superior to BNT. Correlations computed between assessment number and discrepancy scores were significantly negative for this subgroup, but were confounded by negative discrepancy scores following the fourth assessment. Thus, although the discrepancy scores did decrease in the expected direction up until the fourth assessment, after this testing, negative scores were obtained, as mean PRAX performance became superior to mean BNT performance. With respect to the cross-sectional analysis of discrepancy scores across CDR stage, the RAD subgroup displayed an increase in discrepancy scores with advanced stage, a clearly unexpected finding.

Compared to RAD and GAD, the LAD subgroup had a significantly larger initial discrepancy score and maintained this discrepancy spread across time, up until the fifth follow-up assessment. RAD on the other hand, had a mean initial discrepancy score falling between that of LAD and GAD. However, the RAD group did not retain this midway status. From assessment 2 onward, the discrepancy

scores of the RAD group (when in the expected direction) were not significantly different from those of the GAD subgroup. This finding was in stark contradiction to that predicted for the RAD group, as members of this group (as LAD) were expected to retain their initial pattern of discrepancy for a period of time. Clearly, they were not expected to show comparable discrepancy scores to the GAD group. At the 6th and 7th year follow-up examinations, there were no between-subgroup differences in discrepancy scores. This is in accord with the prediction that eventually all three groups would become indistinguishable, as global impairment is reached in the later phases of the disease.

In sum, it appears that whereas the longitudinal findings for the LAD and GAD subgroups were in accord with prediction, the progression patterns of the RAD subgroup did not conform to those expected (Fisher, Rourke, & Bieliauskas, 1997). Nevertheless, it should be pointed out that some members of the RAD subgroup did indeed retain their presenting pattern of normal word-finding ability within the context of impaired visual-construction across time, and did not demonstrate rapid decline in the initially preserved naming domain or an eventual reversal effect. It appears that the RAD group is itself heterogeneous. Indeed, the within-subgroup variability of discrepancy scores was much higher for this subgroup as compared to the others. Clearly, further research on the RAD subgroup in and of itself is necessary to sort out the apparent variability within this group of patients.

The cross-sectional CDR findings also generally supported hypothesis 4 for LAD and GAD but not RAD. Both the LAD and GAD groups showed a mild decline in discrepancy scores with advancing CDR stage. These findings are in accord with prediction for LAD, which was expected to show less of a discrepancy with advancement of cognitive deterioration, as both domains become affected and global impairment eventuates. It was not expected that GAD discrepancy scores would decrease with advancing CDR stage, but post hoc inspection of the data revealed that scores in both domains reached floors at higher CDR stages, decreasing variability and thus leading to lower mean discrepancies. The finding for the RAD group that discrepancy scores increase with successive CDR stage was clearly unexpected and inconsistent with prediction. Research focussing on the RAD group alone, to sort out the variability within this group, should shed light on this seemingly peculiar cross-sectional finding which would appear in discord with the longitudinal findings for this group.

Integration with the Literature

The three patient subgroups identified in this study are consistent with those reported in earlier studies employing similar measures and at times differing methodologies (Becker et al., 1988; Fisher et al., 1996; Martin et al., 1986; Strite et al., 1997), suggesting robustness of these findings. The current finding that the subgroups did not differ in terms of mean duration of illness is also consistent with the results of previous studies (Becker et al., 1988; Fisher et al., 1996; Martin et al., 1986). Similarly, the finding that the GAD subgroup is more impaired in terms of overall dementia severity compared to the other two subgroups is also consistent with earlier reports (Becker et al., 1988; Fisher et al., 1996).

However, there were some findings of this study that are inconsistent with those of earlier similar research. Namely, past studies have reported no differences between the three subgroups with respect to age (Fisher et al., 1996; Martin et al., 1986; Strite et al., 1997) and educational attainment (Fisher et al., 1996; Martin, 1990; Strite et al., 1997). The current study, however, found the LAD group to be older and less educated than the other two subgroups. Previous studies have also reported that the RAD and LAD groups do not differ from each other in terms of MMSE scores (Fisher et al., 1996; Strite et al., 1997) or functional ADL measures (i.e., Blessed Test; Fisher et al., 1996). In contrast, although the current study found that the GAD group was indeed more impaired than both the RAD and LAD groups on the MMSE and Blessed tests, the LAD group was noted to be more impaired on these measures relative to the RAD group.

These discrepancies from past research may be related to the relatively small sample sizes employed in previous studies, which may have failed to detect the above-mentioned intersubgroup differences. The CERAD sample is much larger (i.e., at least six times larger than any previously

employed sample) and more representative (e.g., in terms of geography, age, and educational levels) than past samples, making findings from the current investigation much more powerful. This may perhaps explain the earlier reports of nonsignificant findings regarding age, education, and overall impairment differences between the subgroups, yet occasional mention of trends in the direction consistent with the findings of the current study (e.g., Becker et al., 1988; Fisher et al., 1996).

It should also be mentioned that, in their study of normal elderly persons in which LAD- and RAD-like preclinical AD groups were identified, Mitrushina et al. (1995) found their LAD- like group to have lower MMSE scores and to be less educated and older than any other subgroup. The current finding that the LAD group scored significantly lower compared to the RAD group on the MMSE may be related to the LAD group's lower educational level and older mean age; age and educational attainment have been shown to be related to MMSE scores (Crum, Anthony, Bassett, & Folstein, 1993; Marcopulos, McLain, & Giuliano, 1997; Tombaugh, McDowell, Krisjansson, & Hubley, 1996). This difference may not have been detected in earlier studies due to the higher mean educational levels and more restrictive age ranges of past samples in comparison to the current sample.

The findings of this study also vary with regard to those of earlier studies in terms of the size of each patient subgroup. Strite et al. (1997) made a point of emphasizing a need for incidence data regarding the three AD subgroups. For comparative purposes, percentages of the samples classified into each subgroup in the current and past subgrouping studies are presented in Table 5. It can be seen from this table that typically, in past research, the GAD subgroup was found to be the largest, followed in size by LAD and then RAD. However, in the current study, LAD was the largest subgroup, followed by RAD and then GAD. These inconsistent incidence rates are difficult to explain.

Whereas all of the studies included in Table 5 employed samples of only those individuals diagnosed with *probable* AD, there were differences across studies in the measures and methodologies employed. Namely, none of the studies aside from the current one and the Fisher et al. (1996) investigation removed outliers from their sample, forcing

Table 5. Comparison of Incidence Rates of the Three Subgroups Across Studies.

Subgroup	Becker et al. (1988)		Fisher et al. (1996)		Strite et al. (1997)		Current Sample	
	n/N	%	n/N	%	n/N	%	n/N	%
GAD	71/86	82.60	45/134	33.58	111/153	72.55	161/960	16.77
LAD	11/86	12.79	29/134	21.64	16/153	10.46	312/960	32.50
RAD	4/86	4.65	23/134	17.16	26/153	16.99	247/960	25.73

Note. n = number of subjects assigned to the subgroup; N = total number of subjects in the sample; % = percent of sample classified into each subgroup; GAD = Global Alzheimer's Disease; LAD = Left Alzheimer's Disease; RAD = Right Alzheimer's Disease.
[Data from the Martin et al. (1986) study are not provided here as the sample employed in that research was preselected to include those with focal patterns.]

all subjects into one of the three subgroups. Furthermore, the Becker et al. (1988) and Strite et al. (1997) subgrouping methodologies involved discrepancy indexes, which are not truly objective classification techniques. This may account for some of the variability across studies. However, the methodology employed in the current investigation was identical to that utilized in the Fisher et al. (1996) study, yet the incidence rates across these two studies still vary, with GAD reported as the largest subgroup in the 1996 study, and the smallest subgroup in the current investigation. Thus, these differences must be due to factors other than classificatory methodology.

The current study used neuropsychological measures which were briefer and hence possibly less reliable/valid than those of past studies (Larrain & Cimino, 1999). On the other hand, the current sample was much larger, spanning many geographical regions, perhaps leading to increased accuracy of incidence rates. In support of this possibility, it should be noted that Joanette, Ska, Poissant, and Beland (1992), in reviewing their comprehensive multiple single-subject research on patients with AD, noted homogeneous impairment across cognitive domains as apparent in only a minority of patients. As an alternate explanation, it may be that the GAD group is underrepresented in the current sample due to terms of involvement in the CERAD project. These terms require agreement to return for follow-up evaluations. Those with GAD, being the most impaired, may have been less willing to agree to these terms.

With respect to the relative sizes of the LAD and RAD subgroups, the current findings are in accord with those of two-thirds of past studies

which report that LAD is more prevalent than RAD (see Table 5). This finding is also consistent with neuroimaging reports which suggest that left hemisphere dysfunction is more common than right hemisphere dysfunction among those with AD (Jamieson et al., 1987; Lowenstein et al., 1989). It must be remembered however, as pointed out by Strite et al. (1997), that incidence rates reported in subgrouping studies do not reflect the general AD population at large. Given the nature of the referral patterns to university clinics, it may be that certain presentations of AD are more likely to be referred for evaluation (i.e., those with predominant language impairments). As well, individuals who agree to participate in research studies are clearly not representative of the population at large.

There is little past research with which to compare the longitudinal and stage findings of the current study. Martin et al. (1990) and Fisher et al. (1997) reported stable subgroup patterns in small numbers of patients studied individually, and similar findings were reported herein for the randomly selected cases from each subgroup. No previous attempt has been made to study larger numbers of members from each subgroup over significant time periods. In general, the current findings of stability of the mean GAD and LAD profiles over time are consistent with the earlier case reports.

The longitudinal findings for the RAD patients are less consistent with these earlier case reports, and the reversal effect noted after the fourth testing has not been previously documented. It may be that in the current study, the small numbers of subjects returning after the fourth assessment, and the selective drop-out factors influencing those who did not return, have served to distort the mean profile of the RAD group. It may also be that the PRAX measure has a higher floor than the BNT measure or that the task becomes overlearned. Moreover, it is probable that, as mentioned previously, the RAD group is a heterogeneous group in itself. It is clear from case examples in the current and past investigations that some members of the RAD group retain their initial pattern over the first few years. It appears though from the current findings that many do not, and a GAD pattern may quickly emerge. Thus, there may be a more rapid variant of RAD.

This is a reasonable speculation; there have been several reports in the literature suggesting rapidly and slowly progressive forms or variants of AD (e.g., Jacobs et al., 1994; Salmon, Lineweaver, Galasko, & Hansen, 1998), including a study reporting that patients with temporal lobe presentations (i.e., impaired language functions in the context of spared visual-constructional skills and executive functions, akin to LAD) have a slower rate of dementia progression (Butters, Lopez, & Becker, 1996). In addition, there has been a preliminary report in the literature that as a group, patients classified as "High Verbal" (i.e., akin to RAD), show a greater rate of decline on the BNT as compared to "High Spatial" patients (i.e., akin to LAD) (Norman, Delis, Salmon, & Bigler, 1998). It may be that the High Verbal group's rate of decline in this latter study was influenced by a predominant subset of members having a more rapid variant of RAD.

Whereas no other studies have cross-sectionally investigated stability of subgroup profiles across stages of AD, there is one cross-sectional report in the literature which investigated presence of AD subgroups across stages of dementia. After identifying groups of patients with AD similar to the three subgroups reported herein, Strite et al. (1997) sought to determine whether members of the three subgroups were apparent across stages of the disease. As such, they examined the distribution of subgroup members stratified by MMSE scores into mildly, moderately, and severely demented groups. Inspection of the resultant frequency distribution revealed that members of subgroups comparable to GAD and RAD were identifiable across the different AD stage-stratified groups. However, all of their LAD-like patients ($n = 16$) were classified as moderately demented. Although replication of this result was not an original goal of the current study,

post hoc analyses using CDR ratings and MMSE scores were undertaken in this regard, as it was felt that the absence of LAD members in the mild and severe stratified groups reported by Strite et al. may have been due to the small sample size employed in that study.

Our analysis revealed that members of the three subgroups were apparent across mild, moderate, and severe (i.e., stages 1–3) CDR stages. Because of the potential difference in CDR and MMSE scores – the CDR is clinician rated and the MMSE is psychometric – and the fact that this alone could account for differences between the current findings and those of Strite et al. (1997), it was next decided to repeat the above analysis using MMSE stratification, employing the same criteria for MMSE stratification utilized in the Strite et al. study (i.e., Haxby et al., 1988). Again, patients from each of the three subgroups were classified into all three severity groups. Thus, it would appear that the subgroups are indeed apparent across stages of dementia, regardless of stratification method employed. The fact that Strite et al. found no LAD patients in their mild and severe MMSE classified groups was likely related to their small sample size; they had only 16 LAD patients, as compared to the 312 LAD patients in the current study.

Strite et al. (1997) reported asymmetric (i.e., LAD or RAD) profiles in 17.6%, 35.6%, and 13.3% of their MMSE-classified mildly, moderately, and severely demented patients, respectively. The figures for the same analysis with the current sample were: 93%, 78%, and 51%. Differences in these figures across studies are no doubt related to methodological measurement and subtyping distinctions, differential control of outliers, and sample size differences. However, it is more interesting to note that the above decreases in percentages of asymmetric profiles with successive severity of the dementia (i.e., for the current sample) supports hypothesis 4 of this study. That is, we predicted decreasing asymmetry (i.e., BNT/PRAX discrepancies) with increasing severity of dementia.

The current subgrouping findings for the control group are not inconsistent with those of Mitrushina et al. (1995) although the samples, methodologies, and measures varied, making comparisons difficult. These researchers identified a subgroup of "normals" who performed within the average range on naming and copying tasks yet demonstrated low average to mildly impaired word list recall performance. Mitrushina et al. labelled this group a memory-impaired preclinical form of AD. This group resembles the first subgroup identified in the current study in some respects.

Like the Mitrushina et al. group, the CERAD control Subgroup 1 displayed average performance on the semantic and visual constructional measures but some memory impairment. However, the pattern of memory impairment differed, as members of the CERAD control Subgroup 1 demonstrated moderately impaired immediate recall, low average delayed recall and average recognition performances. Clearly, the neuropsychological measures employed across the 2 studies were not the same and the sample characteristics varied. It is possible that these two groups are manifestations of the same process. However, given the different apparent memory pattern (measurement and sampling differences aside), other explanations are in order. This memory-impaired group in the current study may not be a preclinical form of AD but may represent a group of normals with attentional problems, as their memory pattern of impaired immediate recall performance in the face of normal delayed and recognition performance is commonly interpreted as due to attentional difficulties. This pattern is often noted among depressed elderly individuals as well (Moss & Albert, 1992). Although the normals in the current study were screened for Major Depressive Disorder, it is possible that those with milder depressive conditions were not screened out.

Limitations of Present Study

The referral patterns of the various CERAD sites have been demonstrated to provide largely white, upper-class, well-educated patients and controls (Morris et al., 1989). Hence, the results of this investigation are limited to this specific population. On the other hand, as has been previously pointed out, the large number of subjects available in the CERAD study and the multi-center nature (i.e., geographical representativeness) of the database provides diversity not possible from single center research (Galasko et al., 1995). Thus, although the generalizability of the current findings is limited by the CERAD sample characteristics, the results of studies utilizing this sample are the most representative to date.

The longitudinal portions of this study were subject to the inherent limitations of longitudinal designs (Pyke & Agnew, 1991; Rybash, Roodin, & Hoyer, 1995), namely, attrition due to selective drop out likely affected sample composition at the follow up assessment intervals. This resulted in successively smaller n's, inconsistency in subjects returning at each visit, and unequal cell sizes preventing repeated measures analyses. Practice effects may have also had an impact on the longitudinal results, as alternate test forms were not used at follow-up testing sessions.

The control sample was significantly younger and more highly educated than the patient sample, despite the fact that the ranges and distributions of each group were similar on these variables. Although age and education norms were utilized in calculating T scores for the neuropsychological measures, the current method could be improved upon by reducing the samples to equate the groups in terms of age and education; it is never known for certain whether demographic normative corrections fully control for age and education effects.

Outliers were not removed from the data prior to the cluster analytic replications of the Q-findings. As a result, it is probable that such deviant individuals may have distorted the patterns obtained in the subsequent replications. However, given that the same three patient Q-groups were identifiable across clustering approaches, algorithms, and similarity measures, it is unlikely that the outliers interfered in any significant way. Nevertheless, utilization of only those subjects classified by the Q-analyses in the cluster analytic replication attempts would likely have increased the accuracy of the replication attempts.

Conclusions and Directions for Future Research

Future research should be directed toward improving upon the above-noted limitations of the current investigation. In such a manner, this research requires replication on a more representative (i.e., of minorities and low SES groups) sample. In addition, it would be beneficial to repeat the current analyses utilizing data collected from cognitively intact normal elderly controls who more closely resemble the patients in terms of age and educational attainment, and who are more closely screened for depressive disorders and cognitive impairments. Neuroimaging studies on members of the individual subgroups would allow for external validation of the classification scheme suggested herein.

Another beneficial avenue of research would be longitudinal examination of the stability of AD subgroup profiles quantitatively. This could be accomplished with repeated Q-factor analyses conducted at each follow-up interval. In this manner, it could be determined whether patients classified into one subgroup after the initial evaluation change subgroup membership. Members of the LAD subgroup would be expected to change to a GAD pattern eventually, but the results of this study suggest continued LAD membership for some time. A subset of RAD patients would be expected to show the same pattern over time, whereas the remaining RAD patients would be predicted to quickly demonstrate a GAD pattern. One would predict that GAD patients would remain within the same subgroup throughout the course of the disease.

Given the apparent additional heterogeneity within the RAD subgroup, research efforts should be devoted to further delineating the variants of this group. It would appear that a subset of RAD patients may have a more rapidly advancing form of the disorder. This hypothesis could be evaluated by subclassifying those in the RAD group into those who have stable patterns over time and those who do not, and studying these two RAD groups separately. It would be of value to examine the performances of the variants of RAD, in addition to the performances of the GAD and LAD subgroups, on neuropsychological measures that are not semantic or visual-constructional in nature. This would assist in further elaborating the various subgroups. Yet another area requiring investigation is longitudinal following of normal elderly individuals via yearly neuropsychological evaluations. This would allow monitoring of premorbid strengths and weaknesses and determination of the extent to which such differences predict subgroup assignment with the development of AD.

Concluding Comments: Significance and Implications of the Current Findings

The fact that the three neuropsychological subgroups of patients with AD reported in the past were again identified in this project, utilizing the largest and most geographically/demographically representative AD sample studied to date, provides strong confirmatory evidence for the existence of qualitatively distinct patterns among this heterogeneous group of patients. The subgroups do not differ in terms of duration of illness. Further, they are identifiable across stages of dementia, whether staging criteria are psychometric or based on clinicians' ratings. Moreover, the initially presenting patterns remain over time for the LAD and GAD groups, in addition to a subset of RAD patients. Taken together, such results are in sharp contradiction to a strictly exclusive "stage model" approach to the conceptualization of AD, in which all patients are characterized as exhibiting global decline across domains of functioning. Whereas it is clear that the GAD subgroup does show homogeneous impairment across semantic and visual-constructional domains, members of the LAD and RAD subgroups are identifiable who demonstrate preservation in one of these areas of functioning for a significant period of time. Thus, there is evidence for different patterns of symptom progression across subgroups of patients. As such, it seems appropriate that in conceptualizing the nature of AD, one engages in a theoretical meshing of the stage and subgroup models of the disease.

It appears that the LAD subgroup is older and less educated than the other two groups, suggesting that age at disease onset and educational attainment may have an impact on neuropsychological presentation. In regard to the former, past CERAD research has suggested that those with a younger age of AD onset perform worse on constructional praxis and better on confrontational naming tasks as compared to those with a later age of onset, and that younger patients appear to decline more rapidly on all CERAD neuropsychological measures (Koss et al., 1996).

Non-CERAD studies have also suggested that those with younger age of AD onset evidence more rapid cognitive decline and better baseline naming performance as compared to those with older ages of onset (Jacobs et al., 1994). In addition, neuroimaging and neurochemical investigations have suggested differences between early- and late-onset patients with AD (Koss, Friedland,

Ober, & Jagust, 1985; Rossor, Iversen, Reynolds, Mountjoy & Roth, 1984). For example, Koss et al. (1985) reported a greater likelihood of right than left hemisphere metabolic reductions in early onset cases, and Rossor and colleagues (1984) noted that neurochemical changes in late onset cases were most predominant in the temporal lobe, whereas the neurotransmitter deficits in early onset cases were more diffuse and severe. All of these findings are in accord with the results of the current investigation, and suggest that age of onset is a potentially important subgrouping variable which may overlap with naming/constructional discrepancies.

REFERENCES

Afifi, A.A., & Clark, V. (1990). *Computer-aided multivariate analysis* (2nd ed.). Los Angeles, CA: Van Nostrand Reinhold.

Aldenderfer, M.S., & Blashfield, R.K. (1984). *Cluster analysis.* Beverly Hills: Sage.

Atkinson, R.C., & Shiffrin, R.M. (1971). The control of short-term memory. *Scientific American, 221,* 82–90.

Berg, L. (1984). Clinical dementia rating. *British Journal of Psychiatry, 145,* 339.

Becker, J.T., Huff, J.F., Nebes, R.D., Holland, A., & Boller, F. (1988). Neuropsychological function in Alzheimer's disease: Pattern of impairment and rates of progression. *Archives of Neurology, 45,* 263–268.

Blashfield, R.K., & Aldenderfer, M.S. (1988). The methods and problems of cluster analysis. In J.R. Nesselroade & R.B. Cattell (Eds.), *Handbook of multivariate experimental psychology* (pp. 447–473). (2nd ed.). New York: Plenum Press.

Blessed, G., Tomlinson, B.E., & Roth, M. (1968). The association between quantitative measures of dementia and senile change in the cerebral grey matter of elderly subjects. *British Journal of Psychiatry, 114,* 797–811.

Butters, M.A., Lopez, O.L., & Becker, J.T. (1996). Focal temporal lobe dysfunction in probable Alzheimer's disease predicts a slow rate of cognitive decline. *Neurology, 46,* 687–692.

Campbell, D.T., & Fiske, D.W. (1959). Convergent and discriminant validation by the multitrait-multimethod matrix. *Psychological Bulletin, 56,* 81–105.

Consortium to Establish a Registry for Alzheimer's Disease. (1996). *Manual of operations: Consortium to establish a registry for Alzheimer's disease (CERAD).* Unpublished CD-ROM documentation. Durham, NC: Duke University Medical Center.

Crum, R.M., Anthony, J.C., Bassett, S.S., & Folstein, M.F. (1993). Population-based norms for the Mini-Mental State Examination by age and educational level. *Journal of the American Medical Association, 269,* 2386–2391.

Del Dotto, J.E., & Rourke, B.P. (1985). Subtypes of left-handed learning-disabled children. In B.P. Rourke, *Neuropsychology of learning disabilities: Essentials of subtype analysis* (pp. 89–130). New York: The Guilford Press.

Edelbrock, C. (1979). Mixture model tests of hierarchical clustering algorithms: The problem of classifying everybody. *Multivariate Behavioral Research, 14,* 367–384.

Everitt, B.S., & Dunn, G. (1991). Cluster analysis. In B.S. Everitt & G. Dunn, *Applied multivariate data analysis* (pp. 99–125). London: Edward Arnold.

Fisher, N.J., Rourke, B.P., & Bieliauskas, L.A. (1997). *Heterogeneity of Alzheimer's disease: Literature review and early neuropsychological model building.* Manuscript submitted for publication.

Fisher, N.J., Rourke, B.P., Bieliauskas, L.A., Giordani, B., Berent, S., & Foster, N. (1996). Neuropsychological subgroups of patients with Alzheimer's disease. *Journal of Clinical and Experimental Neuropsychology, 18,* 349–370.

Fisher, N.J., Rourke, B.P., Bieliauskas, L.A., Giordani, B., Berent, S., & Foster, N.L. (1997). Unmasking the heterogeneity of Alzheimer's disease: Case studies of individuals from distinct neuropsychological subgroups. *Journal of Clinical and Experimental Neuropsychology, 19,* 713–754.

Fletcher, J. (1985). External validation of learning disability typologies. In B.P. Rourke (Ed.), *Neuropsychology of learning disabilities: Essentials of subtype analysis* (pp. 187–211). New York: Guilford.

Folstein, M.F., Folstein, S.E., & McHugh, P.R. (1975). "Mini-Mental State": A practical method for grading the cognitive state of patients for the clinician. *Journal of Psychiatric Research, 12,* 189–198.

Fuerst, D.R., Fisk, J.L., & Rourke, B.P. (1989). Psychosocial functioning of learning-disabled children: Replicability of statistically derived subtypes. *Journal of Consulting and Clinical Psychology, 57,* 275–280.

Galasko, D., Edland, S.D., Morris, J.C., Clark, C., Mohs, R., & Koss, E. (1995). The Consortium to Establish a Registry for Alzheimer's Disease (CERAD): Part XI. Clinical milestones in patients with Alzheimer's disease followed over 3 years. *Neurology, 45,* 1451–1455.

Hair, J.F., Anderson, R.E., Tatham, R.L., & Black, W.C. (1992). *Multivariate data analysis* (3rd ed.). New York: Macmillan.

Haxby, J.V., Grady, C.L., Koss, E., Horwitz, B., Schapiro, M., Friedland, R.P., & Rapoport, S.I. (1988). Heterogeneous anterior-posterior patterns in dementia of the Alzheimer type. *Neurology, 38,* 1853–1863.

Heyman, A. (1996). *CERAD 1986–1996: Consortium to establish a registry for Alzheimer's disease* (Archive Rev 1.0) [CD-ROM data]. Seattle, WA: CERAD Methodology and Data Management Center, University of Washington [Producer]. Durham, NC: Duke University Medical Center [Distributor].

Howell, D.C. (1992). *Statistical methods for psychology* (3rd ed.). Belmont, CA: Duxbury Press.

Hughes, C.P., Berg, L., Danziger, W., Coben, L.A., & Martin, R.L. (1982). A new clinical scale for the staging of dementia. *British Journal of Psychiatry, 140*, 566–572.

Isaacs, B., & Kennie, A.T. (1973). The set test as an aid to the detection of dementia in old people. *British Journal of Psychiatry, 123*, 467–470.

Jaccard, J., Becker, M.A., & Wood, G. (1984). Pairwise multiple comparison procedures: A review. *Psychological Bulletin, 96*, 589–596.

Jacobs, D., Sano, M., Marder, K., Bell, K., Bylsma, F., Lafleche, G., Albert, M., Brandt, J., & Stern, Y. (1994). Age at onset of Alzheimer's disease: Relation to pattern of cognitive dysfunction and rate of decline. *Neurology, 44*, 1215–1220.

Jamieson, D.G., Chawluk, J.B., Alavi, A., Hurtig, H.I., Rosen, M., Bais, S., Dann, R., Kushner, M., & Reivich, M. (1987). The effect of disease severity on local cerebral glucose metabolism in Alzheimer's disease. *Journal of Cerebral Blood Flow and Metabolism, 7*, S410.

Joanette, Y., Ska, B., Poissant, A., & Beland, R. (1992). Neuropsychological aspects of Alzheimer's disease: Evidence for inter- and intra-function heterogeneity. In F. Boller, F. Forette, Z. Khachaturian, M. Poncet, & Y. Christen (Eds.), *Heterogeneity of Alzheimer's disease* (pp. 33–42). Berlin: Springer-Verlag.

Kaplan, E.F., Goodglass, H., & Weintraub, S. (1978). *The Boston Naming Test.* Boston, MA: Veterans Administration Medical Center.

Koss, E., Edland, M.S., Fillenbaum, G., Mohs, R., Clark, C., Galasko, D., & Morris, J.C. (1996). Clinical and neuropsychological differences between patients with earlier and later onset of Alzheimer's disease. *Neurology, 46*, 136–141.

Koss, E., Friedland, R.P., Ober, B.A., & Jagust, W.J. (1985). Differentiation of lateral hemispheric asymmetries of glucose utilization between early- and late-onset Alzheimer type dementia. *American Journal of Psychiatry, 142*, 638–640.

Larrain, C., & Cimino, C. (1998a). Factor analysis of CERAD battery in Alzheimer's disease. *Journal of the International Neuropsychological Society, 4*, 30.

Larrain, C., & Cimino, C. (1999). Alternate forms of the Boston Naming Test in Alzheimer's disease. *The Clinical Neuropsychologist, 12*, 525–530.

Lowenstein, D.A., Barker, W.W., Chang, J.Y., Apicella, A., Yoshii, F., Kothari, P., Levin, B., & Duara, R. (1989). Predominant left hemisphere metabolic dysfunction in dementia. *Archives of Neurology, 46*, 146–152.

MacQueen, J.B. (1967). Some methods for classification and analysis of multivariate observations. *Proceedings of the fifth Berkeley Symposium on Mathematical Statistics and Probability, 1*, 281–297.

Marcopulos, B.A., McLain, C.A., & Giuliano, A.J., (1997). Cognitive impairment or inadequate norms? A study of healthy, rural, older adults with limited education. *The Clinical Neuropsychologist, 11*, 111–131.

Martin, A. (1990). Neuropsychology of Alzheimer's disease: The case for subgroups. In M.F. Schwartz (Ed.), *Modular Deficits in Alzheimer-Type Dementia.* (pp. 144–175). Cambridge, MA: The MIT Press.

Martin, A., Brouwers, P., Lalonde, F., Cox, C., Teleska, P., Fedio, P., Foster, N.L., & Chase, T.N. (1986). Towards a behavioral typology of Alzheimer's patients. *Journal of Clinical and Experimental Neuropsychology, 8*, 594–610.

McKeown, B., & Thomas, D. (1988). *Q methodology.* Sage University Paper series on Quantitative Applica- tions in the Social Sciences, 07-066. Beverly Hills, CA: Sage.

McKhann, G., Drachman, D., Folstein, M., Katzman, R., Price, D., & Stadlan, E.M. (1984). Clinical diagnosis of Alzheimer's disease: Report of the NINCDS-ADRDA work group under the auspices of the Department of Health and Human Services Task Force on Alzheimer's disease. *Neurology, 34*, 939–944.

Mitrushina, M., Uchiyama, C., & Satz, P. (1995). Heterogeneity of cognitive profiles in normal aging: Implications for early manifestations of Alzheimer's disease. *Journal of Clinical and Experimental Neuropsychology, 17*, 374–382.

Morris, J.C. (1993). The Clinical Dementia Rating (CDR): Current version and scoring rules. *Neurology, 43*, 2412–2414.

Morris, J.C., Heyman, A., Mohs, R.C., Hughes, J.P., van Belle, G., Fillenbaum, G., Mellits, E.D., & Clark, C. (1989). The Consortium to Establish a Registry for Alzheimer's Disease (CERAD): Part I. Clinical and neuropsychological assessment of Alzheimer's disease. *Neurology, 39*, 1159–1165.

Moss, M.B., & Albert, M.S. (1992). Neuropsychology of Alzheimer's disease. In R.F. White (Ed.), *Clinical syndromes in adult neuropsychology: The practitioner's handbook* (pp. 305–343). Amsterdam: Elsevier.

Norman, M.A., Delis, D.C., Salmon, D., & Bigler, E.D. (1998). Differential rates of cognitive decline in subgroups of Alzheimer's patients. *Journal of the International Neuropsychological Society, 4*, 31.

Price, B.H., Gurvit, H., Weintraub, S., Geula, C., Leimkuhler, E., & Mesulam, M. (1993). Neuropsychological patterns and language deficits in 20 consecutive cases of autopsy-confirmed Alzheimer's disease. *Archives of Neurology, 50*, 931–937.

Pyke, S.W., & Agnew, N.McK. (1991). The science game: An introduction to research in the social sciences. (5th ed.). Hillsdale, NJ: Prentice Hall.

Rosen, W.G., Mohs, R.C., & Davis, K.L. (1984). A new rating scale for Alzheimer's disease. *American Journal of Psychiatry, 141*, 1356–1364.

Rossor, M.N., Iversen, L.L., Reynolds, G.P., Mountjoy, C.Q., & Roth, M. (1984). Neurochemical characteristics of early and late onset types of Alzheimer's disease. *British Medical Journal, 288*, 961–964.

Rybash, J.M., Roodin, P.A., & Hoyer, W.J. (1995). *Adult development and aging* (3rd ed.). Madison, WI: Brown & Benchmark.

Salmon, D.P., Lineweaver, T., Galasko, D., & Hansen, L. (1998). Patterns of cognitive decline in patients with autopsy-verified lewy body variant of Alzheimer's disease. *Journal of the International Neuropsychological Society, 4*, 228.

Sneath, P., & Sokal, R. (1973). *Numerical taxonomy.* San Francisco: Freeman.

Sokal, R., & Michener, C.D. (1958). A statistical method for evaluating systematic relationships. *University of Kansas Scientific Bulletin, 38*, 1409–1438.

Strite, D., Massman, P.J., Cooke, N., & Doody, R.S. (1997). Neuropsychological asymmetry in Alzheimer's disease: Verbal versus visuoconstructional deficits

across stages of dementia. *Journal of the International Neuropsychological Society, 3*, 420–427.

Tabachnick, B.G., & Fidell, L.S. (1989). *Using multivariate statistics* (2nd ed.). New York: Harper-Collins.

Tombaugh, T.N., McDowell, I., Krisjansson, B., & Hubley, A.M. (1996). Mini-Mental State Examination (MMSE) and the Modified MMSE (3MS): A psychometric comparison and normative data. *Psychological Assessment, 8*, 48–59.

Valdois, S., Joanette, Y., Poissant, A., Ska, B., & Dehaut, F. (1990). Heterogeneity in the cognitive profile of normal elderly. *Journal of Clinical and Experimental Neuropsychology, 12*, 587–596.

Ward, J.H. (1963). Hierarchical grouping to optimize on objective function. *Journal of the American Statistical Association, 58*, 236–244.

Welsh, K.A., Butters, N., Hughes, J.P., Mohs, R.C., & Heyman, A. (1992). Detection and staging of dementia in Alzheimer's disease: Use of the neuropsychological measures developed for the Consortium to Establish a Registry for Alzheimer's disease. *Archives of Neurology, 49*, 448–452.

Welsh, K.A., Butters, N., Mohs, R.C., Beekly, D., Edland, S., Fillenbaum, G., & Heyman, A. (1994). The Consortium to Establish a Registry for Alzheimer's Disease (CERAD). Part V. A normative study of the neuropsychological battery. *Neurology, 44*, 609–614.

Child Neuropsychology
1995, Vol. 1, No. 1, pp. 38–55

Psychosocial Functioning of Children with Learning Disabilities at Three Age Levels*

Darren R. Fuerst[1,2] and Byron P. Rourke[2,3]

[1]Harper Hospital, Detroit Michigan, and [2]University of Windsor, and [3]Yale University

ABSTRACT

In this study, the relationship between age and patterns of psychosocial functioning was investigated in a sample of 728 children with learning disabilities (LD). In the first part of the study, Young (7–8 years), Middle (9–10 years), and Old (11–13 years) children were subtyped by cluster analysis applied to scores on the Personality Inventory for Children (PIC). The subtypes that emerged at each age level were similar to those found in our previous research, and were comparable at each age level. In the second part of the study, children were classified within a PIC-based psychosocial typology developed in previous studies. When the subtypes were broken down by age category, the mean PIC profiles of Young, Middle, and Old children did not differ substantially in shape or elevation, and the proportions of Young, Middle, and Old children in each subtype were comparable. These results suggest that patterns of psychosocial functioning of children with LD are stable across ages 7–13 years and, overall, do not show increased psychopathology with increased age.

In a recent review of the literature regarding psychosocial functioning of children with learning disabilities (LD; Rourke & Fuerst, 1991) we noted that, even when our search was restricted to papers published in the last two decades, we uncovered more than 700 articles. Clearly, this is an issue of some interest to both clinicians and researchers. Of those 700 or so papers, most proposed some causal link between LD and socioemotional functioning – specifically, that LD produces disrupted or aberrant psychosocial functioning. This general proposition, dubbed *Hypothesis 2*[1] by Rourke

for historical reasons, has a compelling, tacit appeal for most clinicians. It appears to make good clinical sense to maintain that youngsters with LD who persist in their learning problems throughout the elementary school years will be the unwilling (and, perhaps, unwitting) butt of criticism and negative evaluations by parents, teachers, and age-mates; that these criticisms will serve to render such children more anxious and less self-assured in learning situations; that a vicious circle will develop that increasingly hampers academic success and encourages progressively more debilitating degrees of anxiety and other forms of psychopathology; that this sort of undesirable situation is virtually inevitable and would be expected to increase in severity as the child fails to make advances in learning.

It is clear that *Hypothesis 2* approaches have engendered a remarkable volume of research. Considered overall, however, these studies have added little to our understanding of the psychosocial functioning of children with LD because the results

---

[1] In *Hypothesis 1* approaches, problems with learning are thought to be caused by disordered psychosocial functioning. Note that, in such cases, the problems in learning are not considered to be "learning disabilities" by contemporary definitions. In *Hypothesis 3* approaches, both particular patterns of learning problems and psychosocial problems are thought to result from particular patterns of cognitive deficits and strengths. See Rourke and Fuerst (1991) for details.

---

*Address for reprint requests: Darren R. Fuerst HA1-6204, Psychology Department, Harper Hospital, 3990 John R. Detroit, MI 48201, USA.
Accepted for publication: November 21, 1994.

of most studies are confused, contradictory, and unreplicable (Rourke & Fuerst, 1991). This is due, in part, to failure to take into account the heterogeneity of children with LD beyond post-hoc excuses for unexpected findings. In our own laboratory, we have sought to study heterogeneity of children with LD by examining systematically patterns of personality and psychosocial functioning, and by developing a psychosocial typology through the use of multivariate subtyping methods.

Our previous studies (Fuerst, Fisk, & Rourke, 1989, 1990; Fuerst & Rourke, 1993; Porter & Rourke, 1985) have been detailed in other sources (e.g., Rourke & Fuerst, 1991) and, in the interests of brevity, lengthy descriptions will not be repeated here. Briefly, in our previous studies we have applied multivariate statistical subtyping techniques (Q-factor analysis and cluster analysis) to the Personality Inventory for Children (PIC; Wirt, Lachar, Klinedinst, & Seat, 1977) scores of children with LD. In these studies, we have identified seven subtypes that we refer to as Normal, Mild Anxiety, Mild Hyperactive, Somatic Concern, Conduct Disorder, Internalized Psychopathology, and Externalized Psychopathology. The internal validity (reliability) of this typology has been convincingly established (Fuerst et al., 1989, 1990; Fuerst & Rourke, 1993), and there is growing evidence for external validity of the typology (Fuerst et al., 1990; Fuerst & Rourke, 1993).

One shortcoming in our previous investigations has been a failure to explore the developmental dimension. In these studies, the subjects covered a wide range of ages (6 to 15 years), but were treated as a single sample in the generation of subtypes. However, this may not be appropriate, as several studies have indicated that the nature of the assets and deficits of some children with LD varies with age (e.g., McKinney, Short, & Feagans, 1985; Morris, Blashfield, & Satz, 1986; Ozols & Rourke, 1988; Rourke, Dietrich, & Young, 1973). It would seem reasonable, therefore, to infer that the socioemotional functioning of some children with LD might also vary as a function of age.

The results of a study by Strang (1981) would seem to argue against this supposition. In this investigation, the mean PIC profiles and scores on three PIC factor scales of 20 children with LD at each of three age levels (viz., 8, 10, and 12 years old) were

compared. Overall, there were very few statistically significant differences between the three groups. The parents of younger (8-year-old) children were more concerned about the intellectual functioning of their children than were the parents of older (12-year-old) children. Conversely, the 10-year-old children scored significantly higher (more pathological) on the Delinquency scale of the PIC than did the 8-year-old children. However, the overall mean PIC profiles of the three age groups were very similar in all other respects, and suggested normal psychosocial functioning.

Failure to find an association between psychosocial functioning and age is at variance with *Hypothesis 2* notions of the socioemotional development of children with LD (i.e., cumulative effects of persistent academic failure leading to increased psychosocial disturbance) and evidence from some longitudinal studies (e.g., McGee, Williams, Share, Anderson, & Silva, 1986). It is also contrary to recent formulations of the psychosocial development of children with the nonverbal learning disabilities (NLD) syndrome (Rourke, 1989) that, based on clinical observations and rational extrapolations from theory, predict changes in both the nature and severity of psychopathology manifested by such children. Indeed, in the Strang (1981) study, there were some interesting trends in mean PIC factor scores at the three age levels. Although these trends did not reach commonly accepted levels of statistical significance, perhaps due to the small sample size, there was a tendency towards greater internalized psychopathology and personality deviance, with reduced parental concern over intellectual development and achievement, at higher age levels.

However, the simple contrasting-groups design employed in the Strang (1981) study may have obscured any association between age and socioemotional adjustment. The additional step of separating the pathological from normal PIC profiles (that are typically predominant in LD samples), followed by comparisons of the PIC profiles across the different age levels, might have been more informative.

In the current study, relatively sophisticated techniques for assessing the association between age and psychosocial functioning in children with LD were used. Perhaps of primary importance, a sufficient number of subjects (more than 700) were included in this study to allow a powerful evaluation of potential differences in psychosocial functioning at different age levels. In addition, rather than simply comparing relatively undifferentiated children at different age levels, the relationships between age and *patterns* of psychosocial functioning were explored using two different methods. In the first approach, an attempt was made to derive psychosocial subtypes at three age levels (viz., 7–8, 9–10, and 11–13 years of age) using cluster analysis, allowing comparisons of patterns of psychosocial functioning at different age levels. In the second approach, a profile-matching technique using prototypical PIC profiles developed in our previous research was applied to all subjects; this allowed for age differences in the composition of known subtypes to be assessed.

Given the exploratory nature of this study, it was not possible to predict with precision the subtypes that would emerge within and across the three age levels, or any differences in composition of known subtypes with respect to age. However, we expected the following: (1) There would be some similarities between the subtypes derived by cluster analysis at all age levels – specifically, that subtypes corresponding to the Normal, Internalized Psychopathology, and Externalized Psychopathology subtypes (i.e., the most reliable subtypes) derived in previous research (Fuerst et al., 1989, 1990; Fuerst & Rourke, 1993; Porter & Rourke, 1985) would be found; (2) If *Hypothesis 2* is tenable, with increasing age there should be a greater diversity of psychosocial subtypes, as psychosocial dysfunction or frank pathology becomes manifest; and (3) If *Hypothesis 2* is tenable, with increasing age there should be, overall, a greater level of psychosocial dysfunction manifested.

METHOD

Subjects

The 728 subjects used in this study (564 males and 164 females) were selected from a group of more than 5200 children examined at a large urban clinic. These children had been referred for neuropsychological assessment because of learning or "perceptual" difficulties to which it was suspected that cerebral dysfunction might be a contributing factor. All children had completed an extensive neuropsychological test battery, administered by competent technicians, in the manner recommended by Rourke (1976). This was the first documented neuropsychological assessment for all children, and none of these children's data had been used in our previous psychosocial subtyping research. The selected children met the following criteria: (a) chronological age between 7 and 13 years (inclusive); (b) WISC Full Scale IQ (FSIQ) of 80 or above; (c) at least one WRAT (Jastak & Jastak, 1965) centile score below 30; (d) no evidence of educational or cultural deprivation; (e) complete PIC scale scores available. Detailed information regarding the socioeconomic status of the selected children was not available, although almost all subjects were drawn from a very homogeneous lower to middle class urban/suburban area.

For some analyses, the sample was partitioned into three subgroups based on age. One group (201 subjects) contained subjects between the ages of 7 and 8 years of age (Young); a second subgroup (258 subjects) contained subjects between the ages of 9 and 10 years of age (Middle); a third subgroup (269 subjects) contained subjects between the ages of 11 and 13 years of age (Old). The mean WISC Full Scale, Verbal IQ (VIQ), and Performance IQ (PIQ) scores of the groups are summarized in Table 1. Overall, the WISC FSIQ, VIQ, and PIQ scores were 98.7, 94.0, and 104.2, respectively, for males, 94.6, 90.4, and 100.5, respectively, for females, and 97.8, 93.2, and 103.4, respectively, for the entire sample. Mean standard scores on the WRAT Reading, Spelling, and Arithmetic subtests are also shown in Table 1. The mean Reading, Spelling, and Arithmetic standard scores were 88.6, 83.4, and 84.1, respectively, for males, 88.78, 85.3, and 84.8, respectively, for females, and 88.7, 84.3, and 84.5, respectively, for the complete sample.

Materials

The Personality Inventory for Children (PIC) is comprised of 600 descriptive statements that are answered "true" or "false" according to the respondent's opinion of the child (Wirt et al., 1977). It is administered to the child's primary caretaker, usually the biological mother. While up to 33 separate scales can be derived from the 600 PIC items, only 16 of these scales are typically used. Of these 16 scales, 3 are measures of the validity of the profile (Lie, F, and Defensiveness), one is a general measure of psychological adjustment (Adjustment), and the remaining 12 constitute "clinical" scales measuring specific behavioral domains (Achievement, Intellectual Screening, Development, Somatic Concern, Depression, Family Relations, Delinquency, Withdrawal, Anxiety, Psychosis, Hyperactivity, and Social Skills). A child's profile on these scales is expressed in the form of T scores, with positive elevations above the mean suggesting greater likelihood of pathology.

Table 1. Characteristics of the Sample: Mean Scores on WISC Full Scale IQ (FSIQ), Verbal IQ (VIQ), and Performance IQ (PIQ), and WRAT Reading (RSS), Spelling (SSS), and Arithmetic (ASS) Standard Scores.

Source	FSIQ	VIQ	PIQ	RSS	SSS	ASS
Ages 7–8 (Young, $n = 201$)						
Males	97.9	94.3	102.3	83.6	82.8	89.2
Females	94.6	91.7	99.4	86.7	84.4	90.2
Overall	97.0	93.6	101.6	84.4	83.2	89.4
Ages 9–10 (Middle, $n = 258$)						
Males	99.4	94.5	105.0	89.2	84.7	86.2
Females	94.7	90.7	100.1	89.4	86.8	85.4
Overall	98.4	93.7	104.0	89.2	85.1	86.0
Ages 11–13 (Old, $n = 269$)						
Males	99.0	93.3	104.7	91.5	82.6	78.5
Females	94.6	88.9	102.0	90.1	84.7	79.4
Overall	97.7	92.3	104.1	91.2	83.0	78.7

RESULTS

Subtype Generation by Cluster Analysis – Strategy

In the interests of clarity, and to avoid redundant descriptions of the analytic approach used in this phase of the study, an overview of the methods used to derive clusters is provided first. Note that cluster analysis was performed at each of three different age levels (Young, Middle, and Old). Results are reported separately for each of the age categories. The differences and similarities between the pattern of results that emerged across age ranges are addressed in the Discussion.

Outlier Detection and Deletion

As all of the cluster analysis algorithms used in this study are known to be sensitive to the presence of outliers, a three-step process was used to identify and eliminate outliers. First, each subject's scores on the PIC scales that were to be used to form clusters were standardized so as to eliminate profile elevation and dispersion (the transformation is outlined in detail below). Next, the Euclidean distance between a subject and all other subjects was calculated. As each distance was calculated, it was compared to a pre-selected constant value (the "radius"). A running frequency count of all distances less than or equal to this value was made for each subject. As the radius was constant for all

subjects, the frequency was proportionate to the density of subjects in the space around a particular case. Finally, a percentage of subjects with the lowest frequency counts (i.e., in the lowest density regions) were discarded. The exact percentage of subjects deleted depended on the performance of the hierarchical-agglomerative clustering techniques used in the replication attempts. For each of the three age levels, 5% of subjects were initially deleted as outliers. This percentage was found to be adequate for both the Young and Middle subjects; however, it was increased to 10% of subjects for the Old children when replication attempts using the initial value were unsuccessful.

Initial K-Means Analysis

Subjects were initially clustered using an iterative partitioning method, k-means analysis (MacQueen, 1967), that has demonstrated good performance in previous research (Fuerst et al., 1989; Fuerst & Rourke, 1993) and is algorithmically and computationally well-suited for clustering of large data sets. The subjects' scores on the Development, Somatic Concern, Depression, Family Relations, Delinquency, Withdrawal, Anxiety, Psychosis, Hyperactivity, and Social Skills PIC scales (10 in all) were subjected to k-means clustering using Euclidean distance as the similarity measure. The Achievement and Intellectual Screening scales were not included in this analysis as previous experience has shown that these two scales and the Development scale tend to be very highly correlated in samples of children with LD, and provide little useful information. The SAS Version 5.18 implementation of the k-means algorithm (FAST-CLUS) was used (Sarle, 1985).

As grouping on the basis of similarity of profile shape was of primary concern, and given that SAS clustering software limits similarity measures to Euclidean distance, the elements of profile elevation and dispersion were first eliminated from the data. This was accomplished by standardizing each subject's 10 PIC scale scores across that subject's profile. The transformation used was $z = X - M/SD$, where X is a subject's raw scale score, M and SD are the mean and standard deviation (respectively) of that subject's profile (calculated across the 10 scales), and z is the resulting standard score (Lorr, 1983).

The number of clusters present in the data was determined by examination of R^2 and pseudo-F values, by internal reliability of the solution (see below), and by the interpretability of the resulting mean PIC profiles at various partition levels (from 3 to 10 clusters). While the latter criterion may appear somewhat "subjective" (and indeed it is), it should be noted that none of the quantitative criteria that has been suggested for determining the true number of clusters has proven to be effective across all techniques and samples (e.g., Everitt, 1980). Previous experience with data similar to that used in this study (Fuerst et al., 1989, 1990; Fuerst & Rourke, 1993) has strongly suggested that replicability (reliability) and clinical interpretability are, in general, superior to specific quantitative methods for evaluating the adequacy of a specific cluster solution.

Subtype Replication by Hierarchical Cluster Analysis

To assess the internal validity (reliability) of the subtypes derived using k-means cluster analysis, five additional clustering methods were applied to the same data used in the initial k-means analysis. The rationale behind this approach can be found in Fletcher (1985) and Fuerst et al. (1989). Briefly, reliability is of particular concern when multivariate subtyping techniques are applied in an exploratory fashion. Multivariate subtyping techniques, such as

any of the many forms of cluster analysis, will always produce some grouping of data, even if purely random data are used in the procedures. Furthermore, different statistical subtyping techniques can, and often do, produce disparate solutions when applied to the same data. Replicability of solutions across different samples from the same population, and across different subtyping techniques, is a crucial step in determining the validity of the subtypes so derived.

As has often been pointed out in the cluster analysis literature, there is a wide variety of clustering techniques available, and there is relatively little compelling evidence to suggest the superiority of one particular technique over others, given the complex interaction between methods, measures, and samples (Aldenderfer & Blashfield, 1984; Lorr, 1983). For the replication attempts, we selected four widely used and relatively well understood hierarchical agglomerative clustering methods: Ward's Minimum-Variance method (Ward, 1963), the complete linkage method (Sorensen, 1948), the weighted pair-group method using arithmetic averages (WPGMA, Sokal & Michener, 1958), and the unweighted pair-group method using arithmetic averages (UPGMA, Sokal & Michener, 1958), plus one relatively new technique, equal-variance maximum likelihood method (EML, Sarle, 1985), for which there is little published information. The SAS version 5.18 implementation of these algorithms was used (Sarle, 1985).

One undesirable feature of hierarchical agglomerative clustering techniques is that, once subjects are assigned to a cluster, they are never removed: Clusters can only be joined, never split. To help guard against the effects of fusion errors, the following procedure was used. First, a k-means solution for a large number of clusters (between 50 and 80) was derived using the SAS FASTCLUS algorithm (Sarle, 1985). These initial clusters were then used as input to the Ward's, complete linkage WPGMA, UPGMA and EML hierarchical clustering techniques. The preliminary results of the hierarchical clustering were examined and the optimal number of clusters selected. Finally, a k-means relocation pass, with seeds determined by cluster membership at the chosen level of the hierarchy, was performed using the BMDPK k-means algorithm.

For all hierarchical methods, the level at which the hierarchy was "cut" was set to the number of clusters identified in the initial k-means analysis. An initial k-means solution was deemed reliable if it was replicated by at least three of the five hierarchical methods. The degree to which these five hierarchical clustering methods replicated the initial subtypes derived using k-means analysis was assessed with three external criteria measures: Rand's statistic (Rand, 1971), and the two adjustments to Rand's statistic suggested by Morey and Agresti (1984) and Hubert and Arabie (1985). Rand's statistic is a measure of the agreement between two different cluster solutions as assessed by the extent to which pairs of subjects are clustered together or apart: That is, for there to be agreement, pairs of subjects clustered together in one solution must be clustered together in the second solution, and vice-versa for pairs of subjects not clustered together. The Morey and Agresti (1984) and Hubert and Arabie (1985) adjustments to Rand's statistic are corrections for chance agreement between solutions.

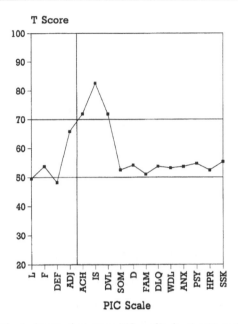

Fig. 1. Prototypical mean PIC profile for the Normal subtype.

Relationship to Known Subtypes

The subtypes that emerged from the k-means cluster analysis were compared to those derived in previous research by Porter and Rourke (1985), Fuerst et al. (1989, 1990), and Fuerst and Rourke (1993). Rather than attempting to intercorrelate all of the subtypes generated in this study and in the previous studies (which would result in a matrix with a few hundred unique correlations), steps were taken to reduce the number of comparisons made. Rourke and Fuerst (1991) reviewed the results of Porter and Rourke (1985), Fuerst et al. (1989, 1990), and Fuerst and Rourke (1993), and, using correlation coefficients, matched corresponding subtypes across studies. The result was seven distinct subtypes (viz., Normal, Mild Hyperactive, Mild Anxiety, Somatic Concern, Conduct Disorder, Internalized Psychopathology, and Externalized Psychopathology). By averaging the PIC scores of corresponding subtypes across studies (e.g., PIC scores of all of the Normal subtypes found in previous studies) "prototypical" mean PIC profiles were generated for the seven subtypes. These profiles are presented in Figures 1 to 7.

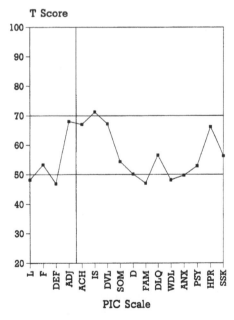

Fig. 2. Prototypical mean PIC profile for the Mild Hyperactive subtype.

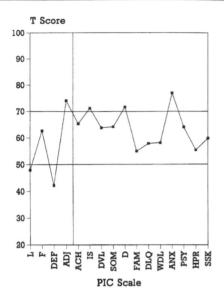

Fig. 3. Prototypical mean PIC profile for the Mild Anxiety subtype.

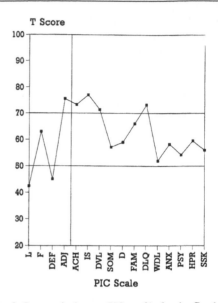

Fig. 5. Prototypical mean PIC profile for the Conduct Disorder subtype.

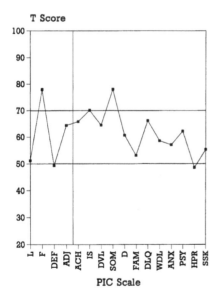

Fig. 4. Prototypical mean PIC profile for the Somatic Concern subtype.

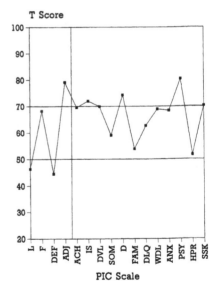

Fig. 6. Prototypical mean PIC profile for the Internalized Psychopathology subtype.

Two methods were used to assess the relations between the cluster analysis derived subtypes in this study and the prototypical subtypes found in previous research. First, and foremost, correlations between the subtypes, using mean PIC scores on all 16 scales, were calculated and compared. These correlations provide a measure of the degree of similarity of mean PIC profile shape between the

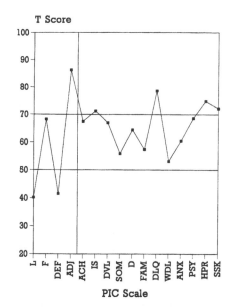

Fig. 7. Prototypical mean PIC profile for the Externalized Psychopathology subtype.

subtypes and prototypes. Second, the subtypes were also compared to the prototypes in terms of relative size (i.e., proportion of assigned subjects falling into each subtype). Note that, as with the prototypical PIC profiles, where multiple instances of a subtype had been found in previous studies, the proportions of assigned subjects were averaged across those studies.

Subtype Generation by Cluster Analysis: Results

Young Children

As outlined above, 5% of Young subjects (11 in all) were deemed to be outliers and were deleted from the sample. With the k-means clustering method, examination of the R^2 and pseudo-F values for 2- to 10-cluster solutions suggested the presence of four subtypes.

These four subtypes were replicated with good accuracy by Ward's, EML, and WPGMA clustering techniques. All versions of Rand's statistic were greater than 0.7. The "pure" Rand's statistic is difficult to interpret directly; theoretically, however, an

adjusted value of 0.0 indicates purely chance-agreement, whereas 1.0 indicates complete agreement. Empirical studies have shown that adjusted values above 0.2 indicate better-than-chance agreement between solutions (Milligan & Cooper, 1986). Finding adjusted values of Rand's statistic greater than 0.7 is indicative of good cluster recovery.

Visual inspection of mean PIC profiles indicated that the subtypes were very similar to four of the seven prototypical PIC subtypes derived in our previous research. To confirm these impressions, the mean PIC profiles of the subtypes were visually matched with those of the prototypes and correlations calculated between corresponding profiles. The prototypical Mild Hyperactive subtype was replicated with excellent accuracy in the Young sample ($r = .95$). The PIC profiles of the Internalized Psychopathology and Externalized Psychopathology subtypes found in the Young sample deviated somewhat from their corresponding prototypes, but were still very similar (for both subtypes $r = .91$).

The Normal subtype of the Young sample was least like its corresponding prototype, with an r of .83. When the profiles of this subtype and prototype were compared, it was apparent that, whereas the prototype showed an essentially flat profile apart from the "cognitive triad" scales (Achievement, Intellectual Screening, and Development), this subtype in the present study evidenced minor peaks on the Somatic Concern and Delinquency scales. Indeed, this subtype was found to correlate .80 and .77 with the Somatic Concern and Conduct Disorder prototypes, respectively. These results suggest that, within the Young sample, the Normal subtype may be somewhat more heterogeneous than has been previously found.

As summarized in Table 2, there were no substantial differences between the proportions of Young subjects assigned to the four subtypes and the proportions for the corresponding prototypes. Thus, in terms of relative size, the four subtypes were very similar to the prototypes.

Middle Children

As outlined above, 5% of Middle subjects (13 in all) were deemed to be outliers and were deleted from the sample. With the k-means clustering

Table 2. Percentages of Assigned Subjects Within Prototypical Subtypes and Subtypes Derived by Cluster Analysis (CA) and Profile Matching.

Source	Subtype						
	Normal	Mild Hpr	Mild Anx	Somatic	Conduct	Internal	External
Prototype	33	26	16	13	10	22	19
Young CA	27	28				25	20
Middle CA	17	20	11	13		23	15
Old CA	27			19		33	22
Profile Matching	28	11	11	11	8	16	16

method, examination of the R^2 and pseudo-F values for 2- to 10-cluster solutions suggested the presence of six subtypes. These six subtypes were replicated with good accuracy by Ward's, EML, and UPGMA clustering techniques. All versions of Rand's statistic were .72 or higher.

Visual inspection of mean PIC profiles indicated that the subtypes appeared very similar to six of the seven prototypical PIC subtypes derived in our previous research, with the exception being the Conduct Disorder prototype. To confirm these impressions, the mean PIC profiles of the subtypes were visually matched with those of the prototypes, and correlations were calculated between corresponding profiles. The prototypical Internalized Psychopathology and Externalized Psychopathology subtypes were replicated with excellent accuracy in the Middle sample ($r = .97$, $r = .99$, respectively). The mean PIC profiles of the Mild Hyperactive and Normal subtypes were also quite similar to their corresponding prototypes ($r = .94$, $r = .89$, respectively). The PIC profiles of the subtypes matching the Mild Anxiety and Somatic Con-cern prototypes, while showing somewhat lower correlations ($r = .87$ in both cases), were, nevertheless, clearly recognizable as instances of these prototypes.

As shown in Table 2, for five of the six subtypes (Mild Hyperactive, Mild Anxiety, Somatic Concern, Internalized Psychopathology, and Externalized Psychopathology) there were no substantial differences between the proportions of subjects assigned to the subtypes and the proportions for the corresponding prototypes. Thus, in terms of relative size, these five subtypes were very similar to the prototypes. However, the Normal subtype was considerably smaller (17%) than the Normal prototype (33%).

Old Children

As outlined above, 10% of Old subjects (27 children in all) were deemed to be outliers and deleted from the sample. With the k-means clustering method, examination of the R^2 and pseudo-F values for 2- to 10-cluster solutions suggested the presence of four subtypes. These four subtypes were replicated with good accuracy by Ward's, UPGMA, and complete linkage clustering techniques. All versions of Rand's statistic were .76 or higher.

Visual inspection of mean PIC profiles indicated that the subtypes appeared very similar to four of the seven prototypical PIC subtypes derived in our previous research. To confirm these impressions, the mean PIC profiles of the subtypes were visually matched with those of the prototypes and correlations calculated between corresponding profiles. The prototypical Normal, Somatic Concern, Internalized Psychopathology, and Externalized Psychopathology subtypes were replicated with excellent accuracy in the Old sample. All correlations between the mean PIC profiles of corresponding subtypes exceeded .96.

As shown in Table 2, for three of the four subtypes (Normal, Mild Hyperactive, and Externalized Psychopathology) there were no substantial differences between the proportions of subjects assigned to the subtypes and the proportions for the corresponding prototypes. Thus, in terms of relative size, these three subtypes were very similar to the prototypes. However, the Internalized Psychopathology subtype was somewhat larger (33%) than the Internalized Psychopathology prototype (22%).

Profile Matching

Our second method of deriving subtypes from the data capitalized on the results of our previous research. As outlined above, by calculating the mean PIC scores on all 16 scales for the seven pre-viously derived subtypes, "prototypical" PIC pro-files for those subtypes were created (see Figures 1 through 7). Correlations between each subject's PIC profile and the seven prototypical PIC profiles were calculated. Subjects were assigned to the subtype to which their PIC profile correlated most strongly (and positively). Subjects showing only negative or trivial correlations (i.e., <.40) with the prototypical profiles were deemed outliers and dropped from subsequent analyses.

In many respects this "profile matching" algo-rithm is similar to k-means cluster analysis. In k-means terminology, the prototypical profiles form the cluster "seeds," with cases being assigned to a cluster on the basis of similarity of profile shape. Some differences between the profile match-ing algorithm and typical implementations of k-means should be noted. First cluster seeds were not selected (randomly or otherwise) from the sample, as the seeds (prototypes) were derived from consid-erable prior research and are the best known defi-nitions of the subtypes. Selection of seeds from the sample data is heuristic and appropriate in exploratory studies, where the underlying struc-ture of the data is unknown. Second, cluster seeds were not updated as cases were assigned to the cluster, as this might perturb these "best" subtype definitions. Third, given the previous point, there was no need to repeat the assignment pass (i.e., the algorithm is not iterative.)

Use of this algorithm resulted in the assignment of 679 subjects to one of the seven subtypes. Forty-nine subjects (6.7% of the total sample) were rejected by the algorithm as outliers. The largest number of subjects, 192 (28.2% of assigned sub-jects) were matched to the Normal prototype. Approximately equal numbers of subjects, 108 and 105 (15.9% and 15.5% of assigned subjects, respectively), were matched to the Externalized Psychopathology and Internalized Psychopath-ology prototypes. Similarly, 77 subjects (11.3% of assigned subjects) were matched to the Somatic Concern prototype, 74 subjects (10.9%) were matched to the Mild Anxiety pro-totype, and 71 subjects (10.5%) were matched with the Mild Hyperactivity prototype. The fewest number of subjects, 52 (7.7% of assigned subjects), were matched to the Conduct Disorder prototype.

Mean PIC profiles for each of the seven subtypes were calculated and used to plot Figures 8 through 14. The visual similarity between the subtypes' PIC profiles and the corresponding prototypical profiles (see Figures 1–7) is obvious. Correlations were cal-culated between the mean PIC profiles of the sub-types and each of the prototypical profiles. As expected, there were very strong relationships between the prototypes and the corresponding sub-types derived by profile matching. All correlations between corresponding prototypes and subtypes were greater than .98, indicating a very high degree of similarity.

The subtypes derived by profile matching were also compared to the prototypes in terms of the proportion of assigned subjects falling into each of the subtypes. These proportions are summ-arized in Table 2. As shown in Table 2, for six of the seven subtypes (Normal, Mild Anxiety, Somatic Concern, Conduct Disorder, Internalized Psychopathology, and Externalized Psychopathol-ogy) there were no substantial differences between the proportions of subjects assigned to the sub-types and the proportions for the corresponding prototypes. Thus, in terms of relative size, these

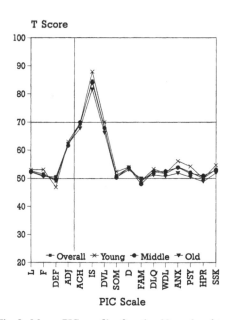

Fig. 8. Mean PIC profile for the Normal subtype derived by profile matching.

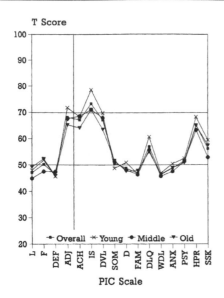

Fig. 9. Mean PIC profile for the Mild Hyperactive subtype derived by profile matching.

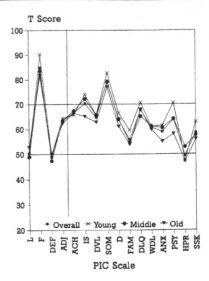

Fig. 11. Mean PIC profile for the Somatic Concern
subtype derived by profile matching.

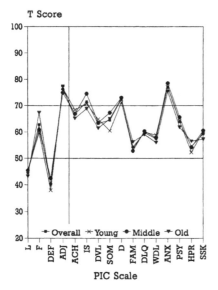

Fig. 10. Mean PIC profile for the Mild Anxiety subtype derived by profile matching.

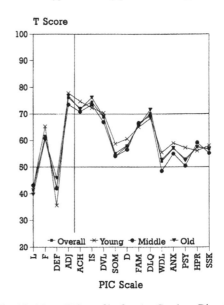

Fig. 12. Mean PIC profile for the Conduct Disorder
subtype derived by profile matching.

six subtypes were very similar to the prototypes.
However, the Mild Hyperactive subtype was somewhat smaller (11%) than the Mild Hyperactive
prototype (26%).

Relationships Between Age and Subtype
Membership

Four methods were used to investigate relationships
between age and subtype membership. First, each

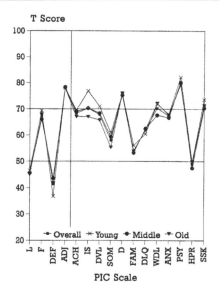

Fig. 13. Mean PIC profile for the Internalized Psychopathology subtype derived by profile matching.

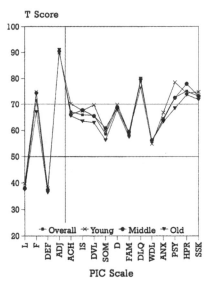

Fig. 14. Mean PIC profile for the Externalized Psychopathology subtype derived by profile matching.

subtype was broken down into the three age categories described above (Young, Middle, and Old). Mean PIC profiles (also found in Figures 8–14) for each of the three age categories within each subtype were calculated and compared. Overall, there were no striking differences between the within-subtypes mean PIC profiles of the Young, Middle, and Old groups. The overall mean PIC profile elevation of the Young children was significantly higher than that of the Old children in the Normal ($F(1,121) = 6.30$, $p < .01$) and Somatic Concern ($F(1,46) = 5.06$, $p < .05$) subtypes. Profile analysis (Harris, 1985) also established that, in the Externalized Psychopathology subtype, the mean PIC profiles of the Young and Old children had significantly different shapes (GCR $= 0.511$, $F(15,60) = 2.046, p < .05$). No other comparisons across age categories within subtypes reached commonly accepted levels of statistical significance.

Second, within each subtype, the frequencies at which each age category achieved the highest mean score on a PIC subscale were determined and compared. There was a tendency for Younger subjects to receive the highest mean scores on more PIC scales relative to the Middle and Older subjects. In the Normal and Internalized Psychopathology

subtypes, Younger children obtained the highest mean scores on 11 of 16 PIC scales, and in the Mild Hyperactive, Somatic Concern, and Conduct Disorder subtypes they received the highest mean scores on 10 of 16 PIC scales. However, the distribution of these frequencies across age categories did not deviate significantly from expected values in any of the subtypes.

Third, frequency cross-tabulations for subtype membership and age categories were also calculated, and used to plot Figure 15. Note that, as there were unequal numbers of subjects at the three age levels, the percentages reported in Figure 15 were calculated relative to the size of the appropriate age group. For example, the percentage associated with Young children in the Mild Hyperactive subtype was about 10%. This percentage does not mean that 10% of the Mild Hyperactive subtype were Young subjects, but rather that 10% of Young subjects were assigned to this subtype. Visual inspection of Figure 15 revealed no striking age differences across subtypes, although three very weak trends were apparent. First, the percentage of subjects classified as Normal tended to decrease with increased age, indicating that, at higher age levels, more children fell into the other

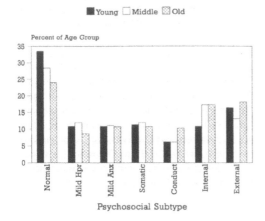

Fig. 15. Percentages of Young, Middle, and Old subjects in the subtypes derived by profile matching.

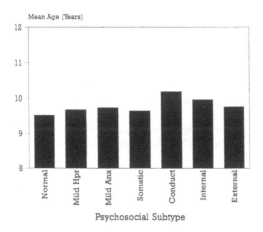

Fig. 16. Mean age of children in the subtypes derived by profile matching.

subtypes. Second, Middle and Old children were slightly more prevalent in the Internalized Psychopathology subtype than were Young children. Third, a somewhat greater proportion of Old subjects were assigned to the Conduct Disorder subtype relative to the Young and Middle subjects.

Finally, the mean ages of subjects assigned to the seven subtypes were calculated and compared. As shown in Figure 16, the mean age of the Conduct Disorder subtype appeared to be slightly higher than that of the Normal subtype; the difference was statistically significant, $t(242) = 2.40$, $p < .05$. While less visually prominent, the mean age of the

Internalized Psychopathology subtype was also significantly higher than that of the Normal subtype ($t(295) = 2.24$, $p < .05$). There were no other significant differences in mean age between subtypes.

Relationships Between Sex and Subtype Membership

As the prevalence of males versus females is known to differ within some clinical populations (e.g., attention deficit disorder), we also examined the proportions of males and females, calculated relative to the size of their respective samples, within each of the seven subtypes. Inspection of the resulting cross-tabulation suggested that females were somewhat more likely to fall within the Normal subtype (37%) than were males (26%), and were also somewhat more likely to fall within the Internalized Psychopathology subtype (20%) than were males (14%). Males, on the other hand, were somewhat more likely to be assigned to the Externalized Psychopathology subtype (17%) than were females (11%). However, note that, overall, the deviations from expected proportions were not statistically significant.

DISCUSSION

At the outset of this study, three predictions were made regarding potential relations between age and psychosocial functioning in children with LD. The first prediction was that Normal, Internalized Psychopathology, and Externalized Psychopathology subtypes would be found at all age levels, as these subtypes have proven to be the most reliable in previous research. Second, it was predicted that, when typologies were compared across age levels, there would be a greater diversity of subtypes with increasing age. The final prediction was that, with increased age, there would be an increase in the level of psychosocial dysfunction evidenced.

Two general approaches were used to test these predictions. In the first approach, subtypes were derived from Young, Middle, and Old samples of children using cluster analysis (referred to as the CAD subtypes). Of the three predictions, only the first was supported by the results. At all three age levels, Normal, Internalized Psychopathology, and Externalized Psychopathology subtypes were found. While there were minor differences between corresponding subtypes across age levels, they were all clearly recognizable as instances of their respective types. However, the finding that the Internalized Psychopathology and Externalized Psychopathology CAD subtypes were very similar across the Young, Middle, and Old samples, also contradicted the third prediction. There was no evidence of greater maladjustment in these two clearly pathological subtypes at higher age levels.

Regarding the second prediction, there was no evidence of greater diversity of subtypes at higher age levels. While more subtypes were found in the Middle sample (six) than in the Young sample (four), only four subtypes could be reliably derived from the Old sample. The discrepancy in the number of subtypes across age levels (four vs. six) was trivial. These results suggest that patterns of psychosocial functioning are quite uniform from ages 7 to 13 years in children with LD.

In the second approach, subjects were assigned to subtypes according to similarity to prototypical PIC profiles derived in previous studies (referred to as the PMD subtypes). While subjects were not "forced" to conform to the prototypical typology, this method did place constraints on the maximum number of subtypes that could be formed (seven), and precluded the derivation of novel subtypes. However, given that the assignment of a child to a subtype was entirely independent of the assignments of other children, this method did allow somewhat more direct tests of the three predictions outlined above, as the formation of subtypes was altogether independent of age level and not subject to sample variations that might perturb traditional methods of cluster analysis.

When the PMD subtypes were broken down by age category, some statistically significant differences between age levels (within subtypes) did emerge. The shapes of the PIC profiles of the Young and Old Externalized Psychopathology subtypes were significantly different; however, inspection of the profiles indicated that the actual deviations were trivial. Similarly, while statistical tests indicated that the PIC profiles of the Young Normal and Somatic Concern subtypes were significantly more elevated than were the profiles of the Old Normal and Somatic Concern subtypes, the actual degree of elevation was extremely small, and in practical terms inconsequential. In addition, while the Young

children tended to score highest on the PIC scales most often in five of the seven subtypes, within none of these subtypes did this trend reach statistical significance. Thus, no evidence was found to support the expectation that greater age would be associated with increased psychosocial dysfunction.

Examination of the relative sizes of the PMD subtypes at the three age levels revealed no striking differences, although three very weak trends were noted: (1) The relative size of the Normal subtype decreased slightly (about 10%) with increasing age; (2) A slightly greater proportion of Old children was assigned to the Conduct Disorder subtype than were Young and Middle children; and (3) Slightly greater proportions of Middle and Old children as compared to the Young children were assigned to the Internalized Psychopathology subtype. The mean age of the Conduct Disorder (and, perhaps, of the Internalized Psychopathology) subtype was slightly higher than the mean age of the Normal subtype.

These trends were not contrary to expectations; however, they were extremely weak. The preponderance of the evidence indicates that there is no change in the diversity of patterns of psychosocial functioning in children with LD with increasing age. Indeed, there was remarkable stability in patterns of functioning across the age ranges examined in this study. No evidence was found to support the notion that children with LD are likely to develop more frank psychopathology as they grow older. Similarly, the results of this study indicate that, given a particular pattern of psychosocial adaptation, there is no substantial change in level of adaptation at higher ages. Thus, overall, as children with LD grow older (within the age ranges explored in this study), they do not show increased risk for the development of pathological patterns of psychosocial adaptation, nor do they show any deterioration in level of psychosocial functioning.

Of course, these conclusions must be tempered with an understanding of the methodological shortcomings of the cross-sectional design used in this study. One concern is that the identification of learning disability (at least as reflected by age at referral for neuropsychological assessment) was at different ages for these children. Thus, it is possible that a child identified as learning disabled at age 13 experienced different psychosocial development than did a child identified as learning disabled at age 8. Perhaps, the latter child exhibited more severe deficits and more opportunities for negative experiences than the former, and thus was at greater risk for the development of psychopathology. This might produce results comparable to those found in this study (i.e., no significant differences in psychopathology in younger and older children with LD). However, this argument overlooks the distinction between *identification* of LD and the *onset* of LD. In the absence of a clear insult to pre- or post-natal CNS development, the onset of the cognitive deficits that produce LD cannot be determined, but likely occurs before the commencement of school. The point at which cognitive deficits are identified, and the moniker of learning disability applied, typically comes later in life and is influenced by a variety of factors (including culture, SES, and the skill of educators and clinicians) not directly related to cognitive and psychosocial development. To further complicate matters, the *expression* of cognitive deficits in academic and psychosocial functioning, and the probability of recognition by educators and clinicians, varies with particular types of LD (Rourke, 1989).

Obviously, the preferred methodology for this type of research is the longitudinal design. However, we must point out that longitudinal designs also have significant shortcomings for the study of children with LD. In most education systems in Western societies, the child with LD, once identified, is subject to numerous and varied interventions. Attempting to equate or otherwise control for interventions that differ in orientation, objective, technique, duration, and quality, even within individual schools, is simply not possible. In this respect, the cross-sectional design is actually superior to longitudinal designs, as children referred for their first neuropsychological assessment have usually had little or no formal treatment.

It is interesting to note that, in the current study, marked differences in the prevalence of males and females within psychosocial subtypes were not found. Males were somewhat more likely to be found in the Externalized Psychopathology subtype, and females were somewhat more likely to be assigned to the Normal and Internalized Psychopathology subtypes. However, these differences were quite small, both in absolute terms, and

relative to the discrepancies frequently reported for some clinical populations (such as attention deficit/hyperactivity). This raises the possibility that the determinants of psychosocial adaptation and the genesis of psychopathology in children with LD may be different than in other clinical populations that do show marked gender discrepancies.

In any case, the results of this study are very much at variance with *Hypothesis 2* formulations of the psychosocial functioning of children with LD. Such formulations generally hold that the negative consequences of having a learning disability (such as frustration, anxiety, or peer rejection due to continued academic failure, or a discrete cognitive deficit that perpetually disrupts psychosocial functioning) over time produce maladjustment by grinding down the child's adaptive abilities. While cumulative negative experiences may be deleterious to some children with LD, the results of this study, and others (e.g., Chapman, 1988; Chapman & Boersma, 1980; Jorm, Share, Matthews, & Maclean, 1986; Strang, 1981) suggest strongly that this is not necessarily the case. It is clear that some children with LD evidence significant maladjustment (e.g., the Internalized Psychopathology and Externalized Psychopathology subtypes); however, the development of pathological patterns of functioning is not more likely with increased age, nor is deterioration in level of adaptation. When such changes are observed in clinical settings, factors other than simple increased age and cumulative exposure to negative experiences, such as a particular constellation of neuropsychological assets and deficits that predisposes the child to maladaptive psychosocial functioning (as in the NLD syndrome), must be considered.

REFERENCES

Aldenderfer, M.S., & Blashfield, R.K. (1984). *Cluster analysis*. Beverly Hills: Sage.

Chapman, J.W. (1988). Cognitive-motivational characteristics and academic achievement of learning disabled children: A longitudinal study. *Journal of Educational Psychology, 80*, 357–365.

Chapman, J.W., & Boersma, F.J. (1980). *Affective correlates of learning disabilities*. Lisse, The Netherlands: Swets & Zeitlinger.

Everitt, B. (1980). *Cluster analysis*. New York: Halsted.

Fletcher, J.M. (1985). External validation of learning disability typologies. In B. P. Rourke (Ed.), *Neuropsychology of learning disabilities: Essentials of sub-type analysis* (pp. 187–211). New York: Guilford Press.

Fuerst, D.R., Fisk, J.L., & Rourke, B.P. (1989). Psychosocial functioning of learning-disabled children: Reliability of statistically derived subtypes. *Journal of Consulting and Clinical Psychology, 57,* 275–280.

Fuerst, D.R., Fisk, J.L., & Rourke, B.P. (1990). Psychosocial functioning of learning-disabled children: Relationships between WISC Verbal IQ – Performance IQ discrepancies and personality subtypes. *Journal of Consulting and Clinical Psychology, 58,* 657–660.

Fuerst, D.R., & Rourke, B.P. (1993). Psychosocial functioning of children: Relations between personality subtypes and academic achievement. *Journal of Abnormal Child Psychology, 21,* 597–607.

Harris, R.J. (1985). *A primer of multivariate statistics* (2nd ed.). Orlando: Academic Press.

Hubert, L., & Arabie, P. (1985). Comparing partitions. *Journal of Classification, 2,* 193–218.

Jastak, J.F., & Jastak, S.R. (1965). *The Wide Range Achievement Test.* Wilmington, DE: Guidance Associates.

Jorm, A.F., Share, D.L., Matthews, R., & Maclean, R. (1986). Behavior problems in specific reading retarded and general reading backward children: A longitudinal study. *Journal of Child Psychology and Psychiatry, 27,* 33–43.

Lorr, M. (1983). *Cluster analysis for social scientists.* San Francisco: Jossey-Bass.

MacQueen, J.B. (1967). Some methods for classification and analysis of multivariate observations. *Proceedings of the Fifth Berkeley Symposium on Mathematical Statistics and Probability, 1,* 281–297.

McGee, R., Williams, S., Share, D.L., Anderson, J., & Silva, P.A. (1986). The relationship between specific reading retardation general reading backwardness, and behavioural problems in a large sample of Dunedin boys: A longitudinal study from five to eleven years. *Journal of Child Psychology and Psychiatry, 27,* 597–610.

McKinney, J.D., Short, E.J., & Feagans, L. (1985). Academic consequences of perceptual-linguistic subtypes of learning disabled children. *Learning Disabilities Research, 1,* 6–17.

Milligan, G.W., & Cooper, M.C. (1986). A study of the comparability of external criteria for hierarchical cluster analysis. *Multivariate Behavioral Research, 21,* 441–458.

Morey, L., & Agresti, A. (1984). The measurement of classification agreement: An adjustment to the Rand statistic for chance agreement. *Educational and Psychological Measurement, 44,* 33–37.

Morris, R., Blashfield, R., & Satz, P. (1986). Developmental classification of reading-disabled children. *Journal of Clinical and Experimental Neuropsychology, 8,* 371–392.

Ozols, E.J., & Rourke, B.P. (1988). Characteristics of young learning-disabled children classified according to patterns of academic achievement: Auditory-perceptual and visual-perceptual abilities. *Journal of Clinical Child Psychology, 17,* 44–52.

Porter, J., & Rourke, B.P. (1985). Socioemotional functioning of learning-disabled children: A subtypal analysis of personality patterns. In B.P. Rourke (Ed.), *Neuropsychology of learning disabilities: Essentials of subtype analysis* (pp. 257–279). New York: Guilford Press.

Rand, W.M. (1971). Objective criteria for the evaluation of clustering methods. *Journal of the American Statistical Association, 66,* 846–850.

Rourke, B.P. (1976). Issues in the neuropsychological assessment of children with learning disabilities. *Canadian Psychological Review, 17,* 89–102.

Rourke, B.P. (1989). *Nonverbal learning disabilities: The syndrome and the model.* New York: Guilford Press.

Rourke, B.P., Dietrich, D.M., & Young, G.C. (1973). Significance of WISC verbal-performance discrepancies for younger children with learning disabilities. *Perceptual and Motor Skills, 36,* 275–282.

Rourke, B.P., & Fuerst, D.R. (1991). *Learning disabilities and psychosocial functioning: A neuropsychological perspective.* New York: Guilford Press.

Sarle, W.S. (1985). The CLUSTER procedure. In S.P. Joyner (Ed.), *SAS user's guide: Statistics, version 5 edition* (pp. 255–315). Cary, North Carolina: SAS Institute, Inc.

Sokal, R., & Michener, C. (1958). A statistical method for evaluating systematic relationships. *University of Kansas Scientific Bulletin, 38,* 1409–1438.

Sorensen, T. (1948). A method of establishing groups of equal amplitude in plant sociology based on similarity of species content and its application to analyses of the vegetation on Danish commons. *Biologiske Skrifter, 5,* 1–34.

Strang, J.D. (1981). *Personality dimensions of learning disabled children: Age and subtype differences.* Unpublished doctoral dissertation, University of Windsor, Windsor, Ontario, Canada.

Ward, J. (1963). Hierarchical grouping to optimize an objective function. *Journal of the American Statistical Association, 58,* 236–244.

Wirt, R.D., Lachar, D., Klinedinst, J.K., & Seat, P.D. (1977). *Multidimensional description of child personality: A manual for the Personality Inventory for Children.* Los Angeles: Western Psychological Services.

Journal of Clinical and Experimental Neuropsychology
2003, Vol. 25, No. 2, pp. 255–273

Comparison of the Psychosocial Typology of Children with Below Average IQ to That of Children with Learning Disabilities

Margaret B. Ralston[1], Darren R. Fuerst[2], and Byron P. Rourke[1,3]

[1]University of Windsor, Windsor, ON, Canada, [2]Wayne State University, Detroit, MI, USA, and
[3]Yale University, New Haven, CT, USA

ABSTRACT

This study investigates the subtypal patterns of psychosocial functioning of children with below average IQ (BAIQ) using the application of both Q-factor analysis and profile-matching. The results suggest that the psychosocial dimensions of children with BAIQ are quite similar to those of children with LD in a general sense. Many of the same subtypes were derived, and the proportions of children displaying normal, mild, and severe levels of psychopathology were not significantly different from those of children with LD. There were some minor differences, however: For example, children with BAIQ exhibited a greater tendency to display psychopathology with internalizing features. Consistent with previous research involving children with LD, there were no changes in either type or severity of psychopathology with advancing years.

Reliable subtypes of psychosocial dimensions have been delineated in children with learning disabilities (LD) using the Personality Inventory for Children (PIC; Wirt, Lachar, Klinedinst, & Seat, 1977, PIC-R; Wirt, Lachar, Klinedinst, & Seat, 1984); [see Rourke and Fuerst (1991) for an extensive review on this topic]. However, children with learning problems who score below average on standardized psychometric tests of intelligence are usually excluded from these studies (e.g., Porter & Rourke, 1985; Speece, McKinney, & Appelbaum, 1985); therefore, previous research results cannot be generalized to include them. The present study examines the psychosocial typology generated from selected PIC scores of children with learning problems who meet other commonly used criteria to define LD (Rourke, 1975) but whose Full Scale Intelligence Quotient (FSIQ) scores on the Wechsler Intelligence Scale for Children (WISC; Wechsler, 1949) fall below average. This typology is then compared to that found previously in children with LD.

The distinction between LD, mental retardation, and general low achievement is somewhat arbitrary and obscured with controversy involving the use of IQ scores as a means of classification (Polloway, Patton, Smith, & Buck, 1997; Siegel, 1988, 1989; Stanovich, 1991). In the current study no attempt is made to classify children with below average IQ (BAIQ) scores into one of these three groups. The children are referred to simply as having BAIQ.

As no previous research of which we are aware has investigated the psychosocial typology of children with BAIQ specifically, the following review focuses on the literature that has contributed to the understanding of the psychosocial typology of children with LD; this information is then related to the expected psychosocial typology of children with BAIQ. The review begins with an examination of the Windsor taxonomic research. Then the literature

Address correspondence to: Byron P. Rourke, FRSC, Department of Psychology, University of Windsor, Windsor, Ontario N9B 3P4, Canada. Tel.: +1-519-253-3000. E-mail: bprourke@aol.com
Accepted for publication: August 12, 2002.

that involves children with below average psychometric intelligence is discussed. Finally, expectations are formulated and rationales are explained.

WINDSOR TAXONOMIC RESEARCH

A series of studies conducted at the University of Windsor by Rourke and his colleagues (e.g., Fuerst, Fisk, & Rourke, 1989, 1990; Porter & Rourke, 1985) investigated the relationship between psychosocial functioning and LD. These studies were distinguished by their systematic consideration of methodological issues, for example: Rigorous criteria were used to select subjects, a standardized psychometric measure was used to examine the subjects' psychosocial profiles, and advanced statistical methods were used to generate a typology of heterogeneous psychosocial functioning.

The first in the series of studies was carried out by Porter and Rourke (1985) using the PIC to examine the psychosocial profiles of children with LD. This measure is composed of 600 true-false questions about the child's behavior, attitudes, and interpersonal relations and is usually administered to the child's parents in an unsupervised setting. There are three validity or response style scales [Lie (L), Frequency (F), and Defensiveness (DEF)], one general screening scale [Adjustment (ADJ)], and 12 clinical scales [Achievement (ACH), Intellectual Screening (IS), Development (DVL), Somatic Concern (SOM), Depression (D), Family Relations (FAM), Delinquency (DLQ), Withdrawal (WDL), Anxiety (ANX), Psychosis (PSY), Hyperactivity (HPR), and Social Skills (SSK)]. A child's profile is expressed in T scores with higher scores suggesting greater likelihood of psychological disturbances.

Porter and Rourke (1985) assessed the sample as a whole for psychosocial difficulties by calculating the mean PIC profile. Results showed that only the scales that reflect development, intellectual functioning, and academic achievement suggested any difficulties. Scales that indicate psychosocial disturbance were found to be within the normal range. However, when Q-type factor analysis was applied to the PIC scores, the results revealed four distinct subtypes that differed significantly from one another with regard to mean PIC profiles. The largest of the four subtypes included 44% of the

classified subjects. This group showed no elevations on scales reflecting psychosocial functioning, indicating no significant psychosocial problems. The second subtype included 26% of those classified. The PIC profiles of these children suggested seriously disturbed internalized psychosocial functioning (e.g., depression, withdrawal, and anxiety). Thirteen percent of classified subjects were included in the third subtype which showed elevations on the scale that reflects somatic concern. The fourth subtype included 17% of the classified subjects and indicated difficulties related to delinquency, hyperactivity, and family relations. These kinds of problems are often thought of as "externalized" psychosocial problems.

The subtypes found in this study were similar, both in proportion of children in each subtype and in patterns of functioning, to the normal and deviant subtypes found by Speece et al. (1985). In agreement with other studies that had examined psychosocial heterogeneity (e.g., Epstein, Bursuck, & Cullinan, 1985; Epstein, Cullinan, & Rosemier, 1983; Speece et al., 1985), Porter and Rourke concluded that children with LD are heterogeneous with regard to psychosocial functioning: There is no one pattern that is characteristic of all children with LD.

Porter and Rourke's (1985) study was replicated using a new and larger sample of children and various cluster-analytic techniques in addition to Q-analysis (Fuerst et al., 1989). The results revealed three subtypes that compared quite favourably to similar subtypes found by Porter and Rourke, and the proportion of children assigned to each subtype was also comparable.

Several more studies of the series were conducted. Utilizing a wider range of PIC scales and more sophisticated clustering methods, Fuerst et al. (1990) and Fuerst and Rourke (1993) recovered six clusters (subtypes) rather than three. Fuerst and Rourke (1995) identified and described seven prototypical subtypes by averaging PIC scores of corresponding subtypes across studies. They also examined the relationship between age and patterns of psychosocial functioning and found that subtypes were comparable at each age level in both shape and in elevation. In addition, the proportion of young, middle, and old subjects in each subtype were similar, indicating that patterns of psychosocial functioning are stable, at least across the ages investigated.

In contrast to the commonly held notion that psychosocial problems increase with age in children with LD, the results of this study indicated that psychopathology does not necessarily increase with age.

Tsatsanis, Fuerst, and Rourke (1997) investigated the external validation of the seven prototypical subtypes described by Fuerst and Rourke (1995) and found that the subtypes could be predictably discriminated and identified on a measure other than the one upon which the typology was generated. In addition, age differences among subtypes were examined and, in agreement with the results by Fuerst and Rourke, no age differences among subtypes were found.

The results of the above investigations indicate clearly that LD, generally considered, does not necessarily lead to secondary problems in psychosocial functioning as is often portrayed. More than half of the children with LD exhibited either normal functioning or very mild disturbances. However, as a group, children with LD do have a tendency to display somewhat more psychosocial problems than do normally achieving children (Rourke, 2000); therefore, it is possible that some other factor is responsible for both LD and psychosocial difficulties. A series of studies examined the relationship between the patterns of central processing assets and deficits that characterize the ability subtypes of LD on one hand and the patterns of psychosocial functioning of children with LD on the other (e.g., Fuerst et al., 1990; Fuerst & Rourke, 1993; Strang & Rourke, 1985). These studies indicate that it does not appear to be LD status per se that predicts psychosocial problems. Rather, particular patterns of neuropsychological assets and deficits appear to predict both the kind of LD and the kind and level of psychosocial problems. It is possible that the level of neuropsychological ability may also be associated with the type and/or level of psychosocial pathology. The following is a review of the research pertaining to below average cognitive ability as measured by psychometric tests of intelligence.

REVIEW OF THE RESEARCH PERTAINING TO BELOW AVERAGE COGNITIVE ABILITY

No previous research of which we are aware has examined the psychosocial functioning of children with below average cognitive ability. However, some researchers have included children who were classified as educably mentally retarded (EMR) in their investigations of psychosocial problems in special education students (e.g., Cullinan, Epstein, & Dembinski, 1979; Gajar, 1979; Richmond & Blagg, 1985). Although the FSIQ score of children classified as EMR is somewhat lower (from 50 to 75) than that used in the present study for the children with BAIQ (from 60 to 85), these studies provide some insight into the psychosocial dimensions of "lower functioning" children.

Gajar (1979) used the Behavior Problem Checklist (BPC; Quay & Peterson, 1975) to compare the behavior problems of children with emotional disorder (ED), LD, and EMR. The criteria that were used to identify the children with LD were unspecified. Three dimensions of the BPC were quantified. Higher scores indicated more severe pathology. The results showed that the children with ED scored significantly higher than the other two groups on Conduct Disorder and Personality Problem dimensions, and the children with ED scored significantly higher than the EMR children on the Immaturity–Inadequacy dimension. The ED group was similar to the LD group on the Immaturity–Inadequacy dimension. The BPC was useful in discriminating ED from LD and EMR, but it was not possible to discriminate children with LD from those with EMR on the basis of these scores.

Using the same instrument as that in above study, Cullinan et al. (1979) compared the behavior patterns of four groups of children: EMR, LD, behavior disordered (BD), and regular class students. On the Conduct Disorder dimension, the BD group scored higher (i.e., in a more pathological direction) than all other groups, and the EMR group scored higher than the regular class group; on the Personality Problem dimension, the BD, EMR, and LD groups each exceeded the regular class group; and on the Inadequacy-Immaturity dimension, the EMR group exceeded the regular class group. The BD group could be discriminated from the other groups on the basis of Conduct Disorder scores. In agreement with the study by Gajar (1979), discrimination of LD and EMR groups was not possible on the basis of BPC scores.

More recently, Richmond and Blagg (1985) compared behavior patterns using the same four groups as did Cullinan et al. (1979). Again, the criteria used to classify LD were unspecified. The results were similar to those of Gajar (1979) and Cullinan et al.; no significant differences were found on the three dimensions of the BPC among the EMR, LD, and regular class groups. However, the children with BD scored higher on all three dimensions than did each of the other three groups.

The results of the above studies suggest that the psychosocial functioning of children with EMR may be similar to that of children with LD. However, these studies did not take into account the heterogeneity of either group; therefore, it is difficult to make any definite conclusions. Although the next study did not investigate psychosocial functioning, it does shed some light on the matter of heterogeneity of low functioning children.

McFadden (1990) examined the effects of FSIQ level on the ability subtype structure of low functioning children and children with LD. Subjects were selected on the basis of the usual LD exclusionary criteria (Rourke, 1975), except that children with below average FSIQ were included. The sample was divided into four groups based on restricted WISC FSIQ ranges (i.e., 101–110, 91–100, 81–90, and 70–80). The neuropsychological test performance data of each group was cluster analyzed. Reliability of the solution was assessed by conducting the analysis with several different cluster analytic methods. Four subtypes were recovered in each of the four groups for a total of 16 subtypes. There was good agreement among the various cluster analytic methods. Although the levels of performance varied with FSIQ range, comparisons of the subtypes across groups revealed two basic profile shapes (Shape A and Shape B) which occurred within all four groups. Shape A was designated as "language disordered" and was characterized by less developed word-definition ability, verbal fluency, and long- and short-term memory for verbal information within a context of better developed simple and complex motor skills, visual-spatial skills, nonverbal problem solving, and abstract reasoning. Shape B was related to less developed speeded hand-eye coordination and verbal expressive tasks within a context of better developed simple motor and visual-spatial abilities, nonverbal problem solving and abstract reasoning, and vocabulary. By elucidating the heterogeneity

of lower functioning children and by demonstrating the similarities between ability subtypes of these children and those of children with average cognitive functioning, McFadden's results provide information that is conducive to the formulation of expectations for the present study.

PREDICTIONS

As no previous investigations specifically examined the psychosocial dimensions of children with BAIQ, the present study is considered to be exploratory in nature. Therefore, some of the hypotheses are more general than specific.

1. It was expected that the psychosocial subtype structure that would emerge from the application of statistical subtyping techniques on selected PIC scores of children with BAIQ would be similar to that of children with LD (Fuerst et al., 1989, 1990; Fuerst & Rourke, 1993). Rationale for this hypothesis: (a) Studies that have examined the psychosocial functioning of children with EMR have not found any consistent differences between children with EMR and those with LD (e.g., Cullinan et al., 1979; Richmond & Blagg, 1985), and (b) McFadden (1990) found that groups with lower than average FSIQ scores contained some of the same skill and ability subtypes that were found in groups with average FSIQ scores. Furthermore, as it has been shown that there is a relationship between ability subtype patterns and psychosocial subtype patterns (e.g., Fuerst et al., 1990; Fuerst & Rourke, 1993; Tsatsanis et al., 1997), it would seem reasonable to infer that psychosocial subtypes would be found in children with BAIQ similar to those previously found in children with LD (e.g., Fuerst et al., 1989, 1990; Fuerst & Rourke, 1993).

   Thus, any or all of the following subtypes were expected to emerge: Normal, Mild Anxiety, Mild Hyperactive, Somatic Concern, Conduct Disorder, Internalized Psychopathology, and Externalized Psychopathology. The three most reliable subtypes (i.e., Normal, Internalized Psychopathology, and Externalized Psychopathology) that have been consistently revealed in previous research (e.g., Fuerst et al., 1989, 1990; Porter & Rourke, 1985) were especially anticipated.

2. It was expected that children with BAIQ would be assigned to subtypes in similar proportions to those found in children with LD (Fuerst & Rourke, 1995; Rourke & Fuerst, 1991). It was expected that one-half to two-thirds or more of the children would exhibit either Normal psychosocial functioning or mild disturbances (i.e., Mild Anxiety, Mild Hyperactive, Somatic Concern, and/or Conduct Disorder). The rest of the children were expected to be divided approximately equally between the more severely disturbed subtypes (i.e., Internalized and Externalized Psychopathology).

3. It was expected that there would be no changes in psychopathological type or severity with advancing age. Rationale: (a) Fuerst and Rourke (1995) compared three age groups of children with LD and found that subtypes were comparable at each age level both in profile shape and in elevation, and that the proportion of young, middle, and old subjects in each subtype was also comparable, indicating that patterns of psychosocial functioning of children with LD are stable across the ages of 7–13; and (b) Tsatsanis et al. (1997) compared age levels among severity of psychopathology groups and found no differences, also indicating stability of psychosocial functioning over this developmental period.

METHODS

Subjects

The participants in this study were 101 children (68 males and 33 females) who were selected from a population of 5296 children who had been referred for neuropsychological assessment because of learning difficulties. Experienced psychometrists administered an extensive neuropsychological test battery to each child. The selection criteria for the subjects were as follows: (a) chronological age between 7.0 and 14.9 years (inclusive); (b) WISC FSIQ score between 60 and 84; (c) at least one Wide Range Achievement Test (WRAT; Jastak & Jastak, 1965) centile score below 25; (d) no educational or cultural deprivation; (e) no primary psychosocial problems (as designated by no known referrals for personality/behavioral problems of the child or family members); and (f) the availability of complete PIC scale

Table 1. Subjects' Age, WISC Full Scale IQ (FSIQ), Verbal IQ (VIQ), and Performance IQ (PIQ) Summary Statistics by Gender.

	M	SD	Range
Males (n = 68)			
Age (years)	10.1	2.1	7.1–14.8
WISC			
FSIQ	78.4	5.8	62–84
VIQ	77.9	7.0	63–92
PIQ	81.6	9.4	57–98
Females (n = 33)			
Age (years)	10.2	2.2	7.2–14.8
WISC			
FSIQ	80.3	5.8	63–84
VIQ	80.3	7.4	63–94
PIQ	80.4	8.3	64–100

Note. WISC = Wechsler Intelligence Scale for Children (Wechsler, 1949), FSIQ = Full Scale Intelligence Quotient, VIQ = Verbal Intelligence Quotient, and PIQ = Performance Intelligence Quotient.

scores. Detailed socioeconomic information was not available for selected children; however, the sample was drawn from a homogeneous lower-to-middle class urban/suburban population. See Table 1 for subjects' age and WISC IQ summary statistics by gender.

Materials

The PIC (described previously) was used as a measure of psychosocial functioning. Scale construction of the PIC involved both empirical and rational strategies. Reported test-retest product-moment correlations ranged from .68 to .97 for all 33 scales (Wirt et al., 1977, 1984).

RESULTS

Q-analysis-Derived Psychosocial Typology of Children with BAIQ

A Q-type factor analysis (using SAS version 6) was applied to selected PIC scores of the participants to determine the psychosocial typology of children with BAIQ. Q-analysis was chosen as the statistical subtyping technique for this study because it has shown good performance in previous research of this type using a similar number of subjects (e.g., Fuerst et al., 1989; Porter & Rourke, 1985). PIC scales were selected for the analysis based on minimizing the amount of interscale overlap and maximizing the representation of dimensions measured by the PIC (Porter & Rourke, 1985). Subjects' scores on 10 of the clinical scales of the PIC were utilized (DVL, SOM, D, FAM, DLQ, WDL, ANX, PSY, HPR, and SSK). ACH and IS scales were not included because according to Fuerst and Rourke (1995), these two scales are highly correlated with the DVL scale and provide little additional information.

Outlier Detection and Deletion

As factor analysis techniques are extremely sensitive to outliers (Tabachnick & Fidell, 1996), the first step in the analysis was to screen for them. The method used in this study is similar to that used by Fuerst and Rourke (1995) and involves a three-step process. First, in order to eliminate profile elevation and dispersion, each subject's scores on the 10 selected PIC scales were standardized across that subject's profile. Next, the Euclidean distances between each subject's scores on the 10 PIC scales and those of all other subjects were calculated. Each distance was compared to a previously selected constant value (the "radius"). A running frequency count was kept for each subject's distances that were less than or equal to the radius. The frequency count is proportionate to the density of other subjects around a particular subject. Cases relatively similar to other cases are found in higher density regions, whereas, cases that are relatively dissimilar to others are found in low density regions and are considered to be outliers. In this manner, 6 subjects (5.9% of the sample) were deemed outliers and were eliminated from subsequent analyses.

The Q-analysis

A data matrix was constructed that contained each remaining subject's PIC scores on the 10 selected scales. This data matrix was transposed and the intercorrelations between subject profiles were calculated. Principal-components solution was used to factor the correlation matrix (Fuerst et al., 1989). Orthogonal rotation to varimax criterion was carried out on factors with eigenvalues equal to or greater than the ratio of the number of subjects to the number of variables (i.e., 9.5) plus one additional factor. The result of this analysis yielded five factors that accounted for 78% of the variance and indicated that the subject sample was comprised

of five subtypes that differed from each other with respect to psychosocial functioning as reflected by the selected PIC variables.

Subjects with factor loadings of greater than or equal to positive .50 on at least one factor with an interval of greater than or equal to .10 between their highest and next highest loading were used to define subtypes based on the factor on which they loaded highest (Fuerst et al., 1989; Porter & Rourke, 1985). Of the 95 subjects used in the analysis, 71 (75%) met the above criteria; 24 (25%) were excluded. Nine of these excluded subjects displayed no loadings of at least .50 on any factor and 15 did not exhibit an interval of at least .10 between their two highest loadings.

The largest number of subjects (30% of those assigned to subtypes; $n = 21$) was assigned to subtype 1 (i.e., the first factor). Subtypes 3 and 4 each contained 15 (21% each, of those assigned) members and Subtypes 2 and 5 each contained 10 (14% each, of those assigned) members. For each Q-analysis-derived subtype, the mean PIC scale scores for all 16 scales were calculated and used to plot PIC profiles displayed in Figures 1, 2, 4, 6, and 8. (For comparison, the figures also show the prototypes that are highly correlated with the Q-analysis-derived subtypes and the results of the profile-matching algorithm; these concepts and results are explained below.)

Relationship to Known LD Psychosocial Subtypes

Mean PIC Profile Similarities and Differences
Visual inspection of the figures suggests distinct similarities between the PIC profiles of the Q-analysis-derived psychosocial subtypes of children with BAIQ and the PIC profiles of some of the prototypical subtypes that have been derived through previous research using children with LD (Fuerst & Rourke, 1995; Rourke & Fuerst, 1991). To confirm this impression, the means of the previously selected 10 clinical PIC scales of each Q-analysis-derived subtype were correlated with corresponding means of the seven prototypical subtypes (i.e., Normal, Mild Anxiety, Mild Hyperactive, Somatic Concern, Conduct Disorder, Internalized Psychopathology, and Externalized Psychopathology). These correlations are an indication of the

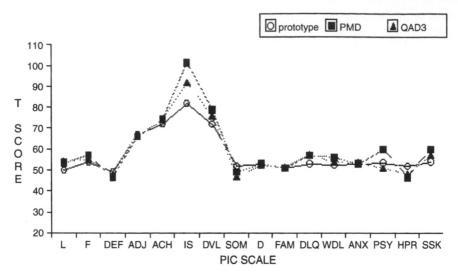

Fig. 1. Mean PIC profile for the Normal subtype. PIC = Personality Inventory for Children (Wirt et al., 1977); PMD = Profile-matching-derived Subtypes; QAD3 = Q-analysis-derived Subtype 3. See text for PIC scale abbreviations.

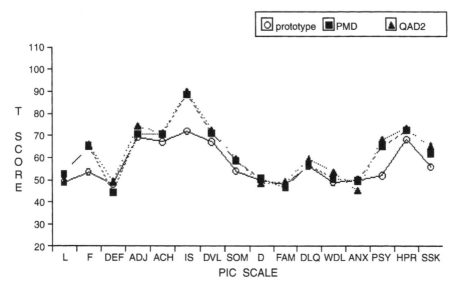

Fig. 2. Mean PIC profile for the Mild Hyperactive subtype. QAD2 = Q-analysis-derived Subtype 2. Other abbreviations are the same as for Figure 1.

degree of similarity between the mean PIC profile shapes of the Q-analysis-derived subtypes and those of the prototypes. The results of the correlation analysis are displayed in Table 2.

As can be seen in Table 2, Q-analysis-derived Subtype 1 is highly correlated ($r = .93$) with only one prototype. Internalized Psychopathology, and represents a good replication of this prototype.

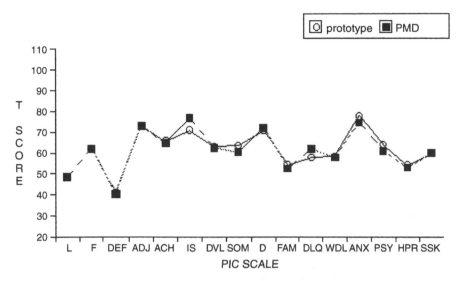

Fig. 3. Mean PIC profile for the Mild Anxiety Subtype. Abbreviations are the same as for Figure 1.

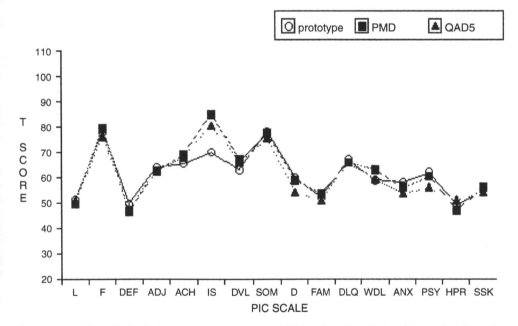

Fig. 4. Mean PIC profile for the Somatic Concern subtype. QAD5 = Q-analysis-derived Subtype 5. Other abbreviations are the same as for Figure 1.

Q-analysis-derived Subtypes 3 and 5 represent good replications of the Normal prototype ($r = .94$) and the Somatic Concern prototype ($r = .93$), respectively. Subtype 2 represents an adequate replication of the Mild Hyperactive prototype ($r = .83$); when the PIC profiles of these two subtypes are compared (see Fig. 2), it is apparent that the main difference is that Subtype 2 exhibits an elevation of

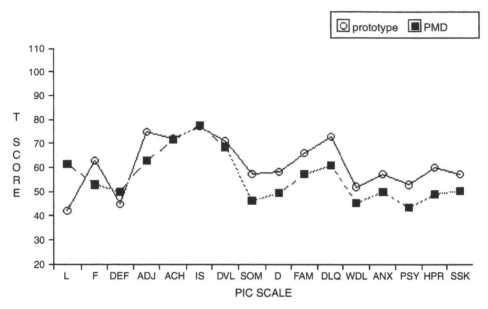

Fig. 5. Mean PIC profile for the Conduct Disorder subtype. Abbreviations are the same as for Figure 1.

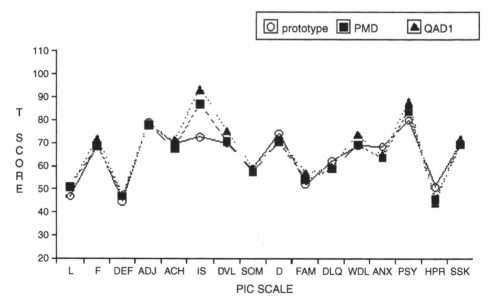

Fig. 6. Mean PIC profile for the Internalized Psychopathology subtype. QAD1 = Q-analysis-derived Subtype 1. Other abbreviations are the same as for Figure 1.

approximately 15 points higher on the PSY scale than does the Mild Hyperactive prototype.

It should also be noted that all five of the Q-analysis-derived subtypes of psychosocial functioning of children with BAIQ evidence much higher elevations on the IS scale than do the prototypical subtypes of children with LD. As the IS scale is a reflection of parental concern that the

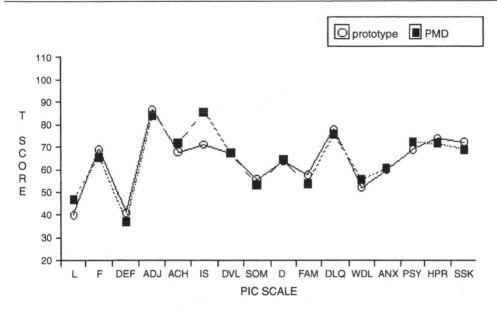

Fig. 7. Mean PIC profile for the Externalized Psychopathology subtype. Abbreviations are the same as for Figure 1.

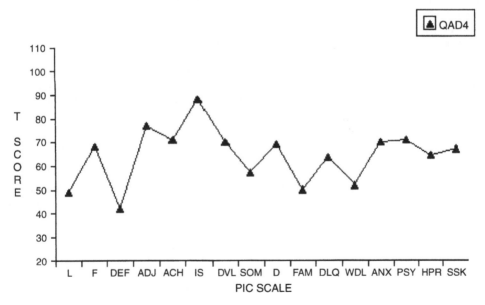

Fig. 8. Mean PIC profile for the Mild Anxiety/Depression subtype. QAD4 = Q-analysis-derived Subtype 4. Other abbreviations are the same as for Figure 1.

child's difficulties may be due to impaired intellectual functioning, it makes intuitive sense that children with BAIQ, on average, exhibit higher elevations on this scale than do children with LD.

Q-analysis-derived Subtype 4 did not correlate highly with any one prototype but showed moderate correlations with three prototypes: Internalized Psychopathology ($r = .59$), Externalized

Table 2. Correlations Between Q-analysis-Derived (QAD) PIC Subtypes and Prototypical PIC Subtypes.

Prototypes	Q-analysis-derived subtypes				
	QAD1	QAD2	QAD3	QAD4	QAD5
N	.34	.47	.94	.41	.31
MH	−.29	.83	.47	.39	.18
MA	.36	−.46	.06	.56	.01
SOM	.20	−.01	.05	−.01	.93
CON	−.33	.18	.57	.04	.26
INT	.93	−.01	.31	.59	−.01
EXT	−.12	.59	.21	.59	−.13

Note. Prototypes: N = Normal, MH = Mild Hyperactive, MA = Mild Anxiety, SOM = Somatic Concern, CON = Conduct Disorder, INT = Internalized Psychopathology, EXT = Externalized Psychopathology.

Table 3. Percentages of Assigned Subjects Within Prototypical, Q-analysis-Derived (QAD), and Profile-Matching-Derived (PMD) Subtypes.

Source	Subtype							
	N	MH	MA	SOM	CON	INT	EXT	MA/D
Prototype	24	19	12	9	7	16	14	
QAD	21	14		14		30		21
PMD	21	12	11	14	3	28	10	

Note. MA/D = Mild Anxiety/Depression. Other abbreviations are the same as for Table 2.

Psychopathology ($r = .59$), and Mild Anxiety ($r = .56$). The PIC profile of Subtype 4 is displayed alone in Figure 8. This subtype has not been found in previous research using children with LD. Based on its most salient features, the subtype was named Mild Anxiety/Depression. The Conduct Disorder, Mild Anxiety, and Externalized Psychopathology prototypes were not adequately replicated in the present sample of children with BAIQ using Q-type factor analysis.

Proportion Similarities and Differences
In addition to the comparison of mean PIC profile shapes to the prototypes, the Q-analysis-derived subtypes were also compared to the prototypes in relation to the proportion of assigned subjects falling into each subtype. Table 3 shows that the percentage of cases assigned to the Normal group (Subtype 3; 21% of those assigned to subtypes) is very similar to that of the Normal prototype (24% of those assigned); however, the Internalized Psychopathology group (Subtype 1) is almost twice as large as the corresponding prototype. The Mild Hyperactive group (Subtype 2) is slightly smaller than the corresponding prototype; whereas, the Somatic Concern group (Subtype 5) is somewhat larger.

A Chi-square test for Goodness-of-Fit (Aron & Aron, 1994) was used to determine significant differences in proportion. As the subtypical structure that emerged from the Q-analysis is quite

different from that of the prototypes, to ease comparison the subtypes were collapsed into three groups for subsequent analyses. This also has the added benefit of increasing the power of the statistical tests. The subtypes were grouped according to degree of severity (i.e., Normal, Mild, and Severe) and according to type of psychopathology (i.e., Normal, Externalized, and Internalized) in a manner similar to that used by Tsatsanis et al. (1997).

The Q-analysis-derived Normal group consisted of children assigned to the Normal subtype; the Mild category contained children assigned to the Mild Hyperactive, Somatic Concern, and Mild Anxiety/Depression subtypes; and the Severe group contained children assigned to the Internalized Psychopathology subtype. The number of members in each of these three groups was the observed frequency for the BAIQ sample and the expected frequency was the number of members in the prototype groups: Normal (Normal), Mild (Mild Hyperactive, Mild Anxiety, Somatic Concern, and Conduct Disorder), and Severe (Internalized Psychopathology and Externalized Psychopathology). Using an alpha level of .05 for all statistical tests, the result of the Chi-square test was not significant, $\chi^2(2) = 0.468$, $p > .05$, suggesting that the proportions of children with BAIQ who exhibited Normal, Mild, and Severe levels of psychopathology was the same as that previously found in children with LD.

Comparisons in type of psychopathology were also made (i.e., Normal, Internalized, and Externalized). The Q-analysis-derived Normal group consisted of children assigned to the Normal subtype. The Externalized group consisted of children

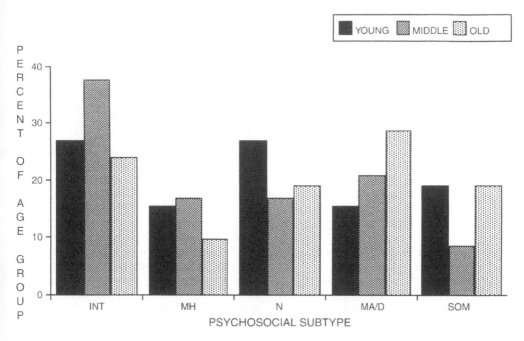

Fig. 9. Percentage of Young, Middle, and Old children assigned to Q-analysis-derived subtypes. INT = Internalized Psychopathology, MH = Mild Hyperactive, N = Normal, MA/D = Mild Anxiety/Depression, SOM = Somatic Concern.

assigned to the Mild Hyperactive subtype and the Internalized group was made up of children assigned to the Internalized Psychopathology subtype. Although the most salient features of the Mild Anxiety/Depression subtype reflect aspects of internalized psychopathology (i.e., Anxiety and Depression), it was not used in this analysis because it also exhibits moderate elevations on features of externalized psychopathology (i.e., Delinquency and Hyperactivity); in fact, it is moderately correlated with both Externalized and Internalized Psychopathology prototypes. The prototypical subtypes were divided as follows: the Normal group consisted of subjects assigned to the Normal prototype; the Externalized group was made up of children assigned to the Mild Hyperactive and Externalized Psychopathology prototypes; and the Internalized group contained those assigned to Mild Anxiety and Internalized Psychopathology prototypes. In this case, the Chi-square test was significant, $\chi^2(2) = 13.102$, $p < .05$, indicating that the proportions of children with BAIQ who

exhibited Normal, Internalized, and Externalized types of psychopathology were significantly different from that found in children with LD. Children with BAIQ appear to be less likely to exhibit external aspects of psychopathology, especially in its more severe form.

Relationship Between Psychosocial Structure and Age

To determine if there were psychopathological changes with increasing age, the cases that were used to define the Q-analysis-derived subtypes ($N = 71$) were divided into three age groups: Young (ages 7.0 to 8.9 years; $n = 26$), Middle (ages 9.0 to 11.9 years; $n = 24$), and Old (age 12.0 to 14.9 years; $n = 21$). Figure 9 displays the percentage of each age group assigned to each of the subtypes. (This means, for example, that of the Middle group, 17% were assigned to the Mild Hyperactive subtype.) To increase power, the subtypes were collapsed into three groups for subsequent analyses: first, according to degree of psychopathology severity (i.e., Normal, Mild, and Severe) and then, according to type of psychopathology (i.e., Normal, Internalized, and Externalized) in the same manner as was described in the section above dealing with proportions. Chi-square tests for Independence (Aron & Aron, 1994) were conducted. The results of the Chi-square test comparing severity of psychopathology and age was nonsignificant, $\chi^2(4) = 1.836, p > .05$, as was the test comparing type of psychopathology and age, $\chi^2(4) = 1.110, p > .05$, indicating that there was no relationship between age and severity or type of psychopathology. In other words, within the age range examined in this study, there were no changes in psychopathological severity or type with advancing years.

Profile-Matching-Derived Psychosocial Typology of Children with BAIQ

A second method of deriving subtypes of psychosocial functioning of children with BAIQ entailed a profile-matching algorithm designed by Fuerst (Fuerst & Rourke, 1995; Rourke & Fuerst, 1991) using SAS macro programming language. Scores of the same 10 PIC scales that were used for the Q-analysis (i.e., DVL, SOM, D, FAM, DLQ, WDL, ANX, PSY, HPR, and SSK) of the entire sample of children with BAIQ ($N = 101$) were used in the analysis which involved the calculation of the correlation between each subject's PIC profile and the PIC profiles of the seven previously mentioned prototypes. Subjects were assigned to the subtype with which their PIC profile correlated most strongly and positively. Those showing only negative or weak correlations (i.e., <.40) with the prototypical profiles and/or an interval of less than .10 between their two highest correlations were considered to be outliers and were dropped from further analyses.

Using this method, 96% ($N = 97$) of the total sample were assigned to one of the seven subtypes. Four subjects (4% of the total sample) were rejected as outliers. The largest number of subjects, 27 (28% of assigned subjects) were matched to the Internalized Psychopathology prototype. The second largest number of subjects, 20 (21% of those assigned) were matched to the Normal prototype. The next largest number of subjects, 14 (14% of those assigned) were matched to the Somatic Concern prototype. Approximately equal

Table 4. Correlations Between Profile-Matching-Derived (PMD) PIC Subtypes and Prototypical PIC Subtypes.

Prototypes	PMD subtypes						
	N	MH	MA	SOM	CON	INT	EXT
N	.91	.39	.07	.14	.40	.51	.20
MH	.52	.89	−.28	−.02	.15	.02	.59
MA	.10	−.27	.95	.32	−.13	.56	−.09
SOM	.26	−.07	.16	.97	.11	.21	−.29
CON	.40	.19	.15	.53	.55	−.13	−.04
INT	.29	−.29	.42	.19	−.36	.97	−.05
EXT	.21	.52	−.11	−.15	.31	.24	.95

Note. Abbreviations are the same as for Table 2.

numbers of subjects, 12, 11, and 10 (12%, 11%, and 10%, respectively) were matched to the Mild Hyperactive, Mild Anxiety, and Externalized Psychopathology prototypes. The smallest number of subjects, 3 (3% of those assigned) were matched to the Conduct Disorder prototype.

Relationship to Prototypes and Q-analysis-Derived subtypes

Mean PIC Profile Similarities and Differences
The mean PIC profiles for each of the seven profile-matching-derived (PMD) subtypes were calculated and are shown in Figures 1–7. Visual inspection of the Figures suggests distinct similarities between the PMD subtypes and the corresponding prototypes. To confirm this impression, the means of the previously selected 10 clinical PIC scales of each PMD subtype were correlated with the corresponding means of the prototypical subtypes. The results of the correlation analysis are displayed in Table 4 which shows that all of the PMD subtypes are correlated .89 or better with their corresponding prototypes with one exception: the PMD Conduct Disorder subtype is only moderately correlated ($r = .55$) with its corresponding prototype. Figure 5 shows that, although the two profiles are virtually the same shape, the PMD subtype evidences lower mean scores (approximately 10 points) on the clinical scales than does the prototype. A few other minor differences between the two typologies were noted, such as the following: the PSY scale of the PMD Normal subtype is slightly elevated compared to the corresponding

prototype, and the PSY scale of PMD Mild Hyperactive subtype is elevated approximately 15 points compared to the corresponding prototype. In addition, almost all of the PMD subtypes of psychosocial functioning of children with BAIQ exhibit substantially higher elevations on the IS scale than do the prototypes.

Figures 1, 2, 4, and 6 show similarities and differences between the PMD subtypes and the corresponding Q-analysis-derived subtypes. The PMD Mild Hyperactive subtype and the Q-analysis-derived Mild Hyperactive subtype are almost identical in both shape and elevation. Both of these subtypes evidence greater elevations on the PSY scale compared as to the prototype. Consistent with comparison between the PMD subtype and the prototype, the PSY scale of the PMD Normal subtype is slightly elevated as compared to the Normal Q-analysis-derived subtype.

Proportion Similarities and Differences
Percentages of subjects assigned to each PMD subtype are displayed in Table 3. The Table shows that there are some proportion similarities and differences between the PMD subtypes and that of the prototypes. For example, the Normal subtypes of both typologies are similar in size. The PMD and prototype Mild Anxiety subtypes are also similar in size. In agreement with the proportion differences between the prototypes and the Q-analysis-derived subtypes, the PMD Mild Hyperactive subtype is smaller than the corresponding prototype, whereas, the Somatic Concern subtype is somewhat larger. Also in agreement with the Q-analysis subtype structure, the PMD Internalized Psychopathology subtype is the largest subtype of the typology and it is much larger than the corresponding prototype. In addition, the PMD Conduct Disorder and Externalized Psychopathology subtypes are both somewhat smaller than those of the prototypes.

A Chi-square test for Goodness-of-Fit (Aron & Aron, 1994) was used to determine if the proportion differences that were noted between the PMD subtypes and the prototypes were significant. Because the subtypical structures of the prototypes and the PMD subtypes are identical, seven groups were used in the analysis. The result was significant, $\chi^2(6) = 18.530$, $p < .05$, indicating that

children with BAIQ were assigned to PMD subtypes in proportions that were significantly different from that of the prototypes.

Table 3 shows that there are some definite similarities between the number of subjects within each PMD subtype and that of the corresponding Q-analysis-derived subtype. The PMD Normal, Mild Hyperactive, Somatic Concern, and Internalized Psychopathology groups are all similar in size as compared to the corresponding Q-analysis-derived subtypes. A Chi-square test was used to determine if there were, in fact, no significant differences between the two typologies in the proportion of members within the various subtypes. Because the subtypical structure that emerged from the Q-analysis is different from that of the profile-matching method, to ease comparison, the subtypes were collapsed into three groups in the same manner as was described above in the section on proportion similarities and differences between the Q-analysis subtypes and the prototypes. Again, the subtypes were grouped according to degree of psychopathology severity (i.e., Normal, Mild, and Severe) and according to type of psychopathology (i.e., Normal, Externalized, and Internalized). The results were nonsignificant in relation to psychopathology severity, $\chi^2(2) = 3.783$, $p > .05$, and in relation to type of psychopathology, $\chi^2(2) = 2.348$, $p > .05$. These results suggest that the proportions of children with BAIQ assigned to the various PMD subtypes were not significantly different than the proportions of children assigned to the various Q-analysis subtypes in relation to both type and severity of psychopathology.

Relationship Between Psychosocial Structure and Age
To determine if there were psychopathological changes with age, the subjects that were used to define PMD subtypes ($N = 97$) were divided into three age groups: Young (ages 7.0–8.9 years; $n = 39$), Middle (ages 9.0–11.9 year; $n = 36$), and Old (ages 12.0–14.9 years; $n = 22$). The power of the statistical tests was increased by collapsing the subtypes into three groups. First, according to severity of psychopathology (i.e., Normal, Mild, and Severe) and then, according to type of psychopathology (i.e., Normal, Internalized, and

Externalized) in a similar manner as described above. A Chi-square test for Independence (Aron & Aron, 1994) comparing severity of psychopathology and age was nonsignificant, $\chi^2(4) = 3.269$, $p > .05$, as was the test comparing type of psychopathology and age, $(4) = 1.306$, $p > .05$. In agreement with the results from the Q-analysis, the PMD results suggest that there was no relationship between age and severity or type of psychopathology. In other words, within the age range examined in this study, there were no changes in psychopathological severity or type with advancing years.

VIQs-PIQs of PMD Subtypes

Previous research that involved children with LD indicated that WISC Verbal IQ-Performance IQ (VIQ-PIQ) discrepancies were related to psychosocial subtype membership (e.g., Fuerst et al., 1990; Rourke & Fuerst, 1991). Namely, that children with VIQ = PIQ and VIQ < PIQ were found mainly in the normal and mildly disturbed subtypes, and children with VIQ > PIQ were found in a higher frequency than expected in the severely disturbed subtypes, especially Internalized Psychopathology.

To determine if IQ trends similar to those of children with LD occurred in this sample of children with BAIQ, the VIQ, PIQ, and FSIQ scores for each PMD subtype were calculated (see Table 5). As can be seen from the Table, there is a tendency towards higher incidence of VIQ < PIQ in the

Table 5. Mean WISC Verbal IQ, Performance IQ, and Full Scale IQ of Profile-Matching-Derived Subtypes.

PMD subtypes	Mean WISC IQs		
	VIQ	PIQ	FSIQ
N	76.8	82.9	77.0
MH	77.3	81.7	77.3
MA	79.1	86.1	81.0
SOM	79.9	81.9	78.9
CON	82.0	77.3	77.7
INT	80.3	76.9	76.6
EXT	78.3	83.3	78.7

Note. WISC = Wechsler Intelligence Scale for Children (Wechsler, 1949), FSIQ = Full Scale Intelligence Quotient, VIQ = Verbal Intelligence Quotient, and PIQ = Performance Intelligence Quotient. Other abbreviations are the same as for Table 2.

normal and mildly disturbed subtypes and higher incidence of VIQ > PIQ in the Internalized psychopathology subtype. To test for significance, the subtypes were divided into two groups: (1) Mild (which included Normal, Mild Hyperactive, Mild Anxiety, and Somatic Concern groups; $n = 57$; the Conduct Disorder group was not included because of its small membership); and (2) Internalized (which included the Internalized Psychopathology group; $n = 27$). A 2×2 with repeated measures ANOVA analysis with mean IQ scores as the dependent variable was conducted. IQ type (VIQ and PIQ) was the within-subject factor and Group (Mild and Internalized) was the between-subject factor. Using an alpha level of .05 for all statistical tests, the main effects of IQ type, $F(1,82) = 0.299$, $p > .05$, and group, $F(1, 82) = 2.214$, $p > .05$, were not significant. However, the IQ type $\times$ Group interaction was highly significant, $F(1, 82) = 8.637$, $p = .004$, and is depicted in Figure 10.

As can be seen in Figure 10, the Mild group exhibited a lower VIQ and higher PIQ than did the Internalized group; this finding is in agreement with previous research results. Tukey's Honestly Significant Difference (HSD) test was conducted to determine if the IQ group means were significantly different: There was a significant difference between the mean PIQ of the Mild group (83.00) and that of the Internalized group (76.89). The Mild group exhibited a significantly higher PIQ than did the Internalized group. However, the difference between the mean VIQ of the Mild group (78.09) and that of the Internalized group (80.26) was not significant.

DISCUSSION

In support of the first prediction, there were clear similarities between the subtype structure of psychosocial functioning of children with BAIQ that emerged from the Q-analysis and the prototypical subtype structure of children with LD. For example, similar to the corresponding prototype, the Q-analysis-derived Normal subtype exhibited elevations only on the PIC scales that reflect developmental, intellectual, and academic achievement. Scales that are suggestive of psychosocial

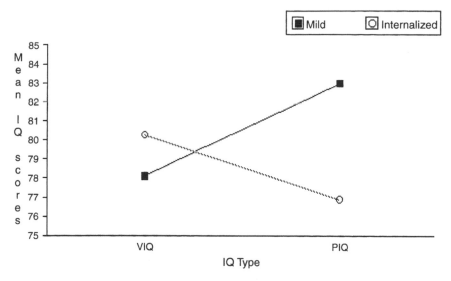

Fig. 10. Mean Verbal IQ (VIQ) and Performance IQ (PIQ) of the PMD Mild group (Normal, Mild Hyperactive, Mild Anxiety, and Somatic Concern groups) versus that of the PMD Internalized group.

difficulties were within normal range. As expected, the other Q-analysis-derived subtypes also exhibited elevations on scales that reflect developmental, intellectual, and academic achievement in addition to elevations on various clinical scales. The Somatic Concern, Internalized Psychopathology, and Mild Hyperactive subtypes represented good replications of the corresponding prototypes. However, the latter subtype was somewhat more elevated on the PSY scale than was the corresponding prototype. It was also noted that the IS scales of all of the Q-analysis-derived subtypes of children with BAIQ were substantially elevated compared to those of the prototypes.

Some unexpected results emerged from the Q-analysis that were not in accord with the first prediction. Of the three most reliable subtypes (i.e., Normal, Internalized Psychopathology, and Externalized Psychopathology) that have been consistently found in previous studies of children with LD (e.g., Fuerst et al., 1989, 1990; Porter & Rourke, 1985), only the Normal and the Internalized Psychopathology subtypes emerged. In addition, a new subtype, Mild Anxiety/Depression, emanated from the data. This new subtype contained features of mild forms of both internalized and externalized types of psychopathology.

The first prediction was also supported by the profile-matching results. The PMD subtype structure of psychosocial functioning of children with BAIQ that arose from this method bore obvious similarities to that of the LD prototypes. All seven prototypical subtypes were derived; although one subtype, Conduct Disorder, was somewhat small. In agreement with the Q-analysis results, the PSY scale of the Mild Hyperactive PMD subtype was somewhat higher in comparison to the corresponding prototype. Also similar to the Q-analysis results, almost all of the PMD subtypes exhibited substantially higher elevations on the IS scales than did the prototypical subtypes.

Some explanation is necessary to account for the fact that the subtype structure that was derived from the profile-matching method was almost identical to the prototypical subtype structure (at least in number, shape, and elevation of the subtypes), whereas, the subtype structure that was derived from the Q-analysis was somewhat different. In this sample of children with BAIQ, the application of the Q-analysis technique resulted in the formation of a new subtype, Mild Anxiety/Depression. The profile-matching algorithm does not allow new subtypes to form (Fuerst & Rourke, 1995); therefore, when this method was applied, the subjects

MARGARET B. RALSTON ET AL.

who were members of the Q-analysis-derived Mild Anxiety/Depression subtype were either matched to one of the seven prototypes or deemed outliers. Examination of the fate of these subjects in the profile-matching results revealed that they were matched to Externalized Psychopathology, Mild Hyperactive, and Mild Anxiety prototypes.

In support of the second prediction, the Q-analysis results revealed that the proportions of children with BAIQ who exhibited Normal, Mild, and Severe levels of psychopathology were not significantly different from those found in children with LD. However, when the proportions of children exhibiting the three main types of psychopathology (i.e., Normal, Externalized, and Internalized) were compared with those of children with LD, significant differences were found.

Regarding the profile-matching results, the PMD Normal and Mild Anxiety subtypes contained similar percentages of subjects as did the corresponding prototypes. The proportion of members within the PMD Mild Hyperactive, Somatic Concern, and Externalized Psychopathology subtypes was somewhat different from that of the prototypes, but not extremely so. An unexpected finding was that the PMD Internalized Psychopathology subtype was the largest subtype of the typology and that it was almost twice as large as its corresponding prototype. In addition, there were definite similarities between the proportion of members falling within the various PMD subtypes and that of the Q-analysis-derived subtypes. In fact, no significant differences were found between the two typologies in relation to both type or severity of psychopathology.

Taken together, the results of the two subtyping methods suggest that children with BAIQ may be more likely to exhibit the more extreme form of psychopathology of the internalizing type (i.e., Internalized Psychopathology) and less likely to exhibit psychopathology of the externalizing type especially in its more extreme form (i.e., Externalized Psychopathology) than are children with LD. However, children with BAIQ appear to exhibit the various levels of psychopathology (i.e., Normal, Mild, and Severe) in similar proportion to those of children with LD. Therefore, it can be concluded that the psychosocial dimensions of children with BAIQ are very similar to those of children with LD

in a general sense, but with some minor differences. This conclusion is consistent with the results of studies that investigated the psychosocial functions of special education students and found no differences between children with LD and those who were classified as EMR (Cullinan et al., 1979; Gajar, 1979; Richmond & Blagg, 1985). As these studies compared undifferentiated groups of children with LD to undifferentiated groups of EMR children, it is conceivable that the minor differences averaged out.

With respect to the third prediction, both methods found no differences in the types or severity of psychopathology within the three age groups examined in this study, indicating that the patterns of psychosocial functioning of children with BAIQ are relatively stable across the ages of 7.0–14.9 years. Although at odds with the notion that children who have learning problems have a tendency to develop more serious types of psychopathology with increasing age because of a progression of anxiety and self-consciousness brought on by criticism from other people, the present finding is consistent with the results of previous research regarding children with LD (Fuerst & Rourke, 1995; Tsatsanis et al., 1997).

An understanding of the principal methodological limitation of the present study should be kept in mind when evaluating the inferences and conclusions that were made. As multivariate subtyping techniques such as Q-analysis will always produce groupings even on random data (Fuerst et al., 1989), the internal validity (reliability) of the solution should have been assessed by applying the subtyping technique to two different sets of subjects. It was not possible to conduct this procedure in the present study because there were not enough subjects available who met the stringent selection criteria. Although the reliability of the solution was not assessed with a different sample, the similarities that were found between the Q-analysis and profile-matching results suggest that the solution may be quite reliable. In addition, potential biases arise with the use of school or clinic-referred samples because these children may be somewhat different from the general population. It is important to keep in mind that the results of this study can be generalized only to children with BAIQ who were referred for neuropsychological assessment due to learning difficulties.

In conclusion, our results appear to indicate that the psychosocial typology of children with BAIQ resembles that of children with LD in a general sense. Similar to children with LD, approximately two-thirds of the children with BAIQ exhibited either normal psychosocial functioning or mild disturbances and one-third exhibited more severe forms of psychopathology. The two groups differed, however, in a specific sense. Although children with BAIQ exhibit many of the same aspects of psychosocial disturbances as do children with LD, they appear to be more inclined to develop psychopathology of the internalizing type and should be assessed regularly for signs of depression, anxiety, and social withdrawal. Moreover, in agreement with previous research results involving children with LD (Fuerst et al., 1990; Rourke & Fuerst, 1991), children with BAIQ who exhibit internalized psychopathology are likely to display more deficient nonverbal skills than are those who exhibit normal functioning or mild disturbances.

REFERENCES

Aron, A., & Aron, E.N. (1994). *Statistics for psychology.* Englewood Cliffs, NJ: Prentice Hall.

Cullinan, D., Epstein, M.H., & Dembinski, R.J. (1979). Behavior problems of educationally handicapped and normal pupils. *Journal of Abnormal Child Psychology, 7,* 495–502.

Epstein, M.H., Bursuck, W., & Cullinan, D. (1985). Patterns of behavior problems among the learning disabled: Boys aged 12–18, girls aged 6–11, and girls aged 12–18. *Learning Disability Quarterly, 8,* 123–129.

Epstein, M.H., Cullinan, D., & Rosemier, R. (1983). Behavior problem patterns among the learning disabled: Boys aged 6–11. *Learning Disability Quarterly, 6,* 305–311.

Fuerst, D.R., Fisk, J.L., & Rourke, B.P. (1989). Psychosocial functioning of learning-disabled children: Replicability of statistically derived subtypes. *Journal of Consulting and Clinical Psychology, 57,* 275–280.

Fuerst, D.R., Fisk, J.L., & Rourke, B.P. (1990). Psychosocial functioning of learning-disabled children: Relations between WISC Verbal IQ-Performance IQ discrepancies and personality subtypes. *Journal of Consulting and Clinical Psychology, 58,* 657–660.

Fuerst, D.R., & Rourke, B.P. (1993). Psychosocial functioning of children: Relations between personality subtypes and academic achievement. *Journal of Abnormal Child Psychology, 21,* 597–607.

Fuerst, D.R., & Rourke, B.P. (1995). Psychosocial functioning of children with learning disabilities at three age levels. *Child Neuropsychology, 1,* 38–55.

Gajar, A. (1979). Educable mentally retarded, learning disabled, emotionally disturbed: Similarities and differences. *Exceptional Children, 45,* 470–472.

Jastak, J.F., & Jastak, S.R. (1965). *The Wide Range Achievement Test.* Wilmington, DE: Guidance Associates.

McFadden, G.T. (1990). *Determination of the Subtypal Composition of Several Samples of Learning Disabled Children Selected on the Basis of WISC FSIQ IQ Level: A Neuropsychological, Multivariate Approach.* Unpublished doctoral dissertation, University of Windsor, Windsor, Ont., Canada.

Polloway, E.A., Patton, J.R., Smith, T.E.C., & Buck, G.H. (1997). Mental retardation and learning disabilities: Conceptual and applied issues. *Journal of Learning Disabilities, 30,* 297–308, 345.

Porter, J.E., & Rourke, B.P. (1985). Socioemotional functioning of learning-disabled children: A subtypal analysis of personality patterns. In B.P. Rourke (Ed.), *Neuropsychology of learning disabilities* (pp. 257–280). New York: Guilford Press.

Quay, H.C., & Peterson, D.R. (1975). *Manual for the Behavior Problem Checklist.* Unpublished manuscript, University of Miami.

Richmond, B.O., & Blagg, D.E. (1985). Adaptive behavior, social adjustment, and academic achievement of regular and special education children. *The Exceptional Child, 32,* 93–98.

Rourke, B.P. (1975). Brain-behavior relationships in children with learning disabilities. *American Psychologist, 30,* 911–920.

Rourke, B.P. (2000). Neuropsychological and psychosocial subtyping: A review of investigations within the University of Windsor laboratory. *Canadian Psychology, 41,* 34–51.

Rourke, B.P., & Fuerst, D.R. (1991). *Learning disabilities and psychosocial functioning: A neuropsychological perspective.* New York: Guilford Press.

Siegel, L.S. (1988). Evidence that IQ scores are irrelevant to the definition and analysis of reading disability. *Canadian Journal of Psychology, 42,* 201–215.

Siegel, L.S. (1989). IQ is irrelevant to the definition of learning disabilities. *Journal of Learning Disabilities, 22,* 469–478, 486.

Speece, D.L., McKinney, J.D., & Appelbaum, M.I. (1985). Classification and validation of behavioral subtypes of learning-disabled children. *Journal of Educational Psychology, 77,* 67–77.

Stanovich, K.E. (1991). Discrepancy definitions of reading disability: Has intelligence led us astray? *Reading Research Quarterly, 26,* 7–29.

Strang, J.D., & Rourke, B.P. (1985). Adaptive behavior of children who exhibit specific arithmetic disabilities and associated neuropsychological abilities and deficits. In B.P. Rourke (Ed.), *Neuropsychology of learning disabilities* (pp. 302–328). New York: Guilford Press.

Tabachnick, B.G., & Fidell, L.S. (1996). *Using multivariate statistics* (3rd ed.). Northridge, CA: Harper Collins College Publishers.

Tsatsanis, K.D., Fuerst, D.R., & Rourke, B.P. (1997). Psychosocial dimensions of learning disabilities: External validation and relationship with age and academic functioning. *Journal of Learning Disabilities, 30,* 490–502.

Wechsler, D. (1949). *Wechsler Intelligence Scale for Children manual.* New York: Psychological Corporation.

Wirt, R.D., Lachar, D., Klinedinst, J.K., & Seat, P.D. (1977). *Multidimensional description of child personality: A manual for the Personality Inventory for Children.* Los Angeles: Western Psychological Services.

Wirt, R.D., Lachar, D., Klinedinst, J.K., & Seat, P.D. (1984). *Multidimensional description of child personality: A manual for the Personality Inventory for Children – Revised 1984.* Los Angeles: Western Psychological Services.

The Clinical Neuropsychologist
2000, Vol. 14, No. 3, pp. 325–340

Limited Accuracy of Premorbid Intelligence Estimators: A Demonstration of Regression to the Mean

Michael R. Basso[1], Robert A. Bornstein[3], Brad L. Roper[2], and Victoria L. McCoy[1]
[1]University of Tulsa, [2]Veterans Affairs Medical Center, Memphis, TN, and [3]Neuropsychology Program,
The Ohio State University

ABSTRACT

Regression-based premorbid intelligence estimators have been devised by Barona, Reynolds, and Chastain (1984), Barona and Chastain (1986), Hamsher (1984), Krull, Scott, and Sherer (1995; the Oklahoma Premorbid Intelligence Estimate: OPIE), and Vanderploeg, Schinka, and Axelrod (1996; BEST-3 approach), but little is known of their relative accuracy, particularly in outer ranges of intellectual ability (e.g., below-average, superior, etc.). Towards this end, the Wechsler Adult Intelligence Scale-Revised (WAIS-R) was administered to 150 neurologically normal adults, and estimated VIQ, PIQ, and FSIQ scores were computed according to each regression method. Results showed that methods based solely on demographic factors were most susceptible to meanward regression, rendering them poor estimators of IQ scores in outer ranges. Although the OPIE and BEST-3 performed somewhat better, their accuracy remained relatively weak. The findings suggest that regression-based estimates of premorbid IQ are very susceptible to error, particularly in outer ranges of intellectual function.

In assessing individuals with known or suspected cerebral dysfunction, a primary goal of the neuropsychologist is to determine the degree to which cognitive impairment is present. In making this decision, the clinician compares a patient's current performance to a presumed premorbid neurobehavioral status. Generally, current cognitive function is readily apparent in the form of neuropsychological test scores. Rarely, however, do premorbid test data exist. Toward this end, methods have been devised to estimate premorbid abilities, especially intellectual capacity.

According to one approach, premorbid intelligence is estimated on the basis of demographic variables. In particular, age, sex, education, occupation, and race are combined in multiple regression equations to predict Wechsler Adult Intelligence Scale-Revised (WAIS-R: Wechsler, 1981) IQ scores. The rationale for basing premorbid estimates on such variables becomes apparent when comparing mean IQ scores across demographic subgroups. For instance, in the WAIS-R normative sample, mean Full Scale IQ scores differ by as much as 33 points across subgroups stratified by education (Kaufman, 1990). Relatively large mean differences across gender, race, and occupation classifications are also present in the WAIS-R norms. Hence, demographic variables may serve as potent predictors of intellectual level.

Among the most commonly used demographic-based regression estimates are those developed by Barona and colleagues (Barona & Chastain, 1986; Barona, Reynolds, & Chastain, 1984) and Hamsher (1984). (The latter method is a revision of the Wilson et al. (1978) equation that was used to estimate WAIS IQs). These equations vary in several respects. For instance, the two approaches have distinct schemes for classifying predictor variables.

Address correspondence to: Michael R. Basso, University of Tulsa, Department of Psychology, 600 South College Avenue, Tulsa, OK 74104-3189, USA. Tel.: ++1 918 631 2248. Fax: ++1 918 631 2833. E-mail: michael-basso@utulsa.edu
Accepted for publication: July 24, 2000.

Specifically, in the Barona et al. (1984) equation, one of six values for education and occupation may be entered into the regression. In contrast, the Hamsher equation permits actual years of education to be entered into the regression, and occupation assumes one value from a 10-point range. Consequently, the Barona et al. (1984) equation has a smaller range of possible predictor values than the Hamsher equation. This, in turn, may cause the Barona estimation method to have a more restricted range of predicted scores than the Hamsher equation.

The Oklahoma Premorbid Intelligence Estimate (OPIE; Krull, Scott, & Sherer, 1995) is a recent permutation of this regression-based approach. Similar to the Barona and Hamsher equations, the OPIE incorporates the demographic predictors of age, education, race, and occupation. However, in contrast to the Barona and Hamsher equations, the OPIE includes current performance on individual subtests from the WAIS-R (Vocabulary [VOC] and Picture Completion [PC]). Incorporating current performance into an estimate of premorbid intelligence may seem counterintuitive. Specifically, if cerebral dysfunction is present, there is a possibility that performance on a cognitive measure will be reduced from previous levels, thereby confounding the premorbid estimate. Yet, the OPIE is predicated on the assumption that abilities assessed by VOC and PC are relatively resilient to brain damage. Consequently, performance on these measures may have a low likelihood of decreasing below premorbid levels. Although data exist that both support (e.g., Alekoumbides, Charter, Adkins, & Seacat, 1987) and refute (e.g., Munder, 1976) this assumption, the intent of including current performance in estimates of premorbid ability is to increase the accuracy of prediction over generic demographic categories.

An estimation method that uses demographic variables and WAIS-R subtests in a best performance fashion is the BEST-3 approach (Vanderploeg, Schinka, & Axelrod, 1996). In addition to VOC and PC, the BEST-3 incorporates scores on the Information subtest. Similar to the rationale of the OPIE, these three subtests were selected because of their high reliability, high correlations with IQ scores, and relative resistance to deterioration after brain injury. Although the BEST-3 approach is similar to the OPIE in its use of the VOC and PC subtests, the approach estimates IQs using any of the three subtests employed (e.g., Picture Completion to estimate VIQ). Further distinguishing the BEST-3 from the OPIE is its strategy of using only one of the three subtests in estimating FSIQ. The subtest that yields the highest premorbid IQ is ultimately used in the BEST-3 approach.

Although each of these estimation methods has been used in applied and scientific contexts, relatively little is known about their relative accuracy. In one study, Paolo and Ryan (1992) compared the original (Barona et al., 1984) and revised (Barona & Chastain, 1986) Barona equations in a sample of normal elderly individuals. The two estimates did not differ from the obtained WAIS-R Full Scale IQs, but both were poor in predicting Performance IQs. Moreover, only the Barona et al. (1984) equation accurately predicted Verbal IQs. In a separate study, Sweet, Moberg, and Tovian (1990) compared the Barona et al. (1984) and Wilson et al. (1978; the predecessor of the Hamsher [1984] equation) methods and found that both significantly over-estimated obtained IQ scores. Furthermore, Vanderploeg et al. (1996) found that the BEST-3 method achieved higher correlations with WAIS-R IQs than did the estimates derived from the Barona et al. (1984) equation. In a later study by the same authors (Axelrod, Vanderploeg, & Schinka, 1999), accuracy of the BEST-3, OPIE, and Barona estimates was compared in samples of neurological patients and normal controls. With logistic regression, they examined how well the estimates discriminated between patients and control subjects, and they found no differential accuracy across methods. Apart from these studies, little is known about the relative accuracy of these premorbid estimates.

An additional uncertainty regarding these estimates is their relative accuracy in predicting IQ scores in outer ranges of intellectual function. Previous studies have failed to address this question and, instead, have tended to examine over-all predictive accuracy for the entire range of IQ scores. Nonetheless, there is reason to believe that accuracy of the premorbid estimators will vary across the spectrum of IQ scores. In particular, because all methods examined are multiple regression procedures, they are subject to regression to the mean and a restricted range of predicted values (Stevens,

1985). Hence, their accuracy in outer ranges of intelligence (i.e., below-average, above-average, superior, etc.) may be poor. In contrast, a proposed advantage using current performance in the OPIE and BEST-3 approaches is that range of predicted values will be less restricted, thereby resulting in better prediction of extreme scores (Krull et al., 1995; Scott, Krull, Williamson, Adams, & Iverson, 1997; Vanderploeg et al., 1996). As yet, however, the relative accuracy of premorbid IQ estimators in outer ranges of intelligence is largely undetermined.

In the present study, we compared the predictive accuracy of the Barona (Barona et al., 1984), Revised Barona (Barona & Chastain, 1986), Hamsher (1984), OPIE (Krull et al., 1995), and BEST-3 (Vanderploeg et al., 1996) methods in a group of normal adults. Furthering previous research, accuracy of predicted scores was examined within the below-average, average, above-average, and superior ranges of intellectual function.

To evaluate the relative accuracy of each prediction method, we followed the advice of Crawford and Howell (1998), and compared their Standard Errors of Estimate (SEE). In evaluating the accuracy of prediction with multiple regression methods, the SEE is usually used (Nunnally, 1978; Wiggins, 1973), and has been particularly recommended in neuropsychological applications (Crawford & Howell, 1998). Because validity coefficients are infrequently perfect, multiple regression typically fails to yield perfect prediction of a single score. As such, the SEE depicts the margin of error expected in predicting a criterion score (Anastasi & Urbina, 1997). Specifically, it indicates a range around the predicted score wherein the actual criterion score is likely to fall. Smaller SEEs reflect greater accuracy of prediction than larger ones (Wiggins, 1973).

METHOD

Participants were 150 volunteers who were recruited from hospital staff and the community. Thirty-seven were women and 113 were men. The sample was composed of 143 Caucasians, 4 Hispanics, and 3 African Americans. Age varied from 17 to 60 years ($M = 31.20$; $SD = 9.20$), and education ranged from 9 to 20 years ($M = 15.00$; $SD = 2.40$). Based on an informal interview conducted by either a doctoral- or a masters-level psychologist, all were screened for history of learning disability, prior

educational difficulties, and neurological or psychiatric illness. None were excluded on this basis.

All participants were examined in a hospital neuropsychology laboratory by a trained and supervised technician. They were administered the WAIS-R according to standardization instructions, and Verbal (VIQ), Performance (PIQ), and Full Scale (FSIQ) IQs were obtained. Estimated IQ scores were obtained using the Barona (Barona et al., 1984), Revised Barona (Barona & Chastain, 1986), Hamsher (1984), OPIE (Krull et al., 1995), and BEST-3 (Vanderploeg et al., 1996) methods. Coding of occupation was made solely by a masters-level psychologist (V.M.) who was trained to do so by a doctoral-level psychologist (M.B.). For instance, coding of occupation for the OPIE and the two Barona equations is made according to occupational categories listed in the WAIS-R manual. Specifications for these occupational codes and instructions for calculating IQ estimates appear in the respective source publications.

RESULTS

Classifications of IQ Ranges

In order to examine the accuracy of the premorbid estimates across multiple ranges of IQ, participants were categorized according to their obtained WAIS-R FSIQs, VIQs, and PIQs. FSIQs ranged from 75 to 137 with a mean of 107.38 ($SD = 11.73$). VIQs ranged from 77 to 131 ($M = 106.66$; $SD = 11.81$), and PIQs ranged from 72 to 136 ($M = 107.05$; $SD = 11.88$). Categories of interest were determined on the basis of clinical relevance and statistical considerations. Regarding the former, Wechsler's (1981) clinical descriptors of intellectual function (e.g., borderline, below-average, average, etc.) were used to increase the utility of the data; due to mea-surement error, many clinicians report WAIS-R performance according to range of intellectual ability rather than an IQ score. With respect to statistical considerations, only three participants had FSIQs below 80, thereby decreasing the possibility that reliable statistical comparisons may be conducted with such a small group. Hence, individuals with borderline and below-average IQs were combined to form a single group. Similarly, too few individuals had IQs in the very superior range to permit meaningful statistical comparisons. Hence, individuals with IQs above 120 were combined to form a single group. Consequently, participants were classified as follows: 89 and lower: below-average; 90–109: average; 110–119: above-average;

120 and above: superior. The sample sizes across the defined ranges are listed in Table 1 for WAIS-R IQ scores and each estimate. In subsequent analyses, data were analyzed according to this grouping strategy.

Analyses of Standard Errors of Estimate (SEE)

SEEs for each estimation method were computed for the entire sample of 150 participants. The method for calculating the SEEs was, according to Wiggins (1973):

$$SEE = \sqrt{\frac{\sum (Y - Y')^2}{n}}$$

In this equation, SQRT indicates the square root, Y reflects the obtained WAIS-R IQ score, Y' denotes the predicted IQ score, and n is the number of participants in the analysis.

In order to determine whether the SEEs differed significantly from one another, we employed an inferential test described by Jensen (1980). The statistic is based upon the F-test sampling distribution, and is computed in the following manner:

$$F = \frac{(SEE_1)^2}{(SEE_2)^2}$$

SEE_1 and SEE_2 are the standard errors of the estimate being compared. Degrees of freedom are computed as $n_1 - 2$ and $n_2 - 2$ for the numerator and denominator terms, respectively. To protect against Type I error, a modified Bonferroni correction was used in computing each comparison of SEEs. Specifically, a nominal p value of .01 was selected to determine statistical significance for all contrasts.

Accuracy Across IQ Ranges

SEEs for each estimation method appear in Figures 1–3. We compared these SEEs across the ranges of IQ scores, and outcomes of these

statistical comparisons appear in Table 2. As shown in Table 2, over the entire range of obtained WAIS-R FSIQ and VIQ scores, the OPIE had the smallest SEE (all $ps < .01$). Regarding the PIQ, the OPIE SEE was significantly smaller than the Revised Barona SEE ($p < .01$). Among the remaining estimation methods for FSIQ, VIQ, and PIQ scores, Table 2 shows that there were no statistically significant differences.

With SEEs, a confidence interval may be computed to indicate the likely proximity of the actual WAIS-R IQ score to the predicted IQ score. To obtain a 95% confidence interval, the SEE is multiplied by 1.96. The resulting product may be added and subtracted from the predicted score to provide the upper and lower limits of the confidence interval, respectively (Wiggins, 1973). With respect to the OPIE, Figure 1 shows that the overall FSIQ estimate had a SEE of 7.7. Accordingly, with 95% confidence, the actual WAIS-R IQ fell within a 30-point range of the predicted OPIE FSIQ score. Figure 1 demonstrates that the SEEs for estimates of the three IQ scores ranged from 7.7 to 11.7. As such, 95% confidence bands for estimated IQs varied across a range of 30.2 to 45.9 points.

Accuracy within IQ Ranges

To examine relative accuracy in the outer ranges of intelligence, SEEs were computed for IQ scores in the below-average, average, above-average, and superior ranges. Table 2 reveals that SEEs in the below-average range were relatively poor for all predictors, and no method was significantly better than another. In the average range, SEEs of the OPIE and Revised Barona FSIQ and VIQ estimates were significantly smaller than the Hamsher and BEST-3 estimates ($ps < .01$). With the PIQ, the OPIE and Revised Barona SEEs were significantly smaller than SEEs of the remaining three estimates ($ps < .01$).

Table 1. Frequencies of IQ Scores in Selected IQ Ranges.

IQ	Below-average[a]	Average[b]	Above-average[c]	Superior[d]
FSIQ	11	78	35	26
VIQ	12	73	43	22
PIQ	10	76	43	21

Note. Ranges defined as follows: [a] 89 and below; [b] 90109; [c] 110119; [d] 120 and above.

In estimating above-average FSIQ, the Revised Barona SEE was significantly larger than all other estimates, and the OPIE SEE was significantly smaller than the Barona SEE ($ps < .01$). For above-average VIQ, the OPIE had the smallest SEE among all estimates, and the Revised Barona SEE was significantly larger than that of the remaining estimation methods ($ps < .01$).

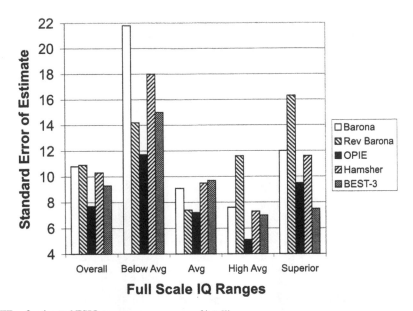

Fig. 1. SEEs of estimated FSIQ scores across ranges of intelligence.

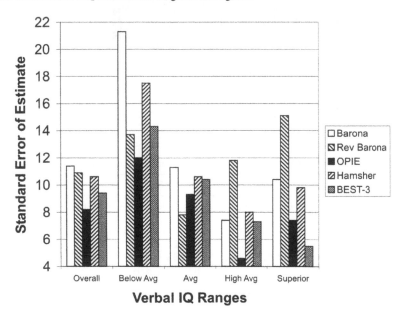

Fig. 2. SEEs of estimated VIQ scores across ranges of intelligence.

Regarding above-average PIQ, the Barona and BEST-3 SEEs were significantly smaller than the Revised Barona SEE ($ps < .01$).

With respect to estimates of superior FSIQ and VIQ, the BEST-3 SEE was significantly smaller than SEEs of the Hamsher, Barona, and Revised Barona estimates. Additionally, the OPIE yielded a SEE that was significantly smaller than was generated by the Revised Barona (all $ps < .01$). There were no significant differences among SEEs

for superior PIQ estimates. Moreover, in no instance did the BEST-3 and OPIE SEEs differ significantly from one another.

Mean Differences between Obtained and Predicted WAIS-R IQs

To delineate the nature of prediction error, mean differences between the obtained and predicted WAIS-R IQs were computed. Mean differences across and within FSIQ, VIQ, and PIQ ranges

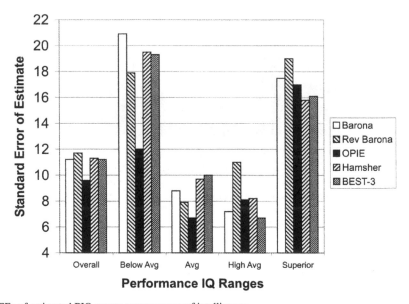

Fig. 3. SEEs of estimated PIQ scores across ranges of intelligence.

Table 2. Comparison of SEEs of B, RB, H, O, and B3 Methods Across and within IQ Ranges.

	FSIQ	VIQ	PIQ
Overall	O < B, RB, H, B3	O < B, RB, H, B3	O < RB
Below average	NS	NS	NS
Average	RB & O < H, B3	RB & O < H, B3	O < B, H, B3
Above average	RB > B, O, H, B3; O < B, RB, H, B3	O < B B & B3 < RB	RB > B, O, H, B3;
Superior	B3 < B, RB, H; O < RB	B3 < B, RB, H	NS

Note. Cell contents indicate significant differences between estimation methods ($ps < .01$).
   B = Barona; RB = Revised Barona; H = Hamsher; O = OPIE; B3 = BEST-3;
   NS = None Significant.

appear in Tables 3–6, respectively. Additionally, the minimum and maximum differences between estimated and actual IQ scores appear in these tables. As revealed in Table 3, except for the Revised Barona, the regression equations slightly overestimated actual IQ scores across the spectrum of intellectual function. Yet, the range of difference scores reveals that substantial inaccuracies were present in the estimated IQ scores for some individuals. In particular, across the regression methods, the maximum overestimates ranged from 18 to 34 points, and the maximum underestimates varied from 13 to 35 points.

As shown in Tables 4–6, the estimated scores tended to deviate markedly from the obtained IQs within the outer ranges of IQ scores. As might be expected, mean estimated IQs in the below-average range exceeded the obtained WAIS-R IQs, with the OPIE displaying the smallest mean deviation from the obtained scores (10 points). In the average range, the estimates again exceeded the obtained IQs, and the Revised Barona estimate had the smallest deviation from the actual WAIS-R IQs (2–4 points). Although these mean differences are relatively small, their standard deviations approximated 7 points. Additionally, there are indications that the Revised Barona equation failed to yield proximal estimates of IQs for some individuals. For instance, its maximum over- and underestimates of FSIQs were 24 and 10 points, respectively. Thus, for some individuals, the prediction was prone to substantial error. In the above-average and superior ranges, WAIS-R IQs were largely underestimated, with the OPIE and BEST-3 methods yielding the smallest deviations from obtained IQs. Again, standard deviations and maximum over- and underestimates were relatively large.

Concordance of Intellectual Classification

Accuracy of the regression equations in predicting Wechsler's ranges of intellectual classification was also evaluated. Based on the WAIS-R standard error of measurement (SEM), we computed the 95% confidence intervals around the obtained IQs. For the VIQ, PIQ, and FSIQ scores, the average SEM is 2.74, 4.14, and 2.53, thereby yielding 95% confidence intervals of ±5, ±8, and ±5 points respectively. We then computed the

frequency with which estimated scores fell within these confidence intervals around the obtained IQ scores. Resulting rates of concordance between estimated and obtained scores appear in Table 7. To determine whether concordance rates differed significantly across estimation procedures, multiple Cochran's Coefficient of Agreement were calculated, and results are also summarized in Table 7. To protect against Type I error, a modified Bonferroni approach was taken, and a nominal p-value of .01 was selected for significance.

As shown, the five estimation methods did not differ significantly in their overall concordance rates for FSIQ, VIQ, or PIQ ($ps > .01$). In general, concordance results suggest that the five estimators are capable of correctly predicting the obtained FSIQ and VIQ scores (within measurement error) only about 30 to 40% of the time. Because the SEM is larger for Wechsler PIQs, the concordance between estimated and obtained PIQs ranged from 45 to approximately 60%.

Because the overall concordance rates are averaged across the entire range of IQ scores, accuracy of prediction within individual IQ categories is obscured. Hence, concordances within each of the previously defined ranges of intelligence were calculated. In contrast to concordances for the entire range of IQ scores, large differences between estimation methods were found. Moreover, concordances were worst in the below-average and superior ranges of intelligence. The Barona and Revised Barona estimates were particularly poor in these ranges, and achieved concordance with WAIS-R IQ scores ranging from 0 to 27%. Nonetheless, there were no significant differences among the estimation methods in the below-average range. In the superior range, the BEST-3 estimate achieved significantly higher concordance rates than the remaining regression methods for FSIQ and VIQ ($ps < .01$). Yet, the BEST-3 estimate demonstrated the worst concordance rates for average FSIQ, VIQ, and PIQ compared to the other regression methods. Collectively, these concordance rates demonstrate that none of the estimation methods is uniformly accurate in predicting intellectual classification, and different estimation methods are relatively better within specific IQ categories.

Table 3. Mean Differences between Estimated and Obtained WAIS-R FSIQ, VIQ, and PIQ Scores Across Ranges of Intellectual Function.

	FSIQ			VIQ			PIQ		
	M	(SD)	Range	M	(SD)	Range	M	(SD)	Range
Barona	2.0	(10.7)	−24.8 to 34.1	3.4	(10.9)	−21.7 to 29.8	0.1	(11.3)	−26.7 to 33.5
Rev. Barona	−2.8	(10.6)	−25.8 to 23.9	−2.5	(10.6)	−25.1 to 23.9	−2.2	(11.6)	−30.6 to 27.1
Hamsher	1.6	(10.2)	−21.4 to 26.8	2.4	(10.3)	−18.8 to 26.9	0.6	(11.3)	−26.3 to 30.1
OPIE	1.3	(7.6)	−18.1 to 20.1	3.3	(7.6)	−13.9 to 21.1	−1.8	(9.4)	−34.4 to 18.5
BEST-3	4.7	(8.0)	−17.0 to 27.2	6.1	(7.2)	−13.3 to 22.9	2.0	(11.0)	−35.3 to 29.6

Note. Values indicate the mean difference between the estimated and obtained WAIS-R IQs. Positive values indicate the magnitude of overestimate, whereas negative values depict the magnitude of underestimate.

Table 4. Mean Differences between Estimated and Obtained WAIS-R FSIQ Scores within Ranges of Intellectual Function.

	Below average[1]			Average[2]			Above average[3]			Superior[4]		
	M	(SD)	Range	M	(SD)	Range	M	(SD)	Range	M	(SD)	Range
Barona	20.4	(7.8)	5.7 to 34.1	6.1	(6.8)	−9.3 to 23.5	−4.1	(6.5)	−24.8 to 4.2	−11.1	(4.8)	−21.5 to −3.9
Rev. Barona	13.0	(6.2)	−2.9 to 18.3	1.9	(7.2)	−11.9 to 23.9	−9.7	(6.4)	−25.7 to 0.65	−15.1	(6.2)	−25.8 to −5.4
Hamsher	16.9	(6.2)	1.7 to 25.7	5.7	(7.6)	−13.3 to 26.8	−4.5	(5.8)	−18.5 to 4.8	−9.9	(6.2)	−21.8 to −0.3
OPIE	9.8	(6.8)	−2.3 to 20.1	4.8	(5.4)	−14.1 to 18.4	−2.4	(4.6)	−16.5 to 5.8	−8.5	(4.4)	−18.1 to −0.8
BEST-3	12.6	(8.5)	3.1 to 27.2	7.4	(6.2)	−17.0 to 20.0	1.3	(7.0)	−13.1 to 21.5	−2.5	(7.2)	−16.1 9.8

Note. WAIS-R IQs are classified, in accordance with Wechsler (1981), as follows: [1] 89 and below; [2] 90–109; [3] 110–119; [4] 120 and above. Values indicate the mean difference between the estimated and obtained WAIS-R IQs. Positive values indicate the magnitude of overestimate, whereas negative values depict the magnitude of underestimate.

Table 5. Mean Differences between Estimated and Obtained WAIS-R VIQ Scores within Ranges of Intellectual Function.

	Below average[1]			Average[2]			Above average[3]			Superior[4]		
	M	(SD)	Range	M	(SD)	Range	M	(SD)	Range	M	(SD)	Range
Barona	18.9	(10.3)	-5.1 to 29.8	9.0	(6.9)	-4.3 to 27.5	-6.3	(6.4)	-21.7 to 6.7	-9.4	(4.5)	-18.6 to -2.4
Rev. Barona	11.3	(8.0)	-0.3 to 22.6	2.9	(7.3)	-12.8 to 23.9	-9.7	(6.8)	-25.0 to 4.1	-14.0	(5.8)	-25.1 to -4.5
Hamsher	15.0	(9.5)	-8.2 to 25.1	7.8	(7.2)	-6.8 to 26.89	-4.6	(6.6)	-16.8 to 10.0	-8.2	(5.5)	-18.9 to -1.5
OPIE	10.0	(6.9)	1.3 to 20.9	7.3	(5.9)	-6.6 to 21.09	-.6	(4.6)	-10.6 to 8.5	-6.2	(4.0)	-13.9 to 0.8
BEST-3	12.7	(6.8)	3.2 to 22.3	8.7	(5.7)	-2.9 to 22.9	2.8	(6.9)	-9.8 to 19.2	0.2	(5.7)	-13.3 to 11.2

Note. WAIS-R IQs are classified, in accordance with Wechsler (1981), as follows: [1]89 and below; [2]90–109; [3]110–119; [4]120 and above. Values indicate the mean difference between the estimated and obtained WAIS-R IQs. Positive values indicate the magnitude of overestimate, whereas negative values depict the magnitude of underestimate.

Table 6. Mean Differences between Estimated and Obtained WAIS-R PIQ Scores within Ranges of Intellectual Function.

	Below average[1]			Average[2]			Above average[3]			Superior[4]		
	M	(SD)	Range	M	(SD)	Range	M	(SD)	Range	M	(SD)	Range
Barona	19.3	(8.4)	6.2 to 33.5	5.8	(6.7)	-14.0 to 21.8	-6.3	(3.5)	-15.1 to 0.2	-16.6	(5.7)	-26.7 to -8.2
Rev. Barona	16.2	(8.1)	0.3 to 27.1	3.9	(6.9)	-10.2 to 17.7	-9.7	(5.3)	-24.5 to 2.4	-17.7	(7.0)	-30.6 to -4.5
Hamsher	17.5	(9.1)	1.7 to 30.1	6.4	(7.2)	-19.2 to 20.3	-6.1	(5.6)	-22.9 to 5.1	-14.6	(6.4)	-26.3 to -2.0
OPIE	10.5	(6.1)	0.6 to 18.5	3.0	(6.1)	-13.7 to 15.7	-6.6	(4.7)	-19.6 to 1.3	-15.3	(7.7)	-34.3 to 3.0
BEST-3	17.4	(8.8)	3.1 to 30.0	7.0	(7.2)	-13.4 to 23.7	-2.6	(6.3)	-16.3 to 9.5	-13.7	(8.6)	-35.3 to -0.2

Note. WAIS-R IQs are classified, in accordance with Wechsler (1981), as follows: [1]89 and below; [2]90–109; [3]110–119; [4]120 and above. Values indicate the mean difference between the estimated and obtained WAIS-R IQs. Positive values indicate the magnitude of overestimate, whereas negative values depict the magnitude of underestimate.

Discriminant Validity of VIQ and PIQ Estimates

Although unrelated to the original hypotheses, it was discovered that the correlations between VIQ and PIQ estimates were extremely high for all methods except the OPIE. Pearson product-moment correlations between VIQ and PIQ estimates for the Barona, Revised Barona, Hamsher, and BEST-3 methods were .99, .94, .98, and .98, respectively. Such extremely high correlations indicate that discriminant validity of VIQ and PIQ estimates is poor. In contrast, the VIQ–PIQ correlation for the OPIE of .52 was quite similar to the WAIS-R VIQ–PIQ correlation of .49. These findings suggest that establishing the discriminant validity of VIQ and PIQ estimates has been largely neglected in the past. The failure of all purely demographic estimators to show discriminant validity raises questions as to the feasibility of providing separate VIQ and PIQ estimates based on demographic factors alone.

DISCUSSION

Previous research concerning the Barona, Revised Barona, Hamsher, OPIE, and BEST-3 methods has generally shown that each method is reasonably accurate in estimating mean WAIS-R IQ scores for groups of individuals. Specifically, estimates tended to overestimate WAIS-R IQs by only a few points. In some respects, the present study is consistent with this prior research. In particular, the mean estimated IQ scores across the entire sample of 150 participants generally exceeded the obtained IQ scores by 5–6 points.

Although comparisons of estimated and obtained mean scores suggest that the estimation methods are reasonably accurate, such analyses fail to indicate the relative error expected in predicting an individual score (cf. Crawford & Howell, 1998). This is the primary contribution of SEEs, and the values generated in the present study suggest that much prediction error may be expected. For instance, when IQ scores were collapsed across the entire sample of 150 participants, the smallest 95% confidence interval of prediction was obtained by the OPIE, and it varied across a range of 30, 32, and 36 points for the FSIQ, VIQ, and

PIQ, respectively. As revealed by the comparison of SEEs, the other estimation methods yielded significantly larger SEEs. Moreover, their 95% confidence intervals had approximate ranges of 40 points. This suggests that, across the range of IQ scores examined in the present study, all of the estimation methods are susceptible to relatively large errors of prediction.

When comparing SEEs within individual ranges of intelligence, there was no single best estimation method. Regarding superior intelligence, the BEST-3 method had significantly smaller SEEs than all estimates save the OPIE. In the above-average range, the Revised Barona FSIQ and VIQ estimates yielded SEEs that were significantly larger than all other estimates. With respect to average FSIQ, VIQ, and PIQ scores, the OPIE had significantly smaller SEEs than the Hamsher and BEST-3 estimates, and the Revised Barona yielded significantly smaller SEEs than these latter methods for FSIQ and VIQ scores. In the below-average range, all estimation methods were equal. Despite these relative differences within ranges, the SEEs remained relatively large. Notably, the SEEs of estimation methods within specific ranges of IQ appeared to be larger than for the entire sample of 150 participants. This is expected, as regression-based predictions tend to yield larger error bands in outer than in middle ranges of score distributions (Crawford & Howell, 1998). For instance, in estimating below-average FSIQ, the smallest SEE was obtained by the OPIE, and approximated 12 points, whereas the largest (22 points) was displayed by the Barona estimate. These SEEs yield respective 95% confidence intervals of ±24 and ±44 points for the OPIE and Barona estimates. These values far exceed those obtained in the average range of intelligence or when scores were collapsed across the below-average, average, above-average, and superior ranges. This suggests that prediction error increases substantially in outer ranges of intelligence.

The nature of the prediction error in outer ranges is apparent when examining mean differences between the actual and predicted IQs. Specifically, the prediction methods grossly overestimated IQ scores in the below-average ranges, and tended to underestimate IQ scores in the above-average and superior ranges. Concordance

Table 7. Concordance between Estimated and Obtained WAIS-R IQ Scores Across Ranges of Intellectual Function.

	Overall			Below average[1]			Average[2]			Above average[3]			Superior[4]		
	FSIQ	VIQ	PIQ	FSIQ	VIQ	PIQ	FSIQ	VIQ	PIQ	FSIQ	VIQ	PIQ	FSIQ	VIQ	PIQ
Barona	39	32	50	0	8	10	45	23	59	57[b]	56[b]	67[b]	12	27	0
Rev. Barona	36	37	45	9	17	10	55[e]	55[acde]	67	29	28	33	0	4	10
Hamsher	40	37	49	9	8	20	41	33	53	54	54[b]	65[b]	30	32	14
OPIE	43	40	58	18	33	20	39	25	77[ace]	74[b]	72[b]	56	27	32	10
BEST-3	37	38	50	27	8	20	28	25	51	54	58[b]	70[b]	46[ab]	59[b]	19

Note. WAIS-R IQs are classified, in accordance with Wechsler (1981), as follows: [1] 89 and below; [2] 90–109; [3] 110–119; [4] 120 and above. Values reflect % concordance within each IQ category. Superscripts show significant differences between estimates according to Cochran's Coefficient of Agreement ($p < .01$); [a] Barona estimate; [b] Revised Barona estimate; [c] Hamsher estimate; [d] OPIE; [e] BEST-3.

rates across and within the ranges of intelligence further delineate this outcome. Specifically, the concordance rates across the 150 participants ranged from 35 to 60%. Yet, within the below-average and superior ranges, nearly all estimates were equally poor. Moreover, within these outer ranges, concordance rates were relatively worse than was obtained across all 150 participants or within the average range. This finding notwithstanding, no estimate of FSIQ or VIQ within the average range of intelligence was accurate more than 55% of the time. Previous research has not examined performance of estimation methods in outer ranges of intelligence. Rather, accuracy across the spectrum of IQ scores was examined. Thus, the findings of earlier studies indicated that the regression equations yielded accurate estimates of premorbid intelligence. The current data imply that the estimation methods are relatively inaccurate overall, and are especially so in outer ranges of intelligence.

This point deserves some elaboration. Among the estimation methods evaluated in this study, the OPIE generally yielded the smallest SEEs. Yet, it yielded 95% confidence intervals with ranges that varied from 20 to 48 points. The magnitude of these confidence intervals suggests that the OPIE's utility is relatively limited. For instance, in the above-average range of FSIQ scores, the OPIE demonstrated a confidence interval that ranged across 20 points. Thus, if the OPIE predicts that an individual had a premorbid FSIQ of 115, the clinician could have confidence that the individual's actual WAIS-R FSIQ fell anywhere from 105 to 125. As such, the individual may have had premorbid intelligence that was either average, above-average, or superior. As another example, consider if the OPIE predicted a premorbid FSIQ of 100. The SEE in the average range was 7.2, yielding a 95% confidence interval that ranged across 28 points. Consequently, the clinician could be reasonably confident that the patient's premorbid FSIQ fell between 86 (below-average) and 114 (above-average). Given that 68% of the WAIS-R normative sample obtained IQs of between 85 and 115, this prediction renders minimal improvement over an estimate based on base-rate information alone. As such, even with the best estimate available, it may be difficult to decide whether a patient's obtained IQ is genuinely less than expected. With

other estimation methods that were more susceptible to prediction error (e.g., Barona or Revised
Barona), this decision will be more difficult.

Notably, it should be acknowledged that the
method used to estimate the SEEs in this study is
relatively conservative. It is based upon sample
statistics, and SEEs for the population will likely
be larger (cf. Crawford & Howell, 1998). Thus,
the confidence intervals detailed in this study are
probably smaller than will be observed within the
population. As such, the prediction methods may
be more inaccurate than observed in the present
study.

Limitations

It is important to recognize some limitations of
the present data that may diminish generalizability of the findings. One such limitation may be
selection of participants. In particular, the sample
included individuals who were volunteers without
cerebral dysfunction, and they were apparently
motivated to give their best performance on the
WAIS-R. Participants also tended to be primarily
Caucasian and male. Potentially, findings based
upon such a sample may not generalize to other
populations, particularly non-Caucasian ethnic
groups. Nonetheless, the range of obtained WAIS-R
IQ scores was broad and ranged from 72 to 137.
Furthermore, demographic variables related to IQ
performance, such as education and occupation,
ranged broadly across the sample, thereby supporting the generalizability of the data to other
samples comprised largely of male Caucasians.

A related limitation of the present findings
is that no participants had IQs within the mentally
retarded range, and relatively few scored within
the borderline or very-superior ranges. Thus,
the study was unable to address accuracy of the
estimation methods in these ranges. Nevertheless,
given the pronounced regression toward the mean
demonstrated by the current data, it seems likely
that accuracy in these outer ranges would be poor.

Finally, the applicability of these data for the
WAIS-III is uncertain. The WAIS-III technical
manual (Tulsky, Zhu, & Ledbetter, 1997) details
that mean WAIS-III IQ scores are 2–4 points lower
than those obtained by the same individuals on the
WAIS-R. It is quite likely that, because of this variation between versions of the WAIS, accuracy of

the estimation methods examined here will worsen
when predicting premorbid WAIS-III IQs.
Specifically, the beta weights for the regression
equations were derived using the WAIS-R as a criterion. Because the WAIS-III and WAIS-R IQs are
not identical, the beta weights are unlikely to yield
accurate prediction of WAIS-III IQs. Additionally,
because discrepancies between WAIS-III and
WAIS-R scores seem to increase in outer ranges of
intelligence, the relatively poor accuracy of the
estimation methods may be exacerbated in below-
average or superior ranges of IQ. Thus, if the estimation methods studied in the present investigation
are used to estimate WAIS-III IQs, extreme caution
should be exercised. Indeed, until research is conducted using these equations to estimate WAIS-III
IQs, it may be prudent not to use them at all.

It seems likely that premorbid estimation
methods for the WAIS-III will be developed to
address these uncertainties. In deriving such estimates, the present findings point to several important considerations. In particular, it seems apparent
that estimation methods based solely upon demographic variables are prone to gross inaccuracy in
outer ranges of function. For instance, the Barona,
Revised Barona, and Hamsher equations tended
to be less accurate than the OPIE and BEST-3
methods. Thus, the former prediction methods
should probably be avoided. Rather, the current
data indicate that, if they are used, demographic
variables should be combined with current performance in new premorbid estimation methods.
It may be best to focus efforts upon current-
performance-based estimators, but care should be
taken to ensure that the current-performance is
genuinely resilient to brain dysfunction.

These considerations notwithstanding, the present study provides important information concerning the relative accuracy of some of the most
commonly used estimates of premorbid intelligence.
Prior to this research, a comprehensive comparison
of all five methods had not been conducted. Moreover, these findings illustrate potential difficulties
that future researchers in this area should address.

REFERENCES

Alekoumbides, A., Charter, R., Adkins, T., & Seacat, G.
(1987). The diagnosis of brain damage by the

WAIS, WMS, and Reitan battery utilizing standardized scores corrected for age and education. *International Journal of Clinical Neuropsychology*, *9*, 11–28.

Anastasi, A., & Urbina, S. (1997). *Psychological testing* (7th ed.). Upper Saddle River, NJ: Prentice-Hall.

Axelrod, B.N., Vanderploeg, R.D., & Schinka, J.A. (1999). Comparing methods for estimating premorbid intellectual functioning. *Archives of Clinical Neuropsychology*, *14*, 341–346.

Barona, A., & Chastain, R.L. (1986). An improved estimate of premorbid IQ for blacks and whites on the WAIS-R. *International Journal of Clinical Neuropsychology*, *8*, 169–173.

Barona, A., Reynolds, C.R., & Chastain, R. (1984). A demographically based index of premorbid intelligence for the WAIS-R. *Journal of Consulting and Clinical Psychology*, *52*, 885–887.

Crawford, J.R., & Howell, D.C. (1998). Regression equations in clinical neuropsychology: An evaluation of statistical methods for comparing predicted and obtained scores. *Journal of Clinical and Experimental Neuropsychology*, *20*, 755–762.

Eppinger, M.G., Craig, P.L., Adams, R.L., & Parsons, O.A. (1987). The WAIS-R index for estimating premorbid intelligence: Cross-validation and clinical utility. *Journal of Consulting and Clinical Psychology*, *55*, 86–90.

Hamsher, K. deS. (1984). Specialized neuropsychological assessment methods. In G. Goldstein & M. Hersen (Eds.), *Handbook of psychological assessment* (pp. 235–258). New York: Pergamon.

Jensen, A.R. (1980). *Bias in mental testing*. New York: Free Press.

Kaufman, A.S. (1990). *Assessing adolescent and adult intelligence*. Boston: Allyn & Bacon.

Krull, K.R., Scott, J.G., & Sherer, M. (1995). Estimation of premorbid intelligence from combined performance and demographic variables. *The Clinical Neuropsychologist*, *9*, 83–88.

Munder, L. (1976). Patterns of deficit in black and white men with brain damage to the left, right, and both hemispheres. *Dissertations Abstracts International*, *37* (1-B), 442–443.

Nunnally, J.C. (1978). *Psychometric theory* (2nd ed.). New York: McGraw-Hill.

Paolo, A.M., & Ryan, J.J. (1992). Generalizability of two methods of estimating premorbid intelligence in the elderly. *Archives of Clinical Neuropsychology*, *7*, 135–143.

Scott, J.G., Krull, K.R., Williamson, D.J.G., Adams, R.L., & Iverson, G.L. (1997). Oklahoma premorbid intelligence estimation (OPIE): Utilization in clinical samples. *The Clinical Neuropsychologist*, *11*, 146–154.

Simpson, C.D., & Vega, A. (1971). Unilateral brain damage and patterns of age-corrected WAIS subtest scores. *Journal of Clinical Psychology*, *43*, 499–504.

Stevens, J. (1985). *Applied multivariate statistics for the social sciences*. Hillsdale, NY: Lawrence Erlbaum.

Sweet, J.J., Moberg, P.J., & Tovian, S.M. (1990). Evaluation of Wechsler Adult Intelligence Scale-Revised premorbid IQ formulas in clinical populations. *Psychological Assessment*, *2*, 41–44.

Tulsky, D., Zhu, J., & Ledbetter, M. (1997). *WAIS-III/WMS-III technical manual*. San Antonio, TX: Psychological Corporation.

Vanderploeg, R.D., & Schinka, J.A. (1995). Predicting WAIS-R IQ premorbid ability: Combining subtest performance and demographic variable predictors. *Archives of Clinical Neuropsychology*, *10*, 225–239.

Vanderploeg, R.D., Schinka, J.A., & Axelrod, B.N. (1996). Estimation of WAIS-R premorbid intelligence: Current ability and demographic data used in a best-performance fashion. *Psychological Assessment*, *8*, 404–411.

Wechsler, D. (1981). *Wechsler Adult Intelligence Scale-Revised manual*. New York: The Psychological Corporation.

Wiggins, J.S. (1973). *Personality and prediction: Principles of personality assessment*. Malabar, FL: Krieger.

Wilson, R.S., Rosenbaum, G., Brown, G., Rourke, D., Whitman, D., & Grisell, J. (1978). An index of premorbid intelligence. *Journal of Consulting and Clinical Psychology*, *46*, 1554–1555.

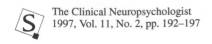
The Clinical Neuropsychologist
1997, Vol. 11, No. 2, pp. 192–197

VIII-F

BRIEF REPORT

Estimating Premorbid WAIS-R IQ with Demographic Variables: Regression Equations Derived from a UK Sample*

J. R. Crawford[1] and K. M. Allan[2]

[1]University of Aberdeen and [2]St. John's Hospital, Livingston, UK

ABSTRACT

A sample of 200 healthy individuals, representative of the adult UK population in terms of age, gender, and occupational classification, completed a full-length WAIS-R. Demographic variables for the participants were recorded (age, gender, years of education, and occupational classification) and used to develop regression equations for the estimation of premorbid WAIS-R IQ. Stepwise multiple regression revealed that occupation was the best predictor of IQ for all three WAIS-R scales (FSIQ, VIQ, and PIQ). Age and years of education significantly increased the variance predicted. Together these three variables accounted for 53%, 53%, and 32% of the variance in FSIQ, VIQ, and PIQ, respectively. The results indicated that the demographic approach to the estimation of premorbid WAIS-R IQ has utility beyond the USA. However, in common with findings for American participants (Barona, Reynolds, & Chastain, 1984) the ability to predict PIQ was markedly inferior to that achieved for FSIQ and VIQ. A frequency table of the discrepancies between estimated premorbid IQ and obtained IQ for the present sample is provided for clinical use.

The detection and quantification of acquired neuropsychological deficits rests upon the comparison of an individual's current cognitive functioning with an estimate of his/her premorbid ability (Crawford, 1992). One approach to obtaining this estimate takes advantage of the well-established relationship between demographic variables (e.g., education, occupational status) and IQ (Kaufman, 1990). Wilson et al. (1978) used the U.S. standardization sample to build regression equations for the prediction of Wechsler Adult Intelligence Scale IQ (WAIS; Wechsler, 1955) from five demographic variables. These equations predicted 54%, 53%, and 42% of the variance in Full Scale (FSIQ), Verbal IQ, (VIQ) and Performance (PIQ), respectively. Subsequently, Barona, Reynolds, and Chastain (1984) and Barona and Chastain (1986) have demonstrated that the demographic approach

can be applied to the Wechsler Adult Intelligence Scale-Revised (WAIS-R; Wechsler, 1981). It should be noted, however, that the predictive power of the WAIS-R regression models was markedly less than that achieved when the WAIS was the criterion measure.

At present, there has been little attempt to employ or evaluate the demographic approach outside of North America. Crawford, Stewart, Cochrane, et al. (1989) used a sample of 151 healthy subjects to build regression equations to estimate premorbid WAIS IQ for the United Kingdom (UK). The regression models incorporated occupational classification, years of education, age, and gender as predictors and accounted for 50%, 50%, and 30% of the variance in FSIQ, VIQ, and PIQ, respectively. However, because virtually all clinical neuropsychologists have now

* This study was partly supported by a grant from the U.K. Mental Health Foundation.
Address correspondence to: John R. Crawford, Department of Psychology, King's College, University of Aberdeen, Aberdeen AB9 2UB, UK.
Accepted for publication: June 2, 1996.

replaced the WAIS with the WAIS-R, these regression equations are now obsolete. The aim of the present study was to determine how successfully demographic variables could be used to predict IQ in the UK when the WAIS-R was used as the criterion variable. To our knowledge, the present study represents the first attempt to employ the demographic approach with the WAIS-R outside of North America.

METHOD

Participants

The sample consisted of 200 Caucasians (104 females, 96 males) screened by interview to exclude any potential participants with a history of neurological, psychiatric, sensory, or systemic disorders. Participants were recruited from a wide variety of sources, that is, local and national businesses, recreational clubs (e.g., senior citizens clubs, angling clubs), community centers, and so forth; all were offered a small honorarium for their participation. Mean age was 44.3 years (SD = 19.2) with a range of 16 to 83 years. Mean years of education was 12.6 (SD = 3.0) with a range of 7 to 21 years. In recording years of education participants were credited with 0.5 of a year for every year spent in part-time education. Part-time education was defined to include day-release courses and evening classes provided that they had led, or were leading to, a qualification. Each participant's occupation was coded using the Office of Population Censuses and Surveys (1980) Classification of Occupations; this classification system consists of five categories which can be defined broadly as follows; 1 = professional, 2 = intermediate, 3 = skilled, 4 = semi-skilled, 5 = unskilled. Retired participants, and those describing themselves as house-husband/house-wives, were coded by their previous occupations as were those currently unemployed. Those who had never worked were coded as 5 (i.e., unskilled).

A goodness-of-fit chi-square test was used to compare the distribution of occupational classifications in the present sample with the census-derived figures for the adult UK population. This revealed that the sample and population distributions did not differ significantly $\chi^2(4, N = 200) = 5.66, p > .05$. A similar procedure was used to examine the representativeness of the sample in terms of age distribution. Nine age bands were formed corresponding to those adopted for the WAIS-R standardization sample, with the exception that the 70–74 age band was replaced with a 70+ age band. A goodness-of-fit test revealed that the sample and population distributions did not differ significantly $\chi^2(8, N = 200) = 7.71, p > .05$; tables of the distributions for occupation and age are available in an extended version of this paper. Finally, the sample's gender distribution was also representative of the adult UK population $\chi^2(1, N = 200) = p > .05$.

Procedure

All participants completed a full-length WAIS-R (UK) according to standardized procedures (Lea, 1986; Wechsler, 1981). Stepwise multiple regression was used to regress the three WAIS-R scales (i.e., FSIQ, VIQ, and PIQ) on the four demographic variables, that is age, gender, years of education, and occupational classification.

RESULTS

The mean score (and SD) for WAIS-R FSIQ was 102.5 (13.12) with a range from 71 to 140. The means for VIQ and PIQ were 102.4 (12.81) and 102.0 (13.40), respectively. The correlation matrix for the three criterion and four predictor variables is presented in Table 1. Stepwise regression revealed that occupational classification was the single best predictor of IQ for all three scales, accounting for 42%, 43%, and 25% of the variance

Table 1. Correlation Matrix for WAIS-R IQ Scores and the Demographic Predictor Variables in a Healthy UK Sample.

	FSIQ	VIQ	PIQ	Age	Gender	Occupation
VIQ	0.94*					
PIQ	0.87*	0.66*				
Age	0.10	0.08	0.11			
Gender	−0.19*	−0.21*	−0.13*	0.19*		
Occupation	−0.65*	−0.65*	−0.50*	0.09	0.19*	
Education	0.58*	0.59*	0.43*	−0.33*	−0.26*	−0.65*

Note. N = 200.
  *$p < .05$.

in FSIQ, VIQ, and PIQ, respectively. Of the three remaining demographic variables, education and age significantly increased the variance predicted at successive steps of the analyses ($p < .001$ for both variables for all three IQ scales). The final regression models predicted 53%, 53%, and 32% of the variance in FSIQ, VIQ, and PIQ, respectively with standard errors of estimate of 9.11, 8.83, and 11.2. The regression equations for each of the three IQ scales are presented below:

Predicted FSIQ = $87.14 - (5.21 \times$ occupation$)$ $+ (1.78 \times$ education$) + (.18 \times$ age$)$

Predicted VIQ = $87.42 - (5.08 \times$ occupation$)$ $+ 1.77 \times$ education$) + (.17 \times$ age$)$

Predicted PIQ = $90.89 - (4.34 \times$ occupation$)$ $+ (1.33 \times$ education$) + (.16 \times$ age$)$

The distribution of discrepancies between predicted IQ and obtained IQ is presented in Table 2.

Table 2. Demographic Prediction of WAIS-R IQ: Distribution of Positive Predicted Minus Obtained IQ Discrepancies in Healthy Participants.

Predicted-obtained Discrepancy	% of Ss when FSIQ Predicted	% of Ss when VIQ Predicted	% of Ss when PIQ Predicted
1	47.5	50.5	46.0
2	42.5	44.5	43.0
3	38.5	40.0	40.0
4	33.5	35.0	37.0
5	28.0	29.0	33.5
6	24.5	27.5	32.0
7	22.0	25.5	29.5
8	19.5	21.5	26.5
9	17.0	16.5	23.5
10	16.0	15.0	20.1
11	14.5	11.5	19.5
12	13.0	11.5	15.0
13	9.5	8.5	13.5
14	8.0	7.5	11.5
15	6.5	6.0	10.0
16	6.5	6.0	8.0
17	3.5	3.0	7.0
18	3.0	1.5	6.5
19	2.0	1.5	5.5
20	2.0	1.0	4.0
21	1.5	1.0	3.5
22	0.5	1.0	2.0
23	0	0.5	0.5
24	0	0.5	0.5
25	0	0.5	0.5
26	0	0.5	0.5
27	0	0.5	0.5
28	0	0.5	0.5
29	0	0.5	0.5
30	0	0.5	0.5
31	0	0.5	0.5
32	0	0.5	0.5

Note. The figures opposite the discrepancy represent the percentage of healthy participants who exhibited that size of positive discrepancy *or larger.* For example, in the case of VIQ, 1% of the sample exhibited a discrepancy of 13 IQ points and a further 7.5% exhibited a discrepancy greater than 13. Therefore the percentage opposite a discrepancy of 13 is 8.5%.

Only positive discrepancies are presented (i.e., cases in which the predicted premorbid IQ exceeded the IQ obtained by testing) because it is this half of the distribution which is of principal concern to clinicians.

DISCUSSION

The present results demonstrate that demographic variables can be employed to predict WAIS-R performance outside of North America. In the case of FSIQ and VIQ, over 50% of the variance in test performance can be accounted for by the three demographic variables of occupation, years of education, and age. Given that the problem of estimating premorbid ability is one commonly faced by all clinical neuro-psychologists, these results should encourage attempts to develop demographic equations in other countries. However, it should be noted that, in common with the U.S. findings, the ability of demographic variables to predict PIQ was markedly inferior to that achieved for FSIQ and VIQ. Although the sample employed in the present study was markedly smaller than the U.S. standardization sample, it was nevertheless representative of the adult UK population in terms of the distributions of age, gender, and occupational classification. Because of this, the equations should have reasonable stability. However, it would be important to examine the accuracy of the present equations in a cross-validation sample.

In clinical practice the predicted IQs derived from the present equations can be compared with the IQs obtained by testing. A substantial discrepancy in favor of the estimated premorbid IQ raises the possibility of cognitive deterioration. The probability of a particular size of discrepancy in favor of the estimated premorbid IQ occurring in the normal population can be assessed by referring to Table 2. For example, in the case of FSIQ, a discrepancy in favor of premorbid IQ of more than 17 points occurred in less than 5% of the present healthy sample. Therefore, a discrepancy of this magnitude is significant at the .05 level and would constitute one source of evidence for the presence of impairment.

The most common formal alternative to the demographic approach to estimating premorbid IQ is through the use of present ability measures, such as the National Adult Reading Test (NART; Nelson, 1982), which are relatively resistant to many forms of cerebral dysfunction. The advantages of this latter approach is that it is liable to be a more powerful predictor of the criterion variable (i.e., WAIS or WAIS-R performance). For example, the healthy sample used to generate the UK demographic equations for the WAIS (Crawford et al., 1989) was also used to cross-validate the NART (Crawford, Stewart, Parker, Besson, & De Lacey, 1989). Therefore, it is possible to compare directly the two methods in the same sample. The NART predicted 66% of FSIQ in comparison with the previously noted figure of 50% for the demographic equation and had a correspondingly smaller standard error of estimate (7.4 vs. 9.1).

The lesser predictive power of demographic methods is potentially offset by their major advantage; namely, that the estimates they provide are independent of an individual's current cognitive status. Because there is evidence for a degree of impairment of NART performance in some neuropsychiatric disorders (see Crawford, 1992), the NART will tend to systematically underestimate premorbid ability. Furthermore, the demographic approach can be employed with clients for whom the NART would clearly be inappropriate (i.e., dysarthric or dyslexic cases).

The principal practical aim of both approaches is to improve the detection and quantification of impairment by providing an individualized comparison standard for a client's current level of functioning. To evaluate the utility of the demographic approach in this regard, studies have examined whether the combination of current ability measures (WAIS or WAIS-R) and demographic estimates of premorbid IQ achieve greater discrimination between healthy and neurological samples than is achieved by current ability measures alone (e.g., Eppinger, Craig, Adams, & Parsons, 1987; Wilson, Rosenbaum, & Brown, 1979). Wilson and colleagues (1979) carried out a discriminant function analysis which demonstrated that the inclusion of the demographic estimate significantly improved discrimination in comparison with WAIS indices alone. Eppinger et al. (1987) found that although the discrepancy between obtained WAIS-R scores and the demographic estimate achieved better classification accuracy than WAIS-R scores alone, the improvement did not achieve statistical significance. The utility of combining current IQ measures with NART-based estimates of premorbid IQ has only been examined in one study. Crawford, Hart, and Nelson (1990) reported that the NART significantly improved discrimination between a healthy sample and samples with either a diagnosis of dementia or CT-scan evidence of cortical atrophy. Unfortunately, there are, as yet, no studies that have directly compared the discrimination achieved when current ability measures are paired with NART versus demographic estimates of premorbid IQ. Such studies would indicate whether or not the superior robustness of demographic estimates outweighs their lesser criterion validity.

Given that a conclusion on the relative utility of the two methods is not yet possible, a reasonable clinical course would be to obtain estimates of premorbid IQ using both methods because neither are time-consuming. Alternatively, a two-stage process could be adopted. Crawford, Allan, Cochrane, and Parker (1990) built a regression equation from a sample of 659 healthy participants that can be used to estimate an individual's expected NART score on the basis of their age, gender, years of education, and occupation. This equation can be used to assess the likelihood that an individual's NART performance is impaired. In cases where the expected and obtained NART scores do not differ significantly, then the NART could be used to provide the primary estimate of premorbid IQ (because of its superior criterion validity). A significant difference between expected and obtained NART scores would be indicative of impaired NART performance. In such circumstances more weight should be placed on demographic estimates of premorbid IQ because there is a danger that the NART systematically underestimates premorbid ability.

REFERENCES

Barona, A., & Chastain, R. L. (1986). An improved estimate of premorbid IQ for blacks and whites on the WAIS-R. *International Journal of Clinical Neuropsychology*, 8, 169–173.

Barona, A., Reynolds, C. R., & Chastain, R. (1984). A demographically based index of premorbid intelligence for the WAIS-R. *Journal of Consulting and Clinical Psychology*, 52, 885–887.

Crawford, J. R. (1992). Current and premorbid intelligence measures in neuropsychological assessment. In J. R. Crawford, W. McKinlay, & D. M. Parker (Eds.), *Handbook of neuropsychological assessment* (pp. 21–49). London: Lawrence Erlbaum.

Crawford, J. R., Allan, K. M., Cochrane, R. H. B., & Parker, D. M. (1990). Assessing the validity of NART estimated premorbid IQs in the individual case. *British Journal of Clinical Psychology*, 29, 435–436.

Crawford, J. R., Hart, S., & Nelson, H. E. (1990). Improved detection of cognitive impairment with the NART: An investigation employing hierarchical discriminant function analysis. *British Journal of Clinical Psychology*, 29, 239–241.

Crawford, J. R., Stewart, L. E., Cochrane, R., Foulds, J., Besson, J. A. O., & Parker, D. M. (1989). Estimating premorbid IQ from demographic variables: A regression equation derived from a UK sample. *British Journal of Clinical Psychology*, 28, 275–278.

Crawford, J. R., Stewart, L. E., Parker, D. M., Besson, J. A. O., & De Lacey, G. (1989). Prediction of WAIS IQ with the National Adult Reading Test: Cross-validation and extension. *British Journal of Clinical Psychology*, 28, 267–273.

Eppinger, M. G., Craig, P. L., Adams, R. L., & Parsons, O. A. (1987). The WAIS-R index for estimating premorbid intelligence: Cross-validation and clinical utility. *Journal of Consulting and Clinical Psychology*, 55, 86–90.

Lea, M. (1986). A *British supplement to the manual for the Wechsler Adult Intelligence Scale – Revised.* San Antonio: Psychological Corporation.

Nelson, H. E. (1982). *National Adult Reading Test (NART): Test Manual.* Windsor: NFER Nelson.

Office of Population, Censuses and Surveys (1980). *Classification of occupations.* London: HMSO.

Wechsler, D. (1955). *Manual for the Wechsler Adult Intelligence Scale.* New York: Psychological Corporation.

Wechsler, D. (1981). *Manual for the Wechsler Adult Intelligence Scale-Revised.* New York: Psychological Corporation.

Wilson, R. S., Rosenbaum, G., & Brown, G. (1979). The problem of premorbid intelligence in neuropsychological assessment. *Journal of Clinical Neuropsychology*, 1, 49–53.

Wilson, R. S., Rosenbaum, G., Brown, G., Rourke, D., Whitman, D., & Grisell, J. (1978). An index of premorbid intelligence. *Journal of Consulting and Clinical Psychology*, 46, 1554–1555.

Journal of Clinical and Experimental Neuropsychology
2000, Vol. 22, No. 3, pp. 316–324

VIII-F

Accuracy of Regression Equation Prediction Across the Range of Estimated Premorbid IQ

Roger E. Graves

Department of Psychology, University of Victoria, Canada

ABSTRACT

Linear regression is often used to predict psychological criterion variables such as premorbid IQ. The prevailing method of evaluating the accuracy of prediction indicates poor accuracy for both high and low criterion values. These results have led to the conclusion that the equations are not applicable for predicting scores beyond about one standard deviation from the mean. The apparent inaccuracy at the extremes, however, is an artifact of inappropriate analysis. An alternative analysis method is described and used to re-analyze two sets of data. Empirical results show that both high and low WAIS-R IQ scores, predicted using versions of the NART, agree with actual measured IQ scores as accurately as do predicted scores near the mean. In addition, confidence intervals were only 5% larger for more extreme predicted values than for values near the mean, which would be of minor clinical consequence. The practical constraint on prediction of extreme values arises not from the regression technique, but from the limited range of the predictor variable(s). The two reviewed IQ prediction equations would, however, have adequate range for a high percentage of individuals.

Linear regression is the primary method used in psychology for predicting a criterion score from one or more predictor scores. A well known example is the prediction of an IQ score on the basis of other scores, such as demographic variables (e.g., Barona, Reynolds, & Chastain, 1984) or reading vocabulary (e.g., Nelson & O'Connell, 1978). Articles describing the results of these regression studies frequently report that prediction accuracy is poor for scores much above or much below the mean score and warn that predictions of extreme scores should be made with caution. Such a limitation would constitute a very major threat to the utility of the prediction method since prediction of scores deviant from the mean is precisely the situation where the method could have practical value. If the actual score is near the mean, then the score can be well predicted by the simple expedient of predicting the mean plus/minus a confidence interval. The main purpose of

this paper is to explain: 1) why prediction of scores with a regression equation appears to have poor accuracy at the extremes when an inappropriate analysis is used, 2) that extreme scores are predicted as well as non-extreme scores, and 3) that regression equation prediction may be considerably more accurate than is sometimes reported. For simplicity, the discussion will focus on prediction of IQ scores, but the argument applies to the use of regression to predict any criterion measure.

Illustrations of the reports of poor accuracy of regression equation prediction at the extremes are seen in the following quotations. The Barona et al. (1984) demographic variable equation is one of the most popular IQ prediction methods. The authors, however, offered this caution:

> In addition, as is true in other uses of regression equations, the regression toward the mean artificially lowers or raises the estimated scores

---

Address correspondence to: Roger E. Graves, Department of Psychology, University of Victoria, PO Box 3050, Victoria, BC, Canada V8W 3P5. Tel. ++1 250 721 7539. Fax: ++1 250 721 8929. E-mail: rgraves@uvic.ca
Accepted for publication: October 19, 1999.

for individual cases falling outside one standard deviation of the population mean. In cases where the premorbid Full Scale IQ was above 120 or below 69, utilization of the formulae might result in a serious under- or overestimation, respectively. (p. 887)

Another popular method of predicting IQ involves use of the National Adult Reading Test (NART) (Nelson & O'Connell, 1978) or one of its variations. Ryan and Paolo (1992) offer this comment on their IQ regression equation method based on NART error scores:

Use of regression procedures have some limitations, including regression towards the mean and limited range of scores. Regression towards the mean will artificially lower or raise estimated scores for individual subjects falling at the extremes of the distribution. (p. 58)

One of the most accurate and well studied of these NART variations (Graves, Carswell, & Snow, 1999) is the revised version (NART-R) developed by Blair and Spreen (Blair, 1988; Blair & Spreen, 1989). Weins, Bryan and Crossen (1993) reported results of a cross-validation study and, while essentially confirming the originally reported accuracy, also offered a warning.

Important limitations were apparent when the Blair and Spreen (1989) prediction equation was used to estimate FSIQ from NART-R errors.

This equation was found to estimate accurately the current FSIQs of the subjects [...] with FSIQ's from 100–109. However, serious estimation errors were found for subjects outside this range. [...] On average it overestimated by about 8 points the obtained FSIQ of those between 90–100, and by as much as 20 points for those between 80–89. [...] The underestimate was about 8 points for those with obtained FSIQ's of 110–119, and an average of 15 or more points for those of 120 and above. (p. 83)

The quotations above appear to set severe restrictions on the utility of the most popular IQ regression prediction methods. It is clear from the quotations above that the authors based their conclusions on results obtained by selecting actual criterion IQ scores in the sample and comparing these to the predicted scores. However, this method of evaluating the accuracy of prediction, while intuitively appealing, will necessarily yield poor apparent accuracy at the extremes. This can be seen from Table 1, which shows the results that this method is expected to yield according to regression theory for a typical situation. For example, if one selects an individual with a measured FSIQ of 126, then Table 1 shows that one should expect (on average) to find that the predicted FSIQ of this individual is 114.9. What is wrong here? Regression theory is supposed to produce equations that predict the criterion accurately,

Table 1. Apparent Prediction Errors, for Selected Values of Observed FSIQ Scores.

Observed FSIQ score ($M = 100, SD = 15$)	Expected predictor score ($M = 100, SD = 15$)	Expected predicted FSIQ	Apparent prediction error
130	122.5	116.9	−13.9
126	119.9	114.9	−11.1
100	100.0	100.0	0
91	93.3	94.9	+3.9
70	77.5	83.1	+13.9

Note. Results expected according to regression theory when there is a correlation of $r = .75$ between FSIQ and the predictor test score. Given the selected observed FSIQ scores (in column 1), the score on a second test is expected to be closer to the mean, the regression to the mean effect. Thus, column 2 shows the expected predictor standard score of an individual when one selects the individual on the basis of his/her measured FSIQ score. Given the score on a predictor variable shown in column 2, the prediction of FSIQ made on the basis of that score is expected to be closer to the mean than the column 2 score. Thus column 3 shows the FSIQ score predicted using the regression equation with the column 2 score as the predictor value. The apparent prediction error is the column 3 score minus the column 1 score.

yet it necessarily produces inaccurate predictions at the extremes according to this manner
of analysis.

The reason for the failure of the above
approach is that, by selecting extreme criterion
scores, the corresponding predictor scores *must*
(by the "regression to the mean" effect) be less
extreme; hence an *apparent* underestimation will
result. The problem lies not with regression theory, but with the above method of assessing accuracy. This method, while deceptively appealing,
provides a correct answer to the wrong question,
namely, "If I have a particular actual IQ score,
does the prediction of that score tend to match the
actual score, or does it tend to fall above or below
the actual score?" Table 1 illustrates the theoretical answer, while the above quotations from
Barona, et al. (1984) and Weins et al. (1993) illustrate empirical answers. The answer to this question, as correctly reported in the quotations, is that
for actual IQ scores near the mean the predictions
match well, while for actual scores much above or
below the mean the predicted scores seriously
diverge from the actual observed scores. This is
not, however, the question that we need to ask. If
we actually had a particular IQ score, then there
would be no practical reason to ask what the prediction of this might be: a prediction would have
no clinical use. The answer to the above question
is not relevant to the issue of whether a prediction
equation is less useful or valid for predictions of
scores away from the mean than it is for scores
near the mean. Conclusions about accuracy of
prediction at the extremes, based on the above
procedure, are inappropriate and misleading.

The practical need for a prediction arises when
we do not have the actual IQ score, but do have a
predicted score. The correct question then to ask
is "If I have a particular predicted IQ score, does
the actual IQ score tend to match the predicted
score, or does it tend to fall above or below the
predicted score?" This latter question can be
answered either theoretically or empirically. Regression theory answers that for any predicted score,
whether it is near the mean or far away, the actual
scores of individuals with that predicted score will
(on average) *exactly* match the predicted score.
The predicted score is the expected actual score,
with no systematic bias to underestimate higher

scores or overestimate lower scores. (The issue of
confidence intervals will be discussed later.)

In view of the apparently widely held belief that
regression prediction equations over- or underestimate extreme scores, and because the empirical
answers to the original question, while technically
irrelevant, still tend to raise doubts about the accuracy of prediction at the extremes, an empirical
answer to the correct question is required. The procedure involves obtaining a sample, making predictions of IQ, measuring actual IQ, selecting
predicted IQ's in specific ranges, and comparing
these to the corresponding measured IQ's. Note
that this procedure, which accords with the practical need for determining how accurate predicted
scores are, is exactly the reverse of the procedure
used by the authors quoted above. The distinction
between the two approaches, as methods of
answering two quite different questions, is cru-
cially important.

The primary purpose of the present studies was
to provide an empirical evaluation of the mean
accuracy of point predictions of IQ regression
equations, for regions above, around, and below
the mean. Results for the old, inappropriate, procedure were first obtained in order to confirm that
the sample data manifest the illusory over- and
underestimation at the extremes described in the
quotations above. Results were then obtained
using the correct approach to determine how
accurate the predictions actually were for the
three regions. Two data samples were analyzed.
Analysis of the first sample shows results for a
prediction equation developed from, and thus
designed to optimally fit, this sample. The second
sample comes from a cross-validation study in
which IQ scores obtained three years before
measurement of the predictor variable were predicted using a previously published equation.
Results for the second sample should provide a
strong test of the accuracy of prediction across the
range of predicted scores.

An additional purpose of the present studies
was to provide an empirical evaluation of the
increase in size of confidence intervals (CI's) for
predicted values above and below the mean.
Crawford and Howell (1998) reported that they
found no published clinical neuropsychological
regression studies that had used the correct

method of calculating CI's. The correct method produces larger intervals for more extreme scores, in contrast to the commonly used method that yields a fixed size CI. (The correct method for calculating CI's replaces the conventional Z value, e.g., 1.645 for a 90% CI, with a $t(N-2)$ value, e.g., 1.669 for a normative sample size of $N = 66$, which makes all CI's larger, and also introduces a scaling factor in the formula for the standard error of prediction, which makes CI's larger the further from the mean they are centered.) While Crawford and Howell (1998) provided results of simulation studies that indicated the increase in magnitude was relatively small, no results for actual regression prediction equations were reported. The present studies provide results for two actual equations and samples to determine whether the increase in CI magnitude affects the practical utility of predictions for more extreme values of predicted IQ.

STUDY 1

METHOD

Sample

The data provided by Blair (1988, Appendix E) were obtained from a sample consisting of 66 normal individuals between the ages of 18–49 (mean = 27 years). The regression equation for these data (Blair, 1988; Blair & Spreen, 1989) predicts WAIS-R FSIQ from the NART-R as: Estimated FSIQ = 127.8 − .78 (NART-R errors), with a standard error of estimate (*SEe*) of 7.63. The reported correlation between the NART-R and FSIQ was $r = .75$.

Procedure

Old question
Observed FSIQ values were selected to comprise three ranges: a range including the highest 16% of observed scores (N.B., for a normal distribution this would include the region beyond one standard deviation above the mean), a range including the lowest 16% of observed scores, and a range including the middle 32% of observed scores. Because of duplication of values, it was not always possible to obtain exactly the desired percentages, but the closest possible range was chosen. The mean of the observed IQ scores within each range was calculated. The mean of the predicted IQ scores corresponding to each of the observed IQ scores in each range was also calculated. The difference between the

predicted and observed mean scores indicates the accuracy with which predicted IQ's match the actual IQ's within each range, providing an answer to the original question.

New question
Predicted IQ values were selected to comprise three ranges: a range including the highest 16% of predicted scores, a range including the lowest 16% of predicted scores, and a range including the middle 32% of predicted scores. Because of duplication of predictor values, it was not possible to obtain exactly the desired percentages, but the closest possible range was used. The mean of the predicted IQ scores within each range was calculated. The mean of the actual measured IQ scores corresponding to each of the predicted IQ scores in each range was also calculated. The difference between the predicted and observed mean scores indicates the accuracy with which actual IQ's match predictions within each range, providing an answer to the new, correct, question.

Confidence intervals
Confidence intervals were calculated, using the formula for the technically correct method (Pedhazur, 1983; Crawford & Howell, 1998), for several values of predicted FSIQ, using Blair's (1988) normative data (NART errors $M = 26.06$, $SD = 10.65$, $N = 66$, $SEe = 7.63$). The conventional, technically incorrect, method for calculating the 90% confidence interval for a predicted FSIQ is $\pm 1.645(7.63)$, or ± 12.6, which is to be centered on the value predicted by the regression equation.

RESULTS

Old Question
Table 2 shows the results. For the top 15% of observed FSIQ scores (mean 126), the predicted mean score was 10.7 points lower. This apparent underestimation is quite close to the theoretically expected 11.1 point underestimation of an observed FSIQ of 126 with interest correlation of $r = .75$ (shown in Table 1). For the lowest 14% of observed FSIQ scores (mean = 91), the predicted mean score was 5.1 points higher. This apparent overestimation is close to the theoretically expected 3.9 point overestimation of an observed FSIQ of 91 (shown in Table 1). The observed apparent prediction errors shown in Table 2 are similar to the theoretically expected values shown in Table 1 and are in accord with the results that Weins et al. (1993) reported for their cross-validation of the Blair equation.

Table 2. Apparent Mean Error of Prediction (Predicted minus Observed) for Three Sets of Cases.

Range of observed FSIQ	Mean observed FSIQ	Mean predicted FSIQ	Apparent mean prediction error
121–134 ($N = 10$)	125.7	115.0	−10.7
101–110 ($N = 22$)	106.1	105.8	+0.3
87–93 ($N = 9$)	90.6	95.7	+5.1

Note. The cases are selected to have the indicated ranges of *observed* FSIQ scores using Blair's (1988, Appendix E) data.

Table 3. Actual Mean Error of Prediction (Predicted minus Observed) for Three Sets of Cases.

Range of predicted FSIQ	Mean predicted FSIQ	Mean observed FSIQ	Observed mean prediction error
115.3–124.7 ($N = 10$)	119.3	121.6	−2.3
105.2–110.6 ($N = 21$)	108.7	104.6	+4.1
86.5–98.2 ($N = 10$)	93.3	93.9	−0.6

Note. The cases are selected to have the indicated ranges of *predicted* FSIQ scores using Blair's (1988, Appendix E) data.

New Question

Table 3 shows the accuracy of the predicted values for three ranges of predictions. The Blair (1988) data show that the regression equation predictions are good for all three ranges and are actually slightly more accurate for the 10 predictions at each extreme than for the 21 predictions centered on the median.

Confidence Intervals

Confidence intervals are shown in Table 4.

STUDY 2

METHOD

Sample

The data provided by Carswell (1995) were obtained from a sample consisting of 49 normal individuals, aged 55–91 (mean = 71 years). On the basis of these data, Carswell (1995) and Carswell, Graves, Snow, and Tierney (1997), reported results of a longitudinal cross-validation of the Ryan and Paolo (1992) regression equation predicting WAIS-R VIQ from the NART. The Ryan and Paolo equation is: Estimated VIQ = 132.3893 − 1.164 (NART errors) with an originally reported SEe of 7.70. The SEe on cross-validation reported by Carswell, et al. (1995) was 7.92.

Procedure

The procedure was the same as in Study 1 except that for calculating the correct confidence intervals the normative data from Ryan and Paolo (1992) were used (NART errors $M = 29.04$, $SD = 8.60$, $N = 126$,

Table 4. Calculated Correct and Conventional 90% Confidence Intervals for Various Values of Predicted FSIQ Scores Using Blair and Spreen's (1989) Normative Data.

Predicted FSIQ	Correct 90% confidence interval	Conventional 90% confidence interval
124.7*	±13.2	±12.6
119.3	±13.0	±12.6
108.7	±12.8	±12.6
100.0	±12.9	±12.6
93.3	±13.1	±12.6
86.4*	±13.4	±12.6

Note. * 124.7 and 86.4 are the highest and lowest predicted FSIQ's in the normative sample corresponding to 4 and 53 errors on the NART. The equation should not be used for clients whose NART score is outside of this range.

$SEe = 7.70$). The conventional, incorrect, method yields a 90% confidence interval for a predicted VIQ of ±1.645(7.70), or ±12.7.

RESULTS

Old Question

Table 5 shows the results. For the top 18% of observed VIQ's, the predictions apparently underestimated the actual scores by 7.5 points; while for the bottom 16% of observed VIQ's, the predictions apparently overestimated the actual VIQ's by 9.6 points. These results are, again, in accord with the claims in the quotations above.

Table 5. Apparent Mean Error of Prediction for Three Sets of Cases.

Range of observed VIQ	Mean observed VIQ	Mean predicted VIQ	Apparent mean prediction error
127–132 ($N = 9$)	128.8	121.3	−7.5
115–122 ($N = 16$)	118.4	116.7	−1.7
91–108 ($N = 8$)	101.8	111.4	+9.6

Note. The cases are selected to have the indicated ranges of *observed* VIQ scores using Carswell's (1995) data.

Table 6. Observed Mean Error of Prediction for Three Sets of Cases Selected to Have the Indicated Ranges of *Predicted* VIQ Scores Using Carswell's (1995) Data.

Range of predicted VIQ	Mean predicted VIQ	Mean observed VIQ	Observed mean prediction error
123.8–126.6 ($N = 7$)	124.2	124.3	−0.1
113.8–119.6 ($N = 21$)	117.0	116.5	+0.5
96.3–109.1 ($N = 8$)	106.1	107.5	−1.4

New Question

Table 6 shows the accuracy of the predicted values for three ranges of predictions. The Carswell (1995) data show that the Ryan and Paolo (1992) regression equation predictions were quite accurate upon cross-validation for all three ranges of predicted VIQ.

Confidence intervals

Confidence intervals are shown in Table 7.

DISCUSSION

Regression equation predictions have been claimed to seriously underestimate high scores and overestimate low scores (Barona et al., 1984; Ryan & Paolo, 1992; Weins et al., 1993). If true, this would greatly limit the clinical utility of regression prediction methods. The claims are based on a procedure that answers the following question, "If I have a particular actual IQ score, does the prediction of that score tend to match the actual score, or does it tend to fall above or below the actual score?" This procedure will necessarily result in large apparent prediction errors, as explained in Table 1. Using this procedure, the present study obtained empirical results from two different data sets that are in accord with the claims: the predicted scores (Tables 2 and 5) deviate seriously from actual IQ scores at both extremes. However, as outlined in the Introduction, this procedure provides an answer to a question that is actually not relevant to the issue

Table 7. Calculated Correct and Conventional 90% Confidence Intervals for Various Values of Predicted VIQ Scores Using Ryan and Paolo's (1992) Regression Equation and Normative Data.

Predicted VIQ	Correct 90% confidence interval	Conventional 90% confidence interval
132.4	±13.4	±12.7
124.2	±13.1	±12.7
117.0	±13.0	±12.7
115.0	±12.9	±12.7
106.1	±12.8	±12.7
100.0	±12.8	±12.7
85.0	±12.9	±12.7

of whether a prediction equation is less useful or valid for predictions of scores away from the mean than it is for scores near the mean. Conclusions about accuracy of prediction at the extremes, based on the above procedure, are therefore inappropriate and misleading.

The correct question to ask is, "If I have a particular predicted IQ, does the actual IQ score tend to match the predicted score, or does it tend to fall above or below the predicted score?" Regression theory answers that the actual scores are expected to match the predicted scores *throughout the range*. The present studies provided empirical answers to this question. Results of the present studies (Tables 3 and 6) indicate that the NART and NART-R regression equations were able to predict actual IQ without serious underestimation for higher predicted values and without overestimation for lower predicted values.

There are two additional issues that affect the potential accuracy of prediction for predictions above and below the mean. The first is that the width of the confidence interval for the predicted value increases as the prediction moves further from the mean (cf. Pedhazur, 1983). In practice a point estimate of IQ has little clinical value and an interval estimate would routinely be required. If the confidence interval were much larger for high and low predicted values, the predictions would be less useful for more extreme values. Recently Crawford and Howell (1998) have discussed this problem and have provided results for simulated data that indicate that, for sample sizes and inter-test correlations typical of actual neuropsychological regression equations, the confidence interval increase is actually quite small. The present studies provided empirical results that confirm the simulation study results: the magnitude of confidence intervals increases only very slightly at the extremes of the prediction range. The amount of increase (5% for the most extreme possible prediction of the Blair equation) would not constitute a practical limitation on the utility of predictions at the extremes. Users of regression equations should, however, routinely calculate confidence intervals using the correct method (Pedhazur, 1982; Crawford & Howell, 1998), rather than with the conventional method that slightly underestimates the size of the interval even at the mean.

One remaining problem for the prediction of extreme values concerns limits in the range of the predictor variables. For example, the Blair (1988) equation should not be used to produce a predicted FSIQ greater than 124.7 (because this was the highest predicted FSIQ in the normative sample). The Ryan and Paolo (1992) equation mathematically can produce a maximum predicted VIQ of 132.4 (with zero NART errors), but it is unclear whether this value would actually be allowed since Ryan and Paolo did not report the range of predicted values in their sample. (Regression equations are not considered to be valid for predictions beyond the range actually found in the normative sample.) While these upper limits are quite high in terms of the small percentage of individuals with IQ scores above the limits, the inability to predict higher values will constrain the utility of the equations for some applications, such as detecting cognitive decline of a person with a true IQ higher than the maximum possible predicted value. The maximum and minimum allowed prediction values should be kept in mind when any regression equation is used.

Of the three issues discussed above that could have an effect on the accuracy and utility of regression equation predictions of values above and below the mean, two can be dismissed. Regression predictions are not, contrary to widespread belief, less accurate at the extremes than in the median range. On the other hand, regression prediction confidence intervals, contrary to the calculation method conventionally used in neuropsychology, actually do increase for more extreme predictions when the proper formula is used. However, the increase is a very small percentage over the error of prediction present in the median range, and this increase would not cause practical problems. The third issue, limits on prediction range due to limited range of the predictor variable(s), can lead to practical constraints, but the range available for the two prediction equations reviewed would be adequate to predict most normal individuals' IQ scores.

The results of these studies indicate that previous warnings against the use of regression equations for prediction of values outside the median range are unwarranted to the extent that the warnings were based on inappropriate statistical analyses. Nevertheless, clinicians should continue to be concerned about the accuracy of the popular prediction equations, since the accuracy of these equations *even within the median range*, may not be adequate (Graves et al., 1999; Hawkins, 1995). Furthermore, predicted scores outside the median range may be less accurate and valid, not because of statistical problems of the regression method, but because the normative sample may not be representative of these individuals. Thus, collateral supportive evidence is especially important for predicting high or low functional status.

REFERENCES

Barona, A., Reynolds, C.R., & Chastain, R. (1984). A demographically based index of premorbid intelligence for the WAIS-R. *Journal of Consulting and Clinical Psychology, 52*, 885–887.

Blair, J.R. (1988). A Revision of the New Adult Reading Test. Master of Science thesis, University of Victoria, Victoria, B.C.

Blair, J.R., & Spreen, O. (1989). Predicting premorbid IQ: a revision of the National Adult Reading Test. *The Clinical Neuropsychologist, 7*, 129–136.

Carswell, L.M. (1995). An examination of the effectiveness of premorbid IQ indices at postdicting IQ scores in normal subjects. Master of Science thesis, University of Victoria, Victoria, B.C.

Carswell, L.M., Graves, R.E., Snow, W.G., & Tierney, M.C. (1997). Postdicting Verbal IQ of elderly individuals. *Journal of Clinical and Experimental Neuropsychology, 19*, 914–921.

Crawford, J.R., & Howell, D.C. (1998). Regression equations in clinical neuropsychology: An evaluation of statistical methods for comparing predicted and obtained scores. *Journal of Clinical and Experimental Neuropsychology, 20*, 755–762.

Graves, R.E., Carswell, L.M., & Snow, W.G. (1999). An evaluation of the sensitivity of premorbid IQ estimator for detecting cognitive decline. *Psychological Assessment, 11*, 29–38.

Hawkins, K.A. (1995). Limitations to the validity of the Barona regression formula and similar demographically-based methods of estimating pre-injury intellectual functioning. *Behavioral Sciences and the Law, 13*, 491–503.

Nelson, H.E., & O'Connell, A. (1978). Dementia: the estimation of premorbid intelligence levels using the New Adult Reading Test. *Cortex, 14*, 234–244.

Pedhazur, E.J. (1982). *Multiple regression in behavioral research.* For Worth: Holt, Rinehart and Winston, pp. 143–146.

Ryan, J.J., & Paolo, A.M. (1992). A screening procedure for estimating premorbid intelligence in the elderly. *The Clinical Neuropsychologist, 6*, 53–62.

Weins, A.N., Bryan, J.E., & Crossen, J.R. (1993). Estimating WAIS-R FSIQ from the National Adult Reading Test-Revised in normal subjects. *The Clinical Neuropsychologist, 7*, 70–84.

The Clinical Neuropsychologist
2000, Vol. 14, No. 2, pp. 181–186

PPVT-R as an Estimate of Premorbid Intelligence in Older adults

Beth E. Snitz[1], Linas A. Bieliauskas[1,2], Alicia Crossland[2], Michael R. Basso[3], and Brad Roper[4]
[1]V.A. Medical Center, [2]University of Michigan, [3]University of Tulsa, Oklahoma, and [4]V.A. Medical Center, Memphis

ABSTRACT

The Peabody Picture Vocabulary Test-Revised (PPVT-R) was examined as an estimate of premorbid intelligence in a clinical sample of elderly patients ($N = 150$) undergoing clinical neuropsychological evaluation. PPVT-R standard scores were compared across grossly cognitively intact, mildly/moderately and severely impaired groups of patients, and compared to a short form of the Wechsler Adult Intelligence Scale-Revised (WAIS-R) and the Barona regression equation. Results indicate that, while the PPVT-R is vulnerable to increasing levels of cognitive impairment among patients with fewer years of education, the PPVT-R is stable across mild to moderate levels of impairment for patients with greater than 12 years of education. In a subsample of grossly cognitively intact patients ($n = 91$), the PPVT-R standard score correlated significantly with estimated WAIS-R FSIQ ($r = .61$). Compared to the Barona equation, the PPVT-R was less likely to over-estimate WAIS-R FSIQ in the grossly cognitively intact patients. These data suggest the PPVT-R to be a useful estimate of premorbid ability for patients with a greater than high-school education.

One of the essential tasks in clinical neuropsychological evaluation of dementia in the elderly is to assess premorbid intelligence in order to make judgments about the presence and degree of cognitive decline. A popular approach for estimating premorbid intelligence has been the use of regression equations based on demographic predictors (e.g., age, education, occupation). Perhaps the most widely used equations are those developed by Barona, Reynolds, and Chastain (1984) to estimate Wechsler Adult Intelligence Scale-Revised IQ scores (WAIS-R; Wechsler, 1981). Although estimates from the Barona equations are highly correlated with WAIS-R IQs, they are limited in several respects. For instance, they are reported to over-estimate IQ scores in neurologically normal (Eppinger, Craig, Adams, & Parsons, 1987) and impaired (Sweet, Moberg, & Tovian, 1990) subjects. The Barona equations have also been

criticized for overgeneralized coding of occupation and education (Eppinger et al., 1987). Furthermore, because of the problem of regression toward the mean, the Barona formulas are inapplicable at the extremes of the normal distribution and generally yield IQ scores only from 69 to 120 (Barona et al., 1984).

Another common method for estimating premorbid IQ has been the use of word-reading measures, based on the rationale that vocabulary is a "hold" ability resilient to the effects of brain damage (cf. Matarazzo, 1977; Nelson & McKenna, 1975). Two such popular tests are the National Adult Reading Test (NART; Nelson, 1982) and the WRAT-R Reading subtest (Jastak & Wilkinson, 1984), both of which are measures of the ability to pronounce irregular English words. There is evidence, however, that word-reading ability may decline in the presence of even mild dementia

Address correspondence to: Linas A. Bieliauskas, Ph.D., Psychology Service (116B), VA Medical Center, 2215 Fuller Road, Ann Arbor, MI 48104, USA. Email: Linas@umich.edu
Accepted for publication: February 13, 2000.

(O'Carroll et al., 1995; Storandt, Stone & LaBarge, 1995), although Schmand, Geerlings, Jonker and Lindeboom (1998) report greater stability with a Dutch version of the NART.

Receptive measures of vocabulary, which do not require any verbal output, have received little attention, to date, with regard to potential utility in estimating premorbid intelligence. One such popular measure is the Peabody Picture Vocabulary Test-Revised (PPVT-R; Dunn & Dunn, 1981). Because the PPVT-R is highly correlated with WAIS-R FSIQ (Carvajal, Shaffer, & Weaver, 1989; Prout & Schwartz, 1984) and requires only a pointing response from subjects, we considered it of interest to evaluate as an estimate of premorbid intelligence in older patients with known or suspected neurologic disease.

The objective of this study was to compare the PPVT-R with the Barona equation across stages of cognitive impairment, using a short-form WAIS-R as a criterion measure. It was hypothesized that, if the PPVT-R provides stable estimates of premorbid IQ, PPVT-R performance decrements across levels of cognitive impairment should be minimal. It was also predicted that, compared to Barona-estimated FSIQ, PPVT-R standard scores would be less vulnerable to over-estimation of short-form WAIS-R FSIQ. Finally, because the Barona equation tends to be over-inclusive in coding of demographic variables, we predicted that PPVT-R would be a more valid measure of estimated premorbid intelligence and therefore more highly correlated with short-form WAIS-R FSIQ in grossly cognitively intact patients.

METHOD

Data were collected retrospectively from 89 women and 61 men with known or suspected brain damage who were consecutively referred for neuropsychological evaluations in a large university medical center. Fifty-nine of the patients had a confirmed neurological condition, such as Alzheimer's disease, Parkinson's disease, cerebrovascular accident, and so forth, while the 91 others did not have a diagnosis suggestive of CNS involvement. Participants ranged in age from 43 to 95, with a mean age of 75.42 ($SD = 7.21$) years. Their level of education ranged from 3 to 22 years, with a mean of 13.35 ($SD = 3.52$) years.

As part of their evaluations, patients were administered the PPVT-R, the Block Design, Arithmetic, Comprehension, and Similarities subtests of the WAIS-R, and the Folstein Mini-Mental Status Examination (MMSE; Folstein, Folstein, & McHugh, 1975). The WAIS-R subtests were combined to estimate FSIQ following the method of Tellegen and Briggs (cited in Sattler, 1992).

Patients' levels of impairment were categorized on the basis of MMSE scores. Those patients with scores of 19 and below were classified as severely impaired, 20 to 23 as mildly/moderately impaired, and 24 and above as grossly cognitively intact.

RESULTS

Table 1 presents demographic variables and the means of the Barona-estimated FSIQ, PPVT-R standard score, and short-form WAIS-R FSIQ, across levels of impairment. One-way ANOVAs indicated that age did not differ significantly among the groups ($F(2, 146) = 2.20$, $p = .12$), but that years of education did differ significantly ($F(2, 144) = 6.52, p < .01$).

To examine the effects of impairment level and education on estimated premorbid IQ, a 3 (impairment) $\times$ 2 (education) $\times$ 3 (estimation method) repeated measures ANOVA was carried out. Years of education were categorized into 12 years or less, and greater than 12 years. Significant between-group main effects for impairment ($F(2, 140) = 13.09, p < .001$) and education ($F(1, 140) = 50.99$, $p < .001$) were observed. As expected, estimated IQ scores were lower for greater levels of impairment and in the lower educational category. A within-group main effect of estimation method was also observed ($F(2, 280) = 88.64, p < .001$). For the entire sample, the mean Barona-estimated IQ (113.59, $SD = 11.77$) and the mean PPVT-R standard score (99.83, $SD = 21.02$) were higher than short-form WAIS-R FSIQ (94.33, $SD = 15.08$). Additionally, significant interactions of Impairment $\times$ Estimation method ($F(4, 280) = 2.98$, $p = .02$) and Impairment $\times$ Education ($F(2, 280) = 8.78, p < .001$) were observed.

To better understand the nature of the Impairment $\times$ Estimation method interaction, the simple effects of method across level of impairment were examined. For the short-form WAIS-R, mean FSIQ differed significantly across levels of

Table 1. Mean (SD) Estimated IQ Scores, Age, and Education by Levels of Cognitive Impairment.

| | Folstein MMSE Score | | | | | |
| | 24 and above (n = 91) | | 20–23 (n = 35) | | 19 and below(n = 24) | |
	M	(SD)	M	(SD)	M	(SD)
Age	74.47	(6.67)	77.34	(6.97)	76.17	(9.00)
Education (years)	13.99	(3.55)	13.26	(3.36)	11.17	(2.82)
WAIS-R FSIQ	99.10	(13.59)	90.96	(14.08)	81.61	(12.30)
Barona FSIQ	115.81	(10.93)	113.26	(10.63)	104.70	(12.08)
PPVT-R (standard score)	104.94	(18.35)	97.26	(20.51)	82.52	(22.03)

Table 2. Mean (SD) Estimated IQ Scores by Levels of Cognitive Impairment and Education.

| Education | Folstein MMSE Score | | | | | |
| 12 years and below | 24 and above (n = 37) | | 20–23 (n = 16) | | 19 and below (n = 19) | |
	M	(SD)	M	(SD)	M	(SD)
WAIS-R FSIQ	93.07	(12.05)	85.56	(10.08)	79.87	(10.77)
Barona FSIQ	106.24	(5.97)	104.00	(7.62)	101.21	(10.17)
PPVT-R (standard score)	96.14	(19.39)	85.63	(16.16)	79.26	(21.92)
13 years and above	(n = 51)		(n = 19)		(n = 5)	
WAIS-R FSIQ	103.47	(13.06)	95.50	(15.56)	88.30	(15.49)
Barona FSIQ	122.75	(8.10)	121.05	(4.95)	121.25	(2.50)
PPVT-R (standard score)	111.33	(14.71)	107.05	(18.86)	97.80	(14.79)

impairment ($F(2, 146) = 16.58$, $p < .001$) (see Table 1). To protect against Type I error, Tukey's honestly significant difference (HSD) comparisons of the intact, mildly/moderately, and severely impaired groups were performed. These analyses revealed that all three groups were significantly different from each other ($ps < .05$).

For the Barona estimate as well, patients differed across levels of impairment ($F(2, 146) = 9.40, p < .001$). Tukey HSD comparisons showed that both the intact and the mildly/moderately impaired groups had higher Barona-estimated FSIQ than the severely impaired group ($ps < .01$).

Patients also differed across levels of impairment with regard to mean PPVT-R scores ($F(2, 147) = 12.51, p < .001$). Follow-up comparisons revealed that the intact and the mildly/moderately impaired groups had higher standard scores than the severely impaired group ($ps < .01$). In addition, there was a trend toward a higher mean score in the intact group compared to the mildly/moderately impaired group ($p = .07$).

Because of the significant education effect, we further divided the sample into two groups, according to the educational categories: patients with 12 years or less of education ($n = 72$), and those with greater than 12 years ($n = 75$; three patients were missing education data). Table 2 reports mean IQ estimates by level of impairment and education.

For the patients with 12 years of education or less, short-form WAIS-R FSIQ decreased significantly with increased impairment level ($F(2, 69) = 8.98, p < .001$) (see Table 2). Tukey HSD comparisons indicated that the intact group differed from the severely impaired group ($p < .001$) and a trend emerged toward the intact group differing from the mildly/moderately impaired group ($p = .08$). For the Barona estimate, patients did not significantly differ between impairment level ($F(2, 69) = 2.76$, $p = .07$). For the PPVT-R, patients differed significantly with respect to levels of impairment ($F(2, 69) = 5.10$, $p < .001$). Follow-up comparisons showed that the intact group had significantly higher scores than the severely impaired group ($p < .01$).

For the patients with greater than 12 years of education, short-form WAIS-R FSIQ decreased significantly with increased impairment level ($F(2, 72) = 4.34, p < .05$). Follow-up comparisons indicated that the intact group differed significantly from the severely impaired group ($p = .05$). Neither the Barona estimate nor the PPVT-R standard score differed significantly among the three impairment groups (one-way ANOVA Fs $> .15$).

Because short-form WAIS-R FSIQ decreased significantly across each level of MMSE scores, we addressed questions of accuracy and validity of premorbid IQ estimation within the grossly cognitively intact group only ($n = 91$). To examine the degree of over-estimation of WAIS-R IQ, difference scores were calculated between short-form WAIS-R FSIQ and the Barona estimate and PPVT-R standard scores, respectively. The mean difference score between the Barona estimate and short-form WAIS-R FSIQ within the grossly cognitively intact group was 16.99 IQ points ($SD = 12.62$). The mean difference score between PPVT-R standard score and short-form WAIS-R FSIQ was 6.24 ($SD = 15.00$).

Pearson correlation coefficients were also computed within the grossly cognitively intact group. The correlation between short-form WAIS-R FSIQ and Barona-estimated FSIQ was .51 (two-tailed $p < .01$), and the correlation between short-form WAIS-R FSIQ and PPVT-R standard score was .61 ($p < .01$). However, these correlations did not differ significantly from each other ($p > .10$)

DISCUSSION

It was presumed that, if the PPVT-R provides stable estimates of premorbid IQ in older adults, PPVT-R performance decrements would be minimal across levels of cognitive impairment. Within the entire sample, there was no statistically significant difference between the grossly intact and mildly/moderately impaired groups, although the p value was close to significance ($p = .07$). There was, however, a significant decline in mean scores between the mildly/moderately impaired and severely impaired groups. Furthermore, the mean

PPVT-R standard score initially declined at a rate almost identical to the short-form WAIS-R (i.e., by a difference between the intact and mildly/moderately impaired group means of approximately 8 points).

The pattern of results, however, changes according to educational level. For patients with a high-school education or less, the mean PPVT-R score declined at a rate comparable to the WAIS-R. By contrast, for patients with greater than a high-school education, mean PPVT-R scores declined at a slower rate than the WAIS-R. Furthermore, PPVT-R scores did not significantly differ between levels of impairment, although lack of power due to the small sample sizes was likely a factor. Mean PPVT-R scores also remained within the average range as MMSE scores decreased, although again it must be pointed out that the group of patients in this educational category with MMSE scores below 20 is small ($n = 5$). These results suggest that the PPVT-R can provide reasonably stable estimates of premorbid intelligence for patients with a greater than high-school education, at least for MMSE scores down to 20.

The tendency for both the Barona equation and the PPVT-R to over-estimate WAIS-R IQ is consistent with reports in the literature of neurologically normal subjects (Eppinger et al., 1987; Mangiaracina & Simon, 1986). In this sample, however, the PPVT-R over-estimated short-form WAIS-R FSIQ to a considerably lesser degree than did the Barona equation in grossly cognitively intact patients. The PPVT-R was also more highly correlated with WAIS-R FSIQ within the grossly intact group than was the Barona equation, as predicted; however, the difference in amount of variance accounted for was small and not statistically significant.

The finding of a slower rate of decline in PPVT-R scores for the higher educational group is consistent with the predictions of Satz (1993) and others (e.g., Berkman, 1986; Mortimer & Graves, 1993) regarding brain reserve capacity. According to this view, given the same degree of brain damage, individuals with higher premorbid intelligence levels are less likely than those with lower premorbid abilities to evidence neuropsychological deficits and dementia. Also consistent with this theory is the finding that the Barona scores, which are based upon demographic variables and not current levels of functioning, were significantly lowered in the severely impaired group within the entire sample.

In sum, the present study supports the use of the PPVT-R to estimate premorbid IQ in older adults with education beyond high school, and before MMSE score falls below 20. For individuals with less than 13 years of education, the use of the Barona equation is more stable, although it still results in a general over-estimate of WAIS-R FSIQ. A limitation of the present findings is that, although the MMSE cut-score of 23 is standard practice in clinical settings, one cannot rule out the possibility that WAIS-R FSIQ was reduced to an unknown degree in what we called our "grossly cognitively intact" group. Therefore, replication of these results using a truly premorbid criterion of premorbid intelligence is certainly warranted. An additional limitation is that the present data are based entirely on a sample of elderly individuals and cannot be generalized to a younger population. Finally, these results were obtained from a sample with relatively heterogeneous neurological presentations. It is possible that specific pathologies may particularly affect PPVT-R performance (e.g., insult to the language dominant hemisphere may not greatly impact MMSE scores, but it may significantly reduce PPVT-R performance). Follow-up research that addresses these questions will help to further clarify and delineate the appropriate uses of the PPVT-R as an estimate of premorbid intelligence.

REFERENCES

Barona, A., Reynolds, C.R., & Chastain, R. (1984). A demographically based index of premorbid intelligence for the WAIS-R. *Journal of Consulting and Clinical Psychology*, *52*, 885–887.

Berkman, L.F. (1986). The association between educational attainment and mental status examinations: Of etiologic significance for senile dementia or not? *Journal of Chronic Diseases*, *39*, 171–174.

Carvajal, H., Shaffer, C., & Weaver, K.A. (1989). Correlation of scores of maximum security inmates on Wechsler Adult Intelligence Scale-Revised and the Peabody Picture Vocabulary Test-Revised. *Psychological Reports*, *65*, 268–270.

Dunn, L.M., & Dunn, L. (1981). *Peabody Picture Vocabulary Test-Revised: Manual for forms L and M*. Circle Pines, MN: American Guidance Service.

Eppinger, M.G., Craig, P.L., Adams, R.L., & Parsons, O.A. (1987). The WAIS-R index for estimating premorbid intelligence: Cross-validation and clinical utility. *Journal of Consulting and Clinical Psychology*, *55*, 86–90.

Folstein, M.F., Folstein, S.E., & McHugh, P.R. (1975). "Mini-Mental State." A practical method for grading the cognitive state of patients for the clinician. *Journal of Psychiatric Research*, *12*, 189–198.

Jastak, S., & Wilkinson, G.S. (1984). *Wide Range Achievement Test-Revised*. Wilmington, DE: Jastak Assessment Systems.

Mangiaracina, J., & Simon, M.J. (1986). Comparison of the PPVT-R and WAIS-R in state hospital psychiatric patients. *Journal of Clinical Psychology*, *42*, 817–820.

Matarazzo, J.D. (1977). *Wechsler's measurement and appraisal of adult intelligence*. New York: Oxford University Press.

Mortimer, J.A., & Graves, A.B. (1993). Education and other socioeconomic determinants of dementia and Alzheimer's disease. *Neurology*, *43*, S39–S44.

Nelson, H.E. (1982). *National Adult Reading Test (NART): Test manual*. Windsor: NFER Nelson.

Nelson, H.E., & McKenna, P. (1975). The use of current reading ability in the assessment of dementia. *British Journal of Social and Clinical Psychology*, *14*, 259–267.

O'Carroll, R.E., Prentice, N., Murray, C., van Beck, M., Ebmeier, K.P., & Goodwin, G.M. (1995). Further evidence that reading ability is not preserved in Alzheimer's disease. *British Journal of Psychiatry*, *167*, 659–662.

Patterson, K.E., Graham, N., & Hodges, J.R. (1994). Reading in dementia of the Alzheimer type: A preserved ability? *Neuropsychology*, *8*, 395–412.

Prout, H.T., & Schwartz, J.F. (1984). Validity of the Peabody Picture Vocabulary Test-Revised with mentally retarded adults. *Journal of Clinical Psychology*, *40*, 584–587.

Sattler, J.M. (1992). *Assessment of children* (3rd ed.). San Diego: Author.

Satz, P. (1993). Brain reserve capacity on symptom onset after brain injury: A formulation and review of evidence for threshold theory. *Neuropsychology*, *7*, 273–285.

Schmand, B., Geerlings, M.I., Jonker, C., & Lindeboom, J. (1998). Reading ability as an estimator of premorbid intelligence: Does it remain stable in emergent dementia? *Journal of Clinical and Experimental Neuropsychology*, *20*, 42–51.

Storandt, M., Stone, K., & LaBarge, E. (1995). Deficits in reading performance in very mild dementia of the Alzheimer type. *Neuropsychology, 9,* 174–176.

Sweet, J.J., Moberg, P.J., & Tovian, S.M. (1990). Evaluation of Wechsler Adult Intelligence Scale-Revised premorbid IQ formulas in clinical populations. *Psychological Assessment: A Journal of Consulting and Clinical Psychology, 2,* 41–44.

Wechsler, D. (1981). *Wechsler Adult Intelligence Scale-Revised manual.* New York: The Psychological Corporation.

Journal of Clinical and Experimental Neuropsychology
1997, Vol. 19, No. 6, pp. 825–837

VIII-F

Predicting Premorbid Neuropsychological Functioning Following Pediatric Traumatic Brain Injury*

Keith Owen Yeates[1] and H. Gerry Taylor[2]

[1]Department of Pediatrics, The Ohio State University and Children's Hospital, Columbus, OH, and
[2]Department of Pediatrics, Case Western Reserve University and Rainbow Babies and Children's Hospital, Cleveland, OH

ABSTRACT

This study examined the prediction of premorbid neuropsychological functioning using data from an ongoing prospective study of traumatic brain injuries (TBI) in children ages 6 to 12 years. Prediction equations were derived based on 80 children with orthopedic injuries (OI), who served as a comparison group for the children with TBI. Collectively, parent ratings of premorbid school performance, maternal ethnicity, family socioeconomic status, and children's word recognition skill predicted from 13% to 45% of the variance in three measures of neuropsychological functioning. The regression equations were used to compute predicted scores among 109 children with TBI. Actual scores fell significantly below predicted scores among children with TBI, and the magnitude of the deficits was correlated with injury severity. Premorbid neuropsychological functioning can be predicted in children with TBI, but with less precision than would be desirable for clinical purposes.

The prediction of premorbid neuropsychological functioning is of critical importance in both clinical and research activities directed toward understanding the consequences of pediatric traumatic brain injury (TBI). Clinicians must estimate premorbid functioning to gauge the magnitude of neuropsychological impairment associated with TBI and to make predictions about children's long-term prognosis. Researchers must estimate premorbid functioning not only to determine the extent to which TBI produces neuropsychological deficits, but also to insure that groups of children who experience TBI were similar premorbidly to children who constitute control groups in their research (e.g., children with orthopedic trauma).

One means of estimating premorbid functioning is to collect pertinent information retrospectively. For instance, school records frequently contain the results of group achievement testing and other indicators of cognitive ability, and might be used to estimate premorbid functioning (Levin & Eisenberg, 1979). Similarly, parent and teacher ratings of premorbid school performance also might yield valid estimates (Richardson, 1963). On the other hand, school records do not always contain relevant information, and the quality of the information will vary

* The research presented here was supported by Grant MCJ-390611 from the Maternal and Child Health Research Bureau (Title V, Social Security Act), Health Resources and Services Administration, Department of Health and Human Services. The authors wish to acknowledge the contributions of Matt Diamond, Nori Mercuri Minich, Madeline Polonia, Barbara Shapero, and Elizabeth Shaver. We also wish to acknowledge the participation of the Children's Hospital Medical Center of Akron and the collaboration of Duane Bishop, Dennis Drotar, Susan Klein, Timothy Mapstone, Scott Maxwell, Terry Stancin, George Thompson, G. Dean Timmons, Shari L. Wade, and Dennis Weiner. A preliminary version of this paper was presented at the Pacific Rim meeting of the International Neuropsychological Society in Cairns, Australia, July 1995.
Address correspondence to: Keith Owen Yeates, Department of Psychology, Children's Hospital, 700 Children's Dr., Columbus, OH 43205, USA.
Accepted for publication: April 30, 1997.

from school to school. Moreover, school records may not always be available, particularly for children who have attended multiple schools. Ratings from previous teachers also may be difficult to obtain after a TBI, particularly if an extended period of time has elapsed since the injury. Thus, parent ratings are likely to be the only retrospective source of information that can be elicited in a routine and standardized manner, especially in research settings.

Rather than relying on retrospective data, contemporary research efforts have focused on methods the use current information to predict premorbid neuropsychological functioning, defined in most cases as premorbid IQ (Klesges & Tröster, 1987). Two methods have received the most attention. The first involves the use of sociodemographic variables such as educational attainment, family income, and ethnic status, which are known to be correlated with IQ. This method has yielded significant results among both children and adults (e.g., Barona, Reynolds, & Chastain, 1984; Karzmark et al., 1985; Klesges & Sanchez, 1980; Reynolds & Gutkin, 1979), although it has been criticized for generating estimates that are not sufficiently accurate to be used in clinical practice (Silverstein, 1987).

The other method, which has been applied almost exclusively to adult samples, involves tests of skills such as vocabulary and word reading that are known to be related to IQ and that are thought to be relatively stable despite acute brain injury. Early research in this tradition using "hold" and "don't hold" subtests from the Wechsler intelligence scales has largely been discredited, because such measures are more vulnerable to brain impairment than first supposed (Klesges & Tröster, 1987). However, more recent efforts using measures of single-word reading ability such as the National Adult Reading Test or the Wide Range Achievement Test have shown more promising results (e.g., Blair & Spreen, 1989; Bryan, Weins, & Crosson, 1992), although such measures also are not immune to the effects of brain impairment (Stebbins, Gilley, Wilson, Bernard, & Fox, 1990; Stebbins, Wilson, Gilley, Bernard, & Fox, 1990).

Recent efforts to predict premorbid IQ have combined the two approaches, using sociodemographic variables and measures of skills such as word recognition in multiple regression analyses to predict premorbid functioning (e.g., Grober &

Sliwinski, 1991; Karekan, Gur, & Saykin, 1995; Krull, Scott, & Sherer, 1995; Willshire, Kinsella, & Prior, 1991). Research combining the two approaches has suggested that both types of variables can make independent contributions to the prediction of IQ, but such research has been conducted only in adult samples. As far as we can determine, there have been no studies of children that have used both sociodemographic variables and tests of concurrent skills to predict premorbid IQ or any other aspect of neuropsychological functioning.

Previous research on the prediction of premorbid functioning in children has also been hampered by a lack of clinical validation. Clinical validation requires that the mean predicted IQs of clinical samples be comparable to the mean actual IQs of matched control groups, and that discrepancies between predicted and actual performance within the clinical samples be correlated with indicators of underlying brain impairment, such as the severity of dementia or TBI. There have been relatively few attempts to satisfy these criteria in samples with documented brain impairment, and they have been concerned exclusively with adults (e.g., Christensen, Hadzi-Pavlovic, & Jacomb, 1991; Grober & Sliwinski, 1991; Hart, Smith, & Swash, 1986; Willshire et al., 1991). We are not aware of any studies that have attempted to validate clinically the prediction of IQ or other neuropsychological test performances in children with documented brain impairment.

We attempted to remedy the limitations of previous research by examining the prediction of premorbid neuropsychological functioning using data from an ongoing prospective study of the effects of TBI on children and their families (Taylor et al., 1995). The study involves two groups of children, one with moderate to severe TBI and a comparison group with orthopedic injuries (OI). Demographic information and retrospective parent ratings of school performance are available for all children, who also have undergone neuropsychological assessments that include standardized measures of word recognition ability.

The goals of the current study were to use retrospective parent ratings, demographic variables, and a measure of word reading skills to assess the prediction of neuropsychological functioning in the OI group, and to validate the resulting prediction equations in the TBI group by comparing predicted to actual performance. We expected that parent ratings, demographic variables, and word reading skills collectively would explain a significant proportion of variance in neuropsychological test performance among the OI group. We also expected that the actual neuropsychological test performance of the TBI group would be lower than their predicted performance, and that the magnitude of the discrepancy would be related to injury severity.

METHOD

Participants

Participants were drawn from a total of 189 children, 109 with TBI and 80 with OI, who were recruited from consecutive admissions to four hospitals in the midwestern United States. All children were between 6 and 12 years of age and used English as their primary language at home. Children were excluded if they had a history of child abuse, previous neurological disorder, or mental retardation. Children were eligible for the TBI group if they sustained a blunt head trauma and their lowest post-resuscitation Glasgow Coma Scale (GCS; Jennett & Bond, 1975) score was 12 or less, or if it was between 13 and 15 but was associated with an intracranial lesion on neuroimaging, skull fracture, neurological deficits, or sustained loss of consciousness (i.e., >15 min).

Children with TBI resulting from causes other than blunt head trauma (e.g., near drowning, gunshot wound) were excluded. Children were eligible for the OI group if they sustained a bone fracture that required at least an overnight hospitalization but did not demonstrate any evidence of loss of consciousness or other indicators of possible brain injury.

Following established conventions, the TBI group was divided into two groups based on injury severity (Fletcher & Levin, 1988). Children whose lowest post-resuscitation GCS scores were 8 or less were considered to have severe injuries, and children with scores of 9 or more were considered to have moderate injuries. Of the 56 children in the moderate TBI group, 47 of them had GCS scores ranging from 13 to 15, but they all demonstrated additional complications indicative of a more severe injury and deemed to necessitate hospitalization (e.g., intracranial lesion on neuroimaging, skull fracture, focal neurological deficits, or loss of consciousness greater than 15 min). Thus, consistent with previous research, their injuries were considered moderate rather than mild in severity (Fletcher & Levin, 1988).

Demographic features of the three groups (i.e., severe TBI, moderate TBI, OI) are summarized in Table 1. The groups did not differ in gender or age at injury. They also did not differ in maternal education, annual family income, or the Duncan occupational status index. The groups did differ in maternal ethnicity, with a significantly higher proportion of non-Whites in the OI group than the TBI groups, $\chi^2(2, N = 189) = 6.64, p < .05$.

Table 1. Demographic Features of Participants.

Variable	Group					
	OI		Moderate TBI		Severe TBI	
n	80		56		53	
Child's gender (% male)	59		73		74	
Maternal ethnic status (% White)*	58		75		75	
	M	(SD)	M	(SD)	M	(SD)
Maternal education[a]	3.67	(1.13)	3.49	(1.12)	3.61	(1.30)
Family income[b]	3.45	(2.77)	4.22	(2.81)	3.65	(2.81)
Duncan occupational status index	32.40	(19.68)	32.44	(18.31)	32.59	(20.62)
Child's age at injury (years)	9.28	(1.91)	9.98	(1.89)	9.37	(2.09)
Child's age at testing (years)	9.33	(1.90)	10.05	(1.89)	9.42	(2.12)
Interval from injury to testing (days)*	20.69	(12.36)	22.55	(10.11)	26.94	(13.86)
Glasgow Coma Scale score*	15.00	(0.00)	14.02	(1.85)	4.83	(1.81)
Injury Severity Score*	7.32	(3.15)	12.47	(5.66)	20.08	(11.91)
Partial Injury Severity Score*	7.32	(3.15)	2.29	(3.64)	8.53	(10.25)
WJ-R Word Identification standard score	99.60	(14.99)	98.30	(15.41)	95.54	(17.32)

Note. OI = Orthopedic injury; TBI = Traumatic brain injury; WJ-R = Woodcock Johnson Test of Achievement-Revised; SES = Socioeconomic status; [a]Scale from 1 ("less than 7 years") to 7 ("graduate degree"); [b]Scale from 1 ("≤$20,000") to 8 ("≥$60,000"); * Groups differ significantly, $p < .05$.

As anticipated, the groups also differed in injury severity. The Injury Severity Score (ISS; Mayer, Matlack, Johnson, & Walker, 1980) presented in Table 1 is based on all injuries that the children sustained, whereas the partial ISS is calculated based only on injuries unrelated to TBI. As Table 1 shows, the severe TBI group suffered more severe injuries overall than either the moderate TBI group or OI group. In turn, the moderate TBI group suffered more severe injuries overall than the OI group. When injury severity was defined based only on injuries not involving the brain, the severe TBI and OI groups were comparable, and were both higher than the moderate TBI group. Thus, the severe TBI group had the most severe injuries overall, but did not differ from the OI group in the severity of injuries not involving the brain.

Procedures

All age-appropriate admissions to the four participating hospitals were monitored for potential eligibility. Once children meeting entry criteria were deemed medically stable, their parents were invited to participate in the study. After informed consent was obtained, family interviews were conducted, during which demographic information and ratings of the children's premorbid school performance were elicited. In most cases, the respondent for interviews and questionnaires was the child's mother.

Baseline assessments of the children's neuropsychological functioning and academic skills were conducted as soon as possible after their injuries. Children in the TBI group were screened for posttraumatic amnesia using the Children's Orientation of Amnesia Test (COAT; Ewing-Cobbs, Levin, Fletcher, Miner, & Eisenberg, 1990); they were not considered eligible for testing until their score on the COAT was within two standard deviations of the mean for their age for 2 consecutive days.

As shown in Table 1, the mean time between injury and baseline assessment differed significantly across the three groups, with somewhat longer intervals in the TBI groups than in OI group. However, the mean interval was less than 1 month for all groups, and the difference between groups in mean interval was less than 1 week. The slightly longer interval in the TBI groups is not likely to affect the results presented here. If it did, it would tend to introduce a bias against the study hypotheses, because the longer interval would permit more recovery among the TBI groups, thereby diminishing any discrepancies between their predicted and actual test scores.

Measures

Predictors

Four variables were used as predictors of neuropsychological functioning among the OI group: parent ratings of premorbid school performance, maternal ethnicity, socioeconomic status, and children's word reading skill.

Parent ratings of children's premorbid school performance were elicited using the Child Behavior Checklist (CBC; Achenbach, 1991). The CBC has been standardized on a large sample of community and clinic-referred children between the ages of 4 and 18, and has demonstrated satisfactory reliability and validity in previous research (Achenbach, 1991). On the CBC, parents are asked to rate children's performance in academic subjects on a 4-point scale from "failing" to "above average." Their ratings are summarized in a T score, which was used as one of the predictors of neuropsychological functioning.

The demographic variables selected for the prediction of neuropsychological functioning were maternal ethnicity (i.e., White vs. non-White) and a composite measure of socioeconomic status. Both maternal ethnicity and socioeconomic status have been consistent predictors of children's intellectual outcomes in previous research (Finkelstein & Ramey, 1980; Ramey, Stedman, Borders-Patterson, & Mengel, 1978). The composite socioeconomic measure was based on three variables: maternal education, coded on a 7-point scale from "less than 7 years" to "graduate degree"; annual family income, coded on an 8-point scale from "≤$20,000" to "≥$60,000"; and the Duncan index, a continuous measure that reflects occupational status (Stevens & Featherman, 1981). Because the three variables were moderately correlated, they were combined in a composite measure that was constructed by averaging z scores computed for each variable across the entire sample.

The measure of word reading skill used for the prediction of neuropsychological functioning was the age-corrected standard score on the Word Identification subtest from the Woodcock-Johnson Tests of Achievement-Revised (WJ-R; Woodcock & Mather, 1989). The Word Identification subtest requires the child to read individual words aloud. The test has satisfactory reliability and correlates well with other measures of word recognition (Woodcock & Mather, 1989).

Dependent Variables

Most previous studies of the prediction of premorbid functioning have been concerned solely with IQ. However, the IQ score is not the only measure of neuropsychological test performance with which clinicians or researchers are concerned, and the IQ score is by no means universally accepted as the benchmark against which other neuropsychological test performances should be compared (Lezak, 1995). Hence, we wanted to determine whether other neuropsychological measures could be predicted as well as IQ and whether the explanatory significance of the four predictors differed across measures.

We selected three measures of neuropsychological functioning from a larger battery as dependent variables. The three measures were chosen because they tap domains of functioning (i.e., nonverbal skills and memory) that have been shown to be particularly sensitive to the effects of TBI in prior research (Levin, Ewing-Cobbs, & Eisenberg, 1995). We chose variables sensitive to TBI because the validity of the prediction of premorbid performance rests on the ability to detect the known effects of TBI. An examination of predictive validity using variables that are not sensitive to TBI would not have been informative, because the severe TBI group would not have been expected to display a discrepancy between predicted and actual performance.

The first measure of neuropsychological functioning was a prorated Performance Scale IQ (PIQ) derived from a short form of the third edition of the Wechsler Intelligence Scale for Children (WISC-III; Wechsler, 1991). The short form included the Block Design and Object Assembly subtests, from which the prorated Performance Scale IQ was derived. Computed using the formula presented by Sattler (1992), the prorated PIQ has a reliability of .85 and validity coefficient of .83. The PIQ is a measure of nonverbal skills sensitive to the acute effects of TBI in children (Fletcher & Levin, 1988).

The second measure of neuropsychological functioning was the age-corrected standard score from the Developmental Test of Visual-Motor Integration (VMI; Beery, 1989). The VMI is a drawing task that requires visuoperceptual, constructional, and graphomotor skills. It has satisfactory reliability and validity, and has been shown to be sensitive to TBI in children (Thompson et al., 1994).

The last measure of neuropsychological functioning was the total number of words recalled across five learning trials on a shortened version of the children's California Verbal Learning Test (CVLT; Delis, Kramer, Kaplan, & Ober, 1994). The CVLT is a word-list learning task that measures verbal memory skills. Total recall on the CVLT is a reliable and valid measure of verbal memory that has been shown to discriminate between children with TBI and matched controls (Yeates, Blumenstein, Patterson, & Delis, 1995). Age-corrected standard scores are not available for this version of the CVLT. Prior to analyses, therefore, age was regressed on the CVLT score in the OI group, and the resulting regression equation was used to compute predicted scores for all participants. Residual scores were standardized based on the standard deviation of the OI group, and transformed into age-corrected standard scores comparable to those for PIQ and the VMI (i.e., $M = 100$, $SD = 15$).

Data Analysis

The first step in data analysis was to regress the parent rating of premorbid school performance, maternal ethnic status, the composite socioeconomic measure, and the WJ-R Word Identification standard score on the actual neuropsychological test scores in the OI group. Analyses including all four predictors were completed first, to assess overall model fit. Stepwise regression analyses were then conducted to select the most economical model, using a forward stepping procedure with a one-tailed p of .05 required for entry and removal. The resulting regression equations were examined not only for their statistical properties, but also for their ability to predict performance for individual children.

Some children in the OI group did not complete all three of the neuropsychological tests, usually because the nature of their injuries prevented test administration (e.g., upper extremity cast, spica cast, traction). For the prediction of PIQ, children who had been tested despite such circumstances were also eliminated from the analysis, because preliminary comparisons indicated that they performed significantly worse than their peers on the subtests used to measure PIQ. In contrast, their performance on the VMI or the CVLT was not affected by the circumstances of testing. Finally, parent ratings on the CBC were not available for a few children. Thus, different numbers of OI children were available for prediction of each of the neuropsychological measures: 30 for PIQ, 62 for the VMI, and 75 for the CVLT. The samples included in each analysis are representative of the entire OI group; preliminary analyses indicated that the children included in each analysis did not differ demographically from children who were excluded.

In the second step in data analysis, the prediction equations derived in the OI group were used to compute predicted scores for the two TBI groups. We first examined the correlation between predicted and actual test scores in the combined TBI groups. Scores representing the discrepancy between predicted and actual scores were next entered into one-way analyses of variance (ANOVA), using group membership (severe TBI, moderate TBI, and OI) as the independent variable. Following omnibus tests, a priori single-degree-of-freedom contrasts were used to determine if the combined TBI groups differed from the OI group, and if the severe TBI group differed from the moderate TBI group. For illustrative purposes, we then compared the proportion of children in each group whose predicted scores were 10 or more points higher than their actual scores, to assess how often each group displayed discrepancies of this magnitude.

Finally, to examine further the relationship between injury severity and the discrepancy between actual and predicted neuropsychological functioning, we correlated the discrepancy scores of the combined TBI groups with continuous measures of injury severity. The measures of injury severity included the lowest post-resuscitation GCS and the duration of impaired consciousness, defined as the number of days after the injury that elapsed before children were able to follow one-step commands

(Fletcher, Ewing-Cobbs, Miner, Levin, & Eisenberg, 1990).

Some children in the TBI group did not complete all three of the neuropsychological tests, either because the nature of their injuries prevented test administration or because they demonstrated prolonged coma or post-traumatic amnesia. For the analysis of PIQ, children who had been tested despite non-optimal circumstances (i.e., upper extremity case, spica cast, traction) also were eliminated from the analysis. Finally, a few children did not have parent ratings on the CBC. Thus, different numbers of TBI children were available for analyses of the three neuropsychological measures: 90 for the PIQ, 97 for the VMI, and 100 for the CVLT.

The significance level for each set of analyses was corrected for multiple comparisons using a Bonferroni procedure. The correction resulted in a p of .017 for the following analyses: The three regressions predicting neuropsychological test performance in the OI group; the three correlations between predicted and actual test scores in the combined TBI groups; the three ANOVAs comparing the groups' mean discrepancies between predicted and actual test scores; and the three comparisons of the proportions of clinically significant discrepancies within groups. A p of .0083 was employed for the six correlations between discrepancy scores and measures of injury severity in the combined TBI group.

RESULTS

Development of Prediction Equations in the OI Group

Taken together, parent ratings of premorbid school performance, maternal ethnicity, socioeconomic status, and word reading skill predicted 45% of the variance in prorated PIQ, with a multiple R of .67, $F(4, 25) = 5.13, p < .005$. The stepwise procedure retained parent ratings and maternal ethnicity as the best predictors, which together accounted for 43% of the variance in PIQ. The regression equation including only parent ratings and maternal ethnicity had a standard error of estimate of 12.07, as compared to a sample standard deviation for PIQ of 15.41.

The predicted PIQs had a more restricted range (82 to 111) than the actual PIQs (58 to 136). Across the entire OI group, 67% of the predicted scores were within 10 points of the actual scores. As expected, the prediction equation systematically underestimated high scores, and systematically overestimated low scores. Thus, when we included only children with actual PIQs between 80 and

120 (i.e., scores from approximately the 10th to 90th centile), accuracy was better, so that the discrepancy between predicted and actual PIQs was 10 points or less for 77% of the sample.

The next analysis involved the prediction of the VMI. The combination of four predictors accounted for 36% of the variance in the VMI standard score, with a multiple R of .60, $F(4, 53) = 7.58$, $p < .001$. In this instance, the stepwise procedure retained maternal ethnicity and children's word reading skills as predictors, without any appreciable reduction in the multiple R. The standard error of estimate for the regression equation including only maternal ethnicity and word reading skill was 11.43, as compared to a sample standard deviation for the VMI of 14.23.

The predicted VMI standard scores had a more restricted range (84 to 116) than the actual scores (74 to 145), particularly at the high end. Across the OI group, only 57% of the predicted scores were within 10 points of the actual scores. When only children with actual scores between 80 and 120 were considered, 66% of the predicted scores fell within 10 points of the actual scores.

The regression equation using all four predictors of the CVLT standard score did not reach significance after Bonferroni correction, accounting for only 13% of the variance, with a multiple R of .37, $F(4, 70) = 2.71, p < .037$. However, the stepwise procedure retained socioeconomic status as a predictor, with only a small reduction in the multiple R, and the resulting model was significant, $F(1, 73) = 8.44, p < .005$. The standard error of estimate for the resulting regression equation was 14.57, which was only slightly better than the sample standard deviation for the CVLT of 15.29.

The predicted CVLT standard scores had a much more restricted range (91 to 111) than the actual scores (41 to 139). Across the entire sample, 64% of the predicted scores were within 10 points of the actual scores. When only children with actual scores between 80 and 120 were considered, however, predicted scores fell within 10 points of the actual scores in 75% of the cases.

Validation of Prediction Equations in the TBI Groups

Table 2 provides the final regression equations that were used to predict performance in the TBI

Table 2. Final Regression Equations.

Outcome Measure	Prediction Equation
PIQ	$82.83 + (0.52 \times$ CBC standard score$) - (16.41 \times$ Ethnicity$)$
VMI standard score	$69.59 + (0.35 \times$ WJ-R standard score$) - (12.98 \times$ Ethnicity$)$
CVLT standard score	$100.47 + (5.64 \times$ SES$)$

Note. PIQ = Prorated Performance IQ; VMI − Developmental Test of Visual-Motor Integration; CVLT = California Verbal Learning Test; CBC = parent rating of school performance, Child Behavior Checklist; SES = Composite measure of socioeconomic status; WJ-R = Word Identification subtest, Woodcock Johnson Test of Achievement-Revised; Ethnicity = dummy variable coded 0 (White) or 1 (non-White).

Table 3. Actual, Predicted, and Discrepancy Scores for Each Outcome by Group.

Group	n	Type of Score					
		Actual		Predicted		Discrepancy	
		M	(SD)	M	(SD)	M	(SD)
PIQ							
OI	30	101.43	(15.41)	101.43	(10.09)	0.00	(11.65)
Moderate TBI	49	98.86	(18.43)	101.74	(9.27)	−2.88	(15.95)
Severe TBI	41	90.39	(18.88)	102.34	(8.46)	−11.95	(17.26)
VMI standard score							
OI	58	101.67	(14.23)	101.67	(8.49)	0.00	(11.42)
Moderate TBI	52	100.54	(17.36)	101.01	(9.24)	−0.47	(15.82)
Severe TBI	45	91.58	(16.73)	100.15	(8.75)	−7.83	(15.15)
CVLT standard score							
OI	75	100.34	(15.29)	100.34	(4.92)	0.00	(14.47)
Moderate TBI	55	99.12	(14.56)	100.99	(4.73)	−1.87	(13.83)
Severe TBI	45	89.75	(18.88)	100.02	(5.00)	−10.27	(17.87)

Note. OI = Orthopedic injury; TBI = Traumatic brain injury; PIQ = Prorated Performance IQ; VMI = Developmental Test of Visual-Motor Integration; CVLT = California Verbal Learning Test.

groups. The correlations between predicted and actual scores in the combined TBI groups were smaller than those in the OI group, but significant: .44 for PIQ; .41 for the VMI; and .31 for the CVLT (all $ps < .001$). Thus, parent ratings, demographic variables, and current measures of academic skills also predict individual differences in neuropsychological functioning among children with TBI, but with less precision than for non-injured children.

Actual, predicted, and discrepancy scores, representing the difference between actual and predicted scores for each of the neuropsychological measures, are displayed for all three groups in Table 3. Notably, the predicted mean scores for the two TBI groups are quite comparable to the actual mean scores obtained by the OI group, suggesting

that the neuropsychological functioning of the TBI and OI groups was similar pre-morbidly.

Discrepancy scores were subjected to ANOVAs, with group as the independent variable. The overall ANOVA for the PIQ discrepancy score was significant, $F(2, 117) = 6.12$, $p < .005$. Planned contrasts revealed a marginally significant difference between the TBI groups and the OI group, $F(1, 117) = 5.12$, $p < .026$, and a significant difference between the severe and moderate TBI groups, $F(1, 117) = 7.65$, $p < .01$. As shown in Table 2, the mean discrepancy was largest in the severe TBI group, which performed more poorly than predicted.

The ANOVA for the VMI discrepancy score also was significant, $F(2, 151) = 4.59$, $p < .012$.

The planned contrast between the TBI groups and the OI group did not reach the Bonferonni-corrected level of significance, $F(1, 151) = 3.13$, $p < .08$, but the contrast between the severe and moderate TBI groups was significant, $F(1, 151) = 6.48$, $p < .012$. The TBI groups tended to show larger discrepancies than the OI group, and the severe TBI group showed a larger discrepancy than the moderate TBI group, again performing more poorly than expected.

The ANOVA for the CVLT discrepancy score also was significant, $F(2, 172) = 6.71$, $p < .005$. Planned contrasts revealed significant differences between the TBI groups and the OI group, $F(1, 172) = 6.77$, $p < .01$, as well as between the severe and moderate TBI group, $F(1, 172) = 7.53$, $p < .01$. Once again, children with TBI performed more poorly than expected, especially those with severe injuries.

The statistically significant group differences were also reflected in the likelihood that children would display discrepancies of 10 points or more favoring their predicted scores over their actual scores. The Figure displays the proportion of children in each group who demonstrated discrepancies of this magnitude on each neuropsychological measure. Group differences were significant for all three measures: PIQ, $\chi^2(2, N = 120) = 8.97$, $p < .011$; VMI, $\chi^2(2, N = 154) = 8.47$, $p < .014$, and CVLT, $\chi^2(2, N = 175) = 8.32$, $p < .016$. In all cases, the severe TBI group showed the highest rate of discrepancy.

Finally, as Table 4 shows, all but one of the correlations between the discrepancy scores for each of the neuropsychological variables and the two

Table 4. Correlations Between Severity of Injury and Discrepancy Scores for Combined TBI Groups.

Injury severity measure	Outcome measure		
	PIQ	VMI	CVLT
Glasgow Coma Scale score	.25	.28*	.34*
Duration of impaired consciousness	−.43*	−.33*	−.43*

Note. Discrepancy scores = Actual − predicted score; PIQ = Prorated Performance IQ; VMI = Developmental Test of Visual-Motor Integration; CVLT = California Verbal Learning Test.
*$p < .008$.

measures of injury severity were significant for the combined TBI groups. Thus, the extent to which the actual scores of children with TBI were lower than their predicted scores was directly related to the severity of their injuries.

DISCUSSION

The results indicate that parent ratings of premorbid school performance, maternal ethnicity, family socioeconomic status, and children's word recognition skills can be combined successfully to predict neuropsychological functioning, capturing between 13% and 45% of the variance in neuropsychological test scores among a sample of children with OI. Moreover, when the resulting prediction equations are used to predict premorbid functioning in children with TBI, the predicted performance of the TBI group is commensurate with the actual performance of the OI group, the TBI group displays significantly larger discrepancies between actual and predicted performance than the OI group, and the magnitude of the discrepancies is related to injury severity.

The results suggest that premorbid neuropsychological functioning can be predicted using retrospective ratings, demographic variables, and measures of concurrent skills. Interestingly, though, the relationship between predictors and outcomes varied across neuropsychological domains. That is, the stepwise regression analyses in the OI group selected different variables as predictors for each of the neuropsychological tests: parent ratings of premorbid school performance and maternal ethnicity for PIQ; maternal ethnicity and children's word reading skills for the VMI; and socioeconomic status for the CVLT. As far as we can determine, ours is the only study in which each of the three approaches outlined in the introduction – retrospective ratings, demographic variables, and concurrent skills – have been applied to the prediction of different aspects of neuropsychological functioning in children. The results indicate that each of the methods may prove useful, although the relative utility of the three methods may depend on the particular outcome under consideration.

The use of three different regression equations may seem to introduce an undesirable degree of

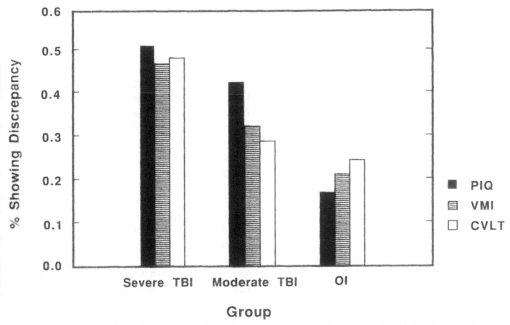

Fig. 1. Percentage of children in each group displaying predicted scores 10 or more points higher than actual scores for each outcome measure.

complexity into the prediction of premorbid functioning. However, we would have been very surprised if the regression equations for the three dependent variables had been the same, because there was no a priori reason to expect the relationships between predictors and outcomes would hold constant across outcomes. We suspect that clinical neuropsychologists would welcome the opportunity to reliably predict premorbid neuropsychological functioning, even if they needed to use separate regression equations for different tests.

On the other hand, when one considers the multicollinearity of the predictors, the variation in predictive relationships is not as great as it might appear. In the OI group, an examination of the correlation matrices involving predictors and outcomes indicated that the predictors were moderately intercorrelated and demonstrated similar relationships to the three outcomes. Moreover, in the regression equations containing all four predictors, the regression coefficients were lower and their standard errors were considerably higher than when the individual predictors were considered in isolation. Thus, the different results obtained in the stepwise

regression analyses may reflect small variations in the correlations among predictors and outcomes, and hence are not likely to be stable from one sample to another. The results therefore provide support for the use of all three methods when predicting premorbid test performance, and do not clearly indicate that one method is more effective than the other.

When the three methods are combined, however, they do not demonstrate the same predictive accuracy across outcomes. The four predictors accounted for the most variance when PIQ was the outcome of interest. They accounted for somewhat less variance in the VMI, and for even less in the CVLT. This is one of the first times that research concerned with the prediction of premorbid functioning has focused on outcomes other than IQ (Klesges & Tröster, 1987). Thus, the reason for the inconsistency in prediction is unclear. However, the results suggest that measures of general cognitive abilities (e.g., PIQ) are more closely related to demographic variables, school performance, and academic skills than are measures of more specific neuropsychological domains (e.g., CVLT). Improved prediction of premorbid neuropsychological abilities is likely to require a search for predictors that are more closely linked to the specific skills in question (e.g., parent ratings of learning and memory as a predictor of CVLT performance).

There is considerable room for improvement in prediction even for measures of general cognitive abilities. Indeed, more than 50% of the variance in PIQ was not accounted for by the four predictors. Thus, although prediction was statistically significant for all three outcomes, the resulting regression equations were not especially accurate for individual children, especially those with the lowest and highest scores. Less than two thirds of the OI group had a predicted score within 10 points of their actual score, regardless of the outcome under consideration. When the analysis was restricted to OI children whose actual scores fell between the 10th and 90th centiles, more than 20% of the group continued to demonstrate large discrepancies between observed and expected scores across all three outcomes. Thus, consistent with prior research in adults (Silverstein, 1987), the regression equations presented here are not sufficiently accurate to provide precise estimates for individual children, but instead can only be used to forecast rather liberal ranges within which a child's score might be expected to fall.

Because a child's predicted score must necessarily be expressed as a range, the use of regression equations such as those presented here in clinical practice must be tempered with considerable caution. Children with severe TBI were two to three times more likely than children in the OI group to demonstrate at least a 10-point deficit in their actual performance when it was compared to their predicted score. However, between 16% and 24% of the children in the OI group also displayed deficits of this magnitude, compared to approximately 50% of the severe TBI group. Thus, a moderate discrepancy between actual and predicted scores is not sufficiently sensitive or specific to guarantee the presence of residual neuropsychological deficits following TBI in individual children. On the other hand, a very large discrepancy is likely to reflect a true deficit in neuropsychological functioning, because it will be relatively uncommon in children without TBI. For instance, 20% to 30% of the severe TBI group showed a 20-point deficit in their actual performance when it was

compared to their predicted score, compared to only 2% to 6% of the OI group. In other words, children with TBI are 5 to 10 times more likely to display such a large discrepancy. Unfortunately, such large discrepancies are likely to occur precisely in cases where the presence of residual deficits is less likely to be in question (i.e., in cases of severe rather than mild TBI).

For clinicians, therefore, the current results are a mixed bag. Although clinicians can use multiple sources of information (i.e., parent ratings, family demographics, concurrent word reading skills) to predict premorbid functioning, the resulting estimates are not likely to be as accurate as would be desirable for individual children. Clinicians can reliably identify children who display very large deficits in their actual performance as compared to their predicted performance, and who consequently are likely to have suffered a true decline in their neuropsychological functioning following a TBI. However, the absence of a large discrepancy between actual and predicted performances cannot be taken as proof that a child's neuropsychological functioning has not deteriorated. Thus, prediction equations such as those presented here are likely to prove applicable primarily to children with severe TBI, for whom the equations can be used to establish an initial estimate of deficit; in contrast, they are not likely to be of much use in cases involving mild TBI.

For researchers, the results are more encouraging. The findings suggest that there are several variables, all relatively easy to measure, that can be used to predict the premorbid level of performance on neuropsychological tests in groups of children with TBI. Individual prediction is not as important in research as opposed to clinical contexts. Instead, researchers need to demonstrate that children with TBI were similar as a group to their non-injured peers premorbidly, and to take into account the variables that predict premorbid neuropsychological functioning in data analyses comparing the two groups. By doing so, the researcher can better isolate the effects of TBI from other, pre-injury influences on outcome. Our findings indicate that the OI and TBI groups in the current research were similar premorbidly, and also suggest that we should covary retrospective parent ratings, demographic variables, and measures of word reading skills in comparative analyses of other neuropsychological outcomes. Similar procedures could be followed by other researchers concerned with the neurobehavioral outcomes of pediatric TBI.

The results presented here must be considered cautiously because of several methodological shortcomings of the research. Perhaps most critically, the sample sizes for the regression analyses in the OI group varied according to which outcome measure was under consideration. Although the smaller samples were representative of the larger OI group, less than 50% of the original sample was available for the regression analysis predicting PIQ, limiting the power of the analysis significantly. The power for the two other regression analyses was acceptable, but the results may nonetheless be unstable because the sample sizes were not large. Hence, all of the analyses are in need of replication using larger samples.

One opportunity for replication would be to draw on normative data collected during the standardization of tests widely used in clinical practice. For example, both the WISC-III and the Wechsler Individual Achievement Test were administered to a representative sample of children as part of their standardization (Psychological Corporation, 1992; Wechsler, 1991). Because demographic information also was collected at the same time, the normative data on the two tests provide an excellent opportunity for future studies of the prediction of premorbid functioning. The construction of tables showing the proportion of normal children showing discrepancies of various magnitudes between actual and predicted IQ scores would be especially beneficial for clinical neuropsychologists working with children with TBI and other forms of acquired brain impairment.

Future research also will be needed to determine if parent ratings of premorbid school performance and concurrent measures of word recognition skills remain valid predictors among children with TBI after longer post-injury intervals. In the current study, parent ratings of premorbid school performance were obtained very soon after children sustained their injuries, and the testing of children's word recognition skills followed soon thereafter. Retrospective parent ratings might be less reliable if they were elicited after a longer post-injury interval,

and hence be less accurate predictors of premorbid functioning. Similarly, more severe TBI might interfere with academic progress and thereby result in lower word recognition skills over time, rendering concurrent measures of reading less accurate predictors as well. In future work, we plan to use data from the prospective study that serves as the basis for the current research to address these issues. In the meantime, the current results suggest that premorbid neuropsychological functioning can be predicted in children with TBI, but with less precision than would be desirable in clinical contexts.

REFERENCES

Achenbach, T.M. (1991). *Manual for the Child Behavior Checklist/4–18 and 1991 profile.* Burlington, VT: Department of Psychiatry, University of Vermont.
Barona, A., Reynolds, C.R., & Chastain, R. (1984). A demographically based index of premorbid intelligence for the WAIS-R. *Journal of Consulting and Clinical Psychology, 52,* 885–887.
Beery, K.E. (1989) *Revised Administration, Scoring, and Teaching Manual for the Developmental Test of Visual-Motor Integration.* Cleveland, OH: Modern Curriculum Press.
Blair, J.R., & Spreen, O. (1989). Predicting premorbid IQ: A revision of the National Adult Reading Test. *The Clinical Neuropsychologist, 3,* 129–136.
Bryan, J., Weins, A., & Crosson, J. (1992). Estimating WAIS-R IQ from the National Adult Reading Test-Revised among normal adults. *Journal of Clinical and Experimental Neuropsychology, 14,* 64.
Christensen, H., Hadzi-Pavlovic, D., & Jacomb, P. (1991). The psychometric differentiation of dementia from normal aging: A meta-analysis. *Psychological Assessment, 3,* 147–155.
Delis, D.C., Kramer, J.H., Kaplan, E., & Ober, B.A. (1994). *Manual for The California Verbal Learning Test for Children.* New York: Psychological Corporation.
Ewing-Cobbs, L., Levin, H.S., Fletcher, J.M., Miner, M.E., & Eisenberg, H.M. (1990). The Children's Orientation and Amnesia Test: Relationship to severity of acute head injury and to recovery of memory. *Neurosurgery, 27,* 683–691.
Finkelstein, N.W., & Ramey, C.T. (1980). Information from birth certificates as a risk index for educational handicap. *American Journal of Mental Deficiency, 84,* 546–552.
Fletcher, J.M., Ewing-Cobbs, L., Miner, M., Levin, H., & Eisenberg, H. (1990). Behavioral changes after

closed-head injury in children. *Journal of Consulting and Clinical Psychology, 58,* 93–98.

Fletcher, J.M., & Levin, H.S. (1988). Neuro-behavioral effects of brain injury in children, In D.K. Routh (Ed.), *Handbook of pediatric psychology* (pp. 258–295). New York: Guilford Press.

Grober, E., & Sliwinski, M. (1991). Development and validation of a model for estimating premorbid verbal intelligence in the elderly. *Journal of Clinical and Experimental Neuropsychology, 13,* 933–949.

Hart, S., Smith, C.M., & Swash, M. (1986). Assessing intellectual deterioration. *British Journal of Clinical Psychology, 25,* 119–124.

Jennett, B., & Bond, M. (1975). Assessment of outcome after severe brain damage. *Lancet, 1,* 480–487.

Karekan, D.A., Gur, R.C., & Saykin, A.J. (1995). Reading on the Wide Range Achievement Test-Revised and parental education as predictors of IQ: Comparison with the Barona formula. *Archives of Clinical Neuropsychology, 10,* 147–157.

Karzmark, P., Heaton, R.K., Grant, I., & Matthews, C.G. (1985). Use of demographic variables to predict Full Scale IQ: A replication and extension. *Journal of Clinical and Experimental Neuropsychology, 7,* 412–420.

Klesges, R.C., & Sanchez, V.C. (1980). Cross-validation of an index of premorbid intellectual functioning in children. *Journal of Consulting and Clinical Psychology, 49,* 141.

Klesges, R.C., & Tröster, R.C. (1987). A review of premorbid indices of intellectual and neuropsychological functioning: What have we learned in the past five years? *The International Journal of Clinical Neuropsychology, 9,* 1–11.

Krull, K.R., Scott, J.G., & Sherer, M. (1995). Estimation of premorbid intelligence from combined performance and demographic variables. *The Clinical Neuropsychologist, 9,* 83–88.

Lezak, M.D. (1995). *Neuropsychological assessment* (3rd ed.). New York: Oxford University Press.

Levin, H.S., & Eisenberg, H.M. (1979). Neuropsychological outcome of closed-head injury in children and adolescents. *Journal of Pediatric Psychology, 4,* 389–402.

Levin, H.S., Ewing-Cobbs, L., & Eisenberg, H.M. (1995). Neurobehavioral outcome of pediatric closed head injury. In S.H. Broman & M.E. Michel (Eds.), *Traumatic head injury in children* (pp. 70–94). New York: Oxford University Press.

Mayer, T., Matlack, M., Johnson, D., & Walker, M. (1980). The Modified Injury Severity Scale in pediatric multiple trauma patients. *Journal of Pediatric Surgery, 15,* 719–726.

Psychological Corporation. (1992). *Wechsler Individual Achievement Test.* San Antonio, TX: Psychological Corporation.

Ramey, C.T., Stedman, D.J., Borders-Patterson, A., & Mengel, W. (1978). Predicting school failure from information available at birth. *American Journal of Mental Deficiency, 82,* 525–534.

Reynolds, C.R., & Gutkin, T.B. (1979). Predicting the premorbid intellectual status of children using demographic data. *Clinical Neuropsychology, 1,* 36–38.

Richardson, F. (1963). Some effects of severe head injury: A follow-up study of children and adolescents after protracted coma. *Developmental Medicine and Child Neurology, 5,* 471–482.

Sattler, J.M. (1992). *Assessment of children* (3rd ed.). San Diego: Jerome M. Sattler.

Silverstein, A. (1987). Accuracy of estimates of premorbid intelligence based on demographic variables. *Journal of Clinical Psychology, 43,* 493–495.

Stebbins, G.T., Gilley, D.W., Wilson, R.S., Bernard, B.A., & Fox, J.H. (1990). Effects of language disturbances on premorbid estimates of IQ in mild dementia. *The Clinical Neuropsychologist, 4,* 64–68.

Stebbins, G.T., Wilson, R.S., Gilley, D.W., Bernard, B.A., & Fox, J.H. (1990). Use of the National Adult Reading Test to estimate premorbid IQ in dementia. *The Clinical Neuropsychologist, 4,* 18–24.

Stevens, G., & Featherman, D.L. (1981). A revised socioeconomic index of occupational status. *Social Science Research, 10,* 364–395.

Taylor, H.G., Drotar, D., Wade, S., Yeates, K.O., Stancin, T., & Klein, S. (1995). Recovery from traumatic brain injury in children: The importance of the family. In S. Broman & M. Michel (Eds.), *Traumatic head injury in children* (pp. 188–218). New York: Oxford.

Thompson, N.M., Francis, D.J., Stuebing, K.K., Fletcher, J.M., Ewing-Cobbs, L., Miner, M.E., Levin, H.S., & Eisenberg, H. (1994). Motor, visual-spatial, and somatosensory skills after closed-head injury in children and adolescents: A study of change. *Neuropsychology, 8,* 333–342.

Wechsler, D. (1991). *Manual for the Wechsler Intelligence Scale for Children – Third Edition.* New York: Psychological Corporation.

Willshire, D., Kinsella, G., & Prior, M. (1991). Estimating WAIS-R IQ from the National Adult Reading Test: A cross-validation. *Journal of Clinical and Experimental Neuropsychology, 13,* 204–216.

Woodcock, R.W. & Mather, N. (1989). *Woodcock-Johnson Tests of Achievement – Revised. Standard and supplemental batteries.* Allen, TX: DLM Teaching Resources.

Yeates, K.O., Blumenstein, E., Patterson, C.M., & Delis, D.C. (1995). Verbal learning and memory following pediatric closed-head injury. *Journal of the International Neuropsychological Society, 1,* 78–87.

The Clinical Neuropsychologist
1993, Vol. 7, No. 4, pp. 454–459

VIII-G

COMPUTERIZING THE CLINICIAN

A Computer Program for Performing Meta-Analyses When the Outcome Variable is Dichotomous: Relevance to Neuropsychology and Biomedical Research

Domenic V. Cicchetti[1], Donald Showalter[1], and Bruce E. Wexler
[1]West Haven VA Medical Center, and [1,2]Yale University

ABSTRACT

The research clinical neuropsychologist is increasingly faced with the critical challenge of deciding whether the corpus of data in a given area of inquiry does or does not produce consistent or replicable findings. For our focus of interest, the most general case involves any clinical problem that can be cast into a 2 × 2 or fourfold table. One specific class of relevant queries would address those studies focusing on the efficacy of two forms of treatment (A or B) on the outcome (success, failure) of a specific type of brain injury. A second class would involve the effects of two treatments on the outcome (positive, negative) of specific types of neuropsychological disorders. This report describes a computer program that performs appropriate meta-analyses by providing statistics of choice that vary according to both the number of studies comprising the meta-analytic research endeavor and to the sample sizes within each study of focus.

Although the science of neuropsychology is relatively young, there are many areas of focus that contain a number of studies that address the same specific research question. Some examples include the relative success or failure in the treatment of frank neuropsychological disorders with distinct neuropsychologic features, such as traumatic brain injury, stroke, or any of a number of neuropsychological disorders with arguably less well-defined neurologic features, such as schizophrenia, alcoholism, or environmentally induced clinical depression.s As the number of well-designed neuropsychological studies addressing the same question continue to be published, it becomes possible to compare the results of the various studies with more methodologic rigor than might have been possible in the prototypic review paper.

One comprehensive tool that renders such rigor possible is the more general technique of meta-analysis. Although a number of variants of this technique are possible when the outcome variable is continuous or dimensional (e.g., Hedges & Olkin, 1985), the computer program we described herein has specific application to the general class of clinical problems whose output can be cast into a 2 × 2 or fourfold contingency table. For example, Fleiss (1981) refers to an application of meta-analysis in which the question of interest was whether data based on three separate studies showed a significant difference in the proportion of patients diagnosed as schizophrenic in the U.S. (New York) and the U.K. (London).

Whether the field of application is biomedical, neuropsychological, or otherwise, the same two

A listing of the C source code, complete documentation, and sample applications can be obtained from Dr. Domenic V. Cicchetti, Senior Research Psychologist and Biostatistician, VA Medical Center and Yale University, 950 Campbell Avenue, West Haven, CT 06516, USA.
Please address reprint requests to: Domenic V. Cicchetti, Ph.D., Senior Research Psychologist and Biostatistician, West Haven VA Medical Center & Yale University, 950 Campbell Avenue, West Haven, Connecticut 06516, USA.
Accepted for publication: June 10, 1993.

fundamental questions need to be addressed. The first, and most basic, is whether the various research investigations are sufficiently alike in design, treatments administered, and criteria for success, so that each of the individual studies can be viewed as a replicate investigation of the same clinical phenomenon.

Note: If this fundamental criterion is not met, any meta-analysis that is performed will be an exercize in futility.

If this criterion is met, one then needs to choose an appropriate meta-analytic approach to the data. Fleiss (1981) discusses three such methods. Whichever is appropriate, the general logic or rationale underlying their usage remains the same. Appropriate variations of the standard chi-squared test result are decomposed into two additive components, namely, the chi-squared test of *homogeneity* (with $g - 1$ degrees of freedom) and the test of *association* (with 1 degree of freedom). When all of the studies of interest go in the *same* direction (say, all indicate that the same treatment is the more efficacious one), then the value of the chi-squared test of *homogeneity* will, depending on sample size, tend toward nonsignificance while the chi-squared test of *association* will point in the direction of statistical significance. In short, the test of homogeneity informs whether it makes clinical sense to perform the test of *association* at all. Specifically, if the results are positive for a given therapy in some studies but prove negative in others, it makes no sense to combine them together. What would make sense, in this situation, would be to undertake a more fine-grained analysis of each of the individual studies toward the goal of understanding better what factors may have played a major role in producing the conflicting evidence.

An Application
In a recently published study, Wexler and Cicchetti (1992) investigated the corpus of literature focusing upon the relative efficacy of individual psychotherapy, pharmacotherapy, or the two in combination as treatment modalities for depressed outpatients.

The specific application that follows involves one of several meta-analyses that we performed, namely, for comparing the efficacy of psychotherapy and pharmacotherapy as treatments for outpatient clinical depression. More generally, Wexler and

Cicchetti (1992) showed that, contrary to what has been believed and reported, combined treatment (psychotherapy plus pharmacotherapy) offers no advantage over psychotherapy alone and only a modest advantage over pharmacotherapy alone.

Five studies were available that met the basic criterion of similarity in research design, treatment modalities, and criteria to define a successful outcome. Specifically: (1) Each study was a clinical trial in which patients were randomized to either psychotherapy or pharmacotherapy; (2) the psychotherapy treatments utilized (cognitive or interpersonal) are considered to be of comparable efficacy (Richelson, 1989) as are the choices of pharmacologic agents, amitriptyline or imipramine (Elkin et al., 1989); (3) all five studies used the same rating scale (The Beck Depression Inventory (BDI), Beck, 1976); and (4) each used highly similar cutoff scores to define treatment success: One of them used a score of 8 or less (McLean & Hakstian, 1979); one used a cutoff of 9 or below (Blackburn, Bishop, Glen, Whalley, & Christie, 1981); and the remaining three studies used 10 or less (Hersen, Bellack, Himmelhock, & Thase, 1984; Murphy, Simons, Wetzel, & Lustman, 1984; and Rush, Beck, Kovacs, & Hollon, 1977). Scores this low are clinically equivalent for two reasons. First, they reflect very substantial remission of depressive symptomatology. Second, they are well within the range of variability that can be expected in any given test-retest reliability study of the BDI. These convincing data provided the necessary rationale for pursuing further the question of whether the combined evidence favored one type of treatment over the other.

The second question is which of three meta-analytic approaches is most appropriate. As noted by Fleiss (1981), this depends on whether the number of studies and the sample sizes within each individual study are considered small, moderately large, or large.

For the number of studies or groups (g), we used 10 or fewer to define small and for individual study sample sizes (N), we used below 30, 30–39 and 40 or above to define, respectively, small, moderately large, and large N. In our application, the number of studies (groups) is small ($g = 5$), but the number of patients in each group ranged between moderately large ($N = 33$) and very large ($N = 135$). Of the three meta-analytic techniques of choice, Fleiss (1981) would recommend the chi-squared method based upon the logarithms of the odds ratios (Gart, 1962, 1970, 1971; Naylor, 1967, Sheehe, 1966).

Note: For other combinations of group and individual study sample sizes, the mathematically very similar methods of either Mantel and Haenszel (1959) or one reported by Cornfield (1956) and extended by Gart (1970), would be appropriate.

Our first question was whether the results favored consistently one type of treatment over the other. For each of the five investigations, treatment success favored psychotherapy over pharmacotherapy. For individual studies, the percentages of treatment success favoring psychotherapy (presented first) were: 83% to 29% (Rush et al., 1977); 73% to 55% (Blackburn et al., 1981); 65% to 56% (Murphy et al., 1984); 55% to 43% (Hersen et al., 1984); and 37% to 24.5% (McLean & Hakstian, 1979).

Consistent with each individual study favoring psychotherapy over pharmacotherapy, the log of the odds ratio chi-squared value, with 4 df (the test of *homogeneity* of results across studies) was only 4.72 (p = NS; with a value of 9.49 required for statistical significance at the .05 level). This result indicates that, since there is a consistency of results across studies (a significant chi-squared test of *homogeneity* would indicate that this was *not* the case), it now makes clinical sense to apply the chi-squared test of *association* to determine whether there is a statistically significant difference between the two treatments, favoring psychotherapy, when the *combined* evidence over the five clinical trials is considered. Again, consistent with the results deriving from each individual study, the chi-squared test of *association* (with 1 df) produced a value of 8.38, which is significant at a probability level of .006.

Thus, we conclude that the available evidence, over the five clinical trials that have compared the two treatments, indicates that psychotherapy is more efficacious for treating outpatient clinical depression than is pharmacotherapy. (For more specific details, the interested reader is referred, once again, to Wexler & Cicchetti, 1992).

Program Features

Input to this computer program is provided by the user and consists of responses to DOS prompts for the following: the number of study groups, in the

format of fourfold tables; cell counts of each table, followed by eight character labels, first for each of the two columns, then for each of the two rows. Once the tables are entered, they are printed on the screen along with their assigned labels and cell frequencies. At this time, the user is given the opportunity to correct any error that may have occurred in data entry. Once the errors have been corrected, the program displays output data, first in terms of each separate study and then for the meta-analyses across the g-(number) of combined studies.

Output includes the following statistics for any *single* fourfold table (individual g study): chi-squared (both uncorrected and using Yates' (1934) correction for continuity); the Phi coefficient (standard Pearson correlation coefficient applied to fourfold tables); Phi/Phi max, to adjust for the usual case, in which a maximum Phi value of +1 is not possible because of unequal marginal frequencies; the odds ratio (using the recommended addition of .5 to each inputed value, i.e., see Fleiss, 1981 for rationale); and a series of statistics relevant to studies in which test outcome (say the results of a screening test [positive or negative]) are compared to a criterion, used as a true outcome (positive/negative). These statistics include: overall accuracy (summed over positive and negative cases); sensitivity; specificity; predicted positive accuracy; predicted negative accuracy; false positive error (based upon the true or criterion outcome); false positive error (based upon the test result); false negative error (based upon the criterion outcome); and the false negative error (based upon the test result).

The next and final set of outputs is preceded by a statement that the analysis of combined tables will be performed, although the (Log Odds ratio, Cornfield/Gart; or Mantel-Haenszel Test) is most appropriate for these data. For each one of the three meta-analyses, both the chi-squared test of *homogeneity* and the chi-squared test of *association* are performed, as well as the level of probability pertaining to each.

Since the *standard* chi-squared test is inappropriate/invalid for performing meta-analyses due to its relative insensitivity to study group results which go in different directions (see again Fleiss, 1981), the program does not perform this incorrect analysis.

REFERENCES

Beck, A.T. (1976). *Cognitive therapy and the emotional disorders.* New York: International Universities Press.

Blackburn, I.M., Bishop, S., Glen, A.I.M., Whalley, L.J., & Christie, J.E. (1991). The efficacy of cognitive therapy in depression: A treatment trial using cognitive therapy and pharmacotherapy, each alone and in combination. *British Journal of Psychiatry, 139,* 181–189.

Cornfield, J. (1956). A statistical problem arising from retrospective studies. In J. Neyman (Ed.), *Proceedings of the third Berkeley symposium on mathematical statistics and probability,* Vol. 4, (pp. 135–148). Berkeley: University of California Press.

Elkin, I., Shea, M.T., Watkins, J.T., Imber, S., Sotsky, S.M., Collins, J., Glass, D., Pilkonis, P., Leber, W., Docherty, J., Fiester, S., & Parloff, M. (1989). National Institute of Mental Health treatment of depression collaborative research program. *Archives of General Psychiatry, 46,* 971–982.

Fleiss, J.L. (1981). *Statistical methods for rates and proportions* (2nd ed.). New York: Wiley.

Gart, J.J. (1962). On the combination of relative risks. *Biometrics, 18,* 601–610.

Gart, J.J. (1970). Point and interval estimation of the common odds ratio in the combination of 2×2 tables with fixed marginals. *Biometrika, 57,* 471–475.

Gart, J.J. (1971). The comparison of proportions: A review of significance tests, confidence intervals and adjustments for stratification. *Reviews of the International Statistical Institute, 39,* 16–37.

Hedges, L.V., & Olkin, I. (1985). *Statistical methods for meta-analysis.* New York: Academic Press.

Hersen, M., Bellack, A.S., Himmelhock, J.M., & Thase, M.E. (1984). Effects of social skill training, amitriptyline, and psychotherapy in unipolar depressed women. *Behavior Therapy, 15,* 21–40.

Mantel, N., & Haenszel, W. (1959). Statistical aspects of the analysis of data from retrospective studies of disease. *Journal of the National Cancer Institute, 22,* 719–748.

McLean, P.D., & Hakstian, A.R. (1979). Clinical depression: Comparitive efficacy of outpatient treatments. *Journal of Consulting and Clinical Psychology, 47,* 818–836.

Murphy, G.E., Simons, A.D., Wetzel, R.D., & Lustman, P.J. (1984). Cognitive therapy and pharmacotherapy: Singly and together in the treatment of depression. *Archives of General Psychiatry, 41,* 33–41.

Naylor, A.F. (1967). Small sample considerations in combining 2×2 tables. *Biometrics, 23,* 349–356.

Richelson, E. (1989). Antidepressants: Pharmacology and clinical use. In American Psychiatric Association, *Treatments of psychiatric disorders: A task force report of the American Psychiatric Association* (pp. 1773–1786). Washington, D.C.: American Psychiatric Association.

Rusk, A.J., Beck, A.T., Kovacs, M., & Hollon, S.D. (1977). Comparitive efficacy of cognitive therapy and pharmacotherapy in the treatment of depressed outpatients. *Cognitive Therapy and Research, 1,* 17–37.

Sheehe, P.R. (1966). Combination of log relative risk in retrospective studies of disease. *American Journal of Public Health, 56,* 1745–1750.

Wexler, B.E., & Cicchetti, D.V. (1992). The outpatient treatment of depression: Implications of outcome research for clinical practice. *Journal of Nervous and Mental Disease, 180,* 277–286.

Yates, F. (1934). Contingency tables involving small numbers and the chi-squared test. *Journal of the Royal Statistical Society (Supplement), 1,* 217–235.

The Clinical Neuropsychologist
1999, Vol. 13, No. 4, pp. 495–508

Normative Clinical Relationship Between Orientation and Memory: Age as an Important Moderator Variable*

Jerry J. Sweet[1], Yana Suchy[2], Brian Leahy[3], Carolyn Abramowitz[4], and Cindy J. Nowinski[5]

[1]Evanston Hospital/Northwestern University Medical School, [2]Evanston Hospital, [3]Illinois Institute of Technology, [4]Finch University of Health Sciences/Chicago Medical School, and [5]Northwestern University Medical School

ABSTRACT

The present study examined the relationship between memory and orientation to time, place, and personal and general information, as moderated by age, education, and simple attentional ability. A heterogeneous sample of 312 clinical referrals was divided into four groups, according to delayed memory functioning. Patients with globally good, globally poor, poor visual, and poor auditory memory were at differential risk of being disoriented, with the globally poor memory patients having the greatest risk. Overall, poorly oriented patients were older and less educated, with worse recall of digits backward. Discriminant Function Analysis selected visual and auditory memory and age as predictors of orientation. Normative tables stratified by age and memory performance are presented.

In clinical settings, orientation to time, place, and personal and general information is one of the most frequently assessed functions. Clinical interpretation of disorientation is generally brief, with no links being made to anatomic substrates or underlying basic cognitive abilities (Varney & Shepherd, 1991). Instead, impaired orientation has simply been used as a general indicator of underlying brain dysfunction (Daniel, Crovitz, & Weiner, 1987). Such interpretation is supported by research that has demonstrated that performance on orientation questions separates patients with and without brain dysfunction (Prigatano, 1977), and patients with head injuries and orthopedic controls (Brooks, 1976). Additionally, decreases in orientation abilities have been found to correlate with increased periods of post-traumatic amnesia, as well as with an increased incidence of Alzheimer's Disease (Small, Viitanen, & Backeman, 1997). However, it is important to note that the vast majority of psychiatric and neurologic patients are well-oriented (Wang, Kaplan, & Rogers, 1975), and

that disorientation alone is not a sensitive marker of dementia (Desmond, Tatemichi, Figueroa, Gropen, & Stern, 1994).

Given the frequency with which orientation is assessed, research on the incidence, mechanisms, and neuropathology of disorientation has occupied a surprisingly negligible position in the literature. Even though it has been suggested that orientation *cannot* be reduced to more basic cognitive functions (Lipowski, 1980), several underlying processes have been implicated. First, it has been proposed that, in disoriented individuals, the ability to store new information has been disrupted, resulting in a failure to continuously update knowledge regarding temporal and environmental circumstances (Benson, Gardner, & Meadows, 1976; Benton, Van Allen, & Fogel, 1964; High, Levin, & Gray, 1990; Mattis, 1988). However, several findings suggest that this interpretation of orientation is incomplete. Specifically, Varney and Shepherd (1991) examined the relationship between memory and orientation in alcohol abusers and found

---

*Address correspondence to: Jerry J. Sweet, Ph.D., Neuropsychology Service, Evanston Northwestern Healthcare, 2650 Ridge Avenue, Evanston, IL 60201. E-mail: j-sweet@nwu.edu.
Accepted for publication: September 22, 1999.

that, even though virtually all participants who were disoriented also had a significantly impaired delayed recall, intact orientation did not guarantee intact memory functioning. Similarly, Guilmette, Tsoh, and Malcolm (1995) did not find orientation to be helpful in predicting memory performance in three patient groups (CVA, Mixed Neurological Group, and TBI). In fact, over one third of elderly patients with CVA who were fully oriented achieved impaired memory scores, and intact orientation was even less predictive of memory functioning with younger patient groups.

Factor analytic investigations also reveal a dissociation between orientation and both verbal and nonverbal memory tests. Skilbeck and Woods (1980) reviewed five factor-analytic studies of the Wechsler Memory Scale (WMS). In four of five investigations, a three-factor solution provided the best fit, yielding a memory/learning/retention factor, an attention/concentration factor, and an orientation factor. This three-factor solution was also shown to be stable in both normal and combined psychiatric/neurologic populations. Subsequent factor analytic study of the WMS by Larrabee, Kane, and Schuck (1983) concluded a greater number of factors, with orientation and personal information as the fifth factor. Similarly, Ferrario, Seccia, Massaia, Fonte, and Molaschi (1998) found that the Logical Memory subtest of the WMS correlated with all domains of the Mini-Mental State Exam (MMSE: Folstein, Folstein, & McHugh, 1975), except orientation. Studies of the Wechsler Memory Scale-Revised (WMS-R) have generally not included the information/orientation subtest (Bornstein & Chelune, 1988; Elwood, 1991; Leonberger, Nicks, Goldfader, & Munz, 1991; Roth, Conboy, Reeder, & Boll, 1990; Woods, 1993).

In an attempt to account for the inconsistencies in the relationship between memory and orientation, Schnider, von Daniken, and Gutbrod (1996) proposed that disorientation may result, not from a failure to store new information, but rather from a confusion in the temporal ordering of remembered information. Disoriented patients may be unable to consistently distinguish between knowledge acquired minutes ago from that acquired in the more distant past, thus failing to select the currently correct response from memory. This explanation could potentially account for fluctuation in orientation level across short intervals of time.

In addition to examining cognitive correlates of orientation, the contribution of demographic variables has been explored. Most studies have found little decline in orientation over the lifespan (Brotchie, Brennan, & Wyke, 1985; Hopp, Dixon, Grut, & Bacekman, 1997; Ishizaki et al., 1998; Margolis & Scialfa, 1984; Natelson, Haupt, Fleischer, & Grey, 1979), with as many as 92% of normal elderly adults (65–84 years) presenting with perfect or near perfect orientation (Benton, Eslinger, & Damasio, 1981). Normative data from the WMS-R indicate that, even though orientation to time, place, and personal and general information remains relatively stable until the age of 70, the variability in performance increases significantly at that point (Wechsler, 1987). When investigated in neurological populations, age typically has not been found to have a significant relationship to the presence of disorientation (Benton, Van Allen, & Fogel, 1964; Margolis & Scialfa, 1984; Zagar, Arbit, Stuckey, & Wengel, 1984). Exceptions have been reported with clinical patients, such as elderly patients who become more severely disoriented after electroconvulsive therapy, even though not for a longer duration, than younger patients (Daniel, Crovitz, & Weiner, 1987).

The possible influence of education on disorientation has also been investigated. Natelson et al. (1979) found a modest relationship between temporal orientation and education level in a nonpatient population. In particular, less educated participants (i.e., those without a high school diploma) were more prone to mistake the day of the week, the day of the month, and the current month, and their errors tended to be more serious. Similarly, Ishizaki et al. (1998) found that performance on the orientation portion of the MMSE declined with education. However, Benton, Van Allen, and Fogel (1964) failed to find a significant relationship between education and orientation.

The purposes of this study were (1) to examine, in a heterogeneous clinical referral population, the apparently complex and multivariate relationships among memory measures, demographic variables, and orientation to time, place, and general and personal information (hereafter referred to as 'orientation'), and (2) to generate normative tables that characterize these relationships in this population. The utility of such tables would be threefold. First, on a purely theoretical level, they could assist in understanding the cognitive underpinnings of orientation. Second, with respect to clinical utility, such tables may help identify, by divergence of findings, atypical performances that may be due to insufficient effort, or that may indicate acute psychiatric (e.g., psychotic) or acute neurologic (e.g., delirium) processes. Finally, knowledge of the expected associations among orientation and other variables may help determine whether, and under what circumstances, orientation alone may be used as a memory screen, thereby improving the efficiency of assessment and potentially decreasing time demands. It should be noted that the present study was not designed to address information performance in non-clinical, normal populations, as this issue has been addressed sufficiently by normative research conducted with the WMS-R (e.g., Wechsler, 1987).

In order to address these relationships, the widely used Information/Orientation (IO) subtest from the WMS-R was selected as a measure of orientation. Memory was assessed using WMS-R Logical Memory II (LMII) and Visual Reproduction II (VRII) as measures of auditory memory and visual memory, respectively. Delayed recall, as opposed to immediate recall, was selected so as to encompass general memory components (i.e., registration, encoding, retention, and retrieval). Memory for logically organized stories (LMII), as opposed to a list learning task, was used, so as to avoid confounding memory by executive abilities and learning. General ability to attend, register information, and concentrate was assessed using WMS-R Digit Span Forward (DSF) and Digit Span Backward (DSB). Although many clinicians are now transitioning to the newer version of WMS, the present results are expected to generalize theoretically, conceptually, and psychometrically to the newer WMS-III version, as the changes in the presently used portions of the test were not dramatic.

METHOD

Participants

The sample consisted of 312 individuals (162 males and 150 females) referred to the Evanston Hospital Neuropsychology Service for clinical assessment. For inclusion in the sample, participants must have completed standard administrations of the instruments in the study. Individuals with potential for secondary gain issues at the time of the assessment (e.g., patients involved in litigation or disability determination processes) were excluded, as were individuals with fewer than eight years of education, because they do not represent a meaningful segment of clinical referrals and often represent outlying performance values of unknown neuropsychological significance. The resulting sample ranged in age from 17 to 92 ($M = 55.5$, $SD = 17.7$) and had 8 to 23 years of education ($M = 14.7$, $SD = 2.7$).

Diagnoses included cerebral vascular accident ($n = 64$), traumatic brain injury (50), probable Alzheimer's Disease (35), Parkinson's Disease (25), intracranial neoplasm (21), seizure disorder (12), multiple sclerosis (3), and other degenerative dementias (3). Additionally, 52 patients had multiple neurological conditions or had cognitive impairment as a result of less frequent conditions in our referral base, such as encephalitis, lupus erythematosus, and HIV. Another 28 individuals appeared to have neurocognitive disorders based on accepted standards of neurological examination, which were further confirmed by the present testing, but etiology of these conditions was unknown. Of the remaining 19 patients, 14 met DSM criteria for major depression (diagnoses made by a board-certified psychiatrist or psychologist) and 5 apparently neurologically normal individuals had non-psychotic psychological conditions for which more specific diagnoses could not be identified. Probable Alzheimer's diagnoses were based on criteria established by the National Institute of eurological and Communicative Disorders and the Alzheimer's Disease and Related Disorders Association (McKhann et al., 1984). All other neurological diagnoses were either based on independent irrefutable medical evaluations (such as magnetic resonance imaging, computerized tomography, or electroencephalogram, or appropriate medical laboratory measures), or were made by a board-certified medical specialist. Because the goal of the study was to characterize IO performances among patients typically referred for neuropsychological evaluations, patients who were found to have no cognitive deficits but were determined to meet diagnostic criteria for a non-psychotic psychiatric disorder (generally depression or Axis II disorder) were included in the study.

Procedure

All participants in the study completed selected subtests of the WMS-R (Wechsler, 1987) as part of a larger neuropsychological evaluation. Tests were administered and scored by doctoral-level psychologists or graduate-student trainees who had been trained on standardized scoring and administration of these instruments.

Materials

The WMS-R (Wechsler, 1987) is an individually administered comprehensive memory assessment instrument. Memory subtests selected for the present study demand the abilities to recall verbally presented logically organized stories (LMII) and to reproduce visually presented abstract designs (VRII), both after a 30-min delay. Attention and concentration subtests selected for this study require that participants repeat strings of digits forward (DSF) and backward (DSB). The Information and Orientation (IO) subtest, used as a measure of orientation, includes 14 scored items, each scored 0 or 1, and does not contribute to the General Memory Index or other WMS-R subscores. As described in the manual (pp. 3–4), IO items pertain to orientation to person, place (locality and place of testing), and time (date, time of day), and "common information from long-term memory," such as age, birthdate, and mother's name (Wechsler, 1987).

Data Analysis

Because examination of frequency distribution demonstrated that IO data were severely skewed, examination of measures of central tendency and variance would not be appropriate and could lead to spurious findings. In order to address this issue, the scores were dichotomized into "Orienters" and "Non-orienters." Orienters were defined as those whose IO scores were within one standard deviation of the mean according to WMS-R norms (Wechsler, 1987), and non-orienters had IO scores that were more than one standard deviation below the mean. Specifically, for individuals below age 70, Orienters had to have a score of 13 or 14, and for those 70 and above, Orienters had to have a score of 12, 13, or 14.

In order to identify cognitive and demographic variables that are most related to one's ability to be oriented, stepwise discriminant function analyses (DFA) were conducted, using dichotomized IO as the independent variable. The predictor variables were LMII, VRII, DSF, DSB, age, and education. Because most individuals remain well oriented into their seventies and eighties (Benton et al., 1981) despite accompanying normal declines in memory, memory and attention raw scores were converted to age-corrected T scores based on appropriate WMS-R norms (Wechsler, 1987). In this manner, the relationship of orientation to *normal* (i.e., age-appropriate) versus *pathologically abnormal* memory abilities could be examined, as well as the role of age as a moderator variable in this clinically relevant context.

RESULTS

Examination of univariate relationships for the four neurocognitive variables and the two demographic variables revealed that Non-orienters were older than Orienters, had fewer years of education, and performed more poorly than Orienters on all assessed neurocognitive measures, except DSF. Independent t-values, probabilities, means, and standard deviations can be seen in Table 1. Correlation coefficients among independent variables are presented in Table 2.

Stepwise discriminant function analysis (DFA) with minimum partial F-to-enter = 3.84 and maximum partial F-to-remove = 2.71 (default for SPSS version 8.0) yielded a function that correctly classified 74.9% of Orienters and 78.8% of Non-orienters, with an overall 76.9% of participants being classified correctly, Chi-square (3) = 103.03, $p = .000$. Variables that entered into the model included VRII, $F(1,310 = 81.36, p = .000$, LMII, $F(1,309) = 53.61, p = .000$, and Age, $F(1,308) = 40,71, p = .000$. Education and Digit Span did not meet statistical criteria for entry into the discriminant function. Standardized canonical discriminant function coefficients were −.36 for age, .52 for LMII, and .48 for VRII, with a canonical correlation of .53.

In order to enhance conceptual understanding of the joint effect of VRII, LMII, and age on the ability to orient, three-way frequency distributions for the three variables that entered into the model and IO raw scores were generated; these data are presented in Figures 1a and 1b. As can be seen, both VRII and LMII T scores were related to IO raw scores in that participants with extremely impaired IO had extremely impaired memory, and participants with above average memory tended to be well oriented. However, participants with extremely impaired memory exhibited all levels of IO scores, and participants with intermediate memory exhibited both intact and somewhat impaired IO scores. Age relationship is apparent from the graphs, with less oriented participants being older.

In an attempt to further characterize the relationships among memory, age, and IO, four memory groups were created: Globally Good Memory (GGM: VRII and LMII both above $T = 40$), Globally Poor Memory (GPM: VRII and LMII both at or below $T = 40$), Poor Visual Memory (PVM: VRII at or below $T = 40$ and LMII above $T = 40$), and Poor Auditory Memory (PAM: LMII

Table 1. Means, Standard Deviations, and Univariate Results of Demographic and Neurocognitive Variables for
Orienters and Non-orienters.

	Orienters ($n = 227$)		Non-orienters ($n = 85$)		Independent t	Significance (p)
	M	(SD)	M	(SD)		
Age (years)	52.07	(17.30)	64.68	(15.21)	5.92	.000
Education (years)	14.98	(2.62)	14.06	(2.27)	2.76	.006
Digit Span Forward	51.33	(11.88)	50.06	(9.63)	0.51	n.s.
Digit Span Backward	50.56	(11.34)	44.94	(9.16)	4.10	.000
Logical Memory II	46.56	(10.76)	34.87	(9.00)	8.91	.000
Visual Reproduction II	47.07	(11.77)	34.42	(8.69)	9.02	.000

Note. Standard deviations are presented in parentheses. All neurocognitive measures are presented as standardized
T scores.

Table 2. Correlation Matrix for Predictor Variables Used in Discriminant Function Analysis.

	Age	Education	Digit Span Forward	Digit Span Backward	Logical Memory II
Education	0.021				
Digit Span Forward	0.082	0.159*			
Digit Span Backward	−0.149*	0.225*	0.516*		
Logical Memory II	−0.252*	0.169*	0.128	0.338*	
Visual Reproduction II	−0.332*	0.199*	0.155*	0.329*	0.599*

Note. Raw scores for all neurocognitive measures were converted to age-corrected T scores prior to analyses.
    *$p < .01$.

at or below $T = 40$ and LM above $T = 40$). The
distribution of IO raw scores and ages in the four
memory groups are presented in Figure 2, demonstrating the combined influences of both auditory
and visual memory.

As can be seen in Figure 2, the GGM group
was characterized by good orientation in an overwhelming majority of participants, with relatively
few impaired performances. In contrast, a much
greater proportion of the PVM and PAM groups
exhibited somewhat impaired IO performance.
The GPM group results were unique in that a substantial proportion of participants had extremely
impaired IO performance. The risk of significant
disorientation by degree of memory impairment is
evident in the following *risk rates* associated with
membership in each group: GGM (14 not ori-
ented/143 oriented) = .097; PVM (11/50) = .220;
PAM (7/39 = .179; GPM (53/81) = .654. The
odds ratio, which can also be referred to as a *relative risk ratio* (Feinstein, 1985), associated with
being disoriented when memory is impaired, can
be computed using orientation status (abnormal

orientation vs. normal) and memory status (using
GPM + PVM + PAM as abnormal memory vs.
GGM as normal), as follows:

$$\frac{71 \text{ (disoriented and memory impaired)} \times 129 \text{ (oriented and intact memory)}}{14 \text{ (disoriented and memory intact)} \times 98 \text{ (oriented and memory impaired)}}$$

$$\text{or } 9{,}158 \div 1{,}372 = 6.68$$

This result demonstrates that individuals with
abnormal memory are 6.68 times more likely to
be disoriented than those with normal memory.

Finally, in order to allow clinicians to identify
expected performances in their patient populations,
normative data based on the present heterogeneous clinical sample are presented in Tables 3a–d.
These tables present typical IO raw scores associated with VRII and LMII performance, both
for the entire sample and for three age groups.
Because IO data were severely skewed, ranges
are presented along with means and standard
deviations. Clinicians are cautioned to consider

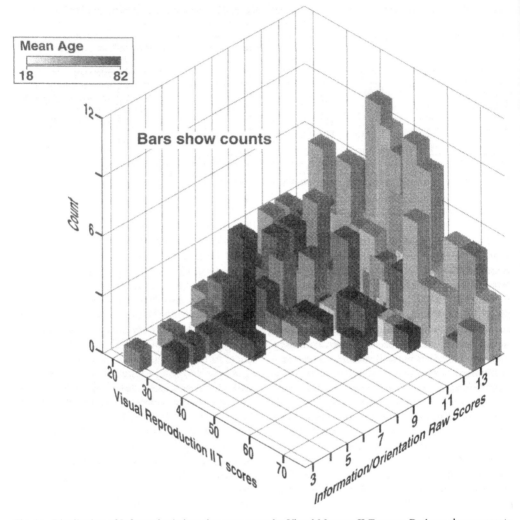

Mean Age

18   82

Fig. 1a. Distribution of Information/orientation raw scores by Visual Memory II *T* scores. Darker color represents higher age.

the means only in the context of the accompanying ranges so as to avoid arriving at misleading conclusions.

DISCUSSION

Present results in a diverse patient sample indicate that poorly oriented patients were significantly older and less educated. However, the contribution of these two demographic factors to orientation status was not comparable. Statistical predictors

of orientation status were delayed visual memory, delayed auditory memory, and age. More specifically, relationships among delayed visual and auditory memory and orientation status appeared to be moderated by age. In all memory groups, poorer orientation was associated with older age. Neither attentional ability, at least as measured by Digit Span, nor education contributed to orientation status independent of age and delayed memory measures, even though both attention and education were significantly different between Orienters and Non-orienters.

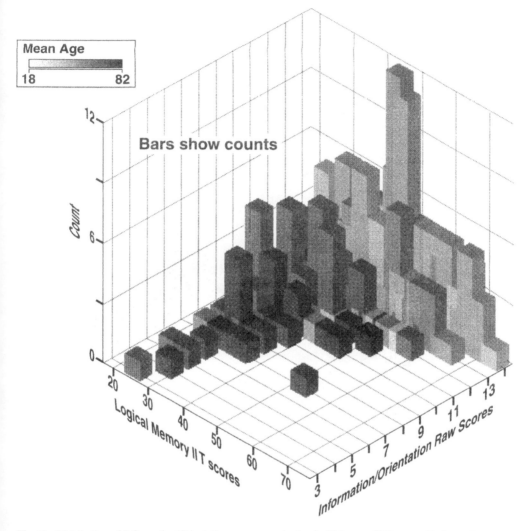

Fig. 1b. Distribution of Information/Orientation raw scores by Logical Memory II *T* scores. Darker color represents higher age.

The present results do not address the contribution of absolute memory abilities, but rather the contribution of age-appropriate (i.e., normal vs. pathological) memory abilities to orientation.

This distinction is demonstrated in the following example. A 50-year-old individual with a VRII raw score of 8 and LMII raw score of 2 is considered to have severely impaired (i.e., $T < 30$) performance in both visual and auditory domains. In contrast, the same raw scores in a 70-year-old would suggest average visual (i.e., $T > 40$) and

mildly impaired auditory ($30 < T < 40$) memory. As the currently presented normative tables for IO show, 70-year-olds who have average visual memory and mildly impaired auditory memory generally have normal orientation (mean = 12.2), although their scores can be as low as 10. In contrast, 50-year-olds with identical memory raw scores, which represent severely impaired visual and auditory memory, have abnormal orientation (mean = 9.5), and their IO raw scores can be as low as 3. This example shows that an abnormal

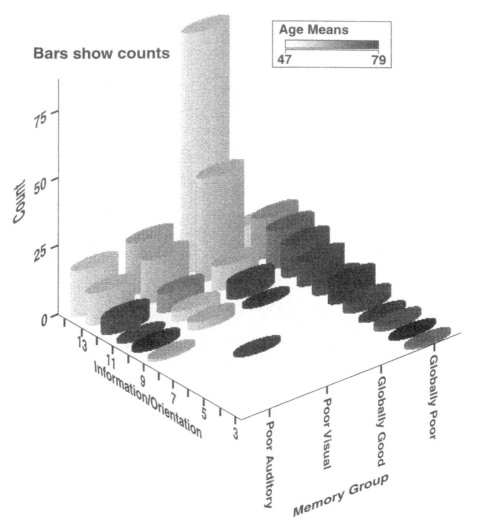

Fig. 2. Distribution of Information/Orientation raw scores for four memory groups. Darker color represents higher age.

pathological process, rather than normal age-related memory decline alone, is likely to be responsible for pathological decline in orientation. At the same time, the tables show that older persons with normal, healthy memory may have mild orientation difficulties. In contrast, younger people with normal memory have virtually no orientation problems.

Irrespective of age, patients with globally good memory, globally poor memory, poor visual memory, and poor auditory memory exhibit different *risk*

rates of being disoriented, with the globally poor memory patients being at much greater risk. For individuals with *globally* poor memory, the rate of poor orientation was more than doubled compared to those with *selectively* poor visual memory, and more than nearly four times greater than those with *selectively* poor auditory memory. Compared to patients who had both good auditory and good visual delayed memory, the memory-impaired patients (globally and selectively) were meaningfully disoriented at a rate six times higher. Odds ratio

Table 3a. Means, Standard Deviations, and Ranges for Information/Orientation Scores by Visual and Verbal Memory for all Participants (Combined Age Groups).

	LMII $T < 30$	LMII $T = 30$–39	LMII $T = 40$–60	LMII $T = 61$–70	LMII $T > 70$
VRII $T < 30$					
n	19	14	3	0	0
M	10	12.21	12.67	n/a	n/a
SD	2.91	1.58	1.53	n/a	n/a
Range	3–13	8–14	11–14	n/a	n/a
VRII T 30–39					
n	26	22	46	0	0
M	10.15	11.18	12.85	n/a	n/a
SD	2.62	2.34	1.41	n/a	n/a
Range	4–14	7–14	7–14	n/a	n/a
VRII T 40–60					
n	6	30	99	16	0
M	12.67	13.03	13.34	13.69	n/a
SD	1.97	1.16	0.96	0.48	n/a
Range	9–14	10–14	10–14	13–14	n/a
VRII T 61–70					
n	0	3	16	6	1
M	n/a	14	13.5	13.83	14
SD	n/a	n/a	0.52	0.41	n/a
Range	n/a	14	13–14	13–14	14
VRII $T > 70$					
n	0	1	2	2	0
M	n/a	14	13	14	n/a
SD	n/a	n.a	0	0	n/a
Range	n/a	14	13	14	n/a

Note. n/a = not applicable; VRII T = standardized T scores for Visual Reproduction II; LMII T = standardized T scores for Logical Memory *II*.

Table 3b. Means, Standard Deviations, and Ranges for Information/orientation Raw Scores by Visual and Verbal Memory T Scores for 72 Participants Aged 17–45.

	LMII $T < 30$	LMII $T = 30$–39	LMII $T = 40$–60
VRII $T < 30$			
n	2	2	1
M	12.5	13	11
SD	2.12	1.41	n/a
Range	11–14	12–14	11
VRII $T = 30$–39			
n	2	4	14
M	13.5	13	12.86'
SD	0.71	0.82	1.23
Range	13–14	12–14	10–14
VRII $T = 40$–60			
n	2	10	35
M	14	13.5	13.46
SD	0	0.53	0.82
Range	14	13–14	11–14

Note. n/a = not applicable; VRII T = standardized T scores for Visual Reproduction II; LMII T-standardized T scores for Logical Memory II.

Table 3c. Means, Standard Deviations, and Ranges for Information/Orientation Raw Scores by Visual and Verbal Memory T Scores for 118 Participants Aged 46–69.

	LMII $T < 30$	LMII $T < 30$–39	LMII $T = 40$–60
VRII $T < 30$			
n	14	11	2
M	9.5	12.09	13.5
SD	3.16	1.7	0.71
Range	3–14	8–14	13–14
VRII $T = 30$–39			
n	6	8	21
M	11.33	12.5	13.33
SD	1.21	1.51	0.97
Range	10–13	9–14	11–14
VRII $T = 40$–60			
n	3	10	43
M	12	12.4	13.63
SD	2.65	0.84	0.66
Range	9–14	12–14	12–14

Note. VRII T = standardized T scores for Visual Reproduction II; LMII T = standardized T scores for Logical Memory II.

Table 3d. Means, Standard Deviations, and Ranges for Information/Orientation Raw Scores by Visual and Verbal Memory T Scores for 75 Participants Aged 70 and above.

	LMII $T < 30$	LMII $T = 30$–39	LMII $T = 40$–60
VRII $T < 30$			
n	3	1	0
M	10.67	12	n/a
SD	0.58	n/a	n/a
Range	10–11	12	n/a
VRII $T = 30$–39			
n	18	10	11
M	9.39	9.4	11.91
SD	2.68	2.07	1.92
Range	4–13	7–13	7–14
VRII $T = 40$–60			
n	1	10	21
M	12	12.2	12.57
SD	n/a	1.48	1.29
Range	12	10–14	10–14

Note. n/a = not applicable; VRII T = standardized T scores for Visual Reproduction II; LMII T = standardized T scores for Logical Memory II.

results indicate that, when considering all conditions together, having an impairment in delayed auditory memory, delayed visual memory, or both increases the *relative risk* of being disoriented by more than six times, compared to individuals with normal memory in both visual and auditory domains.

The phenomenon of abnormal orientation in patients whose delayed memory is good is intriguing. Although it is an infrequent event for patients with adequate memory to have abnormal orientation, this condition deserves further attention in a research context, given the possibility that it could shed light on key variables that determine the presence of abnormal orientation. As can be seen in Figure 2, in patients whose memory functions were *not* globally impaired (i.e., memory was intact or selectively impaired), orientation errors were less serious and occurred in older patients.

Overall results suggest that impaired memory is neither sufficient (i.e., some patients with poor memory maintain orientation) nor necessary (i.e., a small number of patients with intact memory make orientation errors) to produce abnormal orientation. Similarly, previous research also failed to find a straightforward relationship between memory function and orientation (Desmond et al., 1994; Guilmette et al., 1995; Varney & Shepherd, 1991). Rather, the literature is in general agreement with the present findings in indicating that orientation is typically intact in patients with normal memory and may range from normal to abnormal in patients with memory impairment. The present study extends previous research in that it demonstrates the contribution of age, as well as the joint effect of visual and auditory memory impairment to orientation.

Normative tables for heterogeneous clinical populations have been presented with the belief that they could be used to determine expected relationships among age, memory, and orientation in individual clinical cases. However, caution in interpretation should be exercised for individuals with extremely good or extremely poor memory because, as would be expected in a normally distributed heterogeneous sample, normative data for such individuals are based on fewer cases. When predicted expectations appear to be met with initial screening measures on an individual case, it may be possible to conserve time needed for the remainder of the evaluation. Also, with such tables, it may be possible to identify patients whose memory versus orientation performances are statistically unexpected. The tables presented are based upon patient performances that were independent of secondary gain and with an independent confirmation of neurological status. Although only hypothetical at present, future research may be able to demonstrate the utility of such tables for identifying patients whose memory and orientation performances are not in line with expectations, perhaps raising concerns regarding non-neurological

memory phenomena and/or motivational problems secondary either to specific psychiatric condition (e.g., psychosis) or malingering. At present, these tables refer only to expected relationships among age, memory, and orientation in well-motivated patients who have at least eighth-grade education, and either well-defined neurological status or nonpsychotic psychiatric diagnosis. It is not clear whether the statistical relationships among cognitive and demographic variables and orientation would change in a sample with a somewhat different distribution of diagnoses; this question needs to be addressed in future research. Finally, future research may also focus on examining the relationships among the presently examined variables and specific diagnoses. Such extension of the present study would likely lead to even finer characterization of performances, and may enhance the diagnostic decision-making process.

REFERENCES

Bachrach, H., & Mintz, J. (1974). The Wechsler Memory Scale as a tool for the detection of mild cerebral dysfunction. *Journal of Clinical Psychology*, *30*, 58–60.

Benton, A.L., Van Allen, M.W., & Fogel, M.L. (1964). Temporal orientation in cerebral disease. *Journal of Nervous and Mental Disease*, *139*, 110–119.

Benton, A.L., Eslinger, P., & Damasio, A. (1981). Normative observations on neuropsychological test performances in old age. *Journal of Clinical Neuropsychology*, *3*, 33–42.

Bornstein, R., & Chelune, G. (1988). Factor structure of the Wechsler Memory Scale-Revised. *The Clinical Neuropsychologist*, *2*, 107–115.

Brooker, A.E. (1997). Performance on the Wechsler Memory Scale-Revised for patients with mild traumatic brain injury and mild dementia. *Perceptual and Motor Skills*, *84*, 131–138.

Brooks, D.N. (1976). Wechsler Memory Scale performance and its relationship to brain damage after severe closed head injury. *Journal of Neurology, Neurosurgery, and Psychiatry*, *39*, 593–601.

Brotchie, J., Brennan, J., & Wyke, M. (1985). Temporal orientation in the pre-senium and old age. *British Journal of Psychiatry*, *147*, 692–695.

Daniel, W.F., Crovitz, H.F., & Weiner, R.D. (1987). Neuropsychological aspects of disorientation. *Cortex*, *23*, 169–187.

Desmond, D.W., Tatemichi, T.K., Figueroa, M., Gropen, T.I., & Stern, Y. (1994). Disorientation following stroke: Frequency, course, and clinical correlates. *Journal of Neurology, 241,* 585–591.

Elwood, R.E. (1991). Factor structure of the Wechsler Memory Scale-Revised (WMS-R) in a clinical sample: A methodological reappraisal. *The Clinical Neuropsychologist, 5,* 329–337.

Feinstein, A.R. (1970). *Clinical epidemiology: The architecture of clinical research.* Philadelphia: W.B. Saunders Co.

Ferrario, E., Seccia, L., Massaia, M., Fonte, G.F., & Molaschi, M. (1998). Mini-Mental State Examination and Wechsler Memory Scale subtest of logical memory correlation in an over 70-year-old population. *Archives of Gerontology & Geriatrics, 6,* 175–180.

Folstein, M.F., Folstein, S.E., & McHugh, P.R. (1975). Mini-Mental State. *Journal of Psychiatric Research, 12,* 189–198.

Guilmette, T.J., Tsoh, J.Y., & Malcolm, C.D. (1995). Orientation and three-word recall in predicting memory: Age effects and false-negative errors. *Neuropsychiatry, Neuropsychology, and Behavioral Neurology, 8,* 20–25.

High, W.M., Levin, H.S., & Gary, H.E. (1990). Recovery of orientation following closed-head injury. *Journal of Clinical and Experimental Neuropsychology, 12,* 703–714.

Hopp, G.A., Dixon, R.A., Grut, M., Bacekman, L. (1997). Longitudinal and psychometric profiles of two cognitive status tests in very old adults. *Journal of Clinical Psychology, 53,* 673–686.

Ishizaki, J., Meguro, K., Ambo, H., Shimada, M., Yamaguchi, S., Harasaka, C., Komatsu, H., Sekita, Y., & Yamadori, A. (1998). A normative, community-based study of Mini-Mental State in elderly adults: The effect of age and educational level. *Journal of Gerontology: Series B—Psychological Sciences & Social Science, 53,* P539–P363.

Kear-Colwell, J.J. (1973). The structure of the Wechsler Memory Scale and its relationship to "brain damage". *British Journal of Social and Clinical Psychology, 12,* 384–392.

Larrabee, G.J., Kane, R.L., & Schuck, J.R. (1983). Factor analysis of the WAIS and Wechsler Memory Scale: An analysis of the construct validity of the Wechsler Memory Scale. *Journal of Clinical Neuropsychology, 5,* 159–168.

Leonberger, F.T., Nicks, S., Goldfader, P., & Munz, D. (1991). Factor analysis of the Wechsler Memory Scale-Revised and the Halstead-Reitan Neuropsychological Battery. *The Clinical Neuropsychologist, 5,* 83–88.

Margolis, R.B., & Scialfa, C.T. (1984). Age differences in Wechsler Memory Scale performance. *Journal of Clinical Psychology, 40,* 1442–1449.

McKhann, G., Drachman, D., Folstein, M., Katzman, R., Price, D., & Stadlan, E.M. (1984). Clinical diagnosis of Alzheimer's Disease: Report of the NINCDS-ADRDA work group under the auspices of Department of Health and Human Services Task Force on Alzheimer's Disease. *Neurology, 34,* 939–944.

Mattis, S. (1988). *Dementia rating scale.* Odessa, FL: Psychological Assessment Resources.

Meiran, N., Stuss, D., Guzman, A., LaFleche, G., & Willmer, J. (1996). Diagnosis of dementia: Methods for interpretation of scores of 5 neuropsychological tests. *Archives of Neurology, 53,* 1043–1054.

Natelson, B.H., Haupt, E.J., Fleischer, E.J., & Grey, L. (1979). Temporal orientation and education. *Archives of Neurology, 36,* 444–446.

Prigatano, G.P. (1977). Wechsler Memory Scale is a poor screening test for brain dysfunction. *Journal of Clinical Psychology, 33,* 772–777.

Roth, D., Conboy, T., Reeder, K., & Boll, T. (1990). Confirmatory factor analysis of the Wechsler Memory Scale-Revised in a sample of head injured patients. *Journal of Clinical and Experimental Neuropsychology, 12,* 834–842.

Schnider, A., von Daniken, C., & Gutbrod, K. (1996). Disorientation in amnesia: A confusion of memory traces. *Brain, 119,* 1627–1632.

Skilbeck, C.E., & Woods, R.T. (1980). The factorial structure of the Wechsler Memory Scale: Samples of neurological and psychogeriatric patients. *Journal of Clinical Neuropsychology, 2,* 293–300.

Small, B.J., Viitanen, M., & Bacekman, L. (1997). Mini-Mental State Examination item scores as predictors of Alzheimer's Disease: Incidence data from the Kungsholmen Project, Stockholm. *Journals of Gerontology, 52A,* M299–M304.

Varney, N.R., & Shepherd, J.S. (1991). Predicting short-term memory on the basis of temporal orientation. *Neuropsychology, 5,* 13–16.

Wang, P.L., Kaplan, J.R., & Rogers, E.J. (1975). Memory functioning in hemiplegics: A neuropsychological analysis of the Wechsler Memory Scale. *Archives of Physical Medicine and Rehabilitation, 56,* 517–521.

Wechsler, D. (1987). *Wechsler Memory Scale-Revised.* San Antonio, TX: The Psychological Corporation.

Wechsler, D. (1997). *Wechsler Memory Scale* (3rd ed.) San Antonio, TX: The Psychological Corporation.

Woodard, J. (1993). Confirmatory factor analysis of the Wechsler Memory Scale-Revised in a mixed clinical population. *Journal of Clinical and Experimental Neuropsychology, 15,* 968–973.

Zagar, R., Arbit, J., Stuckey, M., & Wengel, W. (1984). Developmental analysis of the Wechsler Memory Scale. *Journal of Clinical Psychology, 40,* 1466–1473.

The Clinical Neuropsychologist
1994, Vol. 8, No. 2, pp. 209–218

CLINICAL ISSUES

Longitudinal Comparison of Alternate Versions of the Symbol Digit Modalities Test: Issues of Form Comparability and Moderating Demographic Variables

Craig Lyons Uchiyama[1,2], Louis F. D'Elia[3], Ann M. Dellinger[4], Ola A. Selnes[6], James T. Becker[5], Jerry E. Wesch[7], Bai Bai Chen[6], Paul Satz[3], Wilfred van Gorp[3], and Eric N. Miller[3]

For the Multicenter AIDS Cohort Study*, [1]UCSF Langley Porter Psychiatric Institute, [2]UCSF Center on Deafness, [3]UCLA School of Medicine, [4]UCLA School of Public Health, [5]University of Pittsburgh Graduate School of Public Health and School of Medicine, [6]Johns Hopkins University School of Hygiene and Public Health, and [7]Howard Brown Memorial Clinic-Northwestern University Medical School

ABSTRACT

A longitudinal examination of the comparability of two alternate versions of the Symbol Digit Modalities Test (SDMT) was undertaken on a large ($N = 3,509$), multiregional, healthy male sample. Significant differences were noted between the test scores of the two forms, both upon initial and longitudinal administration, with higher test scores generally being associated with the original version, and higher recall scores being associated with the alternate version. Due to these differences, it is recommended that comparisons between the forms be made only with standardized scores based on test-specific norms, such as those provided in the present study. It was determined that no significant practice effects were noted over the 2-year retest period, demonstrating the relatively stability of the two versions across time. Finally, the demographic characteristics of age, and estimated IQ were demonstrated to be significantly associated with test performance, emphasizing the importance of the stratification of normative data by these variables in interpreting SDMT performance.

---

*The Multicenter AIDS Cohort Study includes the following investigators: *Baltimore*–The Johns Hopkins University School of Hygiene and Public Health: Alfred J. Saah, Principal Investigator; John Palenicek, Haroutune Armenian, Homayoon Farzadegan, Neil Graham, Joseph Margolick, Justin C. McArthur, Ola A. Selnes. *Chicago*–Howard Brown Memorial Clinic – Northwestern University Medical School: John P. Phair, Principal Investigator; Joan S. Chmiel, Kenneth Bauer, Bruce A. Cohen, Daina Variakojis, Jerry Wesch, Steven M. Wolinsky. *Los Angeles*–University of California, UCLA Schools of Public Health and Medicine and the Jonsson Comprehensive Cancer Center, Los Angeles: Roger Detels, Principal Investigator; Barbara R. Visscher, Jan Dudley, Irvin Chen, John L. Fahey, Janis V. Giorgi, Shelia Jin, Andrew Leuchter, Oto Martinez-Maza, Eric N. Miller, Hal Morgenstern, Pari Nishanian, Marc Nuwer, Paul Satz, Elyse Singer, Jeremy Taylor, Wilfred van Gorp, Jerry Zack. *Pittsburgh* – University of Pittsburgh Graduate School of Public Health and School of Medicine: Charles R. Rinaldo, Jr., Principal Investigator; Lawrence Kingsley, James T. Becker, Mary Amanda Dew, Phalguni Gupta, Monto Ho, Lili Penkower. *Data Coordinating Center* – The Johns Hopkins School of Hygiene and Public Health: Alvaro Muñoz, Principal Investigator; Helena Bacellar, Noya Galai, Leonardo Epstein, Donald R. Hoover, Lisa P. Jacobson, Jill Kirby, Curtis Meinert, Kenrad Nelson, Steven Piantadosi, Sol Su. *National Institutes of Health*–National Institute of Allergy and Infectious Disease: Lewis Schrager, Project Officer; Sten H. Vermund, Richard A. Kaslow, Mark J. VanRaden; National Cancer Institute: Iris Obrams, Daniela Seminara.
Supported by National Institutes of Health contracts N01 AI 72631, AI 72634, AI 32535, AI 72676, and AI 72632.
Requests for reprints should be sent to: Craig Lyons Uchiyama, Ph.D., UCSF, Langley Porter Psychiatric Institute; 401 Parnassus Box CPT; San Francisco, CA 94143-0984 U.S.A.
Accepted for publication: December 21, 1993.

The Symbol Digit Modalities Test (SDMT) is a measure of visual attention (Lezak, 1983; Shum, McFarland, & Bain, 1990), with psychomotor (Polubinski & Melamed, 1986), visuo-perceptual (Lezak, 1983; Polubinski & Melamed, 1986; Royer, Gilmore, & Gruhn, 1981), novel learning, and orthographic components. Impaired performance on this test has been associated with cocaine use (O'Malley, Adamse, Heaton, & Gawin, 1992), involvement in litigation (Lees-Haley, 1990), P3 latency (Emmerson, Dustman, Shearer, & Turner, 1989), Parkinson's disease (Starkstein, Bolduc, Preziosi, & Robinson, 1989), lack of exercise in older adults (Stones & Kozma, 1989), differentiation of organic and psychiatric patients (Arsuaga, Higgins, & Sifre, 1986), anticholinergic medications (Ray et al., 1992), and brain damage in male children (Lewandowski, 1984).

The SDMT also has been used as a screening measure for global pathology (Miller et al., 1988), and has demonstrated high correlations with the similar, but conceptually different, Digit Symbol subtest of the WAIS-R (Bowler, Sudia, Mergler, Harrison, & Cone, 1992). In addition to the standard orthographic version of this test, other versions also have been used, including the oral version (Knuckle & Asbury, 1986; van Dijk, 1987), a computerized version (Skinner, MacDonnell, Glen, & Glen, 1989; Zur & Yule, 1990), and alternate orthographic versions of varying difficulty (Royer, Gilmore, & Gruhn, 1981).

Although the use of alternate versions has, potentially, considerable clinical significance, little research has been done to examine the comparability of such forms from a psychometric viewpoint. Furthermore, because repeated, long-term retesting is frequently required to monitor the course of recovery from acute conditions (such as closed-head injury) or of decline in degenerative conditions (such as a dementing disorder), it must be determined to what extent the practice effects associated with repeated exposure significantly bias test performance.

The purpose of this investigation is to analyze the comparability of the original and an alternate written version of the Symbol Digit Modalities Test, as well as to examine the effects of multiple, long-term administrations on test performance. An orthographic alternate version was chosen for

comparison to circumvent the confounding effects of the different response modalities associated with the oral and computerized versions. In addition to these analyses, the demographic characteristics of the sample – such as age, education, ethnicity, and estimated IQ – were examined to determine if they were associated with test performance and, as such, need to be interpreted when assessing SDMT performance.

METHOD

Subjects

Subjects were recruited from the Multicenter AIDS Cohort Study (MACS), and consisted of 3,509 homosexual and bisexual HIV-seronegative males from sites in Baltimore, Chicago, Los Angeles, and Pittsburgh. The purpose of the MACS is to examine the neurological and neuropsychological functioning of HIV-1 seropositive and seronegative persons within a longitudinal framework. Subjects were excluded from the investigation if they demonstrated a history of learning disability, a prior loss of consciousness, or a non-English primary language. Each center recruited subjects according to a combination of the following procedures: media publicity (including the gay press), personal connections with gay activists and early participants, promotional events (such as raffles), and previous clinical contacts. For complete information on subject recruitment procedures, the reader may refer to the previously published works by Miller and associates (1990), and Kaslow and associates (1987).

The mean age of the sample was 38.13 years ($SD = 7.98$), with a range of 20 to 73 years. Because the exact number of years of education was not obtained on a large portion of the sample, the level of education could not be treated as a continuous variable. However, stratified information concerning educational level was available for all subjects. In this sample, 35% had less than 16 years of education, 27% had 16 years, and 38% had more than 16 years. Ethnically, the sample was made up of 85% non-Hispanic Caucasians, 5% Hispanic Caucasians, 9% non-Hispanic African-Americans, <1% Hispanic African-Americans, <1% Native American, <1% Asian-American, and <1% other. Zachary estimates of WAIS-R IQs obtained from the Shipley-Hartford Test also were available for the subjects. In the present sample, the mean estimated IQ was 108.86 ($SD = 9.13$).

In the normative sample, it was found that 3,281 individuals had received the original version (Form 1) on their first administration of the test. Their mean age was 38.08 years ($SD = 7.90$); and their mean estimated

IQ was 109.04 (SD = 8.95). It was found that 86% were Caucasian and 14% were non-Caucasian; and 35% had less than 16 years education, 27% had 16 years, and 38% had more than 16 years. Two-hundred and twenty-eight subjects were administered the alternate version (Form 2) first. The mean age of this group was 38.91 years (SD = 9.03) and their mean estimated IQ was 107.35 (SD = 10.42). Racially, this sample was 76% Caucasian and 23% non-Caucasian; 34% had less than 16 years of education, 33% had 16 years, and 33% had more than 16 years. When comparing the two normative groups in terms of these demographic characteristics, it was noted that the groups significantly differed in terms of ethnicity. Therefore, this variable was controlled in the manner described in the Results section.

When the data were examined longitudinally, 39 subjects were found to have been administered Form 1 of the test first with successive yearly follow-ups for 2 years. This group had a mean age of 37.62 years (SD = 7.20) and a mean estimated IQ of 109.29 (SD = 10.14); 82% were Caucasian and 18% were non-Caucasian; and 36% had less than 16 years of education, 28% had 16 years, and 36% had more than 16 years. Twenty subjects received Form 2 first, with successive follow-ups for 2 years. This group had a mean age of 40.04 (SD = 7.05) and a mean estimated IQ of 110 (SD = 7.23); all were Caucasian; and 20% had less than 16 years education, 35% had 16 years, and 45% had more than 16 years. Because these samples did not differ statistically in terms of any of their demographic characteristics, these variables were not controlled in the longitudinal analyses.

Procedure

Subjects were tested over 12 data collection periods that were each 6 months in length. Two orthographic forms of the Symbol Digit Modalities Test (SDMT) were administered to the subjects. The first, which will subsequently be referred to as Form 1, was the standard version developed by Smith (1968, 1973). The test consists of symbols that are matched to numbers from 1 to 9 according to a key printed at the top of the test. The subject is presented with a series of figures, and asked to write the numbers with which the figures are associated as quickly as possible in a 90-s period.

The second version, which will be referred to as Form 2, was developed by Selnes and consists of the same symbols as the standard version. Although the symbols are paired with different numbers in the test key, the order in which they are presented in Form 2 is the same as in Form 1. Because of this, and because Form 1 more frequently incorporates smaller numbers at the beginning of the test and gradually exposes the subject to the larger numbers, Form 2 subjects do not have the benefit of such gradated exposure and sequential associative learning, a difference that could potentially limit the comparability of the two versions. Form 1 was administered in Waves 1, 2, 3, 4, 6, 8, 10, and 12; and Form 2 was administered in Waves 5, 7, 9, and 11.

Subjects were administered the test according to standard procedures. Immediately following the test, subjects were administered an unannounced, incidental learning test. This was composed of a line of 15 symbols in which all 9 original symbols were included at least once. The subjects were asked to fill in the number associated with that symbol. In those cases where a symbol was presented more than once, and the subject correctly identified the number on one occasion and incorrectly identified it on another, the subject was given credit for the correct identification. The purpose of this was to assess the automatic learning component of the task.

RESULTS

Normative Analyses

The means and standard deviations from the normative analyses, which were stratified according to age, education, and estimated IQ, are presented in Table 1. Due to the relatively limited non-Caucasian sample size, the data could not be meaningfully stratified for ethnicity.

The normative data were subjected to general linear model analyses to determine the comparability of the two forms, as the number of people receiving the different forms first was highly discrepant. In these analyses, test form was entered as an independent variable. As the two samples showed significant differences in racial make-up, this variable was controlled by dichotomizing it into Caucasian and non-Caucasian, and incorporating it as an independent variable. By doing this, the effects of test form could be examined through the partial sums of squares without the influencing effects of ethnicity.

Because a large portion of the subjects did not receive the recall trial on their first administration, test scores and recall scores were entered as dependent variables in separate analyses, with alpha levels being corrected by dividing them by the number of comparisons. The partial sums of squares revealed that total scores were significantly higher for Form 1 ($F = 7.59$; $df = 1$; $p < .025$; $n = 3,507$), although recall scores were significantly higher for Form 2 ($F = 8.55$; $df = 1$; $p < .025$; $n = 2,024$).

Table 1. Means and Standard Deviations on Alternate Forms of the Symbol Digits Test.

	FORM 1	FORM 1 RECALL	FORM 2	FORM 2 RECALL
TOTAL:	54.91 (9.54)	5.85 (2.46)	52.82 (10.33)	6.39 (2.51)
	(*n* = 3,281)	(*n* = 1,798)	(*n* = 228)	(*n* = 228)
AGE	57.31 (10.11)	6.36 (2.38)	56.12 (11.56)	6.46 (2.42)
(20–29)	(*n* = 481)	(*n* = 212)	(*n* = 26)	(*n* = 26)
AGE	56.11 (9.26)	6.18 (2.39)	53.55 (10.32)	6.52 (2.48)
(30–39)	(*n* = 1,596)	(*n* = 795)	(*n* = 119)	(*n* = 119)
AGE	52.96 (9.26)	5.53 (2.47)	52.21 (9.87)	6.41 (2.49)
(40–49)	(*n* = 952)	(*n* = 600)	(*n* = 58)	(*n* = 58)
AGE	50.14 (8.18)	4.86 (2.42)	46.79 (8.08)	5.04 (2.58)
(>50)	(*n* = 252)	(*n* = 191)	(*n* = 24)	(*n* = 24)
EDUC	53.26 (9.97)	5.67 (2.51)	51.05 (10.54)	5.77 (2.59)
(<16)	(*n* = 1,144)	(*n* = 653)	(*n* = 78)	(*n* = 78)
EDUC	55.90 (8.78)	6.15 (2.39)	53.96 (10.32)	6.72 (2.37)
(16)	(*n* = 875)	(*n* = 441)	(*n* = 74)	(*n* = 74)
EDUC	55.80 (9.43)	5.83 (2.44)	53.51 (10.02)	6.55 (2.47)
(>16)	(*n* = 1,249)	(*n* = 691)	(*n* = 76)	(*n* = 76)
Estimated IQ	47.31 (7.51)	4.19 (2.18)	41.67 (8.69)	4.75 (2.99)
(<90)	(*n* = 71)	(*n* = 31)	(*n* = 12)	(*n* = 12)
Estimated IQ	53.83 (8.73)	5.84 (2.32)	50.86 (9.16)	6.00 (2.52)
(91–110)	(*n* = 792)	(*n* = 251)	(*n* = 92)	(*n* = 92)
Estimated IQ	58.70 (8.95)	6.63 (2.16)	55.30 (10.49)	6.96 (2.18)
(≥111)	(*n* = 877)	(*n* = 248)	(*n* = 91)	(*n* = 91)

The relation of the demographic variables to test score was examined by a multiple linear regression, with test score as the criterion variable and age, estimated IQ, years of education, and ethnicity as predictor variables. Due to the limited non-Caucasian sample size, ethnicity was entered into the analysis as a dichotomized (Caucasian, non-Caucasian) indicator variable. The partial sums of squares revealed significant results for age ($F = 211.02$; $p < .05$), ethnicity ($F = 221.62$; $p < .05$), and estimated IQ ($F = 13.46$; $p < .05$), demonstrating the significant associations of these variables with test scores; higher scores were associated with younger age and higher IQ. The total R-square for the regression model was .229.

Longitudinal Analyses
The means and standard deviations for the longitudinal analyses are presented in Table 2.

The longitudinal data were analyzed by a one-way general linear model analysis, with test form as the independent variable and test scores and recall scores from the 2-year retest period as the dependent variables. The multivariate F ratio for test version ($F = 2.36$; $df = 6$; $p < .05$) revealed significant differences between the forms when used longitudinally. Although no significant practice effects were noted over time ($F = 2.49$; $df = 2$; $p > .05$), what appeared to be a somewhat anomalous drop in performance Form 2 was noted at the 2-year retest. In addition, the time by test form interaction was nonsignificant ($F = 1.86$; $df = 2$; $p > .05$), indicating that any difference noted across time in the two forms was not significant in terms of slope or direction.

Equivalent-Form Reliability
The equivalent-form retest reliability coefficients are presented in Table 3. The retest coefficients were based on comparisons with the initial administration of the test. The coefficients were significant and moderately large for test scores; they were significant and moderate in size for recall scores. Only a minimal discrepancy was noted between the coefficients for the two versions for test scores. However, a moderately large difference

Table 2. Longitudinal Means and Standard Deviations on Alternate Versions of the Symbol Digit Test.

	0 Years	1 Year	2 Years
Form 1 (n = 39)	56.21 (8.69)	56.95 (7.27)	58.18 (10.15)
Form 1 Recall	6.05 (2.31)	7.49 (2.30)	7.13 (2.15)
Form 2 (n = 20)	55.65 (10.71)	58.05 (12.78)	54.90 (12.40)
Form 2 Recall	7.10 (2.10)	7.25 (2.12)	7.45 (2.48)

Table 3. Equivalent-Form Retest Reliability of Alternate Forms of the Symbol Digit Test.

	6-Month	1-Year	2-Year
Form 1	.794** (n = 1,045)	.715** (n = 39)	.717** (n = 39)
Form 1 Recall	.461** (n = 158)	.515** (n = 39)	.709** (n = 39)
Form 2	—	.767** (n = 20)	.721** (n = 20)
Form 2 Recall	—	.678** (n = 20)	.446* (n = 20)

Note. $*p \le .05$ (two-tailed significance)
$**p \le .01$ (two-tailed significance)

was noted between the recall coefficients of the two versions upon 2-year retest, with Form 2 evidencing lower reliability.

Alternate-Form Reliability

The alternate-form 6-month reliability coefficients were significant and relatively large for total scores ($r = .738$; two-tailed $p < .01$), although they were slightly lower for the recall scores ($r = .515$; two-tailed $p < .01$). These findings are comparable to the equivalent-form 6-month reliability for Form 1.

DISCUSSION

The present investigation provides stratified normative data for two versions of the Symbol Digit Modalities Test on a very large, multiregional, healthy male sample. As the current sample was composed of seronegative, healthy gay and bisexual

men, the possibility existed that the validity and normative findings from this investigation may not be reflective of non-gay or non-bisexual male populations. Therefore, the total scores of the original form from the present study were compared to previously published normative findings on males who were not selected according to sexual orientation. Studies were not included in the comparison that were not stratified by sex (Royer, Gilmore, & Gruhn, 1981; Smith, 1982) and age, or whose sample size was too restricted for meaningful comparisons (Gilmore, Royer, & Gruhn, 1983). The one study that was found to meet these criteria was that of Yeudall, Fromm, Reddon, and Stefanyk (1986). The age groups from this study that overlapped those of the present study were selected for comparison.

The mean test score from the Yeudall et al. study was found to be very similar to that of the present one, with only a difference of 1.56 points found between the two investigations. Due to this noteworthy similarity, there does not seem to be compelling evidence for the present findings not to be generalized to non-gay male populations, particularly as there is no a priori reason or previous published findings that would support such a contention.

It was found that, upon initial administration, test scores were significantly higher for Form 1, and recall scores were significantly higher for Form 2, indicating that comparisons between the two versions should be made using only standardized scores based on form-specific normative data, such as those provided herein. Lower test scores may be related with Form 2 because it lacks the gradated exposure and sequential associative learning found in Form 1, making the items of this version more difficult to learn. Due to this increased difficulty, additional effort may be required in cognitively encoding Form 2, making it more accessible on retrieval, as evidenced by its higher recall scores. It is recommended that the psychometric differences of these forms be the focus of future research in order to more fully understand the nature of these versions and their dissimilarities.

When these forms were examined longitudinally over the course of 2 years, significant differences were noted, with slightly higher test scores again generally being associated with Form 1 and slightly higher recall scores with Form 2. As no significant practice effects were noted with long-term repeated exposure, both forms seemed to evidence a relative stability over time that allows for direct comparisons of retest scores with original scores over a 2-year retest period.

The longitudinal reliability coefficients were found to be significant and comparable for the two forms for test scores; however, a markedly lower coefficient was obtained for recall scores for Form 2 upon 2-year retest. This would suggest that the two forms evidence unequal retest reliability for recall scores, and that, given their unreliability, Form 2 recall scores should be interpreted with caution when used longitudinally.

In examining the demographic characteristics of the sample, age, ethnicity, and estimated IQ were found to be significantly associated with SDMT performance, indicating that normative data should be stratified and interpreted according to these variables. The present results revealed that higher scores were associated with younger age and higher IQ. These findings are congruent with previous studies in that age (Emmerson et al., 1989; Stones & Kozma, 1989) and IQ (Waldmann, Dickson, Monahan, & Kazelskis, 1992) have demonstrated a significant association to SDMT performance.

Although ethnicity was found to be significantly associated with test performance, the relatively restricted sample size of non-Caucasian males limited the interpretations that may be made on these findings, and therefore the normative data were not stratified for this variable. However, it is recommended that ethnicity be the focus of future research in which the social, cultural, and economic factors that could potentially moderate the effects of ethnicity may be more carefully scrutinized.

It remains to be demonstrated if the present normative data can be used with females. Although gender effects have not been universally found to be associated with SDMT performance (Gilmore, Royer, & Gruhn, 1983), some studies have suggested that women score higher than men (Knuckle & Asbury, 1986; Laux & Lane, 1985; Polubinski & Melamed, 1986). It is, therefore, not recommended that the present data be used with women until more research can be undertaken examining this question.

In conclusion, the alternate forms of the SDMT showed significant discrepancies both on initial and longitudinal presentation that may limit their comparability. However, when used with the appropriate normative data provided herein, and interpreted in accordance with those demographic variables shown to impact test performance, the alternate versions of the Symbol Digit Modalities Test potentially have substantial clinical and research significance in the long-term assessment of attention and novel learning.

REFERENCES

Arsuaga, E.N., Higgins, J.C., & Sifre, P.A. (1986). Separation of brain-damaged from psychiatric patients with the combined use of an ability and a personality test: A validation study with a Puerto Rican population. *Journal of Clinical Psychology*, *42*, 328–331.

Bowler, R.M., Sudia, S., Mergler, D., Harrison, R., & Cone, J. (1992). Comparison of digit symbol and symbol digit modalities tests for assessing neurotoxic exposure. *Clinical Neuropsychologist*, *6*, 103–104.

Emmerson, E.Y., Dustman, R.E., Shearer, D.E., & Turner, C.W. (1989). P3 latency and symbol digit performance correlations in aging. *Experimental Aging Research*, *15*, 151–159.

Gilmore, G.C., Royer, F.L., & Gruhn, J.J. (1983). Age differences in Symbol-Digit Substitution Task performance. *Journal of Clinical Psychology*, *39*, 114–124.

Kaslow, R.A., Ostrow, D.G., Detels, R., Phair, J.P., Polk, B.F., & Rinaldo, C.R. (1987). The Multicenter AIDS Cohort Study: Rationale, organization, and selected characteristics of the participants. *American Journal of Epidemiology*, *126*, 310–318.

Knuckle, E.P., & Asbury, C.A. (1986). WISC-R discrepancy score directions and gender as reflected in neuropsychological test performance of Black adolescents. *Journal of Research and Development in Education*, *20*, 44–51.

Laux, L.F., & Lane, D.M. (1985). Information processing components of substitution test performance. *Intelligence*, *9*, 111–136.

Lees-Haley, P.R. (1990). Contamination of neuropsychological testing by litigation. *Forensic Reports*, *3*, 421–426.

Lewandowski, L.J. (1984). The Symbol Digit Modalities Test: A screening instrument for brain-damaged children. *Perceptual and Motor Skills*, *59*, 615–618.

Lezak, M.D. (1983). *Neuropsychological assessment* (*2nd ed.*). New York: Oxford University Press.

Miller, E.N., Selnes, O.A., McArthur, J.C., Satz, P., Becker, J.T., Cohen, B.A., Sheridan, K., Machado, A.M., van Gorp, W.G., & Visscher, B. (1990). Neuropsychological performance in HIV-1-infected homosexual men: The Multicenter AIDS Cohort Study (MACS). *Neurology, 40*, 197–203.

Miller, P.S., Richardson, J.S., Jyu, C.A., Lemay, J.S., Hiscock, M., & Keegan, D. L. (1988). Association of low serum anticholinergic levels and cognitive impairment in elderly presurgical patients. *American Journal of Psychiatry, 145*, 342–345.

O'Malley, S., Adamse, M., Heaton, R.K., & Gawin, F.H. (1992). Neuropsychological impairment in chronic cocaine abusers. *American Journal of Drug and Alcohol Abuse, 18*, 131–144.

Polubinski, J.P., & Melamed, L.E. (1986). Examination of the sex difference on a symbol digit substitution test. *Perceptual and Motor Skills, 62*, 975–982.

Ray, P.G., Meador, K.J., Loring, D.W., Zamrini, E.W., Yang, X.H., & Buccafusco, J.J. (1992). Central anticholinergic hypersensitivity in aging. *Journal of Geriatric Psychiatry and Neurology, 5*, 72–77.

Royer, F.L., Gilmore, G.C., & Gruhn, J.J. (1981). Normative data for the Symbol Digit Substitution task. *Journal of Clinical Psychology, 37*, 608–614.

Shum, D.H., McFarland, K.A., & Bain, J.D. (1990). Construct validity of eight tests of attention: Comparison of normal and closed head injured samples. *Clinical Neuropsychologist, 4*, 151–162.

Skinner, F.K., MacDonnell, L.E., Glen, E.M., & Glen, A.I. (1989). Repeated automated assessment of abstinent male alcoholics: Essential fatty acid supplementation and age effects. *Alcohol and Alcoholism, 24*, 129–139.

Smith, A. (1968). The Symbol Digit Modalities Test: A neuropsychologic test for economic screening of learning and other cerebral disorders. *Learning Disorders, 3*, 83–91.

Smith, A. (1973). *Symbol Digit Modalities Test Manual.* Los Angeles: Western Psychological Services.

Smith, A. (1982). *Symbol Digit Modalities Test Manual.* Los Angeles: Western Psychological Services.

Starkstein, S.E., Bolduc, P.L., Preziosi, T.J., & Robinson, R.G. (1989). Cognitive impairments in different stages of Parkinson's disease. *Journal of Neuropsychiatry and Clinical Neurosciences, 1*, 243–248.

Stones, M.J., & Kozma, A. (1989). Age, exercise, and coding performance. *Psychology and Aging, 4*, 190–194.

van Dijk, P.K. (1987). Study of the discriminant ability of the Symbol Digit Modalities Test (SDMT). *Nederlands Tijdschrift voor de Psychologie en haar Grensgebieden, 42*, 262–265.

Waldmann, B.W., Dickson, A.L., Monahan, M.C., & Kazelskis, R. (1992). The relationship between intellectual ability and adult performance on the Trail Making Test and the Symbol Digit Modalities Test. *Journal of Clinical Psychology, 48*, 360–363.

Yeudall, L.T., Fromm, D., Reddon, J.R., & Stefanyk, W.O. (1986). Normative data stratified by age and sex for 12 neuropsychological tests. *Journal of Clinical Psychology, 42*, 918–946.

Zur, J., & Yule, W. (1990). Chronic solvent abuse: I. Cognitive sequelae. *Child Care, Health and Development, 16*, 1–20.

The Clinical Neuropsychologist
1995, Vol. 9, No. 1, pp. 89–92

Post-Concussive Symptoms: Base Rates and Etiology in Psychiatric Patients*

David D. Fox[1], Paul R. Lees-Haley[2], Karen Earnest[3], and Sharon Dolezal-Wood[3]

[1]Glendale, California, [2]Lees-Haley Corporation, Encino, California, [3]Southern California Kaiser Permanente

ABSTRACT

This study was intended to provide a normative comparison base for estimating the rates of neuropsychological symptoms in psychiatric patients. Four hundred individuals seeking psychotherapy were administered a checklist composed of symptoms reported to be common in the post-concussional syndrome (PCS). Of the entire sample, 9% of the patients reported a recent history of bumping their head (BUMP), 3.5% reported being knocked out (LOC), and 9% were involved in a lawsuit (LITS). Many, but not all of the PCS symptoms were as common among the BUMP and LITS groups as the LOC group. There are suggestions that some PCS symptoms are related to head trauma while others reflect situational variables or general psychological distress.

When neuropsychologists rely on self-reported complaints as evidence of neuropsychological impairment in connection with the post-concussion syndrome (PCS), it is essential to differentiate between relevant symptoms and those that occur in other conditions or as normal background. Although there is no precise or universally accepted roster of PCS symptoms, a familiar list of self-reported complaints have come to be associated with closed-head injuries (Binder, 1986; Gouvier, Cubic, Jones, Brantley, & Cutlip, 1992; Levin, Benton, & Grossman, 1982; Lezak, 1983; Oddy, Coughlan, Tyerman, & Jenkins, 1985; Rutherford, Merrett, & McDonald, 1977). Typical symptoms include headaches, memory and concentration problems, dizziness, anxiety, insomnia, depression, irritability, and fatigue.

Rimel, Giordani, Barth, Boll, and Jane, (1981) found that in a sample of 424 patients who had suffered mild brain injury 78% complained of headaches, 59% had memory problems, and 14%

had difficulty doing everyday chores. This and other studies, however, do not separate out the effect of peripheral or psychiatric injuries from those directly caused by injury to the brain. Indeed, there is some controversy regarding the precise etiology of PCS complaints. Some have argued that they are largely psychological (Mackay, 1960) while others believe that the research indicates genuine brain dysfunction (Davidoff, Laibstain, Kessler, & Mark, 1988) or an attempt at monetary compensation (Miller, 1961). Furthermore, Lees-Haley and Brown (1993), have posited that the litigation process often associated with head trauma is likely to increase the rate of endorsement of various psychological and neuropsychological symptoms through response bias or the stress of litigation.

A few studies of PCS have compared the rates of symptoms with non-head-injured patients. Gouvier, Uddo-Crane, and Brown, (1988) found few differences in the rate of reported symptoms of those who had mild head injuries and similar aged students

* Portions of this study were presented at the 1993 Conference of the National Academy of Neuropsychology. A more extensive report with a complete list of item frequencies is available from David D. Fox, Ph.D., 435 Arden Ave, Suite 440, Glendale, CA 91203, USA.
Accepted for publication: May 9, 1994.

who had not. Likewise, 71 normal college students at a medical center (Newman, 1992) had a high rate of symptom endorsement for various symptoms of emotional distress as well as memory problems, headaches, and word finding difficulties. Newman concludes that "it would appear that many of the symptoms characteristic of the post-concussional syndrome are not unique to head injury" (p. 3).

Many PCS complaints are common to a variety of psychological and medical conditions. For example, Rattan, Strom, and Dean (1987) found that there is considerable overlap in reported symptoms between depressed patients and those with neurologic disease including memory problems and confusion. The only complaints to accurately differentiate the neurologic patients from the depressed related to hallucinations, numbness, balance problems, localized sensitivity, and vertigo.

There are important reasons for accurately determining the base rates of various neuropsychological complaints. The validity of a syndrome depends on the occurrence of a group of signs and symptoms that are reasonably unique to that syndrome. Only by specifying the occurrence rates of these signs and symptoms in different patient groups can the sensitivity and specificity of a syndrome be established, thus, making the differential diagnosis of psychological versus neuropsychological syndromes more reliable and valid. It is also important to differentiate the direct effects of a blow to the head from the general distress associated with an injury to the body or other factors secondary to the injury. This is especially true if there are other stressors present such as being involved in a lawsuit.

The purpose of this study was to measure the rate of self-reported PCS complaints in a group of psychiatric outpatients to determine whether the complaints are associated with having general psychological difficulties. The influences of head trauma, with and without loss of consciousness, and of being involved in a lawsuit in this population were ascertained as well.

METHOD

Subjects

Subjects consisted of 400 members of a large Southern California HMO who sought or were referred for outpatient psychological treatment. These patients were being evaluated for treatment of various psychological concerns, typically anxiety, depression, and marital or family problems. Immediately prior to intake interviews, the patients completed a 44-item checklist of symptoms and demographic data. Of the 400 patients, 172 (43%) were male, 219 (55%) female with 9 (2%) of unknown gender. In this sample, 33 subjects (8.3%) were less than 18 years of age, for whom parents may have assisted in completing the checklist. There were no significant differences between males and females in age ($M = 37.48$; $SD = 14.16$; range = 6 to 78) or education ($M = 13.63$; $SD = 3.91$; range = 2 to 25 years).

Materials

The checklist is an extension of the one used by Lees-Haley and Brown (1993) which addressed whether the patient had experienced in the last 2 years any of a list of complaints commonly associated with closed-head injuries. The checklist also contained items concerning common physical problems that do not implicate psychological or neuropsychological dysfunction and information about whether the subjects had been in a lawsuit, had been knocked unconscious, or "bumped" their head. Finally, the list contained three nonsensical items to detect random responding or gross symptom exaggeration. Although such a self-report measure does not assess the severity or etiology of symptoms, as a practical matter, such checklists are often used to support a diagnosis of PCS.

Statistical analysis was performed via SPSS for Windows 6.0.

RESULTS AND DISCUSSION

Of the 400 patients, 36 (9%) indicated that they had been involved in a lawsuit in the past 2 years (LITS). Fourteen patients (3.5%) indicated that they had been knocked unconscious in that period (LOC). Four subjects were in both the LOC and LITS groups. There were 37 subjects (9.3%) who reported bumping their heads (BUMP), of which 29 did not indicate that they had been knocked out. Those with neither LOC nor LITS nor BUMP totaled 329 (82.3%) and constitute the Pure Psych group.

The results yielded conflicting evidence regarding the uniqueness and etiology of PCS symptoms. For virtually every item, regardless of content, the LOC group had equal or greater endorsement rates than those without LOC. Many symptoms had high endorsement rates but were not reported significantly more often among psychiatric patients who have had a LOC than did those who have not; for example, 77% of the entire sample reported anxiety, 64% sleep problems, 55% fatigue, 53% impatience, and 42% feeling disorganized. Even when statistical significance was obtained, the occurrence rate of many of these self-reported symptoms was so high among those without LOC that such a complaint cannot be used to indicate the presence of a post-concussive condition with any precision (the Pure Psych group rates for some items: depression (65%), irritability (51%), and concentration problems (42%)). Examination of item content indicates that psychiatric patients have a high rate of cognitive and physical complaints as well the expected emotional problems.

Equally significant, those who report BUMP without LOC and those in the LITS group had comparable rates of endorsement on many items to the LOC group (e.g., depression, loss of interest, memory problems). Because some subjects were in more than one group it is possible that a single factor was responsible for increased endorsement of any particular item. To evaluate the unique variance contributed by each of these variables, logistic regressions (forward conditional variable entry; .05 criterion) were performed using LOC, LITS, BUMP, and their interaction variables as factors to predict endorsement of each symptom. Because one of the nonsense items (teeth itching) was endorsed more often by both the LOC and BUMP groups, those subjects ($N = 9$) who endorsed that item were removed from the logistic analysis.

The regression results indicate that LOC, LITS, and BUMP predicted some symptoms alone. Those who had hit their heads but did not report being knocked out were more likely to have headaches than either the LITS or LOC subjects. Being in the LITS group uniquely was responsible for restlessness, fatigue, irritability, feelings of disorganization, and health worries. Those with the highest probability of brain injury, the LOC group, were more likely to report having word finding problems, dizziness, numbness, and tremors. Many symptoms were related to more than one factor. For example, memory problems and bumping into things were related to all three investigated variables, LOC, LITS, and BUMP. Interestingly, some of the PCS symptoms were unrelated to any of the factors among these

psychiatric patients (anxiety, concentration, sleep, and reading problems).

Analysis of the total number of items endorsed by each subject reveals that the LOC, LITS, and BUMP groups endorsed more total items than did the Pure Psych group (Means = 23.71, 18.47, 19.95, 10.32, respectively; $p < .05$). Group comparisons reveal that those in the LOC group reported more symptoms than did the LITS or BUMP subjects. Multiple regression analysis to predict total number of complaints revealed that LOC, LITS, and BUMP independently contributed significant variance (Multiple $R = .43$).

Some symptoms are considered "classic" signs of the post-concussion syndrome. These include: headaches, memory problems, dizziness, ears ringing, sensitivity to noise, concentration problems, vision troubles, fatigue, irritability, and impatience. When scores were totaled for these 10 symptoms for each subject, the factors of BUMP, LITS, and LOC all were associated with higher scores than were obtained by the Pure Psych group (means = 5.84, 5.44, 6.86, 3.46, respectively; $p < .05$). Further comparisons of these means reveal that those with LOC had higher scores than did the LITS group but there was no difference between the BUMP and LOC groups. Thus, being knocked out tends to increase these "classic" PCS symptoms but no more so than just bumping of the head, although the reason for this finding requires further study.

CONCLUSIONS

The primary purpose of this study was to establish the base rates of self-reported neuropsychological symptoms in a patient population. The data suggest that PCS symptoms are common among psychiatric patients and that the report of such symptoms should be used cautiously to diagnose a concussion when a psychiatric condition is present. The base rates of many of these symptoms are so large that they provide little unique information regarding the presence of a neuropsychological syndrome. It is still possible that a particular constellation of symptoms may yet have some diagnostic value for such cases. Likewise, there may be qualitative differences in these symptoms which are relatively unique to the post-concussive condition. Further research along these lines is recommended.

The current results imply that several factors contribute to most PCS complaints. Being knocked out, suffering a bump to the head, and being in litigation independently and together seemingly influence different PCS symptoms. Although greater symptom endorsement was associated with being knocked out, many of the symptoms thought to be associated with brain dysfunction (e.g., headaches, impatience, fatigue, irritability) appear to be more strongly related to nonneurological factors such as being in litigation or merely bumping the head. These findings suggest that psychological and social psychological factors need to receive further study to more fully understand the post-concussion syndrome.

The current data are useful because PCS patients often suffer from emotional distress. However, it is important for the base rates of PCS symptoms in other patient groups, such as neurological patients, to be determined as well. The authors are currently engaged in examining such groups.

REFERENCES

Binder, L.M. (1986). Persisting symptoms after mild head injury: A review of the post-concussive syndrome. *Journal of Clinical and Experimental Neuropsychology, 8,* 323–346.

Davidoff, D.A., Laibstain, D.F., Kessler, H.R., & Mark, V.H. (1988 March/April). Neurobehavioral sequelae of minor head injury: A consideration of post- concussive syndrome versus post-traumatic stress disorder. *Cognitive Rehabilitation,* pp. 8–13.

Gouvier, W.D., Cubic, B., Jones, G., Brantley, P., & Cutlip, Q. (1992). Post-concussion symptoms and daily stress in normal and head-injured college populations. *Archives of Clinical Neuropsychology, 7*(3), 193–211.

Gouvier, W.D., Uddo-Crane, M., & Brown, L.M. (1988). Base rates of post-concussional symptoms. *Archives of Clinical Neuropsychology, 3,* 273–278.

Lees-Haley, P., & Brown, R. (1993). Neuropsychological complaint base rates of 170 personal injury claimants. *Archives of Clinical Neuropsychology, 8,* 203–209.

Levin, H., Benton, A., & Grossman, R. (1982). *Neurobehavioral consequences of closed head injury.* New York: Oxford University Press.

Lezak, M. (1983). *Neuropsychological assessment.* (2nd ed.) New York: Oxford University Press.

Mackay, R.P. (1960). Post-traumatic neurosis. *Industrial Medicine and Surgery, 29,* 200–203.

Miller, H. (1961). Accident neurosis. *British Medical Journal, 1,* 919–925; 992–998.

Newman, B. (1992). Research in mild traumatic brain injury. *New York University Medical Center R & T Center News, 4*(1), 3.

Oddy, M., Coughlan, T., Tyerman, A., & Jenkins, D. (1985). Social adjustment after closed-head injury: A further follow-up seven years after injury. *Journal of Neurology, Neurosurgery, and Psychiatry, 48,* 564–568.

Rattan, G., Strom, D., & Dean, R.S. (1987). The efficacy of a neuropsychological symptom inventory in the differential diagnosis of neurological, depressed, and normal patients. *Archives of Clinical Neuropsychology, 2,* 257–264.

Rimel, R.W., Giordani, B., Barth, J.T., Boll, T.J., & Jane, J.A. (1981). Disability caused by minor head injury. *Neurosurgery, 9*(3), 221–228.

Rutherford, W.H., Merrett, J.D., & McDonald, J.R. (1977, January). Sequelae of concussion caused by minor head injuries. *Lancet,* 1–4.

The Clinical Neuropsychologist
1993, Vol. 7, No. 2, pp. 224–233

FORUM

Clinical Discriminations and Neuropsychological Tests: An Appeal to Bayes' Theorem

Richard W. Elwood
Department of Veterans Affairs Medical Center, Tomah, WI

ABSTRACT

Neuropsychological tests are routinely used to make clinical judgements regarding the classification, diagnosis, or prediction of subject variables. The accuracy of those decisions depends on the discriminant validity of the tests used. The traditional method of validating psychological tests by comparing the mean test scores of reference groups is often unrelated to actual clinical discriminations. Alternative measures based on Bayesian probabilities are reviewed, with specific application to neuropsychological assessment.

The discriminant validity of clinical tests is traditionally judged by their ability to discriminate a criterion group of subjects who have a disorder from a reference group of those who do not. The ability to discriminate between groups in turn is usually accepted if statistical group contrasts (e.g., *t* test, ANOVA, MANOVA) are significant. Moreover, group comparisons conducted during the development of a new test are usually based on samples of equal or similar size to maximize their statistical power and make it easier to control for potentially confounding variables. The validation of most neuropsychological tests still rests largely on the traditional contrasting-group method.

Although significant group differences in test scores may be useful in basic research, they are often irrelevant to the clinical decisions they are used to support. Statistical significance merely indicates the likelihood (set by α) that an observed difference is due to chance, *given* that the null hypothesis is true (i.e., that the means of the respective populations are essentially equivalent). However, significance alone does not reflect the magnitude of group differences nor does it imply that the test can discriminate individual patients with sufficient accuracy for clinical use (Elwood, 1991). Further, there is no sound rational basis for reducing a continuum of probabilities to the arbitrary decision of accepting .05 as significant while rejecting .06 (Cohen, 1990; Rosnow & Rosenthal, 1989). Although the effect size *does* measure the extent of between-group differences and is useful for comparing neuropsychological tests (Christensen, Hadzi-Pavlovic, & Jacomb, 1991), it is also a group statistic and does not reflect the accuracy of individual classifications.

CONDITIONAL PROBABILITIES

Sensitivity and specificity are often used in assessment research to overcome the limitation of group

The author gratefully acknowledges the editor and several anonymous reviewers for their helpful comments on an earlier draft of this article.
Address correspondence to: Richard W. Elwood, PhD, Psychology Service (116B), DVA Medical Center, Tomah, WI 54660, USA.
Accepted for publication: August 31, 1992.

comparisons. Sensitivity, or true positive rate, is the proportion of subjects with a target disorder who are identified by a positive test finding (i.e., an abnormal test score). Conversely, specificity, or true negative rate, is the proportion of subjects without the disorder correctly identified by a negative test result (i.e., a normal score).

Although sensitivity and specificity provide important information about how a test performs *in general*, their limitation in classifying individual subjects is apparent when they are expressed in terms of conditional probabilities. Sensitivity is $P(+|d)$, the probability (P) of a positive test result ($+$) given that the subject has the target disorder (d). However, the task which clinicians face is usually just the opposite: determining $P(d|+)$, the probability that a patient has the disorder given that they obtained a positive test result. In the same way, specificity can be expressed as $P(-|-d)$, the probability of a negative test result given that a patient does not have the disorder. Here again, the clinical task is just the opposite: determining $P(-d|-)$, the probability that a patient does not have the disorder given a normal test score. Clinicians often treat $P(d|+)$ as equal to its inverse, $P(+|d)$, although the two expressions are not mathematically equivalent.[1] Rather, by Bayes's theorem

$$P(d|+) = P(+|d) \times P(d)/P(+)$$

where $P(d)$ is the prevalence rate of the disorder and $P(+)$ reflects the proportion of positive test results. The equation shows the probability that a test positive case is true (i.e., a true positive) depends on $P(d)$, the prevalence rate of the target disorder in the population being assessed.

The standard measures of discriminant validity exaggerate the ability of neuropsychological tests to discriminate subjects under actual clinical conditions. First, the tests are used to predict $P(d|+)$ and $P(-d|-)$ but are at best evaluated only by their inverse probabilities, sensitivity and specificity. Secondly, validation studies usually employ

samples of equal size, whereas target disorders are usually far less prevalent in actual clinical settings. Sines (1966) anticipated the problem by arguing that psychological tests should be developed in just the reverse of their usual order. He proposed that we first classify subjects according to their test responses and *then* explore the relationships of those classifications to certain criterion groups. Sines' method has the distinct advantage of assessing $P(d|+)$ at the outset, although it has not been applied to psychological test development.

PREVALENCE AND VALID PREDICTION

In a now classic article, Meehl and Rosen (1955) introduced the base-rate problem to the psychological literature. They showed that the probability of valid test positive classifications depends on the base-rate or prevalence of the criterion disorder and that the base-rate itself represents the proportion of valid test positives due to chance. Meehl and Rosen showed that under certain conditions tests can result in more classification errors than chance alone. They further argued against inflexible cut-off scores, recommending instead that cutoffs be adjusted to local base-rates to optimize the probability of valid test discriminations. Although Meehl and Rosen are widely cited and their conclusions long conceded, Bayesian probabilities are still largely ignored in applied clinical assessment.

Several authors have replaced the cumbersome formulas for Bayesian probabilities by organizing the classification outcomes into a binary table, making it easier to visualize and calculate the respective probabilities (Baldessarini, Finklestein, & Arana, 1983; Griner, 1981; Wiggins, 1973). In this scheme, shown in Table 1, positive predictive power (PPP) is the ratio of true positives to test positives and expresses $P(d|+)$, the probability that a test positive is a true positive. Negative predictive power (NPP) is the ratio of true negatives to all test negatives and states $P(-d|-)$, the probability that a test negative is a true negative. This matrix scheme and the concept of predictive power has been applied to the diagnosis of mental disorders (Widiger, Hurt, Frances, Clarkin, & Gilmore, 1984) and more recently to the validation of psychological tests (Elwood, in press; Gerardi, Keane, & Penk, 1989; Moldin, Gottesman,

---

[1] The conditional probabilities $P(d|+)$ and $P(-d|-)$ are algebraically equivalent to their respective inverse, $P(+|d)$ and $P(-|-d)$, only when $P(d) = P(+)$ [in which case it also follows that $P(-d) = P(-)$]. Although either expression may be equal to its inverse under certain circumstances, their equivalence cannot be presumed.

Table 1. Classifications and Conditional Probabilities.

		criterion		
		+	−	
Test Result	+	a	b	(a + b)
	−	c	d	(c + d)
		a + c	b + d	N

a = true positives   b = false positives
c = false negatives   d = true negatives

$$Prevalence = \frac{a + c}{N}$$

$$\frac{a}{a + c} = sensitivity\ P\ (+|d)$$

$$\frac{d}{b + d} = specificity\ P\ (-|-d)$$

$$\frac{a}{a + b} = PPP\ (Positive\ predictive\ power)\ P\ (d|+)$$

$$\frac{d}{c + d} = NPP\ (Negative\ predictive\ power)\ P\ (-d|-).$$

Rice, & Erlenmeyer-Kimling, 1991; Rapp, Parisi, Walsh, & Wallace, 1988).

Both positive and negative predictive powers are influenced by prevalence, although with reciprocal effect. A lower prevalence results in a loss of PPP and a corresponding gain in NPP. This is an important consideration because tests are often validated with prevalence rates near 50% and will suffer an inherent and often dramatic loss of PPP when applied to typical clinical settings which have a far lower prevalence. Although sensitivity and specificity are independent of prevalence, they are still related to predictive power. PPP is vulnerable to loss in specificity (i.e., an increase in false positives), whereas NPP is reduced by the loss of sensitivity (i.e., an increase in false negatives).

The application of Bayesian probabilities to neuropsychological assessment has long been advocated (Gordon, 1977; Satz, Fennell, & Reilly, 1970) and they were used in several early studies to evaluate clinical predictions (Satz, 1966, 1972). Despite such repeated recommendations, predictive power is seldom considered in the development, validation, or interpretation of neuropsychological tests.

APPLICATIONS OF PREDICTIVE POWER

One reason for the disregard of predictive power in neuropsychological assessment may be the assumption that the base-rate problem applies only to extremely rare disorders. However, a simple example demonstrates that predictive power can be effected by moderate base-rates that are often encountered in clinical practice. Imagine a test is developed to discriminate Alzheimer's dementia and is administered to normative samples of 50 Alzheimer and 50 normal subjects. Assume that the sensitivity and specificity are both found to be .90, certainly respectable parameters for any clinical test. The differences between cells are significant. As shown in Table 2, positive and negative predictive powers are an impressive .90. That is, 90% of the subjects who obtain a positive test score are

Table 2. Hypothetical Test for Alzheimer's Disease.

		Prevalence = 50% Alzheimer's				Prevalence = 10% Alzheimer's		
		+	−			+	−	
Test	+	45	5	50	+	9	9	18
	−	5	45	50	−	1	81	82
		50	50	100		10	90	100

$$\text{PPP} = 45/50 = .90$$
$$\text{NPP} = 45/50 = .90$$

$$\text{PPP} = 9/18 = .50$$
$$\text{NPP} = 81/82 = .99$$

actually demented, far above the 50% that would be predicted by chance alone. However, now assume the test is used to detect Alzheimer's dementia among elderly community residents, where the prevalence is near 10% (Evans et al., 1989). Because sensitivity and specificity are independent of prevalence rate, they remain at .90. The number of valid test negatives is $.90 \times 90 = 81$. The remaining cells and marginals can be obtained by subtraction. In this case, again referring to Table 2, the positive predictive power falls to .50. That is, a subject who obtains a positive test result is no more likely to have Alzheimer's disease than he or she is to be free of the disorder.

Incidentally, even though the hypothetical test fails to predict dementia under these conditions, it correctly classifies 89% of the total subjects. This discrepancy simply reflects the fact that most of the correct classifications ($81/89 = 91\%$) are true negatives. Overall rates of correct classifications, which are often used as evidence for discriminant validity, are deceptive when used with low prevalence disorders. The high rate of true negatives simply obscures the parallel decline in the rate of true positives. In effect, the loss of positive predictive power is masked by the increase in negative predictive power.

Clinical discriminations based on current neuropsychological tests must be considered suspect because their predictive powers are simply unknown. They are not provided in test manuals or stated in validation studies. With few exceptions (Loring, Lee, Martin, & Meador, 1989; Sunderland, et al., 1989; Wolfe-Klein, Silverstone, Levy, Brod, & Breuer, 1989; Zec et al., in press), validation studies do not provide the "hit rates," or correct

classifications, from which predictive power could be calculated.

A notable exception is a study by Masur et al., (1989) that reported the sensitivity, specificity, and predictive powers of the Selective Reminding Test in discriminating normal and demented elderly subjects, based on a realistic prevalence of dementia. Zec et al. (in press) recently evaluated the Alzheimer Disease Assessment Scale and reported the rates of correctly classifying both the presence and the severity of Alzheimer's dementia. From these data one can easily calculate the predictive powers in local situations. Both tests showed sufficient specificity to achieve high predictive powers even when applied to low base-rate disorders.

Other tests may not fair as well. Willis (1984) reanalyzed the data from five studies that claimed to discriminate brain-damaged groups by their scores on common neuropsychological tests. He found that their diagnostic accuracies were highly related to prevalence rate and that many of the hit rates did not exceed the corresponding base rate, in other words, not beyond chance. More recently, desRosiers (1992) reviewed 41 studies that compared depressed and demented subjects and found that with a 38% prevalence rate, positive predictive powers ranged as low as .34.

The clinical decision model has thus far assumed a binary matrix, corresponding to dichotomous clinical predictions of the presence or absence of certain disorders. Of course, the matrix could be expanded to accommodate any k groups of clinical interest, such as multiple stages of Alzheimer's disease (Zec et al., in press), although the matrix becomes more cumbersome. Alternately, multiple reference groups can be collapsed together and compared with a target criterion group. For example, a test designed to detect dementia in a mixed psychiatric setting could be validated by a reference group of nondemented psychiatric patients. This approach keeps the procedure simple (and thus clinically useful) while leaving the diagnosis of the functional mental disorders to other assessment methods.

The clinical decision model can be used to adjust local cutoff scores for optimal predictive power. For example, the scales developed to assess posttraumatic stress disorder (PTSD) among Vietnam veterans were validated on clinical samples in which the incidence of PTSD was around 50%. When the same scales were used in an epidemiological survey (National Vietnam Veterans Readjustment Study; NVVRS) where the prevalence was roughly 14%, cutoff scores had to be substantially adjusted because of the high rate of false positives and corresponding loss of predictive power (Kulka et al., 1988).

SUMMARY AND CLINICAL IMPLICATIONS

To the extent that psychometric instruments are imperfect predictors, decisions based on test results will always reflect implicit conditional probabilities. Although such probabilities are crucial measures of discriminant validity, they are seldom considered in clinical practice. The practical discriminant validity of common neuropsychological tests is largely unknown. Traditional statistical methods of establishing discriminant validity are inadequate for judging the performance of clinical tests. Group comparisons do not measure the extent of group differences or the accuracy of individual discriminations. Effect sizes reflect the magnitude of group differences but they also ignore individual classifications. Sensitivity and specificity are useful because they indicate how well a test detects or rules out a target disorder with individual patients. However, both of these statistics predict test scores, not disorders. Neither addresses the more pressing clinical task: deciding if a target disorder is present on the basis of a test score. That decision ultimately implies predictive power. Clearly, the clinical interpretation of individual test results requires

the joint consideration of predictive power, sensitivity, *and* specificity.

Bayesian probabilities pose major implications for neuropsychological assessment. First, *if we continue to ignore those probabilities, the accuracy of test-based clinical discriminations, even those derived from common and apparently well-validated tests, will remain suspect.* Although this state of affairs is (or ought to be) disconcerting to clinicians, the situation can be easily remedied. If commercial test developers and researchers simply specify the classification outcomes, the corrsponding probabilities can be easily computed. The outcomes can likely be extracted from the existing research data on many current tests, without having to replicate validation studies with new clinical samples.

Secondly, as Meehl and Rosen (1955) demonstrated, cutoff scores should be adjusted according to the base-rate of the target disorder. Local prevalence rates should be compiled from existing records or estimated from clinical or epidemiological studies of similar populations. Whatever method is used, the essential point is that predictive power should be based on reasonable estimates of prevalence in the population being assessed. Obviously, errors of omission and commission may be weighted differently, depending on the purpose of the assessment. Thus the cutoff scores should be selected for a desired compromise between Type I and Type II error rates. Highly sensitive tests may be useful as broad screening devices, even if they are not highly specific whereas tests that are highly specific but not very sensitive are more useful in confirming the positive findings of initial screenings.

Third, test interpretations should not exceed the limit of their predictive power in the clinical setting where they are employed. Some highly specific tests may fulfil this more rigorous standard and continue to be used with confidence. Other tests may have to be interpreted more cautiously or abandoned altogether. Proposing that clinicians themselves are responsible for determining the predictive powers of tests they use is a fairly radical idea. However, the alternative, ignoring predictive power and the effect of base rates, undoubtedly results in substantial clinical errors and is clearly untenable. Moreover, predictive powers can be easily computed on a pocket calculator and the information they provide is directly relevant to routine clinical decisions.

Outcome probabilities are relevant to any test-based clinical decisions, not just to diagnosing the organic mental disorders. For example, predicting a patient's ability to resume a former occupation or to live independently after a head injury both express implicit conditional probabilities. As measures of test performance, Bayesian probabilities are consistent with the shift away from detecting and localizing brain lesions to describing specific components of cognitive functioning or guiding rehabilitation (Leonberger, 1989). Further, the base-rate problem is not just an esoteric statistical issue that applies only to rare disorders. Predictive power is substantially effected by even the moderate base-rates that are typically encountered in clinical practice.

The discriminant validity of neuropsychological tests obviously involves more than the application of Bayes' theorem. First, subjects must be classified by some means independent of the test itself. Whereas reliable diagnostic criteria have been developed for the functional mental disorders (DSM-III-R; American Psychiatric Association, 1987), no similar criteria have been adopted for the organic mental disorders or clinical syndromes. Moreover, whereas structured diagnostic interviews have become the "gold standard" for diagnosing mental disorders, there is no analogous standard for neuropsychological disorders. The closest equivalent to a gold standard in neuropsychological assessment is the NINCDS-ADRDA criteria for the clinical diagnosis of Alzheimer's disease (McKhann et al., 1984). Secondly, predictive power assumes that sensitivity and specificity values from validation studies generalize to the clinical settings in which it is applied. In practice, that is not a major limitation because, as Rorer and Dawes (1982) point out, that assumption is implied by the rational use of any psychological test. Thirdly, the stability of predictive power is a function of test reliability. Tests with low reliability will provide discrepant classifications across subjects or over successive administrations. Replication and cross-validation apply as much to predictive powers as they do to other test charateristics. In summary, although predictive power is a good measure of discriminant validity, it does not replace traditional indices of psychometric performance.

The base-rate problem in psychological assessment has changed little since Meehl and Rosen (1955) first raised the issue four decades ago. Meehl (1960) since wrote, "Personally, I find the cultural lag between what the published research shows and what clinicians persist in claiming to do with their favorite devices even more disheartening than the adverse evidence itself" (p. 27). Some researchers have recently begun to apply Bayesian probabilities to neuropsychological assessment. That encouraging trend is long overdue.

REFERENCES

American Psychiatric Association (1987). *Diagnostic and statistical manual of mental disorders* (3rd ed., rev.). Washington, DC: Author.

Baldessarini, R.J., Finklestein, S., & Arana, G.W. (1983). The predictive power of diagnostic tests and the effect of prevalence of illness. *Archives of General Psychiatry, 40,* 569–573.

Cohen, J. (1990). Things I have learned (so far). *American Psychologist, 45,* 1304–1312.

Clarkin, J.F., Widiger, T.A., Frances, A., Hurt, S.W., & Gilmore, M. (1983). Prototypic typology and the borderline personality disorder. *Journal of Abnormal Psychology, 92,* 263–275.

Christensen, H., Hadzi-Pavlovic, D., & Jacomb, P. (1991). The psychometric differentiation of dementia from normal aging: A meta-analysis. *Psychological Assessment, 3,* 147–155.

desRosiers, G. (1992). Primary or depressive dementia: Psychometric assessment. *Clinical Psychology Review, 12,* 307–343.

Elwood, R.W. (in press). The clinical utility of the MMPI-2 in diagnosing unipolar depression among male alcoholics. *Journal of Personality Assessment.*

Elwood, R.W. (1991). The Wechsler Memory Scale-Revised: Psychometric characteristics and clinical application. *Neuropsychology Review, 2,* 179–201.

Evans, D.A., Funkenstein, H., Albert, M.S., Scherr, P.A., Cook, N.R., Chown, M.J., Heert, L.E., Hennekens, C.H., & Taylor, J.O. (1989). Prevalence of Alzheimer's disease in a community population of older persons. *Journal of the American Medical Association, 262,* 2551–2556.

Gerardi, R., Keane, T.M., & Penk, W. (1989). Sensitivity and specificity in developing diagnostic tests of combat-related post-traumatic stress disorder (PTSD). *Journal of Clinical Psychology, 45,* 691–703.

Gordon, N.G. (1977). Base rates and the decision making model in clinical neuropsychology. *Cortex, 23,* 3–10.

Griner, P.F., Mayewski, R.J., Mushlin, A.I., & Greenland, P. (1981). Selection and interpretation of diagnostic tests and procedures: Principles and applications. *Annals of Internal Medicine, 94*, 557–592.

Kulka, R.A., Schlenger, W.E., Fairbank, J.A., Hough, R.L., Jordan, B.K., Marmar, C.R., & Weiss, D.S. (1988). *Contractual report of findings from the National Vietnam Veterans Readjustment Study*. Research Triangle Park, NC: Research Triangle Institute.

Leonberger, F.T. (1989). The question of organicity: Is it still functional? *Professional Psychology: Research and Practice, 20*, 411–414.

Loring, D.W., Lee, G.P., Martin, R.C., & Meador, K.J. (1989). Verbal and visual memory index discrepancies from the Wechsler Memory Scale-Revised: Cautions in interpretation. *Psychological Assessment, 1*, 198–202.

Masur, D.M., Fuld, P., Blau, A.D., Thal, L.J., Levin, H.S., & Aronson, M.K. (1989). Distinguishing normal and demented elderly with the Selective Reminding Test. *Journal of Clinical and Experimental Neuropsychology, 11*, 615–630.

McKhann, G., Drachman, D., Folstein, M., Katzman, R., Price, D., & Stadlan, E.M. (1984). Clinical diagnosis of Alzheimer's disease: Report of the NINCDS-ADRDA Work Group under the auspices of Department of Health and Human Services Task Force on Alzheimer's Disease. *Neurology, 34*, 939–944.

Meehl, P.E. (1960). The cognitive activity of the clinician. *American Psychologist, 15*, 19–27.

Meehl, P.E., & Rosen, A. (1955). Antecedent probability and the efficiency of psychometric signs, patterns, or cutting scores. *Psychological Bulletin, 52*, 194–216.

Moldin, S.O., Gottesman, I.I., Rice, J.P., & Erlenmeyer-Kimling, L. (1991). Replicated psychometric correlates of schizophrenia. *American Journal of psychiatry, 148*, 762–767.

Rapp, S.R., Parisi, S.A., Walsh, D.A., & Wallace, C.E. (1988). Detecting depression in elderly medical inpatients. *Journal of Consulting and Clinical Psychology, 56*, 509–513.

Rorer, L.G., & Dawes, R.M. (1982). A base-rate bootstrap. *Journal of Consulting and Clinical Psychology, 50*, 419–425.

Rosnow, R.L., & Rosenthal, R. (1989). Statistical procedures and the justification of knowledge in the psychological science. *American Psychologist, 44*, 1276–1284.

Satz, P. (1966). A block rotation task: The application of multivariate and decision theory analysis for the prediction of organic brain disorder. *Psychological Monographs, 80* (21, Whole No. 629).

Satz, P., Fennell, E., & Reilly, C. (1970). The predictive validity of six neurodiagnostic tests: A decision theory analysis. *Journal of Consulting and Clinical Psychology, 34*, 375–381.

Satz, P. (1972). Pathological left-handedness: An exploratory model. *Cortex, 10*, 121–135.

Sines, J.O. (1966). Actuarial methods in personality assessment. In B.A. Maher (Ed.), *Progress in experimental personality research* (pp. 133–193). New York: Academic Press.

Sunderland, T., Hill, J.L., Mellow, A.M., Lawlor, B.A., Gundersheimer, J., Newhouse, P.A., & Grafman, J.H. (1989). Clock drawing in Alzheimer's disease: A novel measure of dementia severity. *Journal of the American Geriatrics Society, 37*, 725–729.

Widiger, T.A., Hurt, S.W., Frances, A., Clarkin, J.F., & Gilmore, M. (1984). Diagnostic efficiency and DSM-III. *Archives of General Psychiatry, 41*, 1005–1012.

Wiggins, J.S. (1973). *Personality and prediction: Principles of personality assessment*. Reading, MA: Addison-Wesley.

Willis, W.G. (1984). Reanalysis of an actuarial approach to neuropsychological diagnosis in consideration of base rates. *Journal of Consulting and Clinical Psychology, 53*, 567–569.

Wolfe-Klein, G.P., Silverstone, F.A., Levy, A.P., Brod, M.S., & Breuer, J. (1989). Screening for Alzheimers' disease by clock drawing. *Journal of the American Geriatrics Society, 37*, 730–734.

Zec, R.F., Landreth, E.S., Vicari, S.K., Feldman, E., Belman, J., Andrise, A., Robbs, R. Kumar, V., & Becker, R. (in press). Alzheimer Disease Assessment Scale: Useful for both early detection and staging of dementia of the Alzheimer type. *Alzheimer Disease and Related Disorders*.

The Clinical Neuropsychologist
1999, Vol. 13, No. 3, pp. 283–292

Practice Effects on Commonly Used Measures of Executive Function Across Twelve Months*

Michael R. Basso[1], Robert A. Bornstein[2], and Jennifer M. Lang
[1]University of Tulsa, OK, and [2]Neuropsychology Program, The Ohio State University, Columbia, OH

ABSTRACT

Fifty men (age $M = 32.50$; education $M = 14.98$ years) were administered the Wisconsin Card Sorting Test (WCST), Ruff Figural Fluency Test (FFT), Verbal Concept Attainment Test (VCAT) Trail Making Test, Parts A and B (TMT), and F-A-S Verbal Fluency at baseline and 12 months later. WCST, FFT, and VCAT scores improved significantly over a 12-month interval. In contrast, TMT and F-A-S scores did not change. Level of intellectual ability failed to moderate the effect of previous testing upon performance. Suggestions concerning the use of these measures in longitudinal research designs and clinical follow-up examinations are offered, and reliable change indices concerning these measures are included.

An important clinical and scientific application of neuropsychological measures is to assess changes in cognitive function across time. In re-examining individuals, inferences may be made regarding disease course, recovery of function, and effects of pharmacologic and rehabilitation interventions (Lezak, 1995). However, because of previous experience taking the tests, performance may improve, thereby obscuring true changes in neuropsychological function. In particular, improvement due to practice may be especially pronounced on measures of executive function.

Measures of executive function tend to present examinees with novel problem-solving contexts, and they assess the capacity to generate appropriate solutions and to recognize abstract concepts. During the course of initial testing, examinees are apt to learn strategies for successful performance.

With repeated exposure, test-taking strategies may be refined (cf. Anastasi & Urbina, 1997), yielding improved test scores across time. Furthermore, responses to test items may become more automatic and require less attention and concentration than during prior administrations (cf. Kaufman, 1990). Thus, what is measured in a re-examination of executive function performance may be quite different from what is assessed during an initial examination.

Despite this potential, relatively little is known about the effects of repeated examinations on measures of executive function. Few studies have detailed the effects of re-testing on such measures (cf. McCaffrey & Westervelt, 1995). Moreover, test manuals and source publications for some commonly used measures such as the Controlled Oral Word Association Test (Benton & Hamsher, 1978),

*We thank A. Harkness, R. Hogan, and B. Roper for their helpful comments regarding previous drafts of this manuscript.

Preparation of this manuscript was supported in part by a grant from the National Institute of Mental Health (MH454649) to R.A. Bornstein.

Portions of this data were presented at the 1996 and 1997 annual conventions of the American Psychological Association.

Address correspondence to: M.R. Basso, Department of Psychology, University of Tulsa, 600 South College Avenue, Tulsa, OK 74104, USA. E-mail: Michael-Basso@utulsa.edu

Accepted for publication: March 23, 1999.

Trail Making Test, Parts A and B (Reitan & Wolfson, 1993), and Verbal Concept Attainment Test (Bornstein & Leason, 1985) do not include data concerning the effects of previous testing. In the manual for the Wisconsin Card Sorting Test (Heaton, Chelune, Talley, Kay, & Curtiss, 1993), a set of adolescents is reported to have been administered the test twice during a month, but the magnitude and significance of change is not reported. In contrast, the Ruff Figural Fluency Test manual (Ruff, 1988) reports data concerning repeated testing across 6 months, and indicates that number of designs increases upon re-testing whereas the perseverative error ratio does not change.

A further factor that has yet to be thoroughly examined concerns the length of intertest interval. Some investigations have examined performance change on measures of attention and new learning across relatively short time intervals such as 1–2 weeks (e.g., Bornstein, Baker, & Douglass, 1987; McCaffrey, Ortega, Orsillo, Nelles, & Haase, 1992). These authors have found substantial improvement on measures of new learning and attention, but similar improvement may not extend to measures of executive function. Furthermore, such short intertest periods may bear little relevance to typical clinical practice or outcome research, wherein repeat examinations often occur in 6- or 12-month intervals (e.g., Dikmen, Machamer, Temkin, & McLean, 1990; Phillips & McGlone, 1995). Yet, little research has examined performance changes over these longer time periods. Hence, the degree to which practice influences performance over long intertest periods remains uncertain.

To address these issues, the present study determined whether performance on measures of executive function is subject to the effects of prior testing, particularly over a relatively long intertest interval. Commonly used measures of executive function were administered at baseline and 12 months later, and performance during both intervals was compared using repeated measures analyses of variance. Performance in a group of neurologically normal individuals was studied rather than a patient group, because performance changes associated with practice would potentially be confounded by genuine clinical improvement in the latter group. By examining performance in a sample of normal individuals only, any significant

improvement in test scores would be attributable to practice and measurement error rather than recovery from illness. In addition to determining whether prior testing yields subsequent increases in test scores, we examined the contributions of measurement error to change in performance. Recent investigations have proposed that it is important to take such error into consideration when deciding whether performance variation is due to genuine change in function or measurement error (Chelune, Naugle, Luders, Sedlak, & Awad, 1993). In so doing, base-rates of change on neuropsychological measures may be estimated. Furthermore, intellectual ability has been shown to moderate the effects of practice on the Wechsler Adult Intelligence Scale-Revised (Rapport, Brines, Axelrod, & Theisen, 1997). Specifically, Rapport et al. showed that individuals with average and above-average IQs display greater improvement upon re-testing than do those with low-average IQs. Regarding executive function, these findings suggest that individuals with above average intellectual ability may show greater improvement than those with a lower level of intelligence. Towards this end, we also examined whether intelligence moderated the magnitude of practice effects.

METHOD

Participants

The participants were 82 men who were recruited from the community through newspaper advertisements, and none was paid for his participation. Only men were recruited due to logistic limitations in recruiting sufficient numbers of women; rather than recruit small numbers of men and women we opted to recruit a relatively large group of men. The group was composed of 78 Caucasians, 2 African Americans, and 2 Hispanics. At baseline, average age of the entire sample was 31.90 years ($SD = 9.00$), and mean education level was 14.56 years ($SD = 2.26$). During each assessment interval, informal interviews were conducted to screen participants for neurological disease, head injury, learning disabilities, or other medical illness. Participants were also screened for psychiatric disorders through a structured clinical interview (Structured Clinical Interview for the DSM-III-R: Spitzer, Williams, Gibbon, & First, 1990). None were excluded on the basis of these screens.

Of the original 82 participants, 50 returned to complete the second assessment interval. To rule out potential bias between those who did and did not complete the protocol, we tested whether significant differences existed between the groups on demographic variables and baseline neuropsychological performance. Univariate analyses of variance (ANOVAs) were computed for age, education, and each test index. The groups differed only with respect to Full Scale IQ, Verbal IQ, and Trail Making Test, Part B performance (p's < .05), with the participants who completed the study having better performance than those who did not. Specifically, those who completed the protocol had mean Full Scale IQs of 109.30 (SD = 12.29), Verbal IQs of 108.28 (SD = 11.99), and Trail Making Test, Part B scores of 48.70 s. (SD = 17.76), whereas those who did not finish the study had average Full Scale IQs of 100.97 (SD = 12.11), Verbal IQs of 98.93 (SD = 12.27), and Trail Making Test, Part B scores of 56.96 s. (SD = 15.31). These findings suggest that there were some slight distinctions in neuropsychological performance between the two groups, although relatively few differences existed on measures of executive function.

Of the 50 participants who completed the two assessment intervals, age ranged from 20 to 59, with a mean of 32.50 years (SD = 9.27). Education ranged from 12 to 19 years, and the mean education level was 14.98 years (SD = 1.93). This group of participants included 48 Caucasians, 1 African American, and 1 Hispanic. All remaining data analyses concern the performance of these 50 participants.

Materials and Procedures

At baseline, subjects were administered the Wechsler Adult Intelligence Scale-Revised (WAIS-R: Wechsler, 1981). The WAIS-R was administered only at baseline due to time limitations. The Wisconsin Card Sorting Test (Heaton et al., 1993), Ruff Figural Fluency Test (Ruff, 1988), Verbal Concept Attainment Test (VCAT: Bornstein & Leason, 1985), F-A-S Verbal Fluency (Benton & Hamsher, 1978), and Trail Making Test, Parts A and B (Reitan & Wolfson, 1993) were administered at baseline and at 12-month follow-up. All tests included in the study were administered in accordance with respective standardization rules by technicians who were employed within a hospital neuropsychology laboratory. Hence, all participants were given the same test instructions, and they were requested to give their best performance across all tasks. Before administering tests to participants, a doctoral-level psychologist trained the psychometrists and judged their test-administration skills as competent. Furthermore, psycho-metrists were periodically monitored to make certain they were administering tests within the parameters of standardization instructions. Moreover, psychometrists were unaware of specific hypotheses related to the present study.

RESULTS

To examine whether intelligence mediated changes in performance across re-administrations, a categorical variable was created based on WAIS-R Full Scale IQ scores. Groups were dichotomized based on a cutoff score of 110 in order to remain consistent with relevant clinical benchmarks. Specifically, IQs of 110 and above comprised above average to very superior intelligence, and IQs of 109 and below were labeled average to borderline normal (Wechsler, 1981). Although some individuals had scores that fell in the below average and superior ranges, there were too few to permit meaningful comparisons. Thus, they were combined with participants having average and above-average intelligence, respectively.

Twenty-six participants had IQs in the range of 110 to 137, and 24 had IQs ranging from 109 to 78. The above average group had a mean Full Scale IQ of 118.73 (SD = 5.86), mean age of 34.56 years (SD = 10.57), and mean education of 15.46 years (SD = 1.75). The average IQ group was comprised of 24 men with a mean Full Scale IQ of 99.08 (SD = 8.67), mean age of 30.38 years (SD = 7.24), and mean education of 14.46 years (SD = 2.02). To test for differences in IQ, age, and education between the two groups, three ANOVAs were completed, and only the difference in Full Scale IQ scores was statistically significant ($F(1, 48)$ = 89.38, p < .001).

To examine the extent to which neuropsychological performance changed as a function of previous testing, all scores were entered into a MANOVA. The multivariate model was chosen to protect against Type I error. The MANOVA consisted of a 2 (IQ Groups) × 2 (Time) × 15 (Scales) mixed-factor design, with Time and Scales being repeated. Significant multivariate effects were succeeded by appropriate univariate analyses. Intelligence level did not appear to mediate performance increments across time, as the interactions of IQ Groups × Time × Scale and IQ Groups × Time were not significant. Consequently, the effect of IQ Groups was not examined in subsequent univariate analyses. In contrast, the interaction of Time × Scales (Hotellings' $F(14, 36)$ = 6.56, p < .001) was significant, indicating that performance changed significantly across time only on some measures. As such, the effect of Time on each Scale was tested in subsequent univariate analyses.

Wisconsin Card Sorting Test Univariate Analyses

As shown in Table 1, re-testing resulted in significantly improved performances on nearly all indices on the Wisconsin Card Sorting Test. The magnitude of change was particularly evident on the number of trials necessary to complete the test. Specifically, on average, 101.12 cards were required at baseline, whereas only 84.74 trials were necessary 12 months later. In addition, the number of perseverative errors and perseverative responses decreased by nearly half upon re-testing.

Ruff Figural Fluency Test Univariate Analyses

Prior to analysis, raw scores on the Ruff Figural Fluency Test were converted to T scores based upon normative tables included in the test manual (Ruff, 1988). As shown in Table 2, number of unique designs increased 7 T-score points (nearly an entire standard deviation) at the 12-month follow-up, whereas there was no change in the ratio of perseverative errors to unique designs. These findings are consistent with those reported by Ruff (1988).

VCAT Univariate Analyses

Regarding VCAT performance, the main effect of time was significant, and as shown in Table 2, VCAT scores increased nearly one point at the

Table 1. Statistical Comparisons of Wisconsin Card Sorting Test Indices Across Time.

Index	Baseline		12 Months		F
	M	(SD)	M	(SD)	
Categories	5.16	(1.38)	5.42	(1.55)	1.70
Number of Trials	101.12	(22.87)	84.74	(18.59)	21.99***
% Correct	76.48	(12.39)	80.99	(12.45)	6.79**
Errors	26.12	(18.04)	16.68	(11.88)	17.65***
Perseverative Errors	14.20	(10.53)	8.44	(6.16)	20.47***
% Perseverative Errors	12.79	(7.52)	9.84	(7.45)	7.37**
% Conceptual Response	70.23	(17.94)	76.10	(18.74)	5.60*
Perseverative Responses	16.02	(12.82)	9.34	(7.70)	17.98***
Learning to Learn	−3.14	(5.76)	−.72	(3.90)	8.32**
Failure to Maintain Set	1.16	(1.67)	.80	(1.16)	1.62

Note. $df = (1, 48)$. * $= p < .05$; ** $= p < .01$; *** $= p < .001$.

Table 2. Statistical Comparisons of Ruff Figural Fluency Test, Trail Making Test, VCAT, and F-A-S Verbal Fluency Performances Across Time.

Index	Baseline		12 Months		F
	M	(SD)	M	(SD)	
Ruff Figural Fluency					
Unique Designs	52.02	(8.59)	58.83	(8.86)	49.39***
Ratio	48.39	(9.84)	49.20	(8.30)	.06
TMT, Part A	21.52	(7.54)	21.32	(7.36)	.41
TMT, Part B	48.70	(17.76)	47.72	(19.33)	.49
VCAT	20.76	(2.45)	21.50	(1.88)	9.54**
F-A-S Verbal Fluency	47.68	(10.82)	48.42	(12.06)	.48

Note. $df = (1, 48)$. Trail Making Test (TMT) performances are reported in seconds. Ruff Figural Fluency performances are reported in T scores. F-A-S performances reflect number of words generated with age, sex, and education corrections added (Benton & Hamsher, 1978). VCAT = Verbal Concept Attainment Test. ** $= p < .01$; *** $= p < .001$.

12-month examination. Although one point may not appear to be a large increase, this likely reflects a ceiling effect; the maximum score on the VCAT is 23, and baseline scores were nearly 21.

Trail Making Test, Parts A and B and F-A-S Verbal Fluency Univariate Analyses
As shown in Table 2, performances on Trail Making Test, Parts A and B did not improve as a result of re-testing. Regarding F-A-S verbal fluency, Table 2 demonstrates that re-testing similarly had no effect on performance.

Reliable Change Intervals
Although the multivariate and univariate analyses show which test scores changed significantly across 12 months, they do not describe the magnitude of change. To address this issue, mean change scores could have been calculated. Nonetheless, such change scores may fail to characterize fully the range of change demonstrated by the sample. Thus, in order to estimate the range of change in a thorough manner, estimates of reliable change were calculated (cf. Jacobson & Truax, 1991). Reliable change indices describe the base-rate range of change on a test while accounting for random fluctuation across time (i.e., measurement error inherent in psychological tests) and the influence of previous testing. Such change estimates have been employed in studies of neuropsychological change in clinical samples, and have been useful in discriminating practice effects from genuine recovery of cognitive function (e.g., Chelune et al., 1993).

One method of computing reliable change was proposed by Jacobson and Truax (1991) and elaborated upon by Chelune et al. (1993). With this strategy, reliable change is calculated on the basis of the standard error of differences (SE_{DIFF}: Anastasi & Urbina, 1997). However, as noted by Charter (1996), this method may be less than ideal for assessing change on measures that are susceptible to the effects of practice. Specifically, the SE_{DIFF} assumes that error between the assessments is uncorrelated, and is intended for use in assessment situations in which practice effects are irrelevant (e.g., attitude scales). In order to compute reliable change on measures in which measurement error is likely correlated, Charter (1996)

suggests using the Standard Error of Prediction (SEP), which is computed as follows:

$$SEP = SD_{Y2}\left(\left(1 - r_{Y1Y2}{}^2\right)^{1/2}\right).$$

In this equation, SD_{Y2} is the standard deviation of scores during the second assessment interval, and r_{Y1Y2} is the correlation between test scores across the assessment intervals. The confidence interval was computed by multiplying the SEP by $+1.64$, and then summing the positive and negative values with the estimated true retest score. Similar to Chelune et al., the 90% confidence interval for each index (permitting a 5% interval at both tails of the sampling distribution of change scores) was used. The estimated true score is calculated as follows (Charter, 1996):

$$Y_{TRUE} = M + r\left(Y_{OBS} - M\right).$$

In this equation, M is the sample mean of the test, Y_{OBS} is the actual score obtained by the individual, and r is the reliability coefficient. In the present study, internal consistency coefficients could not be calculated for the Wisconsin Card Sorting Test and Trail Making Test, because items on these tests are dependent upon one another. Consequently, to estimate reliability for these measures, the test-retest coefficient was used to estimate true scores at 12 months. To remain consistent across indices, this same coefficient was used to estimate true scores for the VCAT, F-A-S Verbal Fluency, and Ruff Figural Fluency Tests. Test-retest coefficients for each index are listed in Tables 3 and 4. Regarding the confidence intervals, if the actual score obtained by the individual falls outside of the computed confidence interval, the obtained test score is significantly different from expected levels, and it is unlikely that the change in score from baseline to 12 months is due to measurement error alone.

In Tables 3 and 4, the mean estimated true scores at 12 months are listed together with the SEP and resulting 90% confidence intervals for each test index. Also listed in these tables are the number of times that obtained scores fell either below or above the expected confidence interval of scores based upon the SEP. Of particular importance, these data indicate that a wide range of retest scores may fall within the 90% confidence interval. For instance, on the Wisconsin Card Sorting Test, an individual's performance could increase or decrease across a range of two obtained categories, 17 errors, 9 perseverative errors, or 11% perseverative errors, and still reflect measurement error rather than meaningful change. Similarly, an individual could increase or decrease performance by as much as 10 T-score units on the Ruff Unique Designs index, 24-s on Trail Making Test, Part B, or 12 words on Verbal Fluency without displaying meaningful changes in performance. These large confidence intervals imply that much variation in executive function performance may be expected across 12 months, and such changes are due entirely to the effects of practice and random measurement error.

An additional implication of the data in Tables 3 and 4 is that normal individuals do not uniformly improve their performance on these measures.

Table 3. Descriptive Statistics and Confidence Intervals for Estimated True Scores at 12-Month Follow-Up on Wisconsin Card Sorting Test Indices.

	M	r_{Y1Y2}	SEP	90% CI	Significant Changes	
					Above	Below
Categories	5.42	.54	1.30	±2	0	3
Number of Trials	84.73	.30	17.71	±29	4	0
Errors	16.68	.50	10.29	±17	0	0
Perseverative Errors	8.43	.52	5.25	±9	2	0
% Perseverative Errors	9.85	.47	6.56	±11	1	0
% Conceptual Response	76.11	.54	15.74	±26	0	2
Perseverative Responses	9.34	.50	6.65	±11	2	0
Learning to Learn	.73	.36	3.63	±6	0	1
Failure to Maintain Set	.80	−.02	1.15	±2	5	0

Note. Mean scores represent the mean estimated true score for the sample at 12-month follow-up. The confidence intervals are at the 90% level (i.e., 1.64 * *SEP*). All confidence interval values are rounded to the nearest whole digit. To use the confidence intervals, the 90% confidence band should be summed with an individual's estimated true score. Significant changes reflect the frequency of obtained scores that fell above or below the confidence interval.

Table 4. Descriptive Statistics and Confidence Intervals for Estimated True Scores at 12-Month Follow-Up on Ruff Figural Fluency Test, Trail Making Test, Verbal Concept Attainment Test, and F-A-S Verbal Fluency.

	M	r_{Y1Y2}	SEP	90% CI	Significant Changes	
					Increases	Decreases
Ruff Figural Fluency						
Unique Designs	58.66	.71	6.22	±10	0	0
Ratio Score	49.20	.39	7.64	±13	0	0
TMT, Part A	21.33	.38	6.80	±11	1	0
TMT, Part B	47.92	.64	14.85	±24	0	0
VCAT	21.50	.63	1.45	±2	0	1
F-A-S	48.41	.80	7.23	±12	0	0

Note. Unique Designs and Ratio scores reflect estimated true T scores at 12 months. Trail Making Test (TMT) estimated mean true scores are reported in seconds. F-A-S estimated mean true scores reflect total words (corrected for age, education, and sex) generated at 12 months. VCAT = Verbal Concept Attainment Test. The confidence intervals are at the 90% level (i.e., 1.64 * *SEP*). All confidence interval values are rounded to the nearest whole digit. To use the confidence intervals, the 90% confidence band should be summed with an individual's estimated true score. Significant changes reflect the frequency of obtained scores that fell above or below the confidence interval.

Although mean performance of the sample tended to improve across time, some individuals showed worsening performance at 12-month follow-up. Notably, with respect to the 90% confidence intervals, no individual obtained a score that reflected significant improvement in performance. Nonetheless, several individuals showed performance declines that exceeded the 90% confidence intervals. Thus, even normal individuals can show significant declines across time without corresponding impairment of brain function.

DISCUSSION

As indicated earlier, the measures studied in the present research are among the most commonly administered tests of executive function. Yet, prior to the current investigation, little was known concerning the degree to which performance on these measures changes as a function of repeated administration, particularly over a long intertest period such as 12 months. The present study shows which of these measures are likely to be influenced by practice, and indicates the magnitude of practice-mediated improvement that might be expected across a 1-year period. Specifically, the results show that test scores on the Wisconsin Card Sorting Test, VCAT, and Ruff Figural Fluency Test improved significantly across 12 months. Moreover, the rate of improvement due to practice was generally quite large, and, as demonstrated by the reliable change indices, wide variation in performance was common within this sample of individuals.

These findings may appear counter-intuitive, as it initially may seem unlikely that a single-exposure to test stimuli would influence subsequent performance after 12 months. Specifically, after such a long time period and brief exposure, test stimuli might be forgotten. Nonetheless, the data suggest that neurologically normal individuals are able to retain knowledge of testing over extended time periods, thereby influencing subsequent performance.

Although performance increments may be due in part to recall of the testing tasks, it is unlikely that specific test elements are remembered such as words included in the VCAT or the specific

progression of rule changes on the Wisconsin Card Sorting Test. Rather, a more probable explanation is that procedural knowledge of test demands and effective test-taking strategies was retained, thereby shaping and enhancing subsequent performance. For example, perhaps during the baseline examinations, participants recognized more efficient figure generation tactics for the Ruff Figural Fluency Test. Additionally, during the baseline examination, examinees may have realized that correct sets shifted in a predictable fashion on the Wisconsin Card Sorting Test. Upon re-examination, recall of these strategies and procedures may have resulted in an overall improvement on test scores.

Along with retention of effective strategies, other aspects of the testing situation may have yielded improved performance. For instance, novelty of testing likely diminished with re-testing, thereby reducing any potential anxiety associated with the examination process (cf. Anastasi & Urbina, 1997). Hence, examinees may have been more comfortable and better able to focus attention to testing tasks during subsequent assessment periods.

Despite probable retention of procedural knowledge of the tests, performance increments were not uniform across all measures. Hence, an additional contribution of the present research is the demonstration that retesting did not yield improved performance on F-A-S verbal fluency and the Trail Making Test, Parts A and B. This suggests that these measures are not subject to significant practice effects across 12 months. Furthermore, interactions involving IQ group and time or IQ group and scale were not significant, thereby implying that the presence and magnitude of practice effects on measures of executive function are similar among individuals of average and above-average intelligence. This finding parallels the results of Rapport et al. (1997). Similar to the present research, Rapport et al. found that average and above-average IQ groups demonstrated equivalent improvement in IQ scores across time. In contrast, these same two groups showed greater improvement on the WAIS-R than individuals with low-average IQ. Perhaps with the inclusion of a low-average IQ group, intelligence level may mediate rate of improvement on these executive function measures.

In accounting for the differential effects of retesting on performance, it seems likely that practice effects are moderated by task complexity. Specifically, the strategies required for successful performance on F-A-S Verbal Fluency and the Trail Making Test, Parts A and B are relatively simple. In comparison, the Wisconsin Card Sorting Test, Ruff Figural Fluency, and VCAT seem to require a more sophisticated degree of strategy generation and hypothesis testing. With these latter measures, effective test-taking strategies may not be apparent to examinees until an initial administration has been completed. Thereafter, examinees may continue to use these strategies, resulting in enhanced outcomes. Hence, the ability to generate solutions in a novel problem-solving context is probably not assessed during a re-examination. Rather, because the test-taking demands are apparently familiar, recollection rather than generation of efficient problem-solving strategies may be what is actually assessed in a re-examination.

These findings have implications for investigations using the Wisconsin Card Sorting Test, VCAT, and Ruff Figural Fluency Test. In particular, a potential application of these measures is to determine the relative benefit of clinical interventions across time. In order to detect true improvement, the current data imply that multiple baselines might be worthwhile to employ. For instance, McCaffrey and Westervelt (1995) suggest using dual baseline assessments. They hypothesize that, upon a second administration, practice effects may plateau, and all subsequent changes in performance will primarily reflect the influence of interventions. Accordingly, this method may provide a more stable and reliable estimate of baseline performance, thereby diminishing the potential confound of practice effects. Alternatively, inclusion of a no-treatment control group in intervention studies might yield indirect estimates of practice effects; any change in performance among a no-treatment control group would be attributable to measurement error, practice effects, and variation associated with disease course. In contrast to the Wisconsin Card Sorting Test, VCAT, and Ruff Figural Fluency Test, no effect of practice was observed on Trail Making Test, Parts A and B or F-A-S verbal fluency, thereby commending their use for serial examinations.

With respect to clinical practice, in which multiple baselines or no-treatment control groups are largely impractical or irrelevant, the reliable change index data may hold some utility. Specifically, the estimates of reliable change indicate that relatively large variations in performance may reflect the confounding effects of practice and measurement error. Towards this end, the reliable change indices may provide a comparison for patient change, thereby granting a means of distinguishing genuine clinical change from measurement error. Nonetheless, certain issues may limit the applicability of these reliable change indices to clinical samples. In particular, practice effects are assumed to reflect memory for prior testing. Owing to potential memory difficulties, patient samples may not recall testing tasks to the same degree as normals. Consequently, the magnitude of practice effects may differ between normal and clinical samples. Further complicating matters, contributions of practice effects and actual clinical change tend to be confounded in certain clinical samples (e.g., head injury, cerebral vascular accidents). For instance, individuals with closed-head injuries tend to experience improved executive function as they recover from acute insult (Dikmen, Reitan, & Temkin, 1983). Because retesting and recovery of function occur during the same time intervals, the distinction of practice effects from genuine improvement may be difficult to make. Hence, the current data may not present an ideal method for estimating reliable change in clinical samples, but they may provide a reasonable option. Accordingly, as performance increments or decrements approximate the upper and lower bounds of the confidence intervals, inferences of genuine change could be made with increasing confidence.

These suggestions for re-assessments notwithstanding, the current data imply that re-testing with these executive function measures may be susceptible to significant error. In particular, the magnitude of the reliable change intervals indicates that measurement error contributes greatly to the variance in re-test scores. Consequently, the capacity of these measures to reflect meaningful changes in executive function seems grossly diminished. To illustrate this point, consider the "number of correct categories" index on the

Wisconsin Card Sorting Test. On this index, the reliable change confidence interval includes fluctuations as large as four categories. Thus nearly two thirds of all score fluctuations possible on this index (possible scores range from 0 to 6) will reflect measurement error rather than genuine changes in function. Although it remains uncertain whether the current results generalize to clinical populations, they do raise questions concerning the meaning of re-test scores on measures of executive function.

Finally, it is important to recognize potential limitations of the present study. Specifically, the participants tended to be predominantly Caucasian males who ranged in age from 20 to 59. They were relatively well educated, and they generally possessed average to above-average intelligence. It remains uncertain whether the current findings would generalize to other demographic groups. For instance, because practice effects appear to diminish with increasing age (Horton, 1992), these data may not generalize to elderly individuals. Regarding gender, there is evidence that men and women have differing patterns of performance, particularly on measures of verbal ability (cf. Halpern, 1992). Thus, the present data concerning F-A-S verbal fluency may not be especially relevant to repeated neuropsychological assessments of women. Nonetheless, according to their source publications, gender does not mediate performance on the Wisconsin Card Sorting Test, Ruff Figural Fluency Test, VCAT, or Trail Making Test, Parts A and B, thereby suggesting that the current findings concerning these tests likely generalize to women. Furthermore, because there tend to be some differences between ethnic groups on measures of neuropsychological function (cf. Kaufman, 1990; Lezak, 1995), these findings may not generalize to non-Caucasians.

Yet, despite these potential limitations, there is little or no published information concerning the influence of repeated testing on executive function measures, particularly over relatively long intertest intervals. Consequently, because these measures are widely used in clinical and scientific applications, the present data may be particularly important to the practitioner and investigator. Notably, these findings indicate which executive function measures are susceptible to practice effects, and they provide compelling evidence that even apparently substantial changes in performance may reflect the confounding effects of practice and measurement error.

REFERENCES

Anastasi, A., & Urbina, S. (1997). *Psychological testing* (7th ed.). Upper Saddle River, NJ: Prentice-Hall.

Benton, A.L., & Hamsher, K. des. (1978). *Multilingual aphasia examination*. Iowa City, IA: University of Iowa.

Bornstein, R.A., Baker, G.B., & Douglass, A.B. (1987). Short-term retest reliability of the Halstead-Reitan Battery in a normal sample. *The Journal of Nervous and Mental Disease, 175*, 229–232.

Bornstein, R.A., & Leason, M. (1985). Effects on localized lesions on the Verbal Concept Attainment Test. *Journal of Clinical and Experimental Neuropsychology, 7*, 421–429.

Charter, R.A. (1996). Revisiting the standard errors of measurement, estimate, and prediction and their application to test scores. *Perceptual and Motor Skills, 82*, 1139–1144.

Chelune, G.J., Naugle, R.I., Luders, H., Sedlak, J., & Awad, I.A. (1993). Individual change after epilepsy surgery: Practice effects and base-rate information. *Neuropsychology, 7*, 41–52.

Dikmen, S., Machamer, J., Temkin, N., & McLean, A. (1990). Neuropsychological recovery in patients with moderate to severe head injury: 2 year follow-up. *Journal of Clinical and Experimental Neuropsychology, 12*, 507–519.

Dikmen, S., Reitan, R.M., & Temkin, N. (1983). Neuropsychological recovery in head injury. *Archives of Neurology, 40*, 333–338.

Halpern, D.F. (1992). *Sex differences in cognitive abilities* (2nd ed.). Hillsdale, NJ: Erlbaum.

Heaton, R.K., Chelune, G.J., Talley, J.L., Kay, G.G., & Curtiss, G. (1993). *Wisconsin Card Sorting Test manual*. Odessa, FL: Psychological Assessment Resources.

Horton, A.M. (1992). Neuropsychological practice effects * age: A brief note. *Perceptual and Motor Skills, 75*, 257–258.

Jacobson, N.S., & Truax, P. (1991). Clinical significance: A statistical approach to defining meaningful change in psychotherapy research. *Journal of Consulting and Clinical Psychology, 59*, 12–19.

Kaufman, A.S. (1990). *Assessing adolescent and adult intelligence*. Boston: Allyn & Bacon.

Lezak, M.D. (1995). *Neuropsychological assessment* (3rd ed.). New York: Oxford University Press.

McCaffrey, R.J., & James, H.J. (1995). Issues associated with repeated neuropsychological assessments. *Neuropsychology Review, 5,* 203–221.

McCaffery, R.J., Ortega, A., Orsillio, S.M., & Niles, W.B. (1992). Practice effects in repeated neuropsychological assessments. *The Clinical Neuropsychologist, 6,* 32–42.

Phillips, N.A., & McGlone, J. (1995). Grouped data do not tell the whole story: Individual analysis of cognitive change after temporal lobectomy. *Journal of Clinical and Experimental Neuropsychology, 17,* 713–724.

Rapport, L.J., Brines, D.B., Axelrod, B.N., & Theisen, M.E. (1997). Full scale IQ as mediator of practice effects: The rich get richer. *The Clinical Neuropsychologist, 11,* 375–380.

Reitan, R.M., & Wolfson, D. (1993). *The Halstead-Reitan Neuropsychological Test Battery.* Tucson, AZ.: Neuropsychology Press.

Ruff, R.M. (1988). *Ruff Figural Fluency Test administration manual.* San Diego: Neuropsychological Resources.

Ruff, R.M., Light, R.H., & Quayhagen, M. (1988). Selective reminding tests: A normative study of verbal learning in adults. *Journal of Clinical and Experimental Neuropsychology, 11,* 539–550.

Spitzer, R.L., Williams, J.B.W., Gibbon, M., & First, M.B. (1990). *Structured Clinical Interview for DSM-III-R.* Washington, DC: American Psychiatric Press.

Wechsler, D. (1981). *Wechsler Adult Intelligence Scale-Revised manual.* New York: The Psychological Corporation.

Journal of Clinical and Experimental Neuropsychology
1997, Vol. 19, No. 4, pp. 543–559

VIII-J

Assessment of Cognitive Deterioration in Individual Patients Following Cardiac Surgery: Correcting for Measurement Error and Practice Effects*

Eline F. Bruggemans[1], Fons J. R. Van de Vijver Hair[2], and Hans A. Huysmans[1]

[1]Department of Cardio-Thoracic Surgery, University Hospital, Leiden, The Netherlands, and [2]Tilburg University, The Netherlands

ABSTRACT

Assessment of cognitive change in individual patients may be confounded by unreliability of test scores and effects of repeated testing. An index correcting for both problems is proposed and compared with change indices that do not or do not adequately deal with measurement error and practice effects. These indices were used to examine cognitive deterioration in a sample of 63 patients undergoing cardiac surgery. It was demonstrated that for test measures with a low reliability, failure to correct for measurement error resulted in overestimation of deterioration rates. For test measures with a high reliability, but showing substantial practice effects, failure to correct for practice effects resulted in underestimation of deterioration rates. With the proposed index, cognitive deterioration shortly after cardiac surgery was most frequently observed for attention and psychomotor speed, less frequently for verbal fluency, and only occasionally for learning and memory.

Medical intervention may be accompanied by changes in cognitive functioning. Negative cognitive effects have been reported, for example, following epilepsy surgery (Chelune, 1992; Naugle, 1992), cardiac surgery involving extra-corporeal circulation (Benedict, 1994; Newman, 1993), intrathecal chemotherapy or central nervous system radiation therapy (Brown & Madan-Swain, 1993; Fletcher & Copeland, 1988; Roman & Sperduto, 1995), and pharmacotherapy of Parkinson's disease (Karayanidis, 1989; Saint-Cyr, Taylor, & Lang, 1993). Positive effects have sometimes been reported after pharmacotherapy of hypertension (Waldstein, Manuck, Ryan, & Muldoon, 1991) and of AIDS or AIDS-related complex (Everall, 1995; Maj, 1990). Cognitive effects of medical intervention are most frequently studied using a pretest-posttest design. Pretest to posttest changes in performance on neuropsychological tests are usually evaluated by means of a statistical test of the changes in group means. This method, however, is often not satisfactory for clinical practice because overall changes in group performance do not disclose changes in individual patients. Assessment of cognitive change at the individual level is important for evaluating individual risks or benefits of medical treatment and informing patients about anticipated outcomes.

Different indices for identifying individual change can be found in the literature. Most of these indices define an individual's test performance as significantly changed if the difference in test scores obtained before and after treatment (i.e., the observed change score) is larger than some criterion measure. For instance, in recent studies of the negative cognitive effects of temporal lobectomy or cardiac surgery, a decline in test performance was defined significant if a

---

* This study was supported by Grant 89.249 from the Netherlands Heart Foundation.
Address correspondence to: Eline F. Bruggemans, Department of Cardio-Thoracic Surgery, University Hospital, P.O. Box 9600, 2300 RC Leiden, The Netherlands.
Accepted for publication: January 29, 1997.

patient's pre- to post-operative test score decrement was at least one standard deviation (SD), the SD being generally determined on the distribution of the preoperative scores in the patient sample (Loring et al., 1995; Phillips & McGlone, 1995; Sellman, Holm, Ivert, & Semb, 1993; Shaw et al., 1986, 1987; Treasure et al., 1989). Such an SD criterion, however, can be criticized because it does not adequately deal with the problem of measurement error (i.e., imperfect reliability of test scores). When an unreliable test is applied, score fluctuations of more than one SD that are entirely due to measurement error will frequently be observed. Moreover, random score fluctuations may cause change scores of less than one SD when intervention effects do exist. Hence, application of the SD criterion may lead to both overestimation and underestimation of incidence rates.

Several suggestions have been made as to how measurement error can be taken into account in the assessment of individual change. Some authors have proposed an index in which the observed change score is divided by the standard error of measurement (SEM) of the pretest scores instead of the SD (e.g., Edwards, Yarvis, Mueller, Zingale, & Wagman, 1978; Jacobson, Follette, & Revenstorf, 1984; Shatz, 1981). More specifically, these authors suggested that a change score larger than 1.96 SEM, or, with rounding, 2 SEM, could be considered as statistically significant (p < .05). At first sight, this SEM criterion seems less arbitrary than the SD criterion because it takes into account test reliability: the less reliable the test, the greater the amount of score change required to be significant. Yet, it does not compensate for all effects of measurement error. A first criticism concerns the fact that the SEM statistic does not make allowance for the unreliability of the posttest scores. Score changes should be corrected for unreliability of the instrument at both the pretest and the posttest. Accordingly, alternative standard error measures have been put forward as a more appropriate denominator in the above change index, such as the standard error of the difference between the observed pre- and post-test scores (e.g., Christensen & Mendoza, 1986; Jacobson & Truax, 1991) and the standard error of prediction (e.g., Hsu, 1989, 1995; Knight, 1983).

A second criticism concerns the use of the observed change score in the numerator of the above change index. Unfortunately, all indices using this numerator can be criticized for having ambiguous statistical properties, irrespective of the type of standard error in the denominator. The reason is that the standard errors make, in effect, reference to estimated true change scores rather than observed change scores. Sampling distributions of statistics that are based on mixtures of observed-score and estimated-true-score characteristics are usually unknown. Consequently, the confidence intervals that are required to judge whether the individual has significantly changed cannot properly be determined. Thus, in order to correct for all effects of measurement error, the numerator of the index has also to be adapted. It is important to note that the recommendation to employ the individual's estimated true pretest score as a substitute for the observed pretest score (e.g., Knight, 1983; Speer, 1992, 1993) does not entirely solve the problem. The numerator should comprise both the estimated true pretest and the estimated true posttest score (e.g., Hageman & Arrindell, 1993). Recently, Zegers and Hafkenscheid (1994) suggested an index that adequately deals with the above criticisms with regard to both numerator and denominator. Their Reliable Change (RC) index is defined as the ratio of the estimated true change score to the estimated standard error of this score (details are given below).

All change indices described thus far have still one problem in common: They do not address the practice effects that frequently arise from repeated neuropsychological testing. In healthy subjects, improved test scores at retesting have been reported for many cognitive performance tests (e.g., Feinstein, Brown, & Ron, 1994; Macciocchi, 1990; Wing, 1980). Practice effects and measurement error should be carefully distinguished. Both reliable and unreliable tests may show practice effects. Some test measures with a high test-retest reliability, such as the Verbal IQ, Performance IQ, and Full Scale IQ of the Wechsler Adult Intelligence Scale (WAIS) or WAIS-Revised, showed a low test-retest stability in absolute test scores (Matarazzo, Carmody, & Jacobs, 1980; Matarazzo & Herman, 1984). Thus, also with a reliable test, practice effects should be dealt with in the assessment of intervention effects in individual patients. Otherwise, negative cognitive effects of intervention could be underestimated and positive effects overestimated.

A method that considers both measurement error and practice effects was recently proposed by Chelune, Naugle, Lüders, Sedlak, and Awad (1993) in a study on cognitive change following temporal lobectomy. These authors subtracted the mean practice effect observed in a control group from the patient's pre- to post-operative change in test scores before applying the RC index as defined by Jacobson and Truax (1991). There are, however, two difficulties associated with this method. First, measurement error is not adequately dealt with because the numerator of the RC index of Jacobson and Truax includes observed change scores rather than estimated true change scores. Second, it is counterintuitive to correct individual change scores by using the mean change score of controls because there is ample evidence of marked individual differences in the magnitude of practice effects (Matarazzo et al., 1980; Matarazzo & Herman, 1984).

A method that makes allowance for individual differences in practice effects and that is more familiar in the literature was employed by the same group of authors in analyzing the same data set (McSweeny, Naugle, Chelune, & Lüders, 1993). In a linear regression model, the posttest scores of the control group were predicted on the basis of their pretest scores. The regression coefficient and intercept of the control group's regression line were then applied to obtain predicted posttest scores for individual patients. A patient was said to be significantly changed at the posttest if the difference between the observed and the predicted posttest score divided by the standard error of prediction was larger than a criterion value. Yet, this method can again be criticized for not adequately dealing with measurement error. The regression model makes the incorrect assumption that the predictor (i.e., the pretest score) has been measured free of error. As a consequence, the unreliability of the pretest scores is not adequately taken into account (cf., Alder, Adam, & Arenberg, 1990; Blomqvist, 1977; Geenen & Van de Vijver, 1993; Jin, 1992; Myrtek & Foerster, 1986). To some extent, this criticism to the regression-based

index adopted by McSweeny et al. mirrors that raised to the SEM index described above because both indices consider the measurement error of one testing occasion only.

In the current study, an alternative technique is proposed that aims to deal with the above criticisms to existing change indices. Because it is an elaboration of the RC index of Zegers and Hafkenscheid (1994), it corrects for measurement error by using estimated true change scores. In addition, it corrects for individual variations in practice effects by contrasting a patient's estimated true change score with the estimated true change scores in a matched control group (i.e., a group of controls with similar pretest scores as the patient). To illustrate the results of this technique, an empirical comparison is made among six change indices, falling into three categories: (a) the SD index, which considers neither measurement error nor practice effects; (b) the RC indices of Jacobson and Truax (1991) and Zegers and Hafkenscheid, correcting for measurement error; and (c) the indices of Chelune et al. (1993) and McSweeny et al. (1993), and the currently proposed index, correcting for both measurement error and practice effects (hereafter called reliability-stability or RST indices). The neuropsychological data analyzed for this purpose were collected in a study performed on cardiac surgery patients. An analysis of the current data in terms of group means has been published elsewhere (Bruggemans, Van Dijk, & Huysmans, 1995).

METHOD

The data used for illustrative analysis were obtained as part of a longitudinal study of the cognitive effects of coronary artery bypass graft (CABG) surgery. A battery of neuropsychological tests was administered to 63 CABG patients 2 weeks preoperatively (T1), and 1 week (T2), 1 month (T3), and 6 months (T4) postoperatively. The effects of practice and relieved distress after surgery were controlled for by including the spouses of these patients, exposed to the same stressors associated with the operation and daily life, as a control group. A more detailed description of the methodology of this study can be found in Bruggemans et al. (1995).

Subjects
The 63 CABG patients (55 men, 8 women) and their 63 spouses were enrolled in the study at the University

Hospital of Leiden, The Netherlands. Exclusion criteria for patients and spouses were previous cardiac surgery with extracorporeal circulation; a history of neurological disorders (including cerebrovascular diseases), psychiatric illness, or alcohol or drug abuse; a preoperative Mini-Mental State Examination (MMSE; Folstein, Folstein, & McHugh, 1975) score lower than 24; and major visual or hearing deficits. Unpaired t tests (two-tailed) revealed no significant differences between patients and spouses for age ($M = 58.98$ years, $SD = 9.16$ vs. $M = 56.22$ years, $SD = 11.00$), $t(124) = 1.53$, $p > .05$; years of education ($M = 10.46$, $SD = 3.34$ vs. $M = 9.63$, $SD = 2.18$), $t(124) = 1.64$, $p > .05$; and MMSE score at entry ($M = 27.50$, $SD = 2.27$ vs. $M = 27.33$, $SD = 2.47$), $t(121) = 0.40$, $p > .05$.

Efficacy of controlling for the effects of changes in distress was evaluated by assessing self-reported mood states in patients and spouses concurrent with the neuropsychological examinations. Changes in mood state scores were not significantly different between the two groups (Bruggemans et al., 1995).

Neuropsychological Test Measures

The following neuropsychological test measures, pertaining to three categories of cognitive functioning, were used in the current analysis: *Learning and memory.* (a) The total score (i.e., Forward plus Backward) of the Digit Span and Visual Memory Span subtests of the Wechsler Memory Scale-Revised (WMS-R; Wechsler, 1987); and (b) the number of words correctly recalled on the first, the fifth, and a 30-min delayed recall trial of the Rey Auditory Verbal Learning Test (RAVLT; Rey, 1964), using a Dutch version with alternate forms (Kingma & Van den Burg, 1985). No interference list was used. *Verbal fluency.* The sum of all admissible words for the letters N, K, and A used in the Controlled Oral Word Association Test (Benton & Hamsher, 1978). *Attention and psychomotor speed.* (a) The average time per line in the Bourdon-Vos Test (Vos, 1988), a cancellation task; (b) the time required for Parts A and B of the Trail Making Test of the Halstead-Reitan Neuropsychological Battery (Reitan, 1958). This test was not included in the test battery for the first nine couples participating in this study; (c) the interference score (i.e., the time required for color-naming of color names printed in nonmatching colored inks minus the time required for color-naming of colored dots) of the Stroop Color-Word Test (Stroop, 1935). The interference score could not be obtained in 2 patients suffering from color blindness; and (d) the number of correctly placed digits in the Symbol Digit Modalities Test (Smith, 1982).

Surgical Parameters

The following surgical parameters were registered: duration of extracorporeal circulation, aortic cross-clamp time, minimum nasopharyngeal temperature, and mean flow and mean arterial pressure during extracorporeal circulation and during aortic cross-clamping (details can be found in Bruggemans et al., 1995).

Statistical Analysis

For the assessment of negative cognitive effects of CABG surgery in individual patients, the raw test scores obtained at times T1 and T2 of the original study were used. Cognitive deterioration in individual patients was defined according to six different change indices:

The Standard Deviation Index

According to this method, cognitive deterioration is expressed by the following formula:

$$C = \frac{X_2 - X_1}{s_1} \tag{1}$$

where X_1 and X_2 are the patient's observed pre- and post-operative test scores, and s_1 is the standard deviation of the distribution of the preoperative scores in the patient sample. As in previous studies on the cognitive effects of cardiac surgery, cognitive deterioration in a patient was said to be significant if $|C| > 1$, the sign of the index being dependent on the denotation of the test score (e.g., Sellman et al., 1993; Shaw et al., 1986, 1987; Treasure et al., 1989).

The Reliable Change Index of Jacobson and Truax (1991)

This index is described by the authors by the following formula:

$$RC_{JT} = \frac{X_2 - X_1}{SE_{diff}} \tag{2}$$

in which X_1 and X_2 are defined as in Equation 1, and SE_{diff} denotes the standard error of the difference between the observed pre- and post-test scores. The SE_{diff} term is computed from $SE_{diff} = [2(SEM)^2]^{1/2}$, where SEM is the standard error of measurement, computed from $SEM = s_1(1 - r_{12})^{1/2}$. The change in a patient's test score from pre- to post-testing is usually taken to be significant if $|RC_{JT}| > z_{\alpha/2}$ (two-tailed), where α is the Type I error rate. In the present study, it was decided to work with a one-tailed significance test ($\alpha = .05$, $z = 1.645$) because the interest was in cognitive deterioration.

The Reliable Change Index of Zegers and Hafkenscheid (1994)

This RC index is given by the following formula:

$$RC_{ZH} = \frac{(X_2 - X_1)r_{DD} + (M_2 - M_1)(1 - r_{DD})}{\sqrt{r_{DD}}\sqrt{(1 - r_{DD})}s_D} \tag{3}$$

in which X_1 and X_2 are defined as in Equation 1, M_1 and M_2 are the observed pre- and post-operative means of the patient sample, r_{DD} denotes the reliability of the pre- to post-test change scores, and s_D denotes the standard deviation of these change scores. The r_{DD} term is computed by the formula:

$$r_{DD} = \frac{r_{11}s_1^2 + r_{22}s_2^2 - 2r_{12}s_1s_2}{s_1^2 + s_2^2 - 2r_{12}s_1s_2} \qquad (4)$$

where r_{11} and r_{22} are the reliabilities of the pre- and post-test scores, r_{12} is the correlation between the pre- and post-test scores (test-retest reliability), and s_1 and s_2 are the standard deviations of the pre- and post-test scores. The s_D term is computed by $s_D = (s_1^2 + s_2^2 - 2r_{12}s_1s_2)^{1/2}$. Because the numerator of Equation 3 expresses the patient's estimated true change score and the denominator represents the error of this estimate (i.e., error of prediction; see also Hsu, 1995), RC_{ZH} is a normally distributed z-score. As for RC_{JT}, the absolute value of RC_{ZH} indicated significant cognitive deterioration when it was larger than 1.645.

In the present study, we used the data of the control group to compute the reliability (r_{DD}) and standard deviation (s_D) of the change scores because large variances in patients' posttest scores may reflect individual differences in surgery effects rather than test score properties. Variability in posttest scores has generally been shown to be substantially larger among cardiac surgery patients than among controls (Benedict, 1994). In order to estimate the reliabilities of the pretest (r_{11}) and posttest (r_{22}) scores in the control group, a factor analysis was carried out on the controls' test scores at times T1 to T4. The estimated communalities of the scores at times T1 and T2 were taken as a measure of r_{11} and r_{22}, respectively (see Crocker & Algina, 1986, p. 295).

The Reliability–Stability Index of Chelune et al. (1993)

Chelune et al. used the above RC index of Jacobson and Truax (1991), with a modification to accommodate for practice effects. Their index can be described by the following formula:

$$RST_{Chel} = \frac{(X_2 - X_1) - (M_2 - M_1)}{SE_{diff}} \qquad (5)$$

in which X_1, X_2, and SE_{diff} are defined as in Equation 2, and M_1 and M_2 are the observed pre- and post-operative means of the control group. The absolute value of RST_{Chel} had to be larger than 1.645 in order to indicate significant cognitive deterioration.

The Reliability–Stability Index of McSweeny et al. (1993)

This index, based on the regression model, deals with individual differences in practice effects. A regression line is fit to the data of the control group, the posttest scores being predicted on the basis of the pretest scores. A patient's predicted posttest score is then calculated on the basis of his or her pretest score, using the regression parameters (i.e., regression coefficient and intercept) for the regression line of the control group. The regression formula for predicting a patient's posttest score, X_2', from his or her pretest score is given by:

$$X_2' = bX_1 + c \qquad (6)$$

where X_1 is defined as in Equation 1, and b and c are the regression coefficient and intercept, respectively, for the regression line to the control group data. The index of McSweeny et al. is given by:

$$RST_{McS} = \frac{X_2 - X_2'}{SE_{pred}} \qquad (7)$$

in which X_2 and X_2' are defined as in Equation 1 and Equation 6, respectively, and SE_{pred} is the standard error of prediction, computed by $SE_{pred} = s_2(1 - r_{12}^2)^{1/2}$. For significant deterioration, the absolute value of RST_{McS} had to be larger than 1.645.

The Proposed Reliability–Stability Index

The currently proposed index is an elaboration of the above RC index of Zegers and Hafkenscheid (1994), purporting to correct for individual differences in practice effects. Each patient is matched with a group of control subjects with similar pretest scores (cf. the above regression-based index of McSweeny et al., 1993). Matching with multiple controls rather than with a single subject is carried out to minimize the effects of irrelevant idiosyncratic variations in the change scores of individual control subjects. Matched control group sizes may vary among patients, depending on the opportunities to find appropriate matches. In the present study, on average 10 matched controls were gathered for each patient. The mean change score of the matched control group is considered to represent the change score of a single ideal control subject. Analogous to the change scores of patients, change scores of ideal controls will be subject to measurement error. Consequently, the RC_{ZH} index (Equation 3) is applied to the observed mean pre- and post-test scores of the matched control (mc) subjects, that is:

$$RC_{mc} = \frac{(M_{mc_2} - M_{mc_1})r_{DD} + (M_2 - M_1)(1 - r_{DD})}{\sqrt{r_{DD}}\sqrt{(1 - r_{DD})}s_D}$$
$$\qquad (8)$$

where M_{mc_1} and M_{mc_2} are the observed mean pre- and post-test scores of the matched controls, M_1 and M_2 are the observed pre- and post-test means for the entire control group, s_D denotes the standard deviation of pre- to post-test change scores of all control subjects, and r_{DD} denotes the reliability of these change scores. The proposed new index (RST_{new}) is then a composite index based on two RC_{ZH} indices:

$$RST_{new} = RC_{pat} - RC_{mc} \qquad (9)$$

where RC_{pat} is the RC_{ZH} index of the patient as described in Equation 3 and RC_{mc} is the RC_{ZH} index of his or her matched controls as given in Equation 8. Because RST_{new} is the difference between two z-scores, like for the other z-score indices, its absolute value had to be larger than 1.645 in order to indicate significant cognitive deterioration.

In addition to comparing the incidence of cognitive deterioration for the six different indices, the question was addressed as to how the indices differ in their relationships with predictor variables, that is patients' age and surgical parameters. In order to answer this question, Pearson correlations were computed between, on the one hand, individual change scores as generated by the indices and, on the other hand, age and surgical parameters. The correlations were subjected to one-tailed t tests on the basis of expectations about the effects of predictor variables on cognitive deterioration.

RESULTS

For each of the neuropsychological test measures, reliabilities and practice effects observed in the control group are reported first as they form the basis of the RC (RC_{JT} and RC_{ZH}) and RST (RST_{Chel}, RST_{McS}, and RST_{new}) indices. Then, the results for the six indices will be presented.

Test Score Reliabilities in the Control Group

For each test measure, the three reliability coefficients (r_{11}, r_{22}, and r_{12}) are presented in Table 1. Only for the immediate memory measure (i.e., Trial I) of the RAVLT, reliabilities were low with coefficients ranging from .32 to .49. Coefficients for the other measures ranged from .61 to .95. Reliability coefficients for the measures of learning and memory (WMS-R and RAVLT) were smaller than those for the measures of verbal fluency (Controlled Oral Word Association) and attention and psychomotor speed (Bourdon-Vos, Trail Making Test, Stroop Interference, and Symbol Digit Modalities). Similar differences in reliability coefficients have been reported in the literature (Spreen & Strauss, 1991).

Practice Effects in the Control Group

In order to evaluate practice effects, paired t tests (one-tailed) were carried out on the pre- to post-test change scores of the entire control group. For change scores (i.e., observed posttest minus observed pretest scores) on each test measure, the mean value, standard deviation, and associated t value

Table 1. Reliability Coefficients of the Neuropsychological Test Measures in the Control Group.

Test measure	Reliability at T1 (r_{11})	Reliability at T2 (r_{22})	Test-retest reliability (r_{12})
Learning and memory			
WMS-R Digit Span	.79	.82	.71
WMS-R Visual Memory Span	.68	.72	.61
RAVLT Trial I	.45	.49	.32
RAVLT Trial V	.62	.78	.62
RAVLT Delayed Recall	.70	.76	.63
Verbal fluency			
Controlled Oral Word Association	.89	.89	.85
Attention and psychomotor speed			
Bourdon-Vos	.89	.95	.89
Trail Making Test, Part A	.76	.80	.73
Trail Making Test, Part B	.80	.89	.79
Stroop Interference	.82	.84	.77
Symbol Digit Modalities	.92	.93	.90

Note. WMS-R = Wechsler Memory Scale-Revised; RAVLT = Rey Auditory Verbal Learning Test.

are presented in Table 2. Significant improvements in performance were found for the verbal fluency measure and for all measures of attention and psychomotor speed, whereas no significant changes were obtained for the learning and memory measures.

The above mean values are the basis of the correction for practice effects as applied in the RST_{Chel} index. The other two RST indices, RST_{McS} and RST_{new}, correct for practice effects using change scores of control subjects with similar pretest scores as the patient. Table 2 presents the change scores for controls matched to the patient with the lowest and the patient with the highest pretest score on each test measure. For the RST_{McS} index, the change scores represent differences between predicted posttest and observed pretest scores. For RST_{new}, the values represent the mean estimated true change scores for the on average 10 matched controls gathered for each patient.

As expected, the change scores used in both indices showed considerable variability among pretest score levels, underlining the necessity to apply level-dependent corrections of patients' scores.

Comparison of Change Indices

Critical Values and Deterioration Rates

Table 3 presents critical values for significant test score deterioration (i.e., observed posttest minus observed pretest scores) for each of the six change indices. For the SD, RC_{JT}, RC_{ZH}, and RST_{Chel} indices, the values apply to the entire patient group. For the RST_{McS} and RST_{new} indices, critical values depend on a patient's pretest score. In Table 3, the values are presented only for the patient with the lowest and the patient with the highest pretest score on each test measure.

The effects of score corrections for measurement error can be examined by comparing the results

Table 2. Change Scores in the Control Group.

Test measure	Entire control group			Matched controls			
	M	SD	t	RST_{McS}		RST_{new}	
				Lowest pretest score	Highest pretest score	Lowest pretest score	Highest pretest score
Learning and memory							
WMS-R Digit Span[a]	0.06	2.02	0.25	1.57	−1.46	0.40	−0.22
WMS-R Visual Memory Span[a]	0.21	2.28	0.72	1.63	−1.90	0.34	−0.09
RAVLT Trial I[a]	−0.40	1.96	−1.60	2.56	−1.79	0.01	−0.68
RAVLT Trial V[a]	0.17	1.74	0.80	2.31	−1.03	0.52	0.09
RAVLT Delayed Recall[a]	−0.38	2.31	−1.31	2.17	−1.55	0.18	−0.71
Verbal fluency							
Controlled Oral Word Association[a]	4.38	6.09	5.71[*]	7.84	2.04	4.75	3.72
Attention and psychomotor speed							
Bourdon-Vos[b]	−0.69	0.94	−5.79[*]	−0.66	−0.76	−0.58	−0.63
Trail Making Test, Part A[b]	−4.91	9.10	−3.96[*]	2.10	−11.14	−4.46	−5.48
Trail Making Test, Part B[b]	−10.06	20.13	−3.67[*]	−0.24	−40.79	−8.13	−14.16
Stroop Interference[b]	−8.13	14.30	−4.51[*]	4.06	−30.65	−5.75	−10.00
Symbol Digit Modalities[a]	3.79	4.56	6.60[*]	4.89	2.56	4.24	4.05

Note. Change scores represent observed posttest minus observed pretest scores for the entire control group, predicted posttest minus observed pretest scores for matched controls in the Reliability–Stability index of McSweeny et al. (RST_{McS}; 1993), and estimated true posttest minus estimated true pretest scores for the matched controls in the currently proposed Reliability–Stability index (RST_{new}); WMS-R = Wechsler Memory Scale-Revised; RAVLT = Rey Auditory Verbal Learning Test.
[a]A positive change score indicates improvement in performance; [b]A negative change score indicates improvement in performance.
*$p < .001$, one-tailed.

Table 3. Critical Values for Significant Test Score Deterioration.

Test measure	SD index	RC indices (Correcting for measurement error)		RST indices (Correcting for measurement error and practice effects)				
		RC_{JT}	RC_{ZH}	RST_{Chel}	RST_{McS}		RST_{new}	
					Lowest pretest score	Highest pretest score	Lowest pretest score	Highest pretest score
Learning and memory								
WMS-R Digit Span[a]	−2.97	−3.18	−4.78	−3.12	−1.63	−4.65	−3.58	−5.45
WMS-R Visual Memory Span[a]	−2.38	−3.64	−5.69	−3.44	−1.85	−5.38	−4.24	−6.07
RAVLT Trial I[a]	−1.52	−3.46	−7.19	−3.86	0.14	−4.21	−7.15	−10.30
RAVLT Trial V[a]	−2.25	−2.74	−4.93	−2.56	−0.38	−3.71	−2.64	−4.54
RAVLT Delayed Recall[a]	−2.74	−3.60	−3.87	−3.98	−1.43	−5.15	−3.22	−6.36
Verbal fluency								
Controlled Oral Word Association[a]	−11.10	−9.77	−20.48	−5.39	−2.06	−7.86	−2.16	−6.13
Attention and psychomotor speed								
Bourdon-Vos[b]	2.38	1.43	1.39	0.75	0.90	0.80	−0.26	−0.43
Trail Making Test, Part A[b]	10.83	14.99	26.31	10.08	16.11	2.87	4.09	−0.96
Trail Making Test, Part B[b]	37.09	33.01	30.17	22.95	31.43	−9.12	1.19	−20.31
Stroop Interference[b]	17.07	24.87	29.13	16.75	20.56	−14.15	13.84	2.54
Symbol Digit Modalities[a]	−9.30	−7.31	−3.74	−3.51	−2.62	−4.94	14.73	13.88

Note. Critical values represent observed posttest minus observed pretest scores. RC_{JT} = Reliable Change index of Jacobson and Truax (1991); RC_{ZH} = Reliable Change index of Zegers and Hafkenscheid (1994); RST_{Chel} = Reliability–Stability index of Chelune et al. (1993); RST_{McS} = Reliability–Stability index of McSweeny et al. (1993); RST_{new} = currently proposed Reliability–Stability index; WMS-R = Wechsler Memory Scale-Revised; RAVLT = Rey Auditory Verbal Learning Test.
[a]A positive change score indicates improvement in performance; [b]A negative change score indicates improvement in performance.

for the SD and RC indices. For the majority of test measures, both RC indices produced larger absolute critical values than the SD index, the RC_{ZH} index tending to be more conservative than the RC_{JT} index. The discrepancies between the SD and RC indices are mainly attributable to the reliability of the test scores: For test measures associated with relatively low reliability coefficients (see Table 1), the RC indices tended to be more conservative than the SD index. This behavior of the RC indices is intuitively appealing in that they correct for the increased uncertainty by enlarging their critical value. In general, for test measures having a low reliability, critical values for the RC indices can become much larger than for the SD index.

Comparison of the results for the RC and RST indices reflects the influence of correcting for practice effects. As could be expected, all three RST indices produced in general much less

conservative critical values than the RC indices for test measures showing significant practice effects (i.e., the measures of verbal fluency and attention and psychomotor speed; see Table 2), the RST_{new} index being less conservative than the RST_{Chel} and RST_{McS} indices. Correction for practice effects may lead to seemingly counter-intuitive behavior of the RST indices. According to the RST_{McS} and RST_{new} indices, for example, a score improvement up to 9 or 20 points, respectively, on the Trail Making Test, Part B, could mean a net worsening. In general, for test measures showing substantial practice effects, even a score improvement might imply a significant cognitive deterioration.

Table 4 presents the deterioration rates for the six indices, based on the critical values in Table 3. In Table 4, once again, the impact of score corrections for measurement error and practice effects is reflected. For test measures having a relatively

Table 4. Deterioration Rates (as percentages).

Test measure	SD index	RC indices (Correcting for measurement error)		RST indices (Correcting for measurement error and practice effects)		
		RC_{JT}	RC_{ZH}	RST_{Chel}	RST_{McS}	RST_{new}
Learning and memory						
WMS-R Digit Span	10	0	0	0	3	0
WMS-R Visual Memory Span	16	7	2	7	5	5
RAVLT Trial I	18	2	0	2	0	0
RAVLT Trial V	14	14	3	14	11	3
RAVLT Delayed Recall	29	18	18	18	21	11
Verbal fluency						
Controlled Oral Word Association	3	6	0	18	16	24
Attention and psychomotor speed						
Bourdon-Vos	11	19	21	35	32	73
Trail Making Test, Part A	15	11	2	15	15	33
Trail Making Test, Part B	15	19	19	28	33	67
Stroop Interference	8	5	5	12	28	25
Symbol Digit Modalities	10	13	48	48	46	100

Note. RC_{JT} = Reliable Change index of Jacobson and Truax (1991); RC_{ZH} = Reliable Change index of Zegers and Hafkenscheid (1994); RST_{Chel} = Reliability–Stability index of Chelune et al. (1993); RST_{McS} = Reliability–Stability index of McSweeny et al. (1993); RST_{new} = currently proposed Reliability–Stability index; WMS-R = Wechsler Memory Scale-Revised; RAVLT = Rey Auditory Verbal Learning Test.

low reliability and not showing significant score improvements due to practice (i.e., the learning and memory measures), the SD index generated larger deterioration rates than the RC and RST indices. On the other hand, for test measures with a relatively high reliability but showing significant practice effects (i.e., the measures of verbal fluency and attention and psychomotor speed), the RST indices revealed in general much larger deterioration rates than the SD and RC indices, with the RST_{new} index by far showing the largest rates. The most salient example of this concerns the Symbol Digit Modalities measure. According to the RST_{new} index, all patients were deteriorated on this test measure.

It can be concluded from Table 4 that the six indices showed different results regarding the negative effects of CABG surgery on cognitive functioning. When using the SD index, moderate deterioration rates were found for the measures of learning and memory and those of attention and psychomotor speed (8–29%), whereas deterioration on verbal fluency occurred in only 3% of the patients. The two RC indices produced generally low deterioration rates for the learning and memory measures and for verbal fluency (0–18%). They showed moderate rates for the measures of attention

and psychomotor speed, the RC_{ZH} index showing a larger variation in rates (2–48%) than the RC_{JT} index (5–19%). Like the RC indices, the RST indices generally resulted in low deterioration rates for the learning and memory measures (0–21%). However, moderate to high rates were obtained for the attention and psychomotor speed measures, with moderate rates (12–48%) for the RST_{Chel} and RST_{McS} indices, and high rates (25–100%) for RST_{new}. Verbal fluency was affected in a moderate number of patients (16–24%) for the RST indices.

Correlations with Age and Surgical Parameters
Table 5 presents the correlations between individual change scores as generated by the six indices and relevant predictor variables. Because intercorrelations among the SD index, the two RC indices, and the RST_{Chel} index by definition are equal to one (since they all imply a linear transformation of the observed change score), their correlations with predictor variables are identical.

The data show that the relationships with age and surgical parameters were essentially similar for all indices. Only a limited number of significant correlations were found. Low mean flow during

Table 5. Correlations between Change Indices and Predictor Variables.

Test measure	Age			ECC			ACC			Temperature		
	SD^a	RST_{McS}	RST_{new}	SD^a	RST_{McS}	RST_{new}	SD^a	RST_{McS}	RST_{new}	SD^a	RST_{McS}	RST_{new}
Learning and memory												
WMS-R Digit Span	.04	.03	.05	-.07	.03	.00	-.04	.03	.00	.13	.04	.06
WMS-R Visual Memory Span	-.09	-.15	-.17	.03	.03	.03	-.02	-.05	-.04	.01	.04	.06
RAVLT Trial I	.06	.08	.09	-.02	-.03	-.05	-.06	-.09	-.10	.22*	.18	.17
RAVLT Trial V	-.18	-.18	-.18	-.03	-.06	-.03	.06	.00	.03	.07	.14	.12
RAVLT Delayed Recall	-.05	-.06	-.14	-.15	-.18	-.22*	-.21*	-.25*	-.29*	.27*	.34**	.42***
Verbal fluency												
Controlled Oral Word Association	-.02	-.03	-.03	-.23*	-.21*	-.23*	-.25*	-.25*	-.26*	.08	.06	.07
Attention and psychomotor speed												
Bourdon-Vos	.18	.19	.17	-.03	-.03	-.01	-.03	-.03	-.01	-.03	-.03	-.03
Trail Making Test, Part A	.15	.24*	.17	-.02	-.06	-.03	.00	-.01	.00	-.27*	-.22	-.22
Trail Making Test, Part B	.20	.24*	.24*	.11	.06	.08	.04	-.01	.03	-.27*	-.22	-.24*
Stroop Interference	-.12	.09	-.02	-.04	-.04	-.06	-.07	-.04	-.08	.01	-.01	-.01
Symbol Digit Modalities	-.07	-.11	-.07	-.15	-.13	-.13	-.15	-.15	-.14	.29*	.29**	.26*

Test measure	Flow 1			Flow 2			Pressure 1			Pressure 2		
	SD^a	RST_{McS}	RST_{new}	SD^a	RST_{McS}	RST_{new}	SD^a	RST_{McS}	RST_{new}	SD^a	RST_{McS}	RST_{new}
Learning and memory												
WMS-R Digit Span	.05	.07	.07	.12	.10	.10	.10	.11	.12	-.07	-.05	-.04
WMS-R Visual Memory Span	.07	.17	.13	.02	.07	.04	-.09	-.13	-.11	-.24	-.20	-.19
RAVLT Trial I	.15	.26*	.23*	.20	.24*	.24*	.03	.10	.11	.12	.11	.15
RAVLT Trial V	.17	.23*	.20	.32*	.36**	.35***	.11	.11	.10	.04	.02	.00
RAVLT Delayed Recall	.21*	.26*	.27*	.22*	.25*	.28*	-.01	.01	.01	-.15	-.14	-.13
Verbal fluency												
Controlled Oral Word Association	.10	.13	.12	.02	.04	.04	.00	.01	.01	.06	.07	.07
Attention and psychomotor speed												
Bourdon-Vos	-.09	-.10	-.08	-.10	-.11	-.09	.25	.24	.23	.12	.11	.10
Trail Making Test, Part A	-.18	-.22	-.23*	-.18	-.18	-.20	.11	.09	.11	.03	.01	.00
Trail Making Test, Part B	-.10	-.11	-.13	-.19	-.18	-.21	.07	.07	.04	.00	-.03	-.05
Stroop Interference	-.13	-.23*	-.19	-.18	-.24*	-.21	.00	-.08	-.04	-.13	-.16	-.15
Symbol Digit Modalities	.36**	.38**	.35**	.37**	.37**	.34**	-.05	-.05	-.09	-.01	-.02	-.05

Note. ECC = duration of extracorporeal circulation; ACC = aortic cross-clamp time; Temperature = minimum nasopharyngeal temperature; Flow 1 and Flow 2 = mean flow during extracorporeal circulation and during aortic cross-clamping, respectively; Pressure 1 and Pressure 2 = mean arterial pressure during extracorporeal circulation and during aortic cross-clamping, respectively; RST_{McS} = Reliability–Stability index of McSweeny et al. (1993); RST_{new} = currently proposed Reliability–Stability index; WMS-R = Wechsler Memory Scale–Revised; RAVLT = Rey Auditory Verbal Learning Test.
^{a}Correlations for the SD, RC_{JT}, RC_{ZH}, and RST_{Chel} indices are identical.
* $p < .05$, ** $p < .01$, *** $p < .001$, one-tailed.

extracorporeal circulation as well as during aortic cross-clamping and low minimum nasopharyngeal temperature appeared to be the most pertinent predictors of cognitive deterioration. The neuropsychological test measures most affected by these surgical parameters were the delayed recall measure of the RAVLT and the Symbol Digit Modalities measure. These two test measures have in common that they make a demand on memory retrieval.

DISCUSSION

The interpretation of individual changes in neuropsychological test scores is hampered by problems of measurement error and practice effects. In this study, six different indices of individual change were applied to assess cognitive deterioration in patients following CABG surgery: the SD index, which considers neither measurement error nor practice effects; the RC indices of Jacobson and Truax (1991) and Zegers and Hafkenscheid (1994), correcting for measurement error; and the RST indices of Chelune et al. (1993) and McSweeny et al. (1993), and the currently proposed RST index, correcting for both measurement error and practice effects. Results for these indices were compared on various neuropsychological test measures. The purpose was to examine the impact of score corrections for measurement error and practice effects in the assessment of individual change and to evaluate the consequences for the incidence of cognitive deterioration in CABG patients.

The indices showed marked differences in deterioration rates on the various test measures due to measurement error and practice effects, as may be expected. For test measures with a relatively low reliability and showing no significant practice effects (the learning and memory measures), the SD index produced higher deterioration rates than did the RC and RST indices. In contrast, for test measures with a relatively high reliability but showing significant score improvements due to practice (the verbal fluency and attention and psychomotor speed measures), the RST indices produced higher deterioration rates than did both the SD index and the RC indices. These findings are consistent with the mathematical differences among the indices that imply that the discordance of the SD index versus

the RC and RST indices will increase when tests become less reliable, and that the discordance of both the SD index and the RC indices versus the RST indices will increase when tests show larger practice effects.

Although the RC_{ZH} index more adequately corrects for measurement error than does the RC_{JT} index, systematic differences in deterioration rates between these two indices were not found in the present study. It should, however, be emphasized that with other data sets the indices may yield a larger discrepancy. This can be explained by the fact that the mathematical difference between the indices is not merely a function of test reliability. In comparison with the RC_{JT} index, the RC_{ZH} index involves additional sample statistics, such as the mean of the observed pretest scores, and the mean and standard deviation of the observed posttest scores. Therefore, the discordance between the two RC indices will depend on the characteristics of the study sample.

Analogous reasoning holds for the behavior of the three RST indices. In the present study, the statistically more adequate RST_{new} index revealed considerably higher deterioration rates than the RST_{Chel} and RST_{McS} indices on the measures of attention and psychomotor speed, the latter two indices showing almost equal rates. As for the RC indices, however, application of the RST indices in other study samples may result in other incongruities. Because the three RST indices employ partially different sample statistics, their discordance may vary with the characteristics of the study sample.

The current results clearly show that conclusions about the incidence of cognitive change after medical intervention strongly depend on the index utilized. Because of their psychometric shortcomings, application of the SD index, the two RC indices, and the RST_{Chel} and RST_{McS} indices may lead to fallacious conclusions. Thus, with the SD index, presumably too many CABG patients in the present sample were considered as significantly deteriorated on learning and memory (i.e., false positives), whereas too few patients were considered as significantly deteriorated on verbal fluency and attention and psychomotor speed (i.e., false negatives). The major problem of the two RC indices concerned false negatives on verbal fluency and attention and psychomotor speed (i.e., false negatives). The major problem of the two RC indices concerned false negatives on verbal fluency and attention and psychomotor speed. Finally, false negatives on attention and psychomotor speed were also observed for the RST_{Chel} and RST_{McS} indices.

Utilization of the RST_{new} index in the analysis of the current data indicated differential effects of CABG surgery on cognitive functioning, with deterioration frequently occurring on attention and psychomotor speed (25–100%), to a smaller degree on verbal fluency (24%), and only occasionally on learning and memory (0–11%). This pattern of early cognitive dysfunctioning (i.e., deterioration detectable 1 week following CABG surgery) is consistent with that quantified in terms of group means for this patient sample (Bruggemans et al., 1995). At 1 week postoperatively, patients' mean scores on attention and psychomotor speed as well as on verbal fluency were significantly deteriorated compared with the mean scores of spouses, whereas mean change scores for memory and learning showed no differences between both groups. This pattern is also consistent with the early pattern revealed by other controlled studies reporting group means (e.g., Hammeke & Hastings, 1988; Townes et al., 1989). On the other hand, there is little agreement with studies that analyzed group means but did not include a control group (e.g., Fish et al., 1987; Zeitlhofer et al., 1993). These studies in general did not show important differences in deterioration among different cognitive functions and sometimes even suggested improvement in functioning, probably due to practice effects.

As mentioned before, the SD index has been commonly used to report on the incidence of cognitive deterioration following CABG surgery. In two studies applying this index, the deterioration rates on the various test measures were inconsistent and also differed considerably from those of the RST_{new} index in the current study. In one study, learning and memory were slightly more often affected than attention and psychomotor speed (Shaw et al., 1986, 1987), whereas this pattern was not replicated in the other study (Harrison et al., 1989). The other studies applying the SD index (see introduction), however, can in general be criticized for underrating the influence of the composition of the test battery. In these studies, cognitive deterioration in a patient was generally said to occur in

case of a drop in test performance of at least one *SD* on two or more of the administered tests (see also Mahanna et al., 1996). Even though using this additional criterion may well reduce the influence of random score fluctuations on the diagnosis of cognitive deterioration, the differential pattern of deterioration is neglected in this definition. Hence, the likelihood of assessing cognitive deterioration will depend on the homogeneity of the test battery.

In the present study, relationships between relevant predictor variables (i.e., patients' age and surgical parameters) and individual change scores showed much correspondence for the six indices, indicating high intercorrelations among the indices. As stated before, the SD index, the two RC indices, and the RST_{Chel} index by definition show a perfect intercorrelation. The corrections for practice effects as applied in the RST_{McS} and RST_{new} indices, however, may entail a nonlinear transformation of the observed change score because these corrections depend on a patient's pretest score. Nevertheless, Pearson correlations between observed change scores and the RST_{McS} and RST_{new} indices were high, ranging from .80 to 1.00 and from .91 to .99, respectively, and thus suggest almost linear corrections for practice effects. Empirical studies have frequently shown that estimated true change scores (RST_{new}) are linearly related to initial scores (e.g., Alder et al., 1990; Fahrenberg, Foerster, & Wilmers, 1995; Myrtek & Foerster, 1986). The same holds probably for residualized change scores (RST_{McS}). It may, therefore, be assumed that individual score corrections for practice effects tend to amount to an almost linear transformation of observed change scores and that, in general, correlations for the RST_{McS} and RST_{new} indices with external variables will only slightly deviate from those for the SD index, the two RC indices, and the RST_{Chel} index.

The above findings have implications for choosing the most appropriate index in the assessment of individual change. If one is interested in the incidence of cognitive change rather than in its prediction, the use of the RST_{new} index is to be preferred over the use of the other indices. Application of this new index will reduce the likelihood of incorrect decisions about the significance of change scores because of the corrections for both measurement error and practice effects. If one is primarily interested in predicting cognitive change on the basis of external variables, then the different indices will frequently yield similar results and, therefore, there is no need to select among the indices.

Three practical problems may be encountered in applying the RST_{new} index. First, the different reliability coefficients (i.e., r_{11}, r_{22}, and r_{12}) may not always be available. When using standardized neuropsychological tests, useful reliability estimates may be found in the test manual or reports in the literature. Here the question may arise as to what types of estimates are appropriate for inclusion in the index. For both r_{11} and r_{22}, one could use one of the various estimates of internal consistency, such as the alpha coefficient, the split-half coefficient, or the communality derived from factor-analysis as employed in the present study. The only meaningful estimate for r_{12} is the test-retest correlation coefficient. It is important to note that the intraclass correlation coefficient as a measure of agreement (cf., McGraw & Wong, 1996; Shrout & Fleiss, 1979), which in other circumstances may be considered a very useful reliability estimate (cf., Brown, Rourke, & Cicchetti, 1989), cannot be employed here. A high value of this coefficient indicates both a reliable and a stable (in absolute test scores) measurement. A low value reflects poor reliability, instability, or both. The RST_{new} index, however, assumes reliability estimates that only reflect the influence of measurement error.

Second, in some cases estimates of internal consistency such as the split-half coefficient will seriously underestimate the true reliability of the instrument. In such cases, the value of the test-retest correlation can be almost as high as the internal consistency estimates and, as a consequence, the reliability of the change score can become close to or even equal to zero. The value of the RST_{new} index will then be mainly determined by the difference in group means at both test occasions, thereby underrating the relevance of the change in the individual. In such a case, however, the use of the other indices may not lead to more appropriate results.

The third problem in applying the RST_{new} index may involve the lack of information about practice effects. As for test reliability, test manuals or reports in the literature may provide useful data on test-retest stability. It is highly unlikely, however, that these will contain data on groups with a pretest score similar to the patient's. Applying corrections for mean practice effects such as those applied in the RST_{Chel} index will then be the only viable option.

In summary, six different indices for assessing individual change, differing in the extent that corrections were made for measurement error and practice effects, have been examined. The present findings suggest that when one is interested in incidence rates, the RST_{new} index will be very useful. This index enables a statistically adequate test of individual change both when measurement error and practice effects jeopardize the validity of classical approaches. The index was applied here to assess the negative cognitive effects of cardiac surgery but the domain of application is broader and includes all pretest-posttest designs in which individual change is examined.

REFERENCES

Alder, A. G., Adam, J., & Arenberg, D. (1990). Individual-differences assessment of the relationship between change in and initial level of adult cognitive functioning. *Psychology and Aging, 5,* 560–568.

Benedict, R. H. B. (1994). Cognitive function after open-heart surgery: Are postoperative neuropsychological deficits caused by cardiopulmonary bypass? *Neuropsychology Review, 4,* 223–255.

Benton, A. L., & Hamsher, K. (1978). *Multilingual Aphasia Examination Manual-Revised.* Iowa City, IA: University of Iowa.

Blomqvist, N. (1977). On the relation between change and initial value. *Journal of the American Statistical Association, 72,* 746–749.

Brown, R. T., & Madan-Swain, A. (1993). Cognitive, neuropsychological, and academic sequelae in children with leukemia. *Journal of Learning Disabilities, 26,* 74–90.

Brown, S. J., Rourke, B. P., & Cicchetti, D. V. (1989). Reliability of tests and measures used in the neuropsychological assessment of children. *The Clinical Neuropsychologist, 3,* 353–368.

Bruggemans, E. F., Van Dijk, J. G., & Huysmans, H. A. (1995). Residual cognitive dysfunctioning at 6 months following coronary artery bypass graft surgery. *European Journal of Cardio-Thoracic Surgery, 9,* 636–643.

Chelune, G. J. (1992). Using neuropsychological data to forecast postsurgical cognitive outcome. In H. O. Lüders (Ed.), *Epilepsy surgery* (pp. 477–485). New York: Raven Press.

Chelune, G. J., Naugle, R. I., Lüders, H., Sedlak, J., & Awad, I. A. (1993). Individual change after epilepsy surgery: Practice effects and base-rate information. *Neuropsychology, 7*, 41–52.

Christensen, L., & Mendoza, J. L. (1986). A method of assessing change in a single subject: An alteration of the RC Index. *Behavior Therapy, 17*, 305–308.

Crocker, L., & Algina, J. (1986). *Introduction to classical and modern test theory.* Orlando, FL: Holt, Rinehart, and Winston.

Edwards, D. W., Yarvis, R. M., Mueller, D. P., Zingale, H. C., & Wagman, W. J. (1978). Test-taking and the stability of adjustment scales. Can we assess patient deterioration? *Evaluation Quarterly, 2*, 275–291.

Everall, I. P. (1995). Neuropsychiatric aspects of HIV infection. *Journal of Neurology, Neurosurgery, and Psychiatry, 58*, 399–402.

Fahrenberg, J., Foerster, F., & Wilmers, F. (1995). Is elevated blood pressure level associated with higher cardiovascular responsiveness in laboratory tasks and with response specificity? *Psychophysiology, 32*, 81–91.

Feinstein, A., Brown, R., & Ron, M. (1994). Effects of practice of serial tests of attention in healthy subjects. *Journal of Clinical and Experimental Neuropsychology, 16*, 436–447.

Fish, K. J., Helms, K. N., Sarnquist, F. H., Van Steennis, C., Linet, O. I., Hilberman, M., Mitchell, R. S., Jamieson, S. W., Miller, D. C., & Tinklenberg, J. S. (1987). A prospective, randomized study of the effects of prostacyclin on neuropsychologic dysfunction after coronary artery operation. *Journal of Thoracic and Cardiovascular Surgery, 93*, 609–615.

Fletcher, J. M., & Copeland, D. R. (1988). Neurobehavioral effects of central nervous system prophylactic treatment of cancer in children. *Journal of Clinical and Experimental Neuropsychology, 10*, 495–538.

Folstein, M. F., Folstein, S. E., & McHugh, P. R. (1975). "Mini-Mental State". A practical method for grading the cognitive state of patients for the clinician. *Journal of Psychiatric Research, 12*, 189–198.

Geenen, R., & Van de Vijver, F. J. R. (1993). A simple test of the Law of Initial Values. *Psychophysiology, 30*, 525–530.

Hageman, W. J. J. M., & Arrindell, W. A. (1993). A further refinement of the Reliable Change (RC) Index by improving the pre-post difference score: Introducing RC_{ID}. *Behaviour Research and Therapy, 31*, 693–700.

Hammeke, T. A., & Hastings, J. E. (1988). Neuropsychologic alterations after cardiac operation. *Journal of Thoracic and Cardiovascular Surgery, 96*, 326–331.

Harrison, M. J. G., Schneidau, A., Ho, R., Smith, P. L. C., Newman, S., & Treasure, T. (1989). Cerebrovascular disease and functional outcome after coronary artery bypass surgery. *Stroke, 20*, 235–237.

Hsu, L. M. (1989). Reliable changes in psychotherapy: Taking into account regression toward the mean. *Behavioral Assessment, 11*, 459–467.

Hsu, L. M. (1995). Regression toward the mean associated with measurement error and the identification of improvement and deterioration in psychotherapy. *Journal of Consulting and Clinical Psychology, 63*, 141–144.

Jacobson, N. S., Follette, W. C., & Revenstorf, D. (1984). Psychotherapy outcome research: Methods for reporting variability and evaluating clinical significance. *Behavior Therapy, 15*, 336–352.

Jacobson, N. S., & Truax, P. (1991). Clinical significance: A statistical approach to defining meaningful change in psychotherapy research. *Journal of Consulting and Clinical Psychology, 59*, 12–19.

Jin, P. (1992). Toward a reconceptualization of the Law of Initial Value. *Psychological Bulletin, 111*, 176–184.

Karayanidis, F. (1989). Parkinson's disease: A conceptualization of neuropsychological deficits within an information-processing framework. *Biological Psychology, 29*, 149–179.

Kingma, A., & Van den Burg, W. (1985). *Vijftien Woorden Test* [Fifteen Words Test]. Groningen, The Netherlands: University Hospital.

Knight, R. G. (1983). On interpreting the several standard errors of the WAIS-R: Some further tables. *Journal of Consulting and Clinical Psychology, 51*, 671–673.

Loring, D. W., Meador, K. J., Lee, G. P., King, D. W., Nichols, M. E., Park, Y. D., Murro, A. M., Gallagher, B. B., & Smith, J. R. (1995). Wada memory asymmetries predict verbal memory decline after anterior temporal lobectomy. *Neurology, 45*, 1329–1333.

Macciocchi, S. N. (1990). "Practice makes perfect": Retest effects in college athletes. *Journal of Clinical Psychology, 46*, 628–631.

Mahanna, E. P., Blumenthal, J. A., White, W. D., Croughwell, N. D., Clancy, C. P., Smith, L. R., & Newman, M. F. (1996). Defining neuropsychological dysfunction after coronary artery bypass grafting. *Annals of Thoracic Surgery, 61*, 1342–1347.

Maj, M. (1990). Psychiatric aspects of HIV-1 infection and AIDS. *Psychological Medicine, 20*, 547–563.

Matarazzo, J. D., Carmody, T. P., & Jacobs, L. D. (1980). Test-retest reliability and stability of the WAIS: A literature review with implications for clinical practice. *Journal of Clinical Neuropsychology, 2*, 89–105.

Matarazzo, J. D., & Herman, D. O. (1984). Base rate data for the WAIS-R: Test-retest stability and VIQ-PIQ differences. *Journal of Clinical Neuropsychology, 6*, 351–366.

McGraw, K. O., & Wong, S. P. (1996). Forming inferences about some intraclass correlation coefficients. *Psychological Methods, 1*, 30–46.

McSweeny, A. J., Naugle, R. I., Chelune, G. J., & Lüders, H. (1993). "T Scores for change": An illustration of a regression approach to depicting change in clinical neuropsychology. *The Clinical Neuropsychologist, 7*, 300–312.

Myrtek, M., & Foerster, F. (1986). The Law of Initial Value: A rare exception. *Biological Psychology, 22*, 227–237.

Naugle, R. I. (1992). Neuropsychological effects of surgery of epilepsy. In H. O. Lüders (Ed.), *Epilepsy surgery* (pp. 637–645). New York: Raven Press.

Newman, S. (1993). Neuropsychological and psychological changes. In P. L. Smith & K. M. Taylor (Eds.), *Cardiac surgery and the brain* (pp. 34–54). London: Hodder & Stoughton.

Phillips, N. A., & McGlone, J. (1995). Grouped data do not tell the whole story: Individual analysis of cognitive change after temporal lobectomy. *Journal of Clinical and Experimental Neuropsychology, 17*, 713–724.

Reitan, R. M. (1958). Validity of the Trail Making Test as an indicator of organic brain damage. *Perceptual and Motor Skills, 8*, 271–276.

Rey, A. (1964). *L'examen clinique en psychologie* [Clinical psychological assessment]. Paris: Presses Universitaires de France.

Roman, D. D., & Sperduto, P. W. (1995). Neuropsychological effects of cranial radiation: Current knowledge and future directions. *International Journal of Radiation Oncology, Biology, Physics, 31*, 983–998.

Saint-Cyr, J. A., Taylor, A. E., & Lang, A. E. (1993). Neuropsychological and psychiatric side effects in the treatment of Parkinson's disease. *Neurology, 43* (Suppl. 6), S47–S52.

Sellman, M., Holm, L., Ivert, T., & Semb, B. K. H. (1993). A randomized study of neuropsychological function in patients undergoing coronary bypass surgery. *Thoracic Cardiovascular Surgeon, 41*, 349–354.

Shatz, M. W. (1981). WAIS practice effects in clinical neuropsychology. *Journal of Clinical Neuropsychology, 3*, 171–179.

Shaw, P. J., Bates, D., Cartlidge, N. E. F., French, J. M., Heaviside, D., Julian, D. G., & Shaw, D. A. (1986). Early intellectual dysfunction following coronary bypass surgery. *Quarterly Journal of Medicine, 225*, 59–68.

Shaw, P. J., Bates, D., Cartlidge, N. E. F., French, J. M., Heaviside, D., Julian, D. G., & Shaw, D. A. (1987). Long-term intellectual dysfunction following coronary artery bypass graft surgery: A six month follow-up study. *Quarterly Journal of Medicine, 239*, 259–268.

Shrout, P. E., & Fleiss, J. L. (1979). Intraclass correlations: Uses in assessing rater reliability. *Psychological Bulletin, 86*, 420–428.

Smith, A. (1982). *Symbol Digit Modalities Test. Manual-Revised 1982.* Los Angeles: Western Psychological Services.

Speer, D. C. (1992). Clinically significant change: Jacobson and Truax (1991) revisited. *Journal of Consulting and Clinical Psychology, 60*, 402–408.

Speer, D. C. (1993). Correction to Speer. *Journal of Consulting and Clinical Psychology, 61*, 27.

Spreen, O., & Strauss, E. (1991). *A compendium of neuropsychological tests: Administration, norms, and commentary.* New York: Oxford University Press.

Stroop, J. R. (1935). Studies of interference in serial verbal reactions. *Journal of Experimental Psychology, 18*, 643–662.

Townes, B. D., Bashein, G., Hornbein, T. F., Coppel, D. B., Goldstein, D. E., Davis, K. B., Nessly, M. L., Bledsoe, S. W., Veith, R. C., Ivey, T. D., & Cohen, M. A. (1989). Neurobehavioral outcomes in cardiac operations: A prospective controlled study. *Journal of Thoracic and Cardiovascular Surgery, 98*, 774–782.

Treasure, T., Smith, P. L. C., Newman, S., Schneidau, A., Joseph, Ph., Ell, P., & Harrison, M. J. G. (1989). Impairment of cerebral function following cardiac and other major surgery. *European Journal of Cardio-Thoracic Surgery, 3*, 216–221.

Vos, P. G. (1988). *Bourdon-Vos Test. Manual.* Lisse, The Netherlands: Swets & Zeitlinger.

Waldstein, S. R., Manuck, S. B., Ryan, C. M., & Muldoon, M. F. (1991). Neuropsychological correlates of hypertension: Review and methodologic considerations. *Psychological Bulletin, 110*, 451–468.

Wechsler, D. (1987). *Wechsler Memory Scale-Revised. Manual.* New York: Psychological Corporation.

Wing, H. (1980). Practice effects with traditional mental test items. *Applied Psychological Measurement, 4*, 141–155.

Zegers, F. E., & Hafkenscheid, A. (1994). *The Ultimate Reliable Change Index: An alternative to the Hageman & Arrindell approach.* (Heymans Bulletins HB-94-1154-EX). Groningen, The Netherlands: University of Groningen.

Zeitlhofer, J., Asenbaum, S., Spiss, C., Wimmer, A., Mayr, N., Wolner, E., & Deecke, L. (1993). Central nervous system function after cardiopulmonary bypass. *European Heart Journal, 14*, 885–890.

The Clinical Neuropsychologist
1997, Vol. 11, No. 4, pp. 375–380

Full Scale IQ as Mediator of Practice Effects: The Rich Get Richer*

Lisa J. Rapport[1], D. Brooke Brines[1], Bradley N. Axelrod[2], and Mary E. Theisen[1]

[1]Wayne State University, and [2]Department of Veterans Affairs Medical Center, Detroit, MI

ABSTRACT

Differential effects of practice over four administrations of the WAIS-R were examined as a function of Full Scale IQ at initial testing ($N = 36$). Twelve education-matched normal adults represented each of three groups: Low-Average (80–90), Average (95–105), and High-Average (110–120) Full Scale IQ. Participants were tested at 2-week intervals. Repeated measures analysis of variance indicated that Average and High-Average groups made greater gains across retest intervals than did the Low-Average group ($p < .002$). Across groups, gains were greater at the first retest than at the second or third retest ($p < .001$). A Scale × Time interaction indicated disproportionate gain in Performance IQ versus Verbal IQ, particularly at the first retest ($p < .001$). Previous exposure to the WAIS-R dramatically alters performance: Traditional interpretations regarding expected gain and profile analysis are not valid at retest.

The effect of repeated administration on the Wechsler Adult Intelligence Scale-Revised (WAIS-R) is well established: In the absence of factors adversely affecting cognitive or motivational status, scores increase with repeated exposure to the battery. In general, instruments that have a speeded component, require an infrequently-practiced response, or that have easily-conceptualized solutions are likely to result in significant practice effects (Dodrill & Troupin, 1975).

Practice effects reflect a combination of memory for item-specific factors of the test and memory for procedural aspects of the task. For instruments such as the WAIS-R that have no alternate forms, these two factors are inextricably confounded. Practice effects associated with memory for specific items are particularly likely to occur on tests that have a single solution that is easily remembered (e.g., object assembly). In contrast, procedural effects of practice reflect memory for general task demands,

in which repeated exposure improves performance through increased facility and familiarity with materials, as well as through the development of more effective problem-solving strategies (e.g., block design). Anastasi (1988) referred to this phenomenon as "test sophistication" and recommended that: (1) data regarding expected gains on retest are provided in test manuals, and (2) adjustment for expected gains are incorporated in the process of interpreting test scores (p. 45).

Few studies have examined test-retest reliability of the WAIS-R in either normal or clinical populations (Rawlings & Crewe, 1992). The existing literature indicates that the WAIS-R maintains robust test-retest reliability; however, these data reflect sizeable test-retest correlations, and do not necessarily indicate the absence of meaningful score change (Sattler, 1988). Individuals may demonstrate substantial change in performance at retest; yet, this phenomenon would have no effect on the

---

* Preliminary results of these data were presented at the 1996 meeting of the American Psychological Association, Toronto, Canada.
Address correspondence to: L. Rapport, Department of Psychology, 71 West Warren, Wayne State University, Detroit, MI 48202, USA.
Accepted for publication: February 12, 1997.

test-retest reliability coefficient were the individuals to maintain the same relative rank order. Thus, it is essential to differentiate the issue of test-retest reliability from that of test-retest *stability*, which reflects the extent to which individual scores remain the same across serial assessments. Information regarding stability of test scores is essential to clinical practice. For example, failure to account for expected gains due to practice may grossly underestimate an individual's level of disability, particularly with regard to deterioration in functioning or motivational change. Conversely, gains in scores at retest due to practice effects also may be misconstrued as recovery of function or improvement in ability.

In their review of test-retest stability for the WAIS, Matarazzo, Carmody, and Jacobs (1980) suggested that Full Scale IQ should be corrected on retest for an expected gain of 5 points due to practice effects. This guideline was later confirmed by an examination of the WAIS-R standardization data (Matarazzo & Herman, 1984). A variety of subsequent studies underscored the importance of differentiating the nature of practice effects for different populations of interest. For example, Horton (1992) reported that normal young adults showed greater improvement on intelligence tests at retest than did normal older persons. Similarly, Ryan, Paolo, and Brundgardt (1992) examined WAIS-R stability in a sample of normal adults aged 75 years or older and concluded that practice effects typically observed among young adult and middle-aged individuals may not occur as reliably in older populations.

Shatz (1981) argued that the criterion for expected gain on retest also varies as a function of brain state: Patients with significant brain damage may not be expected to show any practice effects with a single retesting. More important, Mitrushina and Satz (1991) highlighted the relevance of population-specific expectations by demonstrating differential patterns of gain on retest among old versus very old individuals. These authors reported greater effects of practice on Performance IQ among participants less than 75 years of age compared to their very old counterparts.

Little research has examined the effects of repeated administrations beyond a single retest. Yet, multiple assessments with the WAIS-R are common in clinical practice to document the course of illness and may frequently occur as a byproduct

of the adversarial nature of personal injury litigation (Putnam, Adams, & Schneider, 1992). Catron and Thompson (1979) followed a group of individuals across four retest intervals (1 week, 1 month, 2 months, and 4 months following the initial assessment) and reported gains in Wechsler Adult Intelligence Scale (WAIS) Full Scale IQ of 8, 6, 5, and 4 points, respectively. In an examination of WAIS-R practice effects among 85 patients recovering from traumatic brain injury, Rawlings and Crewe (1992) compared matched groups tested twice (2 and 12 months) and four times (2, 4, 8, and 12 months). Although both groups demonstrated significant gains in IQ scores at the 12-month evaluation, the group receiving four testings demonstrated significantly greater score improvements than did their twice-tested counterparts. Thus, research among neurologically-compromised individuals suggests that multiple assessments with the WAIS-R result in significant score improvements. However, there is also evidence that practice effects interact with brain state, and that cognitively-impaired individuals will benefit less from practice than will normal individuals (Kvale, 1988; Shatz, 1981).

A central and unanswered question relevant to expected gains following repeated administration of the WAIS-R concerns the potential mediating effects of IQ at initial testing on IQ at retest. Given evidence of population-specific differences in gain at retest, it is reasonable to expect that normal individuals obtaining below-average IQs at initial testing may benefit less from repeated exposure to the battery than would their average or above-average counterparts. To date, there are no published reports examining this phenomenon.

METHOD

Participants

The sample consisted of 36 normal adults (11 men and 21 women), ranging in age from 18 to 48 years ($M = 26.7$; $SD = 7.4$). Exclusionary criteria included significant medical history, substance abuse, and use of medications that may alter cognitive status. The present sample excludes one participant who withdrew from the study. Twelve participants, matched for education ($+2$ years), were assigned to each of three groups based on WAIS-R Full Scale IQ at initial testing: Low-Average (80–90),

Average (95–105), and High-Average (110–120). Mean years of education for the three groups were 15.3 (SD = 1.2), 15.5 (SD = 1.5), and 15.0 (SD = 1.6), respectively. The groups were equivalent in age ($F[2, 33]$ = 0.21, p = .81) and in the proportion of men and women, χ^2 (2, N = 36) = 4.05, p = .13.

Measures and Procedure

The WAIS-R was administered in its entirety as part of a larger neuropsychological assessment, using standard procedures described in the test manual (Wechsler, 1981). All participants were evaluated on four occasions, with retest intervals of exactly 2 weeks.

RESULTS

The main analyses were conducted using two analyses of variance (ANOVA) for repeated measures (alpha = .025). To control experiment-wise error, alpha for post hoc tests was set at .005. The first analysis examined change in Full Scale IQ, with Group (Low-Average, Average, and High-Average) as the between-subjects factor and Time of Testing as the within-subject factor. To directly examine differential performance in gains at each retest, the dependent variable was expressed as a difference score between adjacent administrations of the test. Thus, the within-subject factor had three

levels, reflecting gain in Full Scale IQ at Retests 1, 2, and 3. The ANOVA indicated significant main effects of both Group ($F[2, 33]$ = 7.87, p < .002) and Time ($F[2, 66]$ = 11.94, p < .001), but no Group × Time interaction ($F[4, 66]$ = 29.11, p = .24). Post hoc analyses conducted using univariate ANOVA revealed that total gain across the four assessments was significantly lower among the Low-Average group than among the Average and High-Average groups, whose mean gains were statistically equivalent ($F[2, 33]$ = 7.87, p < .002). Paired-sample t tests revealed that significantly greater gains were made at the first retest (M = 8.86, SD = 4.88) than at the second (M = 4.33, SD = 4.22; $t[35]$ = 4.31, p < .001) or third (M = 4.31, SD = 3.99; $t[35]$ = 4.02, p < .001) retest; however, gains made at the second and third retests were equivalent ($t[35]$ = 0.03, p = .49). Figure 1 depicts the cumulative mean gain in Full Scale IQ across the four testings for the three groups. Descriptive statistics for each condition are presented in Table 1.

A second repeated measures ANOVA was conducted to investigate whether the groups demonstrated differential patterns of gain on WAIS-R Verbal versus Performance IQ scales over the repeated administrations. As expected, the Group

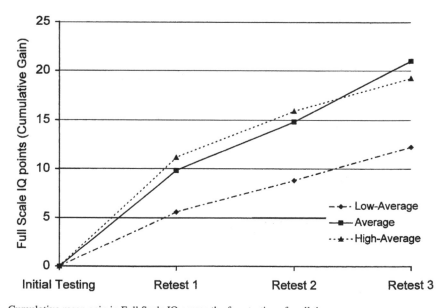

Fig. 1. Cumulative mean gain in Full Scale IQ across the four testings for all three groups.

and Group × Time ANOVAs were no different from the analysis for Full Scale IQ. A significant main effect was found for Scale ($F[1, 34] = 106.36, p < .001$), and the Scale × Time interaction was also significant ($F[2, 66] = 4.09, p < .02$). The Group × Scale ($F[2,33] = 0.11, p = .90$) and Group × Scale × Time ($F[4, 66] = 1.36, p = .26$) interactions were not significant. Post hoc tests of interest for the Scale × Time interaction included comparisons between gains on Verbal versus Performance IQ at similar retest intervals. Paired t tests revealed that, across groups, relative gains in Performance IQ significantly exceeded those observed in Verbal IQ at the first ($t[35] = 6.47, p < .001$), second ($t[35)] = 3.13, p < .002$) and third ($t[35] = 2.73, p < .005$) retest intervals. Moreover, the magnitude of gain in Performance IQ at the first retest ($M = 12.53, SD = 7.13$) was significantly greater than at the second ($M = 6.00, SD = 6.54; t[35] = 3.56, p < .001$) and third

($M = 5.78, SD = 5.13; t[35] = 4.75, p < .001$) retests, whereas gains in Performance IQ at the second and third retests were equivalent ($t[35] = 0.14, p = .45$). Gains in Verbal IQ across the first ($M = 4.06, SD = 4.01$), second ($M = 2.00, SD = 3.84$), and third ($M = 2.56, SD = 4.64$) retesting intervals were not significantly different, given adjustment for experiment-wise error (all $ps > .02$).

At initial testing, 12 participants (33%) displayed Verbal-Performance IQ discrepancies greater than 10 points. At the first retest, however, 21 participants (58%) displayed Verbal-Performance IQ discrepancies of this magnitude, with all but 2 of these individuals demonstrating a pattern of Performance IQ greater than Verbal IQ. By the final assessment, 27 participants (75%) displayed Performance IQ greater than Verbal IQ by 10 points or more, whereas no participant showed a Verbal IQ greater than Performance IQ discrepancy.

Table 1. Descriptive Statistics for WAIS-R Performance Over Four Assessments for Low-Average, Average, and High-Average Initial Full Scale IQ.

	Low-Average		Average		High-Average	
	M	SD	M	SD	M	SD
Full Scale IQ						
Initial testing	85.25	(3.33)	99.01	(2.68)	112.50	(1.93)
Retest 1	90.83	(5.34)	108.92	(6.16)	123.37	(6.80)
Mean gain	5.58	(2.84)	9.83	(4.22)	11.17	(5.59)
Retest 2	94.08	(6.27)	113.92	(8.66)	128.42	(7.38)
Mean gain	3.25	(2.56)	5.00	(4.49)	4.75	(5.29)
Retest 3	97.50	(6.97)	120.08	(8.38)	131.75	(5.45)
Mean gain	3.42	(2.84)	6.17	(4.84)	3.33	(3.70)
Verbal IQ						
Initial testing	85.75	(3.55)	100.08	(3.96)	108.92	(5.14)
Retest 1	87.42	(4.64)	104.83	(4.43)	114.67	(8.33)
Mean gain	1.67	(2.19)	4.75	(3.93)	5.75	(4.59)
Retest 2	90.25	(6.41)	106.00	(6.40)	116.67	(9.33)
Mean gain	2.83	(3.54)	1.17	(5.08)	2.00	(2.66)
Retest 3	91.42	(5.96)	111.00	(8.34)	118.17	(7.42)
Mean gain	1.17	(2.92)	5.00	(5.74)	1.50	(4.15)
Performance IQ						
Initial testing	88.00	(4.88)	98.83	(8.04)	115.42	(4.93)
Retest 1	97.58	(9.23)	113.42	(13.44)	128.83	(8.21)
Mean gain	9.58	(5.50)	14.58	(7.67)	13.42	(7.61)
Retest 2	101.58	(9.32)	121.08	(11.39)	135.17	(7.90)
Mean gain	4.00	(4.45)	7.67	(7.36)	6.33	(7.40)
Retest 3	108.50	(9.52)	126.33	(12.20)	140.33	(7.46)
Mean gain	6.92	(4.25)	5.25	(5.58)	5.17	(5.70)

Note. Retest intervals = 2 weeks. Low-Average, Average, and High Average Initial Full Scale IQ: all $n = 12$.

DISCUSSION

The results suggest that individuals with Average and High-Average Full Scale IQ at initial testing benefit more from prior exposure to the WAIS-R than do individuals with Low-Average IQ at initial testing. In essence, although all subjects improve across the four assessments, the rich get richer. Thus, because practice effects are mediated by initial IQ, clinicians should modify tolerance for expected gains at retest accordingly. This finding is consistent with related reports of population-specific differences in practice effects on the WAIS-R as a function of age (Horton, 1992; Mitrushina & Satz, 1991; Ryan, Paolo, & Brundgardt, 1992) and among clinical populations on the WAIS (Shatz, 1981).

Regardless of initial Full Scale IQ, the pattern of gains on repeated testings was both nonlinear, with the majority of gain occurring at the first retest, as well as asymmetric, with a preponderance of the improvement occurring in Performance versus Verbal IQ. In addition, the discrepancy between gain in Performance versus Verbal IQ was particularly great at the first retest. The disproportionate gain in Performance IQ likely reflects a vulnerability of the WAIS-R performance subtests associated with bonus points awarded for speed of solution. Although the development of alternate forms for these subtests would address practice effects associated with memory for specific items, a solution of this nature would not address increased task familiarity for subtests such as Block Design. Therefore, one possible solution would be to combine the development of a parallel form with restandardization of bonus points awarded for speed at retest.

Clinicians conducting profile interpretations should note that by the first retest, nearly 60% of normal individuals displayed a Verbal-Performance IQ discrepancy that exceeds the 95% confidence interval as provided in the WAIS-R manual. Nearly all of these cases represented a disproportionate gain in Performance IQ. Thus, verbal-performance discrepancies observed at retest far exceeded the base rate of statistically reliable verbal-performance discrepancies observed among individuals tested once in the WAIS-R standardization sample (37%; Matarazzo & Herman, 1984). At initial testing, verbal-performance discrepancies in the present sample (33%) approximated the base rate of that phenomenon in the WAIS-R standardization sample.

In sum, previous exposure to the WAIS-R dramatically alters performance, and traditional methods of calculating expected gain and profile analysis are not valid at retest.

REFERENCES

Anastasi, A. (1988). *Psychological testing* (6th ed.). New York: Macmillan.

Catron, D.W., & Thompson, C.C. (1979). Test-retest gains in WAIS score after four retest intervals. *Journal of Clinical Psychology, 35*, 352–357.

Dodrill, C.B., & Troupin, A.S. (1975). Effects of repeated administrations of a comprehensive neuropsychological battery among chronic epileptics. *The Journal of Nervous and Mental Disease, 161*, 185–190.

Horton, A.M. (1992). Neuropsychological practice effects. Age: A brief note. *Perceptual and Motor Skills, 75*, 257–258.

Kvale, V.I. (1987). WAIS-R practice effects. *Journal of Clinical and Experimental Neuropsychology, 9*, 35.

Matarazzo, J., Carmody, T.P., & Jacobs, L.D. (1980). Test-retest reliability and stability for the WAIS: A literature review with implications for clinical practice. *Journal of Clinical Neuropsychology, 2*, 89–105.

Matarazzo, J., & Herman, D.O. (1984). Base rate data for the WAIS-R: Test-retest stability and VIQ-PIQ differences. *Journal of Clinical Neuropsychology, 6*, 351–366.

Mitrushina, M., & Satz, P. (1991). Effect of repeated administration of a neuropsychological battery in the elderly. *Journal of Clinical Psychology, 47*, 790–801.

Putnam, S.H., Adams, K.M., & Schneider, A.M. (1992). One-day test-retest reliability of neuropsychological tests in a personal injury case. *Psychological Assessment, 4*, 312–316.

Rawlings, D.B., & Crewe, N.M. (1992). Test-retest effects and test score changes of the WAIS-R in recovering traumatically brain-injured survivors. *The Clinical Neuropsychologist, 6*, 415–430.

Ryan, J.J., Paolo, A.M., & Brundgardt, T.M. (1992). WAIS-R test-retest stability in normal persons 75 years and older. *The Clinical Neuropsychologist, 6*, 3–8.

Sattler, J.M. (1988). *Assessment of children* (3rd ed.). San Diego: Sattler.

Shatz, M.W. (1981). WAIS practice effects in clinical neuropsychology. *Journal of Clinical Neuropsychology, 3*, 171–179.

Wechsler, D. (1981). *WAIS-R Manual: Wechsler Adult Intelligence Scale-Revised*. New York: The Psychological Corporation.

Journal of Clinical and Experimental Neuropsychology
1994, Vol. 16, No. 1, pp. 155–161

METHODOLOGICAL NOTE

Multiple Comparison Methods: Establishing Guidelines for their Valid Application in Neuropsychological Research

Domenic V. Cicchetti
West Haven VAMC and Yale University

ABSTRACT

This comment serves to provide a rationale for research clinical neuropsychologists to decide: (1) under what conditions multiple comparison methods are required; and (2) what specific guidelines can be used to distinguish conditions favoring a given multiple comparison technique over its competitors. The topic is discussed both for the parametric and nonparametric case, as well as for post hoc tests following both statistically significant main effects and interactions.

INTRODUCTION

Scientists, in general, and neuropsychologists, in particular, are often faced with the task of deciding the following: first, under which conditions multiple comparison procedures are warranted, and, secondly, which criteria to apply in choosing one available technique over another.

It is the purpose of this report to provide specific guidelines to the research clinical neuropsychologist who must make decisions about these two fundamental issues.

Because the analysis of variance (ANOVA), in one of its variations, usually precedes the question of whether it is necessary to apply multiple comparison methods, it will be discussed first, in terms of main effects, such as in one-way ANOVA, and then, with respect to interactions deriving from a factorial ANOVA. Finally, briefly the issue of performing multiple comparisons when the ANOVA model does not apply are addressed. In summary, then, the issue of multiple comparisons are discussed both for the parametric (ANOVA) and non-parametric case.

THE PROBLEM

In the case of any two-group comparison in which the samples derive from the **same** normal population, Type I or alpha error (falsely claiming statistical significance) will occur at a nominal rate of 5% (e.g., Boneau, 1960). The Type II or beta error (missing statistical significance when it, in fact, exists) can be expected to occur at the same rate. However, the convention is to consider Type I error to be of the order of about four times more serious than Type I error. Therefore, the Type II (beta) error is usually set at about 20% (e.g., Cohen, 1988). Since power $= (1 - $ Beta error), this translates into power of 80%.

TESTS PRECEDING MULTIPLE COMPARISONS: I: THE ANALYSIS OF VARIANCE (ANOVA)

When we speak of the problem of multiple comparisons, we are referring to a minimum of three groups of interest in the frequent case when no

---

Address correspondence to: Domenic V. Cicchetti, Ph.D., Department of Veterans Affairs, Medical Center, 950 Campbell Avenue, West Haven, CT 06516, USA.

specific directional hypothesis is warranted, either on the basis of clinical or research considerations. At least in the case of interval (continuous, or dimensional) data, we are usually referring to a research design involving one of the numerous analysis of variance (or ANOVA) models. This robust procedure dates back to the first paper on this topic which was published by R.A. Fisher and W.A. Mackenzie in 1923. As discussed by Cochran in 1980, the original authors analyzed the results of a $2 \times 12 \times 3$ factorial experiment in which the dependent variable was yield of potatoes. The three factors were: (1) Farmyard manure classified at 2 levels: absent or present; (2) Variety of potato (12 types); and (3) Type of chemical added to the planting soil (3 conditions, namely, none, potassium sulphate, or potassium chloride). The layout was described as a split-plot agricultural design.

In 1947, the statistician, Churchill Eisenhart, published an important theoretical paper, in the third volume of **Biometrics**, entitled "The Assumptions Underlying the Analysis of Variance". Curiously, although Eisenhart discussed briefly the assumption of normality, his treatise focused more upon structural aspects of the ANOVA model such as formulae for deriving components of variance, and mathematical relationships among ANOVA formulae. Over the ensuing four decades and more, a proliferation of articles has focused upon the consequences of violating the basic assumptions underlying the **application** of ANOVA models to research data. Basically, three assumptions were considered: (1) that group sample sizes need to be equal; (2) that the shape of group distributions must be the same or very similar; and (3) that variances shall not vary appreciably (the assumption of homoskedasticity). It should be noted that some statisticians, such as Kerlinger (1973) had made the erroneous implication that interval scale data are necessary for using ANOVA methods. However, as Gaito and others have noted, an examination of the ANOVA requirements reveals that "an assumption of interval scale is nowhere to be found". (Gaito 1974, p. 39).

In my attempt to summarize the results of this vast, varied, and diversified literature, it must be borne in mind that no matter how noble the attempt, there will always be lacunae, voids, missing pieces to the puzzle.

This becomes inevitable in any area of research given the constraints or limitations of time, money, and fundamental knowledge.

Having said that, the best conclusion that can be reached is that the ANOVA is quite robust to violations of assumptions, and will therefore provide adequate protection against both Type I and Type II errors. This holds if the violations of assumptions involve any one of these three conditions:

1. The ns differ appreciably **but** there are no appreciable differences in either variances or shapes of distributions of the groups which are being compared.
2. The shapes of the distributions differ but the sample sizes and variances are quite similar.
3. The variances differ appreciably but the sample sizes as well as the shapes of the sample distributions are quite similar.

There appear to be four classes of **egregious** violations of assumptions underlying the ANOVA-ones that provide **inadequate** protection against Type I (alpha) and Type II (beta) errors, or that provide an unacceptably high risk of either claiming statistical significance when the claim is unwarranted (alpha error) or failing to claim statistical significance when it is, in fact, warranted (beta error). The four classes or conditions of violations are:

1. **Both** the ns and the variances differ appreciably from one sample to the next (i.e., ns 3:1 or greater and S^2s 4:1 or greater).
2. **Both** the ns and the shapes of the sample distributions vary widely from one sample to another (i.e., ns 3:1 or greater and qualitatively different distributions, such as normal vs. exponential, vs. U-shaped vs. rectangular).
3. **Both** the variances and the shapes of the distributions differ considerably (i.e., S^2s 4:1 or greater and qualitatively different shapes of sample distributions).
4. The ns, the variances, and the shapes of the sample distributions differ appreciably (i.e., ns 3:1 or greater and S^2s 4:1 or greater **and** shapes of the distributions **qualitatively** dissimilar).

Under any one of these four conditions, ANOVA procedures cannot be used and appropriate nonparametric analogues of the ANOVA need to be applied (e.g., the recommended statistical tests and multiple comparison procedures published in Leach, 1979). Depending upon the specific group comparisons that are of research interest, one can choose appropriately the multiple comparison method of choice. This is illustrated as follows:

A. The one-way ANOVA case based upon k groups

Specific Group Comparisons	Statistic of Choice	Reference
a) Restricted to a smaller number of the available $k(k-1)/2$ paired comparisons	Bonferroni inequality	Fleiss, 1986, pp. 104–107
b) Restricted to all possible $k(k-1)/2$ paired comparisons	Tukey test	Fleiss, 1986, pp. 58–59
c) Restricted to comparing a Control (C) group to to two or more Experimental (E) groups (with no interest in comparing the E groups to each other)	Dunnett test	Fleiss, 1986, pp. 92–96
d) Generalized to all possible comparisons	Sheffé test	Fleiss, 1986, pp. 55–57

Before proceeding to a consideration of multiple comparison procedures in the Factorial ANOVA case, it should be noted that I have purposely avoided mentioning several other major multiple comparison procedures. These include: (1) multiple application of the standard t test (paired or unpaired) for each comparison of interest; (2) the test due to Duncan (1955); and (3) the Newman-Keuls test, based upon the work of Newman (1939) and Keuls (1952). The reason for these omissions is that each of these tests has been shown empirically to fail to protect adequately at least for Type I error (see, especially the early work of Petrinovich & Hardyck, 1969). Since the tests produce more sample comparison significance than occurs in parent populations, they tend to control well for Type II error. Since Type I error is usually considered far more serious than Type II error, most statisticians recommend that these procedures not be utilized. (For a comprehensive review of available multiple comparison

procedures, the interested reader is referred to Toothaker, 1991.)

B. The factorial ANOVA case

In the preceding one-way ANOVA case, once an appropriate multiple comparison procedure is selected — Bonferroni, Tukey, Dunnett, or Sheffé — there is no problem in interpreting the meaning of the results of a given group comparison, since each group is defined on the basis of a **single** variable of classification, such as diagnostic category. This phenomenon, or unconfounded interpretation of the means deriving from a given one-way ANOVA design, is also more generally true of any statistically significant **main** effect deriving from a factorial ANOVA design. It will present serious problems of interpretation when one attempts to compare the means of the individual cells comprising the interaction table of specific focus. Cicchetti (1972, pp. 405–406) addressed this problem more generally. Thus, in the simplest of the factorial ANOVA designs (Table 1) a statistically significant 2×2 interaction will present with problems of interpretation whenever one intends to compare some of the four group means A_1B_1, A_1B_2, A_2B_1, A_2B_2, to each other. As noted in the 1972 article (again pp. 405–406):

"It is clear that if one compared either Cells A_1B_2 and A_2B_2 or Cells A_2B_1 and A_1B_2, one could not determine how much of the difference to attribute to Factor A, and how much to attribute to Factor B, all other things being equal. This problem of interpretation does not occur in the remaining four paired contrasts.

Table 1. Illustration of Confounded Comparisons in a 2×2 (A $\times$ B) Interaction Table.[1]

Factor	Factor	
	B_1	B_2
A_1	A_1B_1	A_1B_2
A_2	A_2B_1	A_2B_2

Note. [1] The four unconfounded comparisons are A_1B_1 vs. A_1B_2; A_2B_1 vs. A_2B_2; A_1B_1 vs. A_2B_1; and A_1B_2 vs. A_2B_2. The two confounded comparisons are A_1B_1 vs. A_2B_2 and A_1B_2 vs. A_2B_1.
(This information derives from Cicchetti (1972, p. 406.)

Table 2. Illustration of the 12 cells in a 3 × 4 (A × B) Interaction Table.[1]

Factor	Factor			
	B_1	B_2	B_3	B_4
A_1	A_1B_1	A_1B_2	A_1B_3	A_1B_4
A_2	A_2B_1	A_2B_2	A_2B_3	A_2B_4
A_3	A_3B_1	A_3B_2	A_3B_3	A_3B_4

Note. [1] The total number of possible paired comparisons is given by $k(k-1)/2 = (12)(11)/2 = 66$. The number of unconfounded comparisons is given for rows by $R[k(k-1)/2] = 3[(4)(3)/2] = 18$, and, for columns as $C[k(k-1)/2] = 4[(3)(2)/2] = 12$, giving a total of 30 unconfounded comparisons. By subtraction, there are $66-30$ or 36 or 55% confounded comparisons.

The number of confounded comparisons increases the greater the number of cells in a given interaction table. Thus, for the simple 3 × 4 analysis of variance, the proportion of confounded comparisons is about 55%, as shown in Table 2. The importance of this fact is that the more comparisons one is making in any given experiment, the greater the probability that some of these comparisons will be significantly **different** from each other, by **chance** alone. In order to correct for this phenomenon the difference between any set of means, to be judged statistically significant, must **increase** the greater the number of means one is comparing." (pp. 405–406)

The significance of the information provided in Table 2 is that there are $(12 \times 11)/2$ or 66 paired contrasts in all. If one were to apply the standard Tukey multiple range test to actual data deriving from such a 3 × 4 interaction table, one would be "**penalized** by being forced to accept a minimal significant difference based upon 66 comparisons, when only 30 of these can be meaningfully interpreted" (Cicchetti, 1972, p. 406).

The solution to this problem is presented in detail in Cicchetti (1972, pp. 406–408), in both the all $k(k-1)/2$ unconfounded **comparisons** case (the Tukey test adjustment) and the all possible **unconfounded comparisons** case (the Scheffe adjustment). It should be noted that while the less than $k(k-1)/2$ unconfounded comparisons case (the Bonferroni test adjustment) was not considered in

this paper, its application seems self-evident and could easily be applied by utilizing the formulae provided in Fleiss (1986, pp. 104–107). Finally, my adjustment has recently been recommended (with applications for its use) by the multiple comparison specialist (Toothaker, 1991, pp. 122–126).

Before leaving this topic, it is important to note that the scholarly computer simulation study of Petrinovich and Hardyck (1969) provides some crucial information on minimal sample size requirements required for the valid application of appropriate multiple comparison methods. These authors note:

"If sample size is less than 10, it scarcely seems worthwhile to carry out the computations for multiple comparisons since the power of any method to detect differences between small groups is extremely low." (p. 53)

In the final section of this paper, I shall discuss the issue of performing multiple comparisons when the ANOVA model does not apply. This phenomenon would occur, for example, when: (a) violations of assumptions of the ANOVA fit the classification of **Egregious**; (b) the ANOVA is inappropriate for other reasons (e.g., the data are Nominally scaled); or (c) the data are summarized in the form of statistics **other** than the **mean**, such as comparisons of, say, **proportions** of cases (e.g., deriving from previous chi-square(d) analyses).

In such a case, one needs, first, to select an appropriate analogue to the original statistic of choice (say, the Kruskal-Wallis statistic as a substitute for the one-way ANOVA). One then determines the number of comparisons of interest. As an example, one might compare the ranked scores of four groups of subjects and be interested in all six paired contrasts (or $4 \times 3)/2 = 6$). Here, with alpha error set at the conventional .05 level, **adjusted** alpha becomes $.05/6 = .008$. If application of the Kruskal-Wallis test produces a statistically significant result at .006, then one would need to select an appropriate nonparametric test to make each of the six specific paired comparisons. An appropriate test here would be the Rank Sum test (e.g., see Leach, 1979, Chapter 4, pp. 148–168; see also Toothaker, 1991, Chapter 4, pp. 106–109).

In summary, this commentary is a discussion of some of my recent thoughts about the multiple comparison problem in biomedical and behavioral science research. Accompanying this report is a bibliography applicable to this commentary and to the field more generally. Given that the topic is not presented in this format in any of the available general psychology statistical texts with which I am familiar, it is hoped this report fills the resultant void. For a scholarly, more detailed and technical treatise of this topic, the interested reader is referred again to the recent text by Toothaker (1991).

REFERENCES

Algina, J., & Tang, K.L. (1988). Type I error rates for Yao's and James' tests of equality of mean vectors under variance-covariance heteroscedasticity. *Journal of Educational Statistics, 13*, 281–290.

Bevan, M.F., Denton, J.Q., & Myers, J.L. (1974). The robustness of the F test to violations of continuity and form of treatment population. *British Journal of Mathematical and Statistical Psychology, 27*, 199–204.

Bishop, T.A., & Dudewicz, E.J. (1976, March). *Heteroscedastic ANOVA*. (Tech. Rep. No. 143). Columbus: Ohio State University, Department of Statistics.

Bishop, T.A., & Dudewicz, E.J. (1977, March). *Analysis of variance with unequal variances test procedures and tables*. (Tech. Rep. No. 144). Columbus: Ohio State University, Department of Statistics.

Blair, R.C., & Higgins, J.J. (1985). Comparison of the power of the paired samples *t* test to that of Wilcoxon's Signed-Ranks Test under various population shapes. *Psychological Bulletin, 97*, 119–128.

Bohrer, R., Chow, W., Faith, R., Joshi, V.M., & Wu, C.F. (1981). Multiple three-decision rules for factorial simple effects: Bonferroni wins again! *Journal of the American Statistical Association, 76*, 119–124.

Boneau, C.A. (1960). The effects of violations of assumptions underlying the *t* test. *Psychological Bulletin, 57*, 49–64.

Box, G.E.P. (1953). Non-normality and tests on variances. *Biometrika, 40*, 318–335.

Bradley, J.V. (1966). *Studies in research methodology VII: The Central Limit effect for two dozen populations and its correlation with population moments*. (Tech. Rep. (AMRL-TR) No. 66–242). Ohio: Wright-Patterson Air Force Base, Aerospace Medical Research Laboratories.

Bradu, D., & Gabriel, K.R. (1974). Simultaneous statistical inference on interactions in two-way analysis of variance. *Journal of the American Statistical Association, 69*, 428–436.

Breen, L., & Gaito, J. (1970). Comments on Friedman's R_m procedure. *Psychological Bulletin, 73*, 309–310.

Cicchetti, D.V. (1972). Extension of multiple range tests to interaction tables in the analysis of variance: A rapid approximate solution. *Psychological Bulletin, 77*, 405–408.

Cicchetti, D.V. (1974). Reply to Keselman concerning Cicchetti's interpretation of the findings of Petri novich and Hardyck. *Psychological Bulletin, 81*, 896–897.

Cochran, W.G. (1980). Fisher and the analysis of variance. In S.E. Fienberg & D.V. Hinkley (Eds.), *Lecture notes in statistics 1: R.A. Fisher: An appreciation* (pp. 17–34). New York: Springer-Verlag.

Cohen, J. (1988). *Statistical power analysis for the behavioral sciences* (2nd ed.). Hillsdale, NJ: Lawrence Erlbaum.

Dawkins, H.C. (1983). Multiple comparisons misused: Why so frequently in response-curve studies? *Biometrics, 39*, 789–790.

Duncan, D.B. (1955). Multiple range and multiple F tests. *Biometrics, Il*, 1–42.

Duncan D.B., & Bryant, L.J. (1983). Adaptive *t* tests for multiple comparisons. *Biometrics, 39*, 790–794.

Dunn, O.J. (1961). Multiple comparisons among means. *Journal of the American Statistical Association, 56*, 52–64.

Dunnett, C.W. (1955). A multiple comparison procedure for comparing several treatments with a control. *American Statistical Association Journal, 50*, 1096–1121.

Dunnett, C.W. (1964). New tables for multiple comparisons with a control. *Biometrics, 20*, 482–491.

Dunnett, C.W. (1980). Pairwise multiple comparisons in the homogeneous variance, unequal sample size case. *Journal of the American Statistical Association, 75*, 789–795.

Dunnett, C.W. (1980). Pairwise multiple comparisons in the unequal variance case. *Journal of the American Statistical Association, 75*, 796–800.

Eisenhart, C. (1947). The assumptions underlying the analysis of variance. *Biometrics, 3*, 1–21.

Fisher, R.A., & Mackenzie, W.A. (1923). Studies in crop variation. II. The manurial response of different potato varieties. *Journal of Agricultural Science, 13*, 311–320.

Fleiss, J.L. (1986). *The design and analysis of clinical experiments*. New York: John Wiley & Sons.

Friedman, M. (1937). The use of ranks to avoid the assumption of normality implicit in the analysis of variance. *Journal of the American Statistical Association, 32*, 675–701.

Gabriel, K.R. (1963). *A computer program for testing the homogeneity of all sets of means in analysis of variance*. Unpublished manuscript.

Gabriel, K.R. (1964). A procedure for testing the homogeneity of all sets of means in the analysis of variance. *Biometrics, 20*, 459–477.

Gabriel, K.R. (1978). A simple method of multiple comparisons of means. *Journal of the American Statistical Association, 73*, 724–729.

Gaito, J. (1974). A review of F.N. Kerlinger's *Foundations of behavioral research* (2nd ed.). New York: Holt, Rinehart, & Winston, 1973. *Psychometrika, 39*, 273–274.

Grove, W.M., & Andreasen, N.C. (1982). Simultaneous tests of many hypotheses in exploratory research. *Journal of Nervous and Mental Disease, 170*, 3–8.

Harris, R.J. (1975). *A primer of multivariate statistics.* New York: Academic Press.

Harter, H.L. (1960). Tables of range and studentized range. *Annals of Mathematical Statistics, 31*, 1122–1147.

Harter, H.L. (1970). Multiple comparison procedures for interaction. *The American Statistician, 24*, 30–32.

Higazi, S.M.F., & Dayton, C.M. (1988). Tables for a multivariate extension of the Dunnett test when the control group and balanced experimental groups have different sample sizes. *Communications in Statistics: Simulations, 17*, 85–101.

Hollingsworth, H.H. (1980, March). *Estimating strength of levels of main, simple main and interaction effects in ANOVA.* Paper presented at the joint meeting of the American Statistical Association.

Horsnell, G. (1953). The effect of unequal group variances on the F test for the homogeneity of group means. *Biometrika, 40*, 128–136.

Jaccard, J., Becker, M.A., & Wood, G. (1984). Pairwise multiple comparison procedures: A review. *Psychological Bulletin, 96*, 589–596.

Johnson, D.E. (1976). Some new multiple comparison procedures for the two-way ANOVA Model with interaction. *Biometrics, 32*, 929–934.

Kerlinger, F.N. (1973). *Foundations of behavioral research* (2nd ed). New York: Holt, Rinehart, & Winston.

Keselman, H.J. (1974). Cicchetti's reversal of Petrinovich and Hardyck's major conclusions. *Psychological Bulletin, 81*, 896–897.

Keselman, H.J. (1976). A power investigation of the Tukey multiple comparison statistic. *Educational and Psychological Measurement, 36*, 97–104.

Keselman, H.J., Games, P.A., & Clinch, J.J. (1979). Tests for homogeneity of variance. *Communications in Statistics: Simulations and Computations, 138*, 113–129.

Keselman, H.J., Games, P.A., & Rogan, J.C. (1980). Type I and Type II errors in simultaneous and two-stage multiple comparison procedures. *Psychological Bulletin, 88*, 356–358.

Keselman, H.J., & Keselman, J.C. (1988). Repeated measures multiple comparison procedures: Effects of violating multisample sphericity in unbalanced designs. *Journal of Educational Statistics, 13*, 215–226.

Keselman, H.J., Murray, R., & Rogan, J. (1976). Effect of very unequal group sizes on Tukey's multiple comparison test. *Educational and Psychological Measurement, 36*, 263–270.

Keselman, H.J., & Rogan, J.C. (1977). The Tukey multiple comparison test: 1953–1976. *Psychological Bulletin, 84*, 1050–1056.

Keselman, H.J., & Toothaker, L.E. (1973). Error rates for multiple comparison methods: Some evidence concerning the misleading conclusions of Petrinovich and Hardyck. *Psychological Bulletin, 80*, 31–32.

Keselman, H.J., & Toothaker, L.E. (1974). Comparison of Tukey's T-method and Sheffé's S-method for various numbers of all possible differences of averages contrasts under violation of assumptions. *Educational and Psychological Measurement, 34*, 511–519.

Keuls, M. (1952). The use of the "studentized range" in connection with an analysis of variance. *Euphytica, 1*, 112–122.

Kramer, C.Y. (1956). Extension of multiple range tests to group means with unequal numbers of replications. *Biometrics, 12*, 307–310.

Leach, C. (1979). *Introduction to statistics: A nonparametric approach for the social sciences.* New York: John Wiley & Sons.

Lehmann, E.L., & Shaffer, J.P. (1977). On a fundamental theorem in multiple comparisons. *Journal of the American Statistical Association, 72*, 576–578.

Marascuilo, L.A. (1966). Large-sample multiple comparisons. *Psychological Bulletin, 65*, 280–290.

Maxwell, S.E. (1980). Pairwise multiple comparisons in repeated measures designs. *Journal of Educational Statistics, 5*, 269–287.

Miller, R.G. (1976). *Advances in multiple comparisons in the last decade* (Tech. Rep. No. 26). California: Stanford University.

Miller, R.P. (1977). Developments in multiple comparisons: 1966–1976. *Journal of the American Statistical Association, 72*, 779–788.

Milligan, G.W. (1980). Factors that affect Type I and Type II error rates in the analysis of multidimensional contingency tables. *Psychological Bulletin, 87*, 238–244.

Newman, D. (1939). The distribution of range in samples from a normal population, expressed in terms of independent estimate of a standard deviation. *Biometrika, 31*, 20–30.

O'Brien, P.C. (1983). The appropriateness of analysis of variance and multiple comparison procedures. *Biometrics, 39*, 787–794.

O'Grady, K.E. (1982). Measures of explained variance: Cautions and limitations. *Psychological Bulletin, 92*, 766–777.

Permutter, J., & Myers, J.L. (1973). A comparison of two procedures for testing multiple contrasts. *Psychological Bulletin, 79*, 181–184.

Petrinovich, L.F., & Hardyck, C.D. (1969). Error rates for multiple comparison methods: Some evidence concerning the frequency of erroneous conclusions. *Psychological Bulletin, 71*, 43–54.

Rodger, R.S. (1974). Multiple contrasts, factors, error rate and power. *British Journal of Mathematical and Statistical Psychology, 27*, 179–198.

Rosenthal, R., & Rubin, D.B. (1983). Ensemble-adjusted p values. *Psychological Bulletin, 94*, 540–541.

Ryan, T.A. (1959). Multiple comparisons in psychological research. *Psychological Bulletin, 56*, 26–47.

Ryan, T.A. (1960). Significance tests for multiple comparison of proportions, variances, and other statistics. *Psychological Bulletin, 57*, 318–328.

Ryan, T.A. (1980). Comment on "protecting the overall rate of Type I errors for pairwise comparisons with an omnibus statistic." *Psychological Bulletin, 88*, 354–355.

Ryan, T.A. (1985). "Ensemble adjusted p values": How are they to be weighted? *Psychological Bulletin, 97*, 521–526.

Schafer, W.D., & Macready, G.B. (1975). A modification of the Bonferroni procedure on contrasts which are grouped into internally independent sets. *Biometrics, 31*, 227–228.

Scheffé, H. (1953). A method for judging all contrasts in the analysis of variance. *Biometrica, 40*, 87–104.

Shaffer, J.P. (1977). Multiple comparisons emphasizing selected contrasts: An extension and generalization of Dunnett's procedure. *Biometrics, 33*, 293–303.

Sirotnik, B.W.Q., & Beaver, R.J. (1984). Paired comparison experiments involving all possible pairs. *British Journal of Mathematical and Statistical Psychology, 37*, 22–33.

Smith, R.A. (1971). The effect of unequal group size on Tukey's HSD procedure. *Psychometrika, 36*, 31–34.

Stoline, M.R., & Ury, H.K. (1979). Tables of the studentized maximum modulus distribution and an application to multiple comparisons among means. *Technometrics, 21*, 87–93.

Toothaker, L.E. (1991). *Multiple comparisons for researchers.* Newbury Park, CA: Sage.

Ury, H.K., & Wiggins, A.D. (1974). Use of the Bonferroni inequality for multiple comparisons among means with post hoc contrasts. *British Journal of Mathematical and Statistical Psychology, 27*, 176–178.

Journal of Clinical and Experimental Neuropsychology
1992, Vol. 14, No. 6, pp. 981–982

VIII-K

COMMENT

Adjusting for Demographic Covariates by the Analysis of Covariance

Nancy C. Berman[1] and Samuel W. Greenhouse[2]

[1] Harbor-UCLA Medical Center, and [2] George Washington University

A paper by Adams, Brown, and Grant (1985), appearing in this Journal, advised against adjusting for demographic covariates by the analysis of covariance (ANCOVA). This paper came to our attention because one of us (NB) is a co-author on a paper submitted to a journal that was rejected by one referee on the basis of the cited paper. The article has also been cited in grant reviews. We thus deduce that the Adams et al. paper has had a big impact on the scientific community that constitutes the readership of *JCEN*.

We find several points made by Adams et al. of questionable validity, for the most part obscuring the major thesis the authors are trying to make, and leading to questionable interpretations by their readers. According to our reading, the main point made by the authors is that the classical (Fisherian) ANCOVA should not be carried out when the rather rigorous assumptions necessary for the validity of that procedure are violated. We agree. No amounts of pseudo-simulations are needed to establish this conclusion. However, these assumptions apply to any type of covariate not merely to demographic ones and do not imply that ANCOVA should be uniformly avoided for all possible demographic covariates. We must point out that Adams et al. discuss or construct examples using education as the covariate where associations between the dependent variable and education within the patient and control groups were different, or where this relationship within the two groups was the same but was different between the two groups, thereby obtaining "anomalous" results.

Since these are violations of one of the major assumptions of ANCOVA, the result is not surprising. We remark that any kind of a covariate, not only demographic ones, might lead to anomalous results when ANCOVA is applied incorrectly.

Our most serious concern, however, is that the Adams et al. paper has led many readers to the conclusion that no analysis of the effects of imbalances in important covariates should be made at all, whether or not mean values ought to be adjusted. As an illustration, assume with corresponding difference in some dependent variable Y between two groups:

Less than 8 yrs	+30
8 yrs	+20
9–12 yrs	(−20)
12 or more yrs	(−30)

We may not want to adjust the average difference in order to arrive at an overall difference, but every investigator should be interested in exploring and understanding these strata results. We also note that, unlike Fisher's ANCOVA, such analyses are carried out without the necessity of constructing models of the data. We let the data speak for themselves.

REFERENCE

Adams, K.M., Brown, G.C., & Grant I. (1985). Analysis of covariance as a remedy for demographic mismatch of research subject groups: Some sobering simulations. *Journal of Clinical and Experimental Neuropsychology, 7*, 445–462.

Authors address for reprints: Nancy G. Berman, Ph.D. Assistant Professor Harbor-UCLA Medical Center, 1000 West Carson Street, Torrance, CA 90509, USA.
Accepted for publication: March 3, 1992.

Journal of Clinical and Experimental Neuropsychology
1992, Vol. 14, No. 6, pp. 983–985

VIII-K

COMMENT

Covariance is Not the Culprit: Adams, Brown, and Grant Reply

Kenneth M. Adams[1], Gregory G. Brown[2], and Igor Grant[3]

[1]Veterans Affairs Medical Center and The University of Michigan, Ann Arbor, [2]Henry Ford Hospital, and [3]University of California and Veterans Affairs Medical Center, San Diego

Berman and Greenhouse (1992) have suggested that our 1985 JCEN paper (Adams, Brown, & Grant, 1985) somehow misleads readers and has had a negative impact upon the ability of investigators to utilize analysis of covariance (ANCOVA) as a tool in neuropsychological research. Let us first say that our intent in writing the paper was constructive and didactic in nature. We are gratified that the paper has merited attention by colleagues in the field; but we regret any misapplication of our contribution. The epitome of our message has been aired fully in the statistical literature for some time. Our goal in bringing the issue to JCEN readers' attention with some original simulations was to alert colleagues to a misuse of covariance that had been appearing in published reports with increasing frequency.

The common sense problem leading to the misuse is simple. Unfortunate situations occur in neuropsychological research wherein the investigator has carefully marshalled data on a clinical group or procedure of interest, only to find at the time of analysis that the control or comparison group differs on one or more variables that are of key importance (usually – but not always – age and education). This situation is made more complex by more general problems inherent in the role of attribute variables in neuropsychological research (Tupper & Rosenblood, 1984).

After-the-fact remedies for the problem of demographic mismatch are rarely easy or methodologically without risk. It is difficult to know how the practice started, but some neuropsychological researchers in the mid 1970's began to use analysis of covariance to examine the effect of such demographic mismatches on the dependent variable(s) of interest. Doubtless this occurred in part because of the increased accessibility to such statistical procedures that occurred at that time. However, this increased availability of computer mainframe software was not always accompanied by full documentation of the real indications for, and limits of, such analysis (cf., Rourke & Adams, 1984).

Neuropsychological researchers employing such ANCOVA programs apparently became persuaded that the results from an analysis of covariance somehow corrected the demographic mismatch or permitted them to exclude demographic mismatch as a cause for their findings. Especially problematic was the use of ANCOVA to adjust for systematic group differences in a covariate when the differences were produced by a sampling bias. Our paper simply informed readers that such adjustments were not adequate with some illustrative examples from our own research. Mean adjustments were not the central point of the paper, as most statistical experts

Address correspondence to: Kenneth M. Adams, Ph.D., Department of Psychiatry (Box 0704), University of Michigan Medical Center, Ann Arbor, MI, 48109-0704, USA.
Accepted for publication: April 18, 1992.

would agree; but these "adjusted means" aided in illustrating the absurd outcomes of some of our simulations employing the misapplication.

Several points are also worth additional emphasis in light of the Berman and Greenhouse (1992) critique. Our paper addressed itself to *ex-post-facto* use of ANCOVA. Carefully conceptualized protocols that build covariance corrections into the design as structural elements are a rather different case when combined with appropriate power and parametric expectancies. With reference to the contention by Berman and Greenhouse (1992) that we have implicitly or explicitly discouraged applications of ANCOVA, a complete reading of our original paper will bear no such interpretation; in point of fact we recapitulated a number of valid and useful ways in which ANCOVA can deal with needs of investigators other than that of sanction-ing direct causal effects that are more wish than fact (cf., Adams et al., 1985, p. 446). Adjustments using ANCOVA can deal with such significant issues as baseline effects on outcome performance, and more precise within-cell regression adjustments on demographic variables where there are **not** differences between groups on these variables and there are *a priori* reasons to make these adjustments.

The ANCOVA technique is simply not the problem here. Rather, the issue is more the misguided deployment of the technique to falsely reassure the investigator that the results of a memory tests pitting less well-educated alcoholics against far better-educated nonalcoholic controls can somehow dismiss education as a viable main explanation for the results.

As to the example offered by Berman and Greenhouse (1992), one can only suggest that it is highly unlikely that real-world neuropsychological test measures would array themselves in this way. It is a statistical curiosity to create such data, but it is rather another matter to link it to the ways in which demographic variables typically influence neuropsychological performance measures. Perhaps one might want to reflect on a representative experimental outcome suggested by the imaginary data offered by Berman and Greenhouse (1992):

	Memory Attainment	
	Group 1	Group 2
Less than 8 years	30	60
8 years	25	45
9–12 years	20	40
12 or more years	15	45

Does this make sense? Even if the data had some resemblance to a likely neuropsychological research outcome, the issue was and is that of demographic mismatch. If the groups *differ* in level of education through differing frequencies of recruitment within these strata, ANCOVA will **not** eliminate education as a viable full explanation for the group difference. If the groups *do not differ*, one might wish to "examine strata" to heart's content – a point clear made in our paper (Adams et al., 1985, p. 446).

Our point was rather different than that of Berman and Greenhouse. To call to mind Lord (1967) to repeat our focused message yet again, "... there is simply no logical statistical procedure that can be counted on to make proper allowances for uncontrolled preexisting differences between groups" (Lord, 1967, p. 305).

REFERENCES

Adams, K.M., Brown, G.G., & Grant, I. (1985). Analysis of covariance as a remedy for demographic mismatch of research subject groups: Some sobering simulations. *Journal of Clinical and Experimental Neuropsychology*, 7, 445–462.

Berman, N.G., & Greenhouse, S.W. (1992). Adjusting for demographic covariates by the analysis of covariance. *Journal of Clinical and Experimental Neuropsychology*, 14, 000–000.

Lord, F.M. (1967). A paradox in the interpretation of group comparisons. *Psychological Bulletin*, 68, 304–305.

Rourke, B.P., & Adams, K.M. (1984). Quantitative approaches to the neuropsychological assessment of children. In R. Tarter & G. Goldstein (Eds.) *Advances in clinical neuropsychology*, Vol. 2 (pp. 79–108). New York: Plenum Press.

Tupper, D.E., & Rosenblood, L.K. (1984). Methodological considerations in the use of attribute variables in neuropsychological research. *Journal of Clinical Neuropsychology*, 6, 441–453.

Journal of Clinical and Experimental Neuropsychology
1994, Vol. 16, No. 3, pp. 339–343

Re-examining Threats to the Reliability and Validity of Putative Brain-Behavior Relationships: New Guidelines for Assessing The Effect of Patients Lost to Follow-up

Domenic V. Cicchetti[1] and Linda D. Nelson[2]

[1]WHVAMC and Yale University West Haven, CT and [2]University of California, Irvine

ABSTRACT

It often happens in behavioral and biomedical research that subjects in prospective, multiple assessment investigations, including clinical trials, are lost to follow-up evaluations. The purpose of this report is to outline a model that will enable the investigators to determine the extent to which results based upon the maintained cohort can be generalized to the attrited cohort, or those subjects lost to follow-up. While our proposed model derives from a specific application pertaining to changes in personality and affect behaviors following left and right hemisphere stroke, it should apply, with appropriate study-specific modifications, to a wide range of follow-up research designs in neuropsychology, behavioral science more generally, and other areas of biomedical research.

In the field of biomedical research, Feinstein (1977) pointed an accusatory finger at biostatisticians for not being sensitive to the potential biases that can occur when study conclusions are based upon an inadequate follow-up sample. Thus, he notes the following:

> ... suppose an investigator has satisfactory follow-up data for 60 members of a cohort of 100 people, and finds that 30 of those 60 people survived. If he ignores the 40 people who are 'lost,' he concludes that the survival rate is 50% (=30/60). Suppose he tracked down those 40 missing people, however, and found that only 5 of them had survived. The true survival rate would now be 35% (=35/100). (Feinstein, 1977, p. 101)

Feinstein's sage and primary recommendation is for the investigator to perform the critical scientific role of what he refers to as the TOLPER, an acronym for *Tracer Of Lost Persons*. But suppose one, despite Herculean attempts at "Tolpery," is still unable to produce suitable follow-up information on the study sample? Feinstein is quite correct in rejecting the somewhat common life-table adjustment procedure since it is founded on the untested assumption that the remaining and attrited study subjects have experienced the *same* rates of the outcome variable (here, of course, the rate of death).

Feinstein's advice is again most appropriate. Thus, he recommends that the investigator's best method of 'compensation' for bias is not recourse to a life-table analysis but to the performance of a prognostic stratification for the lost members of the cohort. If the prognostic distribution of the lost group is essentially similar to that of the maintained group, the investigator can be justified in assuming that the outcome rates of the two groups

Please address reprint requests to: Domenic V. Cicchetti, Ph.D., Senior Research Psychologist and Biostatistician, West Haven VA Medical Center & Yale University, 950 Campbell Avenue, West Haven, CT, O65 16, USA.
Accepted for publication: June 10, 1993.

would have been similar (Feinstein, 1977, pp. 101–102).

RELEVANCE TO NEUROPSYCHOLOGICAL RESEARCH

When the outcome variable is dichotomous and poses no observer variability or questions of reliability or validity of measurement (such as rate of death), Feinstein's solution is readily applicable. Examples in neuropsychological research would include rates of death due to one of many possible alterations in brain-behavior relationships, such as brain dysfunction, traumatic and severe closed-head injury, diabetic coma, and stroke. For a given area of biomedical or behavioral science research in which the outcome variable is survival rate, and Tolpery fails, it seems cogent to perform the required prognostic stratifications on age, educational level, and gender in order to draw reasonable conclusions about similarities between the attrited and maintained study subjects. This reasoning rests upon the knowledge that these three variables have been shown consistently to affect survival rates. Being younger, better-educated, and female each enhances survival rates while being older, less well-educated, and male each favors somewhat earlier mortality.

However, when the outcome variable is not dichotomous and may be subject to observer variability and/or questions of validity, then the advice of Feinstein needs to be modified appropriately in order to do justice to the accurate assessment of both the reliability and validity of study conclusions caused by patients or other members of a cohort who are lost to follow-up.

We were presented recently with the problem of patients lost to follow-up and its potential impact upon the reliability and validity of study outcomes and conclusions. The problem, the model we derived and tested, and its general applicability to other follow-up investigations are discussed next in terms of: (1) study objectives; (2) the proposed model; (3) evidence for reliability and validity; (4) comparison of attrited and maintained groups on (a) each relevant stratification variable and (b) each major outcome variable; (5) results; and (6) conclusions.

STUDY OBJECTIVES

Using the UCLA Neuropsychology and Affect Profile (NBAP-Nelson et al., 1989), with the patient's "significant other" as the informant, we were interested in assessing personality/mood changes in male **first** stroke, right- (RH) and left- (LH) hemisphere lesioned patients at 2 weeks, 2 months, and 6 months post stroke. Personality/mood variables were: **indifference, inappropriateness, pragnosia, depression,** and **mania.** NBAP item examples include: (1) **indifference:** "seeming unconcerned about events around one"; (2) **inappropriateness:** "childish, immature, self-centered behavior"; (3) **pragnosia** (a defect in the pragmatics of communicative style); for example, "missing the point of a discussion"; (4) **depression:** "often seeming unhappy"; and (5) **mania:** "feeling unrealistically empowered to accomplish great things."

THE PROPOSED MODEL

Our model consists of: first, identifying independent groups having a single assessment (about 2 weeks post stroke), two assessments (2 weeks and 2 months post stroke) or all three assessments (2 weeks, 2 months, and 6 months post stroke). Next, the model requires comparing the three assessment groups on each relevant patient and informant stratification variable. These include the patient variables age, educational level, gender, mental status (Folstein, Folstein, & McHugh, 1978) and aphasia screening exam results (Wheeler & Reitan, 1962). The informant variable is level of reported depression, as measured by the Beck Depression Inventory (Beck, Ward, Mendelsohn, Mock, & Erbaugh, 1961).

The next step in the process is to compare the three assessment groups on each of the aforementioned personality/mood outcome variables. On the basis of all these evaluations, it is possible to determine whether conclusions based upon the retained cohort should be generalized to the attrited sample.

The complete cohort consisted of 70 first stroke male patients with CT and neurologic confirmation of **right** ($n = 27$), **left** ($n = 29$), or **bilaterial** ($n = 14$) stroke. In this phase of the research, interest focused upon the right (RH) and left (LH) patients because of the hypothesized mechanisms controlling emotional responsivity in RH and LH stroke patients (notably, the work of Kinsbourne & Bemporad, 1984; Robinson & Starkstein, 1991).

IDENTIFYING GROUPS WITH ONE, TWO, OR ALL THREE ASSESSMENTS

Of the 56 RH and LH stroke patients, the significant other (spouse, relative, friend) was available for the following: 25 patients for the first assessment (2 weeks post stroke only); 12 patients for the first two assessments (2 weeks and 2 months); and 19 patients for all three assessments (2 weeks, 2 months, and 6 months). A further analysis revealed that attrition was not biased by patient's side of stroke. Thus, of the 25 single assessment patients, 12 were RH and 13 were LH; the two-assessment group divided evenly into 6 RH and 6 LH patients; and the three-assessment group divided, as closely as possible, into 9 RH and 10 LH patients. Rationale was, therefore, available for combining RH and LH patients to produce sample sizes of 25, 12, and 19 to comprise the single-, two-, and three-assessment groups, respectively.

ASSESSING RELIABILITY/VALIDITY OF OUTCOME VARIABLES

Reliability Assessments of the NBAP

A previous investigation showed test-retest reliability of informant responses concerning dementia patients' ($n = 66$) pre-stroke personality/mood status to be exceedingly high, with intraclass r values ranging between .97 (for **indifference**) to .99 (for **mania**). (For example, see Nelson et al., 1989).

With respect to our stroke study, test-retest NBAP data were available (first assessment vs. second assessment pre-stroke status) for 38 patients (15 RH, 16 LH and 7 bilateral stroke). Results, expressed again as intraclass r values, were as follows: **indifference** (.75), **inappropriateness** (.65), **pragnosia** (.65), **depression** (.75), and **mania** (.63). While not as high as the R_I values

demonstrated for dementia patients, these values still fit the classification of **good** (.60–.74) to **excellent** (.75 and higher), according to the interpretive guidelines introduced earlier by Cicchetti and Sparrow (1981) and Fleiss (1981).

Validity Assessments of the NBAP

Several sources of information support claims for the validity of the five NBAP personality and affect categories: **indifference, inappropriateness, pragnosia, depression,** and **mania**.

Content validation or relevance (i.e., Fitzpatrick, 1983) was demonstrated by Nelson et al. (1989) in that the retained items for each of the five NBAP categories were agreed upon by at least five of six independent judges' ratings.

Discriminant validity was achieved in two separate investigations. In the first, Nelson et al. (1989) confirmed the hypothesis that evaluations of each of the five NBAP personality and affect categories would not significantly differentiate 65 dementia outpatients, **premorbidly**, from 88 elderly controls equated for age, gender, and education with the dementia patients. However, as also hypothesized, reassessments of NBAP variables following the onset of dementia did significantly differentiate the two groups. Specifically, more pathology was demonstrated by the dementia patients on four of the five personality and affect categories, namely, **indifference, inappropriateness, pragnosia,** and **depression**.

In the second investigation (Nelson et al., in press) we showed differences between RH and LH patients that were consistent with the theoretical writings of both Kinsbourne and Bemporad (1983) and Robinson and Starkstein (1991). The major findings indicated that, 2 weeks post stroke, LH relative to RH patients showed significantly elevated levels for **depression** and **inappropriate** and **indifferent** behaviors.

Comparing Attrited and Maintained Groups on Stratification Variables

Data were available for the following relevant stratification (demographic) variables: (1) the patient variables age, educational level, mental status exam findings (Folstein et al., 1978) and the results of aphasia screening (Wheeler & Reitan,

1962); and (2) the level of informants' reported depression (Beck et al., 1961). Analyses of variance showed no statistically significant differences (at or beyond the conventional .05 level) on any of the patient/informant stratification (demographic) variables.

Thus, the groups were comparable on all stratification (demographic) variables that were considered relevant to an assessment of personality/ mood differences in RH and LH patients.

Comparing Attrited and Maintained Groups on Outcome Variables

Since NBAP data were available for **each** of the three groups 2 weeks post stroke, they were compared in a 3 × 2 × 5 factorial analysis of variance (ANOVA) design with one between-groups factor at three levels (0, 1, or 2 follow-up sessions) and two within-group factors (assessment periods, at two levels: **before** stroke and 2 weeks **after** stroke) and type of mood or affect scale at **five** levels: **indifference, inappropriateness, pragnosia, depression**, and **mania**.

Results indicated no statistically significant differences between groups on NBAP scales. Since there were no statistically significant differences between the three assessment groups on any of the relevant stratification (demographic) or outcome variables, this increased the probability that whatever results will be obtained on the maintained sample (for whom all three post-stroke assessments were available) can be generalized to the attrited sample (those for whom only one post-stroke assessment was available).

The proposed model derived from a specific brain-behavior application pertaining to post stroke changes in personality and affect behaviors. With proper adjustments, the general model should apply to a wide range of assessment problems in research. In this sense, the arguments presented in this initial investigation should apply to diverse areas of neuropsychological, general behavioral, and biomedical research. The model is especially relevant when the outcome variables are not as clear-cut and distinct as life or death, and an appreciable proportion of the initial study cohort is lost to follow-up assessment.

In closing, several caveats are in order. First, the proposed model fits a follow-up study design

in which the full cohort (or mostly all of the eligible subjects) provide data on the first assessment. A prime example would be clinic samples in which refusal rates tend to be extremely low.

Second, it should be understood that similarity in scores on the dependent measures for independent groups of subjects receiving one, two, or more assessments will not guarantee generalizability of results from the maintained sample to the full cohort of subjects. It will, however, increase the probability that this is so above and beyond the demonstration of no significant assessment group differences on relevant demographic variables (the current standard procedure for assessing the effects of subjects lost to follow-up).

Third, although the issue of minimal sample size requirements will, of course, depend on the variability of subject performance on the dependent measures, the empirically based caveat of Petrinovich and Hardyck (1969, p. 53) bears repeating: "If sample size is less than 10, it scarcely seems worthwhile to carry out the computations for multiple comparisons, since the power of any method to detect differences between small groups is extremely low."

Fourth, although none of our comparisons of subjects receiving one, two, or all three NBAP assessments showed differences on the demographic variables that were statistically significant at the conventional .05 level, it should be noted that, even if this were the case, it would not in and of itself rule out the possibility of generalizing from the maintained sample to the full cohort. It would still be necessary to show that the demographic variable under examination correlated in a statistically and clinically meaningful manner with each of the dependent measures.

Finally, it should be stressed that the analysis we presented happened to produce favorable results that increase our confidence concerning similarities between results based upon the maintained and full cohort. Future studies can and will produce findings indicating the opposite, namely, that results cannot be safely generalized from the maintained to the full cohort. In either case, the only purpose of applying the suggested guidelines is to increase one's confidence that the conclusions based upon the maintained sample are derived in a valid manner.

REFERENCES

Beck, A.T., Ward, C.H., Mendelsohn, M., Mock, J., & Erbaugh, J. (1961). An inventory for measuring depression. *Archives of General Psychiatry, 4*, 53–63.

Cicchetti, D.V., & Sparrow, S.S. (1981). Developing criteria for establishing interrater reliability of specific items: Applications to assessment of adaptive behavior. *American Journal of Mental Deficiency, 86*, 127–137.

Feinstein, A.R. (1977). *Clinical biostatistics*. St Louis, MO: Mosby.

Fitzpatrick, A.R. (1983). The meaning of content validity. *Applied Psychological Measurement, 7*, 3–13.

Fleiss, J.L. (1981). *Statistical methods for rates and proportions* (2nd ed.). New York: Wiley.

Folstein, M., Folstein, S., & McHugh, P. (1978). Mini mental state. *Journal of Psychiatric Research, 12*, 189–198.

Kinsbourne, M., & Bemporad, B. (1984). Lateralization of emotion: A model and the evidence. In N. Fox & R. Davidson (Eds.), *The Psychobiology of affect* (pp. 259–292). Hillsdale, NJ: Erlbaum Associates, Inc.

Nelson, L.D., Satz, P., Mitrushina, M., Van Gorp, W., Cicchetti, D., Lewis, R., & Van Lancker, D. (1989). Development and validation of the Neuropsychology Behavior and Affect Profile. *Psychological Assessment: A Journal of Consulting and Clinical Psychology, 1*, 266–272.

Nelson, L., Cicchetti, D.V., Satz, P., Stern, S., Sowa, M., Metrushina, M., & Van Gorp, W. (1993). Emotional sequelae of stroke. *Neuropsychology, 1*, 553–560.

Petrinovich, L.F., & Hardyck, L.F. (1969). Error rates for multiple comparison methods: Some evidence concerning the frequency of erroneous conclusions. *Psychological Bulletin, 71*, 43–54.

Robinson, R.G., & Starkstein, S.E. (1991). Heterogeneity in clinical presentation following stroke: Neuropathological correlates. *Neuropsychiatry, Neuropsychology, and Behavioral Neurology, 4*, 4–11.

Wheeler, L., & Reitan, R.A. (1962). The presence and laterality of brain damage predicted from responses to a short aphasia screening test. *Perceptual and Motor Skills, 15*, 783–799.

Child Neuropsychology
1995, Vol. 1, No. 2, pp. 128–139

Prenatal Cocaine Exposure and Neurobehavioral Development: How Subjects Lost to Follow-up Bias Study Results*

Linda C. Mayes and Domenic V. Cicchetti
Yale Child Study Center, New Haven, CT

ABSTRACT

Ninety-four prenatally cocaine-exposed and 50 non-cocaine-exposed infants were enrolled at birth and seen at 3, 6, and 12 months. Applying a recently developed model (Cicchetti & Nelson, 1994) produced four independent groups: those infants assessed at birth only ($n = 61$), those returning for at least one ($n = 29$) or two ($n = 15$) assessments after birth, and those returning for all three ($n = 35$). Among those infants having all follow-up assessments, cocaine-exposed infants showed significantly lower psychomotor performance on the Bayley Scales of Infant Development (BSID) than did non-exposed infants. Results approached statistical significance for mental development. Except for birthweight (cocaine-exposed infants weighed significantly less), none of a wide range of maternal, perinatal, or neurobehavioral demographic variables biased study results or the generalization of findings to the total sample from those who returned for all visits.

Studies of the effects of prenatal or postnatal exposure to drugs such as cocaine, marijuana, or heroin often involve repeated assessments of developmental performance or of more specific functions such as attention, neuromotor maturation, or adaptive behaviors (e.g., Chasnoff, Griffith, Freier, & Murray, 1992; Griffith, Azuma, & Chasnoff, 1994; Mayes, Bornstein, Chawarska, & Granger, 1995). These repeated measures of developmental and neuropsychological capacities are important for understanding the stability of early differences between exposed and non-exposed groups, the pattern of maturational changes in both groups, and the potential expression of later differences that are not apparent in the immediate postnatal period. To date, several studies have reported no differences between cocaine-exposed and non-cocaine-exposed infants on general measures of developmental competency or intelligence (Chasnoff et al., 1992; Griffith et al., 1994). In contrast, on measures of attention and specific aspects of information processing, cocaine-exposed infants in general show more impaired performance (summarized in Mayes & Bornstein, 1995a, 1995b, 1995c).

However, findings such as these are based on longitudinal cohorts with incomplete follow-up rates. Assuring compliance with repeated follow-up visits and maintaining a cohort is a major problem in studies of prenatal drug exposure because of the disruptive effects of substance abuse on family and parental functioning (Mayes, in press). For example, in a 2-year follow-up of cocaine and other

* The authors gratefully acknowledge our many collaborators in the present ongoing study of the effects of prenatal cocaine addiction. These include Donald Cohen, Marc Bornstein, Colleen Sullivan, Kasia Chawarska, and Richard Schottenfeld. This research is supported by the Smith-Richardson Foundation, the Robert Wood Johnson Foundation, the March of Dimes Birth Defects Foundation, and The National Institute on Drug Abuse (NIDA). Additionally, the mothers are part of an ongoing project supported by NIDA, and Linda C. Mayes is supported through a Research Scientist Development Award (NIDA).
Address correspondence to: Linda C. Mayes, M.D., Yale Child Study Center, 230 S. Frontage Road, New Haven, CT 06510, USA.
Accepted for publication: February 15, 1995.

drug use in pregnancy, Chasnoff and colleagues (1992) began with 106 infants in the cocaine-exposed group at 3 months but were able to assess only 29 (27%) by 24 months. Attrition in the non-drug and alcohol/marijuana comparison groups was 62% (50/81) and 31% (14/45), respectively. In a cohort of children exposed to cocaine and other drugs, those exposed to other drugs without cocaine, and a non-drug exposed group, Griffith et al., (1994) reported on the 3-year outcome of 142 children in three groups available from "more than 300" (p. 21) originally enrolled. Similarly, Mayes et al., (1995) reported on the habituation performance of 108 three-month-old infants out of 163 enrolled at birth.

Attrition from the initially enrolled cohort is not unexpected in studies of very high-risk samples. The greater the number of environmental risk factors (e.g., homelessness, polydrug abuse, chronic illness in the parent), the more likely it is that a family will drop out of a follow-up study. While a number of strategies, such as reimbursement, frequent home visits or telephone contacts, cards and letters on holidays, and addresses of friends and relatives, are necessary devices to improve cohort maintenance, it is often the case that even intensive tracking maintains only 70 to 75% of the original cohort (Gainey, Wells, Hawkins, & Catalano, 1993).

That attrition introduces a *potential* bias in interpreting the results of longitudinal assessment is a well-recognized fact and presents a problem for generalizing results to those infants who are not followed (Feinstein, 1977). For example, those families who are able to return for all visits may be better organized and more motivated with the attendant potentially positive effects on infant outcome. In this instance, measures of developmental competency of those drug-exposed infants maintained in the sample may overestimate the developmental performance of those not maintained and who may be at much greater risk for impairment and delay. Conversely, those families who remain involved in a follow-up study may be those who are most concerned about their child's apparent delays or impairments and, thus, data on the maintained cohort may overestimate the severity of impairment of prenatally exposed children.

How to determine whether or not such *potential* biases introduced by subject attrition are indeed

real biases and threats to generalizability has been an important methodologic endeavor. One strategy for dealing with missed visits in a longitudinal design is to include in the final analyses only infants who have completed all visits. However, such a strategy not only requires recruiting more infants in the initial cohort but also potentially overlooks the possibility that subjects who miss one or more visits may be different from those who complete all assessments. Moreover, it is assumed that such differences are important for understanding maturation, individual stability, and possible later expression of an exposure-related effect. This first strategy also assumes that drop-out occurs randomly and that those subjects maintained are not systematically different from those who are lost.

A second strategy involves the performance of a prognostic stratification for those subjects who drop out and are lost to follow-up on salient baseline variables. If the distribution of baseline variables for the subjects who have not completed the follow-up visits is similar to those who have completed all visits, it is assumed that there are no systematic differences between those who were maintained in the sample and those who were maintained in the sample and those who were lost (Feinstein, 1977). However, two problems obtain with this second, commonly employed strategy (Cicchetti & Nelson, 1994).

The first involves the nature of the outcome variable. When the outcome variable is dichotomous and poses no questions of reliability, observer variability, or measurement validity, a prognostic stratification solution is sufficient. Examples of such variables include rates of survival or rates of a specific neurologic complication following an identifiable event such as a perinatal infection. In such cases, selecting those baseline variables that are assumed to affect survival or neurologic outcome, such as gestational age or obstetric complications, and demonstrating similarities between the maintained and lost subjects is a sufficient strategy for studying potential biases introduced by an incomplete follow-up.

But most developmental outcome studies do not involve these types of outcomes. Rather, more commonly, studies of high-risk infants, such as those prenatally cocaine-exposed, employ neurobehavioral assessments of motor or mental capacities, for example, the Bayley Mental and Psychomotor Developmental Indices (Bayley, 1969, 1993). These types of outcomes are subject to observer variability and to individual differences in rates of change month-to-month that may or may not be related to baseline variables commonly obtained, including parental education or socioeconomic level, or perinatal variables such as birthweight, gestational age, or obstetric complications.

The second problem with the prognostic stratification strategy involves the pattern of subject attrition in the majority of longitudinal studies of infants, but particularly in studies of high-risk families. While a certain proportion of infants do not return after one or two visits, a more common pattern is for infants to miss one or two visits in a follow-up protocol due, for example, to weather conditions or illness or, in the case of substance abuse, to increased parental drug use and acute dysfunction. When visits are separated by only weeks or a few months, a missed visit due to illness may be rescheduled in the next follow-up visit period. The infant is not lost to follow-up but has missed one or more visits in the overall follow-up design. Similarly, even for assessments spaced at intervals of 6 and 12 months or 12 and 18 months, it is not uncommon that one visit in the schedule is missed but the subject remains in the study. In these instances, comparing those lost – that is, those who have not completed consecutive visits – to those maintained obscures considerable variability in the so-called "lost" sample.

Assuring that those infants who complete the full follow-up protocol are no different from those who miss one or more visits is crucial to evaluating the representativeness and generalizability of the sample. If this is true and there are no differences in the group who complete the full follow-up protocol and the entire sample, this increases the probability of successfully generalizing study results to the full cohort. To the extent that this sequence of events does not hold, the potential for bias exists and needs to be examined in more detail. In this paper, the method introduced by Cicchetti and Nelson (1994) is applied for examining the impact of missed visits on the reliability and validity of multiple measures of infant capacities and for assessing the presence of potential biases introduced by different patterns of visit participation.

METHODS

Study Sample

Subjects included 144 infants (94 prenatally cocaine-exposed and 50 non-cocaine-exposed) and their mothers who were recruited over a 14-month period through the prenatal clinic and the postpartum ward of Yale-New Haven Hospital. All mothers presenting for prenatal care at the Women's Center, or at delivery if they delivered without prenatal care, were asked about substance abuse in a screening interview conducted by skilled interviewers trained in a substance abuse clinic that serves pregnant women. Urine was screened on all women for cocaine, heroin, methamphetamine, and tetrahydrocannabinol. Cocaine-exposure status was determined either by self-report or by a positive urine screen at a prenatal visit or at delivery.

Following determination of cocaine use, written consent was obtained and a more detailed history of other drug use (alcohol, tobacco, marijuana, opiates, amphetamines, and sedatives) was obtained. Cocaine use at any time during pregnancy resulted in inclusion in the cocaine-exposed group. A history or positive urine screen for opioids resulted in exclusion.

The mothers of infants in the control group were interviewed prenatally about drug use in a fashion similar to that employed for mothers in the cocaine-using group. Those who reported no cocaine or opiate use and who had negative urine screens were invited to participate. Infants in the control group were not enrolled until the time of delivery when a brief substance use interview and maternal urine screens were again performed. Mothers were not excluded from either the cocaine-exposed or non-cocaine-exposed groups if they reported use of alcohol, tobacco, or marijuana alone or in any combination.

At the time of delivery, every infant was seen for administration of the Brazelton Neonatal Behavioral Assessment Scales (NBAS; Brazelton, 1984). On the basis of 27 behavioral items and 20 reflexes, the NBAS evaluates the infant's neurological intactness, behavioral organization (e.g., state regulation and autonomic reactivity), and interactiveness and responsiveness with both animate and inanimate stimuli.

Lester and colleagues (Lester, Als, & Brazelton, 1982) have summarized the behavioral items into six clusters and use the neurological reflex behaviors to define a seventh cluster. Each of the seven clusters yields a numerical score describing the infant's performance in that area. The six behavioral clusters are habituation, orientation, motor, range of state, regulation of state, and autonomic regulation. A higher score on any one of the six behavioral clusters indicates better, or more mature, newborn performance. The reflex cluster is the total number of deviant reflex scores so that, in the case of the reflex cluster, a higher number indicates a more deviant neurological exam. We have previously reported on the results of the NBAS in cocaine-exposed as compared to non-cocaine-exposed infants (Mayes, Granger, Frank, Schottenfeld, & Bornstein, 1993).

While infants were still on the postpartum ward, the NBAS was administered between 24 and 48 hours of age by one of two pediatricians or a pediatric nurse practitioner. Ratings on the NBAS demonstrate adequate interobserver reliability (Brazelton, 1984). Additional information collected at the time of delivery included a measure of prenatal and perinatal complications. These were obtained from the hospital and obstetric clinic records of mothers and infants and were quantified using the Obstetric Complications Scale (OCS; Littman & Parmelee, 1978). Following the assessment at birth, infants were evaluated at 3, 6, and 12 months of age. At those times, infants were assessed using the Bayley Scales of Infant Development (BSID; Bayley, 1969, 1993).

The BSID was administered by a tester blind to the infant's drug-exposure status. Performance on the BSID was expressed in terms of the Mental Developmental Index (MDI) and the Psychomotor Developmental Index (PDI) corrected, when applicable, for gestational age < 36 weeks. A developmentally trained pediatric nurse practiner and two psychologists administered the Bayley Scales. Acceptable interobserver reliability has been demonstrated for the BSID (Bayley, 1993).

Proposed Model
The model for assessing the impact of missed visits consists of first identifying independent groups of the 144 infants with the following breakdown of visits: birth only ($n = 61$); at least one visit at 3, 6, or 12 months after birth ($n = 29$); at least two visits after birth (3 and 6, 6 and 12, or 3 and 12 months) ($n = 19$); and completing three visits after birth ($n = 35$). Using these groups, interactions between visit participation and relevant independent variables are examined for the cocaine-exposed and non-cocaine-exposed group.

For the purposes of illustrating the model for assessing the effects of sample attrition and different patterns of visit participation, the following measures were considered as baseline or independent variables: (1) maternal demographic measures, including maternal age, ethnicity, education, and associated use of tobacco, alcohol, and marijuana (Over 90% of mothers in both the cocaine-using and non-cocaine-using groups were unemployed and single. Thus, these measures of maternal demographic status were not considered.); (2) perinatal demographic measures, including infant gender, gestational age, birthweight, head circumference, and OCS scores; (3) neurobehavioral demographic variables as measured by the seven NBAS clusters. The outcome or dependent variables were the motor (PDI) and mental (MDI) scores on the BSID.

A variable was defined to represent a potential bias and threat to generalizability if there was a statistically significant difference between the cocaine-exposed and non-cocaine-exposed groups on that variable (1) for the total sample, and (2) for any one or all of the four visit participation patterns. If a variable was defined as potentially biasing, then the relation between that variable and the outcome measure was examined for both the cocaine-exposed and non-cocaine-exposed groups separately. This is important in order to prevent the possible masking of a different relationship for each group (e.g., positive for cocaine, negative for non-cocaine, resulting in no relation when the total group is examined).

Failure to find a significant relation between the potentially biasing variable and the outcome measure for either drug-exposure group indicated that this independent variable did not represent a bias and that the results of the cohort returning for all visits might be generalized to the total sample. On the other hand, if there were a significant relation between the potentially biasing independent variable and the outcome measure for the cocaine-exposed and non-cocaine-exposed groups, then there would be bias. Hence, results from those infants returning for all visits may not be generalizable to the total sample.

RESULTS

Outcome Measure for the Sample Returning for All Visits
Table 1 shows the mean MDI and PDI scores for the sample of 35 infants who returned for all visits. Repeated measures analysis of variance showed a

Table 1. Relation of Prenatal Cocaine Exposure to Outcome Variables. Infants Returning for All Visits ($N = 35$).

Months	MDI Cocaine exposure		PDI Cocaine exposure	
	No ($n = 18$)	Yes ($n = 17$)	No ($n = 18$)	Yes ($n = 17$)
	Mean (SD)	Mean (SD)	Mean (SD)	Mean (SD)
3	108.9 (27.2)	91.8 (30.0)	106.0 (25.1)	82.2 (30.2)
6	98.5 (15.3)	96.5 (10.8)	107.9 (14.9)	98.5 (13.0)
12	99.7 (12.2)	93.2 (8.6)	101.9 (19.4)	97.7 (13.2)

main effect approaching significance for cocaine-exposure status for both the MDI and PDI (for MDI, $F(1,33) = 3.6$, $p = .07$ and for PDI, $F(1,33) = 3.3$, $p = .08$). There were no main effects for time of evaluation for either the MDI or PDI (for MDI, $F(2,66) = .5$ and for PDI, $F(2,66) = 1.3$). However, there was a significant interaction between group exposure and time of evaluation for the PDI but not the MDI (for MDI, $F(2,66) = 1.8$ and for PDI, $F(2,66) = 3.4$, $p = 0.04$). Using multiple range tests reported by Dunn (1961), Cicchetti (1972, 1994), Toothaker (1991), and Tukey (1953), a significant difference was found between the cocaine-exposed and non-cocaine-exposed infants on the PDI at the 3-month visit only. Whether or not these findings can be generalized to the larger sample of infants who did

not return for all visits, however, depends on the relation between the outcome measure and independent variables that are identified as potentially biasing.

Identifying Potentially Biasing Variables
The comparison of the three categories of baseline information for the total sample of cocaine-exposed and non-cocaine-exposed infants is reported in Table 2. For the *maternal demographic variables*, the mothers of cocaine-exposed infants were significantly older, less likely to have completed high school, and more likely to have used tobacco, alcohol, and marijuana during their pregnancy. There were no differences in maternal ethnicity between the cocaine-exposed and non-cocaine-exposed groups. For the *perinatal demographic variables*, the infants of cocaine-using mothers were more

Table 2. Relation of Prenatal Cocaine Exposure to Baseline Variables. Total Sample.

	Cocaine exposure status		
	No ($n = 50$)	Yes ($n = 94$)	
Maternal demographics			
Maternal Age (mean yrs (SD))	25.0 (4.5)	27.3 (4.4)	$F(1,142) = 8.6$**
Maternal Ethnicity (% African-American)	82	76	$\chi_c^2 = .23$
Maternal Education			
(% Completed High School)	82	39	$\chi_c^2 = 21.9$***
Maternal Use of			
Tobacco (% = yes)	28	82	$\chi_c^2 = 33.7$***
Alcohol (% = yes)	40	78	$\chi_c^2 = 17.6$***
Marijuana (% = yes)	31	67	$\chi_c^2 = 14.8$***
Perinatal demographics			
Infant Gender (% male)	46	50	$\chi_c^2 = .08$
	M (SD)	M (SD)	$F(1,142)$
Infant Gestational Age (weeks)	39.5 (1.1)	38.9 (1.6)	4.5*
Birthweight (grams)	3322 (496)	2913 (459)	24.5***
Head Circumference (cm)	33.5 (1.7)	32.8 (1.5)	7.5**
OCS scores	102.9 (22.9)	94.8 (18.6)	5.2*
Neurobehavioral demographics (NBAS scores)			
Habituation	6.7 (1.7)	5.5 (1.9)	11.0***
Orientation	5.4 (1.6)	4.8 (1.7)	3.7
Motor Maturity	4.6 (.9)	4.3 (.9)	3.5
Range of State	3.6 (.7)	3.3 (1.1)	2.4
Regulation of State	5.6 (1.7)	5.3 (1.8)	.7
Autonomic Reactivity	5.7 (1.8)	5.3 (1.9)	1.6
Reflex	3.9 (3.0)	3.9 (2.7)	.04

Note. *$p \leq .05$; **$p \leq .01$; ***$p \leq .001$.

likely to show lower birthweights, gestational age, and head circumference, and to have been born after more complicated pregnancies and deliveries (lower OCS scores). Finally, for the *neurobehavioral demographic variables*, only the habituation cluster of the NBAS significantly differentiated between the two groups, with cocaine-exposed infants showing depressed habituation performance.

Demographic Categories and Visit Participation Patterns

The relations among the three groups of independent variables (maternal and infant demographic and neurobehavioral variables), cocaine-exposure status, and the four visit participation groups are displayed in Tables 3 and 4. For the maternal demographic variables, there was a significant main effect for maternal age for cocaine-exposure $(F(1, 142) = 7.8, p < .01)$, with the mothers of cocaine-exposed infants being consistently older across all visit groups (Table 3). For maternal education (Table 4), cocaine-using mothers were less likely to complete high school for two of the four visit patterns ($\chi_c^2 = 8.6$ for birth only and 7.3 for any one visit). Cocaine-using mothers were also significantly more likely to use tobacco or alcohol for at least two of the visit groups (Table 4; for tobacco $\chi_c^2 = 7.5$ for birth only and 13.4 for all four visits; for alcohol, $\chi_c^2 = 5.1$ for any two visits and 3.6 for all four visits). There were no significant differences in marijuana use for any of the visit patterns.

For the perinatal demographic variables (Table 3), there was a significant main effect for cocaine-exposure for gestational age $(F(1, 142) = 4.0, p < .05)$, birthweight $(F(1, 142) = 23.9, p < .001)$, head circumference $(F(1, 142) = 10.8, p < .001)$, and OCS scores $(F(1, 142) = 5.0, p < .05)$. For the neurodevelopmental demographic scores (Table 3), there were significant main effects for the habituation $(F(1, 142) = 10.5, p < .01)$ and range of state clusters $(F(1, 142) = 4.1, p < .05)$.

Thus, maternal age and education, use of tobacco and alcohol, infant gestational age, birthweight, head circumference, OCS scores, and neurobehavioral performance on the habituation and range of state clusters represented potentially biasing variables for generalizing the results of findings from the group returning for all visits to the total sample. The third step was to evaluate the effect of such potentially biasing variables on two outcome variables, MDI and PDI, for the total sample of cocaine-exposed and non-cocaine-exposed infants.

Relation between Biasing Variables and Outcome Measures

Tables 5 and 6 show the relation between the potentially biasing demographic variables and the MDI and PDI scores for the first assessment after birth for the cocaine-exposed and non-cocaine-exposed groups. For the maternal demographic category, the correlations between maternal age and the MDI or PDI ranged between $-.01$ and $.10$ (Table 5). When cocaine-using and non-cocaine-using mothers were divided into those who did and did not complete high school, there were no significant differences in the mean MDI or PDI scores (Table 6). Similarly, for maternal tobacco and alcohol use, there were no differences in MDI or PDI scores between those who did and did not use these two drugs for either the cocaine-using or non-cocaine-using groups (Table 6). Thus, none of the maternal demographic variables significantly biased PDI or MDI performance.

For the infant demographic variables, there were no significant correlations between gestational age or OCS scores with the MDI or PDI for the non-cocaine or cocaine-exposed group (Table 5). Head circumference was not significantly correlated with the PDI for either the non-cocaine-exposed or cocaine-exposed groups but was significantly related to the MDI for the non-cocaine-group only $(r = .51)$. Birthweight was significantly related to both MDI and PDI performance for the non-cocaine group $(r = .43$ and $.47$ for MDI and PDI, respectively) but not for the cocaine-exposed group $(r = .10$ and $-.02$ for MDI and PDI, respectively).

In order to explore this relationship further, infants from the two exposed groups were divided into those with birthweights above and below the mean for that group, and an Exposure Group (2) X Birthweight Group (2) ANOVA was performed (Table 7). Birthweight group was significantly related to both MDI and PDI for the non-cocaine-exposed infants only. Similar analyses were carried out for head circumference, and no significant

Table 3. Comparison Among Patterns of Participation for Continuous Baseline Variables. Means (SD).

Baseline variables	Birth only		Any 1 visit		Any 2 visits		All visits		Main effect
	Cocaine		Cocaine		Cocaine		Cocaine		Cocaine exposure
	Neg	Pos	Neg	Pos	Neg	Pos	Neg	Pos	$F(1, 142)$
N	17	44	7	22	8	11	18	17	
Maternal demographics									
Maternal Age (yrs)	25.2 (4.2)	27.1 (4.8)	29.6 (5.9)	27.2 (3.5)	23.2 (2.6)	28.4 (4.7)	24.9 (4.7)	24.9 (4.8)	7.8**
Perinatal demographics									
Gestational age (wk)	39.4 (1.4)	38.9 (1.8)	40.0 (0)	38.9 (1.8)	39.6 (1.1)	39.1 (1.7)	39.4 (1.1)	39.2 (1.2)	4.0*
Birthweight (gm)	3292 (431)	3003 (492)	3474 (432)	2817 (466)	3191 (407)	2836 (366)	3349 (617)	2853 (404)	23.9***
Head Circum (cm)	33.4 (1.3)	32.9 (1.6)	34.7 (1.6)	32.3 (1.4)	33.3 (1.3)	32.3 (1.3)	33.3 (2.1)	33.1 (1.4)	10.8***
OCS scores	95.4 (20.5)	92.6 (17.9)	110.6 (19.3)	98.2 (17.8)	101.7 (30.1)	89.7 (21.1)	107.5 (22.5)	99.6 (19.5)	5.0*
Neurobehavioral demographics									
Habituation	6.3 (1.9)	5.4 (2.1)	7.2 (1.8)	5.7 (1.8)	7.2 (1.1)	5.5 (.9)	6.7 (1.9)	5.6 (1.9)	10.5**
Orientation	5.3 (1.6)	4.5 (1.8)	5.8 (1.4)	5.1 (1.4)	5.1 (2.5)	5.2 (1.2)	5.5 (1.5)	4.8 (2.2)	1.9
Motor Maturity	4.6 (.9)	4.3 (.9)	4.6 (.9)	4.2 (.8)	4.5 (.7)	4.5 (.6)	4.5 (.9)	4.0 (1.4)	2.3
Range of State	3.5 (.9)	3.4 (1.1)	3.8 (.5)	3.4 (1.2)	3.7 (.8)	3.0 (.7)	3.5 (.5)	3.0 (1.2)	4.1*
Regulation of State	6.2 (1.6)	5.2 (1.8)	5.7 (2.0)	5.7 (1.4)	4.7 (1.8)	5.3 (2.1)	5.3 (1.4)	5.3 (2.2)	.2
Autonomic Reactivity	5.8 (1.6)	5.0 (2.0)	6.4 (2.6)	5.3 (1.9)	4.9 (2.2)	5.8 (1.2)	5.7 (1.4)	5.5 (2.2)	.5
Reflex	4.4 (3.7)	4.1 (2.6)	3.4 (2.8)	4.3 (3.2)	4.2 (2.7)	3.4 (2.3)	3.4 (2.6)	3.6 (2.4)	0

Note. * $p \leq .05$, ** $p \leq .01$, *** $p \leq .001$.

Table 4. Comparison Among Patterns of Participation for Dichotomous Variables.

	Birth only			Any 1 visit			Any 2 visits			All visits		
	Cocaine exposure			Cocaine exposure			Cocaine exposure			Cocaine exposure		
	No	Yes	χ^2_c	No	Yes	χ^2_c	No	Yes	χ^2_c	No	Yes	χ^2_c
Maternal demographics												
Maternal Ethnicity (% African American)	94	75	1.7	71	86	.1	87	27	.04	72	70	0
Maternal Education (% High School)	82	36	8.6**	100	32	7.3**	62	45	.1	83	53	2.5
Maternal Drug Use¹ (% Yes)												
Tobacco	23	75	7.5**	33	82	3.3	43	91	2.8	18	88	13.4***
Alcohol	54	79	2.2	33	68	1.2	43	100	5.1**	31	70	3.6*
Marijuana	31	64	3.2	33	64	.7	28	73	1.8	31	76	1.8
Perinatal demographics												
Infant Gender %m	47	45	.06	57	50	0	25	54	.2	55	41	.3

Note. ¹Data are not available on other drug use for 8 mothers.
*$p \leq .05$, **$p \leq .01$, ***$p \leq .001$.

Table 5. Correlations Between Biasing Variables and Outcome Measures.

	No cocaine		Cocaine	
	MDI	PDI	MDI	PDI
Maternal demographics				
Maternal Age	.10	−.01	.01	.03
Perinatal demographics				
Gestational Age	.14	.28	−.22	−.01
Birthweight	.43*	.47**	.10	−.02
Head Circumference	.51**	.27	.01	−.04
OCS Scores	−.11	.10	−.02	.10
Neurobehavioral clusters				
Habituation	.39*	.38*	−.20	−.19
Range of State	−.25	−.11	−.02	−.06

Note. $*p \leq .05$, $**p \leq .01$, $***p \leq .001$.

relations were found for the MDI or PDI for the non-cocaine or cocaine-exposed groups. Thus, birth-weight is a biasing variable and poses a threat to generalizing from the group returning for all visits to the total sample.

For neurobehavioral demographic measures (Table 5), there were no significant relations between range of state performance and the MDI or PDI for either the non-cocaine-exposed or cocaine-exposed groups. However, similar to the findings for birthweight, performance on the habituation cluster was significantly related to both the MDI and PDI for the non-cocaine-exposed group only ($r = .39$ and $.38$ for the MDI and PDI, respectively). There were no significant relations between the habituation cluster performance and the MDI or the PDI for the cocaine-exposed group ($r = -.19$).

In order to explore this relationship further, infants from the two exposed groups were divided into those with habituation cluster scores above and below the mean for that group and an Exposure Group (2) X Birthweight Group (2) ANOVA was performed (Table 7). The habituation cluster grouping was not significantly related to the MDI or the PDI for either the non-cocaine or cocaine-exposed groups. Thus, performance on the habituation cluster in the newborn period does not appear to represent a biasing variable that limits generalizations to the total sample from the sample that returned for all visits.

CONCLUSIONS

In the present sample, birthweight was a significant biasing variable that limited generalization from the sample of infants returning for all visits to the total sample. One caveat is important to note. Differences in birthweight between cocaine-exposed and non-cocaine-exposed infants may also reflect a direct effect of cocaine on fetal growth (Zuckerman, Frank, Hingson, & Amaro, 1989). However, because maternal cocaine use is also associated with many other factors (e.g., poor prenatal care, maternal alcohol and tobacco use) that may also contribute to reduced birthweight, it cannot be assumed that differences in birthweight are attributable to cocaine alone and, thus, it should be examined as a potentially biasing variable. The proposed model is particularly relevant to studies of high-risk infants in which continuous measures of development and psychological functions are the standard and in instances where an appreciable proportion of the initial cohort is likely to be lost to follow-up or to miss one or more visits in a follow-up schedule. The key feature of this model is the comparison of *independent* groups of subjects defined by their patterns of participation in the follow-up schedule (Cicchetti & Nelson, 1994). However, one caveat is in order. The proposed model is a strategy for evaluating the generalizability of data from those subjects who complete follow-up to those with incomplete visit participation and those subjects

Table 6. Relation Between Potentially Biasing Maternal Demographic Variables and Outcome Measures.

Maternal Demographics	No cocaine					Cocaine				
	n	MDI Mean (SD)	F	PDI Mean (SD)	F	n	MDI Mean (SD)	F	PDI Mean (SD)	F
Education										
High School										
No	6	96.3 (20.9)	1.7	94.5 (28.5)	1.7	29	91.5 (16.2)	1.7	93.9 (19.2)	.9
Yes	21	104.4 (11.9)		104.9 (14.7)		21	96.6 (8.4)		97.6 (11.3)	
Tobacco Use										
No	21	104.9 (13.0)	.7	105.9 (14.4)	1.6	7	85.9 (21.4)	2.7	94.0 (24.4)	.02
Yes	8	99.9 (17.5)		96.4 (2.5)		43	94.9 (11.8)		95.1 (15.5)	
Alcohol Use										
No	19	100.9 (13.3)	1.9	101.4 (19.5)	.6	12	96.2 (13.2)	.6	96.9 (17.7)	.2
Yes	10	108.4 (15.3)		106.8 (15.6)		38	92.8 (13.8)		94.3 (16.6)	

Table 7. Relation Between Potentially Biasing Neurobehavioral Variables and MDI and PDI Scores for Total Sample.

	No cocaine			Cocaine		
	<Mean	>Mean	F	<Mean	>Mean	F
Birthweight						
MDI	97.5 (11.0)	106.9 (14.8)	4.0*	92.5 (12.7)	94.8 (14.8)	.3
PDI	92.4 (17.7)	110.8 (13.8)	11.3**	93.8 (17.1)	96.1 (16.6)	.2
Head Circumference						
MDI	98.0 (14.5)	107.4 (12.9)	3.6	91.3 (11.6)	95.3 (15.2)	1.1
PDI	99.8 (22.7)	106.8 (12.0)	1.1	93.2 (16.1)	96.8 (16.3)	.6
Habituation Cluster						
MDI	96.7 (14.2)	107.4 (14.9)	3.5	96.9 (11.4)	90.6 (15.7)	2.3
PDI	99.2 (24.1)	106.4 (14.5)	.9	97.8 (19.1)	89.6 (14.3)	2.5

Note. * $p \leqslant .05$, ** $p \leqslant .01$.

who are lost to follow-up. It does not address the problem of missing data in a repeated measures design (Jennrich & Schluchter, 1986).

In general, and depending upon the specific research design and questions of interest, there are a number of ways to control for biasing variables in longitudinal research. These would include randomization to treatment and control conditions where this might apply. Failing in this attempt, because of small sample sizes, one could apply appropriate analysis of covariance procedures. If the sample size is large enough, a third strategy would be to delete those subjects in either group that contribute most to the biasing effect and then reanalyze the data based on the redefined samples.

However, these particular strategies were not applicable in the current study for the following reasons: (1) the design did not allow for randomization procedures; (2) the fact that biases occurred in one group but not in the other (e.g., the PDI) – meaning that the correlation between the covariate and the outcome variable was positive for one group and negative for the other group – in fact violated one of the assumptions underlying covariance, namely, that the regression lines for the two groups were not parallel. A final strategy would be to increase efforts to successfully track subjects who are "loss-to-follow-up" or, in Feinstein's (1977) terminology, to increase the role of the TOLPER (tracer of lost persons).

More generally, to the extent that one is focusing upon high-risk samples such as cocaine-abusing mothers and cocaine-exposed infants, the probability increases that "tolpery" will fail. A significant number of subjects will be lost-to-follow-up, and almost inevitable biases will be introduced. This inevitable problem thereby necessitates a technique similar to the one described, in order to determine the effect of subjects lost-to-follow-up upon the reliability and validity of study results.

To date, studies of prenatal cocaine-exposure have reported contradictory findings regarding the specificity and severity of developmental impairments in cocaine-exposed infants (summarized in Mayes & Bornstein, 1995a, 1995b, 1995c). In part, aspects of these controversies may reflect biases introduced by incomplete follow-up or by subjects completely lost to follow-up. In substance-abusing samples, the frequency of multiple, interactive

risk factors for impaired developmental outcome (e.g., prenatal cocaine exposure and intrauterine growth retardation, or maternal substance abuse and a history of depression) make it more likely that significant attrition or irregular visit patterns will introduce important differences between those infants maintained in follow-up and those who are not. The proposed model presents an approach for evaluating the severity of the threat of such biases to the study results.

REFERENCES

Bayley, N. (1969). *Bayley Scales of Infant Development*. New York, NY: Psychological Corporation.

Bayley, N. (1993). *Bayley Scales of Infant Development*. New York, NY: Psychological Corporation.

Brazelton, T.B. (1984). *Neonatal Behavior Assessment Scale*. (Clinics in Developmental Medicine, No. 88, 2nd ed.). Philadelphia, PA: Lippincott.

Chasnoff, I., Griffith, D.R., Freier, C., & Murray, J. (1992). Cocaine/polydrug use in pregnancy: Two-year follow-up. *Pediatrics, 89*, 284–289.

Cicchetti, D.V. (1972). Extension of multiple range tests to interaction tables in the analysis of variance: A rapid approximate solution. *Psychological Bulletin, 77*, 405–408.

Cicchetti, D.V. (1994). Multiple comparison methods: Establishing guidelines for their valid application in neuropsychological research. *Journal of Clinical and Experimental Neuropsychology, 16*, 155–161.

Cicchetti, D.V., & Nelson, L.D. (1994). Re-examining threats to the reliability and validity of putative brain-behavior relationships: New guidelines for assessing the effect of patients lost to follow-up. *Journal of Clinical and Experimental Neuropsychology, 16*, 339–343.

Dunn, O.J. (1961). Multiple comparisons among means. *Journal of the American Statistical Association, 56*, 52–64.

Feinstein, A.R. (1977). *Clinical biostatistics*. St. Louis, MO: Mosby.

Gainey, R.R., Wells, E.A., Hawkins, J.D., & Catalano, R.F. (1993). Predicting treatment retention among cocaine users. *International Journal of the Addictions, 28*, 487–505.

Griffith, D.R., Azuma, S.D., & Chasnoff, I.J. (1994). Three-year outcome of children exposed prenatally to drugs. *Journal of American Academy of Child Psychiatry, 33*, 20–27.

Jennrich, R.I., & Schluchter, M.D. (1986). Unbalanced repeated measures models with structured covariance matrices. *Biometrics, 42*, 805–820.

Lester, B., Als, H., & Brazelton, T.B. (1982). Regional obstetric anesthesia and newborn behavior: A reanalysis toward synergistic effects. *Child Development, 53,* 687–692.

Littman, D., & Parmelee, A. (1978). Medical correlates of infant development. *Pediatrics, 77,* 209–211.

Mayes, L.C. (in press). Substance abuse and parenting. In M.H. Bornstein (Ed.), *The handbook of parenting.* Hillsdale, NJ: Erlbaum.

Mayes, L.C., Bornstein, M.H., Chawarska, K., & Granger, R.H. (1995). Information processing and developmental assessments in three-month-old infants exposed prenatally to cocaine. *Pediatrics, 95,* 539–545.

Mayes, L.C., Granger, R.H., Frank, M.A., Schottenfeld, R., & Bornstein, M. (1993). Neurobehavioral profiles of infants exposed to cocaine prenatally. *Pediatrics, 91,* 778–783.

Mayes, L.C., & Bornstein, M. (1995a). Attention regulation in infants born at risk: Preterm and prenatally cocaine-exposed infants. In J. Burak & J. Enns (Eds.), *Development, attention, and psychopathology.* New York: Guilford Publications.

Mayes, L.C., & Bornstein, M. (1995b). Developmental dilemmas for cocaine abusing parents and their children. In M. Lewis, & M. Bendersky, (Eds.), *Cocaine mother and cocaine babies: The role of toxins in development.* Hillsdale, NJ: Lawrence Erlbaum Associates.

Mayes, L.C., & Bornstein, M. (1995c). The context of development for young children from cocaine-abusing families. In P. Kato & T. Mann, (Eds.), *Health psychology of special populations.* New York: Plenum Press.

Toothaker, L.E. (1991). *Multiple comparisons for researchers.* Newbury Park, CA: Sage.

Tukey, J.W. (1953). *The problem of multiples comparisons.* Unpublished monograph.

Zuckerman, B., Frank, D.A., Hingson, R., & Amaro, H. (1989). Effects of maternal marijuana and cocaine use on fetal growth. *New England Journal of Medicine, 320,* 762–768.

Child Neuropsychology
1995, Vol. 1, No. 3, pp. 211–223

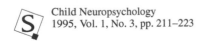

VIII-L

Assessment of Children's Receptive Vocabulary Using Event-Related Brain Potentials: Development of a Clinically Valid Test*

Joseph M. Byrne[1,2], Christopher A. Dywan[3], and John F. Connolly[4,5]

[1]IWK Children's Hospital, Halifax, Nova Scotia, [2]Department of Pediatrics, Dalhousie University School of Medicine, [3]Dalhousie University, [4]Dalhousie University, Department of Psychiatry, and [5]Dalhousie University School of Medicine

ABSTRACT

The combined verbal and motor impairments characteristic of children with disorders such as Cerebral Palsy (CP) frequently compromise the accuracy of standard psychometric assessments. What is needed is a test to measure language that does not require verbal or motor responses. This study was designed to determine whether single-word receptive vocabulary could be assessed in young children without CP, using an ERP-compatible test based on Form M of the Peabody Picture Vocabulary Test – Revised (PPVT-R). Fifteen 10-year-old children with normal levels of psychometric intelligence participated. Ninety pictures were selected from the PPVT-R (Form M), representing three levels of single-word receptive vocabulary (Preschool, Child-Adolescent, Adult). Each picture was presented twice (pseudo-random), once paired with a spoken word that was semantically congruent with the picture and once paired with a semantically incongruent word. The children's N400 was significantly larger to incongruent than to congruent pairs, but only when the vocabulary was within their repertoire. The results are discussed in terms of electrophysiologic correlates of acquired language and the clinical use of this ERP test as an adjunct to assessing patients with moderate to severe communication and/or motor impairments (e.g., cerebral palsy, autism, head injury).

Researchers have recently been developing ERP paradigms to *directly* assess the cognitive or neurolinguistic status of difficult-to-assess patient populations (Byrne, Dywan, & Connolly, 1995; Connolly, Byrne, & Dywan, in press; Molfese, Morris, & Romski, 1990). We have been developing an ERP paradigm to aid in the assessment of receptive vocabulary in clinic populations for whom traditional motor or language responses would be extremely difficult. This paradigm has been developed with the needs of young patients with moderate to severe cerebral palsy (CP) serving as a conceptual framework. The eventual test battery using this paradigm will be more inclusive

*This study was supported, in part, by an IWK Research Investigatorship Award (JMB), and by grants from the Hospital for Sick Children – Toronto (JMB, JFC), the Natural Sciences and Engineering Research Council of Canada (NSERC) (JFC), the Scottish Rite Schizophrenia Research Foundation (JFC), a NSERC Postgraduate Scholarship and an honourary IWK Memorial Scholarship awarded to CD. A preliminary report of these data was made at the International Neuropsychological Society Meeting, Seattle, February, 1995. The participation of the children, and their families is appreciated. The cooperation of the childrens' schools is greatly appreciated, as is the assistance of Shannon MacLean, research assistant. Thanks are also extended to the Dr. Lloyd M. Dunn and Leota M. Dunn, authors of the Peabody Picture Vocabulary Test – Revised, for granting permission to reproduce three of the PPVT-R items. Finally, we would like to acknowledge the very helpful technical assistance of the staff at Neuroscan Inc., El Paso, TX. Correspondence can be made to either JMB, Department of Psychology, IWK Children's Hospital, 5850 University Avenue, Halifax, Nova Scotia, Canada or JFC, Department of Psychology, Dalhousie University, Halifax, Nova Scotia, Canada, B3H 4J1.
Accepted for publication: August 2, 1995.

(e.g., attention, memory, language comprehension, problem solving). However, we decided to concentrate on the application of this paradigm to receptive language, as this is the most frequently chosen mode of interaction with these patients (e.g., following instructions).

CP is a chronic disorder that can have a pervasive impact on every aspect of a person's life. It is estimated that, by early school age, CP is diagnosed in 1.2 to 2.3 children per 1000 (Blair & Stanley, 1985; Paneth, 1986). For children with moderate to severe CP, eventual quality of life is greatly determined by level of cognitive functioning (Nelson, 1989) and, therefore, an accurate assessment of this dimension is of paramount importance. However, CP represents one of the largest clinic populations for whom formal psychometric testing is notoriously difficult because of the possible severity of the combined motor and language impairments characteristic of the condition. Accuracy of assessment depends greatly on the severity of these impairments, as well as on the level of frustration experienced by patients when trying to complete standardized tests with their limited verbal and motor abilities (McCarty, St. James, Berninger, & Gans, 1986; Miller & Rosenfeld, 1952; Nelson, 1989; Sattler, 1988; Strother, 1952). Even experienced clinicians, using a patchwork of test protocols, are often able to assess only a limited repertoire of cognitive functioning because of their patients' difficulties in providing oral or written answers or in executing object manipulation (McCarty et al., 1986).

Three main strategies have been pursued to facilitate the assessment of patients with CP. Each of these strategies has met with only limited success (Byrne et al., 1995). A preferred alternative strategy for assessing individuals with moderate to severe verbal and motor impairments should facilitate the assessment of a wide range of cognitive functioning, over a wide age range, and with minimal reliance on motor or expressive language functioning. Byrne et al. (1995) have proposed one such strategy that incorporates the use of ERPs to provide an on-line measure of cortical processing (Brandeis & Lehmann, 1986). ERPs have several advantages for clinical assessment. *First*, more than one modality (e.g., auditory, visual) can be *directly* assessed. *Second*, compared to the other

perceptual-cognitive paradigms (previously noted), typical ERP paradigms (e.g., odd-ball paradigm) entail a larger sampling of responses from each patient. This sampling feature allows for the recording of a more characteristic response pattern, and reduces the negative impact of inattention or interfering behaviour (e.g., motor spasm) on the assessment. *Third*, ERPs are less susceptible to the effects of habituation (Ritter, Vaughan, & Costa, 1968) compared to visual attention/EKG paradigms (Berg & Berg, 1987). *Fourth*, traditional ERP paradigms allow for rapid presentation of stimuli, thus increasing the range of cognitive tasks that can be presented within a single testing session (i.e., testing different levels and/or types of cognition). *Fifth*, some ERP paradigms do not require a behavioural response, a particularly important feature for the patient with CP.

There have been few studies using ERPs as a method to assess language directly in populations with verbal and/or motoric impairments. Molfese and his colleagues have carried out extensive studies of the language abilities of normal preverbal infants using ERP paradigms (e.g., for review see Molfese & Betz, 1988). For example, Molfese, Wetzel, and Gill (1993) demonstrated that infants as young as 12 months of age were able to discriminate between known and unknown words reliably, as reflected in their ERP responses. On the basis of such results, Molfese and his coworkers advanced the development of ERP paradigms for testing language processing *without* the need for the young participants to respond overtly (e.g., verbal answer, depress button). The young infants (12–16 months) studied by Molfese and his colleagues actually share many important characteristics with older children who have moderate to severe CP; neither can typically provide rapid and reliable verbal or motor responses. Therefore, their ERP technology has direct application to such clinic populations.

Using a similar approach, Molfese et al. (1990) conducted one of the first studies demonstrating the clinical application of ERPs to the assessment of difficult-to-assess patient populations. Auditory ERPs were used to test adolescents with moderate or severe mental handicap. They found that auditory ERPs systematically varied as a function of meaningful versus unknown symbols, suggesting that this method of assessment could be used to infer neurolinguistic processes in this difficult-to-assess patient population. However, since the stimuli used were arbitrary visual-graphic symbols, the Molfese et al. (1990) paradigm could not be used to obtain an age-equivalent approximation of the participants' level of neurolinguistic functioning, nor could it provide an estimate of routine, functional receptive language (e.g., vocabulary), thereby limiting its clinical value.

Recently we addressed several of these methodological issues with difficult-to-assess populations (Byrne et al., 1995). First, given the motor and language impairments characteristic of children with moderate to severe CP, we designed an ERP-compatible test that required only that the patient visually attend to a computer screen while listening to meaningful words over headphones. No overt behavioural response (e.g., verbal answer, pointing) was required. Second, the ERP test was based on a computerized version of Form M of the PPVT-R (Dunn & Dunn, 1981). By using stimuli directly adapted from a standardized test we could move closer to deriving an estimate of *age-appropriate* single-word vocabulary. This would extend the clinical application of previous ERP paradigms that have relied upon either arbitrary sound-symbol stimuli (Molfese et al., 1990) or, more recently, upon words of unspecified difficulty (Molfese et al., 1993).

An initial clinical test of this ERP-compatible test of receptive vocabulary was thought best achieved by testing an adolescent patient with severe CP (Byrne et al., 1995). It was reasoned that an older patient would more likely be cooperative and, compared to younger patients, might be able to better control extraneous movement that might have compromised the recording of ERPs. We administered our ERP test to a male adolescent with severe spastic quadriplegia and to three matched controls (age, gender). Each participant was seated before a computer monitor upon which pictures, electronically scanned from the PPVT-R (Form M), were presented individually in a pseudo-random fashion. Once the picture was presented on the monitor, the participants heard (over headphones) a semantically correct (congruent condition) or semantically incorrect (incongruent condition) naming of that picture. For example, when the

picture of a "bus" appeared it was correctly named ("bus"), followed at a later time in the testing by an incorrect naming of the bus ("watch"). A 180-trial session was conducted during which 90 pictures were presented (pseudo-randomly) on two separate occasions, once paired with a semantically congruent word, and once with a semantically incongruent word.

The main ERP component of interest was the N400, a negativity that has been firmly linked to violations of semantic expectancies both in sentence contexts (e.g., Connolly & Phillips, 1994; Connolly, Phillips, & Forbes, 1995) and in a wide variety of priming paradigms (e.g., Holcomb & Anderson, 1993; Holcomb & Neville, 1990, 1991). In particular, the N400 has been the focus of investigation in a cross-form, cross-modal priming paradigm identical to the present approach using an adult population (Connolly et al., in press). The N400 is typically manifested as the most negative point between 350 to 600 ms post-word onset (for reviews: Kutas & Van Petten, 1988; Pritchard, Shappell, & Brandt, 1991).

The results of our initial single-case, multiple control study showed that, as predicted, the *N400* ERP component was substantially larger when the picture-word pairs were semantically incongruent as compared to when the picture-word pairs were semantically congruent. Furthermore, it was demonstrated that this differential ERP pattern was confined to vocabulary that was within the participants' psychometrically determined repertoire established prior to the ERP testing using Form L of the PPVT-R. When the receptive vocabulary was above the participants' vocabulary level, the *N400* ERP component for congruent and incongruent picture-word pairs did not differ significantly. Most important the findings were evident on an individual basis. That is, in contrast to previous studies that report the ERP components based on group performance, this study demonstrated that, for individuals, ERP waveforms could be reliably altered as a function of the congruency between the picture-word pairs. Therefore, the clinical use of this test was particularly noteworthy.

Our next step in developing this ERP-compatible version of the PPVT (Form M) was twofold: (a) to determine more specifically the scalp site distribution of the ERP patterns in response to these stimuli;

and (b) to determine whether additional ERP components are present during the processing of these stimuli. We chose adults as the test group for the larger ERP study because the potentially confounding issues of noncompliance and extraneous movement would be of minimal concern, and they have a more established receptive vocabulary, thus allowing a more stringent test of this new paradigm. The results of this second study revealed, once again, a significantly larger posteriorly distributed *N400* to the incongruent than to the congruent picture-word pairs for the vocabulary *within* the participant's acquired vocabulary level (Connolly et al., in press). This differential pattern was absent for incongruent picture-word pairs at vocabulary levels *above* the adults' psychometrically determined repertoire. Instead, the advanced vocabulary level elicited an equivalent *N400* response to both congruent and incongruent pairs. In this study, two earlier components (PMN, P300) were also found to be sensitive to the phonemic manipulations of the paradigm, but the N400 was the most reliable component, for both the group and individual profiles.

The results of these two preliminary studies were encouraging and provided empirical support for the validity of our ERP-compatible test of receptive vocabulary. However, the long-term goal of this line of research was to develop the ERP test for use in assessing the single-word receptive vocabulary of young children with moderate to severe CP. It is clear that children are more challenging to test, particularly those with special needs (e.g., CP) (Sattler, 1988). Therefore, we sought to determine whether our ERP-compatible test of receptive vocabulary, which was shown to be useful with linguistically mature adolescents and adults (17–34 years), could be successfully used with school-aged children (9–10 years). This would establish the foundation for future assessments of school-aged children who exhibit moderate to severe CP.

METHOD

Participants

Fifteen children (7 males and 8 females) who spoke English as their first language were recruited from schools in a large metropolitan area. The children ranged in age from 9 to 11 years ($M = 10.27$, $SD = .59$ years)

and were in age-appropriate grades (i.e., grades 4 to 6). None of the children had a history of a developmental disability, head trauma, or learning disability. Handedness was determined by self-report (writing/drawing, combing hair), and was confirmed by parental report. Twelve children were right-handed, 2 were left-handed, and 1 child was ambidextrous. On Form L of the PPVT-R the children's standard scores ranged from 93 to 123 ($M = 106.73$, $SD = 8.09$). These scores reflect performance within the normal range. Data collected from an additional 5 children were not included in this analysis because of their failure to satisfy all inclusion criteria, equipment difficulties, or poor co-operation.

Procedure

Computerized PPVT-R
A 180-trial computerized version of Form M of the PPVT-R was developed (see Byrne et al., 1995; Connolly et al., in press). Each trial consisted of a line drawing presented on a high resolution computer screen and a word heard over headphones. The pictures ($N = 90$) were selected from the PPVT-R to correspond with three levels of single-word receptive vocabulary: Level 1 ($n = 25$): Preschooler (2½–5 years); Level 2 ($n = 40$): Child-Adolescent (10–17 years); Level 3 ($n = 25$): Adult (>17 years; advanced vocabulary). Each picture had been electronically scanned, using the Complete Half-Page Scanner™ and the SmartScan Software™, and subtended a visual angle of approximately 7 degrees.

Each word ($N = 180$) either correctly ($n = 90$) or incorrectly ($n = 90$) named it's corresponding picture. For example, for a congruent or match trial, a picture of a "ball" would be paired with the word "ball". For an incongruent trial, a picture of a "ball" would be paired with the word "wagon". Examples of picture-word pairs typical of all three vocabulary levels are provided in Figure 1.

The words had been digitally recorded in stereo at 12 Khz in a male voice using the Neuroscan Sound Program™ and were between 750 and 1000 ms in duration. A curser-sampling program provided a graphic display of each word's digitized waveform so that word onset could be determined visually by placing a trigger at the beginning of the waveform. Trigger placement was verified auditorially and was used to time-lock EEG sampling to word onset.

The timing and sequence of the visual and auditory stimuli were computer-controlled using the Neuroscan Gentask Program™. During each trial, a picture appeared 700 ms prior to word onset. The picture then remained visible until 1000 ms after completion of the word. This sequence ensured that ERP offset responses to picture termination would not interfere with the recording of auditory ERPs. The order of trial presentation was

Vocabulary Level	Picture	Congruent Word	Incongruent Word
1 Preschool (2.5 - 5)	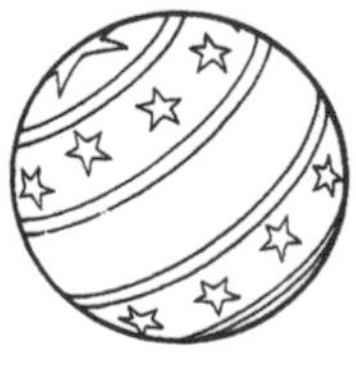	*"Ball"*	*"Wagon"*
2 Child/ Adolescent (10 - 17)	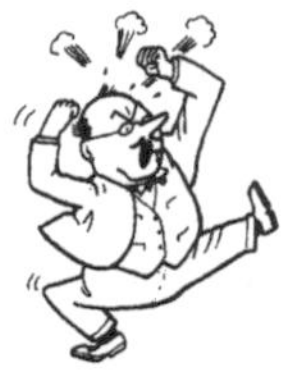	*"Furious"*	*"Pleased"*
3 Adult (Advanced)	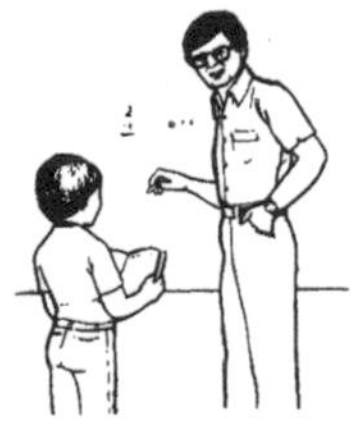	*"Pedagogue"*	*"Potentiate"*

Fig. 1. Examples of picture-word pairs for the ERP-compatible computerized version of the PPVT-R (Form M).

randomized for both level of difficulty and congruency, with the stipulation that trials containing the same picture be separated by at least one other trial. During the 5.2-s intertrial interval, the screen was blank except for a small central fixation point (a plus sign).

The children were tested individually in a sound-attenuated testing booth, and sat approximately 84 cm from the computer screen. They were provided with a two-button response pad and were instructed to depress the right button (blue) for congruent or matching picture-word pairs and the left button (red) for incongruent or mismatching picture-word pairs. They were asked to guess when uncertain. The children were asked to avoid blinking while the picture was visible on the screen, and to blink between trials, if needed. Short breaks (1–2 min) were given to reduce subject fatigue or eye strain.

Electrophysiological recordings
Auditory ERPs time-locked to word onset were recorded from Fz, Cz, Pz, T5, and T6 (International 10–20 System)

using Ag/AgCl electrodes (Invivo Metric™) with linked ears as the reference and a ground placed on the back of the neck. Vertical and horizontal eye movements (EOG) were recorded with electrodes placed supraorbitally and over the outer canthus of the right eye (Connolly & Kleinman, 1978). Electrode impedance was maintained at or below 5 K Ohms. Recordings were made using a band pass of 0.01–70 Hz and were sampled at 250 Hz for 500 ms before and 1350 ms after word onset. EEG data were recorded on a Nihon Kohden Neurofax – 4418A™ and acquired through the NeuroScan Acquisition™ software, through which EEG analog-digital conversion and EEG artifact editing were conducted.

Trials with EOG greater than 75 μv (100 ms before to 1000 ms after word onset) were tagged for rejection from the analysis and confirmed as unacceptable by visual inspection. The percentage of artifact-free trials was very good (80%). Trials were not sorted into correct/incorrect categories on the basis of behavioural responses, because the long-term objective of our research program is to use this ERP-compatible vocabulary test with clinic populations for whom reliable language or motor responses are not possible (e.g., cerebral palsy).

The ERP component of interest was the N400. Its amplitude was scored in the conventional manner (μv difference between prestimulus level and poststimulus ERP component peak) (e.g., Byrne et al., 1995; Connolly et al., 1995; in press). The N400 amplitude was scored as the most negative peak between 350–600 ms after word onset.

RESULTS

For all analyses, conservative Greenhouse-Geisser degrees of freedom and Tukey's post hoc analyses were employed as indicated.

Behavioural Response Data

Comparability of PPVT-R Form L and computerized Form M

As noted earlier, standard administration of the PPVT-R (Form L) was conducted prior to the ERP testing. The children's standard scores ranged from 93 to 123 ($M = 106.7$, $SD = 8.1$), reflecting normal performance. The mean percentage of correct responses for the three levels of vocabulary on the standardized (Form L) and computerized (Form M) versions of the PPVT-R are displayed in Figure 2. The behavioural data from two children could not be included due to malfunctioning of the response pad during ERP testing.

A one-way ANOVA, with percentage of correct responses as a repeated measure, confirmed expectation that the children's behavioural responses on the computerized version of the PPVT-R were significantly influenced by the vocabulary level, $F(2) = 213.86$, $p < .01$. Tukey's post hoc analyses revealed the difference to involve higher percentages of correct responses in Level 1 ($M = 93.7$, $SD = 4.4$), and Level 2 ($M = 83.7$, $SD = 10.4$) vocabulary, compared to Level 3 ($M = 50.2$, $SD = 10.6$), the adult vocabulary (advanced), $F(2) = 213.86$, $p < .05$.

Of the three levels of vocabulary, only Level 2 vocabulary items fell within the psychometrically determined range of the children. In comparing Form L and M, reference to baseline and ceiling was necessary for Form L (standard presentation). Given the mean chronological age of 10 years,

it was reasonable to assume: (a) near perfect performance for Level 1 (Preschool: 2½–5 yr); and (b) chance performance for Level 3 (Adult: > 17 yr). An examination of the percentage of correct responses at Level 1 (93.7%, $SD = 4.4$) and Level 3 (50.2%, $SD = 10.6$) of the computerized PPVT-R are similar to the levels of performance assumed for the standardized administration of the test (see Figure 2). At Level 2 (Child–Adolescent) vocabulary, a paired t test comparing the percentage correct obtained during administration of the computerized (83.7%, $SD = 10.4$) and standardized (80.3%) PPVT-R versions revealed no sig-nificant difference. This compatibility between the computerized and standardized versions of the PPVT-R indicates that the integrity of the PPVT-R (Form M) was not compromised when trans-ferred to the computer and presented within our ERP test.

Response latency

The children's latency to respond behaviourally (depress button) on the computerized PPVT-R (Form M) was examined using a 2 (Congruency) $\times$ 3 (Vocabulary Level) repeated measures MANOVA. A main effect was found for Congruency, $F(10, 1) = 5.77$, $p < .05$, with shorter mean behavioural response latencies for incongruent picture-word pairs ($M = 1399$ ms), as compared to congruent pairs ($M = 1460$ ms). A main effect for Vocabulary Level was found, $F(20,2) = 41.89$, $p < .001$. The Tukey post hoc analyses revealed: Level 1 ($M = 1205$ ms) to have significantly shorter latency than Level 2 ($M = 1466$ ms) $F(2) = 261$, $p < .05$), and Level 3 ($M = 1618$ ms), $F(2) = 413$, $p < .05$, and Level 2 to have a significantly shorter latency than Level 3, $F(2) = 152$, $p < .05$.

N400 Amplitude

Consistent with our findings for adolescents and adults, there was a main effect for Electrode Site, $F(4, 56) = 4.74$, $p < .05$. However, in contrast to the centro-parietal distribution established by these older participants (Connolly et al., in press), the children exhibited a more tempro-parietal distribution (see Figure 3). Compared to the frontal site (Fz), larger N400 amplitudes were exhibited at the posterior sites: Pz, $F(4,56) = 10.01$, $p < .05$; T6, $F(4, 56) = 8.08$, $p < .05$. A significant Electrode Site $\times$ Congruency interaction was also found,

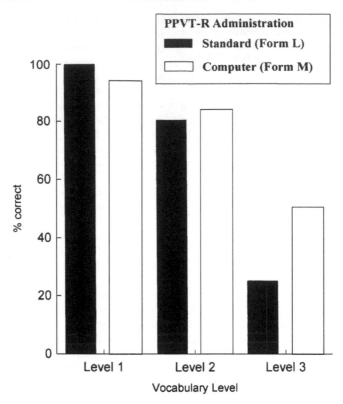

Fig. 2. Percentage of correct responses for Form L (Standard form) and Form M (ERP-compatible computer form) calculated according to level of single-word receptive vocabulary (Level 1: Preschool; Level 2: Child-Adolescent; Level 3: Adult).

$F(4, 56) = 4.66$, $p < .01$, consistent with the above-noted distribution.

As predicted, a main effect for Congruency was found, $F(1, 14) = 5.86, p < .05$, with significantly larger N400 amplitudes to semantically incongruent than to semantically congruent picture-word pairs. There was also a Vocabulary Level × Congruency effect, $F(2, 28) = 4.15, p < .05$. Post hoc analyses revealed a differential pattern of N400 amplitude that could be used to differentiate between the congruent and incongruent conditions for Level 1 vocabulary only. The Level 1 incongruent condition produced a significantly larger N400 amplitude compared to the Level 1 congruent condition, $F(2, 28) = 5.9, p < .05$. This differential N400 pattern was confined to Level 1 vocabulary. At Level 2 and Level 3 vocabulary, no significant difference was found between N400

amplitude to the incongruent and congruent pairs. Comparison across levels showed that the incongruent conditions of both Level 2 [$F(2, 28) = 5.06$, $p < .05$] and Level 3 [$F(2, 28) = 6.39, p < .05$] were significantly larger than the congruent condition of Level 1. This pattern of findings provides convergent evidence that the absence of a significant difference between the incongruent and congruent conditions at Level 2 and Level 3 is due primarily to the overall increased N400 amplitude of the congruent condition, rather than to attenuation of the N400 amplitude in the incongruent condition. This pattern of results is consistent with our earlier findings (Connolly et al., in press) that the absence of a significant difference between congruent and incongruent pairs at relatively advanced levels of vocabulary is due primarily to an overall elevation of the N400 in the congruent condition

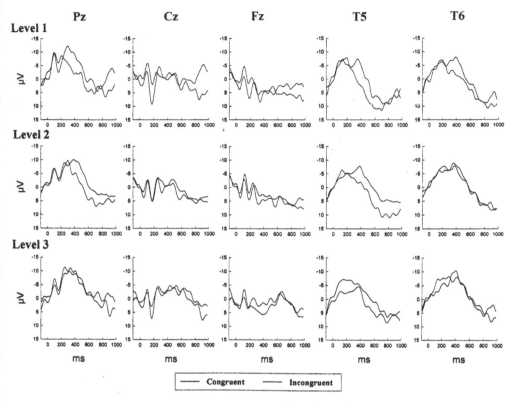

Fig. 3. Grand average ERP waveforms recorded at the three midline and two temporal sites (Pz, Cz, Fz, T5, T6) at each of the three levels of single-word receptive vocabulary (Level 1: Preschool; Level 2: Child-Adolescent; Level 3: Adult). The solid line depicts the responses to the incongruent picture-word pairs, and the dotted line depicts the responses to the congruent pairs. The N400 is demarcated by the downward arrow.

and not to attenuation of the N400 amplitude in the incongruent condition. This interpretation is supported by a main effect for Vocabulary Level, $F(2, 28) = 7.37, p < .01$, with significantly larger N400 amplitudes (when collapsed across congruency) at Level 3 versus Level 1, $F(2, 28) = 3.77$, $p < .05$, and Level 2, $F(2, 28) = 2.52, p < .05$.

Reanalysis of Level 2 Vocabulary

It was initially hypothesized that the N400 amplitude would be significantly larger to the incongruent than to congruent picture-word pairs at Level 2. This hypothesis was based on the finding that it was exhibited by adolescents (Byrne et al., 1995) and adults (Connolly et al., in press), and was based on the assumption that the majority of the vocabulary at Level 2 was age appropriate for

school-aged children (9–11 years). One interpretation for the absence of a differential N400 was that the Level 2 vocabulary (10–17 years) was indeed *within* the range for adolescents and adults but not within the range for the younger children (9–11 years). Because the ERP components are summed over the *entire* cluster of picture-word pairs, it is possible that the more difficult pairs, representing vocabulary outside the child's repertoire (upper limit, Level 2), masked differential ERP patterns (congruent vs. incongruent) for vocabulary within the child's repertoire. To test the hypothesis that the more difficult items from Level 2 vocabulary were outside the age-equivalent vocabulary range for the school children, Level 2 was divided into two sublevels, Level 2A (10–14 years) and Level 2B (15–17 years).

Analyses were conducted on both behavioural and ERP patterns.

Behavioural response pattern

The results confirmed that, on Form L of the PPVT-R (administered in the standard format prior to ERP testing) the children's performance dropped from 91% correct at Level 2A to 63% correct at Level 2B (or the more challenging vocabulary). On Form M of the PPVT-R (computerized form), the children's performance dropped from 87% correct at Level 2A to 76% correct at Level 2B. This same downward trend, albeit a smaller difference, will be discussed later.

Further support for the hypothesis that Level 2B vocabulary was more challenging for the children was obtained from analysis of the behavioural response latency data. A 2 (Vocabulary Sublevel: Level 2A, Level 2B) × 2 (Congruency) repeated measures ANOVA revealed a main effect for Vocabulary Sublevel. There was a significantly longer response latency at Level 2B, ($M_A = 1443$, $M_B = 1546$ ms; $F(10, 1) = 6.56$, $p < .05$). The children's behavioural response latency significantly increased as the difficulty of the vocabulary increased. These results suggest that the more challenging vocabulary items were associated with greater levels of uncertainty and were manifested in longer behavioural response latencies.

N400 Amplitude

A 2 (Vocabulary Level: Level 2A, Level 2B) × 2 (Congruency) × 5 (Electrode Site) repeated measures ANOVA was conducted, with conservative Greenhouse-Geisser degrees of freedom and Tukey's post hoc analyses ($p < .05$) employed as indicated. The anticipated main effect for Vocabulary Level did not reach statistical significance, but the effect did approach significance, $F(1, 14) = 4.19, p = .06$, reflecting the anticipated higher N400 amplitudes (both congruent and incongruent) in the more difficult sublevel of vocabulary (Level 2B). A main effect for Electrode Site was found $F(4, 56) = 4.34$, $p = .02$, with the lowest amplitudes found at the frontal (FZ) site relative to the more posterior sites.

Comparison of ERP and PPVT-R Performance

The children's ERP performance (Form M) and their PPVT-R performance (Form L) were compared using multiple regression analyses. For each level of vocabulary, the magnitude of the children's N400 amplitudes for the incongruent conditions was used to predict their previously established PPVT-R (Form L) raw scores, after covarying for the size of their N400 amplitudes in the congruent conditions. These analyses achieved significance for Level 2 vocabulary, $F(2, 12) = 7.13$, $p = .02$. The N400 residuals were negatively correlated with the raw scores, and accounted for approximately 30% of the variance in predicting the raw scores (see Figure 4, $r^2 = -.60$).

The absence of a significant prediction at Level 1 and 3 is not unexpected given the range restriction and ceiling effect associated with the children's performance at Levels 1 and 3, respectively. These results suggest that, at least for the Level 2 vocabulary (representing sufficient range of performance), it is possible to estimate a child's level of acquired vocabulary based on N400 amplitude data.

DISCUSSION

The primary aim of the present study was to determine whether our recently developed brain ERP-compatible test of single-word receptive vocabulary, used successfully with older participants (17–34 years) (Byrne et al., 1995; Connolly et al., in press), could be used with younger school-aged children. The findings of this study are very encouraging. First, as for older participants, children 10 years of age were able to understand and complete the task. Second, their behavioural response patterns indicated that the basic integrity of Form M of the PPVT (computerized version) was maintained, consistent with the findings with older participants (Connolly et al., in press). Third, as predicted, the 10-year-olds exhibited a significantly larger N400 to incongruent picture-word pairs, as compared to the congruent pairs, but only if the pairs represented vocabulary *within* the children's repertoire. That is, the 10-year-olds exhibited a significantly larger N400 to vocabulary in Level 1 (Preschool), but not at Level 3 (Adult).

The ERP findings at Level 2 (Child-Adolescent) were, initially, less clear. Unlike adolescents and adults (Byrne et al., 1995; Connolly et al., in press),

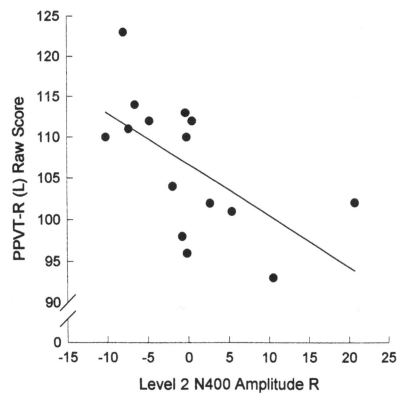

Fig. 4. Correlation between the children's raw scores on Form L of the PPVT-R and the N400 residual data collected from the ERP-compatible version of the PPVT-R (Form M).

the 10-year-olds did not exhibit a significantly larger N400 to the incongruent picture-word pairs at Level 2. However, it would be reasonable to assume that children with a mean age of 10 years would have difficulty with Level 2, as it contained picture-word pairs that covered the age range of 10–17 years, a range not too difficult for the 17- to 34-year-olds tested in our previous studies. In fact, a review of the percentage of correct answers on Form L (administered *prior* to the ERP test), divided into Level 2A (10–14 years) and 2B (15–17 years), revealed that the children had 91% correct behavioural responses at Level 2A and only 63% correct responses at Level 2B.

Consistent with this pattern, a reanalysis of the N400 revealed there was a larger N400 response to the incongruent versus congruent pairs at Level 2A ($p < .06$), but not at Level 2B. These results offer tentative support for the hypothesis, as in Level 3, that the upper portion of Level 2 (Level 2B) represented vocabulary predominantly beyond the repertoire of the 10-year-old participants. It is expected that, in future studies, if additional picture-word pairs were presented in Level 2A and 2B, a more characteristic response profile would emerge, and that the difference would reach statistical significance.

With respect to the integrity of the computerized PPVT-R (Form M), the results showed that school-aged children exhibited a comparable number of correct behavioural responses on both forms at Level 2 (83.7%, 80.3%), with a decreased rate of correct responses as the vocabulary became more challenging (Level 3) (50%, 25%). In addition, the children exhibited significantly longer response latencies (button depression) with increasingly more challenging vocabulary, possibly reflecting more cognitive processing and uncertainty.

The reanalysis of Level 2 vocabulary (Level 2A, 2B) confirmed that, on Form L, the children had 91% correct responses at Level 2A vocabulary and only 63% correct responses at Level 2B (more challenging vocabulary). On Form M of the PPVT-R (computerized form), the trend was in the same direction, but the children performed at 87% at Level 2A and at 76% at Level 2B. The magnitude of percentage correct was not as great for Form M as compared to Form L.

There are at least two reasons for this finding. First, there is a difference between the two forms in regard to probability of a correct answer. For Form M, there are only two response choices, in that the spoken word is either congruent or incongruent with the picture on the computer screen. In contrast for Form L, there are four response choices in that the spoken word matches one of four possible pictures (four stimuli per test plate). Therefore, by chance, a correct response on Form M is 50%, but on Form L it is 25%.

Second, there is a difference between the two forms in regard to method of test administration. Form M was presented in a pseudo-random fashion such that the picture-word pairs did not progressively increase in difficulty from the preschool, child-adolescent, to adult levels of vocabulary. In contrast, the standard presentation of Form L is such that the vocabulary levels increase in difficulty in a linear fashion. Therefore, Form M presentation may promote more uncertainty in responding, and this uncertainty coupled with a higher chance rate of correct responding (25% vs. 50%) may have resulted in a slightly higher (possibly artificial) rate of "correct" behavioural responding at Level 2B.

Nonetheless, these behavioural data still support the hypothesis that the children were, possibly, engaged in greater cognitive effort for Level 2B items that are representative of the upper end of Level 2 vocabulary. This hypothesis, discussed in our previous work (Connolly et al., in press), is also seen in the N400 pattern. That is, as the vocabulary became more challenging (Level 2, 3), the children exerted more cognitive effort and, possibly, became less certain as to the accuracy of their response. This cognitive effort manifested itself in an overall increased N400 amplitude to *both* incongruent and congruent conditions, thereby reducing the difference between the conditions.

Further support for this hypothesis of cognitive effort comes from the behavioural response latency data. The findings revealed that there was a virtual stepwise increase in response latency as the level of vocabulary increased in difficulty (Level 1: $M = 1205$ ms; Level 2: $M = 1466$ ms; Level 3: $M = 1618$ ms). This increase in latency cannot be attributed to response fatigue, such as might be seen with linear progression (easy-difficult) through the test in the standard administration (e.g., Form L). The picture-word pairs were presented in a pseudo-random fashion. This would suggest that, regardless of order of presentation, the more difficult pairs required additional time to allow a decision as to whether the words were congruent.

A residual of the N400 amplitude data (Level 2 vocabulary) was found to predict the children's raw scores on the standardized PPVT-R (Form L). This result provides additional support for the clinical validity our ERP-compatible version of the PPVT-R in the assessment of receptive vocabulary in children with severe communication and motor impairments.

In summary, this test, which has been shown to be a valid measure of adolescent and adult single-word receptive vocabulary, can also measure receptive vocabulary in the young school-aged child. As with adolescents and adults, this ERP-compatible receptive vocabulary test has promise as an adjunct to the assessment protocol for the pediatric population presenting with cerebral palsy, stroke, head injury, or autism. These disorders may be characterized, to a varying degree, by impaired language and/or motor skills, thereby detrimentally affecting the administration of standardized assessment protocols. The use of such ERP tests offers possible adjuncts to the assessment of language skills in patient populations with language/communication and motor impairments. Many of the clinic populations for whom such an application would be appropriate would likely have some degree of acquired brain damage or developmental abnormality.

Further study would have to include an examination of whether the N400 component is substantially affected by the underlying cerebral structure abnormalities probably present in such populations. Such studies would include testing clinic patients with moderate to severe CP with an expanded version of this ERP-compatible vocabulary test, using a wider range of age-appropriate vocabulary. This would allow for an assessment yielding a closer estimate of actual receptive vocabulary.

REFERENCES

Berg, W.K., & Berg, K.M. (1987). Psychophysiological development in infancy: State, startle, and attention. In J.D. Osofsky (Ed.), *Handbook of infant development*. (2nd ed.), (pp. 238–317). New York: Wiley.

Blair, E., & Stanley, F. (1985). Inter-observer reliability in the classification of cerebral palsy. *Developmental Medicine and Child Neurology, 27*, 615.

Brandeis, D., & Lehmann, D. (1986). Event-related potentials of the brain and cognitive processes: Approaches and applications. *Neuropsychologia, 24*, 151–168.

Byrne, J.M. (1984). Cognitive-perceptual abilities of the neurologically impaired infant: An alternative assessment strategy. *Developmental Medicine and Child Neurology, 26*, 391–400.

Byrne, J.M., Dywan, C., & Connolly, J.F. (1995). An innovative method to assess the receptive vocabulary of children with cerebral palsy using event-related brain potentials. *Journal of Experimental and Clinical Neuropsychology, 17*, 9–19.

Connolly, J.F., Byrne, J.M., & Dywan, C.A. (in press). Assessment of receptive vocabulary with event-related brain potentials: An investigation of cross-modal and cross-form priming. *Journal of Clinical and Experimental Neuropsychology.*

Connolly, J.F., & Kleinman, K.M. (1978). A single channel method for recording vertical and lateral eye movements. *Electroencephalography and Clinical Neurophysiology, 45*, 128–129.

Connolly, J.F., & Phillips, N.A. (1994). Event-related potential components reflect phonological and semantic processing of the terminal word of spoken sentences. *Journal of Cognitive Neuroscience, 6*, 256–266.

Connolly, J.F., Phillips, N.A., & Forbes, K.A.K. (1995). The effects of phonological and semantic features of sentence-ending words on visual event-related brain potentials. *Electroencephalography and Clinical Neurophysiology, 94*, 276–287.

Dunn, L.M., & Dunn, L.M. (1981). *Peabody Picture Vocabulary Test-Revised*. Circle Pines, MN: American Guidance Service.

Greenhouse, S.W., & Geisser, S. (1959). On methods in the analysis of profile data. *Psychometrika, 24*, 95–112.

Holcomb, P.J., & Anderson, J.E. (1993). Cross-modal semantic priming: A time-course analysis using event-related brain potentials. *Language and Cognitive Processes, 8*, 379–411.

Holcomb, P.J., & Neville, H.J. (1990). Auditory and visual sematic priming in lexical decision: A comparison using evoked potentials. *Language and Cognitive Processes, 5*, 281–312.

Holcomb, P.J., & Neville, H.J. (1991). The electrophysiology of spoken sentence processing. *Psychobiology, 19*, 286–300.

Kutas, M., & Van Petten, C. (1988). Event-related brain potential studies of language. In P.K. Ackles, J.R. Jennings, & M.G.H. Coles (Eds.), *Advances in psychophysiology*. (pp. 139–187). Greenwich, CT: JAI Press.

McCarty, S.M., St. James, P., Berninger, V.W., & Gans, B. (1986). Assessment of intellectual functioning across the life span in severe cerebral palsy. *Developmental Medicine and Child Neurology, 28*, 369–372.

Miller, E., & Rosenfeld, G.B. (1952). Psychological evaluation of children with cerebral palsy and its implications in treatment. *Journal of Pediatrics, 41*, 613.

Molfese, D.L., & Betz, J.C. (1988). Electrophysiological indices of early development of lateralization for language and cognition, and their implications for predicting later development. In D.L. Molfese & S. Segalowitz (Eds.), *Lateralization in children: Developmental implications* (pp. 171–190). New York: Guilford Press

Molfese, D.L., Morris, R.D., & Romski, M.A. (1990). Semantic discrimination in nonspeaking youngsters with moderate or severe retardation: Electrophysiological correlates. *Brain and Language, 38*, 61–74.

Molfese, D.L., Wetzel, W.F., & Gill, L.A. (1993). Known versus unknown word discriminations in 12-month-old human infants: Electrophysiological correlates. *Developmental Neuropsychology, 9* (3 & 4), 241–258.

Nelson, K.B. (1989). Cerebral palsy. In K.F. Swaiman (Ed.), *Pediatric neurology: Principles and practice* (pp. 363–371). St. Louis: CV Mosby.

Paneth, N. (1986). Birth and the origins of cerebral palsy. *New England Journal of Medicine, 315*, 124.

Pritchard, W.S., Shappell, S.A., & Brandt, M.E. (1991). Psychophysiology of N200/N400: A review and classification scheme. In P.K. Ackles, J.R. Jennings, & M.G.H. Coles (Eds.), *Advances in psychophysiology*, Vol. 4. (pp. 43–106) Greenwich, CT: JAI Press.

Ritter, W., Vaughan, H.G., Jr., & Costa, L.D. (1968). Orienting and habituation to auditory stimuli: A study of short-term changes in average evoked responses. *Electroencephalography and Clinical Neurophysiology, 25*, 550–556.

Sattler, J.M. (1988). *Assessment of children*. (3rd ed.). San Diego: Author.

The Clinical Neuropsychologist
1996, Vol. 10, No. 1, pp. 80–89

VIII-L

Development and Psychometric Properties of the Brief Test of Attention*

David Schretlen[1], Julie Hoida Bobholz[2], and Jason Brandt[3]

[1]Johns Hopkins University School of Medicine, [2]Chicago Medical School, and
[3]Johns Hopkins University School of Medicine

ABSTRACT

The development and preliminary psychometric properties of a new instrument called the Brief Test of Attention (BTA) are described. In terms of the conceptual model proposed by Cooley and Morris (1990), the BTA is best described as a measure of auditory divided attention. The test consists of two parallel forms that require less than 5 minutes each to administer and score. The results of testing 926 patients and normal control subjects support the BTA's reliability, equivalence of forms, and construct validity. Coefficients alpha for the entire test range from .82 to .91, while between-form correlations range from .69 to .81. Neither practice nor interference effects were found to influence performance from the first to second form administered. Correlation and principal components analyses showed that the BTA correlates more strongly with widely accepted measures of attention than with other cognitive tasks, and more strongly with complex than simple attention tasks.

Impairments of attention characterize most neuropsychiatric disorders. Attentional deficits are central to attention-deficit hyperactivity disorder (Barkley, Grodzinsky, & DuPaul, 1992) and delirium (Mesulam, 1985), but also have been associated with schizophrenia (Braff, 1993), depression (Hartlage, Alloy, Vasquez, & Dykman, 1993), traumatic brain injury (Stuss & Gow, 1992), learning disabilities (Fleisher, Soodak, & Jelin, 1984), cortical and subcortical dementia syndromes (Cummings & Benson, 1992), epilepsy (Mirsky, 1989), and alcohol abuse (Oscar-Berman & Bonner, 1985), to name just a few.

The majority of widely used clinical tests of attention were developed without respect to theories of attention. Elegant cognitive and neuroanatomical models of attention, such as those proposed by Triesman (1964), Atkinson and Shiffrin (1968), Gibson (1969), Posner and Snyder (1975), Wickens (1984), and Mesulam (1985), captured scientific attention long after most attention tests enjoyed a secure place in clinical neuropsychology. Few experts would question the clinical utility of the Digit Span and Digit Symbol (Wechsler, 1939), Trail Making (Reitan, 1958), Stroop Color-Word (Stroop, 1935), or continuous performance tests. However, aside from Mirsky's (1989) factor analytic approach to defining components of attention, clinical tests rarely are described in terms of these conceptual models.

One possible explanation for this dissociation between clinical practice and experimental neuropsychology is that accepted clinical measures mix different components of attention, and confound attention with other, often complex cognitive processes. Cooley and Morris (1990) described a

* The Brief Test of Attention© may be obtained by contacting the first author. The authors wish to thank two anonymous reviewers for their helpful comments on an earlier draft of this manuscript. Address correspondence to: David Schretlen, Ph.D., Johns Hopkins Hospital, 600 N. Wolfe St., Meyer 218, Baltimore, MD 21287-7218, tel: (410) 955-3268, USA.
Accepted for publication: April 26, 1995.

framework for conceptualizing the task demands of various clinically accepted measures of attention. They argue that both sustained and divided attention tasks can be conceptualized as special cases of a basic selective attention process. Every selective attention task involves two components: target identification (attend) and distractor inhibition (inhibit). According to this model, *sustained* attention tasks are conceptualized as the extension of these two component processes over time. *Divided* attention is understood as requiring the performance of two simultaneous selective attention tasks. Cooley and Morris conceptualize factors that influence the "inhibit" and "attend" components in terms of four levels of processing. At the most basic level, tonic arousal regulates general information processing (Mesulam, 1985). Modality-linked sensory registration processes, as required by the detection of light flashes or buzzes, define the second level of processing. Modality-specific perceptual processes, such as matching designs or letters, define the third level. The fourth level involves conceptual processing. Relevant tasks typically involve the use of multiple cognitive processing systems, cross-modal comparisons, and/or the allocation of processes between systems. Finally, Cooley and Morris argue that each of the above levels of processing may be represented within five (verbal, spatial, memory, motor, and executive) functional neuropsychological systems.

In this article, we use the model proposed by Cooley and Morris (1990) to describe a new measure of auditory divided attention called the Brief Test of Attention (Schretlen, 1989). We examine its psychometric properties, and compare its processing requirements to those of other tests of attention.

BRIEF TEST OF ATTENTION

Development of the Brief Test of Attention (BTA) began in 1989. The primary aim was to devise a brief, relatively simple and easily administered test of auditory divided attention that would be sensitive to subtle attentional impairments. A secondary goal was to reduce confounding task demands such as psychomotor speed or conceptual reasoning.

The Brief Test of Attention consists of two parallel forms that are presented via audio cassette. Subjects are administered both forms; each requires 4 minutes to administer and score. On Form N, a voice reads 10 lists of letters and numbers (e.g., "M-6-3-R-2") that increase in length from 4 to 18 items. The subject's task is to disregard the letters and count how many *numbers* are read aloud. Each list is followed by 5 s of silence, during which the subject reports how many numbers were recited. The *same* 10 lists are presented as Form L, for which the subject's task is to disregard the numbers and count how many *letters* are read aloud. Unlike digit span tests, the subject is not asked to recall which numbers (or letters) are presented. The number of correctly monitored lists is summed across forms; thus, total BTA scores can range from 0 to 20.

The BTA was tape recorded in a sound-attenuated studio. The voice is that of a female radio broadcast professional who read test stimuli at the rate of one letter or number per second. Each trial is followed by 5 s of silence. After all 10 lists were recorded, the resulting production was re-mastered using digital audio recording to filter out noise between trials. The first 10 trials are introduced on tape as, "Brief Test of Attention, Part A." However, the same 10 trials are duplicated on the tape and subsequently introduced as, "Brief Test of Attention, Part B." In this way, either form N or L can be presented first. The effect of order of presentation is discussed below. Prior to beginning the tape, directions are read to the subject by the examiner. The examiner also reads two short sample lists. If the respondent fails all three trials of both sample lists, the test is discontinued; otherwise, the entire form is administered. The tape is never stopped during the administration of a given form. However, in some circumstances, the use of only one form will yield reliably interpretable results.

STUDY 1: RELIABILITY AND DEMOGRAPHIC CORRELATIONS

The purpose of this study was to document basic psychometric properties of the Brief Test of Attention in normal and clinical samples.

METHOD

Subjects

Normal sample
This sample consisted of 275 adults and 74 children who served as normal control subjects in one of five separate studies. The children included all second ($n =$ 24), fifth ($n = 25$), and eighth ($n = 25$) grade students of a local elementary school. Although the elementary ($n = 74$) and college ($n = 62$) students, as well as 45 adult normal control subjects did not undergo any particular screening procedures, the remaining ($n = 213$) adult subjects were screened for dementia, severe psychiatric disorders, and current substance abuse.

Clinical sample
This sample consisted of 577 patients drawn from studies and clinics conducted at the Johns Hopkins University and Hospital. Included were patients with schizophrenic ($n = 55$), affective ($n = 105$), sexual ($n = 24$), substance abuse ($n = 16$), eating ($n = 14$), mental retardation ($n = 16$), and other ($n = 40$) psychiatric disorders, as well as Huntington's disease ($n = 56$), dementia ($n = 32$), traumatic brain injury ($n = 44$) and adrenoleukodystrophy ($n = 51$). The primary diagnosis was either unavailable or not recorded for 124 patients. Demographic characteristics of both normal and patient samples are shown in Table 1.

Procedure
After giving voluntary informed consent, control subjects were administered the BTA along with whatever other measures were included in the protocol in which they served. Patients referred for clinical evaluations were administered the BTA as part of their examinations. The BTA was not administered in a systematic order relative to other tests. Although demographic information was obtained for most subjects, the available psychometric data varied greatly, depending on research protocols and patient referral questions.

RESULTS

Internal Consistency
Based on the 349 normal adults and children, internal consistency analyses yielded a coefficient alpha of .82 for the BTA (.71 for Form L and .66 for Form N). When these data were pooled with those of 480 patients for whom item scores were recorded, and internal consistency analyses were repeated using this combined sample ($n = 829$), the coefficient alpha increased to .91 for the BTA (.83 for Form L and .84 for Form N).

Form Equivalence
Based on the 349 normal adults and children, the Pearson correlation (r) between forms N and L was .69. However, the between-forms correlation increased to .81 for the combined ($n = 926$) normal and clinical samples. Despite the modest correlation between forms, paired-sample t-tests revealed that normal adults produced virtually identical scores on Forms L and N (8.5, $SD = 1.6$ vs. 8.5, $SD = 1.5$; $t_{(274)} = 0.67; p = .50$). The patients produced lower and more variable scores overall, but they also showed virtually identical performance on Forms L and N (5.6, $SD = 2.9$ vs. 5.5, $SD = 2.9$; $t_{(596)} = 1.02; p = .31$), as did the normal children ($t_{(73)} = -0.62; p = .54$).

The effect of order of administration was examined by subtracting each subject's score on whichever form was administered first from that obtained on the form administered second. A practice effect should result in positive difference scores; an interference effect should lead to negative difference scores. However, if intra-individual variability across forms is random, then the difference scores should be normally distributed with a central tendency that approaches zero. In fact,

Table 1. Demographic Characteristics of Normal and Clinical Samples.

Demographic Variable	n	Age M (SD)	Sex M/F	Race W/B/O[1]	Education M (SD)[2]
Normal Samples					
Adults	275	47.1 (19.3)	112/163	205/30/0[3]	14.4 (2.7)
Children	74	10.1 (2.5)	38/36	70/4/0	4.0 (2.5)
Clinical Sample	577	40.4 (15.7)	327/250	336/201/7[3]	12.2 (3.2)[4]

Note. [1]Race: W = White; B = Black; O = Other. [2]Education expressed in years completed. [3]Race was not recorded for 40 normal control subjects and 33 patients. [4]Education not recorded for 37 patients.

the mean difference score of the 765 patients and normal subjects for whom order was recorded did approach zero ($M = .15$, $SD = 1.8$ points). The distribution of difference scores was mildly leptokurtic (.30), indicating that more subjects than expected produced difference scores of zero. The distribution showed negligible skewness ($-.07$), suggesting that exposure to the first form given neither facilitated nor impeded performance on the second form. In fact, over 97% of normal subjects and 93% of patients produced scores that differed by 3 points between Forms L and N.

Impact of Demographic Characteristics

Among the 74 second, fifth, and eighth grade children, BTA scores were highly correlated with both age ($r = .65$) and education ($r = .62$), which were very highly correlated with one another ($r = .98$). The 38 boys produced significantly lower BTA scores than the 36 girls (11.2, $SD = 3.9$ vs. 13.3, $SD = 3.8$: $t_{(72)} = -2.37$; $p = .021$). In order to examine further the impact of demographic characteristics on test performance, BTA scores were regressed on age, sex, and education (race was ignored because only 4 subjects were not White). Using stepwise multiple regression with forward variable selection, age and sex each met entry criteria for inclusion in a highly significant model (Adjusted $R^2 = .45$; $p < .0001$).

In the sample of normal adults, both age ($r = -.32$, $p < .001$) and education ($r = .13$, $p < .05$) were correlated with BTA scores. Women scored marginally higher than men ($t_{(273)} = -2.18$; $p = .03$), but the men were nearly 10 years older on average, a difference that was highly significant ($t_{(273)} = 3.86$; $p < .001$). When age was entered as the covariate in an analysis of covariance, the main effect of sex disappeared ($F_{(1,272)} = 1.12$; $p = .29$). Among the normal adult sample were 30 African-Americans who were significantly older ($t_{(194)} = -4.36$; $p < .001$) and less educated ($t_{(188)} = 2.72$; $p < .01$) than White subjects in the same age range. Nevertheless, White and Black subjects did not produce significantly different BTA scores (17.2, $SD = 2.5$ vs. 16.3, $SD = 3.2$: $t_{(194)} = 1.68$; $p = .094$). When BTA scores were regressed on age, sex, race, and education using stepwise multiple regression, only age accounted for significant variance in the BTA performance of normal adults (Adjusted $R^2 = .085$; $p < .0001$).

Cumulative frequency data for the BTA are presented in Table 2.

Within the sample of 577 psychiatric patients, BTA scores correlated with both age ($r = -.36$, $p < .001$) and education ($r = .32$, $p < .001$). Male and female patients did not differ in their total BTA scores (11.4, $SD = 5.4$ vs. 10.6, $SD = 5.7$, respectively; $t_{(595)} = 1.81$; $p = .07$). Total BTA scores were regressed on age, sex, education, and race using stepwise multiple regression with forward variable selection. Three predictors each accounted for significant unique variance in BTA scores, as demonstrated by the incremental adjusted R^2s associated with each: age (.141), education (.114), and race (.037). The final model was associated with an overall adjusted R^2 of .292, which was highly significant ($F_{(3,526)} = 73.6$; $p < .0001$). Education and race were confounded in the clinical sample, but ANCOVA revealed that the main effect of race ($F_{(1,549)} = 23.0$; $p < .001$) remained significant after age, sex, and education were entered as covariates. When patients were grouped according to years of education (< 9, 9–11, 12, 13–16), examination of BTA scores revealed that Black patients scored 1.5 to 2.0 points lower than White patients in each of the three upper education subgroups, although race-related differences were not found among patients with less than 9 years of education (Blacks, 7.6, $SD = 4.8$; Whites, 7.2, $SD = 5.8$; $p = .79$).

Only 3 (1%) of the normal adults scored less than 4 on either Form L or Form N. Based on this finding, a series of frequency analyses was conducted using all *clinical* cases for whom the order of test administration was recorded ($n = 548$). First, patients who scored $<4/10$ on the first form given were identified. Their protocols then were examined to determine how many of these patients produced *abnormal* scores (i.e., more than two *SD*s below the normal age group mean) on the *total* test. Altogether, 142 (98%) of the 145 patients who scored <4 on the first form given also produced abnormal total BTA scores. The remaining 3 patients all were 75 years old. Conversely, when those patients who scored $>7/10$ on the first form given were identified ($n = 155$), and their total BTA scores were examined, not one produced an

Table 2. Percent Cumulative Frequency of BTA Scores for Normal Control Subjects by Age Group.

BTA Score	Age range							
	6–8 $n = 24$	9–11 $n = 25$	12–14 $n = 25$	17–19 $n = 24$	20–39 $n = 89$	40–59 $n = 54$	60–69 $n = 68$	70–81 $n = 40$
20			100	100	100	100	100	100
19			96	67	75	82	82	93
18		100	84	50	55	67	68	78
17		96	84	46	40	44	60	65
16		88	72	29	23	35	47	55
15		76	68	17	15	26	38	40
14	100	72	36	4	9	17	24	35
13	96	52	24		3	13	16	30
12	88	44	20			9	9	23
11	75	36	12			4	4	15
10	63	28	8			2	3	15
9	58	12	8				3	10
8	50	8	4				2	5
7	33	8						3
6	21							
5	13							
4	8							
3	4							
2	4							
1	4							
0	4							

abnormal total BTA score. As shown in Table 1, performance on the BTA is highly age-dependent. For those who are 70 or older, total scores of 8/20 are within normal limits. Thus, any elderly subject who scores >7/10 on the first form given thereby demonstrates normal performance. However, the present analyses indicate that, regardless of age, *no* patient who earned >7/10 points on the first form given produced an abnormal total BTA score.

DISCUSSION

The results of this study indicate that the Brief Test of Attention has adequate internal consistency. Correlations between Forms N and L ranged from .69 to .81. Between-form difference scores were normally distributed with a near-zero mean, and were 3 points for 93–97% of subjects. Among normal adults, age alone accounted for significant unique variance in BTA performance, although age and sex both contributed significantly to the BTA performance of children. Among the more heterogeneous patients, age, education, and race all made significant contributions to the final regression model. Sex did not account for significant variance in BTA performance in either adult sample. Overall, the BTA score frequency distributions observed in these normal subjects must be viewed as preliminary, as they are based on samples of convenience. Cutoff scores used to identify attentional impairment might need to be lowered by 1–2 points for persons with less than 12 years of schooling, but verification of this will require further study. Further study also is needed to establish test-retest reliability of the BTA; such research is in progress.

STUDY 2: CONSTRUCT VALIDITY

An analysis of the BTA based on the model of Cooley and Morris (1990) clearly places it within the verbal/linguistic functional system. On Form L, the subject listens to alpha-numeric lists and must detect letters (attend) while ignoring numbers (inhibit). This selective attention process is extended to a lesser degree (the longest list is 18 s) than is the complexity of simultaneous processing. That is, after each target is detected, the subject must reallocate attention to the cumulative sum of previously reported letters and increase it by one. Therefore, the BTA is conceptualized as an auditory perception task that requires divided attention to a much greater extent than sustained attention. Both the perceptual (i.e., distinguishing letters from numbers) and conceptual (counting from 1 to 12) requirements of the BTA are simple. The BTA is designed to reveal impairments of the ability to divide attentional resources between these simultaneous tasks. Implicit in the model is the assumption that impairments of tonic arousal, sensory registration, or the underlying perceptual abilities will also impede performance.

For purposes of comparison, consider digit recall. Digit repetition involves a prototypic selective attention process within the verbal/linguistic functional system. Like the BTA, output is verbal rather than motoric. Until one's immediate storage capacity is reached, repeating digits forward would appear to represent an uncomplicated selective attention test. Repeating digits backward, on the other hand, introduces a requirement of simultaneous processing at the end of each digit string presented. Thus, we predicted that BTA performance would correlate more highly with backward than forward digit span.

Part A of the Trail Making Test (Reitan, 1958) can be viewed as a selective attention task in which the targets are presented visually and output is motoric. Part B of this test is better described as requiring divided attention because it involves two simultaneous selective attention tasks (i.e., monitoring two series to identify targets). Consequently, we predicted that the BTA would correlate more highly with Part B than Part A of this test.

Word reading and color naming portions of the Stroop paradigm (Stroop, 1935) both require simple selective attention at the perceptual level of processing, but also require involvement of both visual and verbal functional systems. The interference portion of the Stroop involves naming the color ink in which (different) color words are printed. This can be conceptualized as requiring either a form of selectivity (i.e., inhibiting the bias to read color

words), or as requiring divided attention (i.e., perceiving both the color ink and color word, then selecting the former). In either case, we predicted that BTA performance would correlate more highly with the interference trial than with color naming or word reading.

METHOD

Subjects and Procedure

Subsamples for this study were drawn from the 926 subjects described in Study 1. Prior to each analysis, a brief description of the relevant subsample is provided. Because the subjects either served as normal controls in one of several studies, or were patients referred for clinical evaluations, the subsamples used for each analysis differ (albeit with some overlap) based on the specific neuropsychological measures administered.

RESULTS

Digit Span

Pearson correlations between BTA scores and digit span (Wechsler, 1981) were based on a subsample of 452 patients and 149 normal subjects, of whom 314 (52.2%) were male. The subjects ranged from 6 to 86 years of age ($M = 38.1$, $SD = 19.7$). Of the 572 subjects for whom race was recorded, 59% were White, 40% were Black, and 1% were "Other". The subjects had completed a mean of 11.0, $SD = 4.0$ years of schooling. The actual number of digits recalled, both forward and backward, was used to compute correlations. As predicted, BTA scores correlated more highly with backward ($r = .53$, $p < .001$) than forward ($r = .43, p < .001$) digit span.[1] A test for the difference between dependent correlations (Bruning & Kintz, 1987) revealed that the disparity between these two correlations is statistically significant ($t_{(597)} = 3.12, p < .01$).

Trail Making Test

Pearson correlations between BTA scores and the Trail Making Test (Reitan, 1958) were based on a

---

[1] When the results of normal subjects and patients were analyzed separately, BTA scores consistently correlated more highly with digits backward than digits forward.

subsample of 311 patients and 73 normal adults, of whom 59% were men. Of the 348 subjects for whom race was recorded, 83% were White, 16% were African-American, and 1% were "Other". Their ages ranged from 15 to 86 (41.1, $SD = 15.4$) years. As compared to the group used to examine correlations with digit span, this subsample contained more normal subjects, fewer patients with severe mental disorders, and fewer African-American subjects. As predicted, total BTA scores correlated more highly with Part B ($r = -.55$, $p < .001$) than Part A ($r = -.48$, $p = .001$) of the Trail Making Test.[2] Again, the difference between these correlations was statistically significant ($t_{(381)} = 2.42, p < .02$).

Stroop Color-Word Test

Correlations between BTA scores and the Stroop Color-Word Test (Golden, 1978) were based on a subsample of 227 adults, which included 183 patients and 44 normal control subjects, of whom 53% were men. Race was not recorded for one subject, but the remaining sample included 117 (52%) White subjects, 105 (47%) African-Americans, and 4 (2%) "Others." Subjects ranged in age from 15 to 72 ($M = 37.9, SD = 11.7$) years. They had an average of 12.1, $SD = 3.3$ years of education. As expected, BTA scores correlated significantly with all three parts of the Stroop (word reading, $r = .66$; color naming, $r = .68$; color-word naming, $r = 67$; all $ps < .001$). However, BTA scores did not correlate more strongly with the interference trial than with word reading or color naming trials.[3]

Factor Analysis

To examine further the construct-related validity of the BTA, we conducted a principal components analysis based on a subsample of 107 psychiatric patients who completed a battery of neuropsycho-

logical tests. The patients ranged from 19 to 68 years of age, and included 62 (58%) men. Ninety patients (84%) were African-American, 13 (12%) were White, and the remaining 4 (4%) belonged to other races. They completed a mean of 10.7, $SD = 2.6$ years of school.

All 107 patients completed a neuropsychological test battery from which 13 (raw scores) test variables were selected for entry into principal components analysis. The scores of six WAIS-R subtests were chosen a priori and combined to create three composite scores: Verbal (Information + Similarities), Perceptual (Picture Completion + Block Design), and Attention (Digit Span + Digit Symbol). In addition to BTA total scores, nine other cognitive test scores were entered as variables in principal components analysis. These were Logical Memory and Visual Reproduction (immediate recall) from the Wechsler Memory Scale-Revised (Wechsler, 1987), a 30-item short form of the Boston Naming Test (Kaplan, Goodglass, & Weintraub, 1978), total words recalled on the Hopkins Verbal Learning Test (Brandt, 1991), the Rey-Osterrieth complex figure drawing (Osterrieth, 1944), average time to complete two trials of the Grooved Pegboard test (Kløve, 1963) with the dominant hand, and all three trials of the Stroop Color-Word Test (Golden, 1978). Principal components analysis with varimax rotation yielded three factors with eigenvalues greater than unity (7.26, 1.08, and 1.01, respectively). This three-factor solution accounted for 71.9% of the total variance and is highly interpretable. As shown in Table 2, Factor 1 accounted for the largest proportion of variance. This factor is aptly described as reflecting *general and verbal mental abilities*. Factor 2 clearly reflects *attentional* abilities, as the BTA, WAIS-R Digit Span, and Digit Symbol composite scores, and all three Stroop scores loaded most highly on it. Factor 3 appears to be defined by *perceptual abilities and psychomotor speed*.

---

[2] When the results of normal subjects and patients were analyzed separately, BTA scores consistently correlated more highly with Trails B than Trails A.

[3] When the results of patients were analyzed separately, BTA scores correlated more highly with performance on the interference trial than with performances on the word reading and color naming trials. This was not the case for normal subjects.

DISCUSSION

The results of this study suggest that the Brief Test of Attention does, in fact, measure attention. The task demands of the BTA are consistent with the

Table 3. Variable Loadings on Each Factor Derived from Principal Components Analysis.

Variable	Factor 1	Factor 2	Factor 3
WAIS-R Verbal (Inf. + Sim.)	**.70**[1]	.30	.35
WAIS-R Attention (DSp. + DSym.)	.47	**.60**	.37
WAIS-R Perceptual (PC + BD)	.51	.15	**.74**
Boston Naming Test	**.68**	.22	.25
Hopkins Verbal Learning Test	**.74**	.22	.26
WMS-R Logical Memory	**.78**	.32	.12
WMS-R Visual Reproduction	.46	.13	**.77**
Brief Test of Attention	.46	**.61**	.22
Stroop A (word reading)	.36	**.81**	.09
Stroop B (color naming)	.23	**.84**	.27
Stroop C (color-word interference)	.15	**.61**	.50
Grooved Pegboard (dom. hand)	.01	−.45	**−.71**
Rey-Osterrieth (copy)	.35	.25	**.71**

[1] The highest factor loading for each measure is shown in bold.

description of auditory divided attention offered by Cooley and Morris (1990). The BTA was found to correlate more strongly with the complex than simple components of two accepted tests of attention that involve different functional neuropsychological systems. Thus, the BTA may tap an aspect of attention that is modality-independent in operation. This would appear to involve the shifting of attentional resources back and forth between two simultaneous but relatively simple cognitive processes.

CONCLUSIONS

As shown in Study 1, the Brief Test of Attention and its two constituent forms have acceptable internal consistency based on the results of 829 patients and normal control subjects. Despite the modest correlations (.69 to .81) between Forms L and N, group mean scores differed by less than .15 points in every sample examined, indicating that the two forms are equally difficult. Further, individual between-forms difference scores were normally distributed with a central tendency of zero, suggesting that neither practice nor interference effects influenced performance from the first to second form administered. Test-retest reliability estimates are not yet available, but these data are being collected. The distribution of scores produced by normal subjects, as shown in Table 1, must be regarded as provisional because the sample does not represent the U.S. population as a whole.

Study 2 provides initial validation the BTA as a measure of auditory divided attention. Like most neuropsychological tests, the BTA measures general mental ability, as shown by its substantial loading (.46) on the first factor that emerged from principal components analysis. However, like all three parts of the Stroop test and the sum of WAIS-R Digit Span and Digit Symbol, the BTA loaded most highly (.61) on a factor that clearly is defined by attentional abilities. Further evidence of the construct and criterion validity of the BTA is presented in a companion article (Schretlen, Brandt, & Bobholz, 1996).

When applied to patients who are demographically similar to the normal subjects used in this study, the Brief Test of Attention appears to provide a reliable and valid appraisal of auditory divided attention. The entire test requires less than 10 minutes to administer and score, and when patients score <4/10 or >7/10 on the first form given, the second form may be omitted without compromising the reliability of clinical judgements regarding the presence or absence of impaired attention. Until more broadly representative normative data become available, this report is intended to provide preliminary psychometric information that will enable others to use the BTA for research and, with appropriate caution, for clinical applications.

REFERENCES

Atkinson, R.C., & Shiffrin, R.M. (1968). Human memory: A proposed system and its control processes. In K.W. Spence & J.T. Spence (Eds.), *The psychology of learning & motivation: Advances in research & theory* (Vol. 2, pp. 89–195). New York: Academic Press.

Barkley, R.A., Grodzinsky, G., & DuPaul, G.J. (1992). Frontal lobe functions in attention deficit disorder with and without hyperactivity: A review and research report. *Journal of Abnormal Child Psychology, 20,* 163–188.

Braff, D.L. (1993). Information processing and attention dysfunctions in schizophrenia. *Schizophrenia Bulletin, 19,* 233–259.

Brandt, J. (1991). The Hopkins Verbal Learning Test: Development of a new memory test with six equivalent forms. *The Clinical Neuropsychologist, 5,* 125–142.

Bruning, J.L., & Kintz, B.L. (1987). *Computational handbook of statistics.* Glenview, IL: Harper Collins Publishers.

Cooley, E.L., & Morris, R.D. (1990). Attention in children: A neuropsychologically based model for assessment. *Developmental Neuropsychology, 6,* 239–274.

Cummings, J.L., & Benson, D.F. (1992). *Dementia: A clinical approach* (2nd ed.). Boston: Butters-worth.

Fleisher, L.S., Soodak, L.C., & Jelin, M.A. (1984). Selective attention deficits in learning disabled children: Analysis of the data base. *Exceptional Children, 51,* 136–141.

Gibson, E.J. (1969). *Principles of perceptual learning and development.* New York: Appleton-Century-Crofts.

Golden, C.J. (1978). *Stroop Color and Word Test.* Wood Dale, IL: Stoelting Co.

Hartlage, S., Alloy, L.B., Vasquez, C., & Dykman, B. (1993). Automatic and effortful processing in depression. *Psychological Bulletin, 113,* 247–278.

Kaplan, E.F., Goodglass, H., & Weintraub, S. (1978). *The Boston Naming Test.* Boston: E. Kaplan & H. Goodglass.

Kløve, H. (1963). Clinical neuropsychology. In F.M. Forster (Ed.), *The medical clinics of North America.* New York: Saunders.

Mesulam, M.M. (1985). Attention, confusional states, and neglect. In M-M Mesulam (Ed.), *Principles of behavioral neurology* (pp. 125–168). Philadelphia: F.A. Davis Company.

Mirsky, A.F. (1989). The neuropsychology of attention: Elements of a complex behavior. In E. Perecman (Ed.), *Integrating theory and practice in clinical neuropsychology* (pp. 75–91). Hillsdale, NJ: Lawrence Erlbaum Associates.

Oscar-Berman, M., & Bonner, R.T. (1985). Matching- and delayed matching-to-sample performance as measures of visual processing, selective attention, and memory in aging and alcoholic individuals. *Neuropsychologia, 23,* 639–651.

Osterrieth, P.A. (1944). Le test de copie d'une figure complexe. *Archives de Psychologie, 30,* 206–356.

Posner, M.I., & Snyder, C.R.R. (1975). Attention and cognitive control. In R.L. Solso (Ed.), *Information processing and cognition* (pp. 55–85). Hillsdale, NJ: Erlbaum.

Reitan, R.M. (1958). Validity of the Trail Making Test as an indication of organic brain damage. *Perceptual and Motor Skills, 8,* 271–276.

Schretlen, D. (1989). *The Brief Test of Attention.* Baltimore, MD: Author.

Schretlen, D., Brandt, J., & Bobholz, J.H. (1996). Validation of the Brief Test of Attention in patients with Huntington's disease and amnesia. *The Clinical Neuropsychologist.* This issue.

Stroop, J.R. (1935). Studies of interference in serial verbal reactions. *Journal of Experimental Psychology, 18,* 643–662.

Stuss, D.T., & Gow, C.A. (1992). "Frontal dysfunction" after traumatic brain injury. *Neuropsychiatry, Neuropsychology, and Behavioral Neurology, 5,* 272–282.

Triesman, A.M. (1964). Selective attention in man. *British Medical Bulletin, 20,* 12–16.

Wechsler, D. (1939). *Measurement of adult intelligence.* Baltimore: Williams & Wilkins.

Wechsler, D. (1981). *The Wechsler Adult Intelligence Scale-Revised manual.* San Antonio: The Psychological Corporation.

Wechsler, D. (1987). *Wechsler Memory Scale-Revised manual.* San Antonio: The Psychological Corporation.

Wickens, C.D. (1984) Processing resources in attention. In R. Parasuraman & D.R. Davies (Eds.), *Varieties of attention* (pp. 63–102). Orlando, FL: Academic.

The Clinical Neuropsychologist
1996, Vol. 10, No. 1, pp. 90–95

VIII-L

Validation of the Brief Test of Attention in Patients with Huntington's Disease and Amnesia*

David Schretlen,[1] Jason Brandt,[1] and Julie Hoida Bobholz[2]

[1]Johns Hopkins University School of Medicine, and [2]Chicago Medical School

ABSTRACT

We report two studies of auditory divided attention in patients with Huntington's disease (HD) and organic amnesia using the Brief Test of Attention (BTA). In the first study, 27 patients with HD were individually matched with 27 normal control subjects on the basis of age and Mini-Mental State Examination (MMSE) scores. The patients and normal adults also did not differ in sex, race, or education. Despite the fact that mean MMSE scores were 28.8 ($SD = 1.0$) for both groups, the HD patients scored three SDs below the mean of normal adults on the BTA. In the second study, 9 nondemented amnesic patients and 9 normal adults who were individually matched for age, sex, race, and education produced no significant group differences on the Brief Test of Attention. These results show that BTA performance in impaired in a group known to have severe defects in attention, and that it does not require intact memory for successful performance.

In a companion paper (Schretlen, Bobholz, & Brandt, 1996), the development and preliminary psychometric properties of a new instrument called the Brief Test of Attention (BTA) are described (Schretlen, 1989). The BTA consists of two parallel forms that are presented via audio-cassette. On Form N, a voice reads 10 lists of letters and numbers (e.g., "M-6-3-R-2") that increase in length from 4 to 18 items. The subject's task is to disregard the letters and count how many *numbers* were read aloud. The same 10 lists are presented as Form L, wherein the subject must disregard the numbers and count how many *letters* were read aloud. The number of correctly monitored lists is summed across forms. Thus, total scores for the BTA can range from 0 to 20. The entire test requires about 9 minutes to administer and score. Based on the combined results of 926 patients and normal control subjects, who ranged from 6 to 86 years of age,

the BTA was found to have a coefficient alpha of .91 and a between-forms correlation of .81. When each subject's score on the first form administered was subtracted from his or her score on the second form administered, the resulting distribution was Gaussian in form with a central tendency of zero ($M = .15$, $SD = 1.8$), suggesting that between-form differences were due to random error rather than to interference or practice effects. Moreover, scores on Form L differed from scores on Form N by 3 points for 95% of all subjects.

Consideration of the task demands and comparison of this instrument with other measures of attention suggest that the BTA is best conceptualized as a measure of auditory divided attention, as described by Cooley and Morris (1990). As such, one would predict that patients with impaired attention (e.g., Huntington's disease) would perform poorly on the BTA, whereas cognitively

* This research was supported, in part, by NIH Grant NS 16375 and the John Boogher Fund for Memory Disorders Research. The authors wish to thank Dr. Frederick Bylsma and Dr. Jill Rich for their assistance with data collection. The Brief Test of Attention© may be obtained by contacting the first author. Address correspondence to: David Schretlen, Ph.D., Johns Hopkins Hospital, 600 North Wolfe Street, Meyer 218, Baltimore, MD 21287-7218, (410) 955-3268, USA.
Accepted for publication: April 26, 1995.

impaired patients whose deficits do not include
attention (e.g., amnesics) would perform normally.
If the BTA distinguishes patients with known
attention impairment from matched control
subjects, this would support the construct- and
criterion-related validity of the BTA. If amnesic
patients with intact attention perform normally on
the BTA, this would support the test's discriminant validity.

STUDY 1: HUNTINGTON'S DISEASE

Huntington's disease (HD) is a progressive neu-
rodegenerative disease that is characterized by
neuronal loss and gliosis in the striatum and globus
pallidus. It is inherited as an autosomal dominant
trait with complete lifetime penetrance, and the
onset of symptoms typically occurs around age 40.
Patients with HD suffer from progressively worsening choreiform movements, impaired voluntary
movement, and cognitive decline. Because of the
prominence of basal ganglia pathology, the cognitive deficits associated with HD have been considered prototypic of the subcortical dementias
(Cummings, 1990; McHugh & Folstein, 1975). In
particular, impaired attention and executive functions are among the most prominent cognitive
deficits associated with the dementia of HD, even
in its early stages (Brandt & Bylsma, 1993). Butters
et al. (1988) administered the Wechsler Memory Scale-Revised (WMS-R; Wechsler, 1987) to
patients with amnesia and various dementing illnesses, including HD. They found that, whereas
HD patients and amnesics produced equally abnormal scores on the WMS-R General Memory Index,
only the HD patients produced abnormally low
scores on the WMS-R Attention/Concentration
Index. Based on these findings, we hypothesized
that patients with HD would perform more poorly
on the BTA than normal control subjects.

METHOD

Subjects and Procedure

Included in this study were 27 HD patients and 27
normal adults who were matched individually on the
basis of age and Mini-Mental State Exam (MMSE:
Folstein, Folstein, & McHugh, 1975) scores. Patients
were drawn from a sample of 55 adults with HD who
are being followed prospectively through the Baltimore
Huntington's Disease Project at Johns Hopkins
University. All HD patients had movement disorders
and at least one other affected family member. In most
cases the diagnosis has been confirmed by genetic
analysis at the IT-15 locus. The matched normal subjects were drawn from a pool of 106 healthy adults who
had been given both the MMSE and the BTA. Only
patients and normal adults who scored 27/30 on the
MMSE were considered for inclusion in the present
study. HD patients and normal subjects who produced
identical MMSE scores and were reasonably close in
age comprised the 27 subject pairs included in this
study. As shown in Table 1, the patient and normal control groups produced mean (SD) MMSE scores of 28.8
(SD = 1.0). Based on paired-sample t tests and chi-
square analyses, the two groups did not differ in age,
sex, race, or education. Each patient's (but not each normal subject's) Full Scale IQ was estimated using a two-
subtest WAIS-R short form that yields reasonably
reliable and valid estimates of Full Scale IQ (Benedict,
Schretlen, & Bobholz, 1992; Schretlen, Bobholz, &
Benedict, 1994; Silverstein, 1982). The mildly affected
HD patients produced a mean estimated IQ of 97.9
(SD = 14.8). Subjects completed the BTA along with
whatever other measures comprised the study protocols
in which they served.

Table 1. Study 1 Sample Characteristics.

	HD patients	Normal control	Statistic	p
Age	42.7 ± 10.7	41.5 ± 9.0	$t_{(26)} = .67$	.51
Sex (M/F)	14/13	17/10	$\chi^2_{(1)} = .68$	.41
Race (Wht/Other)	24/2	23/3	$\chi^2_{(1)} = .22$	.64
Education (yrs)	14.6 ± 2.6	14.4 ± 2.3	$t_{(26)} = .32$	.75
MMSE	28.8 ± 1.0	28.8 ± 1.0	$t_{(26)} = .0$	1.0
Estimated IQ[1]	97.9 ± 14.8	–	–	–

Note. [1] Based on Silverstein's (1982) two-subtest short form of the WAIS-R.

RESULTS

As shown in Figure 1, paired-sample t tests revealed that HD patients scored significantly lower than did normal control subjects on the Brief Test of Attention ($M = 12.0$, $SD = 3.5$ vs. $M = 17.5$, $SD = 1.8$; $t_{(26)} = -6.89$; $p < .0001$). Essentially identical results were found when each form of the BTA (Letters and Numbers) was examined separately. Between-form difference scores (Form L minus Form N) were near-zero for each group, and did not differ between HD patients and normal adults.

DISCUSSION

In this study, patients with HD scored significantly lower on the Brief Test of Attention than did normal adults who were matched individually on age and MMSE scores, and who were indistinguishable from the patients in terms of sex, race, and education. This large group effect on the BTA is particularly striking because only HD patients with MMSE scores of 27/30 were included, and because their mean estimated IQ was 98. However, the obtained results are consistent with previous findings that the dementia of HD, a disease with

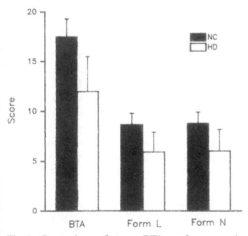

Fig. 1. Comparison of mean BTA performances by normal adults and patients with Huntington's disease. Error bars denote standard deviations. The HD patients scored lower than normal controls on every BTA measure (all $ps < .0001$).

known frontal subcortical pathology, is characterized by impairments of attention and other executive abilities (Bamford, Caine, Kido, Plassche, & Shoulson, 1989; Brandt & Bylsma, 1993; Butters, Sax, Montgomery, & Tarlow, 1978).

STUDY 2: AMNESIA

Amnesia refers to severe memory impairment in the absence of dementia. As shown by Butters et al. (1988), amnesics can be differentiated from demented patients with equally impaired memory by their WMS-R performances. While amnesic and demented patients both produce abnormally low General Memory Index (GMI) and Delayed Recall Index (DRI) scores, only the amnesics produced normal Attention/Concentration Index (ACI) scores. Thus, the anterograde memory impairment appears to be more circumscribed in amnesia than in dementia.

Elsewhere, BTA scores were shown to correlate moderately highly with various measures of attention, and more highly with complex than simple attention tests (Schretlen et al., 1996). These findings suggest that the BTA is sensitive to individual differences in attentional abilities. However, discriminant validity requires that a proposed psychological test be both sensitive *and* specific with respect to the construct it purports to measure. In performing the BTA task, subjects must remember how many letters (or numbers) were recited aloud during each test trial. This raises the question of whether the BTA requires not only intact attention but also intact learning and memory for successful performance. If the BTA measures attention only, then patients with severe memory impairment only should perform this task normally. In this study we examine attention and memory in 9 amnestic patients, and compare their BTA performance to that of 9 individually matched normal adults.

METHOD

Subjects and Procedure

The 9 amnesics included in this study consisted of 2 patients with alcoholic Korsakoff's syndrome and

Table 2. Study 2 Sample Characteristics.

	Amnesic patients	Normal control	Statistic	p
Age	66.7 ± 12.5	66.7 ± 12.9	$t_{(7)}$ = 0.0	1.0
Sex (M/F)	5/4	5/4	$\chi^2_{(1)}$ = 0.0	1.0
Race (Wht/Other)[1]	8/1	8/1	$\chi^2_{(1)}$ = 0.0	1.0
Education (yrs)	16.0 ± 4.4	15.3 ± 3.5	$t_{(7)}$ = 1.26	.24
Full Scale IQ	114.6 ± 10.7	–	–	–

Note. [1]One Hispanic patient with amnesia was matched with an African-American control subject.

7 patients with presumed medial temporal damage due to hypoxia (2), viral encephalitis (1), or cerebrovascular disease (4). All patients demonstrated severe anterograde and retrograde memory impairment on clinical examination. They could not remember the names of their physicians for more than a few minutes, and were unable to recall experiences that occurred 1 hr earlier. Patients' WMS-R Delayed Recall Index scores were 56 points lower on average (range: 43–76 points) than their WAIS-R Full Scale IQ scores.

For the present study, 9 normal adult subjects were matched individually to each amnesic subject in terms of age, sex, race, and education. No other variables were considered when matching patients to normal control subjects. All normal control subjects gave voluntary informed consent to participate.

RESULTS

As shown in Table 2, comparison of the amnesic and normal control subjects, with matched-sample t tests and chi-square analyses, revealed that the two groups were virtually identical in terms of age, sex, race, and years of education. The amnesic patients produced WAIS-R Full Scale IQ scores that ranged from 96 to 132 ($M = 114.6$, $SD = 10.7$). Their scores on the three most relevant WMS-R indices were as follows: General Memory Index (GMI: $M = 74.0$, $SD = 15.8$); Delayed Recall Index (DRI: $M = 58.6$, $SD = 10.5$), and Attention/Concentration Index (ACI: $M = 109.9$, $SD = 10.7$). These scores are nearly identical to those reported by Butters et al. (1988) for a comparable group of amnesics.

The amnesic patients and control subjects did not differ on any BTA measure. The mean BTA score for amnesic patients ($M = 14.3$, $SD = 3.5$)

was marginally lower than that of the normal controls ($M = 15.7$, $SD = 3.0$), although this difference did not approach statistical significance ($t_{(8)} = -1.26$; $p = .24$). Equally small group differences between amnesics and matched control subjects were observed for BTA Form L ($M = 7.1$, $SD = 1.8$ vs. $M = 7.7$, $SD = 1.6$) and Form N ($M = 7.2$, $SD = 2.1$ vs. $M = 8.0$, $SD = 1.9$).

If the BTA measures attention independently of learning and memory, then it should correlate more highly with the WMS-R Attention/Cencentration Index (ACI) than with the WMS-R Memory Index scores. Due to the small sample size and limited score variance observed in this sample, Spearman rank-order correlation coefficients were computed. The BTA did not correlate significantly with any WMS-R index, including the ACI ($\varrho = .27$), GMI ($\varrho = .26$), or DRI ($\varrho = .32$). However, as shown in Figure 2, the 2 patients with alcoholic Korsakoff's syndrome produced the lowest BTA scores. Because Korsakoff amnesics typically demonstrate impaired executive abilities, possibly reflecting frontal systems dysfunction (Squire, 1982), correlations between the BTA and WMS-R indices were recomputed after excluding the Korsakoff amnesics. Based on the remaining 7 amnesics, the BTA showed a significant Spearman correlation with the ACI ($\varrho = .77$; $p = .02$), but not with either the GMI ($\varrho = .00$) or DRI ($\varrho = .45$). Figure 2 also shows that one non-Korsakoff amnesic produced an unusually low score on the ACI. A final reanalysis of the data after excluding this patient as an "outlier" reduced Spearman's rho between ACI and BTA scores to .63, which falls short of statistical significance for this sub-sample of 6 patients ($p = .09$).

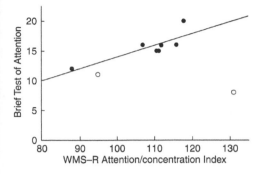

Fig. 2. Scatterplot depicting the relationship between BTA and WMS-R Attention/Concentration Index scores among 2 Korsakoff ( ) and 7 non-Korsakoff (•) amnesics. Regression line is based on data produced by the non-Korsakoff amnesics (Spearman $\varrho = .77, p = .02$).

DISCUSSION

This study demonstrates that patients with severe but circumscribed memory impairment, both clinically and on neuropsychological testing, can perform the Brief Test of Attention successfully. These findings indicate that the BTA effectively discriminates intact attention from the impaired learning and memory of patients with organic amnesia. Finding that BTA scores correlated positively with the WMS-R Attention/Concentration Index scores of non-Korsakoff amnesics supports the convergent validity of this instrument for the construct of attention. The smaller, nonsignificant correlations between BTA and WMS-R memory index scores support the discriminant validity of the BTA.

CONCLUSION

The two studies reported here help define what cognitive processes are required for successful performance of the Brief Test of Attention, and clarify the processing deficits which characterize the dementia of HD and amnesia. In Study 1, very mildly affected patients with Huntington's disease scored three standard deviations below the mean BTA score of individually matched normal control subjects with identical MMSE scores. Huntington's disease thus appears to cripple some component of attentional processing required by the BTA. Whether the vulnerable component primarily involves attentional capacity (e.g., working memory), selective attention (e.g., resisting distraction), or divided attention (e.g., the allocation of attention among simultaneous demands) cannot be answered by this present study, although patients with HD have been shown to perform poorly on tasks that involve each of these aspects of attention (Brandt & Bylsma, 1993).

In Study 2, nondemented but severely amnesic patients were found to be as accurate as normal persons on the BTA, thereby confirming the hypothesis that successful performance of this task does not require intact learning or memory. Particularly in light of the deficient BTA performance by HD patients, the dissociation of intact attention from impaired memory among amnesic patients has several implications. First, this dissociation supports the discriminant validity of the Brief Test of Attention. Second, it provides additional evidence that the failure of the HD patients on the BTA is due to impaired attention rather than deficient learning or memory. Third, it raises the question of whether the explicit memory deficits shown by patients with HD might be an artifact of impaired attention. Fourth, it supports the hypothesis that medial temporal structures play a minor or easily circumvented role in auditory divided attention, whereas the striatum plays a crucial role in the same process.

REFERENCES

Bamford, K.A., Caine, E.D., Kido, D.K., Plassche, W.M., & Shoulson, I. (1989). Clinical-pathological correlation in Huntington's disease: A neuropsychological and computed tomography study. *Neurology, 39*, 796–801.

Benedict, R.H.B., Schretlen, D., & Bobholz, J.H. (1992). Concurrent validity of three WAIS-R short forms in psychiatric patients. *Psychological Assessment, 4*, 322–328.

Brandt, J., & Bylsma, F.W. (1993). The dementia of Huntington's disease. In R.W. Parks, R.F. Zec, & R.S. Wilson (Eds.), *Neuropsychology of Alzheimer's disease and other dementias* (pp. 265–282). New York: Oxford University Press.

Butters, N., Salmon, D.P., Cullum, C.M., Cairns, P., Troster, A.I, Jacobs, D., Moss, M., & Cermak, L.S. (1988). Differentiation of amnesic and demented patients with the Wechsler Memory Scale-Revised. *The Clinical Neuropsychologist, 2*, 133–148.

Butters, N., Sax, D.S., Montgomery, K., & Tarlow, S. (1978). Comparison of neuropsychological deficits associated with early and advanced Huntington's disease. *Archives of Neurology, 35*, 585–589.

Cooley, E.L., & Morris, R.D. (1990). Attention in children: A neuropsychologically based model for assessment. *Developmental Neuropsychology, 6*, 239–274.

Cummings, J.L. (1990). *Subcortical dementia.* New York: Oxford University Press.

Folstein, M.F., Folstein, S.E., & McHugh, P.R. (1975). 'Mini-Mental State': A practical method for grading the cognitive state of patients for the clinician. *Journal of Psychiatric Research, 12*, 189–198.

McHugh, P., & Folstein, M.F. (1975). Psychiatric syndromes of Huntington's chorea: A clinical and phenomenologic study. In D.F. Benson & D. Blumer (Eds.), *Psychiatric aspects of neurologic disease* (pp. 267–286) New York: Grune & Stratton.

Schretlen, D. (1989). *The Brief Test of Attention.* Baltimore: Author.

Schretlen, D., Benedict, R.H.B., & Bobholz, J.H. (1994). Composite reliability and standard errors of measurement for a seven-subtest short form of the Wechsler Adult Intelligence Scale-Revised. *Psychological Assessment, 6*, 188–190.

Schretlen, D., Bobholz, J.H., & Brandt, J. (1996). Development and psychometric properties of the Brief Test of Attention. *The Clinical Neuropsychologist*, this issue.

Silverstein, A.B. (1982). Two- and four-subtest short forms of the Wechsler Adult Intelligence Scale-Revised. *Journal of Consulting and Clinical Psychology, 50*, 415–418.

Squire, L.R. (1982). Comparisons between forms of amnesia: Some deficits are unique to Korsakoff's Syndrome. *Journal of Experimental Psychology: Learning, Memory, and Cognition, 8*, 560–571.

Wechsler, D. (1987) *Wechsler Memory Scale-Revised Manual.* San Antonio: The Psychological Corporation.

Journal of Clinical and Experimental Neuropsychology
1998, Vol. 20, No. 2, pp. 293–295

VIII-M

THE EDITOR'S CORNER

Role of Null Hypothesis Significance Testing (NHST) in the Design of Neuropsychologic Research

Domenic V. Cicchetti
Yale University Child Study Center

A BRIEF REVIEW OF THE PROBLEM

In an earlier publication of *JCEN* (Cicchetti, 1997), I commented extensively on Veiel's (1997) critique of the Wilde, Boake, and Sherer article that was published in this journal, in 1995.

The substance of this paper focuses on a major issue that was introduced by Veiel (1997), but which did not receive the attention it deserves, especially in the context of the readership of this Journal, and for experimental research more broadly defined. I am referring specifically to the role of null hypothesis significance testing (NHST) in the design of research investigations.

Because the role of NHST has very broad research implications, the overarching objective of this brief commentary is to provide information to the readership of this Journal that will hopefully insure that the relevance of the dispute reaches well beyond its present content focus.

SOME NECESSARY BACKGROUND INFORMATION

In my previous critique of Veiel (1997), I pointed out that of three specific experimental hypotheses put forth by Wilde, Boake & Sherer (1995), one was confirmed and the remaining two were not.

Speaking directly to this issue, Veiel, in his reply, states the following: "The only specified condition in the Wilde et al. (1995) study was that of no difference between individuals with and

without recognition-recall discrepancies, and this was the null hypothesis they tested by means of analysis of variance." In commenting on this issue, Fuerst (1997) notes the following:

> I should point out that Wilde et al. did not claim that their findings disproved the hypothesis that in patients with CHI recall-recognition discrepancies are due to retrieval deficits. They concluded only that (consistent with at least one prior study) their results did not support it. This is a far cry from Veiel's assertion that Wilde et al. concluded that recall-recognition discrepancies 'do not reflect a specific retrieval deficit.' It would appear that Veiel has taken the liberty of accepting the null hypothesis on their behalf (p. 151).

Quite apart from the validity of Fuerst's critique, there is another critical scientific issue that involves the proper role of NHST in the design of neuropsychological research, in particular, and in behavioral and biomedical research, more broadly.

THE ROLE OF NHST IN THE DESIGN OF RESEARCH INVESTIGATIONS

Some investigators focus on NHST as an end, in and of itself. Unfortunately, the Null Hypothesis, in this specific context, is used to mean no difference whatsoever, or, as Cohen (1994, p. 1000) states it, as representing an effect size or ES of exactly zero. This, Cohen refers to as the

Address correspondence to: Domenic V. Cicchetti, Yale Child Study Center Home Office, 94 Linsley Lake Road, North Branford, CT 06471, USA. E-mail: dom.cicchetti@yale.edu

Nil Hypothesis (NIL). To be more specific, Cohen (1990) wrote that his work in power analysis forced him to conclude that the NIL must *always be false*. More specifically:

It can only be true in the bowels of a computer processor running a Monte Carlo study (and even then a stray electron may make it false). If it is false, even to a tiny degree, it must be the case that a large enough sample will produce a significant result and lead to its rejection. So if the null hypothesis is always false, what's the big deal about rejecting it? (p. 1308).

Cohen is not alone in his comments on the role of NHST in science. The prominent statistician John W. Tukey (1991) wrote the following: "It is foolish to ask 'Are the effects of A and B different?' They are always different – for some decimal place" (p. 100, as referenced in Cohen, 1994, p. 1000). As early as 1951, the statistician Frank Yates, he of the famed 1934 correction to the chi-square (d) test (with 1 degree of freedom), wrote a scathing review of Fisher's (1951) well-known *Statistical Methods for Research Workers*, specifically, that: "It has caused scientific research workers to pay undue attention to the results of the tests of significance they perform on their data ... and too little to the effects they are estimating" (p. 32, as referenced in Cohen, 1994, p. 1001).

So what is the solution to this conundrum? As Cohen (1994, also p. 1001) puts it: "First, don't look for a magic alternative to NHST, some other objective mechanical ritual to replace it. It doesn't exist." Second, Cohen and many others, (including Tukey (1977), in his ground-breaking text, *Exploratory Data Analysis*), focuses upon "simple, flexible, informal, and largely graphic techniques for understanding the data set in hand" (Cohen, 1994, p. 1001).

Since Tukey's seminal work, numerous others have contributed to the burgeoning field of computer graphics (e.g., Cleveland, 1993; Tufte, 1983; Wainer & Thissen, 1993). The third recommendation of Cohen (1994) is that effect sizes (ES) be routinely reported in the context of the familiar, but under-used confidence limits. Cohen's final recommendation, most recently, in his August 1997 American Psychological Association Master Lecture Series Invited Address (cleverly named

"Much Ado About Nothing," since it focused on null hypothesis significance testing) is for us as scientists to never forget to *replicate* our research efforts, this, in the time-honored tradition of the physical sciences. (See also, Rourke & Costa, 1979.)

SUMMARY AND RECOMMENDATIONS

Let me conclude with the following observations and thoughts for the future of clinical and experimental neuropsychology and science, more generally:

(1) In trying to make the most sense of one's data, the innovative graphical techniques that have been published over the last two decades do indeed support the adage that one picture is worth perhaps a thousand words and

(2) Null or Nil Hypothesis Significance Testing (NHST) is, in and of itself, not a very meaningful scientific activity; it needs, rather, to be understood in the much broader context of issues of power and, especially, replication. In this important regard, Cohen's suggestion (1994, 1997) that confidence intervals be employed, as a matter of routine, especially when issues of power are at stake, as well as a low probability of replication, is, in my opinion, an excellent recommendation for the continued progress and advancement of clinical and experimental neuropsychology, and for science more generally. It is noteworthy that a computer program has just been released that provides power analyses and confidence intervals in a variety of research contexts. Moreover, the resulting tables and graphs may also be inserted into word processing documents and programs. For more specific information, the interested reader is referred to Borenstein, Cohen, and Rothstein (1997).

REFERENCES

Borenstein, M., Cohen, J., & Rothstein, H. (1997). *Power and precision*. Mahwah, NJ: Lawrence Erlbaum.

Cicchetti, D.V. (1997). Do recognition-free recall discrepancies detect retrieval deficits in closed-head injury? Demonstrating the inaccuracies of a reviewer's critique. *Journal of Clinical and Experimental Neuropsychology, 19*, 144–148.

Cleveland, W.S. (1993). *Visualizing data*. Summit, NJ: Hobart.

Cohen, J. (1990). Things I have learned (so far). *American Psychologist, 45*, 1304–1312.

Cohen, J. (1994). The earth is round ($p < .05$). *American Psychologist, 49*, 997–1003.

Cohen, J. (1997, August). *Much ado about nothing. Invited Address: Master Lecture Series*. Annual Meeting of American Psychological Association, Chicago, Illinois.

Fisher, R.A. (1951). *Statistical methods for research workers*. Edinborough, Scotland: Oliver & Boyd.

Fuerst, D.R. (1997). Some critical remarks regarding Veiel's comment on Wilde et al. (1995). *Journal of Clinical and Experimental Neuropsychology, 19*, 149–152.

Rourke, B.P., & Costa, L. (1979). Editorial policy II: *Journal of Clinical Neuropsychology, 1*, 93–96.

Tufte, E.R. (1983). *The visual display of quantitative information*. Cheshire, CT: Graphics Press.

Tukey, J.W. (1977). *Exploratory data analysis*. Reading, MA: Addison-Wesley.

Tukey, J.W. (1991). The philosophy of multiple comparisons. *Statistical Science*, 100–116.

Veiel, H.O.F. (1997). CVLT Recognition-recall discrepancies and retrieval deficits: A comment on

Wilde et al. (1995). *Journal of Clinical and Experimental Neuropsychology, 19*, 141–143.

Wainer, H., & Thissen, D. (1993). Graphical data analysis. In G. Keren & C. Lewis (Eds.), *A handbook for data analysis in the behavioral sciences: Statistical issues* (pp. 391–457). Hillsdale, NJ: Lawrence Erlbaum.

Wilde, M.C., Boake, C., & Sherer, M. (1995). Do recognition-free recall discrepancies detect retrieval deficits in closed-head injury? An exploratory study with the California Verbal Learning Test. *Journal of Clinical and Experimental Neuropsychology, 17*, 849–855.

Wilde, M.C., Boake, C., & Sherer, M. (1997). Do recognition-free recall discrepancies detect retrieval deficits? A response to Veiel. *Journal of Clinical and Experimental Neuropsychology, 19*, 153–155.

Yates, F. (1934). Contingency tables involving small numbers and the χ^2 test. *Journal of the Royal Statistical Society (Supplement), 1*, 217–235.

Yates, F. (1951). The influence of statistical methods for research workers on the development of the science of statistics. *Journal of the American Statistical Association, 46*, 19–34.

Journal of Clinical and Experimental Neuropsychology
1999, Vol. 21, No. 4, pp. 567–570

VIII-M

METHODOLOGICAL COMMENTARY

Sample Size Requirements for Increasing the Precision of Reliability Estimates: Problems and Proposed Solutions

Domenic V. Cicchetti
Yale University Child Study Center, North Branford, CT

The purpose of this report is to challenge the view that a minimum of 400 subjects is required to obtain adequately precise estimates of reliability coefficients, whether pertaining to split-half, alpha, test-retest, alternate-form, or interrater classifications (Charter, 1999).

In determining sample size requirements for precise estimates of reliability, there are two fundamental issues to consider: the one most frequently cited is *power*; the second, and most often neglected or minimized is *precision*.

THE POWER DECISION

The power decision is often settled by choosing a sample size that will provide power of 80% (Type II error rate of .20) to detect a meaningful difference between group means when it really exists; this arbitrary criterion, usually in context with the equally arbitrary Type I or alpha error set at the conventional .05 level is, in the late Jacob Cohen's own words, "chosen with the idea that the general relative seriousness of these two kinds of errors is of the order of (.20/.05), i.e., Type I errors are of the order of four times as serious as Type II errors" (Cohen, 1965, pp. 98–99). On the other hand, Cohen also advised that these conventions should be abandoned whenever "an investigator can find a basis in his specific research investigation to choose a value ad hoc" (Cohen, p. 56).

THE PRECISION DECISION

The precision decision refers to the *reproducibility of the power estimate*, or the expected effect size, again following the terminology set forth by Cohen in a series of classic publications. It follows that the narrower the confidence intervals that contain the desired effect size, the more reliable, or reproducible the estimate.

This all makes sense in the usual context in which these issues are discussed, namely, one in which the investigators are interested in *maximizing* the difference between the two study groups; obviously, the greater the desired difference (measured as an effect size) then the greater the required sample size. It also follows that one would prefer an estimate that is reliable or rather highly reproducible. Put in more technical terminology, the desideratum is for one's effect size to be quite precise. Unfortunately, despite our ardent wishes, we usually have little control over whether the effects we desire will, in fact, occur. So we test the best state-of-the-art medication, as one example; and we appropriately determine Type I and Type II errors. Finally, we determine on the basis of the best laid pilot study plans of man, both the power and expected precision we can *hope* to get in exchange for the time and effort involved in running the appropriately designed clinical trial. I say "hope" because the research investigator has no control whatsoever over the problem of individual

Address correspondence to: Domenic V. Cicchetti, Yale Child Study Center Home Office, 94 Linsley Lake Road, North Branford, CT 06471, USA. E-mail: dom.cicchetti@yale.edu.
Accepted for publication: April 30, 1999.

differences in the characteristics of the study subjects in both groups of interest. And so we walk the researcher's tightrope hoping that the sample size will be large enough for the between group differences to override any preponderance of within group variability, or the extent of individual differences.

POWER AND PRECISION IN THE CONTEXT OF THE RELIABILITY PROBLEM

Let us now contrast this situation with power and precision estimates in the context of the reliability problem. Conceptually, the objective is the complete *opposite* of the group means contrast situation just discussed. There the desideratum was to *maximize* group differences over which we had little experimenter control. In the reliability situation, in very distinct contrast, the desideratum is to produce as close to *zero difference* in the mean ratings as is possible; and here, one does have quite a bit of control over the outcome.

If we restrict it to the author's two-rater problem, we can still train the raters according to very specific criteria and produce extremely high levels of inter-examiner reliability, with rather small sample sizes (certainly well under 100); As research scientists, we have done this ourselves on more than one occasion. Thus, the first and most fundamental research maneuver is to train the raters sufficiently, in order to minimize the number of subjects required to produce acceptable levels of reliability. Dr. Charter has ignored this critical element in his sample size estimates.

The question that follows is: What if this first maneuver does not produce acceptable levels of test reliability? One trains the raters as best as one is able and the results of pilot research indicate a sample size that's too large to obtain, for very practical reasons. What additional maneuvers can be employed? To answer this critical question, a second important strategy, also missing in Charter's equations, is the effect upon the power of a given reliability assessment of increasing the number of independent raters (clinical examiners) beyond the minimal number of two. At any given sample size, when the addition of mere numbers of subjects fails to increase power (we have reached an asymptote), we can easily increase power by simply adding a few more raters. This will be elucidated in somewhat more detail.

The excellent work of Donner and Eliasziw (1987) (which Charter has also cited) illustrates this problem quite clearly. In fact, if power is the primary concern, then there is a rather interesting and *limiting* factor that enters the "equation." To be more specific, these two investigators have shown convincingly, by the application of exact power curves, that a *decrease* in the number of examiners below 10 results in a steep *increase* in the number of subjects required to maintain power at the conventional desideratum of 80%. And here is the solution to this problem: Rather than increasing the number of subjects dramatically, the same level of power can be achieved by a very *modest increase* in the number of independent clinical examiners.

The point here is that Donner and Eliasziw (1987) have demonstrated convincingly, by the application of exact power curves, the following: (1) that rather than increasing the number of subjects dramatically, the same level of power can be achieved by a very modest increase in the number of clinical examiners; and (2) this desideratum can be achieved using no more than 50 subjects. The implications of this reasoning were recently emphasized in Cicchetti, Showalter and Rosenheck (1997, p. 53). The critical message is that: "in designing an appropriate interexaminer reliability study, it is cost-effective to strike an optimal balance between the required numbers of independent examiners and the numbers of subjects that they are required to rate". The important work of Donner and Eliasziw (1987) indicates that an increase in the number of subjects will increase power, in an incremental fashion up to a maximum or optimal level *beyond which no increase in power can be achieved by adding more subjects*. In this sense, beyond a certain limit, more is not only not better, but can be cost-inefficient. At this juncture, one can still increase power, but this can only occur by increasing the number of independent examiners. Because the author's argument is restricted to the two-independent-examiners case, it allows for the cost-inefficient strategy of increasing N dramatically, well beyond its potential for actually increasing power.

The specific combination of the number of examiners and the number of subjects to employ will depend largely upon the objectives of a given reliability study. Finally, there is much for neuropsychologists to learn from reliable ratings obtained by multiple clinical examiners in the independent assessment of a *single subject* alone (e.g., the recent work of Cicchetti, Showalter, & Rosenheck, 1997 and Cicchetti & Showalter, 1997).

A fourth issue that is also notable for its absence in the author's conceptualization of the problem is that reliability levels are very much influenced by the *developmental level* of the subjects under assessment. For example, *lower* levels of test-retest reliability can be expected, on average, for children in the normal range of intelligence than for youngsters who are severely or profoundly mentally retarded.

Finally, because of the known *imprecision* of the measuring instruments that we use in behavioral and biomedical research, biostatisticians have provided rather broad ranges of criteria defining poor, fair, good and excellent levels of test-retest and inter-examiner reliability. As one example, Fleiss (1981) defines poor levels of chance-corrected agreement as below .40; fair to good as between .40 and .74; and excellent as between .75 and 1.00. These criteria were modified in the same year by Cicchetti and Sparrow (1981), to define the fair range to be between .40 and .59, and the good range to vary between .60 and .74; and these sets of criteria are rather widely accepted in both the biostatistical and clinical research communities alike.

Applying these accepted criteria to the author's own data, why would one not be satisfied with the r of .85 deriving from a sample size of 25, with a range between .75 (excellent agreement) and .92 (also excellent agreement); and choose to *increase* the N to 400 to reduce the "confidence interval endpoints" to between .83 (excellent) and .87 (also excellent)? For an even more dramatic example, consider Charter's argument with respect to the effects of sample size on split-half reliability estimates. We are informed that "a split-half r of .90, based on an N of 50, has a 95% confidence interval with lower and upper bounds of .823 and .944 respectively, a range of .121 points. At an N of 300 the 95% confidence interval has bounds of .874 and .920, a range of .046 points." Charter concludes,

rather surprisingly that "One can easily see that there is greater precision with a larger N." Let us reflect for a moment on the practical or clinical meaning of Charter's argument. One needs to increase the number of subjects by 600% to increase the lower bound from .82 to .87 and to decrease the upper bound from .94 to .92!

I cannot conclude, as does Charter, that the added cost and time to increase N by 600% would really be worth the clinically meaningless decrease in the width of the confidence interval. Practically speaking, values of .82 and .87 (not materially different) can be considered in the good range and those between .92 and .94 (also not materially different) are both considered to be in the excellent range of split-half reliability. Specifically, both Cicchetti (1994, p. 286) and Cicchetti and Sparrow (1990) recommend the following guidelines (taking into account the usual caveats involving possible floor and ceiling effects and the need to consider measures of internal consistency in the broader context of other types of reliability assessments, such as inter-examiner): "When the size of the coefficient alpha or other measure of internal consistency is below .70, the level of clinical significance is poor or unacceptable; when it is between .70 and .79, the level of clinical significance is fair; when between .80 and .89, the level is good; and when it is .90 and above, the level of clinical significance can be taken to be excellent." Similarly, more than two decades ago, Jum Nunnaly (1978, p. 245), in providing what he refers to as "standards of reliability" notes that "for basic research, it can be argued that increasing reliabilities much beyond .80 is often wasteful of time and funds. At that level correlations are attenuated very little by measurement error. To obtain a higher reliability, say of .90, strenuous efforts at standardization in addition to increasing the number of items might be required. Thus the more reliable test might be excessively time consuming to construct, administer, and score."

SUMMARY

There are a number of cogent arguments to indicate that the investment of time and resources required to render reliability estimates more precise in the usual two-independent-examiner model is simply not worth the time and effort involved. Rather than increasing N dramatically (e.g., from 25 to 400, as the author recommends in one application) one should simply (a) pay attention to the type of subject being assessed and, (b) as required, increase modestly the number of independent examiners (e.g., from 2 to 4 makes a dramatic difference), and (c) above all, train, train, train the examiners!

REFERENCES

Charter, R.A. (in press). Sample size requirements for precise estimates of reliability, generalizability, and validity coefficients. *Journal of Clinical and Experimental Neuropsychology.*

Cicchetti, D.V. (1994). Guidelines, criteria, and rules of thumb for evaluating normed and standardized assessment instruments in psychology. *Psychological Assessment, 6,* 284–290.

Cicchetti, D.V., & Showalter, D. (1997). A computer program for assessing interexaminer agreement when multiple ratings are made on a single subject. *Psychiatric Research, 72,* 65–68.

Cicchetti, D.V., Showalter, D., & Rosenheck, R. (1997). A new method for assessing interexaminer agreement when multiple ratings are made on a single subject: Applications to the assessment of neuropsychiatric symptomatology. *Psychiatry Research, 72,* 51–63.

Cicchetti, D.V., & Sparrow, S.S. (1981). Developing criteria for establishing interrater reliability of specific items: Applications to assessment of adaptive behavior. *American Journal of Mental Deficiency, 86,* 127–137.

Cicchetti, D.V., & Sparrow, S.S. (1990). Assessment of adaptive behavior in young children. In J.J. Johnson & J. Goldman (Eds.), *Developmental assessment in clinical child psychology:* A handbook. (pp. 173–196). New York: Pergammon.

Cohen, J. (1965). Some statistical issues in psychological research. In B.B. Wolman (Ed.). *Handbook of clinical psychology* (pp. 95–121). New York: McGraw-Hill.

Donner, A., & Eliasziw, M. (1987). Sample size requirements for reliability studies. *Statistics in Medicine, 6,* 441–448.

Fleiss, J.L. (1981). Statistical methods for rates and proportions (2nd ed.). New York: Wiley.

Nunnaly, J.C. (1978). *Psychometric theory* (2nd ed.). New York: McGraw-Hill.

Journal of Clinical and Experimental Neuropsychology
2001, Vol. 23, No. 5, pp. 695–700

METHODOLOGICAL COMMENTARY

The Precision of Reliability and Validity Estimates Re-Visited: Distinguishing Between Clinical and Statistical Significance of Sample Size Requirements

Domenic V. Cicchetti
Yale University Child Study Center Home Office, North Branford, CT, USA

In a previous *JCEN* Methodological Commentary (Cicchetti, 1999), I proposed very specific and cogent arguments to question the clinical meaningfulness of Charter's (1999) recommendations to the wider community of clinical and experimental neuropsychologists of a minimum of 400 subjects for determining precise split-half, coefficient alpha, test-retest, alternate forms, and inter-examiner reliability assessment procedures, and validity coefficients. To refresh the reader's memory, and using Charter's own example, I concluded unabashedly that to increase sample size N from 50 to 300 (a factor of 600%) was simply not worth the considerable added cost and time, to 'increase' a lower-bound precision reliability estimate from .82 to .87, while simulta-neously 'decreasing' the upper bound reliability estimate from .94 to .92. I stand firmly behind that statement, and would add to it that Charter's further conclusion of an N, in fact of '400 or more' in both his earlier and current Methodological Commentary strains credulity even more.

Unfortunately, the content of Charter's reply, or rebuttal to my comments uses precisely the same arguments as previously, and the interested reader is referred, once again, to my earlier critique of his work (Cicchetti, 1999).

This critique will stress the inappropriateness of considering precision solely in the context of increasing N, or using sample sizes of 400 and more, as appears to be Charter's main objective or desideratum. This will be discussed in the broader context of both the necessity to consider the practical or clinical meaningfulness of precision estimates, and the underlying rationale for calculating confidence intervals (CIs) around these estimates, in the first place. Other less critical issues will also be raised, as required.

A PRELIMINARY CLARIFICATION

Charter begins by noting, with obvious pride, that his previous article, appearing in *JCEN*, last year, was 'rejected by some of the finest journals in America,' this spanning a 5-year period between 1993 and 1998. He asks, 'What did *JCEN* know that the others [read journals] didn't?'

In trying to make sense of this phenomenon, Charter chooses to believe that his paper was accepted by *JCEN* because he removed 'the equations and added Part II (Practical Application to Test Scores), which may have been the selling points for the *JCEN* editors.'

I believe a more plausible reason that the Editors concluded that Charter's arguments should not go unchallenged, and therefore I was invited to publish

Address correspondence to: Domentic V. Cicchetti, Yale University Child Study Center, Home Office, North Branford, CT, USA. E-mail: dom.cicchetti@yale.uni
Accepted for publication: November 28, 2000.

my critique of his work alongside his. Not by accident, I have again been invited to do the same with Charter's rejoinder.

CRITICAL COMMENTARY

1. Charter challenges my reference to the earlier Donner and Eliasziw's (1987) paper suggesting that no more than 50 subjects are required for obtaining acceptable reliability coefficients, when the obtained coefficient (Ri, an intra class correlation coefficient) is compared, to an expected Ri of 0, .2, .3, or .4. respectively, Charter then counters with a more recent Feldt and Ankenmann (1999) article (not appearing in the list of references), which, depending upon power level (.50, .75, .90) suggests sample sizes between 30 and 1,056, 'making Charter's N look wimpy.'

Let me refer to an even more recent article, in which the authors used Monte Carlo computer simulation methodology to construct large-sample confidence intervals (CIs) for reliability and validity coefficients, deriving from both random and selected samples. The resulting CIs were at least 90% accurate when N was at least 100 (Mendoza, Stafford, & Stauffer, 2000).

2. The precision decision, as I referred to it in my earlier critique (Cicchetti, 1999), refers specifically to the reproducibility of the power estimate, which, in turn, refers to the effect size (ES), which in the present arena of discourse, refers simply to the size of the reliability coefficient itself (e.g., an intra-class R, coefficient alpha, retest or inter-examiner reliability coefficient). And, of course, the extent of the reproducibility of the precision estimate is reflected in the width of the confidence interval that serves as a lower and upper bound of the estimate. And, of course, there is an inverse relationship between N and CI, so that the larger the N, the narrower the CI, and the more precise the estimate.

But these are technical issues, and, as such, are devoid of the *content* of the issue.

3. Specifically, the conceptual question that has to be asked here (and is also ignored in the reasoning of Charter) is, What is the concept that *underlies* the construction of confidence

intervals around a given reliability or other of the multitude of ES estimates? What is precisely involved here is the idea that if the reliability/validity 'experiment' were to be repeated, say, 100 or 1000 times, then we should expect that with a stated or given size N, we should expect the estimate to fall, say 95% of the time within certain specified confidence limits. But this is only an *indirect* answer to the question. The CI is nothing more than a rough estimate of the actual size of the reliability/validity coefficient itself. What is really critical here is that wherever and whenever possible, one needs to perform a *direct* test of the reliability/validity coefficient and that can only be obtained by performing replication studies. Thus, while the late Jacob Cohen (1994) recognized well and recommended that the ESs be routinely reported in the context of what he referred to as the familiar but under-utilized CIs, he reminded us, more recently (Cohen, 1997) as scientists, to always remember to *replicate our research efforts*, this, then, in the time – honored tradition of the physical scientists. Unfortunately, today's journals, both biomedical and behavioral, tend, mainly, to look asking at the importance of the replication enterprise in research. We are fortunate, in this respect, that this was not lost sight of in the editorial policy of the predecessor of *JCEN*, namely the *Journal of Clinical Neuropsychology* (Rourke & Costa, 1979).

Expanding a bit more on the still broader issue here, namely, the importance of focusing on clinical issues and differentiating them from purely statistical ones, let me say first that the precision of a reliability/validity estimate that one can hope or strive for or, in fact, consider worth pursuing, will, for sure, vary from investigator to investigator and from one content area to another. For Example, for an extremely rare disorder or disease process, one does not have the liberty of choosing an N much larger than the one that is already available to us. Here the reliability estimate and the CI placed around it is about all that we have to examine. In the case of life and death issues, we would want much more precise estimates than if we were focusing on areas not of such great moment. This would involve obtaining larger sample sizes and more precise measurements, but *only to the extent possible.* One cannot magically increase N from 50 to 300 to 400 to 1,000, by simply wishing it to be so, as Charter is able to 'accomplish' in his apochryphal example involving the estimated precision of medical decisions involving whether or not to select a particular treatment modality for a loved one. It is tantamount to Charter's telling the reader something akin to, "So you don't like the results based on 50 cases? Why, we'll just magically increase it to 1,000 and you'll have your desired answer, this in terms of a much narrower CI." Would it be so simple! Charter's approach here bespeaks of one who may have not spent sufficient time toiling in the clinical research vineyards, in order to have a better understanding and appreciation of the time, effort, and financial commitment involved in making appropriate and relevant power and precision decisions. It is one matter (and an easy one at that), to utilize samples of data deriving from the files in a large Veterans Affairs Medical Center's Psychology Testing Laboratory that 'contained manuals and reliability studies for 131 tests (24 personality, 11 intelligence, 42 neuropsychological, and 36 vocational ... in order to gather data 'on a total of 6,322 r's.' It is far different (as well as much more challenging and time-consuming), to develop the new clinical tests and assess their clinical, administrative, and psychometric properties.

4. As one who has worked on testing the accuracy of standard errors and confidence intervals of inter-rater reliability statistics (Fleiss & Cicchetti, 1978); and has been responsible for consulting and collaborating on development and testing of the psychometric properties of a number of clinical instruments (some of which have become standards in the field), I understand not only the importance of distinguishing between statistical and clinical relevance of reliability and validity estimates, but also the limitations of the further examination of materials deriving from already published and sometimes outdated test manuals.

5. Charter, in his relentless pursuit of ever more precise reliability and validity estimates by simply increasing N to 400 and beyond, loses much in the process. First, and foremost, one needs to ask, What is the clinical relevance of an obtained reliability or validity estimate, or ES, in general? Charter seems to believe that the only criterion is N. Prominent bio-statisticians would certainly disagree. As Borenstein, Rothstein, and Cohen (1997, p. 22) describe the phenomenon, "As a rule, the effect size should be based on the user's knowledge of the field and should reflect the smallest effect that would be important to detect in the planned study."

6. Following up on this important theme, one needs to have some useful guidelines or rules-of-thumb to decide just what we are going to accept as sufficiently reliable or valid, for our purposes. I did provide guidelines for establishing the clinical significance of values of coefficient alpha and inter-rater reliability estimates in my earlier critique of Charter (Cicchetti, 1999, pp. 569–570).

What was left out of that critique were rules of thumb for evaluating validity estimates in the basic context of the sensitivity/specificity model. These would apply to levels of overall diagnostic accuracy, sensitivity, specificity, positive predictive accuracy, and negative predictive accuracy, and can be classified as the following: 90–100% = Excellent; 80–89% = Good; 70–79% = Fair, and <70% = Poor (Cicchetti, Volkmar, Klin, & Showalter, 1995). It should be noted that these rules of thumb can also be used to classify the level of observed agreement in the calculation of kappa, weighted kappa, and Ri reliability statistics. Putting together the classification of both observed and chance-corrected levels of inter-examiner agreement, in terms of practical or clinical significance, one derives the following:

Levels of kappa weighted kappa, or R intra-class	Levels of observed agreement (%)	Levels of clinical or practical significance
<.40	<70	Poor
.40–.59	70–79	Fair
.60–.74	80–89	Good
.75–1.00	90–100	Excellent

Both Charter and I have also been arguing about what constitutes acceptably high levels of reliability/validity, as measured by the size of their respective coefficients or indexes. (See also the published and conceptually similar guidelines of Fleiss (1981) and of Landis & Koch (1977) e.g., the latter argue for a similar cut-point for Excellent, theirs at .80, rather than the .75 of both Fleiss (1981) & Cicchetti & Sparrow, (1981) Charter would prefer a minimum of .90 and above. In this context, it bears repeating the sage comment of Nunnally (1978, p. 245) that in terms of so-called 'standards of reliability' it can be argued that to increase reliabilities much beyond .80 (say, in fact, to .90), is often wasteful of time, funds, and human efforts), a point which Charter chooses to respond to by the somewhat irrelevant point that "one does not increase reliability by increasing N, one increases reliability by increasing the number of homogeneous test items (or number of raters for the inter-raterreliability)." How this contradicts my and Nunnally's sage argument is not immediately obvious.

7. Finally, let me give several examples of a less talked about phenomenon, namely, the high practical or clinical value of very low levels of correlation, as they can be interpreted in the context of measuring the importance of some independent variable (say, some form of treatment or therapy) upon some dependent, or outcome variable (say the measured success of that treatment). As a concrete example, adapted from Rosenthal and Rubin (1979) suppose in a randomized clinical trial, half of the patients are randomly assigned to the standard treatment for a particular pernicious disease, while the remainder are assigned to a new treatment. Suppose, further, that success is measured in terms of 5-year survival rates, and that at the end of that period, 70% are still alive in the new treatment group, as compared to only 30% in the standard treatment group. One would be forced to conclude that the treatment, all things considered equal, had proven its effectiveness. Yet, if one were to examine the correlation between treatment and effect (as a validity measure), it would (quite irrespective of the number of cases involved) produce a value of

only .40. In statistical terms, this would mean that only 16% of the variation in survival rates could be explained in terms of the type of treatment the patient received. As Rosenthal and Rubin (1979, p. 395) correctly conclude:

"The conclusion that the treatment is unimportant because it accounts for only 16% of the variance is simply wrong. Percent variance explained can, in some cases, then, be a very deceptive measure." In a more recent publication, Rosenthal (1993) uses the same paradigm to show that even much smaller correlations have characterized the relationship between specific treatments used in actual clinical trials such as the relationship between psychotherapy and patient improvement ($R = .32$); AZT and death rates ($R = .23$); Cyclosporine and death ($R = .15$); Testosterone and adult delinquency ($R = .12$); Vietnam veteran status and alcohol problems ($R = .07$); Propanolol and death ($R = .04$); and Aspirin and heart attacks ($R = .03$).

In commenting on one of these studies (although the same general explanation would hold for all of them), Rosenthal (1993, p. 135) concludes:

"... the propranolol study was discontinued for an effect accounting for 1/5th of 1% of the variance! ... As behavioral researchers we are not accustomed to thinking of r's of .04 as reflecting effect sizes of practical importance. If we were among the 4 per 100 who moved from one outcome to the other, we might well revise our view of the practical import of small effects!"

Well, how do we summarize all of this?

SUMMARY, CONCLUSIONS, AND RECOMMENDATIONS

1. First and foremost, the work of Charter notwithstanding, the issue of assessing appropriate levels of both power and precision and reliability and validity estimates involves much more than simply plugging numbers into confidence interval formulas, applying them to data deriving from already published test manuals

and then using them as a benchmark for sample size requirements. It should also be noted here that the development of valid reliability and validity standard errors and CIs is by no means a trivial matter (Fleiss, Nee, & Landis, 1979; and, very recently, Mendoza et al., 2000). Moreover, more than one pproach to the problem is available and defended by various statistical workers in the field (Dunlap and Silver, 1986), who provide a program for implementing Fieller's theorem; the simpler approach based on the Bonferroni inequality, vdue to Johnson and Wichern (1992), as utilized in the aforementioned Mendoza et al. (2000) investigation; the formulas used by Charter and colleagues. This being the case, one needs to consider the specific formulae used to construct the CIs as themselves another source of variation that would impact upon the obtained results and sample size recommendations.

2. Although, N is the driving force behind precision, it in itself cannot be meaningfully interpreted without a full understanding of the clinical meaningfulness of the results. It will always be true, for example, that it is simply not clinically meaningful to increase the number of subjects from 50 to 300 to increase a lower CI bound from .82 to .87 and to decrease the upper bound from .94 to .92. By any reasonable standards, the two pairs of reliability estimates are not clinically different.

3. One needs to understand that the size of a reliability or validity coefficient alone cannot be meaningfully interpreted without looking deeper into the phenomenon. Thus, a treatment response of 70% improvement in the new treatment group versus only 30% improvement in the standard treatment group (an impressive result that is seldom found in biomedical research (Rosenthal & Rubin, 1979) cannot be meaningfully interpreted in terms of the R of only .40 between treatment and response.

4. In the specific context of reliability assessment, the mere increase in N will increase the power and precision of reliability estimates, only up to a certain extent, beyond that no improvement will occur. Here the only meaningful strategy is to increase the number of independent examiners (Donner & Eliasziw, 1987).

5. While the necessity of placing CIs around effect sizes (ES) in general and around reliability/validity estimates, in particular, is both warranted and, I would add, quite necessary, one must realize that the CI merely serves as a rough ersatz proxy for the sine qua non of research which is replication, replication, replication!

6. In the context of inter-examiner reliability estimation, the role of training on the size of and precision of reliability/validity estimates cannot be underestimated.

REFERENCES

Borenstein, M., Rothstein, H., & Cohen, J. (1997). *Power and precision*. Mahwah, NJ: Lawrence Erlbaum.

Charter, R. (1999). Sample size requirements for precise estimates of reliability, generalizability, and validity coefficients. *Journal of Clinical and Experimental Neuropsychology, 21*, 559–566.

Cicchetti, D.V. (1999). Sample size requirements for increasing the precision of reliability estimates: Problems and proposed solutions. *Journal of Clinical and Experimental Neuropsychology, 21*, 567–570.

Cicchetti, D.V., & Sparrow, S.S. (1981). Developing criteria for establishing interrater reliability of specific items: Applications to assessment of adaptive behavior. *American Journal of Mental Deficiency, 86*, 127–137.

Cicchetti, D.V., Volkmar, F., Klin, A., & Showalter, D. (1995). Diagnosing autism using ICD-10 criteria: A comparison of neural networks and standard multivariate procedures. *Child Neuropsychology, 1*, 26–37.

Cohen, J. (1994). The earth is round ($p < .05$). *American Psychologist, 49*, 997–1003.

Cohen, J. (1997, August). *Much ado about nothing. Invited Address: Master Lecture Series*. Annual Meeting of American Psychological Association, Chicago, IL.

Donner, A., & Eliasziw, M. (1987). Sample size requirements for reliability studies. *Statistics in Medicine, 6*, 441–448.

Dunlap, & Silver, N.C. (1986). Confidence intervals and standard errors for ratios of normal variables. *Behavioral Research Methods, Instruments, & Computers, 18*, 469–471.

Feldt & Ankenmann (1999), cited in text, but not in Charter's Reference list.

Fleiss, J.L. (1981). *Statistical methods for rates and proportions* (2nd ed.). NY: Wiley.

Fleiss, J., & Cicchetti, D.V. (1978). Inference about weighted kappa in the non-null case. *Applied Psychological Measurement, 2*, 113–117.

Fleiss, J.L., Nee, J.C.M., & Landis, J.R. (1979). Large sample variance of kappa in the case of different sets of raters. *Psychological Bulletin, 86*, 974–977.

Johnson, R.A., & Wichern, D.W. (1992). *Applied multivariate statistical analysis.* Englewood Cliffs, NJ: Prentice Hall.

Landis, R.J., & Koch, G.G. (1977). The measurement of observer agreement for categorical data. *Biometrics, 33*, 159–174.

Mendoza, J.L., Stafford, K.L., & Stauffer, J.M. (2000). Large-sample confidence intervals for validity and reliability coefficients for validity and reliability coefficients. *Psychological Methods, 5*, 356–369.

Rosenthal, R. (1993). *Meta-Analytic procedures for social research.* Newbury Park, CA: Sage publications (2nd ed.). Chapter 7, pp. 127–136.

Rosenthal, R., & Rubin, D.B. (1979). A note on percent variance explained as a measure of the importance of effects. *Journal of Applied Social Psychology, 9*, 395–396.

Rourke, B.P., & Costa, L. (1979). Editorial policy II. *Journal of Clinical Neuropsychology, 1*, 93–96.

Child Neuropsychology
1995, Vol. 1, No. 2, pp. 93–105

White Matter Changes on CT Brain Scan Are Associated With Neurobehavioral Dysfunction in Children with Symptomatic HIV Disease*

Pim Brouwers[1], Harry van der Vlugt[2], Howard Moss[1,3], Pamela Wolters[1,3], and Philip Pizzo[1]

[1]Pediatric Branch, National Cancer Institute, Bethesda, Maryland, [2]Department of Psychology, University of Tilburg, The Netherlands, and [3]Medical Illness Counseling Center, Chevy Chase, Maryland

ABSTRACT

The effect of white matter abnormalities on neurobehavioral dysfunction was investigated in 58 children with symptomatic HIV-1 disease, 28 with CT white matter abnormalities and 30 matched (for age, gender, route of infection, and stage of disease) control patients with comparable levels of cortical atrophy, but no white matter abnormalities. Children with white matter abnormalities were more impaired on measures of general level of mental functioning (standard scores of 70.3 vs. 86.1; $p < .05$). They also scored lower than the group without white matter abnormalities on activities of daily living (76.9 vs. 87.4; $p < .05$), particularly those requiring self-help skills, and in socialization (79.5 vs. 89.3; $p < .05$). Furthermore, patients with white matter abnormalities exhibited higher levels of attention deficit/hyperactive behaviors ($p < .05$) and more severe autistic symptoms ($p < .05$). White matter abnormalities by themselves were, thus, associated with deficits in cognitive function and socio-emotional behavior. These findings are in partial agreement with the nonverbal learning disabilities (NLD) model. Although NLD profiles, in general, have been described in older children, the current results seem to suggest that antecedents for these behavior patterns can be found in much younger children with white matter abnormalities.

Central nervous system (CNS) compromise is a significant complication of infection with the human immunodeficiency virus (HIV-1) in infants and children. HIV-1 related CNS disease is a clinical syndrome manifested by varying and sometimes discordant degrees of cognitive, motor, and behavioral impairment (Aylward, Butz, Hutton, Joyner, & Vogelhut, 1992; Belman, Brouwers, & Moss, 1992; Epstein et al., 1986; Hittelman, 1990). Aberrant social-emotional behavior patterns, including depression and autistic symptoms, have been described in children with evidence of progressive HIV encephalopathy and these behaviors appear to be related to CT brain scan abnormalities (Moss et al., 1994).

Because opportunistic infections and lymphoma of the CNS are rather uncommon in infants and children, the predominant cause of the neurological deficits seems directly related to the effects of HIV infection on the CNS (Brouwers, Belman, & Epstein, 1994). The exact timing of CNS invasion is not known and may be different from case to case, but possible early invasion after HIV infection has been indicated by synthesis of HIV antibodies (Epstein et al., 1986; Epstein et al., 1987) and isolation of HIV-1 from the CSF at about the time of

* We wish to express our appreciation for the time and effort given by the children and their caregivers who participated in this research. We also wish to thank Drs. Charles DeCarli and Lucy Civitello for their evaluation of the CT brain scans, and Eugene Tassone, Renee Smith, Debra El-Amin, Nancy Heilman, and Gayl Selkin-Gutman for their assistance during the various phases of this project.

Send requests for reprints to: Dr. Pim Brouwers, Pediatric Branch, National Cancer Institute, NIH Clinical Center, Rm. 10/13N240, Bethesda, MD 20892-1928, U.S.A.

Accepted for publication: October 20, 1994.

seroconversion (Ho et al., 1985). Moreover, as early as 2 weeks after experimental inoculation with simian immunodeficiency virus, evidence of infection of brain parenchyma could be demonstrated in Rhesus macaques (Sharer et al., 1991).

It has been suggested that HIV infection in the CNS causes "white matter disease" with significant effects on myelin. White matter changes with reactive astrocytosis and myelin pallor are found in more than 80% of the pediatric cases at autopsy (Budka, 1991; Epstein et al., 1986; Sharer et al., 1986). Seizures, an indicator of gray matter disorders, are uncommon in pediatric AIDS, even in cases with encephalopathy and advanced disease (Civitello, Brouwers, & Pizzo, 1993).

Computed tomography (CT) and magnetic resonance imaging (MRI) have demonstrated a high incidence of structural brain abnormalities in children with symptomatic HIV infection (Chamberlain, Nichols, & Chase, 1991; DeCarli, Civitello, Brouwers, & Pizzo, 1993; Kauffman et al., 1992; Price et al., 1988). The most common CT abnormal-ity observed in a consecutive series of 100 previously untreated children with symptomatic HIV disease was cortical atrophy. White matter abnormalities, frequently associated with cortical atrophy, were observed in about 25% of all patients (DeCarli et al., 1993). In children with symptomatic HIV infection, CT brain scan abnormalities, even though mild, were related to levels of neurocognitive and socio-emotional dysfunction (Brouwers et al., 1995).

Abnormalities in the white matter may be caused as a consequence of the effects of HIV on myelin, either indirectly through the actions of cytokines and neurotoxins or through possible infection of the oligodendrocites (Mizrachi et al., 1991). White matter connections in the CNS can be divided into three types projection, association, and commissural fibers (Kinney, Brody, Kloman, & Gilles, 1988). Myelination of these types of fibers occurs at different rates and at different periods during most of the child's early development (van der Knaap et al., 1991). The effect of HIV is expected to be global and thus affect all three types of white matter connections. The timing of entry of HIV into the CNS and the periods of maximal replication, that is, interference with CNS processes, may result in different patterns and degrees of abnormalities based on connections that are most vulnerable during that time, that is, those still being formed.

It would be predicted that the effect of HIV on white matter would be more evident in children (particularly those infected from birth) as compared to patients infected after myelogenesis was largely completed, for example, adolescents and adults. In fact, in a previous study we used a stepwise regression model to predict the degree of neurobehavioral dysfunction from CT brain scan abnormalities in children with symptomatic HIV disease. White matter abnormalities entered the equation as the final predictor (after ventricular enlargement and calcifications) for vertically infected children (i.e., children who acquired their infection from their HIV-positive mothers). In contrast, white matter abnormalities were not associated with dysfunction in children who had acquired their infections postpartum, later in life, by transfusion of contaminated blood products (Brouwers et al., 1995).

Intermodal integration defects associated with white matter abnormalities, particularly involving commissural connections, have been implicated as causative factors in the development of Nonverbal Learning Disabilities (NLD; Rourke, 1989). Behavioral abnormalities reported for children with symptomatic HIV infection, such as poor adaptive skills (Wolters, Brouwers, Moss, & Pizzo, 1994), a tendency to social withdrawal (Bose, Moss, Brouwers, Pizzo, & Lorian, 1994; Moss et al., 1994), perceptual-motor deficits (Epstein et al., 1986; Brouwers et al., 1992), and developmental language delays in the very young (Wolters, Brouwers, Moss, & Pizzo, 1994, 1995) seem similar to abnormalities associated with NLD or early signs of the syndrome (Rourke, 1989).

The purpose of the current study was to evaluate the specific contribution of white matter abnormalities to possible dysfunction in the cognitive and/or socio-emotional domains of children with symptomatic HIV disease. That is, we evaluated whether children with white matter abnormalities on CT scan had differential abnormalities in adaptive and socio-emotional behavior and intellectual functioning as compared to children with comparable degree of cortical atrophy but with no white matter abnormalities.

METHODS

Subjects

Patients with symptomatic HIV disease (Class P-2 of Centers for Disease Control and Prevention classification criteria, 1987; see Belman, Brouwers, & Moss, 1992) who were followed by the Pediatric Branch of the National Cancer Institute (NCI) on Phase I–II clinical trials of anti-retroviral agents such as Zidovudine (AZT), ddC, and ddI either alone or in combination (Butler et al., 1991; Husson et al., 1994; Pizzo et al., 1988; Pizzo et al., 1990) were eligible. As part of comprehensive medical monitoring, patients were evaluated with CT brain scans and age-appropriate neuropsychological tests. At the time of evaluation, children were afebrile and were not suffering from another infection.

Twenty-eight patients with white matter abnormalities on CT brain scan were identified. If more than one CT scan showing white matter abnormalities on the same patient was available, then the first scan to show such abnormalities was used with the associated psychological evaluation. Because white matter abnormalities tend to correlate with presence and degree of cortical atrophy, a contrast group ($n = 30$) was selected which matched the index group in overall degree of atrophy, but did not have white matter abnormalities (See Figure 1). In addition, the contrast group was matched for route of infection, age, gender, and parental education. The groups were also matched for severity of disease as reflected by their age-normed z scores for C D4% values (Brouwers, DeCarli, et al., 1994; European Collaborative Study, 1992). Table 1 shows demographics of this sample, divided by presence or absence of white matter abnormalities.

Imaging Study Evaluation

Two neurologists, blind to the clinical status of the patient, independently rated the scans for the presence

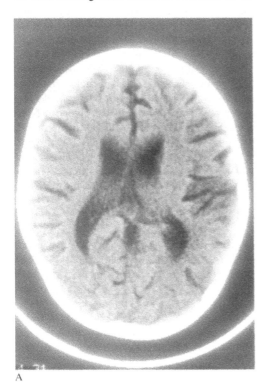

A

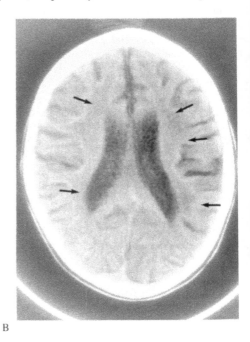

B

Fig. 1. Illustration of CT brain scans of two comparable patients from the two subgroups: (A) an 8.9-year-old male with transfusion acquired symptomatic HIV infection, without white matter abnormalities and a cortical atrophy rating in the severe range (72). (B) an 8-year-old male with transfusion acquired symptomatic HIV infection in the neonatal period, and with white matter abnormalities in the periventricular region of the lateral ventricle (see arrows), as well as other regions, rated in the mild to moderate range (32), and a cortical atrophy rating in the severe range (66).

Table 1. Demographics of Sample.

| | CT brain scan classification | | |
	Total sample	White matter	No white matter
Gender (Male/Female)	33/25	18/10	15/15
Route HIV (Transfusion/Vertical)	15/43	8/20	7/23
Age (years)	4.53 (.47)	4.34 (.62)	4.70 (.70)
Parental education (years)	13.4 (.3)	13.5 (.5)	13.2 (.4)
Cortical atrophy (ratings)	43.6 (2.3)	47.6 (3.2)	40.0 (3.3)
CD4% Levels age-adjusted z score	−3.19 (.20)	−3.18 (.27)	−3.20 (.29)

Note. Indicated are the mean and standard error of the mean.

and severity of ventricular dilatation, subarachnoid enlargement, white matter abnormalities, intracerebral calcifications, and possible other lesions on a 100mm analog scale. Reliabilities between the two raters for both presence and severity of abnormalities were high (intraclass correlations between .84 and .95). The methodology of the CT scan evaluation has been reported in more detail elsewhere (DeCarli et al., 1993). The average of the two ratings was used in our analysis. In Figure 1, two CT brain scans, one with and one without white matter abnormalities, but both with comparable degree of cortical atrophy, illustrate the matching of patients.

Psychological Evaluation

Cognition
Overall cognitive function was assessed with the psychometric instrument appropriate for the child's age and level of functioning: The Wechsler Intelligence Scale for Children-Revised (Wechsler, 1974; $n = 19$), the McCarthy Scales of Children's Abilities (McCarthy, 1972; $n = 14$), and the Bayley Scales of Infant Development (Bayley, 1969; $n = 25$). For children and infants who scored below the deviation scale cut-off on the Bayley and McCarthy Scales, ratio IQs were calculated as described elsewhere (Brouwers et al., 1990) based on age-equivalence and chronological age. All scores less than 40 (on the WISC-R, McCarthy, or Bayley) were set to 39 for equivalence and computational purposes ($n = 6$). In addition, the Peabody Picture Vocabulary Test-Revised (Dunn & Dunn, 1981; $n = 34$), the Gardner Expressive One-Word Picture Vocabulary Test (Gardner, 1979; $n = 26$), and the Developmental Test of Visual Motor Integration (Beery VMI, 1989; $n = 23$) were administered in standard fashion to assess receptive and expressive language and visuomotor abilities.

Adaptive behavior
Adaptive functioning was evaluated in 56 children with the Vineland Adaptive Behavior Scales (Sparrow,

Balla, & Cicchetti, 1984), a semistructured interview administered to the child's parent (or caregiver). Two parts of the test, measuring the domains of daily living (with subdomains for personal, domestic, and community living skills) and socialization (with subdomains for interpersonal, play/leisure, and coping skills) were administered as described previously (Wolters et al., 1994). Standard scores for the two domains were analyzed. For the subdomains, age-equivalent scores were transformed into ratio scores [(age-equivalent/chronological age) × 100] and analyzed as well. Correlations between subdomain and domain scores were all highly significant (range of $r = .64$ to .83; all $p < .0001$), partially justifying our transformation of subdomain scores. All scores less than 40 were set to 39 and all scores greater than 130 were set to 131 for equivalence.

Socio-emotional behavior
In addition, the psychologist administering the cognitive tests also rated the child's socio-emotional behavior during the psychometric evaluation using the NIH Q-sort behavior rating procedure (Moss et al., 1994; $n = 55$). This is a forced-choice rating procedure resulting in item scores between 1 and 7. Scaled scores are calculated based on an average equal weight computation of items loading on derived factors from a factor analysis. The Q-sort procedure generates a severity score, which is an overall measure of the child's aberrant socio-emotional behavior. In addition, depending on the child's age, scores on a number of different scales are obtained. For children less than 2 years of age, the five scales reflect unsocial, apathetic, immature/poorly integrated, flaccid/self-stimulating behaviors, and attention problems. For children older than 2 years, the four scales represent depression, hyperactivity/attention deficit, autistic, and low frustration/irritable behaviors.

Statistics
Psychological and CT scan data were analyzed with analysis of variance (ANOVA), linear regression analysis,

Fisher exact test, Pearson correlations, and partial correlations correcting for degree of cortical atrophy (Waternaux, 1991). Differences between individual means were evaluated using the Bonferroni correction. A minimal two-tailed alpha level of .05 was used in all analyses.

RESULTS

General Sample Description

Demographics (see also Table 1)
The mean age of the sample was 4.5 years ($SE = .5$) with no difference between children with white matter abnormalities (mean $= 4.3$, $SE = .6$) as compared to children without white matter abnormalities (mean $= 4.7$, $SE = .7$). Average parental education was 13.4 ($SE = .3$) years, with no difference between the two groups (means of 13.5, $SE = .5$ and 13.2, $SE = .4$, respectively). There were also no differences in gender distribution or in route of infection.

Neurocognitive and behavioral
The general level of neuropsychological functioning for this sample of pediatric HIV patients was significantly below the published norm ($p < .001$); the mean cognitive index (i.e., MDI, GCI, or FSIQ) was 78.5 ($SE = 3.5$), with a range from 39 to 131. Furthermore, the level of adaptive functioning was also significantly below the published norm ($p < .001$) but comparable to the cognitive index: for Daily Living, the mean standard score was 82.3 ($SE = 2.5$), with a range from 39 to 116; for Socialization, the mean was 84.6 ($SE = 2.2$), with a range from 39 to 114.

Neuroimaging (CT scan)
Every patient with white matter abnormalities also had evidence of cortical atrophy. Therefore, due to our selection procedures for matching, all 58 patients evidenced at least one CT brain scan abnormality, most frequently ventricular enlargement or subarachnoid space dilatation. The mean overall rating for cortical atrophy (combination of ventricular and subarachnoid dilatation, possible range of scores between 0 and 100) was not significantly different ($p > .10$) between those patients without or with white matter abnormalities (means

of 40.0, $SE = 3.3$ and 47.6, $SE = 3.2$). In addition, the incidence of intracerebral calcifications was not significantly different between these two groups.

Immunology
There were no differences between the two groups in age-corrected CD4 percent measures. The mean for the overall sample was a z score of -3.20 ($SE = .20$, range -4.63 to .03), while the means for the two subgroups were -3.18 and -3.20. These z scores correspond to an approximate CD4 percent value of 10% in a 4-year-old.

Group Comparisons

Cognitive functions
Comparison of the overall levels of cognitive function, reflected by the MDI, GCI, and FSIQ, indicated a significant ($p < .05$) difference between the group with white matter abnormalities (mean $= 70.3$, $SE = 4.8$) and the group without such abnormalities (mean $= 86.1$, $SE = 4.8$). For the older children (tested with the McCarthy or WISC-R), mean differences between the two groups in verbal and performance scores failed to reach conventional levels of statistical significance (Verbal means 79.9, $SE = 6.6$ vs. 95.4, $SE = 4.9$; $p = .067$; and Performance means 83.3, $SE = 6.7$ vs. 98.2, $SE = 5.8$; $p = .101$), nor were differences between verbal and performance scores significant within either group. Partial correlation between white matter severity ratings (adjusted for degree of cortical atrophy) and the general cognitive index ($r = -.291$; $p < .05$) was significant, reflecting the earlier noted group difference. Furthermore, a significant partial correlation was found for verbal functioning ($r = -.401$; $p < .05$), and a borderline effect for visual perceptual functioning ($r = -.339$; $p < .07$).

On the additional cognitive tests, the white matter group scored significantly lower than the group without white matter abnormalities on the PPVT-R (76.0, $SE = 6.9$ vs. 96.4, $SE = 5.7$; $p < .05$). Differences on the Gardner and on the Beery VMI did not reach statistical significance. The partial correlation between white matter severity and the Gardner score, however, approached significance ($r = -.387$; $p < .06$).

Socio-Emotional Functions

Vineland measures

Patients with white matter abnormalities had significantly ($p < .05$) lower mean values on the summary domain scores of the Vineland (76.9, $SE =$ 3.8 for Daily Living and 79.5, $SE = 3.2$ for Socialization) as compared to the group without white matter abnormalities (mean values of 87.4, $SE = 3.0$ and 89.3, $SE = 2.8$ respectively; see Figure 2). Further evaluation within the Daily Living domain revealed a significant difference for the Personal subdomain (means of 64.9, $SE =$ 4.9 vs. 80.5, $SE = 4.5; p < .05$), but differences for the other subdomains (Domestic and Community) failed to reach statistical significance. Further evaluation of the subdomains within the Socialization domain showed significant ($p < .05$) differences for all three measures: Interpersonal (61.7, $SE = 3.8$ vs. 75.0, $SE = 4.6$), Play/Leisure (62.1, $SE = 3.6$ vs. 77.7, $SE = 5.7$), and Coping (62.1, $SE = 4.6$ vs. 78.0, $SE = 5.9$).

Using ANOVA, we also investigated whether the effects of white matter abnormality were differentially associated with the age at testing of the child. This was possible for Vineland measures since the same test was administered across the whole age range. Patients were classified as younger or older than 36 months: This divided both the white matter and non-white matter groups about equally (N's of 13, 14, 15, and 14, respectively). This even distribution allowed the evaluation of group by age interactions. Main effects for white matter abnormality remained the same as reported above. None of the age by group interactions was statistically significant (most F's < 1).

Q-sort measures

The Q-sort procedure is different for children less than 2 years of age and children older than 2 years. The overall severity scale, however, can be obtained across all ages. The difference between the two groups on this measure was not significant (means of 3.40, $SE = .30$ vs. 3.23, $SE = .25$, for the white matter and non-white matter groups, respectively) nor was there a significant correlation with white matter severity.

In the older group, significant differences were noted between the two groups on the Hyperactivity/Attention Deficit scale (means of 3.88, $SE = .42$ vs. 2.75, $SE = .35; p < .05$) and on the Autistic scale (means of 2.70, $SE = .36$ vs. 1.68, $SE = .19$; $p < .05$) for the white matter ($n = 18$) and non-white matter ($n = 16$) groups, respectively (see

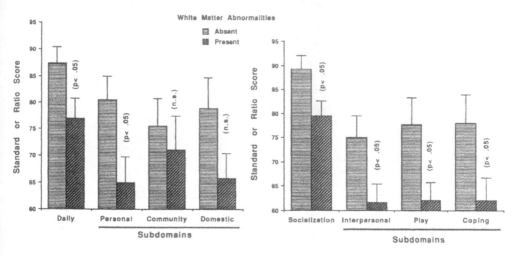

Fig. 2. Comparison of levels of adaptive behavior between patients with white matter abnormalities ($n = 27$) and patients without white matter abnormalities ($n = 29$), but with comparable degree of cortical atrophy on CT brain scan using the Vineland Scales. Illustrated are the scores for the Daily Living domain (standard score) and its subdomains (ratio scores), as well as the Socialization domain (standard score) and its subdomains (ratio scores).

Figure 3). In addition, there was a significant partial correlation between the white matter severity rating and the score on the Autism scale (partial $r = .44$; $p < .01$), but not for the Hyperactivity scale. Differences on the Depression scale and the Irritability scale did not approach statistical significance.

For the younger group, differences between the white matter ($n = 9$) and the non-white matter ($n = 12$) groups did not approach statistical significance on any of the five scales (p at least $>.20$).

DISCUSSION

We have previously demonstrated that CT brain scan abnormalities, although sometimes minimal, are common in children with symptomatic HIV-1 infection (DeCarli et al., 1993). Moreover, these structural lesions, even when mild, were correlated

with both cognitive and socio-emotional dysfunction, suggesting that they had clinical significance (Brouwers et al., 1995). In our consecutive series of 100 previously untreated children with symptomatic HIV disease, white matter abnormalities were noted in approximately 25% of the patients. White matter abnormalities tended to be found around the horns of the lateral ventricles; sometimes the lesions extended anteriorly into the frontal white matter. However, no relation was found between anterior/posterior gradient and severity of leukoaraiosis, nor was any left-right asymmetry noted (DeCarli et al., 1993). We did not investigate at that time, however, the extent to which these abnormalities were, by themselves, associated with specific patterns of cognitive or behavioral dysfunction (Brouwers et al., 1995).

The present study shows that white matter abnormalities on CT brain scans were associated with cognitive and socio-emotional dysfunction.

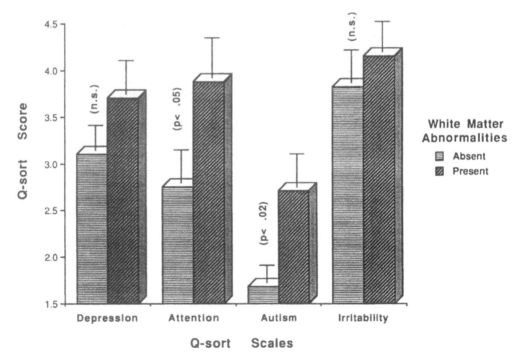

Fig. 3. Comparison of the degree of aberrant socio-emotional behavior between patients with white matter abnormalities ($n = 18$) and patients without white matter abnormalities ($n = 16$), but with comparable degree of cortical atrophy on CT brain scan, using the Q-sort technique. Illustrated are the scores for the older age group (older than 2 years of age) on the four derived factor scales: Depression, Hyperactivity/Attention deficit, Autism, and Irritability/Low frustration threshold.

Specifically, in terms of cognitive function, patients with white matter abnormalities, compared to patients with a similar degree of cortical atrophy but without white matter changes, scored lower on tests that assess general levels of mental functioning. Moreover, the greater the degree of white matter abnormality, the more impaired cognitive functioning. White matter abnormalities were further associated with higher ratings of attention deficit and hyperactivity as well as with autistic symptomatology using the Q-sort technique. In terms of adaptive functioning, the group with white matter abnormalities as compared to the group without the white matter abnormalities exhibited significantly lower scores (i.e., less age-appropriate activities) on the Daily Living and Socialization scales.

There are three types of white matter connections in the CNS that develop at different rates and during different post conception periods. Complete mature myelination is first achieved in the projection fibers. For association fibers myelination occurs later, progressing from the region around the central sulcus towards the poles of the parieto-occipital, temporal, and frontal lobes. Similarly, for the commissural fibers myelination occurs later and over a longer period; the body of corpus callosum is the first area to achieve complete mature myelination, the outer anterior commissure the last (Dietrich et al., 1988; Kinney, Brody, Kloman, & Gilles, 1988). Thus, the period during which a disease process is active or most damaging to myelination could be of critical developmental importance, assuming that connections are most vulnerable when they are still being formed. Very early interference, that is, perinatal, could affect projection fibers as well as association and commissural connections resulting in global patterns of deficits with motor abnormalities. Later interference would largely affect the commissural connections and the connections with the poles of the cerebral lobes (particularly frontal and temporal). Such a pattern of abnormalities may result in defects in intermodal integration that have been implicated as causative factors in the development of Nonverbal Learning Disabilities (NLD; Rourke, 1989).

The effect of HIV is expected to be global and thus affect all three types of white matter connections. It is difficult to determine, however, at which post-infection times active HIV replication within the CNS is occurring that would lead to presumed maximum interference, and this may vary from case to case. One way of monitoring HIV activity could be by the serial examination of potential markers of viral neurotoxicity, such as the exitotoxin quinolinic acid (Brouwers et al., 1993) or tumor necrosis factor alpha (Mintz et al., 1989).

Behaviors characteristic of the NLD syndrome (Rourke, 1989) have been noted in previous research with school-age children, the majority of whom acquired HIV infection through blood or blood-product transfusion. Parents rated these children as lower in social competence, as exhibiting fewer social interactions and less involvement in school and peer activities, and as displaying increased levels of anxiety (Bose et al., 1994). In a study of profiles of neurocognitive dysfunction in school-age children with HIV disease, the general pattern indicated a global step-wise decline for most of the children. A subgroup with differentially poor visuo-spatial abilities was identified; however, no similar subgroup with differentially impaired verbal-linguistic abilities was detected (Brouwers et al., 1992). Few abnormalities in cognitive function were noted in cohorts of HIV positive and HIV negative children with hemophilia (Loveland et al., 1994; Whitt et al., 1993). Deficits were found on timed tasks of visual-motor performance; however, these measures did not discriminate between the two groups (Whitt et al., 1993). HIV interference with CNS processes in these cases with transfusion-acquired HIV infection may have been at a time that most structures and functions, particularly those associated with language skills, had already been formed and, thus, were less susceptible to disruption.

In another study (Wolters et al., 1995) language development was evaluated in infants and children with symptomatic HIV disease, the majority of whom were vertically infected. Compared to uninfected siblings, children with HIV had significantly delayed language function; abnormalities in expressive language were more pronounced than those in receptive language (Wolters et al., 1995). These deficits in verbal function may reflect the fact that HIV interference with CNS processes was at a very early age, prior to the development of most language functions and the myelination of associated structures.

White matter abnormalities were associated with neurobehavioral dysfunction in our current study. Activities of daily living, particularly those requiring self-help skills, were significantly more impaired in children with white matter abnormalities. Similarly, the white matter group also exhibited significantly less age-appropriate socialization behaviors, and these were of comparable magnitude for the interpersonal relationships, the play and leisure time, and the coping skills subdomains. The magnitude of these deficits did not seem to be differentially affected by age at testing. However, one has to take into consideration that these behaviors may be inhibited by psychosocial reactions and changes in life-style for the child and family living with a chronic life-threatening disease such as HIV (Wolters et al., 1994); that is, frequent hospitalizations and/or parents who may become overprotective and/or lenient.

On the Q-sort scales, white matter abnormalities were associated with higher ratings of attention deficit and hyperactivity as well as with autistic symptomatology but only for the group of children older than 2 years of age. We have previously suggested that the Q-sort procedure may be less sensitive in identifying and measuring aberrant behaviors that are associated with the progression of HIV-1 associated encephalopathy in the group of children less than 2 years age (Moss et al., 1994). It is of interest that the attention deficit and autistic scales in this sample (as well as in the original study) were not significantly related. The actual correlation was, in fact, negative ($r = -.158$). This suggests that these are two rather independent behavior patterns that may be associated with different types of white matter abnormalities.

Further evaluation of these behaviors showed that the hyperactivity rating did not correlate with any of the other socio-emotional or cognitive scores. It did show a moderate positive correlation with a marker of HIV disease status, the age adjusted z score of CD4% ($r = .38; p < .05$), suggesting that higher ratings of hyperactivity were associated with less advanced disease. A similar finding was obtained earlier, when a negative correlation between overall degree of CT brain scan abnormality and score on this hyperactivity scale was found (Brouwers et al., 1995). It was then suggested that lower ratings on the hyperactivity/

attention difficulty scale for children with more severe CT brain scan abnormalities may reflect the pervasive activity limiting motor defects in progressive encephalopathy.

The autism rating, on the other hand, correlated with almost all other measures, both in the behavioral and the cognitive domain as well as with the degree of white matter abnormality. The presence of autistic symptoms clearly is associated with generalized compromise of the CNS. Autistic behaviors that seemed most differentially associated with white matter abnormalities were as follows: difficulty in engaging in social interaction, avoidance of physical/social contact, and, to a lesser extent, repetitive rocking and language delays. The correlation with zCD4% ($r = -.19; p > .25$) indicated that these behaviors were not significantly associated with only end-stage disease. Autistic symptomatology has been linked to white matter abnormalities within the NLD model (Rourke, 1989). Our data are supportive of the hypotheses of this model that autistic behaviors would be associated with severe and early white matter damage.

Children with white matter abnormalities also exhibited greater degrees of cognitive dysfunction than did children with only evidence of global cortical atrophy. Differences between verbal-linguistic and perceptual-motor functioning were, however, not significant. This could indicate that most of the HIV infected infants and children in our sample were too young and the brain lesions too early, prior to the acquisition of most neurobehavioral function, to differentially affect the development of abilities. Hence, verbal and perceptual-motor functioning were equally affected. In contrast, children who acquire their white matter abnormalities after age 3–5 typically exhibit differential deficits in visual-motor skill and psychomotor efficiency (Taylor, 1987).

Our behavioral and cognitive findings seem in partial agreement with the NLD model (Rourke, 1989). Some children with white matter abnormalities in this relatively young sample exhibited behaviors that may be considered early behavioral signs of the NLD syndrome. Other infants and children displayed behavior and cognitive profiles that would be indicative of more extensive and earlier white matter damage resulting in patterns of more generalized defects. In children less than 2 years of age however, we could not demonstrate differences in socio-emotional function with the Q-sort technique. It is possible that these behaviors are not yet sufficiently developed by this age to be rated as aberrant and, therefore, that white matter abnormalities are not expressed (Rourke, 1989).

Infectious diseases, such as HIV-1, which may not directly infect neurons in the CNS can still result in acute or delayed aberrant behavioral manifestations. Host-and/or viral-mediated indirect factors are thought to play an important role (Brouwers, Belman, & Epstein, 1994). For example, infection with influenza A-type during the second trimester of pregnancy has been associated with schizophrenia in the offspring (Murray et al., 1992). Autistic-like behaviors have been reported in children and adults following herpes simplex encephalitis (Ghaziuddin, Tsai, Eilers, & Ghaziuddin, 1992; Gillberg, 1991). Group A [beta]-hemolytic streptococcal infections have been linked with obsessive–compulsive symptoms as well as with choreiform movement disorders in children (Swedo, Leonard, & Kiessling, 1994).

It should be noted that MRI technology may be more sensitive to white matter abnormalities of the brain than is CT scan in HIV disease (Brouwers, Belman, & Epstein, 1994), whereas CT scan may be more sensitive to intracerebral calcifications. In an MRI study of vertically infected children (Tardieu, Blanche, & Brunelle, 1991), white matter abnormalities were detected in 40% of the children, but the abnormalities were frequently transient, and the clinical significance of these lesions could not be established. Similar findings have been reported for adults with HIV infection (Bornstein et al., 1992). Using CT scan technology, one may, in fact, establish a severity threshold for recognition of these abnormalities. When detected using CT scan, these lesions may have progressed sufficiently to reflect clinically significant outcome as was shown in this study.

Although NLD profiles have been described in older children, the current results seem to suggest that antecedents for these behavior patterns can be found in much younger children with possible long-standing white matter abnormalities. We have previously suggested that living for many years with HIV infection may have a significant effect on personality development in children (Brouwers,

Moss, Wolters, & Schmitt, 1994). Rourke (1989) has also suggested that if the early behavioral "signs" of NLD are not treated, the child very likely will exhibit the full-blown syndrome later in life. Early interventions that focus on attacking the deficits, rather than on looking for compensatory mechanisms are thus necessary for these young children (Rourke, 1989). A laissez-faire attitude towards these behaviors may arise out of a negativistic outlook for children with HIV-1 disease, which, in turn, may further condemn them to their neuropsychologically and socially isolated worlds.

REFERENCES

Aylward, E.H., Butz, A.M., Hutton, N., Joyner, M.L., & Vogelhut, J.W. (1992). Cognitive and motor development in infants at risk for human immunodeficiency virus. *American Journal of Diseases of Children, 146*, 218–222.

Bayley, N. (1969). *Manual for the Bayley Scales of Infant Development*. San Antonio, TX: The Psychological Corporation.

Beery, K.E. (1989). *The developmental test of Visual-Motor Integration, VMI*; (3rd ed. rev.). Cleveland, OH: Modern Curriculum Press.

Belman, A.L., Brouwers, P., & Moss, H. (1992). HIV-1 and the central nervous system. In D.M. Kaufman, G.E. Solomon, & C.R. Pfeffer, (Eds.), Child and adolescent neurology for psychiatrists, (pp. 238–253), Baltimore: Williams & Wilkins.

Bose, S., Moss, H., Brouwers, P., Pizzo, P., & Lorion, R. (1994). Psychological adjustment of HIV-infected school age children. *Journal of Developmental and Behavioral Pediatrics, 15*, S26–S33.

Bornstein, R.A., Chakeres, D., Brogan, M., Nasrallah, H., Fass, R.J., Para, M., & Whitacre, C. (1992). Magnetic Resonance Imaging of white matter lesions in HIV infection. *Journal of Neuropsychiatry and Clinical Neurosciences, 4*, 174–178.

Brouwers, P., Belman, A., & Epstein, L. (1994). Organ specific complications: Central nervous system involvement: Manifestations, evaluation, and pathogenesis. In P.A. Pizzo & C.M. Wilfert, (Eds.), *Pediatric AIDS; The challenge of HIV Infection in infants, children, and adolescents*. (2nd ed.). (pp. 433–455). Baltimore: Williams & Wilkins.

Brouwers, P., DeCarli, C., Tudor-Williams, G., Civitello, L., Moss, H., & Pizzo, P. (1994). Interrelations among patterns of change in neurocognitive, CT brain imaging, and CD4 measures associated with antiretroviral therapy in children with symptomatic HIV infection. *Advances in Neuroimmunology, 4*, 223–231.

Brouwers, P., DeCarli, C., Civitello, L., Moss, H., Wolters, P., & Pizzo, P. (1995). Correlation between CT-Brain scan abnormalities and neuropsychological function in children with symptomatic HIV disease. *Archives of Neurology, 52,* 39–44.

Brouwers, P., Heyes, M., Moss, H., Wolters, P., Poplack, D., Markey, S., & Pizzo, P. (1993). Quinolinic acid in the cerebrospinal fluid of children with symptomatic HIV-1 Disease: Relationships to clinical status and therapeutic response, *The Journal of Infectious Diseases, 168,* 1380–1386.

Brouwers, P., Moss, H., Wolters, P., Eddy, J., Balis, F., Poplack, D., & Pizzo, P.A. (1990). Effect of continuous-infusion Zidovudine therapy on neuropsychologic functioning in children with symptomatic human immuno-deficiency virus infection. *Journal of Pediatrics, 117,* 980–985.

Brouwers, P., Moss, H., Wolters, P., El-Amin, D., Tassone, E., & Pizzo, P. (1992). Neuro-behavioral typology of school-age children with symptomatic HIV disease [Abstract]. *Journal of Clinical and Experimental Neuropsychology, 14,* 113.

Brouwers, P., Moss, H., Wolters, P., & Schmitt, F. (1994). Developmental deficits and behavioral change in pediatric AIDS. In I. Grant & A. Martin (Eds.), *Neuropsychology of HIV infection: Current research and new directions.* (pp. 310–338). New York: Oxford University Press.

Budka, H. (1991). Neuropathology of human immunodeficiency virus infection. *Brain Pathology, 1,* 163–175.

Butler, K.M., Husson, R.N., Balis, F.M., Brouwers, P., Eddy, J., El-Amin, D., Gress, J., Hawkins, M., Jarosinski, P., Moss, H., Poplack, D., Santacroce, S., Venzon, D., Wiener, L., Wolters, P., & Pizzo, P.A. (1991). Dideoxyinosine (ddI) in symptomatic HIV-infected children: A phase I–II study. *New England Journal of Medicine, 324,* 137–144.

Chamberlain, M.C., Nichols, S.L., & Chase, C.H. (1991). Pediatric AIDS: Comparative cranial MRI and CT scans. *Pediatric Neurology, 7,* 357–362.

Civitello, L.A., Brouwers, P., & Pizzo, P.A. (1993). Neurological and neuropsychological manifestations in 120 children with symptomatic Human Immunodeficiency Virus infection [Abstract]. *Annals of Neurology, 34,* 481.

DeCarli, C., Civitello, L.A., Brouwers, P., & Pizzo, P.A. (1993). The prevalence of computed axial tomographic abnormalities of the cerebrum in 100 consecutive children symptomatic with the human immunodeficiency virus. *Annals of Neurology, 34,* 198–205.

Dietrich, R.B., Bradley, W.G., Zaragoza, E.J., Otto, R.J., Taira, R.K., Wilson, G.H., & Kangarloo, H. (1988). MR evaluation of early myelination patterns in normal and developmentally delayed infants. *American Journal of Neuroradiology, 9,* 69–76.

Dunn, L.M., & Dunn, L.M. (1981). *Peabody Picture Vocabulary Test-Revised.* Circle Pines, MN: American Guidance Service.

Epstein, L.G., Goudsmit, J., Paul, D.A., Morrison, S.H., Connor, E.M., Oleske, J.M., & Holland, B. (1987). Expression of human immunodeficiency virus in cerebrospinal fluid of children with progressive encephalopathy. *Annals of Neurology, 2,* 397–401.

Epstein, L.G., Sharer, L.R., Oleske, J.M., Connor, E.M., Goudsmit, J., Bagdon, L., Robert-Guroff, M., & Koenigsberger, M.R. (1986). Neurologic manifestations of human immunodeficiency virus infection in children. *Pediatrics, 78,* 678–687.

European Collaborative Study. (1992). Age-related standards for T lymphocyte subsets based on uninfected children born to human immunodeficiency virus infected women. *Pediatric Infectious Disease Journal, 11,* 1018–1026.

Gardner, M.F. (1979). *Expressive One-Word Picture Vocabulary Test.* Novato, CA: Academic Therapy Publications.

Ghaziuddin, M., Tsai, L., Eilers, L., & Ghaziuddin, N. (1992). Autism and herpes simplex encephalitis. *Journal of Autism and Developmental Disorders, 22,* 107–113.

Gillberg, C. (1991). Autistic Syndrome with onset at age 31; Herpes encephalitis as a possible model for childhood autism. *Developmental Medicine and Child Neurology, 33,* 920–924.

Hittelman, J. (1990). Neurodevelopmental aspects of HIV infection. In P.B. Kozlowski, D.A. Snider, P.M. Vietze, & H.M. Wisneiwski, (Eds.), *Brain in pediatric AIDS* (pp. 64–71). Basel: Karger.

Ho, D.D., Rota, T.R., Schooley, R.T., Kaplan, J.C., Allan, J.D., Groopman, J.E., Resnick, L., Flesenstein, D., Andrews, C.A., & Hirsch, M.S. (1985). Isolation of HTLV-III from cerebrospinal fluid and neural tissues of patients with neurologic syndromes related to the acquired nimmunodeficiency syndrome. *The New England Journal of Medicine, 313,* 1493–1497.

Husson, R.N., Mueller, B.U., Farley, M., Woods, L. Goldsmith, J., Kovacs, A., Ono, J., Lewis, L.L., Balis, F.M., Brouwers, P., Avramis, V., Church, J., Butler, K.M., Rasheed, S., Jarosinski, P., Venzon, D., & Pizzo, P.A. (1994). Zidovudine and didanosine combination therapy in children with Human Immunodeficiency Virus Infection. *Pediatrics, 93,* 316–322.

Kauffman, W.M., Sivit, C.J., Fitz, C.R., Rakusan, T.A., Herzog, K., & Chandra, R.S. (1992). CT and MR evaluation of intracranial involvement in pediatric HIV infection: A clinical-imaging correlation. *American Journal of Neuroradiology, 13,* 949–957.

Kinney, H.C., Brody, B.A., Kloman, A.S., & Gilles, F.H. (1988). Sequence of central nervous system myelination in human infancy: Patterns of myelination in autopsied infants. *Journal of Neuropathology and Experimental Neurology, 47*, 217–234.

Loveland, K.A., Stehbens, J., Contant, C., Bordeaux, J.D., Sirois, P., Bell, T.E., & Hill, S. (1994). Hemophilia growth and development study: Baseline neurodevelopmental findings. *Journal of Pediatric Psychology, 19*, 223–239.

McCarthy, D. (1972). *The McCarthy Scales of Children's Abilities*. New York: Psychological Corporation.

Mintz, M., Rapaport, R., Oleske, J.M., Connor, E.M., Koenigsberger, M.R., Denny, T., & Epstein, L.G. (1989). Elevated serum levels of tumor necrosis factor are associated with progressive encephalopathy in children with acquired immunodeficiency syndrome. *American Journal of Disease of Children, 143*, 771–774.

Mizrachi, Y., Zeira, M., Shahabuddin, M., Li, G., Sinangil, F., & Volsky, D.J. (1991). Efficient binding, fusion and entry of HIV-1 into CD4-negative neural cells: A mechanism for neuropathogenesis in AIDS. *Bulletin d' Institute Pasteur, 89*, 81–96.

Moss, H.A., Brouwers, P., Wolters, P.L., Wiener, L., Hersh, S.P., & Pizzo, P.A. (1994). The development of a Q-sort behavior rating procedure for pediatric HIV patients. *Journal of Pediatric Psychology, 19*, 27–46.

Murray, R.M., Jones, P., O'Callaghan, E., Takei, N., & Sham, P. (1992). Genes, viruses and neuro-developmental schizophrenia. *Journal of Psychiatric Research, 26*, 225–235.

Pizzo, P., Eddy, J., Falloon, J., Balis, F., Murphy, R., Moss, H., Wolters, P., Brouwers, P., Jarosinski, P., Rubin, M., Broder, S., Yarchoan, R., Brunetti, A., Maha, M., Nusinoff-Lehrman, S., & Poplack, D. (1988). Effect of continuous intravenous infusion of zidovudine (AZT) in children with symptomatic HIV infection. *New England Journal of Medicine, 319*, 889–896.

Pizzo, P., Butler, K., Balis, F., Brouwers, E., Hawkins, M., Eddy, J., Einloth, M., Falloon, J., Husson, R., Jarosinski, P., Meer, J., Moss, H., Poplack, D., Santacroce, S., Wiener, L., & Wolters, P. (1990). Dideoxycytidine alone and in an alternating schedule with zidovudine in children with symptomatic human immunodeficiency virus infection. *The Journal of Pediatrics, 117*, 799–808.

Price, D.B., Inglese, C.M., Jacobs, J., Haller, J.O., Kramer, J., Hotson, G.C., Loh, J.P., Schlusselberg, D., Menez-Bautista, R., Rose, A.L., & Fikrig, S. (1988). Pediatric AIDS: Neuroradiologic and neurodevelopmental findings. *Pediatric Radiology, 18*, 445–448.

Rourke, B.P. (1989). *Nonverbal learning disabilities: The syndrome and the model*. New York: Guilford Press.

Sharer, L.R., Epstein, L.G., Cho, E.S., Joshi, V.V., Meyenhofer, M.F., Rankin, L. F., & Petito, C.K. (1986). Pathologic features of AIDS encephalopathy in children: Evidence for LAV/HTLV-III infection of the brain. *Human Pathology, 17*, 271–284.

Sharer, L.R., Michaels, J., Murphey-Corb, M., Hu, F.-S., Kuebler, D.J., Martin, L.N., & Baskin, G.B. (1991). Serial pathogenesis study of SIV brain infection. *Journal of Medical Primatology, 20*, 211–217.

Sparrow, S., Balla, D., & Cicchetti, D. (1984). *Vineland Adaptive Behavior Scales*. Circle Pines, MN: American Guidance Service.

Swedo, S.E., Leonard, H.L., & Kiessling, L.S. (1994). Speculations on antineuronal antibody-mediated neuropsychiatric disorders of childhood. *Pediatrics, 93*, 323–326.

Tardieu, M., Blanche, S., & Brunelle, F. (1991). Cerebral magnetic resonance imaging studies in HIV-1 infected children born to seropositive mothers. *Neuroscience of HIV-1 infection*, Satellite to VII International Conference on AIDS, Padova, *60* [Abstract].

Taylor, H.G. (1987). Childhood sequelae of early neurological disorders: A contemporary perspective. *Developmental Neuropsychology, 3*, 153–164.

van der Knaap, M.S., Valk, J., Bakker, C.J., Schooneveld, M., Faber, J.A., Willemse, J., & Gooskens, R.H. (1991). Myelination as an expression of the functional maturity of the brain. *Developmental Medicine & Child Neurology, 33*, 849–57.

Waternaux, C. (1991). Statistical considerations for the analysis of neurobehavioral trials. In E. Mohr & P. Brouwers (Eds.), *Handbook of clinical trials, The neurobehavioral approach* (pp. 81–86). Amsterdam/Lisse: Swets & Zeitlinger.

Wechsler, D. (1974). *Manual for the Wechsler Intelligence Scale for Children*. New York: Psychological Corporation.

Whitt, J.K., Hooper, S.R., Tennison, M.B., Robertson, W.T., Golds, S.H., Burchinal, M., Wells, R., McMillan, C., Whaley, R.A., Combest, J., & Hall, C.D. (1993). Neuropsychologic functioning of human immunodeficiency virus-infected children with hemophilia. *Journal of Pediatrics, 122*, 52–59.

Wolters, P. L., Brouwers, P., Moss, H., & Pizzo, P. (1994). Adaptive behavior of children with symptomatic HIV infection before and after Zidovudine therapy. *Journal of Pediatric Psychology, 19*, 47–61.

Wolters, P.L., Brouwers, P., Moss, H.A., & Pizzo, P.A. (1995). Differential receptive and expressive language functioning of children with symptomatic HIV disease and relation to CT scan brain abnormalities. *Pediatrics, 95*, 112–119.

Child Neuropsychology
1998, Vol. 4, No. 2, pp. 144–157

COMMENT

Evidence for the Syndrome of Nonverbal Learning Disabilities in Children with Brain Tumors*

Lauren A. Buono[1], Mary K. Morris[1], Robin D. Morris[1], Nicolas Krawiecki[2], Fran H. Norris[1], Martha A. Foster[1], and Donna R. Copeland[3]

[1]Georgia State University, Atlanta, GA, [2]Emory University School of Medicine, Atlanta, GA, and [3]University of Texas, M.D. Anderson Cancer Center, Houston, TX

ABSTRACT

This study examined the predicted utility of the Nonverbal Learning Disabilities syndrome (NLD) (Rourke, 1995) for characterizing neurocognitive and psychosocial outcomes in 123 children with brain tumors. Children with brain tumors were found to be at high risk of having a specific academic deficit, particularly in arithmetic. Children with arithmetic deficit evidence a higher rate of impairment on nonverbal tasks than on verbal tasks, whereas children with reading deficit evidenced a higher rate of impairment on verbal tasks than on nonverbal tasks. However, significant differences between children with arithmetic and reading deficits were not found for all of the component features of the NLD syndrome, and arithmetic deficit was not related to treatment with irradiation.

Intracranial tumors account for 20% of pediatric cancer diagnoses, with an estimated incidence of 1,200 cases per year in the United States (Cohen & Duffner, 1984; Mulhern, Krisco, & Kun, 1983). Because of increasing survival rates for these children, long-term behavioral and cognitive sequelae of pediatric brain tumors and their treatments have received increased attention. Several factors appear to have a negative impact on outcomes in children with brain tumors, including younger age at diagnosis (Ellenberg, McComb, Siegel, & Stowe, 1987; Glauser & Packer, 1991; Mulhern et al., 1983; Radcliffe, Bunin, Sutton, Goldwein, & Phillips, 1994; Ris & Noll, 1994) and treatment (Ellenberg et al., 1987; Radcliffe et al., 1994), treatment type, particularly radiation (Duffner, Cohen, & Parker, 1988; Duffner, Cohen, & Thomas, 1983; Ellenberg et al., 1987; Glauser & Packer; Hirsch, Renier,

Czernichow, Benveniste, & Pierre-Kahn, 1979; Mulhern et al., 1983; Ris & Noll, 1994; Roman & Sperduto, 1995), tumor location, particularly supratentorial tumors (Danoff, Cowchock, Marquette, Mulgrew, & Kramer, 1982; Glauser & Packer, 1991; Hirsch et al., 1979; Jannoun & Bloom, 1990; Mulhern et al., 1983), and follow-up intervals of greater than one year (Duffner et al., 1988; Ellenberg et al., 1987; Ris & Noll, 1994; Roman & Sperduto, 1995). Overall, the incidence of neuropsychological dysfunction within this population has been estimated to include 40% to 100% of long-term survivors. Our investigation addresses the nature of these deficits.

When the results of outcome studies are evaluated for consistency of reported cognitive deficits, it becomes apparent that decline in intellectual functioning over time, as measured by standardized

---

* This study was supported by NIH/NCI CA 33097 and the Brain Tumor Foundation for Children, Inc. and was submitted in partial fulfillment of the doctoral degree requirements of the first author.
Address correspondence to: Mary K. Morris, Department of Psychology, Georgia State University, University Plaza, Atlanta, GA 30303-3083, USA.
Accepted for publication: August 7, 1997.

intelligence tests, as well as deficits in nonlanguage abilities, relative to language abilities, have been frequently found (Broadbent, Barnes, & Wheeler, 1981; Danoff et al., 1982; Duffner et al., 1983; Duffner et al., 1988; Ellenberg et al., 1987; Glauser & Packer, 1991; Moore, Copeland, Ried, & Levy, 1992; Mulhern et al., 1983; Spunberg, Chang, Goldman, Auricchio, & Bell, 1981; Ris & Noll, 1994; Roman & Sperduto, 1995). More specifically, children diagnosed and treated for brain tumors frequently have been found to demonstrate a pattern of deficits in nonverbal processing, visuo-perceptual and visuo-spatial ability, visual-motor integration, visuo-spatial memory, planning and organizational skills, mechanical arithmetic, attention/concentration, and fine-motor skills. Despite these nonverbal deficits, these children have evidenced relative strengths in verbal skills. These findings suggest the existence of a distinct intellectual, academic, and neuropsychological profile associated with childhood brain tumors and their treatment.

The learning disabilities model proposed by Rourke (1989, 1991, 1995) may provide a useful framework for understanding the specific pattern of cognitive deficits seen in children with brain tumors. This model proposes a pattern of nonverbal processing deficits that includes relative strengths in verbal skills. Rourke proposes a hierarchical, developmental model of Nonverbal Learning Disabilities (NLD) that outlines the relationships among academic, neuropsychological, and socio-emotional assets and deficits found in this subset of children with learning disabilities. The NLD model posits core deficits in attending to, perceiving, and recalling visual and tactile information, and in integrating visual and tactile information with motor output. These nonverbal deficits are hypothesized to impair the development of higher order cognitive skills such as visual attention, visual memory, visual-motor integration, concept formation, problem solving, reading comprehension, and mechanical arithmetic.

Rourke (1988b, 1989) and colleagues (Rourke & Fisk, 1981; Rourke & Fuerst, 1991) have hypothesized that children with NLD are at particular risk for the development of socio-emotional problems due to: (1) difficulties in adapting to novel and complex situations; (2) deficits in social perception,

social judgement, and social interaction skills; (3) poor pragmatic language skills and lack of verbal prosody; and (4) awkward tactile-perceptual and psychomotor abilities that prevent smooth affectional and interpersonal encounters.

Rourke (1987, 1989) has also hypothesized that lesions of the right hemisphere, or white matter pathways that carry information to the right hemisphere, underlie the specific pattern of deficits found in children with NLD and have a more deleterious effect on cognitive functions that require synthetic, integrative processing, especially inter-modal integration. Rourke has also predicted that the NLD syndrome should be prevalent in children with brain tumors who have received large doses of cranial irradiation because white matter is more sensitive to the deleterious effects of radiation than is grey matter, and there is a greater ratio of white matter to grey matter in the right hemisphere (Goldberg & Costa, 1981).

The NLD pattern of deficits is strikingly similar to the pattern of deficits suggested in the outcome studies of children with brain tumors, many of whom have received radiation treatment. Given the inclusion of a broad range of cognitive and psychosocial factors in Rourke's NLD model, it is possible that the NLD model could explain the specific cognitive deficits already described in the literature on childhood brain tumors, as well as predict other deficits that have not been demonstrated empirically in this population. The present study was designed to assess the utility of Rourke's (1989) NLD model for characterizing the neurocognitive and psychosocial outcomes of children with brain tumors.

METHOD

Participants

Data for this study were drawn from a longitudinal research project designed to assess the effects of brain tumors and their treatment on aspects of child and family functioning. The subjects were recruited from two pediatric medical centers in a large urban area. Tumor pathology distribution in this sample was similar to previous reports of the prevalence of brain tumor diagnoses in children (Black, 1991). Extensive intellectual, academic, neuropsychological, and psychological testing was conducted with each child at specific intervals as follows: (1) at diagnosis when possible, (2) six months from diagnosis, and (3) on each anniversary of the diagnosis until the child achieved age 18. The number of evaluations conducted for each child ranged from 1 to 11 ($M = 3.7$, $SD = 2.6$). At each assessment point, parents also completed measures to evaluate child and family functioning.

A total of 123 children diagnosed with brain tumors were selected for the present study on the criteria that they had been evaluated with the Wide Range Achievement Test-Revised (WRAT-R; Jastak & Wilkinson, 1984) on at least one occasion and had completed both the Reading and Arithmetic subtests.

Overall Design
As a first step, the sample of children with brain tumors was subtyped according to patterns of academic strengths and weaknesses in arithmetic and reading achievement. These subtypes were compared on demographic and medical variables. Next, the proportion of children in each subtype who were impaired on measures of general intelligence, specific neuropsychological abilities, and psychosocial functioning was determined, using both an absolute cut-off score and a regression-defined discrepancy from expected performance, based on IQ. Statistical techniques were applied to detect differences among subtypes and to predict subtype membership based on demographic, medical, general intellectual, specific neuropsychological, and psychosocial measures. All analyses for this study were run under SAS Version 6.08 for the PC (SAS Institute, 1989).

Measures
In addition to the WRAT-R, a battery of intellectual, neuropsychological, and psychosocial measures had also been administered at each assessment point. These measures were used to form 13 outcome variables on which the identified subtypes were compared. In some cases, subscales or sub-tests of measures of global intellectual ability were analyzed as separate outcome variables to permit the assessment of specific neuropsychological domains. A subset of these same variables served as predictors of subtype membership in logistic regression analyses. Individual measures and their associated outcome variables appear in Table 1.

Subtype Identification
WRAT-R results for all subjects were categorized based on discrepancies between the Arithmetic and the Reading subtest standard scores, consistent with previous investigations that led to the identification of a subtype of learning-disabled children who exhibited the NLD syndrome (Rourke & Finlayson, 1978; Rourke & Strang, 1978; Strang & Rourke, 1983). An 11-point discrepancy

between reading and arithmetic achievement scores on the WRAT-R is significant for identifying subjects with relative academic deficits. This discrepancy represents the standard error of the difference at the 95% confidence interval between the Arithmetic and Reading standard score distributions (Anastasi, 1988; pp. 136–137).

Given the longitudinal design from which data for this study were drawn, multiple assessments with the WRAT-R were available for the majority of subjects, ranging from two to nine consecutive assessments. Examination of the longitudinal pattern of WRAT-R scores revealed that the performance of individual subjects varied over time. Therefore, to maximize subtype stability, a stable academic discrepancy was defined as the two consecutive evaluations, furthest from diagnosis, that consistently classified a subject with an arithmetic deficit (AD), a reading deficit (RD), or no discrepancy (ND). If subjects with multiple evaluations met the criteria for either AD or RD at one point in time, and also met the criteria for ND at another point in time, classification as either AD or RD was given priority over classification as ND. Outcome variables were drawn from the second evaluation of each set. A subset of subjects, for whom only one evaluation was available, were classified based on that single evaluation ($n = 34$).

In the classification process, a small number of subjects ($n = 4$) who demonstrated unstable classification such that they switched from AD to RD or RD to AD over time were deleted from the analyses. A small proportion of subjects did not meet any of the classification criteria denoted above and were also deleted from the analyses (17 subjects, 14% of sample). One hundred and two subjects were classified into three subtypes as follows: AD ($n = 42$), RD ($n = 16$), and ND ($n = 44$).

When compared to the *expected* proportion (5%) under the normal probability curve for the distribution of the difference between Arithmetic and Reading standard scores, the *observed* proportion of children with significant achievement discrepancies in either direction (57%) was found to be statistically significant ($Z = 26.00$, $p < .001$). The *observed* proportion of children with AD (41%) ($Z = 19.25$, $p < .001$) was determined to be 16 times greater than the *expected* proportion (2.5%) and the *observed* proportion of children with RD (16%) was determined to be 6 times greater than the *expected* proportion (2.5%) ($Z = 6.75$, $p < .001$).

RESULTS

Demographic and Medical Variables
Subtype characteristics on demographic and medical variables for the AD, RD, and ND groups are presented in Tables 2 and 3. Previous studies of this sample have documented a relationship between

Table 1. Assessment Battery.

Outcome variable	Measures
Intellectual	
Composite IQ	Stanford-Binet Intelligence Scale: Fourth Edition (Thorndike, Hagen, & Sattler, 1986)
Verbal IQ[a]	Stanford-Binet: Vocabulary, Comprehension, Memory for Sentences
Nonverbal IQ[a]	Stanford-Binet: Pattern Analysis, Quantitative, Bead Memory
Specific Neuropsychological Abilities	
Visual Motor	Developmental Test of Visual-Motor Integration (Beery & Buktenica, 1967; Beery, 1989)
Visual Attention	Letter Cancellation Task – Omission Errors[b] (Mesulam, 1985) Trail Making Test, Part A (Reitan & Wolfson, 1985)
Visual Memory	Stanford-Binet: Bead Memory
Language	Peabody Picture Vocabulary Test-Revised (Dunn & Dunn, 1981) Stanford-Binet: Verbal Reasoning (Vocabulary, Comprehension)
Verbal Memory	Rey Auditory Verbal Learning Test Total Recall[c] (Bishop, Knights, & Stoddart, 1990; Rey, 1964) Buschke Selective Reminding Test – Consistent Long-Term Retrieval (CLTR)[c] (Buschke, 1973; Buschke & Fuld, 1974) Stanford-Binet: Memory for Sentences
Executive	Trail Making Test, Part B (Reitan & Wolfson, 1985)
Fine Motor	
Simple	Finger Tapping Test[d] (Reitan & Wolfson, 1985)
Complex	Grooved Pegboard[d] (Kløve, 1963)
Right Motor	Finger Tapping Right Hand Score Grooved Pegboard Right Hand Score
Left Motor	Finger Tapping Left Hand Score Grooved Pegboard Left Hand Score
Psychosocial	
Adaptive Behavior	Vineland Adaptive Behavior Scales Composite (Sparrow, Balla, & Cicchetti, 1984)

Note. All measures converted to standard scores. For outcome variables with multiple measures listed, the variable is based on the mean standard score across measures.
[a] Sattler, 1988. [b] Normative data (Talley & Morris, 1994). [c] Subjects received either the Rey Auditory Verbal Learning Test or the Buschke Selective Reminding Test. Correlation between the Rey Total Recall score and the Buschke CLTR ($r = .67$) (Macartney-Filgate & Vriezen, 1988). [d] Mean of right- and left-hand scores.

receiving multiple treatments and poorer intellectual and academic outcomes at 2- to 4-years post diagnosis (Carlson-Green, Morris, & Krawiecki, 1995; Moon, 1995). To explore this question in the present study, extensiveness of treatment following diagnosis was dichotomized, comparing children having multiple treatments in various combinations (surgery, radiation, chemotherapy) with children having single or no treatment. Treatment was also dichotomized based on the presence or absence of radiation.

Chi-square comparisons on categorical variables of gender (Female/Male), race (Non-Caucasian/Caucasian), socioeconomic status (Low/Middle-High) (Hollingshead, 1957), handedness (Non-Right/Right), number of treatments (Multiple/Single), radiation treatment (Radiation/No Radiation), tumor pathology (Glioma/PNET/Other),

Table 2. Demographic Characteristics.

Variable	Sample	AD	RD	ND
n	102	42	16	44
Gender (% Female)	46.1	40.5	68.8	43.2
Race (% Non-Caucasian)	22.5	19.0	31.3	22.7
SES (% Low)	40.6	40.5	50.0	37.2
Handedness (% Non-Right)	29.4	28.6	25.0	31.8
Age Eval. M (SD)	11.5 (4.0)	12.7* (3.8)	11.1 (4.3)	10.6* (3.7)

Note. AD = Arithmetic Deficit; RD = Reading Deficit; ND = No Discrepancy; SES = Socioeconomic Status (% Low; Hollingshead, 1957); Age Eval. = Age in years at Evaluation with WRAT-R.
$*p < .05$.

Table 3. Medical Characteristics.

	Sample	AD	RD	ND
n	102	42	16	44
Age Dx				
M (SD)	7.8 (4.0)	8.6 (4.8)	7.1 (3.9)	7.2 (3.3)
Illness Duration (years)				
M (SD)	3.7 (3.2)	4.1 (3.6)	3.9 (3.9)	3.3 (2.3)
Tumor Pathology (%)				
Glioma	50.5	46.3	50.0	54.5
PNET	31.7	36.6	31.3	27.3
Other	17.8	17.1	18.7	18.2
Tumor Localization (%)				
Posterior Fossa	40.0	41.5	40.0	38.6
Subcortical	29.0	31.7	26.7	27.3
Cortical	31.0	26.8	33.3	34.1
Treatment (%)				
Multiple	54.9	57.1	68.8	47.7
Radiation	67.6	71.4	68.8	63.6

Note. AD = Arithmetic Deficit; RD = Reading Deficit; ND = No discrepancy; Age Dx = Age at diagnosis; PNET = Primitive Neuroectodermal Tumor; Multiple = Treatment with more than one of the following modalities: surgery, radiation, chemotherapy; Radiation = Treatment included radiation.

and tumor localization (Posterior Fossa/Subcortical/Cortical) failed to yield group differnces. Analysis of variance was used to compare subtypes on age at diagnosis and duration of illness; no differences were present. The only significant difference found was for age at WRAT-R evaluation: specifically, children with AD were significantly older than children with ND $(F(2,101) = 3.40, p < .05)$.

Intellectual, Neuropsychological, and Psychosocial Measures

Inspection of the distributions of scores for the general intellectual, specific neuropsychological, and psychosocial outcome variables yielded deviations from normality that suggested possible complications for the use of parametric statistics. Therefore, all variables (in the form of standard scores with a mean of 100 [$SD = 15$]) were dichotomized to yield deficit-no deficit scores, with deficits defined as >1.0 SD below the normative test means. Subtype differences in rates of deficit for these 13 variables were analyzed through Chi-square analyses. Results are presented in Table 4.

Significant differences were revealed on both psychometric intelligence and neuropsychological outcome variables. For Composite IQ, the rate of impairment was found to be highest in the children

Table 4. Rates of Deficit Based on Absolute Cutoff Definition.

| | % | | | |
	Sample (N = 102)	AD (n = 42)	RD (n = 16)	ND (n = 44)
Intellectual				
Composite IQ*	34.7	47.6	33.3	22.7
Verbal IQ	27.6	29.3	40.0	21.4
Nonverbal IQ*	34.0	50.0[a]	20.0	23.8
Specific Neuropsychological				
Visual Motor	48.0	61.0	40.0	38.1
Visual Attention	38.2	42.9	50.0	29.6
Visual Memory	41.0	48.8	26.7	38.6
Language	31.4	26.2	56.3	27.3
Verbal Memory	30.7	33.3	26.7	29.6
Executive	50.0	54.8	46.7	46.5
Fine Motor**	61.6	72.5	81.3	44.2
Right Motor***	55.1	70.0	68.8	32.7[a]
Left Motor	52.6	60.5	62.5	41.9
Psychosocial				
Adaptive Behavior	46.9	57.1	40.0	39.0

[a] Individual cell contributes significantly to overall chi square.
*$p < .05$; **$p < .01$; ***$p < .001$.

with AD, and appeared to be related to their deficits on the nonverbal subtests that contributed to this global IQ score (Nonverbal IQ). Significant subtype differences were also observed in fine motor skills. Children with RD exhibited the highest rate of fine motor impairment, although the significant difference across subtypes was primarily due to the low rate of impairment in the ND group, as compared to both the AD and RD groups. When fine motor skills were divided into right and left motor, to explore possible lateralized differences, a similar pattern of subtype differences was found for each comparison, with a lower rate of deficit in the ND group, although only right motor skills significantly differentiated the groups.

Although other Chi-square analyses did not yield significant subtype differences, trends for rates of impairment tended to fall in the expected direction with the children with RD faring more poorly on verbal tasks (with the exception of verbal memory) and the children with AD faring more poorly on nonverbal tasks (with the exception of visual attention). The children with AD also tended toward slightly higher rates of deficit in the executive and adaptive behavior domains. The ND subtype, as a comparison group, tended to have the lowest rates of impairment.

Examination of the level and pattern of mean standard scores on measures of intelligence, neuropsychological abilities, and psychosocial functioning revealed performance below the normative mean across all measures for all subtypes, as presented in Figure 1.

It was deemed important to differentiate deficits that were a result of generally low functioning from deficits that were significant beyond a given IQ level. Therefore, an alternative definition of deficit was employed that took into account the child's overall level of functioning in determining what constituted a deficit. This definition used a regression approach for computing the score that would be predicted on the neuropsychological and psychosocial outcome variables, given the child's overall intellectual level as measured by the Composite IQ Score. The residual, or discrepancy, between the predicted composite area score and the actual composite area score divided by the standard error, was subjected to a cutoff of >1.0 SD, with impairment scores assigned a "1" or "0" value as described above.

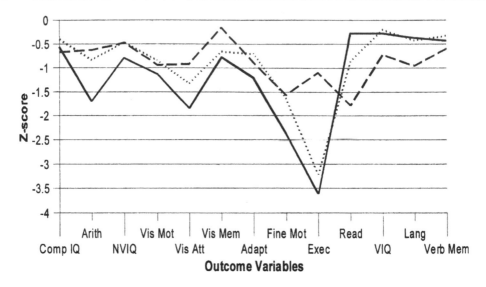

Fig. 1. Mean standard scores on intelligence, academic, neuropsychological and psychosocial outcome variables for three subtypes of children with brain tumors. WRAT-R, Wide Range Achievement Test-Revised; Comp IQ, Stanford-Binet Composite IQ; Arith, WRAT-R Arithmetic subtest; NVIQ, Stanford-Binet Nonverbal Factor (Pattern Analysis, Quantitative, Bead Memory); Vis Mot, Visual Motor (Developmental Test of Visual-Motor Integration); Vis Att, Visual Attention Composite (Mean score: Letter Cancellation Task Omissions, Trail Making Test, Part A); Vis Mem, Visual Memory (Stanford-Binet Bead Memory); Adapt, Adaptive Behavior (Vineland Adaptive Behavior Scales Composite; Fine Mot, Fine Motor Composite (Mean score: Finger Tapping Test, Grooved Pegboard); Exec, Executive (Trail Making Test, Part B); Read, WRAT-R Reading subtest; VIQ, Stanford-Binet Verbal Factor (Vocabulary, Comprehension, Memory for Sentences); Lang, Language Composite (Mean score: Peabody Picture Vocabulary Test, Stanford-Binet Verbal Reasoning); Verb Mem, Verbal Memory (Rey Auditory Verbal Learning Test or Buschke Selective Reminding Test). AD: ___; RD: —; ND: ...

The use of a regression-defined discrepancy definition of deficit resulted in marked reductions in the rates of specific deficit across all variables in comparison to the absolute cut-off criterion (Table 5).

A statistically significant difference between subtypes was obtained on only the language variable. The observed high rate of impairment for children with RD and the observed low rate of impairment for children with AD on this measure was significantly different than would be expected by chance. Children with AD also evidenced greater rates of deficit than did children with RD on the visual memory variable. Twenty-four percent of the AD group were impaired on this measure, while not a single child with RD fell in the impaired range. The zero cell count for the RD

group prevented chi-square analysis; thus, the statistical significance of this difference could not be ascertained. Taken together, these results suggest a dissociation between verbal (Language) and nonverbal (Visual Memory) functioning for the AD and RD subtypes.

Prediction of Subtype Membership

Logistic regression analyses were used to predict subtype membership from a subset of demographic, medical, intellectual, and neuropsychological variables. The applied model-building procedures outlined in Hosmer and Lemeshow (1989) were followed for these analyses. Deletion of cases with missing values resulted in the following sample sizes for three separate logistic regression analyses: AD ($n = 37$) versus ND ($n = 40$); RD ($n = 15$)

Table 5. Rates of Deficit Based on IQ-Discrepancy Definition.

	%			
	Sample (N = 102)	AD (n = 42)	RD (n = 16)	ND (n = 44)
Specific Neuropsychological				
Visual Motor[b]	11.3	14.6	14.3	7.1
Visual Attention	14.9	19.1	6.7	13.6
Visual Memory[c]	19.0	24.4	0	20.5
Language***	15.8	2.4[a]	46.7[a]	18.2
Verbal Memory	12.9	16.7	13.3	9.1
Executive	18.2	14.3	7.1	25.6
Fine Motor	15.3	25.0	6.7	9.3
Psychosocial				
Adaptive Behavior	13.3	14.3	20.0	9.8

[a] Individual cell contributes significantly to overall Chi-square.
[b] Low expected cell counts invalidated the Chi-square comparison.
[c] Although not testable, inspection of frequencies strongly suggests subtype differences.
*** $p < .001$.

versus ND ($n = 43$); and AD ($n = 40$) versus RD ($n = 15$).

Univariate analyses were used to select demographic and medical variables for entry into a multivariate model. Only those variables that significantly discriminated the two subtypes were retained. Measures of intelligence and specific neuropsychological abilities, for which pair-wise Chi-square analyses revealed significant differences in rate of impairment between subtypes, were also entered as predictors of subtype membership. In addition, Composite IQ was entered to explore whether additional variance might be attributable to overall level of psychometric intelligence, after all other predictors had been entered.

AD vs. ND Comparison

Individual demographic and medical variables did not differentiate the AD and ND subtypes, with the exception of the Age at WRAT-R Evaluation variable, where children with AD were found to be older than children with ND. Three measures of intelligence and specific neuropsychological abilities (Nonverbal IQ, Fine Motor, Visual Motor) differentiated the subtypes and were included in the multivariate model.

Results of logistic regression model-building steps for the AD versus ND comparison are presented in Table 6. Only Nonverbal IQ and Age at

WRAT-R Evaluation contributed significantly to the prediction of subtype membership. These results indicate that the most parsimonious model includes two variables, and predicts subtype membership (AD vs. ND) correctly for 70% of the cases in this sample. Impairment in Nonverbal IQ is associated with a four-fold (4.03) greater risk of membership in the AD group. Additionally, for every 5-year increment in age at evaluation, a child in this sample has a two-fold (2.20) greater risk of AD.

RD vs. ND Comparison

Individual demographic and medical variables did not differentiate the RD and ND subtypes. However, it is interesting to note that the number of medical treatments approached significance ($p = .07$) in predicting RD subtype membership. Two specific neuropsychological measures (Language, Fine Motor) differentiated the subtypes and were included in the model.

Results of logistic regression model-building steps for the RD versus ND comparison are presented in Table 7. When added in step-wise fashion, Fine Motor contributed significantly to the prediction of subtype membership, over and above the Language measure; the addition of the Composite IQ failed to explain significant additional variance. These results suggest that the most parsimonious model for prediction of RD versus ND subtype

Table 6. AD versus ND Logistic Regression Analyses: Stepwise Model Building (Adjusted).

Variable	B	SE(B)	Odds ratio	95% CI	−2 Log likelihood	G
NV IQ	1.183	0.502	3.26	(1.22–8.72)	100.78	5.85*
FM	1.007	0.528	2.74	(0.97–7.70)	97.07	3.70
VM	0.769	0.524	2.16	(0.77–6.02)	94.92	2.15
Age Eval.	0.192	0.075	1.21	(1.05–1.40)	87.64	7.28**
Comp IQ	0.617	0.899	1.85	(0.32–10.79)	87.16	0.48

Note. AD = Arithmetic Deficit; ND = No Discrepancy; 95% CI = 95% Confidence interval for the odds ratio; G = Likelihood Ratio Test Statistic; NV IQ = Stanford Binet Nonverbal IQ; FM = Fine Motor; VM = Visual Motor; Age Eval. = Age in years at WRAT-R Evaluation; Comp IQ = Stanford Binet Composite IQ. Adjusted odds ratios are the odds of having AD. The G statistic may differ from actual difference values due to rounding errors.
$*p < .05; **p < .01.$

Table 7. RD versus ND Logistic Regression Analyses: Stepwise Model Building (Adjusted).

Variable	B	SE(B)	Odds ratio	95% CI	−2 Log likelihood	G
Language	1.355	0.627	3.88	(1.13–13.25)	61.48	4.83*
FM	1.806	0.872	6.09	(1.10–33.62)	56.32	5.16*
Comp IQ	−0.057	0.800	0.95	(0.20–4.53)	56.31	0.01

Note. RD = Reading Deficit; ND = No Discrepancy; 95% CI = 95% Confidence interval for the odds ratio; G = Likelihood Ratio Test Statistic; FM = Fine Motor; Comp IQ = Stanford Binet Composite IQ. Adjusted odds ratios are the odds of having RD. The G statistic may differ from actual difference values due to rounding errors.
$*p < .05.$

membership includes two variables and predicts group membership correctly for 63% of the cases in this sample. In this model, Language and Fine Motor impairments are associated with a two-fold (2.00) to six-fold (6.08) greater risk of RD.

AD vs. RD Comparison
Individual demographic and medical variables did not differentiate the AD and RD subtypes. Both Nonverbal IQ and Language differentiated the subtypes and were entered into the multivariate model.

Results of logistic regression model-building steps for the AD versus RD subtypes are presented in Table 8. When added in step-wise fashion, both Nonverbal IQ and Language contributed significant variance. The Composite IQ was not entered due to its substantial overlap with the other two predictors. These results indicate that the most parsimonious model for prediction of AD versus RD subtype membership includes two variables, Nonverbal IQ and Language, and predicts group membership

correctly for 64% of the cases in this sample. Impairment in Nonverbal IQ was associated with a 24-fold (24.59) greater risk of AD, whereas impairment on the Language measure was associated with almost no (.04) risk of AD, thus, predicting RD subtype membership.

DISCUSSION

This study investigated the prevalence of specific academic deficits in children with brain tumors and explored the neurocognitive and psychosocial correlates of different patterns of academic achievement in this population. The utility of Rourke's (1989) NLD model in characterizing the outcome of children with brain tumors was also assessed. Fifty-seven percent of these children were found to have a specific academic deficit. The proportion of children with AD was 16 times greater than expected and the proportion of children with RD

Table 8. AD versus RD Logistic Regression Analyses: Stepwise Model Building (Adjusted).

Variable	B	SE(B)	Odds ratio	95% CI	−2 Log likelihood	G
NV IQ	1.386	0.719	4.00	(0.98–16.37)	60.15	4.30*
Language	−3.124	1.139	0.04	(0.00–0.41)	47.62	12.53**
Comp IQ	Resulted in singularity					

Note. AD = Arithmetic Deficit; RD = Reading Deficit; 95% CI = 95% Confidence interval for the odds ratio; G = Likelihood Ratio Test Statistic; NV IQ = Stanford Binet Nonverbal IQ; Comp IQ = Stanford Binet Composite IQ. Adjusted odds ratios are the odds of having AD. The G statistic may differ from actual difference values due to rounding errors.
$*p < .05; **p < .01$.

was 6 times greater than expected. Thus, although both types of academic deficits were present at greater than expected frequencies, AD was significantly more common. Whereas mathematics disorder accounts for approximately one of every five cases of learning disorder in the U.S. public schools (American Psychiatric Association, 1994), in this sample, AD accounts for approximately three of every four children with brain tumors who have specific academic deficits.

Examination of mean scores on intellectual measures revealed that all subtypes were functioning below expected levels. Children with AD were found to have the highest rate of deficit in overall psychometric intelligence, whereas children without specific academic deficits were found to have the lowest rate. When components of the global IQ score were explored, Nonverbal IQ discriminated the groups whereas Verbal IQ did not. Children with AD had a significantly higher rate of deficit in Nonverbal IQ as compared to children with RD and ND, consistent with the predictions of the NLD model. Children with RD evidenced the highest rate of deficit in Verbal IQ, although not significantly higher than the other two subtypes.

Consistent with the findings on measures of psychometric intelligence, examination of the mean standard scores for the neuropsychological and psychosocial outcome variables across subtypes also revealed below-average functioning across all measures. Thus, deficient performance on specific measures was defined using two different criteria, an absolute cutoff and a regression-defined discrepancy from expectation, based on IQ.

When rates of deficit for specific neuropsychological and psychosocial measures were compared

across subtypes, several differences were found. In general, children with AD had higher rates of impairment on nonverbal tasks requiring visual-motor skills and visual memory. They also were more likely to exhibit problems with adaptive behavior. However, these differences were not statistically significant. Children with AD had significantly lower rates of deficit on verbal tasks requiring receptive and expressive language skills and verbal reasoning ability, whereas children with RD had the highest rate of deficit on this set of measures. Both children with AD and RD had significantly higher rates of impairment of fine motor tasks, particularly with the right hand, relative to children without specific academic deficits. There were no subtype differences in rate of impairment on measures of visual attention or executive skills.

These results support a significant relationship between arithmetic deficits and a subset of the neuropsychological and adaptive strengths and weaknesses associated with the NLD syndrome. Although not all children with brain tumors exhibit arithmetic deficits, those who do so also show a phenotypic resemblance to children with NLD. Impairment in nonverbal intellectual functioning, with relative sparing of verbal intellectual abilities was strongly associated with arithmetic deficits. However, not all features of the NLD syndrome significantly discriminated the groups. Those aspects of the NLD model that did not differentiate the AD group from other groups included impairments in visual-motor skills, visual attention, executive skills, and psychosocial functioning, as well as strength in verbal memory. Measures of executive function (Trail Making Test, Part B) and complex psychomotor skill (Grooved Pegboard), which were

previously found to be most significant in discriminating children with NLD from children
with reading and spelling disabilities (Harnadek
& Rourke, 1994), did not differentiate AD and RD
subtypes in this sample. In some cases, limitations
of the specific measures used to represent a cognitive domain may have contributed to the failure to
find subtype differences. For example, the Trail
Making Test, Part B, the single measure used to
assess executive function, does not adequately
measure all of the complex abilities associated
with this domain.

The failure to identify all of the attributes of
the NLD syndrome in this population may also be
related to the fact that children with brain tumors
have acquired cognitive and behavioral deficits following a period of normal development. Children
with acquired aspects of NLD syndrome are likely
to have had the affordances of a normal sensorimotor period of development to form the basic building
blocks of cause-and-effect relationships that support later learning (Rourke, 1988a, 1995). In contrast, children with "developmental presentation"
of the NLD syndrome, have had early months and
years of compromised sensorimotor, tactile, and
visual-perceptual exploration.

Results of logistic regression analyses indicate
that a discrete set of variables, primarily indexing
verbal and nonverbal abilities, are strongly associated with subtype membership. These analyses
provide further evidence of a dissociation between
nonverbal and verbal abilities in the AD and RD
groups. However, it is important to consider the
impact of base rates on the sensitivity of the prediction models. In this study, due to the low base
rate of RD ($n = 16$), one could have predicted AD
membership ($n = 42$) or ND membership ($n = 44$)
correctly 75% of the time if, in all pair-wise comparisons involving the RD group, the more prevalent outcome were predicted. However, the ability
to discriminate AD and ND groups, which have
similar base rates, using nonverbal IQ and age at
evaluation, represents a 20% improvement from
prediction on the basis of chance alone.

Rourke (1987) has conceptualized a biological
substrate involving white matter damage to explain
the specific pattern of deficits found in children
with NLD, with cranial irradiation as the primary
mechanism resulting in white matter damage in

children with brain tumors. This study explored
a number of medical variables, including radiation
treatment, in the search for possible illness- and
treatment-related factors that would differentiate
subtypes. Tumor location, tumor pathology, exposure to radiation treatment, and exposure to multiple
treatments, all failed to differentiate the academic
deficit groups. However, power to detect such
differences was limited by sample size. Although
not significant, the results were in the predicted
direction: Children with AD had a slightly greater
proportion of subcortical tumors and radiation
treatment in comparison to other subtypes. However, the amount of radiation received and extent
of brain affected varied across subjects and no
measurements of amount of white matter damage
were obtained. Future studies might utilize neuroimaging techniques, such as magnetic resonance
spectroscopy, to link the extent of white matter
damage/dysfunction to specific cognitive deficits
and/or profiles in children with brain tumors. It
is also possible that illess-and treatment-related
variables might have shown a stronger relationship
to features of the NLD syndrome if classification
criteria other than academic achievement patterns had been used to define subgroups. For
example, the presence of specific constellations
of neuropsychological assets and deficits or of
medical factors (e.g., diagnosis before age 7, in
conjunction with radiation treatment more than
2 years prior to evaluation) might have been used
to identify other subgroups of children with brain
tumors.

There was also no relationship between age of
brain tumor diagnosis or time since diagnosis and
subtype membership. However, the AD group was
significantly older than the ND group at the time of
evaluation with the WRAT-R. Regression analyses indicated that every 5-year increment in age at
evaluation is associated with a two-fold greater
risk of having an arithmetic deficit. The emergence
of arithmetic deficits in the AD group at an older
age implies specific difficulties in meeting the
increasing cognitive-developmental demands for
successful performance on the WRAT-R Arithmetic
subtest. These findings are consistent with previous
research indicating that early damage can have
consequences that are only fully manifested later
in development, as the child faces demands for

increased cognitive complexity (Goldman, 1971). They are also consistent with Rourke's developmental hypothesis that children with NLD evidence greater difficulty in mathematics and other nonverbal skills with increasing age (Rourke, Del Dotto, Rourke, & Casey, 1990). A cross-sectional study of children with the NLD syndrome has documented relative declines in mechanical arithmetic and complex visul-perceptual-organizational skills, and relative stability of verbal abilities from middle childhood to early adolescence (Casey, Rourke, & Picard, 1991).

A final direction for future research relates to the developmental pattern and progression of academic deficits in children with brain tumors. The longitudinal examination of achievement test scores for children in this sample raised questions about the stability of achievement patterns over time. A longitudinal exploration of individual achievement patterns, using techniques such as growth curve analysis, would be helpful to tease apart the developmental, illness, and treatment factors that affect recovery from childhood brain tumors. It is possible, as Rourke (1995) has hypothesized for children with NLD, that children with brain tumors may look increasingly more disabled over time, and that the pattern of their disability will evidence increasing similarity to the NLD syndrome. That is, as Rourke and others have suggested, they may "grow into their lesions".

REFERENCES

American Psychiatric Association (1994). *Diagnostic and statistical manual of mental disorders* (4th ed.). Washington, DC: Author.

Anastasi, A. (1988). *Psychological testing.* New York: Macmillan.

Beery, K.E. (1989). *Revised Administration, Scoring, and Teaching Manual for the Developmental Test of Visual-Motor Integration.* Cleveland, OH: Modern Curriculum Press.

Beery, K.E., & Buktenica, N. (1967). *Developmental Test of Visual-Motor Integration.* Student Test Booklet, Chicago: Follet.

Bishop, J., Knights, R.M., & Stoddart, C. (1990). Rey Auditory Verbal Learning Test: Performance of English and French children aged 5 to 16. *The Clinical Neuropsychologist, 4,* 133–140.

Black, P.M. (1991). Brain tumors: Part II. *The New England Journal of Medicine, 324,* 1155–1164.

Broadbent, V.A., Barnes, N.D., & Wheeler, T.K. (1981). Medulloblastoma in childhood: Long-term results of treatment. *Cancer, 48,* 26–30.

Buschke, H. (1973). Selective reminding for analysis of memory and learning. *Journal of Verbal Learning and Verbal Behavior, 12,* 543–550.

Buschke, H., & Fuld, P.A. (1974). Evaluation of storage, retention, and retrieval in disordered memory and learning. *Neurology, 24,* 1019–1025.

Carlson-Green, B., Morris, R.D., & Krawiecki, N. (1995). Family and illness predictors of outcome in children with brain tumors. *Journal of Pediatric Psychology, 20,* 769–784.

Casey, J.E., Rourke, B.P., & Picard, E.M. (1991). Syndrome of nonverbal learning disabilities: Age differences in neuropsychological, academic, and socioemotional functioning. *Development and Psychopathology, 3,* 329–345.

Cohen, M.E., & Duffner, P.K. (1984). *Brain tumors in children.* New York: Raven Press.

Danoff, B.F., Cowchock, F.S., Marquette, C., Mulgrew, L., & Kramer, S. (1982). Assessment of the long-term effects of primary radiation therapy for brain tumors in children. *Cancer, 49,* 1580–1586.

Duffner, P.K., Cohen, M.E., & Parker, M.S. (1988). Prospective intellectual testing in children with brain tumors. *Annals of Neurology, 23,* 575–579.

Duffner, P.K., Cohen, M.E., & Thomas, P. (1983). Late effects of treatment on the intelligence of children with posterior fossa tumors. *Cancer, 51,* 233–237.

Dunn, L.M., & Dunn, L.M. (1981). *Peabody Picture Vocabulary Test-Revised (PPVT-R).* Circle Pines, MN: American Guidance Service.

Ellenberg, L., McComb, J.G., Siegel, S.E., & Stowe, S. (1987). Factors affecting intellectual outcome in pediatric brain tumor patients. *Neurosurgery, 21,* 638–644.

Glauser, T.A., & Packer, R.J. (1991). Cognitive deficits in long-term survivors of childhood brain tumors. *Child's Nervous System, 7,* 2–12.

Goldberg, E., & Costa, L.D. (1981). Hemisphere differences in the acquisition and use of descriptive systems. *Brain and Language, 14,* 144–173.

Goldman, P.S. (1971). Functional development of the prefrontal cortex in early life and the problem of neuronal plasticity. *Experimental Neurology, 32,* 366–387.

Harnedek, M.C.S., & Rourke, B.P. (1994). Principal identifying features of the syndrome of nonverbal learning disabilities in children. *Journal of Learning Disabilities, 27,* 144–154.

Hirsch, J.F., Renier, D., Czernichow, P., Benveniste, L., & Pierre-Kahn, A. (1979). Medulloblastoma in childhood: Survival and functional results. *Acta Neurochirurgica, 48,* 1–15.

Hollingshead, A.B. (1957). *Two-factor model of social position.* New Haven, CT: Author.

Hosmer, D.W., & Lemeshow, S. (1989). *Applied logistic regression*. New York: John Wiley.

Jannoun, L., & Bloom, H.J.G. (1990). Long-term psychological effects in children treated for intracranial tumors. *International Journal of Radiation, Oncology, and Physics, 18*, 747–753.

Jastak, S., & Wilkinson, G.S. (1984). *Wide Range Achievement Test-Revised*. Wilmington, DE: Jastak.

Kløve, H. (1963). Clinical neuropsychology. In F.M. Forster (Ed.), *The medical clinics of North America* (pp. 1069–1077). New York: Saunders.

Macartney-Filgate, M.S., & Vriezen, E.R. (1988). Intercorrelation of clinical tests of verbal memory. *Archives of Clinical Neuropsychology, 3*, 121–126.

Mesulam, M.M. (1985). *Principles of behavioral neurology*. Philadelphia: F.A. Davis.

Moon, F. (1995). *The effects of acquired memory disorders on academic performance*. Unpublished doctoral dissertation, Georgia State University, Atlanta.

Moore, B.D., Copeland, D.R., Ried, H., & Levy, B. (1992). Neurophysiological basis of cognitive deficits in long-term survivors of childhood cancer. *Archives of Neurology, 49*, 809–817.

Mulhern, R.K., Crisco, J.J., & Kun, L.E. (1983). Neuropsychological sequelae of childhood brain tumors: A review. *Journal of Clinical Child Psychology, 12*, 66–73.

Radcliffe, J., Bunin, G.R., Sutton, L.N., Goldwein, J.W., & Phillips, P.C. (1994). Cognitive deficits in long-term survivors of childhood medulloblastoma and other noncortical tumors: Age-dependent effects of whole brain radiation. *International Journal of Developmental Neuroscience, 12*, 327–334.

Reitan, R.M., & Wolfson, D. (1985). *The Halstead-Reitan Neuropsychological Test Battery*. Tucson, AZ: Neuropsychology Press.

Rey, A. (1964). *L'examen clinique en psychologie*. Paris: Press Universitaire de France.

Ris, M.D., & Noll, R.B. (1994). Long-term neurobehavioral outcome in pediatric brain-tumor patients: Review and methodological critique. *Journal of Clinical and Experimental Neuropsychology, 16*, 21–42.

Roman, D.D., & Sperduto, P.W. (1995). Neuropsychological effects of cranial radiation: Current knowledge and future directions. *International Journal of Radiation Oncology, Biology, and Physics, 31*, 983–998.

Rourke, B.P. (1987). Syndrome of nonverbal learning disabilities: The final common pathway of white-matter disease/dysfunction? *The Clinical Neuropsychologist, 1*, 209–234.

Rourke, B.P. (1988a). The syndrome of nonverbal learning-disabilities: Developmental manifestations in neurological disease, disorder, and dysfunction. *The Clinical Neuropsychologist, 2*, 293–330.

Rourke, B.P. (1988b). Socioemotional disturbances of learning-disabled children. *Journal of Consulting and Clinical Psychology, 56*, 801–810.

Rourke, B.P. (1989). *Nonverbal learning disabilities: The syndrome and the model*. New York: Guilford Press.

Rourke, B.P. (Ed.). (1991). *Neuropsychological validation of learning disability subtypes*. New York: Guilford Press.

Rourke, B.P. (1995). Introduction: The NLD syndrome and the white matter model. In B.P. Rourke (Ed.), *Syndrome of nonverbal learning disabilities: Neurodevelopmental manifestations* (pp. 1–25). New York: Guilford Press.

Rourke, B.P., Del Dotto, J.E., Rourke, S.B., & Casey, J.E. (1990). Nonverbal learning disabilities: The syndrome and a case study. *Journal of School Psychology, 28*, 361–385.

Rourke, B.P., & Finlayson, M.A.J. (1978). Neuropsychological significance of variations in patterns of academic performance: Verbal and visual-spatial abilities. *Journal of Abnormal Child Psychology, 6*, 121–133.

Rourke, B.P., & Fisk, J.L. (1981). Socio-emotional disturbances of learning-disabled children: The role of central processing deficits. *Bulletin of The Orton Society, 31*, 77–88.

Rourke, B.P., & Fuerst, D.R. (1991). *Learning disabilities and psychosocial functioning: A neuropsychological perspective*. New York: Guilford Press.

Rourke, B.P., & Strang, J.D. (1978). Neuropsychological significance of variations in patterns of academic performance: Motor, psychomotor, and tactile-perceptual abilities. *Journal of Pediatric Psychology, 3*, 62–66.

Sattler, J.M. (1988). *Assessment of children*. San Diego, CA: Jerome M. Sattler.

Sparrow, S.S., Balla, D.A., & Cicchetti, D.V. (1984). *Vineland Adaptive Behavior Scale Survey Form Manual*. Circle Pines, MN: American Guidance Service.

Spunberg, J.J., Chang, C.H., Goldman, M., Auricchio, E., & Bell, J.J. (1981). Quality of long-term survival following irradiation for intracranial tumors in children under the age of two. *International Journal of Radiation Oncology, Biology, Physiology, 7*, 727–736.

Strang, J.D., & Rourke, B.P. (1983). Concept formation/non-verbal reasoning abilities of children who exhibit specific academic problems with arithmetic. *Journal of Clinical Child Psychology, 12*, 33–39.

Talley, J., & Morris, R. (1994). *The verbal cancellation task: Children's norms*. Unpublished doctoral dissertation, Georgia State University, Atlanta.

Thorndike, R.L., Hagen, E.P., & Sattler, J.M. (1986). *Stanford-Binet* (4th ed.). Chicago: Riverside Publishing.

Child Neuropsychology
1999, Vol. 5, No. 3, pp. 154–170

Music and Language Skills of Children with Williams Syndrome*

Audrey J. Don[1], E. Glenn Schellenberg[2], and Byron P. Rourke[3,4]

[1]The Children's Seashore House of the Children's Hospital of Philadelphia, PA, [2]University of Toronto, Canada,
[3]University of Windsor, Canada, and [4]Yale University, New Haven, CT

ABSTRACT

We examined music and language abilities in a group of children with Williams syndrome (WS, $n = 19$) and a comparison group of normal children ($n = 19$) equivalent for receptive vocabulary. Consistent with previous reports and the model of Nonverbal Learning Disabilities (Rourke, 1989), the children with WS scored better on verbal than performance measures of the WISC-III, and performance on simpler verbal tasks (e.g., receptive vocabulary) was superior to performance on more complex verbal tasks (e.g., comprehension). Performance on music tests was *relatively* good, being comparable to mental age based on receptive vocabulary and similar to that of the comparison group. Music and language abilities were moderately correlated for both groups of children. Compared to normal children, the WS group expressed greater liking of music and a greater range of emotional responses to music.

The unusual constellation of characteristics that typifies individuals with Williams syndrome (WS) has captured the attention of scientists (e.g., Bellugi, Bihrle, Neville, Jernigan, & Doherty, 1992; Levitin & Bellugi, 1998; Mervis, Morris, Bertrand, & Robinson, 1999) and the popular media (e.g., the television program *60 Minutes*). Children with WS have 'elfin' facial features and are often described as friendly and talkative (Lowe, Henderson, Park, & McGreal, 1954; Mervis et al., 1999; Udwin, Yule, & Martin, 1987). Although these children are mentally retarded, they have an unusual cognitive profile with relatively preserved verbal abilities that contrast markedly with their extremely poor visuospatial skills (Bellugi et al., 1992; Lowe et al., 1954; Mervis et al., 1999; Udwin & Yule, 1991). Clinical, experimental, and anecdotal reports suggest that these children may also be relatively musical (Anonymous, 1985; Lenhoff, 1996; Levine, 1992; Levitin & Bellugi, 1998; Udwin et al., 1987; von Arnim & Engel, 1964).

For example, early descriptive studies reported that children with WS have good singing skills (von Arnim and Engel, 1964) and can easily learn songs (Udwin et al. 1987). More recently, Lenhoff (1996) provided a qualitative examination of the music skills of individuals attending a 'Music and Arts' camp for children with WS. The attendees displayed heightened levels of interest and emotional responsivity toward music, facility learning complex rhythms, excellent memory for lyrics, ease in composing song lyrics, ability with harmony, and an unusual number had absolute (perfect) pitch. In another study conducted at the same camp,

* This article is based on a doctoral dissertation submitted by the first author to the Department of Psychology at the University of Windsor.

Funding was provided by a grant awarded to the second author from the Natural Sciences and Engineering Research Council of Canada.

Address correspondence to: Audrey Don, Children's Seashore House, 3405 Civic Center Blvd., Philadelphia, PA 19104, USA. E-mail: adon@mail.med.upenn.edu

Accepted for publication: December 28, 1998.

Levitin and Bellugi (1998) administered a rhythm production test to 8 children with WS (mean age = 13.4 years, SD = 3.6 years) and compared their performance to a control group of children 5 to 7 years of age. Although the groups were equivalent on the rhythm measure, the individuals with WS were more likely to produce musically 'compatible' rhythms when they responded in error.

Unfortunately, the WS group was a select cohort (music camp attendees) and groups were matched using reported norms on Piagetian conservation tasks without verifying that the groups were actually equivalent on these tasks. Thus, one cannot draw firm conclusions about the rhythm abilities of children with WS on the basis of this study. Nonetheless, the presence of relatively intact verbal skills combined with the possibility that such skills are accompanied by relatively intact musical skills provided the impetus for our research questions: (1) Are children with WS more musical than one would expect based on their overall cognitive abilities? and (2) How do the music skills of children with WS compare to their relatively intact language skills?

WS is a rare genetic anomaly characterized by a submicroscopic deletion on chromosome 7, which contains the genes for elastin, LIMK, and other genes (Ashkenas, 1996; Ewart, Jin, Atkinson, Morris, & Keating, 1994; Morris, Thomas, & Greenberg, 1993; Tassabehji et al., 1996). Individuals with WS exhibit vascular problems, such as supravalvar aortic stenosis and hypertension, that are associated with the loss of the elastin gene. The LIMK gene has been implicated in neural-cell development and is believed to be related to the deficits in visuospatial and visuoconstruction skills associated with WS. The overwhelming majority of children with WS (86 to 96%) also exhibit *hyperacusis,* which is characterized by aversive reactions to sounds that do not cause such reactions in normal individuals (Arnold, Yule, & Martin, 1985; Klein, Armstrong, Greer, & Brown, 1990; Udwin et al., 1987).

Although the neuropsychological profile associated with WS suggests right-hemisphere dysfunction, brain-imaging studies show mild microcephaly without specific lateralized structural lesions or anomalies (Jernigan, Doherty, Hesselink, & Bellugi, 1993). Neocerebellar volumes and limbic structures

are *relatively* large, however, and comparable to normal controls (Jernigan et al., 1993; Jernigan & Bellugi, 1990).

Exaggerated left-sided asymmetry of the planum temporale has been reported in professional musicians, particularly those with absolute pitch (Schlaug, Janke, Hunag, & Steinmetz, 1995). Because absolute pitch and relatively good musical skills have also been identified as possible characteristics associated with WS, Bellugi, Hickock, Jones, and Jernigan (1996) examined the planum temporale of individuals with WS. For the majority of their sample, the leftward asymmetry fell between the two groups of professional musicians (i.e., those with or without absolute pitch). Replication and extension of this finding could provide an anatomical basis for the reported musicality of individuals with WS.

Music

Musical skills are *not* typically associated with specific brain structures. *Amusia,* or the loss of music perception or performance abilities due to brain damage, is often accompanied by aphasia (Marin, 1982). In a review of 314 historical cases, Henschen (1920, cited in Judd, Gardner, & Geschwind, 1983) found that left-hemisphere damage and aphasia were present in 97% of cases of amusia. Because the cases of amusia included a wide range of deficits (music performance, composition, reading, music perception), the association with aphasia is too general to implicate localization of musical functioning. Indeed, results of neuropsychological investigations of musical abilities are often contradictory (Hodges, 1999), a likely consequence of the complex nature of music.

Nevertheless, research based on listening tasks, infant development, and lesion analysis reveals clues to the neurobiology and neuroanatomy of music processing. For example, perception of melodic contours (changes in pitch direction) is reliably associated with right-hemisphere functioning for both brain-damaged and normal individuals (see McKinnon & Schellenberg, 1997). By contrast, rhythmic processing has been associated with left-hemisphere functioning, although such findings are inconsistent across studies (Peretz, 1990; Peretz & Morais, 1989). Despite the apparent links between aphasia and amusia, dissociations have also been reported. In a review of lesion studies, Sergent (1993) hypothesized that widely distributed, locally specialized neural substrates subserving music are proximate to, but distinct from, verbal areas. It is also possible that specific aspects of music and language share a common processor, with other aspects being independent. Indeed, a study of patients with amusia without aphasia demonstrated that processing of linguistic prosody and music were linked (Patel & Peretz, 1997).

In normal development, prosodic and melodic elements of speech and song directed to infants and young children are similar (Trehub & Trainor, 1998). Speech to infants typically involves exaggerated prosody with relatively slow and regular rhythmic patterns, shorter phrases, and greater repetition than adult-directed speech (Papousek & Papousek, 1981). It is also higher in pitch with simple pitch contours that span a greater range. Infant-directed singing is similarly slow, high-pitched, and rhythmically exaggerated (Trainor, Clark, Huntley, & Adams, 1997). Moreover, young infants prefer infant-over adult-directed speech (Cooper & Aslin, 1990; Fernald, 1985; Werker & McLeod, 1989), just as they prefer infant- over adult-directed singing (Trainor, 1996). Thus, adults' style of communicating in the auditory domain with very young listeners appears to capitalize on innate perceptual biases and preferences for particular auditory patterns. These similarities across domains are consistent with suggestions of a link between language and musical skills.

An explanatory framework for the unusual cognitive profile associated with WS is provided by Rourke (1989, 1995), who describes the syndrome of *Nonverbal Learning Disabilities* (NLD). NLD is thought to arise as the developmental outcome of an interaction between primary *assets* in auditory perception, rote learning, and simple motor skills, and primary *deficits* in tactile and visual perception, complex psychomotor skills, and adaptation to novelty. During early development, a child typically explores the world through touching, feeling, seeing, and hearing. For a child with NLD, however, weak tactile and visual perception accompanied by difficulty with complex psychomotor skills render the world too confusing to assimilate through nonverbal processes. Instead, the child with NLD explores the world primarily with an auditory and

verbally based approach. This unbalanced development results in an individual who has relative strength in skills subserved primarily by systems within the left cerebral hemisphere (e.g., simple language skills and auditory memory). By contrast, deficits are observed in skills that are thought to be subserved primarily by systems within the right hemisphere as well as in skills that require intermodal processing (e.g., nonverbal, fluid, or creative reasoning, abstract thinking, complex language comprehension, and prosody).

Although the overall level of abilities is lower for children with WS than for the typical child diagnosed with NLD, the pattern of assets and deficits is similar. Children with WS display relative strengths in auditory perception, verbal memory, speech articulation, and quantity of speech, but deficits in psychomotor coordination, visual-spatial-organization, and adaptation to novelty (Mervis et al., 1999). If one assumes that some aspects of auditory processing for language and music are shared, the NLD model also provides a framework for explaining relative strength in music as well as language. In other words, children with WS should demonstrate relatively good memory for simple and repetitive musical patterns in addition to their relatively good language abilities. Moreover, performance on simple language and music measures should be superior to performance on more complex measures. Some areas of reported strength for children with WS, however, such as facial memory and the perception and production of speech prosody (Udwin & Yule, 1991; Bellugi et al., 1988; Bellugi et al., 1994), are not consistent with the NLD profile and suggestive of relatively intact nonverbal functioning for this population in specific areas. Regardless, because these children appear to be 'tuned into' the melodies of speech (i.e., prosody), it is reasonable to expect that their music-perception abilities might also be relatively good.

The linguistic abilities of children with WS are well established, yet their musical skills have not been empirically validated. On the one hand, some aspects of music abilities may be spared in this population relative to their overall level of cognitive functioning, as are some aspects of language use. Indeed, music skills in WS might even stand out as a strength in comparison to the normal population; if demonstrated, this would imply that WS comprises a group of musical *savants*. On the other hand, music may appear to be a relative strength simply because these children often respond enthusiastically to music.

The purpose of the present study was to examine the language and music abilities of children with WS. Because little is known specifically about music skills in individuals with WS, we focused on quantitative measurement of such skills. We expected that music and language skills would be correlated and that both would be better than nonverbal abilities. In addition, children with WS were expected to be similar to normal children of equivalent verbal level in terms of their musical abilities. Finally, if the cognitive profile associated with WS arises in the manner proposed for NLD (Rourke, 1989), intact auditory processing should be a primary means by which children with WS develop an understanding of the world. Thus, *interest* in music might also be greater for children with WS than for normal children.

To test the hypothesis that music and language skills represent areas of relative strength in children with WS, a comparison group with equivalent language skills was chosen. The choice of a language measure on which to equate groups was particularly important because children with WS are relatively strong in *simple* language skills yet weak in more complex areas such as language comprehension and pragmatics (Anderson & Rourke, 1995; Mervis et al., 1999; Rourke & Tsatsanis, 1996). For example, Verbal IQ as defined by the *Wechsler Intelligence Scale for Children, Third Edition (WISC-III;* Wechsler, 1991) measures simple and complex language skills and is unlikely to provide an appropriate basis for comparison. By contrast, receptive vocabulary – a relatively simple verbal skill – better reflects the language strengths observed in children with WS. Thus, a measure of receptive vocabulary was chosen as the basis for establishing between-group equivalence.

METHOD

Participants
Children for the WS group were recruited from Williams Syndrome Associations in Canada and the United States through organization newsletters or meetings. Children for the comparison group were recruited through fliers posted at the University of Windsor and at local churches. All participants spoke English as their primary language and were without significant sensory or physical handicaps.

The study group consisted of 19 children with WS between 8 and 13 years of age (10 boys and 9 girls). Mean chronological age was 10 years, 6 months ($SD = 1$ year, 10 months) and mean mental age – calculated using scores on the *Peabody Picture Vocabulary Test-Revised (PPVT-R*; Dunn & Dunn, 1981) – was 8 years, 1 month ($SD = 2$ years, 2 months). The comparison group – equivalent for mental age on the PPVT-R – was selected from a larger group of 32 normal children between 5 and 12 years of age. Specifically, only children with PPVT-R standard scores between 85 and 115 (average range) were included. The resulting group of 19 children (11 boys and 8 girls) had a mean chronological age of 7 years, 11 months ($SD = 2$ years, 4 months) and mean mental age of 8 years, 1 month ($SD = 2$ years, 5 months), which was identical to that of the WS group.

Measures
Language and music skills were assessed through standardized measures, a questionnaire, and a semi-structured interview. Four language measures (in addition to the PPVT-R) were selected to evaluate a variety of skills – ranging from relatively simple to complex – in both groups of children. The *Auditory Closure Test* (Kass, 1964), arguably the least complex task, was included as a simple measure of sound blending. On this task, the child hears segmented sounds of a word and is asked to blend the sounds to produce the corresponding word. Verbal fluency, another relatively simple verbal task, was assessed through the *Controlled Oral Word Association* to category (Animals) (Halperin, Healy, Zwitchik, Ludman, & Weinstein, 1989, as cited in Spreen & Strauss, 1991), which also provides a measure of *perseverations*. More complex aspects of verbal skill requiring auditory attention and working memory were measured with the *Digit Span* subtest from the WISC-III and *Sentence Repetition* (Spreen & Strauss, 1991). For the WS group only, overall verbal and nonverbal intellectual functioning was measured with the complete WISC-III. The *Comprehension* subtest of the WISC-III provided the most complex measure of language skills for the children with WS.

Our choice of measures to assess musical skills was limited because most music tests are designed to examine the skills of individuals undergoing formal music training. For our purposes, only skills present in infancy or acquired implicitly through exposure to music could provide a basis for the evaluation of general auditory pattern processing abilities. *Gordon's Primary Measures of Music Audiation (PMMA)* (Gordon, 1980) for children in kindergarden through third grade met our criteria. The test was standardized in 1978 on a sample of 873 children residing in suburban New York state. Test-retest reliabilities ranged from .73 to .76 with split-half reliabilities ranging from .72 to .86. The test has also been used to assess the music abilities of mentally retarded adults, with test-retest reliabilities at .81 or higher (Hoskins, Kvet, & Oubre, 1988).

The PMMA comprises *Tonal* and *Rhythm* subtests for which centile scores are computed. Each subtest has 40 taped trials. Each trial (both subtests) consists of a pair of short, monophonic melodic or rhythmic phrases, and children are asked to indicate whether the paired sequences are the same or different. *Standard* and *comparison* phrases are identical on *same* trials but not on *different* trials. *Tonal* phrases have 2 to 5 pure tones (sine waves) that differ in pitch but not in duration on 'different' trials; phrases are presented in either major or minor tonality. *Rhythm* phrases have 2 to 11 pure tones that vary in duration but not in pitch on 'different' trials; 'macro' or 'tempo' tones are included to help establish the meter but these are presented at a relatively low dynamic level and with a different timbre. Practice items are provided with each subtest.

A *Child Music Interest Interview* and a *Parent Music Questionnaire* were constructed for this study. Both contained questions pertaining to the children's musical interests, activities, knowledge, and environment. The parent questionnaire included additional items asking about the child's history of otitis media and hyperacusis.

Procedure

Participants were interviewed and tested at their convenience, either at their homes or at the University of Windsor. After children were interviewed about their musical background and interests, the two music and five language tests were administered in standardized order (i.e., Tonal, Sentence Repetition, Auditory Closure, Controlled Oral Word Association, Digit Span, Rhythm, and PPVT-R). When necessary, test order was modified to maintain the child's interest, but the Tonal subtest always preceded the Rhythm subtest. Parents completed a questionnaire concerning their child's musical and auditory history. For all but two of the WS group, a second session was required for administration of the WISC-III. For one child with WS, results from a recent psychological assessment (1 week prior to testing) were used; another child declined WISC-III testing. All children received a gift of a small toy upon completion of each session.

Administration of the Tonal and Rhythm subtests of the PMMA was adapted slightly to ensure understanding and to maintain interest. The subtests were introduced as 'Mr. Gordon's tests' and the child was asked, 'When is Mr. Gordon going to start?' before the tests began.

Subtests were administered after five practice trials or perfect completion of one practice trial. For children who failed to understand the concepts of *same* and *different* (i.e., 4 children in the WS group, 2 children in the comparison group), *right* and *wrong* were substituted. Because of attentional difficulties, children in the WS group received more breaks and cues to attend than did children in the comparison group.

The Rhythm subtest proved to be especially difficult for a few children. Indeed, for 3 children with WS and 1 comparison child, the measure was unscoreable because of numerous 'don't know' responses or multiple responses per item. Accordingly, these children were given a score of 50% correct (chance level). No child scored below chance on the Tonal subtest.

RESULTS

Verbal Tests

The first set of analyses sought to confirm previously reported patterns of better verbal than visuospatial performance in children with WS. Table 1 provides means, standard deviations, and ranges for the WS group on WISC-III Factors, WISC-III IQ scores, and the PPVT-R. Consistent with previous findings, a paired t test revealed a superiority for verbal over visuospatial skills as measured by the WISC-III Verbal Comprehension and Perceptual Organization Factors, respectively, $t(17) = 7.42$, $p < .001$. The Verbal Comprehension and Perceptual Organization Factors of the WISC-III were used as additional measures of overall verbal and visuospatial functioning because they eliminate extraneous factors (e.g., mental arithmetic, graphomotor speed) present in the more commonly used

Table 1. Scores of Children with Williams Syndrome.

	n	M	(SD)	Range
PPVT-R	19	77.53	(18.33)	48–109
Verbal Comprehension Factor*	18	65.44	(9.65)	50–84
Perceptual Organization Factor*	18	52.56	(3.94)	50–62
VIQ*	18	61.83	(10.27)	46–81
PIQ*	18	50.61	(4.84)	45–62
FSIQ*	18	52.72	(7.60)	40–69

Note. PPVT-R = Peabody Picture Vocabulary Test-Revised; * From the Wechsler Intelligence Scale for Children.

VIQ and PIQ. Nonetheless, a comparison of VIQ and PIQ scores provided additional confirmation that the verbal skills of children with WS were superior to their visuospatial skills, $t(17) = 6.03$, $p < .001$. Indeed, the pattern of higher verbal than nonverbal performance was evident for all children with WS but one, for whom verbal and nonverbal performance were equal.

Additional analyses compared performance on the PPVT-R (a measure of relatively simple verbal skills) with performance on measures of more comprehensive and complex verbal skills, and with performance on nonverbal measures. Consistent with predictions, PPVT-R scores were significantly higher than Verbal Comprehension scores, $t(17) = 4.27$, $p < .001$, and VIQ scores, $t(17) = 5.53$, $p < .001$. Scores on the PPVT-R were also higher than Perceptual-Organization and PIQ scores, $t(17) = 6.43, p < .001$, and $t(17) = 7.35, p < .001$, respectively. Pairwise correlations between PPVT-R and WISC-III scores are provided in Table 2. Although correlations among Factor and related IQ scores and Full Scale IQ were expected, all correlations were significant, which implies that psychometric intelligence accounts for at least some of the variance across measures.

The next set of analyses tested further the hypothesis that the language abilities of the WS group would be inversely related to the complexity of the specific language task. Table 3 provides means and standard deviations for the nine verbal measures administered to the children with WS. A repeated-measures analysis of variance (ANOVA) on standardized scores confirmed that performance varied widely across measures, $F(8, 128) = 17.28$, $p < .001$, from within normal limits on the Auditory Closure task (the simplest task), to almost 3 standard deviations below the norm on the most complex language measure (WISC-III Comprehension).

By contrast, mean levels of performance for the comparison group (see Table 4) were within one standard deviation of the norm for each of the four verbal measures on which they were tested. A repeated-measures ANOVA with one within-subjects factor (standardized scores on the four verbal tests completed by both groups) and one between-subjects factor (WS vs. comparison group) revealed a significant interaction effect, $F(3,90) = 3.63$, $p = .016$, which confirmed that the WS and comparison groups exhibited different patterns of responding across the measures. Follow-up tests examined between-group differences separately for each of the four verbal measures. As shown in Table 4, the WS and comparison groups did not differ on the simplest tests (Auditory Closure and Controlled Oral Word Association). On measures requiring additional mental processing that involved attention and working memory (Sentence Memory and Digit Span), the comparison group's performance was superior to that of the WS group, $t(36) = 2.42$, $p = .021$, and $t(36) = 3.51, p = .001$, respectively. Because of previously reported strengths in

Table 2. Correlations between the Peabody Picture Vocabulary Test-Revised (PPVT-R) and the WISC-III Measures for Children with Williams Syndrome ($n = 18$).

	VC	PO	VIQ	PIQ	FSIQ
PPVT-R	.768	.490	.763	.628	.792
VC		.713	.982	.726	.969
PO			.649	.939	.783
VIQ				.669	.964
PIQ					.835

Note. VC = Verbal Comprehension factor; PO = Perceptual Organization factor. All correlations were significant, $p < .05$.

Table 3. Descriptive Statistics for Children with Williams Syndrome on the Verbal Measures.

	n	M	(SD)
Auditory Closure	19	−0.27	(1.13)
Controlled Oral Word Association	18	−0.78	(1.15)
PPVT-R	19	−1.50	(1.22)
Similarities*	18	−1.87	(0.88)
Digit Span*	19	−1.88	(0.75)
Vocabulary*	18	−1.98	(0.84)
Information*	18	−1.98	(0.85)
Sentence Memory	19	−2.25	(0.98)
Comprehension*	18	−2.74	(0.47)

Note. For comparison purposes, scores are converted to z-scores (number of standard deviations from the mean for normal children of the same mental age).
* WISC-III subtest.

auditory memory (Anderson & Rourke, 1995; Mervis et al., 1999), performance on the Digit Span subtest was further analyzed to examine group differences on the less complex *forward* condition and the more complex *backward* condition. On both tasks, the comparison group's performance was significantly better than the WS group [forward: $t(36) = 3.14$, $p = .003$; backward: $t(36) = 3.10$, $p = .004$].

Music Tests

Means on the Tonal and Rhythm subtests of the PMMA are also provided in Table 4 for both groups of children. A repeated-measures ANOVA with one within-subjects factor (Tonal vs. Rhythm subtest) and one between subject-factor (WS vs. comparison group) revealed a main effect of subtest, $F(1,34) = 45.59$, $p < .001$. Both groups performed better on the Tonal subtest than on the Rhythm subtest [WS group: $t(17) = 6.19$, $p < .001$; comparison group: $t(17) = 3.45$, $p = .003$]. Consistent with predictions, the WS and comparison groups did not differ in their overall performance on the music tests. Although the interaction between group and subtest fell short of statistical significance, $F(1, 34) = 2.92$, $p = .097$, between-group comparisons revealed similar scores on the Tonal subtest but a disadvantage for the WS group on the Rhythm subtest, $t(35) = 2.19$, $p = .036$. Performance on the Tonal and Rhythm subtests was highly correlated for the children with WS, $r = .702$, $N = 18$, $p = .001$, as it was for the children in the comparison group, $r = .773$, $N = 18$, $p < .001$.

Table 4. Scores on the Verbal and Music Measures.

	Williams		Comparison	
	M	(SD)	M	(SD)
Auditory Closure	12.90	(5.03)	10.68	(6.16)
Controlled Oral Word Association	11.79	(4.24)	13.90	(5.22)
Sentence Memory	10.48	(2.44)	12.84	(3.50)*
Digit Span	7.53	(2.50)	10.79	(3.19)*
Digit Span Forward	5.42	(1.35)	7.00	(1.73)*
Digit Span Backward	2.10	(1.37)	3.79	(1.93)*
Tonal	31.94	(5.80)	33.00	(6.17)
Rhythm	25.95	(4.38)	30.11	(6.99)*

Note. * Groups differed significantly, $p < .05$.

To compare performance of the WS group on music measures with their performance on other measures, mental-age based z scores for the Tonal and Rhythm subtests of the PMMA were calculated for the 14 children whose mental age fell within the range of established norms (5.5–9.5 years). These children with WS had a mean mental age (based on PPVT-R performance) of 7 years, 5 months. Mean scores on the Tonal subtest (mental age z-score equivalent = .29) and the Rhythm subtest (mental age z-score equivalent = −.11) were not significantly different from 0, and, thus, typical for mental age. This finding provides additional confirmation that overall performance on the music subtests of the PMMA was consistent with simple verbal abilities, as predicted.

To compare performance of the WS group on music tests with their performance on other verbal and visuospatial measures, z scores for chronological age were *estimated* because test norms did not extend to the chronological age of the WS sample. To illustrate, consider a hypothetical child whose Tonal and Rhythm subtest scores were 0.5 standard deviations above the norm for mental age and 0.2 standard deviations below the norm, respectively, and whose raw PPVT-R score (from which mental age was derived) was 1.5 standard deviations below the norm for chronological age. For chronological age, then, this child's Tonal score was higher than her PPVT-R score but her Rhythm score was lower. To estimate her music abilities relative to chronological age, departures from the norm (i.e., z scores, or *SD* units) were summed. Thus, we estimated that this child would perform 1 $(-1.5 + .5)$ standard deviation below the norm for chronological age on the Tonal subtest, and $-1.7 (-1.5 + -.2)$ standard deviations below the norm for chronological age on the Rhythm subtest.

Mean estimated z scores for the Tonal and Rhythm subtests were -1.17 $(SD = 1.19)$ and $-1.75 (SD = 1.08)$, respectively, both of which are significantly lower than average (i.e., z score = 0), $t(13) = 3.69$, $p = .003$, and $t(13) = 6.06$, $p < .001$, respectively. The finding that tonal and rhythmic discrimination abilities – considered to be indicators of musical aptitude – are well below average for chronological age makes it clear that, as a group, children with WS are *not* musical savants. Rather, their music skills are *relatively* strong when compared to their marked deficits in other areas. Indeed, paired t tests confirmed that estimated z scores on the Tonal subtest were significantly higher than z scores on the WISC-III measures [Verbal Comprehension: $t(12) = 4.19$, $p = .001$; VIQ: $t(12) = 5.45$, $p < .001$; Perceptual Organization: $t(12) = 6.02$, $p < .001$; PIQ: $t(12) = -6.7$, $p < .001$; and FSIQ: $t(12) = 7.02$, $p < .001$]. Similarly, estimated z scores on the Rhythm subtest were significantly higher than Verbal Comprehension scores, $t(12) = 2.83$, $p = .015$, VIQ scores, $t(12) = 4.22$, $p = .001$, Perceptual Organization scores, $t(12) = 4.71, p = .001$, PIQ scores, $t(12) = 5.37$, $p < .001$, and FSIQ scores, $t(12) = 5.83$, $p < .001$. (Thirteen of the children in the WS group had WISC-III results and z scores on the Tonal and Rhythm subtests.)

The next set of analyses evaluated the hypothesis that language and music skills would be correlated.

Table 5. Correlations Between Standardized Scores on the Music and WISC-III Measures for Children with Williams Syndrome ($n = 13$).

	Tonal Subtest	Rhythm Subtest
Verbal Comprehension Factor	.465*	.599**
VIQ	.511**	.618**
Perceptual Organization Factor	.245	.193
PIQ	.364	.287
FSIQ	.552**	.603**

$*p = .055$, $**p < .05$ (one-tailed tests).

Correlations between estimated z scores on the music tests and WISC-III scores for the WS group are provided in Table 5. Despite the relatively small sample, significant positive correlations were evident for the Tonal subtest (i.e., with FSIQ and VIQ) and the Rhythm subtest (i.e., with FSIQ, VIQ, and the Verbal Comprehension factor). In general, music abilities in our relatively small sample of children with WS were significantly associated with verbal abilities and overall intelligence but not with visuospatial abilities.

Correlations for the language measures completed by both groups are provided in Table 6. *Perseverations* on the Controlled Oral Word Association Test (considered pathological) are also included. Although the values in Table 6 provide suggestive evidence that the data from the WS group were somewhat more variable and less strongly correlated than those from the comparison group, statistical comparisons of the magnitude of the correlations revealed no differences between groups. For the groups combined, all measures of language were moderately correlated with the Tonal and Rhythm subtests of the PMMA. Subsequent analyses examined whether the observed associations between language and music skills may have been influenced by mediating variables. Specifically, a series of multiple regressions confirmed that associations between language and music were still evident when differences in age, past history of otitis media, history of ear infection in the past year, past history of hearing loss, current or past history of music lessons, months of music study,

Table 6. Correlations Between Raw Scores on Music and Language Measures for the Williams Syndrome Group, the Control Group, and the Groups Combined.

	Williams Syndrome Group		Control Group		Groups Combined	
	Tonal Subtest	Rhythm Subtest	Tonal Subtest	Rhythm Subtest	Tonal Subtest	Rhythm Subtest
PPVT-R	.374*	.395**	.736**	.507**	.579**	.436**
Auditory Closure	.375*	.426**	.684**	.490**	.520**	.373**
Digit Span	.386*	.261	.643**	.586**	.501**	.551**
Controlled Oral Word Association	.243	.167	.634**	.608**	.465**	.489**
Perseverations	−.740**	−.364*	−.358*	−.339*	−.606**	−.349**
Sentence Memory	.461**	.472**	.671**	.586**	.572**	.611**

$*p < .05$, $**p < .01$ (one-tailed tests).

or hours per week spent listening to music were held constant. In sum, moderately positive correlations between music and language skills were evident, as predicted, and such correlations were equivalent for both groups.

Musical Experience and Interest

Responses on the Child Music Interest Interviews and the Parent Language and Music Questionnaires were used to evaluate and compare groups in terms of their interest in music and their auditory characteristics. The groups did not differ in musical background or environment, or in their history of creating music. In both groups, almost all children (100% of the WS group and 84% of the comparison group) reported that music could make them feel happy. One child in the WS group responded negatively when asked if music could make him happy, but his response was scored affirmatively after he explained that music could not make him happy because it made him *more* than happy. Children in the WS and comparison groups differed, however, when asked if music could make them feel sad. Whereas 79% of the WS group responded affirmatively, only 47% of the comparison group made the same response, $\chi^2(1, N = 36) = 3.95, p = .047$.

Just as children with WS were moved to a greater range of emotions by music than children in the comparison group, they were also more extravagant in rating their overall feelings for music. When asked to describe their interest in music on a scale from 1 (no interest) to 5 (love it), children in the WS group responded more enthusiastically ($M = 4.63$, $SD = .76$) than did those in the comparison group ($M = 3.95$, $SD = 1.08$), $t(36) = 2.26, p = .030$.

The data also corroborated previous reports of hyperacusis in children with WS. Indeed, a history of hyperacusis was evident for *all* of the WS group but for only 10% of the comparison group, $\chi^2(1, N = 38) = 30.76, p < .001$. Unusual fearfulness toward sound was also evident in *all* of the children with WS. Although this characteristic distinguished them from the comparison group, $\chi^2(1, N = 38) = 13.57, p < .001$, a substantial number of comparison children (47%) also had a history of unusual fear for certain sounds. Unusual liking for specific sounds also distinguished the

groups, $\chi^2(1, N = 34) = 17.30, p < .001$; 75% of the children with WS but only one child in the comparison group exhibited an unusual liking for specific sounds. Because otitis media can affect auditory characteristics, the groups were compared on the basis of their history of otitis media, tubes in ears, and hearing loss. No differences between groups were found.

DISCUSSION

We examined the music and language skills of a group of children with WS and compared them to those of a group of normal children with equivalent levels of receptive vocabulary (as measured by the PPVT-R). The findings confirmed previous reports that children with WS perform better on verbal than on nonverbal tasks. In fact, performance on *all* nonverbal tasks, except for Picture Completion (a non-motor visuoperceptual task), was below performance on *all* verbal tasks. We also discovered that children with WS did particularly well (i.e., within the normal range) on tasks measuring relatively simple verbal abilities, but far less well (i.e., about 3 *SD*s below the mean) on measures of more complex language skills. In fact, performance of the children with WS on verbal measures was negatively associated with the complexity of the particular measure, a pattern that distinguished the two groups of children. These findings are completely consonant with predictions arising from the NLD model (Rourke, 1989).

Although it could be argued that the contrast between groups is simply a reflection of the difference in overall intellectual functioning (mentally retarded children are presumed to have difficulty with complexity), the pattern of performance for the WS group is also different from that of the majority of mentally retarded children, who typically perform better on nonverbal than on verbal tasks (Sattler, 1992).

A summary of the WS group's performance across all tasks (as assessed by z scores) is provided in Figure 1. Quantitative measures of music skills revealed that children with WS are relatively 'musical' – much like they are relatively 'linguistic' – with superior performance on the music tests compared to *all* nonverbal tasks and measures of

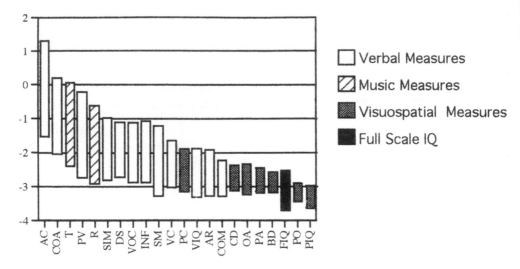

Fig. 1. Mean performance (±1 Standard Deviation) for the WS group on language, music, and visuospatial measures.

complex verbal abilities. Within the limited range of music skills tested, the performance of children with WS was substantially better than one would predict based on their Full Scale, Verbal, or Performance IQs. Indeed, the music skills of children with WS were commensurate with their relatively strong receptive vocabulary (a relatively simple language skill). Moderate correlations between language and music skills were similar for both groups, which implies that simpler aspects of language and music skills are subserved by a common mechanism that is used to process auditory patterns in the general population as well as in the WS population. The present results also suggest that for children with WS, *basic* pattern-perception skills in the auditory modality are stronger than their auditory rote-learning or working-memory abilities, despite the fact that auditory working memory tends to be a relative strength in the WS population (Mervis et al., 1999).

The findings of the present investigation are relevant to contemporary notions of *modularity* (Fodor, 1983; Jackendoff, 1987). According to Fodor (1983), the human mind consists of several *modules*, which are hard-wired areas specified for functioning in a particular domain. One obvious candidate for modularity is language (e.g., Chomsky's Language Acquisition Device). Whereas children with WS have relatively good language skills

despite mild to moderate mental retardation in most cases, aphasics often exhibit good nonverbal skills despite their loss of language. As such, children with WS have often been viewed as the missing link in the search for a double dissociation between language and other abilities (e.g., Levitin & Bellugi, 1998). Although it is possible that *separate* music and language modules (see Jackendoff, 1987) are *both* relatively spared in WS, we find it more parsimonious to speculate that basic abilities to process auditory patterns *in general* underlie the relatively good language *and* music abilities of children with WS. Indeed, because basic, general abilities are antithetical to the modularity concept, we interpret our results as providing rather strong evidence against the idea that WS is characterized by an intact language module or the idea that music and language are distinct modules.

Positive pairwise associations between verbal and nonverbal measures of the WISC-III and PPVT-R provided additional evidence against the idea of modularity of functioning in WS. Rather, the results indicated a role for psychometric intelligence, sometimes hypothesized to reflect general intelligence (*g*), such that children with better verbal and music skills tended to be less impaired overall, even on nonverbal measures. The somewhat greater variability on verbal measures compared to nonverbal measures could stem from floor effects on the nonverbal measures. Alternatively, there could be a greater range of ability in areas where children with WS often perform relatively well.

Even though absolute levels of performance were significantly lower, the WS group's pattern of performance largely paralleled that described by Rourke (1989) for individuals with NLD. Children in the WS group were functioning within the Moderately Mentally Retarded range for Full Scale IQ, Performance IQ, and the Perceptual Organization Factor (see Fig. 1). Scores on the VIQ and Verbal Comprehension Factor were slightly higher, in the Mildly Mentally Retarded Range. Performance on the less complex verbal measure of receptive vocabulary (PPVT-R) was even higher, with a mean score in the upper half of the Borderline range. Thus, our use of mental-age scores based on the PPVT-R – which gave relatively high estimates of verbal functioning – provided a conservative test of our hypothesis that music and verbal abilities would be equivalent.

Performance across language measures was related to task complexity, as predicted on the basis of the NLD model (Rourke, 1989). For the WS group, performance on the Auditory Closure test – arguably the least complex language measure – was closest to the norm. Basic auditory pattern perception is required for this task because it requires children to identify words that are presented in phonemic segments or clusters. Nonetheless, familiarity with the lexicon also affects performance. For example, when the segmented version of the word 'caterpillar' was presented, some children in both the WS and comparison groups identified the word before the last two sounds, 'l' and 'ar' were presented. Because 'caterpillar' is the only English word beginning with the sound pattern 'caterpi,' familiarity with the lexicon allowed these children to identify the word early.

Interestingly, some children in the WS group, but none in the comparison group, provided evidence of accurately synthesizing sound patterns despite lack of familiarity with the word. For example, one child, after correctly responding, 'tractor', asked, 'what is a tractor?' Another child, after responding correctly, asked, 'is that a word?' Children with WS may attend disproportionately to basic phonemic patterns compared to normal children, who may be more likely to rely on word

familiarity. Recent reports of relative strength in phonological fluency among children with WS (Finegan et al., 1996; Mervis et al., 1996; Vicari et al., 1996; Volterra et al., 1996) lend support to the hypothesis that basic auditory pattern perception is intact in these children. Good phonological processing could also help to explain some parents' amazement at how fast their children with WS 'learn' to speak or sing in foreign languages. It is likely, however, that understanding of a foreign language would be very limited for these children.

According to the model of NLD (Rourke, 1989), secondary assets in auditory attention and memory are expected as an outcome of the over-reliance on primary assets in auditory perception and rote learning. For the WS group, performance levels on the Controlled Oral Word Association Test (Animal) were relatively good and similar to levels on the Auditory Closure Test (i.e., within 1 SD of the norm for chronological age). Because rote learning and basic auditory perception are considered primary assets within the NLD model, relatively good performance on this measure was expected.

Although semantic fluency on the word-association task was within the average range, performance of the WS group was inferior to that of the comparison group. This finding implies that semantic fluency and rote learning are less developed in children with WS compared to their basic auditory pattern perception skills. Indeed, poorer performance on measures that place even greater demands on auditory attention or working memory (i.e., Digit Span, Sentence Memory) provides further support for our suggestion that auditory memory is not as strong as simple auditory perception among children with WS. In individuals with WS, their overall level of cognitive functioning may limit the full development of the NLD syndrome such that skills dependent on primary assets in auditory perception are more fully developed than skills dependent on secondary and tertiary assets of auditory attention and rote memory. Nonetheless, the wide range of performance exhibited by the WS group on these measures leaves this speculation open to further investigation.

The present study is the first to provide compelling empirical evidence that music skills represent areas of relative strength for children with WS. Although music skills were at a level typical for mental age based on receptive vocabulary (also a relative strength), they were well below that expected for normal children of equivalent chronological age. In other words, musicality in children with WS may stand out in some instances to clinicians, parents, and teachers because of its *relative* strength, rather than because of high, absolute or savant-like levels of skill.

Although the performance of children with WS on the Tonal and Rhythm subtests was consistent with their mental age, scores on the Rhythm subtest were significantly lower than those for the comparison group. One explanation for this result concerns test order. In compliance with a standardized testing procedure, the Tonal subtest always preceded the Rhythm subtest. Unfortunately, children with WS exhibited notably increased attention difficulties on the Rhythm subtest that were not evident on the Tonal subtest. Similar problems were not observed in the comparison group. Thus, the decrease in Rhythm subtest scores for the WS group relative to the comparison group may have been caused by test order. This hypothesis could be examined in future research by counterbalancing the music subtests with testing order.

The relatively strong music skills of children with WS and the moderate correlations between music and language measures provide support for the hypothesis that relatively intact pattern-perception abilities in the auditory domain underlie *both* music and language skills in children with WS. For the WS group, this interpretation was further supported by the finding of relatively weak correlations between the music tests and measures of visuospatial or visuomotor abilities. It is also important to note, however, that the moderate correlations between language and music skills were equivalent for both groups, which implies that basic auditory-processing abilities underlie some aspects of music and language skills in the general population as well as in the WS population.

The overwhelming prevalence of hyperacusis among children with WS could mean that some aspects of their relatively normal music and language abilities are actually the product of *atypical* auditory processing. Unusual emotional responses to specific sounds were also characteristic of the children with WS and distinguished them from normal children. Specifically, all children in the WS group exhibited unusual fear of specific sounds, and almost two thirds exhibited unusual liking for specific sounds. Moreover, interest in music was higher in the WS group than in the comparison group, as we predicted. One possibility is that relatively intact auditory-perception abilities combined with large visuospatial deficits make auditory stimuli especially salient compared to other stimuli for children with WS. Such increased salience could make it relatively likely for children with WS to have unusual and strong emotional responses to specific sounds, or abnormal sensitivity to particular auditory stimuli. This perspective is similar to the developmental trajectory described by Rourke (1989) for children with NLD.

Questionnaire and interview responses provided additional evidence that emotional responsivity to music may be related to emotional responsivity to sound in general. Although not questioned specifically, 37% of children in the WS group were described by their parents as having an ambivalent relationship with certain sounds. For example, despite extreme fear and anxiety regarding the school fire alarm reported for one child, this same child had an extreme fascination with the same sound when he was placed in charge of initiating the alarm for fire drills. Intense emotional reactions to music were also reported for some children in the WS group. For 2 of the children with WS, a specific love/hate relationship with music was described. For 7 children, an unusual love and fascination with music were reported. Unusual negative reactions to music were described for another 4 children. As babies, these children were reported to scream or cry uncontrollably when they heard lullabies or slow 'relaxing' music. Thus, the music skills of children with WS may develop along a pathway assisted by relatively intact auditory perception abilities, accompanied by fascination and heightened emotional sensitivity.

Implications for Musical Development in Children with WS

The enthusiasm and emotional responsivity to music demonstrated by children in the WS group combined with their relatively intact music abilities raises the possibility that purposeful development of musical skills could help to enrich the lives of these children. It should be noted, however, that there was considerable individual variability in responses toward music. Although most children in the WS group responded enthusiastically toward music, 2 children were notably indifferent toward music and 1 child expressed intense dislike of music. Thus, it would be unwise to apply suggestions for musical development indiscriminately to all children with WS.

In general, physical and cognitive limitations of children with WS are expected to impede skill development in many areas, including music performance. For example, difficulties with fine motor coordination would limit the choices of an appropriate musical instrument for such a child. Bowed stringed instruments generally require high levels of fine motor control to produce even the simplest recognizable song and would be particularly poor choices for instrumental instruction. Guitars require fewer fine motor skills (fretting aids finger placement) and have been a successful choice of instrument for some children with WS when alternative (open) tunings and bar chords were used (National Williams Syndrome Association, 1997); additional instruments reported to be played successfully by children with WS include keyboards, pianos, drums, harmonicas, and trombones. Alternatively, because articulation skills are intact, singing might be an excellent route for the development of musical skill.

Because most children with WS are mentally retarded and because their cognitive profile parallels that of children with NLD (Rourke, 1989), we speculate that music instruction would be most useful if it involved simple tasks, imitation, and an abundance of repetition. Visuospatial-visuomotor impairments and difficulties with complexity are likely to make reading music an unrealistic goal. The fatigue and attentional difficulties noted during testing indicate that teaching sessions should be kept short with breaks provided as necessary. Minimizing distractions and establishing a predictable sequence of events during the music lesson could help to focus and maintain the child's attention.

Findings of creativity and emotional responsivity toward music in children with WS provide additional sources of potential on which musical instruction could be based. For example, challenging a child to create a song using a specific sound, feeling, or technique may help to motivate musical growth. In addition, focusing attention on the sound quality and the emotional aspects of music may help the child to develop productive *and* receptive musical-expression abilities. Because sound preferences, aversions, and emotional responses to music were quite personalized in our sample, these suggestions for teaching may need to be individualized to help each child gain the most from his or her musical experiences.

Limitations

Because our primary goal was to evaluate the level of music skills among children with WS, it was necessary to use standardized measures of such skills. Only a few measures proved to be appropriate for assessing musically untrained children. Consequently, only very basic melodic and rhythmic discrimination skills were assessed. Two limitations involving the administration of the music tests were also observed. One concerned the standardized testing order for the subtests noted earlier. In addition, all children received additional (non-standardized) practice trials when necessary to ensure understanding of the task. Repeated practice trials may have influenced results by inducing practice or fatigue effects. Although between-group comparisons were not affected by this adaptation, comparison with normative data may be less valid than would otherwise be the case.

In a small clinical study such as this, sample size and subject selection are always limitations. Self-selection of subjects is a particularly serious limitation in the present context because the decision to participate in the study might have depended upon the child's interest in music. The possibility that this was an especially 'musical' subgroup from the WS population could not be assessed. Nonetheless, the WS and comparison groups were equivalent in musical background and environment. Moreover, because few children in either group had taken formal music lessons, 'formalized' musicality does not appear to have influenced interest in participating. Indeed, the possibility of self-selection based on musical interest applies equally to both groups and could not be eliminated without random sampling, which is virtually impossible in a study of this sort.

Conclusion

In conclusion, the present study provided an investigation of both a relatively well known and a new area of auditory processing in children with WS – language and music, respectively. The findings yielded evidence of relative strength in both simple music and language skills as predicted based on deductions from the NLD model. The overall pattern of results across verbal tests suggests that skills dependent on primary assets of auditory perception were superior to skills requiring secondary and tertiary assets in auditory attention and memory Overall, findings suggest that intact, basic auditory-processing abilities may underlie the music and language skills observed among these children. In addition, findings suggest that the NLD model may be extended to include relative proficiencies in some simple musical skills.

REFERENCES

Anonymous (1985). Case history of a child with Williams syndrome. *Pediatrics, 75*, 962–968.

Anderson & Rourke (1995). Williams syndrome. In Rourke B.P. (Ed.), *Syndrome of nonverbal learning disabilities: The syndrome and the model* (pp. 138–170). New York: Guilford Publications.

Arnold, R., Yule, W., & Martin, N. (1985). The psychological characteristics of infantile hypercalcaemia: A preliminary investigation. *Developmental Medicine and Child Neurology, 27*, 49–59.

Ashkenas, J. (1996). Williams syndrome starts making sense. *American Journal of Human Genetics, 59*, (756–761).

Bellugi, U., Bihrle, A., Neville, H., Jernigan, T., & Doherty, S. (1992). Language, cognition, and brain organization in a neurodevelopmental disorder. In M. Gunnar & C. Nelson (Eds.), *Developmental behavioral neuroscience* (pp. 201–232). Hillsdale, NJ: Erlbaum.

Bellugi, U., Hickock, G., Jones, W., Jernigan, T. (1996). *The neurological basis of Williams syndrome: Linking brain and behavior.* Paper presented at the seventh international professional Williams syndrome conference, Valley Forge, PA.

Bellugi, U., Marks, S., Bihrle, A., & Sabo, H. (1988). Dissociation between language and cognitive functions in Williams syndrome. In D. Bishop & K. Mogford (Eds.), *Language development in exceptional circumstances* (pp. 177–189). London: Churchill Livingstone.

Bellugi, U., Wang, P., & Jernigan, T. (1994). Williams syndrome: An unusual neuropsychological profile. In S. Broman & J. Grafman (Eds.), *Atypical cognitive deficits in developmental disorders: Implications for brain function* (pp. 23–56). Hillsdale, NJ: Erlbaum.

Cooper, R.P., & Aslin, R.N. (1990). Preference for infant-directed speech in the first month after birth. *Child Development, 61*, 1584–1595.

Dunn, E.S. & Dunn, L.M. (1981). *Peabody Picture Vocabulary Test – Revised.* Circle Pines, MN: American Guidance Service.

Ewart, A.K., Jin, W., Atkinsons, D., Morris, C.A., Keating, M.T. (1994). Supravalvular aortic stenosis associated with a deletion disrupting the elastin gene. *Journal of Clinical Investigation, 93*, 1071–1077.

Fernald, A. (1985). Four-month-old infants prefer to listen to motherese. *Infant Behavior and Development, 8*, 181–195.

Fodor, J.A. (1983). *The modularity of mind.* Cambridge, MA: The MIT Press.

Gordon, E.E., (1980). *Manual for the Primary Measures of Music Audition and the Intermediate Measures of Music Audiation.* Chicago: G.I.A.

Greenberg, F. (1989). Williams syndrome. *Pediatrics, 84*, 922–923.

Hodges, D.A. (1999). Neuromusical research: A review of the literature. In D.A. Hodges (Ed.), *Handbook of music psychology, 2nd ed.* (pp. 197–284). San Antonio: IMR Press.

Jackendoff, R. (1987). *Consciousness and the computational mind.* Cambridge, MA: The MIT press.

Jernigan, T.L., & Bellugi, U. (1990). Anomalous brain morphology on magnetic resonance images in Williams syndrome and Down syndrome. *Archives of Neurology, 47*, 529–533.

Jernigan, T.L., Bellugi, U., Sowell, E., Doherty, S., & Hesselink, J.R. (1993). Cerebral morphologic distinctions between Williams and Down syndromes. *Archives of Neurology, 50*, 186–191.

Judd, H., Gardner, H., & Geschwind, N. (1983). Alexia without agraphia in a composer. *Brain, 106*, 435–457.

Kass, C.E. (1964). Auditory Closure Test. In J.J. Olson & J.L. Olson (Eds.), *Validity studies on the Illinois Test of Psycholinguistic Abilities.* Madison, WI: Photo.

Klein, A.J., Armstrong, B.L., Greer, M.K., & Brown, F.R. (1990). Hyperacusis and otitis media in individuals with Williams syndrome. *Journal of Speech and Hearing Disorders, 55*, 339–344.

Lenhoff, H.M. (1996). *Music and Williams syndrome: A status report and goals.* Paper presented at the seventh international professional Williams syndrome conference, Valley Forge, PA.

Levine, K., (1992). *Information for teachers.* Clawson, MI: The Williams Syndrome Association.

Levitin, D.J., & Bellugi, U. (1998). Musical abilities in Individuals with Williams syndrome. *Music perception, 15*, (357–389).

Lowe, K.G., Henderson, J.L., Park, W.W., & McGreal, D.A. (1954). The idiopathic hypercalcaemic syndromes of infancy. *Lancet, ii*, 101–110.

Marın, O.S.M. (1982). Neurological aspects of music perception and performance. In D. Deutsch (Ed.), *The psychology of music* (pp. 453–477). New York: Academic Press.

McKinnon, M.C., & Schellenberg, E.G. (1997). A left-ear advantage for forced-choice judgements of melodic contour. *Canadian Journal of Experimental Psychology, 51*, 171–175.

Mervis, C.B., Morris, C.A., Bertrand, J., & Robinson, B.F. (1999). Williams Syndrome: Findings from an integrated program of research. To appear in H. Tager-Flusberg (Ed.), *Neurodevelopmental disorders: Contributions to a new framework from the cognitive neurosciences*. Cambridge, MA: MIT Press.

Morris, C.A., Thomas, I.T., Greenberg, F. (1993). Williams syndrome: Autosomal dominant inheritance. *American Journal of Medical Genetics, 47*, 478–81.

Papousek, M., & Papousek, H. (1981). Musical elements in the infant's vocalization: their significance for communication, cognition, and creativity. In L.P. Lipsitt (Ed.), *Advances in infancy research*, (pp. 163–224). Norwood, NJ: Ablex.

Patel, A.D., & Peretz, I. (1997). Is music autonomous from language? A neuropsychological appraisal. In I. Deliege and J. Sloboda (Eds.), *Perception and cognition of music* (pp. 191–215). East Sussex, UK: Psychology Press.

Peretz, I. (1990). Processing of local and global musical information by unilateral brain-damaged patients. *Brain, 113*, 1185–1205.

Peretz, I., & Morais, J. (1989). Music and modularity. *Contemporary Music Review, 4*, 279–293.

Rourke, B.P. (1989). *Nonverbal learning disabilities: The syndrome and the model*. New York: Guilford Press.

Rourke, B.P. (1995). Introduction: The NLD syndrome and the white matter model. In Rourke B.P. (Ed.), *Syndrome of nonverbal learning disabilities: The syndrome and the model* (pp. 1–26). New York: Guilford Publications.

Rourke, B.P. & Tsatsanis, K. (1996). Syndrome of nonverbal learning disabilities: Psycholinguistic assets and deficits. *Topics on Language Disorders, 16(2)*, 30–44.

Sattler, J.M. (1992). *Assessment of children* (3rd ed.). San Diego, CA: Publisher, Inc.

Schlaug, G., Janke, L., Huang, Y., Steinmetz, H. (1995). In vivo evidence of structural brain asymmetry in musicians. *Science, 267*, 699–701.

Sergent, J. (1993). Mapping the musician brain. *Human Brain Mapping 1*, (20–38).

Spreen, O., & Strauss, E. (1991). *A compendium of neuropsychological tests: Administration, norms, and commentary*. New York: Oxford University Press.

Tassabehji, M., Metcalfe, K., Mao, X., Proschel, C., Gutowski, N.J., Fergusson, W.D., Carette, M.J., Dore, J.K., Donnai, D., Read, A.P., & Sheer, D. (1996). *The LIMK gene is deleted in patients with Williams syndrome*. Paper presented at the seventh international professional Williams syndrome conference, Valley Forge, PA.

Trainor, L.J. (1996). Infant preferences for infant-directed versus non-infant-directed play songs and lullabies. *Infant Behavior and Development, 19*, 83–92.

Trainor, L.J., Clark, E.D., Huntley, A., & Adams, B. (1997). The acoustic basis of preferences for infant-directed singing. *Infant Behavior and Development, 20*, 383–396.

Trehub, S.E., & Trainor, L.J. (1998). Singing to infants: Lullabies and play songs. In C. Rovee-Collier, L. Lipsitt, & H. Hayne (Eds.), *Advances in Infancy Research* (pp. 43–77). Stamford, CT: Ablex.

Udwin, O., & Yule, W. (1991). A cognitive and behavioral phenotype in Williams syndrome. *Journal of Clinical and Experimental Neuropsychology, 13*, 232–244.

Udwin, O., Yule, W., & Martin, N. (1987). Cognitive abilities and behavioral characteristics of children with idiopathic infantile hypercalcaemia. *Journal of Child Psychology and Psychiatry, 28*, 297–309.

Von Arnim, G., & Engel, P. (1964). Mental retardation related to hypercalcaemia. *Developmental Medicine and Child Neurology, 6*, 366–377.

Wechsler, D. (1991). *Manual for the Wechsler Intelligence Scale for Children* (3rd ed.). San Antonio, TX: The Psychological Corporation.

Werker, J.F., & McLeod, P.J. (1989). Infant preference for both male and female infant-directed talk: A developmental study of attentional and affective responses. *Canadian Journal of Psychology, 43*, 230–246.

Child Neuropsychology
1997, Vol. 3, No. 3, pp. 192–198

Verbal Learning Strategies of Adolescents and Adults with the Syndrome of Nonverbal Learning Disabilities*

Nancy J. Fisher[1,2] and John W. DeLuca[2]

[1] University of Windsor, Ontario, Canada, and [2] Wayne State University School of Medicine, Detroit, MI

ABSTRACT

Although many psychometric studies of individuals with the syndrome of nonverbal learning disabilities (NLD) have been conducted, one relatively neglected area has been the study of their performance on explicit verbal memory measures. We examined the performance of adolescents and adults with NLD on the California Verbal Learning Test, a measure allowing analysis of self-initiated learning strategies, and compared their performance to age- and Full Scale IQ-matched verbal learning-disabled (VLD) controls. Mean performance of the NLD sample on the semantic clustering index fell one standard deviation below the normative mean, whereas their serial clustering score was within normal limits. Additionally, the serial clustering score for our NLD sample was significantly greater than their semantic clustering score, suggesting that these individuals are more likely to spontaneously employ serial verbal learning strategies as opposed to those that are semantically driven. This difference in serial versus semantic clustering scores was not seen in our VLD controls, who performed equally well, and within normal limits, on both indices.

Adolescents and adults with the syndrome of nonverbal learning disabilities (NLD) display a well-documented pattern of neuropsychological strengths and deficits (Rourke, 1982, 1989, 1995; Rourke & Fisk, 1992). Most notably, such individuals display highly developed rote verbal skills within the context of poor psychomotor, tactile-perceptual, visual-spatial, organizational, and nonverbal problem-solving abilities (Harnadek & Rourke, 1994). Previous studies have shown deficient incidental nonverbal memory (i.e., in terms of Tactual Performance Test *Memory* and *Location* scores [Harnadek & Rourke, 1994] and number of errors on the memory subtest of the Halstead Category Test [Fisher, DeLuca & Rourke, 1997; Strang & Rourke, 1983]) and deficient nonverbal as opposed to verbal memory (e.g., Fletcher, 1985) among those with the syndrome of NLD.

However, detailed analysis of individuals with NLD on specific clinical memory measures such as those assessing explicit memory as distinct from attentional and incidental learning abilities is lacking in the literature. Among child and adolescent samples, these distinct dimensions of memory functioning have been identified in the literature as independent modalities (Sillanpaa & DeLuca, 1995, 1996).

We examined the performances of adolescents and adults diagnosed with the syndrome of NLD on the California Verbal Learning Test (CVLT-C [Children's version]; Delis, Kramer, Kaplan and Ober, 1994; CVLT [Adult version]; Delis, Kramer, Kaplan & Ober, 1987), a well-known explicit learning measure. This instrument is a great contribution to the neuropsychologist's arsenal of measurement tools as it allows: (1) assessment of the

* A preliminary version of this paper was presented at the 8th Annual Meeting of the American Neuropsychiatric Association. Orlando, FL. February 4th, 1997.
Address correspondence to: John W. DeLuca, Wayne State University School of Medicine, Department of Psychiatry, University Psychiatric Center, 2751 E. Jefferson Avenue, Suite 200, Detroit, MI 48207, USA.
Accepted for publication: May 16, 1997.

component skills required for successful retention of verbal material in a rote learning context; and (2) analysis of spontaneous, self-initiated verbal learning strategies, among other dimensions. On the basis of the NLD model (Rourke, 1982, 1989, 1995), we hypothesized that due to poor organizational but well-developed rote skills, a serial clustering strategy as opposed to a semantic clustering learning strategy would predominate for our NLD sample. Indeed, in outlining the linguistic assets and deficits of the NLD syndrome, Rourke and Tsatsanis (1996) note well-developed verbatim encoding, or automatization skills, but reduced appreciation of contextual/conceptual semantic cues. Consistent with these features of the syndrome, we expected that our NLD subjects would demonstrate impairment in terms of their semantic clustering score, yet perform within the average to high-average range in terms of their serial clustering performance. To provide control in testing these hypotheses, we compared our NLD sample with an age- and Full Scale IQ-matched verbal learning-disabled (VLD) control group. Based on past CVLT research involving VLD children (Shear, Tallal & Delis, 1992), we predicted that, unlike our NLD sample, the VLD group would evince no significant difference between their use of serial and semantic verbal learning strategies,

performing in a manner analogous to cognitively normal individuals on these two indices.

METHOD

Subjects

Archival CVLT data (i.e., CVLT-C or CVLT) from 7 individuals with NLD (4 children/adolescents, 3 adults) and 7 individuals with VLD (4 children/adolescents, 3 adults) were utilized in this investigation. All subjects were diagnosed by the same licensed clinical neuropsychologist (J.W.D.), between the years 1987 and 1996, after having been administered an extended Halstead-Reitan neuropsychological test battery. All had been referred to one of three metropolitan outpatient clinics for evaluation regarding academic/cognitive, behavioral, and/or socio-emotional difficulties. Sixty-four percent of the participants were male and right-handed. The NLD and VLD groups did not differ significantly in terms of mean Full Scale IQ (WISC-R, WISC-III, or WAIS-R; Wechsler, 1974, 1981, 1991) [$t(12) = .572$, $p = .578$] or age [$t(12) = .189, p = .854$].

All NLD participants met the majority of neuropsychological test performance criteria for classification of potential NLD subjects outlined by Harnadek and Rourke (1994) (see Table 1). All displayed a Wechsler Intelligence Scale (WISC-R, WISC-III, or WAIS-R; Wechsler, 1974, 1981, 1991), VIQ > PIQ pattern; the mean VIQ > PIQ difference was 11.57 ($SD = 9.31$). Additionally, all demonstrated inferior performances

Table 1. Criteria for Potential NLD Subjects (Harnadek & Rourke, 1994) Met by the Current Sample.

Harnadek & Rourke (1994) Criteria for Potential NLD Subjects	Subject Number						
	1	2	3	4	5	6	7
WISC VIQ > 79	$-^1$	+	+	+	+	+	+
SSPT[a] or Auditory Closure[b] ≤ 1 SD below the mean	+	+	+	+	+	+	+
WRAT Reading & Spelling > Arithmetic by 10 or more SS	+	$-^3$	+	+	+	+	+
Target Test[a] ≥ 1 SD below the mean	N/A	N/A	N/A	N/A	N/A	N/A	N/A
VIQ > PIQ by 10 or more points	$-^2$	+	+	−	−	−	+
Grooved Pegboard (# errors; either hand)[c] ≥ 1 SD below the mean	+	+	+	+	+	+	+
Dysgraphesthesia, finger agnosia, or astereognosis (# errors)[a] ≥ 1 SD below the mean	+	+	−	−	+	+	N/A
Percent of available criteria met	67	83	83	67	83	83	100

Note. N/A = not administered; NLD = Nonverbal Learning Disabled; PIQ = Performance Intelligence Quotient; SD = Standard Deviation; SS = Scaled Score; SSPT = Speech Sounds Perception Test; VIQ = Verbal Intelligence Quotient; WISC = Wechsler Intelligence Scale for Children; WRAT = Wide Range Achievement Test; + = meets criterion; − = does not meet criterion; [1] VIQ = 78; [2] VIQ > PIQ by 9 points; [3] Reading = 105, Spelling = 129, Arithmetic = 96.
[a] Reitan & Davison, 1974, [b] Kass, 1964, [c] Kløve, 1963.

on academic achievement tests of arithmetic as compared to their performances on achievement tests of spelling and reading (i.e., Wide Range Achievement Test-2nd or 3rd version; Jastak & Wilkinson, 1984; Wilkinson, 1993).

The VLD controls were diagnosed with language, speech, reading, or other primarily verbally-based learning or output disorders. They were specifically selected to match the NLD participants in terms of Full Scale IQ and age. All VLD subjects displayed a PIQ > VIQ pattern; the mean PIQ minus VIQ difference was 11.71 (SD = 4.61). (See Table 2 for descriptive demographic and neuropsychological data of interest.)

Measures

The California Verbal Learning Test for Children (CVLT-C; Delis et al., 1994) involves two shopping lists of 15 items each (i.e., List A and List B). List A is composed of five different types of fruit, toys, and articles of clothing; List B comprises five different types of fruit, desserts, and household items. On neither list are items from the same semantic category ever presented consecutively. In administering the test, the child is first told that s/he will be read a list of items to buy on a pretend Monday shopping trip, and instructed to listen

carefully and try to remember as many items from the list as possible, in any order. The examiner then proceeds to read List A at a speed of one word per second. Following this, the examiner records the child's responses verbatim; no reminder cues are given. Next, List A is reread, and once again the child is asked to recall as many items from the list as s/he can in any order, including those reported on the first trial. Again the examiner records the child's responses verbatim. This procedure is repeated for three more learning trials. On each of the five learning trials, the items are read in the same order.

Following the above List A free recall learning trials, the child is informed that s/he will now be read a new shopping list of things to buy on Tuesday (i.e., List B). Again the examinee is instructed to listen carefully while the list is read, and to try to remember as many of the items on the list as possible, in any order. After the list is read, the examiner records the child's responses verbatim.

Immediately upon completion of the List B free recall trial, the child is asked to list as many items as possible from the Monday list (i.e., List A), without List A being reread in the interim. Following this, a List A category cued recall trial is given, in which the child

Table 2. Descriptive Demographic and Psychometric Data.

Variable	M(SD)				Range		n	
	NLD		VLD		NLD	VLD	NLD	VLD
Demographics (Raw)								
Age (years)	19.00	(10.89)	20.43	(16.83)	11–42	10–58	7	7
Male							5	4
Female							2	3
Right-Handed							5	4
Left-Handed							2	3
CVLT (T scores)								
Semantic Clustering	40.00	(7.64)	47.14	(8.59)	30–50	40–65	7	7
Serial Clustering	48.57	(7.48)	44.29	(4.50)	40–60	40–50	7	7
WISC-R/WISC-III/WAIS-R (SS)								
FSIQ	79.43	(3.60)	80.57	(3.87)	73–85	76–88	7	7
PIQ*	74.14	(5.67)	88.14	(5.30)	67–82	84–98	7	7
VIQ*	85.71	(5.65)	76.43	(3.87)	77–93	72–83	7	7
WRAT-R/WRAT-III (SS)								
Reading	99.29	(6.18)	82.57	(18.95)	87–105	53–106	7	7
Spelling*	101.00	(16.73)	79.86	(11.48)	78–129	68–103	7	7
Arithmetic	76.86	(16.84)	74.29	(8.79)	45–95	63–89	7	7

Note. FSIQ = Full Scale Intelligence Quotient; NLD = Nonverbal Learning Disabled; PIQ = Performance Intelligence Quotient; SS = Standard Scores; VIQ = Verbal Intelligence Quotient; VLD = Verbal Learning Disabled; WAIS-R = Wechsler Adult Intelligence Scale Revised; WISC-R = Wechsler Intelligence Scale for Children; WISC-III = Wechsler Intelligence Scale for Children 3rd Revision; WRAT-R = Wide Range Achievement Test Revised; WRAT-III = Wide Range Achievement Test 3rd Revision.

*p < .05 (indicates significant between-group [i.e., NLD vs. VLD] differences).

is asked to list all the items on the Monday list that were "things to wear," then "things to play with," and finally "fruit." After this trial, other nonmemory or nonverbal tests are administered for a 20-min period. Then, without the list being reread, the child is again asked to list as many items from the Monday shopping list as s/he is able. Next, a List A long delay cued recall trial is administered with the same category cues given as in the short delay cued-recall trial. Finally, the child is read a list of shopping items comprised of the List A items, some List B items, and new (yet sometimes phonemically or semantically similar) distractor items, and asked after each item to say "yes" if the object was on the Monday list and "no" if it was not on the Monday list.

The adult version of the CVLT is analogous to the children's version, except there are four semantic categories of four items each, rather than three categories of five items (see Delis et al., 1987, for a complete description). The variables of interest in this study are the serial and semantic clustering scores.

The *serial clustering* score refers to the number of instances in which the examinee reports two consecutive items in the same order as they had appeared on the word list. This score is calculated as the ratio of observed serial clustering instances to those expected by chance (Delis et al., 1987, 1994).

The *semantic clustering* score refers to the number of instances in which the examinee reports two consecutive responses from the same semantic category. This score is the ratio of the observed versus expected number of semantic category related pairs reported, taking into account the total number of responses for each trial and the number of categories from which the examinee has given responses (Delis et al., 1987, 1994).

RESULTS

Scores on the CVLT-C and CVLT semantic and serial clustering variables were converted to T scores ($M = 50$, $SD = 10$; higher scores indicating better performance) using normative data generated by the CVLT and the CVLT-C scoring assistant software (Fridlund & Delis, 1987, 1994). The performance of the NLD group in terms of mean serial clustering T score was within normal limits ($M = 48.57$, $SD = 7.48$), whereas their mean semantic clustering T score fell within the mildly impaired range ($M = 40.00$, $SD = 7.64$). On the other hand, the performance of the VLD group in terms of both mean serial ($M = 44.29$, $SD = 4.5$) and semantic ($M = 47.14$, $SD = 8.59$) clustering T scores were within normal limits.

Within-group paired samples t tests comparing serial to semantic clustering scores indicated significantly greater use of serial as compared to semantic clustering in the NLD group [$t(6) = 3.286$, $p < .05$], but no significant differences between the serial and semantic clustering scores of the VLD group [$t(6) = .703, p = .51$] (see Figure 1).

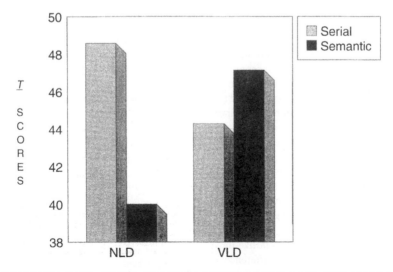

Fig. 1. Mean serial and semantic clustering T scores for the NLD and VLD groups. NLD = Nonverbal Learning Disabled; VLD = Verbal Learning Disabled.

A one-way ANOVA with diagnostic group serving as the independent variable and the mean difference between the serial and semantic clustering T scores (i.e., mean of serial clustering T score minus semantic clustering T score) serving as the dependent variable, revealed a significant main effect of group, with the NLD group showing a significant discrepancy between the two scores, and the VLD group showing only a minimal mean difference score $[F (1,12) = 5.606, p < .05; \eta^2 = .318]$. The effect size, f, obtained for this difference was .683 which is, according to Cohen (1977, p. 284), considered to be a "very large" effect size for an ANOVA result. Given our small sample size, the power for this ANOVA was calculated by reference to tables provided by Cohen (1977) and Howell (1992) (and subsequent linear interpolation) to be approximately .654, indicating a 65.4% probability of correctly rejecting a false H_0. Of note, assuming the effect size remains constant, simply increasing the current sample size to 18 (i.e., adding 2 subjects to each group) would give us a more substantial power figure of .80 (Cohen, p. 384).

DISCUSSION

Within the context of the CVLT, we investigated the verbal learning strategies spontaneously employed by those with the syndrome of NLD, predicting on the basis of the Rourke (1982, 1989, 1995) model that due to poor conceptual/organizational but well-developed rote skills, a serial clustering strategy as opposed to a semantic clustering strategy would predominate. We also expected that our NLD subjects would demonstrate impairment in terms of their semantic clustering score, yet perform within the average to high average range in terms of their serial clustering performance.

As predicted, the mean serial clustering T score for our NLD sample was significantly greater than their semantic clustering T score, suggesting that individuals with this type of learning disability are more likely to spontaneously employ serial verbal learning strategies and less likely to utilize those that are semantic in nature. This difference in mean serial versus semantic clustering T scores was not present for our VLD controls.

With respect to our second hypothesis, the mean performance of our NLD group on the semantic clustering index fell one standard deviation below the normative mean, although their serial clustering score was within normal limits. This pattern of performance differed from that of the VLD group, which performed equally well and within normal limits on both the serial and semantic clustering indices.

The results of this study imply that individuals with NLD are more likely to spontaneously employ serial verbal learning strategies as opposed to those that are semantically driven, suggesting a passive approach unreliant upon organizational abilities (Delis et al., 1994) or the appreciation of contextual cues (Rourke & Tsatsanis, 1996). These findings provide support for Rourke's (1982, 1989, 1995) NLD model, suggesting that those with the syndrome of NLD are not apt to utilize semantic content as a memory aid. Our VLD findings are consistent with those of Shear, Tallal, and Delis (1992) who employed the earlier research version of the CVLT and found no difference in terms of serial or semantic clustering performance between cognitively normal children and those with developmental verbal learning disabilities.

Given the small sample size, the findings reported herein are preliminary and investigations employing larger samples are encouraged. Enlarging the sample size in this manner would allow greater power, reducing the chances of Type II error. Nevertheless, the large effect size we obtained suggests that despite our limited sample, the results reported here are of significant magnitude, likely reflecting substantial serial versus semantic performance differences in the NLD population at large.

REFERENCES

Cohen, J. (1977). *Statistical power analysis for the behavioral sciences* (Rev. ed.). New York: Academic Press.

Delis, D.C., Kramer, J.H., Kaplan, E., & Ober, B.A. (1987). *California Verbal Learning Test Adult Version-manual*. San Antonio, TX: The Psychological Corporation.

Delis, D.C., Kramer, J.H., Kaplan, E., & Ober, B.A. (1994). *California Verbal Learning Test for*

Children-manual. San Antonio, TX: The Psychological Corporation.

Fisher, N.J., DeLuca, J.W., & Rourke, B.P. (1997). Wisconsin Card Sorting Test and Halstead Category Test performances of children and adolescents who exhibit the nonverbal learning disabilities syndrome. *Child Neuropsychology, 3,* 61–70.

Fletcher, J.M. (1985). External validation of learning disability typologies. In B.P. Rourke (Ed.), *Neuropsychology of learning disabilities: Essentials of subtype analysis* (pp. 187–211). New York: Guilford Press.

Fridlund, A.J., & Delis, D.C. (1987). *Administration and scoring software program and user's guide for the California Verbal Learning Test.* San Antonio, TX: The Psychological Corporation.

Fridlund, A.J., & Delis, D.C. (1994). *California Verbal Learning Test-Children's Version (CVLT-C) scoring assistant software.* San Antonio, TX: The Psychological Corporation.

Harnadek, M.C.S., & Rourke, B.P. (1994). Principal identifying features of the syndrome of nonverbal learning disabilities in children. *Journal of Learning Disabilities, 27,* 144–154.

Howell, D.C. (1992). *Statistical methods for psychology* (3rd ed.). Belmont, CA: Duxbury Press.

Jastak, S., & Wilkinson, G. (1984). *Wide Range Achievement Test-Revised.* Wilmington, DE: Jastak Associates.

Kass, C.E. (1964). Auditory Closure Test. In J.J. Olson & J.L. Olson (Eds.), *Validity studies on the Illinois Test of Psycholinguistic Abilities.* Madison, WI: Photo.

Kløve, H. (1963). Clinical neuropsychology. In F.M. Forster (Ed.), *The medical clinics of North America* (pp. 1647–1658). New York: Saunders.

Reitan, R.M., & Davison, L.A. (1974). *Clinical neuropsychology: Current status and applications.* Washington, DC: V.H. Winston.

Rourke, B.P. (1982). Central processing deficiencies in children: Toward a developmental neuropsychological model. *Journal of Clinical Neuropsychology, 4,* 1–18.

Rourke, B.P. (1989). *Nonverbal learning disabilities: The syndrome and the model.* New York: Guilford Press.

Rourke, B.P. (1995). Introduction and overview: The NLD/white matter model. In B.P. Rourke (Ed.), *Syndrome of nonverbal learning disabilities: Neurodevelopmental manifestations* (pp. 1–26). New York: Guilford Press.

Rourke, B.P., & Fisk, J.L. (1992). Adult presentations of learning disabilities. In R.F. White (Ed.), *Clinical syndromes in adult neuropsychology: The practitioner's handbook* (pp. 451–473). Amsterdam: Elsevier.

Rourke, B.P., & Tsatsanis, K.D. (1996). Syndrome of nonverbal learning disabilities: Psycholinguistic assets and deficits. *Topics of Language Disorders, 16,* 30–44.

Shear, P.K., Tallal, P., & Delis, D.C. (1992). Verbal learning and memory in language impaired children. *Neuropsychologia, 30,* 451–458.

Sillanpaa, M.C., & DeLuca, J.W. (1995). Dimensions and patterns of memory functioning in children and adolescents. *The Clinical Neuropsychologist, 9,* 268.

Sillanpaa, M.C., & DeLuca, J.W. (1996). *Dimensions and patterns of memory functioning in children and adolescents.* Manuscript submitted for publication.

Strang, J.D., & Rourke, B.P. (1983). Concept-formation/nonverbal reasoning abilities of children who exhibit specific academic problems with arithmetic. *Journal of Clinical Child Psychology, 12,* 33–39.

Wechsler, D. (1974). *Manual for the Wechsler Intelligence Scale for Children-Revised.* San Antonio, TX: The Psychological Corporation.

Wechsler, D. (1981). *Manual for the Wechsler Adult Intelligence Scale-Revised (WAIS-R).* San Antonio, TX: The Psychological Corporation.

Wechsler, D. (1991). *Manual for the Wechsler Intelligence Scale for Children-III.* San Antonio, TX: The Psychological Corporation.

Wilkinson, G.S. (1993). *Wide Range Achievement Test-3 Manual.* Wilmington, DE: Wide Range.

Journal of Clinical and Experimental Neuropsychology
1993, Vol. 15, No. 1, pp. 40–41

Relationships of Cognitive Skills and Cerebral White Matter in Hydrocephalic Children

J.M. Fletcher, T.P. Bohan, M. Brant, S.R. Beaver, K. Thorstad, B.L. Brookshire, D.J. Francis, K.C. Davidson, and N.M. Thompson

ABSTRACT

Fletcher et al. reported that quantitative MRI measurements of cerebral white matter structures, particularly the corpus callosum, of hydrocephalic children, were strongly correlated with nonverbal cognitive skills. This study provided quantitative measurement of the corpus callosum, lateral ventricles, and internal capsules in a much larger sample of children with diverse etiologies of hydrocephalus and nonhydrocephalic comparison children. Results continued to show that corpus callosum size correlated significantly higher with nonverbal than verbal skills. Relationships of cognitive skills with the size of the lateral ventricles were less robust, reflecting the inclusion of diverse etiologies of hydrocephalus. Internal capsule measurements also showed stronger relationships with nonverbal than verbal cognitive skills. These findings support the relationship between early malformations of the corpus callosum, other white matter changes, and subsequent reductions in nonverbal cognitive skills.

Child Neuropsychology
2000, Vol. 6, No. 4, pp. 262–273

Visual Integration Difficulties in a 9-year-old Girl With Turner Syndrome: Parallel Verbal Disabilities?

Sandra L. Hepworth[1,3] and Joanne F. Rovet[1,2]

[1]Brain and Behaviour Program, The Hospital for Sick Children, [2]Department of Pediatrics, and [3]Department of Psychology, The University of Toronto, Toronto, Canada

ABSTRACT

Turner syndrome (TS) is a genetic disorder in females that arises from the loss of X chromosome material. Affected individuals demonstrate a characteristic neuropsychological profile of strengths in verbal processing and weaknesses in visuospatial processing, consistent with the Nonverbal Learning Disabilities syndrome. Previous research has described a wide range of visuospatial deficits in TS; however, their verbal abilities are less extensively studied. The present paper describes the processing difficulties of a 9-year-old girl with TS who demonstrated problems in integrating details of a complex visual display and using organizational terms to describe visual scenes or events. Her specific cognitive disabilities were thought to underlie some of the social and behavioral problems she was currently experiencing. Her pattern of results is consonant with the neuropsychological pattern that others have attributed to right hemisphere dysfunction and/or white matter abnormality.

Turner syndrome (TS), a genetic condition affecting only females, is typically associated with a deficit in processing visuospatial information and intact verbal abilities. The visuospatial difficulties of affected individuals include problems in direction and route finding (Money & Alexander, 1966), construction (McGlone, 1985; Murphy et al., 1994), design copying (Waber, 1979), drawing (Temple & Carney, 1995), mazes (Nielsen, Nyborg, & Dahl, 1977), mental rotation (Berch & Kirkendall, 1986; Rovet & Netley, 1982), puzzle assembly (Temple & Carney, 1995), visual memory (Bishop et al., 2000; Buchanan, Pavlovic, & Rovet, 1998; Murphy et al., 1994; Ross, Roeltgen, & Cutler, 1995), visual-motor integration (Lewandowski, Costenbader, & Richman, 1985), and also part–whole perception (Silbert, Wolff, & Lilienthal, 1977). Despite reports of early speech and language difficulties (Robinson et al., 1986), subsequent verbal abilities

are usually considered to be normal (Money, 1993; Rovet, 1990). However, their profile of specific language abilities has not been adequately studied. In addition to the selective cognitive deficits just mentioned, individuals with TS often also manifest problems processing social information and have difficulty with social communication (McCauley, 1990; McCauley, Ross, Kushner, & Cutler, 1995; Rovet & Ireland, 1994). As well, they show academic difficulties in arithmetic (Rovet, Szekely, & Hockenberry, 1994; Temple & Carney, 1993), especially calculations and fact retrieval (Temple & Marriott, 1998). In contrast, their reading skills are normal, if not advanced. Overall, their pattern of strengths and weaknesses is consistent with Rourke's depiction of the syndrome of Nonverbal Learning Disabilities (Rourke, 1989). We describe here our findings on a 9-year-old girl with TS who showed a selective

Address correspondence to: Sandra Hepworth, Psychology Department, The Hospital for Sick Children, 555 University Avenue, Toronto, Ont., Canada M5G 1X8. Tel.: +1-416-813-8283. Fax: +1-416-813-8839. E-mail: sandra.hepworth@sickkids.on.ca
Accepted for publication: February 12, 2001.

visuospatial impairment in integrating details of a complex visual scene into a meaningful whole. This difficulty was also evident in her processing of verbal information, despite her seemingly strong verbal abilities. Moreover, this cognitive difficulty also seemed to impact on her social and behavioral functioning.

Turner syndrome (TS) is a genetic disorder that affects about 1 in 5,000 females (Hook & Warburton, 1983; Murphy et al., 1993; Nielsen et al., 1977). It arises as a consequence of a loss of X chromosome material. In about 50% of cases, an entire X chromosome is missing, which is designated as the 45,X karyotype. The remainder of individuals with TS have either a mosaic karyotype with cells containing both the normal 46,XX and the 45,X complement or a structural rearrangement of one or both X chromosomes (Hook & Warburton, 1983; Simpson, 1975). The molecular basis of TS, including identification of candidate genes (Zinn & Ross, 1998), is the focus of considerable research in this field. The physical phenotype involves short stature, mild skeletal abnormalities, and gonadal dysgenesis that leads to a lack of estrogen production and abnormal development of secondary sexual characteristics (Simpson, 1975). Generally, the severity and type of stigmata observable depend upon the specific karyotype, with more severe presentations being associated with the 45,X karyotype (Ross, 1990). Although, estrogen therapy facilitates pubertal development, the majority of females remain infertile. Furthermore, treatment with growth hormone provides moderate increases in ultimate stature (Siegel, Clopper, & Stabler, 1998).

The selective cognitive difficulties of TS have been attributed to both estrogen insufficiency (Ross, Roeltgen, Feuillan, Kushner, & Cutler, 1998, 2000) and genetic factors (Zinn & Ross, 1998). More recently, different specific disabilities have also been attributed to a phenomenon known as genetic imprinting, or the parental origin of the single X chromosome (Jacobs et al., 1997; Skuse et al., 1997). Bishop et al. (2000), for example, reported that females with maternal genotypes (i.e. lack of paternal X chromosome material) had poor verbal memory, whereas females with paternal genotypes had poor visuospatial memory. As with their physical stigmata, the cognitive and behavioral

deficits of individuals with TS are generally more severe in individuals with the 45,X than a mosaic karyotype (Bender, Linden, & Robinson, 1990; O'Neill, Ghelani, Rovet, & Chitiyat, 2000; Rovet & Ireland, 1994; Swillen et al., 1993; Temple & Carney, 1993). Estrogen therapy (Ross et al., 1998), but not growth-hormone therapy (Siegel et al., 1998), is associated with improved outcome in nonverbal processing.

A number of investigators have attempted to identify the neuroanatomic basis of the cognitive deficit in TS. The earliest studies used laterality and neuropsychological tasks to determine whether hemispheric organization for verbal and spatial information was atypical in these individuals (McGlone, 1985; Netley, 1977). The findings of impaired spatial processing were interpreted as evidence of right hemisphere dysfunction (Netley & Rovet, 1983). Because of the resemblance between the TS cognitive profile and the Nonverbal Learning Disabilities syndrome, Rourke's white matter hypothesis was subsequently invoked to account for these findings (Rovet, 1995). According to this hypothesis, visual-spatial impairments result from white matter or myelin deficiencies, which impact to a greater degree on right than left hemisphere processing because of the greater proportion of white matter within the right hemisphere. Recent structural neuroimaging studies have not fully supported this model demonstrating different regional distribution in both gray and white matter (Murphy et al., 1993; Reiss et al., 1993; Ross, Reiss, Freund, Roeltgen, & Cutler, 1993) with white matter reductions in the right and left parietal lobes and increases in the right inferior parietal–occipital region (Reiss, Mazzocco, Greenlaw, Freund, & Ross, 1995). Studies using positron emission tomography have also demonstrated atypical activation of left and right occipital and/or parietal cortices (Clark, Klonoff, & Hayden, 1990; Murphy et al., 1997). In light of findings that functional specialization appears to be altered in genetic syndromes (Karmiloff-Smith, 1998) and that effects tend to impact low-level cognitive processes (Donnai & Karmiloff-Smith, 2000), further studies are required to identify the core deficit in TS.

The present report describes our findings on a girl with TS who underwent an extensive neuropsychological investigation for reported school and social difficulties. As expected, she demonstrated the classic profile of the syndrome reflecting a nonverbal learning deficit with well-developed verbal skills in most areas examined. Her difficulty processing visuospatial information seemed to arise from an inability to process the global aspects of visual arrays, which she instead processed in a strictly local manner with little integration of details. Interestingly, this approach was also observed in her processing of verbal material and was thought to underlie some of the difficulties she was experiencing in social interactions and social communication.

METHOD

Participant

CB (fictitious initials) is a 9-year-old girl who was diagnosed with TS 1 year previously. Her genetic karyotype was found to be 45,X. She began growth hormone treatment shortly after diagnosis. During her pregnancy, CB's mother suffered from nausea and migraines, which were treated with Tylenol and acupuncture. In addition, she experienced toxemia toward the end of the pregnancy. Otherwise, the pregnancy and birth were unremarkable. As an infant, CB had some feeding difficulties, probably related to her high arched palate. At 18 months of age, CB was diagnosed with an atrial-septal defect heart condition. However, developmental milestones were reportedly attained within normal limits. She was in grade 4 at the time of testing.

The present assessment was requested because of reported academic and social difficulties. While her reading was good, she was said to be struggling with math, French language learning, spelling, and writing, and had memory and attention difficulties. CB reportedly has shown significant social and emotional distress beginning as early as grade 1, at which time she was seen by a psychiatrist. In addition to her academic struggles, she has had difficulty in making and keeping friends. Combined with her chronic anxiety, these social problems are also thought to be contributing to her difficulty at school.

Neuropsychological Assessment

CB was administered a battery of neuropsychological tests that included portions of the Wechsler Intelligence Test for Children – III (Wechsler, 1991), the Children's Memory Scale (Cohen, 1997), the Test of Everyday Attention for Children (Manly, Robertson, Anderson, & Nimmo-Smith, 1999), NEPSY (Korkman, Kirk, &

Kemp, 1998), the Wechsler Individual Achievement Test (The Psychological Corporation, 1992), the Wide Range Assessment of Visual Motor Abilities (Adams & Sheslow, 1995), the Complex Figure of the Denman Neuropsychological Memory Scale[1] (Denman, 1984), and the Conners' Continuous Performance Test (Conners, 1992). She also completed the Piers-Harris Children's Self-Concept Scale – Revised (Piers, 1984) and projective drawing tests (Draw-a-Person, Draw-a-Family, and Draw-a-Clock).

Her parents completed the Conners' Rating Scale (Conners, 1997) and the Achenbach Child Behavior Checklist (Achenbach, 1991a). Her teacher completed the Conners' Rating Scale (1997) and the Teachers Report Form (Achenbach, 1991b).

RESULTS

Neuropsychological test results are shown in Table 1 as both Index scores (all with a mean of 100 and a standard deviation of 15) and percentiles (with the average range extending from the 25th to 75th percentile) wherever possible. Of particular note is CB's profile of strengths and weaknesses. She showed a significant discrepancy between her above average Verbal IQ and her below average Performance IQ. On the Children's Memory Scale, CB's global performance was within the average range; however, she demonstrated a disparity between her better verbal than visual memory skills. In addition, while her visual memory skills appeared to be adequate for simple visual displays (i.e. Dot Location), they were considerably weaker when complex visual configurations such as faces were involved. On the NEPSY Visuospatial Index, it is noteworthy that CB performed in the superior range on Design Copy, but was significantly weaker on Arrows and Route Finding, where she performed in the low and below average ranges, respectively. Similarly, on the Wide Range Assessment of Visual Motor Abilities, CB performed in the deficient range on the Matching and Pegboard subtests. On tests of attention, she showed average performance on Map Mission and atypical

---

[1] Although normative values for the Complex Figure for 9-year-old children are only available from Bernstein & Waber (1996), CB was given a 40 min delay, consistent with the Denman Neuropsychological Memory Scale (1984), whose normative values begin at age 10.

Table 1. CB's Neuropsychological Test Results.

Test	Index score[a]	Percentile[b]
Wechsler Intelligence Scale for Children – III		
Verbal IQ	113	81
Performance IQ	83	13
Full Scale IQ	99	47
Verbal Comprehension Index	113	81
Perceptual Organization Index	80	10
Freedom from Distractibility Index	106	66
Children's Memory Scale		
Visual Immediate Index	94	34
Visual Delay Index	94	34
Verbal Immediate Index	112	79
Verbal Delay Index	106	66
General Memory Index	103	58
Attention/Concentration Index	106	66
Learning Index	106	66
Delayed Recognition Index	97	42
NEPSY		
Attention/Executive Functioning Index	104	61
Language Index	103	58
Sensorimotor Index	95	37
Visuospatial Index	106	66
Wechsler Individual Achievement Test		
Reading Index	113	81
Mathematics Index	99	47
Wide Range Assessment of Visual Motor Abilities		
Matching Index	72	3
Pegboard Index	72	3
Test of Everyday Attention for Children		
Map Mission	NA	50
Complex Figure[c]		
Copying	NA	1
Immediate recall	NA	1
Delayed recall	NA	1
Continuous Performance Test[d]		
Hits (%)	NA	92.0
Commission errors	51.2	54.8
Hit RT	40.7	20.3
Hit RT SE	73.9	99.0
Attentiveness	58.0	78.9
Risk taking	76.6	99.0

Note. [a] All index scores are based on a mean of 100 and a standard deviation of 15. Index scores were not available for the Test of Everyday Attention for Children and Complex Figure.
[b] For percentile scores, the average range extends from the 25th to the 75th percentile.
[c] For the Complex Figure, results from the Denman Neuropsychological Memory Scale are reported; however, immediate and delayed scores using Bernstein & Waber's (1996) criteria were also calculated with performance similarly at the 1st percentile using a part-oriented approach.
[d] Continuous Performance Test results are presented as T-scores ($M = 50$; $SD = 10$); T-score for hits is not provided by test (RT: reaction time, SE: standard error).

performance on several of the Continuous Performance Test parameters. In particular, CB committed more than normal omission errors (i.e., fewer than normal hits) and had increased variability of reaction time and an atypically low risk-taking index. In contrast, her levels of impulsivity (commission errors), response time, and attentiveness were within normal limits.

Figure 1 shows CB's copy, immediate, and delayed drawing of the Complex Figure. She adopted a piece-meal strategy that resulted in poor integration of details in the end product. In addition,

Copy

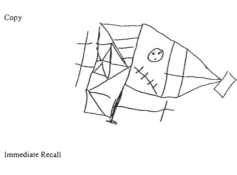

Immediate Recall

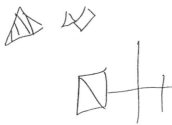

Delayed Recall

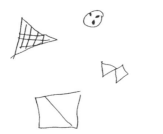

Fig. 1. CB's productions on the copy and immediate and delayed recall components of the Complex Figure of the Denman Neuropsychological Memory Scale.

she worked very slowly and was not able to complete the drawing in the allotted time (6 min). Her recollection of the figure, both immediate and delayed, demonstrated a significant degree of mental disorganization. She did not seem to remember how the pieces went together and therefore drew each of the components separately.

In terms of CB's academic achievement, the Wechsler Individual Achievement Test results indicated above average ability in reading and language and average ability in mathematics and writing. However, when her reading and language scores were examined more closely, CB performed at a superior level in the receptive language domain, whereas her expressive language skills were solidly average and therefore below expectation. Oral and written responses revealed an inability to describe the configural aspects of the picture. She elicited multiple details to describe a scene, but could not integrate these details into a meaningful whole, similar to her deficit in visuospatial ability. For example, when shown a picture of a playground, CB provided detailed descriptions about what the children were wearing and doing and the exact number of bushes in the scene; however, she never provided any global descriptors of the scene such as 'playground', 'park', or 'schoolyard'. Similarly, the written description of her ideal house was poorly organized and conveyed different parts of the house in a list-like fashion.

Tables 2–4 provide the results from the parent, self, and teacher report questionnaires examining aspects of CB's socioemotional and behavioral functioning. Results presented as T-scores ($M = 50, SD = 10$) indicate clinically elevated levels on a number of scales. Parents endorsed attention and attention deficit hyperactivity disorder items as problematic, as well as items concerning cognitive, anxiety, social, and psychosomatic problems. CB herself indicated concerns about her physical appearance and lack of popularity. CB's teacher reported attention problems, particularly in the area of hyperactivity–impulsivity, as well as anxiety and social problems.

Finally, CB's Draw-A-Person picture is shown in Figure 2. Her figure indicated many features characteristic of anxiety and impulsivity, including excessive detailing, shading, and erasures.

Table 2. CB's Results from Parent Report Questionnaires.

Questionnaire	T-Score
Achenbach Child Behavior Checklist (4–18)	
Social competence	39
School performance	33
Activities	49
Withdrawn	68
Somatic complaints	80++
Anxious/depressed	69+
Social problems	70+
Thought problems	76++
Attention problems	79++
Delinquent behavior	57
Aggressive behavior	61
Internalizing	74++
Externalizing	60+
Total score	74++
Conners' Parent Rating Scales	
Oppositional	52
Cognitive problems	>90++
Hyperactivity	>90++
Anxious–shy	76++
Perfectionism	83++
Social problems	>90++
Psychosomatic	>90++
ADHD Index	89++
Restless–impulsive	90++
Emotional lability	71++
Global: total	88++
DSMIV inattentive	>90++
DSMIV hyper-impulsive	>90++
DSMIV total	>90++

Note. All scores represent T-scores, which are standardized scores based on a distribution with a mean of 50 and a standard deviation of 10.
+Borderline.
++Clinical range.

DISCUSSION

The present paper describes the findings of a neuropsychological assessment on a young girl with TS who displayed classic characteristics of the Nonverbal Learning Disabilities syndrome (Rourke, 1989), as is typical for this syndrome (Rovet, 1995; Ross, Stefanatos, Roeltgen, Kushner, & Cutler, 1995). In particular, this child demonstrated relatively intact verbal abilities in contrast to her significantly weaker nonverbal abilities, and she also showed difficulties in attention and visual

Table 3. CB's Results From the Piers–Harris Children's Self-Concept Scale.

Scale	T-Score
Behavior	66
Intellectual and school status	55
Physical appearance and attributes	49+
Anxiety	55
Popularity	39++
Happiness and satisfaction	63
Total score	56

Note. T-scores are standardized scores based on a distribution with a mean of 50 and a standard deviation of 10.
+Borderline range.
++Clinical range.

memory. In addition, while her achievement in mathematics on the Wechsler Individual Achievement Test was within the average range, it was significantly poorer than her achievement in reading. Although CB's verbal abilities were much stronger than her nonverbal abilities, she scored below expectation in her expressive verbal skills compared to her superior-range receptive skills. Moreover, both her visuospatial and verbal difficulties appeared to reflect a difficulty in processing the global or configurational aspects of the information provided. Overall, her profile was suggestive of a selective difficulty in integration processing that affected her abilities in both visuospatial and verbal domains. While CB's visuospatial deficits are comparable to those reported in recent studies of individuals with TS (Temple & Carney, 1995; Ross, Kushner, & Zinn, 1997), the specific verbal difficulties associated with the syndrome have not been previously considered.

On the nonverbal subtests, CB experienced the greatest difficulty when she was required to integrate pieces to form a structural or meaningful whole, as in Object Assembly (1st percentile) or picture arrangement (16th percentile). Her difficulty in integrating was also evident in her deficient performance on the Complex Figure Test (1st percentile), in which she copied and remembered the figure in a very piecemeal fashion but could not integrate the pieces to complete the picture and consequently had difficulty remembering the figure. Similarly, CB indicated difficulty choosing the correct 'piece' to complete each picture in the Matching

Table 4. CB's Results From Teacher Report Questionnaires.

Questionnaire	T-Score
Conners' Teacher Ratin Scale	
Oppositional	60
Cognitive problems	62
Hyperactivity	>90[++]
Anxious–Shy	86[++]
Perfectionism	58
Social problems	84[++]
ADHD Index	84[++]
Restless–impulsive	87[++]
Emotional lability	90[++]
Global: total	>90[++]
DSMIV inattentive	59
DSMIV hyper–impulsive	88[++]
DSMIV total	72[++]
Teacher's Report Form	
Academic performance	37[++]
Working hard	57
Behaving appropriately	37[++]
Learning	35[++]
Happy	35[++]
Sum	37[++]
Withdrawn	60
Somatic complaints	50
Anxious/depressed	80[++]
Social problems	78[++]
Thought problems	50
Attention problems	67[+]
Delinquent behavior	56
Aggressive behavior	68[+]
Total T-score	71[++]
Internal T-score	70[++]
External T-score	68[++]

Note. T-scores are standardized scores based on a distribution with a mean of 50 and a standard deviation of 10.
[+] Borderline range.
[++] Clinical range.

subtest of the Wide Range Assessment of Visual Motor Ability (3rd percentile). In contrast, CB performed within the average range on the Block Design subtest (50th percentile) of the Wechsler Intelligence Scale for Children – III, consistent with other studies of TS (McGlone, 1985; Ross & Zinn, 1999; Silbert et al., 1977; Waber, 1979). However, unlike other individuals with TS (Ross et al., 1997; Waber, 1979), she performed in the superior range on design copying (91st percentile) of the NEPSY. Close analysis of CB's profile of

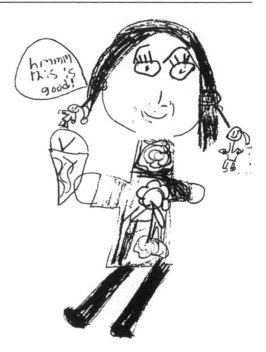

Fig. 2. CB's production on the Draw-A-Person Projective Test.

performance on visuospatial tasks suggests a difficulty in determining the global structure of visually presented information. For example, her performance was satisfactory on Block Design and Design Copying, which provide a model, whereas her performance was deficient on Object Assembly and Picture Arrangement, which do not provide a model.

CB demonstrated strong receptive language skills with superior comprehension, in contrast to average expressive language skill on the Wechsler Individual Achievement Test. In particular, she scored at the 95th percentile on Reading Comprehension and at the 98th percentile on Listening Comprehension. These scores were significantly higher than her performance on Basic Reading (61st percentile) and Oral Expression (53rd percentile). On other expressive language subtests, she also showed average performance (i.e., Spelling at 45th percentile and Written Expression at 50th percentile). When her responses on the expressive language tasks were examined more closely, an interesting pattern emerged.

In both Oral and Written Expression, CB elicited many details but had difficulty in describing the overall picture. As reported above, she described multiple details of the playground scene including what the child was wearing and the number of bushes, but she never provided an organizational term such as 'playground' or 'schoolyard'. This characteristic was also noted in her writing, which was list-like in composition rather than thematic. While CB's visuospatial processing difficulties were to be expected, her difficulty with verbal expression was somewhat surprising since verbal deficits are not typically reported as problematic in TS. However, because affected individuals are believed to have intact verbal abilities, this aspect of their cognitive profile is seldom studied in detail (Van Borsel, Dhooge, Verhoye, Derde, & Curfs, 1999).

Our findings presently suggest that CB has an integration difficulty that affects her ability to process visuospatial and verbal materials and may also be related to her difficulties socially. As a consequence of not adequately integrating information, she may not be able to express herself in an organized manner in social communication and this in turn may contribute to the ostracization and social difficulties she is experiencing (Swillen et al., 1993). In addition, this difficulty may have led in part to the significant anxiety problems she has been experiencing from an early age. Indeed, social and behavioral difficulties are typically observed in older children and adolescents with Nonverbal Learning Disabilities (Rourke, 1989).

Like most cognitive abilities, visuospatial processing is considered multifaceted in nature with several known distinctions (e.g. object versus location processing, global versus local processing). Recently, we examined the TS visuospatial deficit in terms of object versus location aspects of cognitive processing and showed that processing location information, which is thought to implicate the dorsal visual pathway in the brain (Ungerleider & Mishkin, 1982), is selectively affected in these individuals (Rovet & Buchanan, 1999). We now show that this deficit may also be related to poor global or configural processing with spared local or featural processing. While Silbert and colleagues first described difficulties in part – whole perception in individuals with TS in 1977, this specific deficit has

not been studied further, including its impact on verbal functioning.

It is interesting to note that in Williams syndrome, which is a genetic disorder also characterized by Nonverbal Learning Disabilities (Anderson & Rourke, 1995), affected children show a similar pattern of assets and deficits to TS, although children with Williams syndrome are generally lower functioning overall. Like TS, Williams syndrome is characterized by poor visuospatial and other nonverbal skills but relatively spared verbal skills (Anderson & Rourke, 1995). Selective deficits in verbal ability have been described in individuals with Williams syndrome, including delayed language acquisition (Karmiloff-Smith et al., 1998), hyperverbal speech (Udwin & Yule, 1990) that is unstructured and disorganized, and greater facility with expressive than receptive language (Arnold, Yule, & Martin, 1985). These verbal deficits have been attributed to the primary, secondary, and tertiary assets and deficits of the syndrome of Nonverbal Learning Disabilities (Rourke & Tsatsanis, 1996). Some of the features of CB's language described presently are similar to these characteristics in Williams syndrome, although her level of functioning was much higher. In contrast to CB and other individuals with TS (Ross et al., 1997), children with Williams syndrome indicate relatively good face processing skills. Nevertheless, recent evidence on Williams syndrome indicates they process faces atypically, in a manner suggestive of difficulties in global processing. According to Karmiloff-Smith (1997), they are equally proficient on tasks of upright versus inverted face recognition, signifying that they are processing features of faces not facial configurations.

Recently, Donnai and Karmiloff-Smith (2000) attributed the cognitive deficits in Williams syndrome to a problem in global processing, which is similar to CB and consistent with right hemisphere dysfunction (Delis, Kiefner, & Friedlund, 1988; Doricchi & Incoccia, 1998; Lassonde et al., 1999; Robertson & Lamb, 1991). However, according to Karmiloff-Smith (1998), genetics alone cannot account for the good verbal and face processing skills versus poor spatial ability in Williams syndrome. Rather, she claims that changes in their developmental course perturb all aspects of cognitive functioning and that this occurs at a basic low level of processing (Donnai & Karmiloff-Smith, 2000). If this also applies to CB, it is not surprising that she struggles with multiple aspects of cognitive and social processing. Thus, her deficit may not be restricted to right hemisphere deficit but may rather reflect a more global redistribution of functioning in her brain, as has been described in Williams syndrome.

Unlike Williams syndrome, verbal abilities are infrequently studied in TS (Van-Borsel et al., 1999), as with the distinction between global and config- ural processing. Neuroanatomic studies on these individuals have revealed generalized brain abnor- malities (Clark et al., 1990; Murphy et al., 1993; Reiss et al., 1995; Ross et al., 1993) suggestive of atypical hemispheric organization for both verbal and spatial information (McGlone, 1985; Netley, 1977). Despite these findings, the majority of stud- ies focusing on the spatial deficit have emphasized abilities preferentially subserved by the right hemi- sphere. As the present findings showed that some areas of verbal ability may also be compromised in TS, usually ascribed to the left hemisphere dysfunc- tion, explanations other than white matter defi- ciency may hold. In fact, neuroimaging evidence to date does not consistently demonstrate white matter dysfunction. Given that functional magnetic reso- nance imaging studies have been used to dissociate global and local processing in the right and left hemispheres, respectively (Martinez et al., 1997), we eagerly await the findings from functional imag- ing studies examining whether the sites specifically relevant for configural processing are dysfunctional in this population.

The present paper describes our anecdotal find- ings on a single patient. It remains to be determined whether CB's specific deficit in integrating visual information characterizes others with this condi- tion. Furthermore, our findings may be specific to the clinical tasks we used. On the Wechsler Individual Achievement Test, for example, the Reading Comprehension subtest does not require elaborate organization of output, and rote repetition is often sufficient for success. Therefore, the pos- sibility remains that CB may experience reading comprehension difficulties in more complex situa- tions (Rourke & Tsatsanis, 1996). There is also a great need to test the phenomenon more directly using laboratory-based tasks that directly tap and

manipulate global–local processing (Martinez et al., 1997). However, despite these limitations, the pres- ent findings have implications for treatment of chil- dren with TS. As noted by Rourke (1995), they may benefit from parts-to-whole instruction. In addition, it is important that they be provided with the structure of the situation, as seen in Block Design and Design Copying tasks. Moreover, their strength in rote repetition may serve to enhance their learning in any situation.

In summary, the present paper describes a spe- cific cognitive disorder in a 9-year-old girl with TS who was unable to integrate details into a mean- ingful whole. Her deficit was not exclusive to the visuospatial processing domain but also affected her processing of verbal information. Moreover, her specific integration deficit is thought to underlie her social and behavioral difficulties, which are characteristic of children with TS. As the same pat- tern of deficit has been described in children with Nonverbal Learning Disabilities, which has been attributed to right hemisphere dysfunction, CB's difficulties may similarly reflect right hemisphere dysfunction. However, given the left hemisphere's potential involvement, as suggested by deficits in verbal ability and neuroimaging results, future research examining specific language skills as well as aspects of global versus local processing is needed in TS.

REFERENCES

Achenbach, T.M. (1991a). *Child behavior checklist for ages 4–18*. Burlington, VT: Author.

Achenbach, T.M. (1991b). *Teacher's report form for ages 5–18*. Burlington, VT: Author.

Adams, W., & Sheslow, D. (1995). *Wide range assess- ment of visual motor abilities*. Wilmington, DE: Wide Range Inc.

Anderson, P.E., & Rourke, B.P. (1995). Williams syn- drome. In B.P. Rourke (Ed.), *Syndrome of nonverbal learning disabilities: Neurodevelopmental manifesta- tions* (pp. 138–170). New York: The Guilford Press.

Arnold, R., Yule, W., & Martin, N. (1985). The psycho- logical characteristics of infantile hypercalcaemia: A preliminary investigation. *Developmental Medicine and Child Neurology, 27*, 49–59.

Bender, B., Linden, M., & Robinson, A. (1990). SCA: In search of developmental patterns. In D. Berch & B. Bender (Eds.), *Sex chromosome abnormalities and human behavior: Psychological studies* (pp. 20–37). Boulder, CO: Westview Press.

Berch, D.B., & Kirkendall, K.L. (1986). Spatial information processing in 45,X children. In A. Robinson (Chair), Cognitive and psychosocial dysfunctions associated with sex chromosome abnormalities. *Proceedings of the Symposium presented at the meeting of the American Association for the Advancement of Science, Philadelphia.*

Bernstein, J.H., & Waber, D.P. (1996). *Developmental scoring system for the Rey-Osterrieth Complex Figure.* Odessa, FL: Psychological Assessment Resources Inc.

Bishop, D.V.M., Canning, E., Elgar, K., Morris, E., Jacobs, P.A., & Skuse, D.H. (2000). Distinctive patterns of memory function in subgroups of females with Turner syndrome: Evidence for imprinted loci on the X-chromosome affecting neurodevelopment. *Neuropsychologia, 38,* 712–721.

Buchanan, L., Pavlovic, J., & Rovet, J. (1998). A reexamination of the visuospatial deficit in Turner syndrome: Contributions of working memory. *Developmental Neuropsychology, 14,* 341–367.

Clark, C., Klonoff, H., & Hayden, M. (1990). Regional cerebral glucose metabolism in Turner syndrome. *Canadian Journal of Neurological Sciences, 17,* 140–144.

Cohen, M.J. (1997). *Children's Memory Scale.* New York: The Psychological Corporation, Harcourt Brace & Company.

Conners, C.K. (1992). *Manual for the Conners' continuous performance test.* Toronto: Multi-Health Systems Inc.

Conners, C.K. (1997). *Conners' rating scales* (Rev. ed.). Toronto: Multi-Health Systems Inc.

Delis, D.C., Kiefner, M.G., & Friedlund, A.J. (1988). Visuospatial dysfunction following unilateral brain damage: Dissociations in hierarchical hemispatial analysis. *Journal of Clinical and Experimental Neuropsychology, 10,* 421–431.

Denman, S.B. (1984). *Denman neuropsychology memory scale: A clinical assessment of immediate recall, short-term memory, and long-term memory in verbal and non-verbal areas.* Charleston, SC: Author.

Donnai, D., & Karmiloff-Smith, A. (2000). Williams syndrome: From genotype through to the cognitive phenotype. *American Journal of Medical Genetics, 97,* 164–171.

Doricchi, F., & Incoccia, C. (1998). Seeing only the right half of the forest but cutting down all the trees? *Nature, 394* (6688), 75–78.

Hook, E.B., & Warburton, D. (1983). The distribution of chromosomal genotypes associated with Turner's syndrome: Livebirth prevalence rates and evidence for diminished fetal mortality and severity in genotypes associated with structural abnormalities or mosaicism. *Human Genetics, 64,* 24–27.

Jacobs, P., Dalton, P., James, R., Mosse, K., Power, M., Robinson, D., & Skuse, D. (1997). Turner syndrome: A cytogenetic and molecular study. *Journal of American Human Genetics, U,* 471–483.

Karmiloff-Smith, A. (1997). Crucial differences between developmental cognitive neuroscience and adult neuropsychology. *Developmental Neuropsychology, 13,* 513–524.

Karmiloff-Smith, A. (1998). Development itself is the key to understanding developmental disorders. *Trends in Cognitive Sciences, 2,* 389–398.

Karmiloff-Smith, A., Tyler, L.K., Voice, K., Sims, K., Udwin, O., Howlin, P., & Davies, M. (1998). Linguistic dissociations in Williams syndrome: Evaluating receptive syntax in on-line and off-line tasks. *Neuropsychologia, 36,* 343–351.

Korkman, M., Kirk, U., & Kemp, S. (1998). *NEPSY: A developmental neuropsychological assessment.* Toronto: Harcourt Brace & Company.

Lassonde, M., Mottron, L., Peretz, I., Schiavetto, A., Hébert, S., & Décarie, J.-C. (1999). Loss of global visual and auditory processing following right temporal lobe lesion. *Brain and Cognition, 40,* 162–166.

Lewandowski, L., Costenbader, V., & Richman, R. (1985). Neuropsychological aspects of Turner syndrome. *International Journal of Neuropsychology, 1,* 144–147.

Manly, T., Robertson, I.H., Anderson, V., & Nimmo-Smith, I. (1999). *The test of everyday attention for children.* Bury St Edmunds, UK: Thames Valley Test Company Ltd.

Martinez, A., Moses, P., Frank, L., Buxton, R., Wong, E., & Stiles, J. (1997). Hemispheric asymmetries in global and local processing: Evidence from fMRI. *Neuroreport, 6,* 1685–1689.

McCauley, E. (1990). Psychosocial and emotional aspects of Turner syndrome. In D. Berch & B. Bender (Eds.), *Sex chromosome abnormalities and human behavior: Psychological studies* (pp. 78–100). Boulder, CO: Westview Press.

McGlone, J. (1985). Can spatial deficits in Turner's syndrome be explained by focal CNS dysfunction or atypical speech lateralization? *Journal of Clinical and Experimental Neuropsychology, 7,* 375–394.

McCauley, E., Ross, J.L., Kushner, H., & Cutler, G. (1995). Self-esteem and behavior in girls with Turner Syndrome. *Developmental and Behavioral Pediatrics, 16,* 82–88.

Money, J. (1993). Specific neurocognitional impairments associated with Turner (45,X) and Klinefelter (47,XXY) syndromes: A review. *Social Biology, 40,* 147–151.

Money, J., & Alexander, D. (1966). Turner's syndrome: Further demonstration of the presence of specific cognitional deficiencies. *Journal of Medical Genetics, 3,* 47–48.

Murphy, D., Allen, G., Haxby, J., Largay, K., Daly, E., White, B., Powell, C., & Schapiro, M. (1994). The effects of sex steroids, and the X chromosome, on the female brain function: A study of the neuropsychology of adult Turner syndrome. *Neuropsychologia*, *32*, 1309–1323.

Murphy, D., DeCarli, C., Daly, E., Haxby, J., Allen, G., White, B., McIntosh, A., Powell, C., Horwitz, B., Rapoport, S., & Schapiro, M. (1993). X-chromosome effects on female brain: A magnetic resonance imaging study of Turner's syndrome. *Lancet*, *342*, 1197–1200.

Murphy, D.G.M., Mentis, M.J., Pietrini, P., Grady, C., Daly, E., Haxby, J.V., De La Granja, M., Allen, G., Largay, K., White, B.J., Powell, C.M., Horwitz, B., Rapoport, S.I., & Schapiro, M.J. (1997). A PET study of Turner's syndrome: Effects of sex steroids and the X chromosome on brain. *Biological Psychiatry*, *41*, 285–298.

Netley, C. (1977). Dichotic listening of callosal agenesis and Turner's syndrome patients. In C. Netley (Ed.), *Language and development and neurological theory* (pp. 133–143). New York: Academic Press.

Netley, C., & Rovet, J. (1983). Atypical hemisphere lateralization in Turner's Syndrome. *Cortex*, *18*, 377–384.

Nielsen, J., Nyborg, H., & Dahl, G. (1977). Turner's syndrome: A psychiatric–psychological study of 45 women with Turner's syndrome, compared with their sisters and women of normal karyotypes, growth retardation, and primary amenorrhea. *Acta Jutlandica*, *45* (Medicine Series 21), 190.

O'Neill, S., Ghelani, K., Rovet, J., Chitayat, D. (2000). Physical and psychological development of individuals prenatally diagnosed with 45,X/46,XX. *The American Journal of Human Genetics*, *67* (4, Suppl. 2), 135 (Abstract).

Piers, E.V. (1984). *Piers-Harris children's self-concept scale* (Rev. ed.). Los Angeles, CA: Western Psychological Services.

Reiss, A.L., Freund, L., Plotnick, L., Baumgardner, T., Green, K., Sozer, A.C., Reader, M., Boehm, C., & Denckla, M.B. (1993). The effects of X monosomy on brain development: Monozygotic twins discordant for Turner's syndrome. *Annals of Neurology*, *34*, 95–107.

Reiss, A.L., Mazzocco, M.M., Greenlaw, R., Freund, L., & Ross, J.L. (1995). Neurodevelopmental effects of X monosomy: A volumetric imaging study. *Annals of Neurology*, *38*, 731–738.

Robertson, L.C., & Lamb, M.R. (1991). Neuropsychological contributions to theories of part/whole organization. *Cognitive Psychology*, *23*, 299–330.

Robinson, A., Bender, B., Borelli, J., Puck, M., Salbenblatt, J., & Winter, J. (1986). Sex chromosome aneuploidy: Prospective and longitudinal studies. In S. Ratcliffe & N. Paul (Eds.), *Prospective studies on*

children with sex chromosomal aneuploidy (pp. 23–73). New York: Liss.

Ross, J.L. (1990). Disorders of the sex chromosome: Medical overview. In C.S. Holmes (Ed.), *Psychoneuroendocrinology: Brain, behavior, and hormonal interactions* (pp. 127–137). New York: Springer.

Ross, J.L., Kushner, H., & Zinn, A.R. (1997). Discriminant analysis of the Ullrich–Turner syndrome neurocognitive profile. *American Journal of Medical Genetics*, *72*, 275–280.

Ross, J.L., Reiss, A.L., Freund, L., Roeltgen, D., & Cutler, G.B. (1993). Neurocognitive function and brain imaging in Turner syndrome: Preliminary results. *Hormone Research*, *39* (Suppl. 2), 65–69.

Ross, J.L., Roeltgen, D., & Cutler, G.B. (1995). The neurodevelopmental transition between childhood and adolescence in girls with Turner syndrome. In K.A. Albertsson-Wickland & M.B. Ranke (Eds.), *Turner syndrome in a life span perspective: Research and clinical aspects* (pp. 297–308). Amsterdam: Elsevier.

Ross, J.L., Roeltgen, D., Feuillan, P., Kushner, H., & Cutler, G.B. (1998). Effects of estrogen on non-verbal processing speed and motor function in girls with Turner's syndrome. *Journal of Clinical Endocrinology and Metabolism*, *83*, 3198–3204.

Ross, J.L., Roeltgen, D., Feuillan, P., Kushner, H., & Cutler, G.B. (2000). Use of estrogen in young girls with Turner syndrome: Effects on memory. *Neurology*, *54*, 164–170.

Ross, J., Stefanatos, G., Roeltgen, D., Kushner, H., & Cutler, G. (1995). Ullrich–Turner syndrome: Neurodevelopmental changes from childhood through adolescence. *American Journal of Medical Genetics*, *58*, 74–82.

Ross, J.L., & Zinn, A. (1999). Turner syndrome: Potential hormonal and genetic influences on the neurocognitive profile. In H. Tager-Flusberg (Ed.), *Neurodevelopmental disorders: Developmental cognitive neuroscience* (pp. 251–268). Cambridge, MA: The MIT Press.

Rourke, B.P. (1989). *Nonverbal learning disabilities: The syndrome and the model*. New York: Guilford Press.

Rourke, B.P. (1995). Treatment program for children with NLD. In B.P. Rourke (Ed.), *Syndrome of nonverbal learning disabilities: Neurodevelopmental manifestations* (pp. 497–508). New York: Guilford Press.

Rourke, B.P., & Tsatsanis, K.D. (1996). Syndrome of nonverbal learning disabilities: Psycholinguistic assets and deficits. *Topics in Language Disorders*, *16* (2), 30–44.

Rovet, J. (1990). The cognitive and neuropsychological characteristics of children with Turner syndrome. In D. Berch & B. Bender (Eds.), *Sex chromosome abnormalities and human behavior: Psychological studies* (pp. 38–77). Boulder, CO: Westview.

Rovet, J. (1995). Turner syndrome. In B.P. Rourke (Ed.), *Syndrome of nonverbal learning disabilities: Neurodevelopmental manifestations* (pp. 351–371). New York: Guilford Press.

Rovet, J., & Buchanan, L. (1999). Turner syndrome: A cognitive neuroscience approach. In H. Tager-Flusberg (Ed.), *Neurodevelopmental disorders: Contributions to a new perspective from the cognitive neurosciences* (pp. 223–250). Cambridge, MA: MIT Press.

Rovet, J., & Ireland, L. (1994). The behavioral phenotype of children with Turner syndrome. *Journal of Pediatric Psychology, 19*, 779–790.

Rovet, J., & Netley, C. (1982). Processing deficits in Turner's syndrome. *Developmental Psychology, 18*, 77–94.

Rovet, J., Szekely, C., & Hockenberry, M. (1994). Specific arithmetic deficits in children with Turner syndrome. *Journal of Clinical and Experimental Neuropsychology, 16*, 820–839.

Siegel, P.T., Clopper, R., & Stabler, B. (1998). The psychological consequences of Turner syndrome and review of the National Cooperative Growth Study psychological substudy. *Pediatrics, 102*, 488–491.

Silbert, A., Wolff, P., & Lilienthal, J. (1977). Spatial and temporal processing in patients with Turner's syndrome. *Behavior Genetics, 7*, 11–21.

Simpson, J. (1975). Gonadal dysgenesis and abnormalities of the human sex chromosomes: Current status of phenotypic – karyotypic correlations. *Birth Defects: Original Articles Series, 11*, 23–55.

Skuse, D.H., James, R.S., Bishop, D.V.M., Copin, B., Dalton, P., Aamodt-Leeper, G., Bacarese-Hamilton, M., Cresswell, C., McGurk, R., & Jacops, P. (1997). Evidence from Turner syndrome of an imprinted X-linked locus affecting cognitive function. *Nature, 387*, 705–708.

Swillen, A., Fryns, J.P., Kleczkowska, A., Massa, G., Vanderschueren-Lodeweyckx, M., & Van Den Berghe, H. (1993). Intelligence, behavior, and psychosocial development in Turner syndrome: A cross-sectional study of 50 pre-adolescent and adolescent girls (4–20 years). *Genetic Counseling, 4*, 7–18.

Temple, C.M., & Carney, R.A. (1993). Intellectual functioning of children with Turner syndrome: A comparison of behavioral phenotypes. *Developmental Medicine and Child Neurology, 35*, 691–698.

Temple, C.M., & Carney, R.A. (1995). Patterns of spatial functioning in Turner's Syndrome. *Cortex, 21*, 109–118.

Temple, C.M., & Marriott, A.J. (1998). Arithmetical ability and disability in Turner's Syndrome: A cognitive neuropsychological analysis. *Developmental Neuropsychology, 14*, 47–67.

The Psychological Corporation. (1992). *Wechsler Individual Achievement Test*. Toronto: Harcourt Brace & Company.

Udwin, O., & Yule, W. (1990). Expressive language of children with Williams syndrome. *American Journal of Medical Genetics, 6*, 108–114.

Ungerleider, L.G., & Mishkin, M. (1982). Two cortical visual systems. In D.J. Ingle, M.A. Goodale, & R.J.W. Mansfield (Eds.), *Analysis of visual behavior* (pp. 549–586). Cambridge, MA: MIT Press.

Van Borsel, J., Dhooge, I., Verhoye, K., Derde, K., Curfs, L. (1999). Communication problems in Turner syndrome: A sample survey. *Journal of Communication Disorders, 32*, 435–446.

Waber, D. (1979). Neuropsychological aspects of Turner syndrome. *Developmental Medicine and Child Neurology, 21*, 58–70.

Wechsler, D. (1991). *Manual for the Wechsler Intelligence Scale for Children* (3rd ed.). New York: Psychological Corporation.

Zinn, A.R., & Ross, J.L. (1998). Turner syndrome and haploinsufficiency. *Current Opinion in Genetics and Development, 8*, 322–327.

Child Neuropsychology
1998, Vol. 4, No. 3, pp. 225–232

A Case of Triple X Syndrome Manifesting with the Syndrome of Nonverbal Learning Disabilities

Thomas V. Ryan[1,2], W. David Crews Jr.[1], Lawrence Cowen[3], Aaron M. Goering[1], and Jeffrey T. Barth[1]

[1]University of Virginia Health Sciences Center, Charlottesville, [2]Woodrow Wilson Rehabilitation Center, Fisherville, VA, and [3]Private Practice, Staunton, VA

ABSTRACT

There has been a relative absence of studies that have examined comprehensively the neuropsychological profiles of females with Triple X Syndrome across a battery of tests and measures. A case is reported of a 9 1/2-year-old female with Triple X Syndrome whose neuropsychological test results were suggestive of greater right-versus left-cerebral hemisphere dysfunction. Overall, the patient's neuropsychological profile was indicative of the syndrome of Nonverbal Learning Disabilities (NLD) as proposed by Rourke (Rourke 1987, 1988, 1995; Rourke & Tsatsanis, 1996). The results are discussed in light of Rourke's NLD Syndrome and the related white matter model.

By definition, Triple X Syndrome (47XXX) is a sex chromosome abnormality occurring in females that is characterized by the presence of an extra X chromosome (Walzer, 1985). It was first identified by Jacobs and his colleagues in 1959 (Jacobs et al., 1959). The incidence rate of the syndrome has been reported to vary between 0.73 (see Tennes, Puck, Bryant, Frankenburg, & Robinson, 1975) and 1.0 (Nielsen & Wohlert, 1991a) per 1000 female births.

Although the majority of females with Triple X Syndrome appear normal at birth, and without specific congenital malformations or identifying physical characteristics (Cohen & Durham, 1985; Fryns, Kleczkowska, Petit, & Van Den Berghe, 1983; Linden, Bender, Harmon, Mrazek, & Robinson, 1988; Robinson, Lubs, Nielsen, & Sorensen, 1979), they do seem to be at risk for later development of neuropsychological deficits. Specifically, females with Triple X Syndrome have been found to exhibit lower Verbal IQs (as compared to their nonverbal IQs) (Netley & Rovet, 1982; Nielsen, 1991; Nielsen, Sorenson, & Sorenson, 1981, 1982; Rovet & Netley, 1983), deficient verbal achievement (Rovet & Netley), decreased verbal processing (Rovet & Netley), and compromised auditory memory (Rovet & Netley) as compared to matched controls. Studies have also indicated that females with Triple X Syndrome may exhibit lower levels of overall general intelligence as compared to controls (Pennington, Bender, Puck, Salbenblatt, & Robinson, 1982; Robinson et al., 1982).

In contrast to those studies that have found lower IQs and occasional reports of mental retardation in these individuals (Fryns et al., 1983), other studies have found that the majority of females with Triple X have relatively normal intelligence (i.e., mean IQs between 80 and 120; Tennes et al., 1975), and do not always exhibit significant differences between their Verbal and Performance IQs (Pennington et al., 1982). It has also been

*Address correspondence to: Jeffrey T. Barth, Division of Neuropsychology, Department of Psychiatric Medicine, Box 203, University of Virginia Health Sciences Center, Charlottesville, VA 22908, USA. E-mail: jtb4y@virginia.edu.
Accepted for publication: October 22, 1997.

shown that the Performance IQs of some females with Triple X are near or above the mean as compared to controls (Nielsen et al., 1981, 1982).

Other investigations have demonstrated that children with Triple X Syndrome are at increased risk for the development of speech and language problems/delays (Bender et al., 1983; Linden et al., 1988; Robinson et al., 1979; Robinson et al., 1982; Tennes et al., 1975) and neuromotor/ sensory-motor difficulties (e.g., lack of motor coordination; Linden et al., 1988; Nielsen et al., 1982; Robinson et al., 1982). These children may display both receptive and expressive language difficulties, which have been hypothesized to be related to their decreased intellectual abilities (Bender et al., 1983, Robinson et al., 1979). Females with Triple X have also been found to exhibit learning disabilities/disorders (Hier, Atkins, & Perlo, 1980; Pennington et al., 1982), to have academic achievement and school adjustment problems (Robinson et al., 1982; Nielsen et al., 1981), and to require remedial teaching (Nielsen & Wohlert, 1991b).

Psychosocial problems have also been associated with Triple X Syndrome. The incidence of Triple X has been found to be higher in psychiatric inpatients as compared to rates in the general population (Olanders, 1967). A diversity of psychiatric disorders has been reported in such individuals, ranging from psychosis (Wood-house, Holland, McLean, & Reveley, 1992) to Antisocial Personality Disorder (Kazamatsuri, Nanko, & Mato, 1985). Linden et al. (1988) found that 7 of 11 females with Triple X in their study had diagnosable (according to DSM-III criteria) psychiatric disorders, including depression, conduct disorders, undersocialization, and psychoso-matism, and that two other individuals were thought to be at risk for future diagnoses. In comparison, none of the subjects in the control group met DSM-III criteria. Other research has reported the presence of emotional immaturity (Rustagi & Fine, 1987), remoteness, and disturbances in interpersonal contacts/relationships (Tennes et al., 1975). Nielsen and colleagues (1981, 1982), in their examination of 25 children between the ages of 7 and 11 with an extra X or Y chromosome, found that fits of anger, feelings of inferiority, lack of self-confidence, sensitiveness, and emotional vulnerability were present significantly more often in these individuals, as compared to same-age controls. In contrast, in a follow-up study of 17 females with Triple X, aged 15.2 to 18.8 years, Nielsen and Wohlert (1991b) reported that none of these individuals exhibited any signs of mental illness or behavioral problems.

Although a number of studies have examined discrete cognitive and behavioral variables, there appears to be a relative absence of studies that have examined the neuropsychological profiles of females with Triple X Syndrome utilizing a comprehensive battery of tests and measures. This paper presents the case of a female with Triple X Syndrome who was administered a comprehensive neuropsychological assessment and exhibited a pattern of performance suggestive of the syndrome of Nonverbal Learning Disabilities (NLD) as proposed by Rourke (1987, 1988, 1995).

METHOD

Patient and Case History
The child was a 9½-year-old, right-handed female with a history of Triple X Syndrome that had been diagnosed prenatally during amniocentesis. Her mother reported an uneventful pregnancy and delivery that required usage of only low forceps. The child reportedly received high APGAR scores at the time of birth.

Developmentally, the child achieved milestones such as sitting, walking, and speech, within expected time frames. In contrast, the child's physical development, such as her coordination of gross motor movements (e.g., swimming), was clearly delayed, although she demonstrated acceleration of her physical skills following this initial lag. She was described as a happy child, with a good sense of humor. She was friendly and affectionate, and received a good deal of attention from her parents. She tended to think of herself as "dumb," but struggled to maintain a positive self-image.

The child was enrolled in a private school from her preschool years through third grade, at which time she transferred to a public elementary school. Her parents indicated that she exhibited generalized academic difficulties that became increasingly apparent during the second grade. Specifically, she was observed by teachers in the second grade to perform below grade level relative to her reading skills. Interestingly, however, current individualized reading testing revealed average reading abilities. When she continued to have academic difficulties in the third grade, she was referred to the school psychologist for a psycho-educational evaluation.

A battery of tests was administered consisting of the Wechsler Intelligence Scale for Children – Revised (WISC-R; Wechsler, 1974), the Peabody Individual Achievement Test (Dunn & Markwardt, 1970), and the Draw-A-Person Test (Machover, 1949). She achieved a Verbal IQ of 100, a Performance IQ of 88, and a Full Scale IQ of 93. These findings contrast sharply with most reports of females with Triple X who usually exhibit lower verbal than performance scores. She did, however, have trouble expressing herself verbally, but not enough to lower test scores significantly. She was distractible, exhibited some attention problems, gave up easily when confronted with difficult tasks, and demonstrated perceptual/motor processing problems. These deficiencies were most notable on the human figure drawing task where she demonstrated three common indicants of visual-perceptual/visual-motor difficulties in children: closure and overlapping problems, single line body formation (the whole body is drawn in one continuous line from one side of the neck to the other), and extreme lack of symmetry between the two sides of the body. She also constructed several of the Object Assembly items of the WISC-R upside down.

The results of achievement testing revealed grade level or slightly higher functioning in all areas of arithmetic, reading, spelling, and general information. This suggested that she could test at a grade-appropriate level (50th centile for middle third grade), even though she was having observable difficulties in the classroom. Her reading comprehension was marked by many inefficiencies even though she scored only slightly below grade level. Her arithmetic achievement (37th centile) for middle third graders was her lowest score. On this particular measure, mathematical reasoning was evaluated rather than computational skills.

At the time of evaluation, she tended to discontinue challenging cognitive tasks such as completion of homework assignments. She also experienced difficulties in copying sentences, and tended to focus more on the mechanics of reading and, in consequence, exhibited deficient reading comprehension.

The child's medical, psychiatric, and academic histories were otherwise unremarkable. There was no history of seizures, loss of consciousness associated with head trauma, or other neurologic difficulties. At the time of neurocognitive testing, the child was not taking any prescription medications.

Comprehensive neuropsychological assessment
The child was referred for neuropsychological evaluation to determine her current level of functioning and to formulate academically related recommendations. She presented as a well-groomed female and appeared her stated age. Although initially somewhat shy and withdrawn, she rapidly appeared more comfortable, and interacted spontaneously with the examiner once rapport

had been established. She easily separated from her father who accompanied her to the assessment. The child attempted to minimize her involvement with more challenging and difficult tasks, and tended to give up easily on these measures. She appeared to fatigue as the evaluation progressed. A low level of frustration tolerance was also noted and she was easily distracted by extraneous auditory and visual stimuli. Although she seemed to have no difficulty comprehending directions, she required frequent reminders to pay close attention to instructions. Occasional impulsivity was evident in her test-taking style as she often began performance of tasks prior to the completion of instructions. Maximum test performance was enhanced via several testing intermissions. Overall, the results of her neuropsychological evaluation appeared to be a valid estimation of her actual cognitive status as she seemed to exhibit a desire to perform to the best of her abilities when actively engaged in testing.

All testing was conducted in a sound-attenuated examination room by an experienced neuropsychological test technician. The standardized administration and scoring procedures of each test were strictly followed. After a brief rapport-building session and clinical interview, the following tests were administered: the Halstead-Reitan Neuropsychological Battery for Older Children (Reitan, 1979; Reitan & Wolfson, 1993); Kaufman Brief Intelligence Test (K-BIT; Kaufman & Kaufman, 1990); Test of Memory and Learning (TOMAL; Reynolds & Bigler, 1994); and portions of the Wechsler Individual Achievement Test (WIAT; Psychological Corporation, 1992).

RESULTS

An overview of the neuropsychological test data is shown in Table 1. On the KBIT (Kaufman & Kaufman, 1990), she obtained a Vocabulary IQ Standard Score (92) that fell within the average range. In contrast, her Matrices IQ Standard Score (76) was borderline compromised. Her composite IQ Standard Score (82) was in the low average range. There was a significant difference between her Verbal and Matrices IQ Standard Scores in favor of her verbal abilities.

On the WIAT Spelling and Listening Comprehension subtests, her skills were average for someone of her grade level (i.e., 4), whereas her score on the Basic Reading subtest was below average. Alternatively, performance on the WIAT Mathematics Reasoning subtest was significantly below average for this child.

Table 1. Neuropsychological Test Data.

Test	Score/Scaled Score
Kaufman Brief Intelligence Test	
Vocabulary IQ Standard Score	92+
Matrices IQ Standard Score	76+
Composite IQ Standard Score	82
Wechsler Individual Achievement Test (SS,GE)	
Basic Reading	92,3.2
Mathematics Reasoning	81,2.1*
Spelling	99,4.0
Listening Comprehension	102,3.9
Aphasia Screening Examination (errors)	22*
Category Test (errors)	61
Trail Making Test (time in s, errors)	
Part A	22,1
Part B	47,1
Speech Perception Test (errors)	24*
Seashore Rhythm Test (correct)	21
Finger Tapping Test (taps/10 s, D, ND)	32.0,26.4*
Dynamometer (grip strength in kg, D, ND)	7.0*,7.0*
Grooved Pegboard Test (time in s, D, ND)	110*,102*
Sensory-Perception Examination	
Finger Agnosia (errors, D, ND)	2/20*,1/20
Finger-Tip Writing (errors, D, ND)	5/20*,13/20*
Tactile Form Recognition (errors, D, ND)	0,0
Unilateral errors (D, ND)	
Tactile, hand	0,0
Tactile, face	0,0
Auditory	0,0
Visual	0,0
Suppression errors (D, ND)	
Tactile, hand	1,0
Tactile, face	0,0
Auditory	0,0
Visual	1,3*
Tactual Performance Test	
Dominant hand (total time, blocks placed)	5.0,3*
Nondominant hand (total time, blocks placed)	5.0,2*
Both hands (total time, blocks placed)	5.0,6*
Total (total time, blocks placed)	15.0,11*
Memory for blocks (number)	2*
Memory for location of blocks (number)	0*
Test of Memory and Learning (SS)	
Memory of Stories	13
Word Selective Reminding	12
Object Recall	7
Digits Forward	8
Paired Recall	7
Letters Forward	16
Digits Backward	5*
Letters Backward	6*
Verbal Memory Index	131+
Facial Memory	8
Visual Selective Reminding	7
Abstract Visual Memory	9
Visual Sequential Memory	5*
Memory for Location	9
Manual Imitation	9
Test	Score/Scaled Score
Nonverbal Memory Index	96+
Composite Memory Index	115
Delayed Recall Index	93

Note. SS = scaled score; D = dominant hand; GE = grade equivalent; ND = nondominant hand; + = significant difference between scores; * = impaired.

On the Aphasia Screening Examination (Reitan, 1984; Reitan & Wolfson, 1993) she exhibited constructional and enunciatory dyspraxia, and dyscalculia, as well as naming, spelling, and reading difficulties. Her performances on measures of nonverbal abstract reasoning and complex concept formation (i.e., Category Test) and cognitive processing speed/visuo-motor tracking (i.e., Trail Making Tests, Parts A & B) were within normal limits. Her perfomance on a test of immediate attention and sequencing of nonverbal auditory stimuli (i.e., Seashore Rhythm Test) was above average. In contrast, she displayed severe impairment on the Speech-Sounds Perception Test, a measure of auditory concentration and perception of verbal stimuli. On the Finger Tapping Test, her upper extremity motor speed was within normal limits for the right (dominant) hand, and mildly impaired with the left hand. Her hand grip strength (i.e., Hand Dynamometer Test) was below average bilaterally. The child also demonstrated deficient bilateral manual dexterity/eye-hand coordination on the Grooved Pegboard Test (Kløve, 1963).

On the Sensory-Perceptual Examination stereognosis was intact. However, the child exhibited bilateral finger agnosia (more errors with the right hand) and dysgraphythesia (significantly more errors with the left hand). She also displayed one tactile error with the right hand, and bilateral visual field suppressions (greater on the left side).

On the Tactual Performance Test (TPT), she exhibited significant impairment of her complex problem-solving skills when she used her right hand, left hand, and both hands simultaneously. She displayed somewhat greater left, versus right, upper extremity impairment as she was only able to correctly place two of six blocks with the left hand, as compared to three of six blocks with her right hand, in 5 min. Her spatial memory for the shapes utilized in this task, as well as their proper locations, was moderately to severely impaired.

On the TOMAL the child obtained a Verbal Memory Index (131) in the superior range. Her Nonverbal Memory Index (96), in contrast, was in the average range. Her Composite Memory Index (115) was in the above average range, whereas her Delayed Recall Index (93) was average. She also exhibited strengths on the following verbal subtests: Memory for Stories (i.e., contextual memory),

Word Selective Reminding (i.e., unrelated auditory verbal learning), and Letters Forward (i.e., immediate auditory attentional capabilities), although she displayed significant deficiencies on the Digits Backwards and Letters Backwards (i.e., mental control) verbal subtests. She exhibited a deficient performance on a nonverbal subtest, Visual Sequential Memory. All other verbal and non-verbal subtest scores were low average to average.

DISCUSSION

The current study has presented the neuropsychological profile of a 9 1/2-year-old female with Triple X Syndrome. This child exhibited mild to moderate deficiencies involving reading, naming, spelling, and articulation abilities, tactile finger perception with the right hand, and concentration and perception of verbal stimuli, which suggests left cerebral hemisphere dysfunction and is generally consistent with previous research that has found verbally based deficiencies in females with Triple X Syndrome. Overall, however, her neuropsychological profile was more indicative of greater right cerebral hemisphere dysfunction. Specifically, the child displayed a borderline compromised level of nonverbal intelligence on the KBIT (i.e., 76 IQ), (as compared to her average, i.e., 92 IQ verbal intelligence), impaired mathematical reasoning, constructional dyspraxia, deficient motor speed with the left hand, kinesthetic problem solving and tactile discrimination impairment greater with the left than the right hand, deficient visual-spatial memory, and primarily left versus right visual field suppression errors. Similar to the difference between the child's verbal and nonverbal IQs, there was also a highly significant difference between her Verbal and Nonverbal Memory Indexes on the TOMAL in favor of her verbal mnestic abilities. Taken together, these findings are suggestive of more normally developed left (i.e., verbal) versus right (i.e., nonverbal) cerebral hemisphere abilities.

The child's neuropsychological profile/presentation was clearly suggestive of the syndrome of Nonverbal Learning Disabilities (NLD) as proposed by Rourke et al. (Casey, Rourke, & Picard, 1991; Rourke 1987, 1988, 1995; Rourke & Tsatsanis,

1996; Tsatsanis & Rourke, 1995). According to Rourke and his colleagues, the NLD Syndrome is characterized by a series of neuropsychological deficits and assets. Primary areas of impairments include deficiencies in tactile perception, visual perception (including visual-spatial-organizational abilities), complex psychomotor skills, and the effective processing of novel material. These impairments are theorized to lead to secondary deficits that include impaired attention to tactile and visual inputs, and limited exploratory behavior. Similarly, tertiary neuropsychological deficits have been proposed that are hypothesized to result from the secondary deficits. These include deficient tactile and visual (non-verbal) memory, and compromised concept-formation and problem-solving skills. With advancing age, a diversity of verbal deficits may also be observed in the NLD Syndrome, including oral-motor praxis difficulties, limited speech prosody, and verbosity that tends to be repetitive, rote, and deficient in context and pragmatics (function) (Rourke & Tsatsanis, 1996).

The NLD Syndrome has been characterized by a diversity of primary neuropsychological assets, including simple repetitive motor skills, well developed auditory-perceptual capabilities, and mastery of rote material (Casey et al., 1991; Rourke 1987, 1988, 1995; Rourke & Tsatsanis, 1996; Tsatsanis & Rourke, 1995). These abilities are theorized to lead to well-developed attention for simple verbal material (i.e., secondary assets), and eventually good rote verbal memory (i.e., tertiary assets). Verbal assets that become more pronounced with age may include well-developed receptive and rote language/verbal skills.

Rourke and his colleagues have also proposed that individuals with the NLD syndrome eventually exhibit graphomotor, reading comprehension, mechanical arithmetic, mathematics, and science academic deficits (Casey et al., 1991; Rourke 1987, 1988, 1995; Tsatsanis & Rourke, 1995). Alternatively, academic assets may include spelling abilities, verbatim memory, single word reading (i.e., decoding), and improved graphomotor skills (i.e., for words) with advancing age. Furthermore, from a socio-emotional/adaptive perspective, individuals with the NLD syndrome may display difficulty adapting to novel situations, impaired social competence (resulting from diminished social judgement

and affective comprehension), and psychosocial disturbance (e.g., internalized psychopathology) especially during late childhood and adolescence (Casey et al., 1991; Rourke 1987, 1988, 1995; Tsatsanis & Rourke, 1995).

Upon comparison of the principal neuropsychological, academic, and socio-emotional characteristics of the NLD syndrome to this child's neuropsychological profile/presentation in the current study, the resemblances appeared quite striking. Overall, the child's neuropsychological results were consistent with the majority of the hypothesized manifestations (i.e., both deficits and assets) of the NLD syndrome. Hence, it appeared that dual diagnoses of both Triple X and NLD syndromes were appropriate in the present case.

Although a comprehensive discussion of the hypothesized mechanisms that are thought to underlie the NLD syndrome is beyond the scope of this paper (see Rourke, 1987, 1988, 1995; Rourke & Tsatsanis, 1996; Tsatsanis & Rourke, 1995 for reviews), it has been proposed that this syndrome is due to white matter dysfunction/destruction that would be especially debilitating for right hemisphere systems, as the ratio of white to gray matter is much greater in the right, as compared to the left, cerebral hemisphere. The effect of this dysfunction/destruction has been hypothesized to result in altered patterns of axonal connections that, in turn, lead to both structural and functional reorganization. It should be noted, however, that although the NLD syndrome has been reported in conjunction with other X chromosomal abnormalities (e.g., Turner's Syndrome; Rovet, 1995; Tsatsanis & Rourke, 1995; see also edited book by Rourke, 1995, for reviews), as in the present case, the actual underlying neural mechanisms responsible for the NLD syndrome remain speculative and largely unknown. Within the present case, it could be inferred that there was significant right cerebral hemisphere dysfunction that was sufficient to produce the NLD syndrome. Rourke's model also quite explicity states that significant perturbation of white matter (e.g., of the corpus callosum) is also sufficient to produce the NLD syndrome. This child's performance on the TPT may reflect the latter as suggested by her poorer performances on the TPT during the second trial. In essence, this may suggest impaired interhemisphere transfer of information via the corpus callosum. Nonetheless, future research is required through multiple case studies or group studies to delineate the underlying neural mechanisms responsible for the NLD syndrome, especially in children such as the one presented in this study.

In summary, whereas a number of previous studies have suggested that females with Triple X Syndrome tend to exhibit poor left cerebral hemisphere (e.g., verbal) abilities, relative to their right (e.g., nonverbal) hemisphere functions, the present study provides evidence that Triple X Syndrome may also be associated with the syndrome of NLD and, possibly greater right hemisphere dysfunction. Thus, although females with Triple X Syndrome may be genotypically similar, from a neuropsychological and psycho-educational perspective, they may be phenotypically diverse. Such findings argue for the importance of comprehensive neuropsychological evaluations of females with Triple X Syndrome who are referred for assessments of their cognitive and behavioral status versus preconceived neuropsychological classifications (e.g., left hemisphere/verbal dysfunction) of these individuals based solely on their chromosomal makeup and the findings of a number of previous studies. With an incidence of roughly one in every 1,000 female births, it is quite likely that there are a number of individuals in the population with this chromosomal abnormality who are experiencing varying degrees of academic, social, and emotional dysfunction.

REFERENCES

Bender, B., Fry, E., Pennington, B., Puck, M., Salbenblatt, J., & Robinson, A. (1983). Speech and language development in 41 children with sex chromosome anomalies. *Pediatrics, 71*, 262–267.

Casey, J.E., Rourke, B.P., & Picard, E.M. (1991). Syndrome of nonverbal learning disabilities: Age differences in neuropsychological, academic, and socioemotional functioning. *Developmental Psychopathology, 3*, 329–345.

Cohen, F.L., & Durham, J.D. (1985). Sex chromosome variations in school-age children. *Journal of School Health, 55*, 99–102.

Dunn, L.M., & Markwardt, F.C. (1970). *Manual for the Peabody Individual Achievement Test.* Circle Pines, MN: American Guidance Service.

Fryns, J.P., Kleczkowska, A., Petit, P., & Van Den Berghe, H. (1983). X-Chromosome polysomy in the female: Personal experience and review of the literature. *Clinical Genetics, 23*, 341–349.

Hier, D.B., Atkins, L., & Perlo, V.P. (1980). Learning disorders and sex chromosome aberrations. *Journal of Mental Deficiency Research, 24*, 17–26.

Jacobs, P.A., Baikie, A.G., Court-Brown, W.N., MacGregor, T.N., MacLean, N., & Harnden, D.G. (1959). Evidence for the existence of the human superfemale. *Lancet, 2*, 423–425.

Kaufman, A.S., & Kaufman, N.C. (1990). *Kaufman Brief Intelligence Test.* Circle Pines, MN: American Guidance Service.

Kazamatsuri, H., Nanko, S., & Mato, Y. (1985). Homicidality in a woman with a 47 XXX karyo-type. *Journal of Clinical Psychiatry, 46*, 346–347.

Kløve, H. (1963). Clinical neuropsychology. In F.M. Forster (Ed.), *The medical clinics of North America* (pp. 1647–1658). New York: Saunders.

Linden, M.G., Bender, B.G., Harmon, R.J., Mrazek, D.A., & Robinson, A. (1988). 47 XXX: What is the prognosis? *Pediatrics, 82*, 610–630.

Machover, K. (1949). *Personality Projection in the Drawing of the Human Figure.* Springfield, IL: Clark C. Thomas.

Netley, C., & Rovet, J. (1982). Verbal deficits in children with 47 XXY and 47 XXX karyotypes: A descriptive and experimental study. *Brain and Language, 17*, 58–72.

Nielson, J. (1991). Follow-up of 25 unselected children with sex chromosome abnormalities to age 12. *Birth Defects, 26*, 201–207.

Nielson, J., Sorensen, A.M., & Sorensen, K. (1981). Mental development of unselected children with sex chromosome abnormalities. *Human Genetics, 59*, 324–332.

Nielson, J., Sorensen, A.M., & Sorensen, K. (1982). Follow-up until age 7 to 11 of 25 unselected children with sex chromosome abnormalities. *Birth Defects, 18*, 61–97.

Nielson, J., & Wohlert, M. (1991a). Chromosome abnormalities found among 34910 newborn children: Results from a 13-year incidence study in Arhus, Denmark. *Human Genetics, 87*, 81–83.

Nielson, J., & Wohlert, M. (1991b). Sex chromosome abnormalities found among 34910 newborn children: Results from a 13-year incidence study in Arhus, Denmark. *Birth Defects: Original Articles Series, 26*, 209–223.

Olanders, S. (1967). Double barr bodies in women in mental hospitals. *British Journal of Psychiatry, 113*, 1097–1099.

Pennington, B.F., Bender, B., Puck, M., Salbenblatt, J., & Robinson, A. (1982). Learning disabilities in children with sex chromosome anomalies. *Child Development, 53,* 1182–1192.

Psychological Corporation (1992). *Wechsler Individual Achievement Test.* New York: Author.

Reitan, R.M. (1979). Manual for administration of neuropsychological test batteries for adults and children. Tucson, AZ: Reitan Neuropsychological Laboratory.

Reitan, R.M. (1984). *Aphasia and sensory-perceptual deficits in adults.* Tucson, AZ: Neuropsychology Press.

Reitan, R.M., & Wolfson, D. (1993). *Halstead-Reitan Neuropsychological Test Battery: Theory and clinical interpretation* (2nd ed.). Tucson, AZ: Neuropsychology Press.

Reynolds, C.R., & Bigler, E.D. (1994). *Test of Memory and Learning.* Austin, TX: PRO-ED.

Robinson, A., Bender, B., Borelli, J., Puck, M., Salbenblatt, J., & Webber, M.L., (1982). Sex chromosomal abnormalities (SCA): A prospective and longitudinal study of newborns identified in an unbiased manner. *Birth defects: Original article series, 18,* 7–39.

Robinson, A., Lubs, H.A., Nielsen, J., & Sorensen, K. (1979). Summary of clinical findings: Profiles of children with 47 XXX and 47 XYY karyotypes. *Birth defects: Original article series, 15,* 261–266.

Rourke, B.P. (1987). Syndrome of nonverbal learning disabilities: The final common pathway of white-matter disease/dysfunction? *The Clinical Neuropsychologist, 1,* 209–234.

Rourke, B.P. (1988). The syndrome of nonverbal learning disabilities: Developmental manifestations in neurological disease, disorder, and dysfunction. *The Clinical Neuropsychologist, 2,* 293–330.

Rourke, B.P. (1995). Introduction: The NLD Syndrome and the white matter model. In B.P. Rourke (Ed.), *Syndrome of nonverbal learning disabilities: Neurodevelopmental manifestations* (pp. 1–26). New York: Guilford Press.

Rourke, B.P., & Tsatsanis, K.D. (1996). Syndrome of nonverbal learning disabilities: Psycholinguistic assets and deficits. *Topics in Language Disorders, 16,* 30–44.

Rovet, J. (1995). Turner syndrome. In B.P. Rourke (Ed.), *Syndrome of nonverbal learning disabilities,* (pp. 351–371). New York: Guilford Press.

Rovet, J., & Netley, C. (1983). The Triple X chromosome syndrome in childhood: Recent empirical findings. *Child Development, 54,* 831–845.

Rustagi, P.K., & Fine, P.M. (1987). Diagnosis and treatment of a child with X-polysomy. *The Journal of the American Academy of Child and Adolescent Psychiatry, 26,* 593–594.

Tennes, K., Puck, M., Bryant, K., Frankenburg, W., & Robinson, A. (1975). A developmental study of girls with Trisomy X. *The American Journal of Human Genetics, 27,* 71–80.

Tsatsanis, K.D., & Rourke, B.P. (1995). Conclusions and future directions. In B.P. Rourke (Ed.), *Syndrome of nonverbal learning disabilities,* (pp. 476–496). New York: Guilford Press.

Waltzer, S. (1985). X chromosome abnormalities and cognitive development: Implications for understanding normal human development. *Journal of Child Psychology and Psychiatry, 26,* 177–184.

Wechsler, D. (1974). Wechsler Intelligence Scale for *Children – Revised.* New York: Psychological Corporation.

Woodhouse, W.J., Holland, A.J., McLean, G., & Reveley, A.M. (1992). The association between Triple X and psychosis. *The British Journal of Psychiatry, 160,* 554–557.

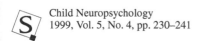
Child Neuropsychology
1999, Vol. 5, No. 4, pp. 230–241

Neuropsychological, Learning, and Psychosocial Profile of Primary School Aged Children with the Velo-Cardio-Facial Syndrome (22q11 Deletion): Evidence for a Nonverbal Learning Disability?

Ann Swillen[1], Leen Vandeputte[1], Joris Cracco[2], Bea Maes[3], Pol Ghesquière[3], Koen Devriendt[1], and Jean-Pierre Fryns[1]

[1]Center for Human Genetics Leuven, University Hospital Gasthuisberg, Leuven, Belgium, [2]Revalidatiecentrum "De Klinker", Knokke-Heist, Belgium, and [3]Department of Educational Sciences, University of Leuven, Leuven, Belgium

ABSTRACT

In this exploratory study, the neuropsychological and learning profile of nine primary school age children with velo-cardio-facial syndrome (VCFS) was studied by systematic neuropsychological testing. In five out of nine children, the following profile was found: a VIQ-PIQ discrepancy (in favor of the VIQ), significantly better scores (.05 level) for reading (decoding) and spelling compared to arithmetic, deficient tactile-perceptual skills (difficulties mainly on the left side of the body), weak but not deficient visual-perceptual abilities, deficient visual-spatial skills, extremely poor psychomotor skills (gross motor skills more deficient than fine motor skills), problems with processing of new and complex material, poor visual attention, good auditory memory and relatively good language skills. These findings correspond to the pattern of neuropsychological assets and deficits that has been described for the syndrome of nonverbal learning disabilities (NLD) (Rourke, 1987, 1988, 1989, 1995). The psychosocial profile of all nine children with VCFS also correspond to that of children with NLD.

Further studies on the relationship between cognitive function, behavior, psychiatric disorder and abnormalities in brain anatomy in young people with VCFS will be needed. In clinical practice, it is worthwhile exploring in greater depth the neuropsychological functions of children with VCFS to rule out NLD, since they may benefit from specific remediation following the learning principles of the NLD-treatment.

Velo-cardio-facial syndrome, also known as Shprintzen syndrome (Shprintzen et al., 1978), is a relatively common congenital anomaly syndrome estimated to affect between 1 in 4000 to 1 in 5000 individuals (Devriendt et al., 1998). Its major features are a cleft palate or velo-pharyngeal insufficiency (with hypernasal speech as the most common presenting symptom), cardiac anomalies, a characteristic facial appearance, learning disabilities or mental retardation. The discovery of a submicroscopic deletion in chromosome 22q11 (Scambler, Kelly, & Lindsay, 1992) in the majority

of patients has confirmed that VCFS is a specific syndrome. In most patients the deletion occurs *de novo*, but familial occurrence with an affected parent is noted in 15% of the patients (Swillen et al., 1998). Marked variability in the associated somatic anomalies and in intelligence has been found. Learning difficulties have been reported frequently. Mental retardation (defined as Full Scale IQ <70 or >2 Standard Deviations below the mean) is found in 45% of the cases, and the incidence of mental retardation is significantly higher in individuals with a familial deletion

Address correspondence to: Ann Swillen, Centre for Human Genetics Leuven, University Hospital Gasthuisberg, Herestraat 49, B-3000 Leuven, Belgium. E-mail: ann.swillen@med.kuleuven.ac.be
Accepted for publication: November 18, 1999.

than in individuals with a *de novo* deletion (Swillen et al., 1997).

In the group of children with learning difficulties (FSIQ > 70), higher verbal IQ than performance IQ (Swillen et al., 1997; Golding-Kushner, Weller, & Shprintzen, 1985; Moss et al., 1995), problems with arithmetic, deficits in attention and concentration, and deficits in visual-spatial-motor abilities have been reported (Golding-Kushner et al., 1985; Swillen et al., 1997; Moss et al., 1999). This pattern of deficits seems to be similar to patterns observed in children who have been identified with nonverbal learning disabilities (NLD). Children and adolescents with NLD syndrome display a pattern of neuropsychological assets and deficits characterized by well developed rote verbal skills within the context of relatively poor psychomotor, tactile-perceptual, visual-spatial-organizational, and non-verbal problem-solving abilities (Harnadak & Rourke, 1994; Rourke, 1989; Rourke, 1995). Problems with social perception, judgement and interactive skills are also reported in children with NLD.

Since the original description of the syndrome (Shprintzen et al., 1978), there is now substantial insight into the medical aspects of the condition. However, we are at an early stage in understanding the complex mechanisms in which the learning difficulties arise in this syndrome. In the present study we examined the neuropsychological abilities, academic achievement and psychosocial profile of primary school age children with VCFS.

The research-project has an explorative character.

METHOD

Subjects
Subjects of the study group were recruited from a group of 134 patients followed by the multidisciplinary team for persons with VCFS at the Center for Human Genetics in Leuven.

Inclusion criteria for the study group were: (a) VCFS confirmed by a 22q11 deletion (shown by FISH: fluorescence *in situ* hybridization using probe DO832); (b) age between 6–12 years (primary school age); (c) Full Scale IQ (FSIQ) > 70 on the most recent intelligence test available.

Thirteen children met the three criteria. Children were recruited by letter and by telephone. Two families did not wish to participate in the study. The original group

studied consisted of eleven children. However, at retesting of intelligence, two children had a FSIQ below 70 and were excluded for further analysis. So, nine children (4 boys, 5 girls) remained who fulfilled the three criteria. Their age varied from 6 years 10 months to 12 years 10 months (mean age: 10, 5).

Table 1 gives a summary of age at the time of testing, sex, origin of the deletion (familial or *de novo*), important medical data, and FSIQ of the nine subjects.

In all nine children the 22q11 deletion occurred *de novo*, and all nine had a heart defect. In seven of the children the heart defect was successfully corrected; in two children (patient no. 3 and patient no. 7) residual cyanosis remained which limited physical exercise.

One child (patient no. 8) had a cleft palate which was surgically repaired and one child (patient no. 9) had a pharyngoplasty for severe velopharyngeal insufficiency.

Procedures
The children were evaluated individually using an assessment battery including measures of intellectual, neuropsychological, linguistic and academic functioning. Children were tested by experienced examiners, and the test battery was presented in a standardized fashion. Parents filled out a form concerning the behavior and psychosocial functioning of their child. The following measures were administered in order to assess neuropsychological abilities and academic skills:

1. Intelligence – The Wechsler Intelligence Scale for Children-Revised (WISC-R) (Van Haasen et al., 1986);
2. Visual Perceptual Skills – Test of Visual Perceptual Skills (TVPS) (Gardner, 1982);
3. Visual Attention – Bourdon-Vos dot-test (Vos, 1988);
4. Auditory Memory – 15 words from Rey (Rey, 1958);
5. Intermodal (visual and auditory) Memory – subtest Name Learning of the Revised Amsterdam Child Intelligence test (RAKIT) (Bleichrodt, Drenth, Zaal, & Resing, 1984);
6. Tactile Perceptual Skills – Finger localization (Benton, Sivan, de Hamsher, Varney & Spreen, 1994);
7. Motor Skills – Bruininks-Oseretzky test of Motor Proficiency (Bruininks, 1978);
8. Visual-motor construction – Visual Motor Integration Test (Beery, 1982):
9. Executive function – Wisconsin Card Sorting Test (WCST) (Heaton, 1981);
10. Language – Language Tests for Children (TVK) (Van Bon, 1982);
11. Academic Skills
    • Reading (decoding) – Brus-One Minute Test (Brus-EMT) (Brus & Voeten, 1979); Klepel – pseudo-word-test (Van den Bos, Spelberg, Scheepstra, & De Vries, 1994);

Table 1. Medical-Data of the Nine Children.

Subject n°	Age (y;m)	Sex	Origin of the deletion	Heart defect	VPI	Other medical problems	FSIQ
1	6;10	F	De novo	Truncus arteriosus	+ +	Feeding problems in infancy; Hypocalcemia; Bilateral VUR;	81
2	7;1	F	De novo	VSD + P.S.	+	Nasal reflux	75
3	7;9	M	De novo	Extreme TOF + right aortic arch	+		73
4	10;2	M	De novo	TOF	−	Constipation; Feeding problems in infancy	71
5	11;6	F	De novo	TOF + right aortic arch	−		70
6	12;0	M	De novo	Extreme TOF	−		70
7	12;5	M	De novo	TOF + right aortic arch	+	Constipation; Laryngomalacie	73
8	12;6	F	De novo	TOF + right aortic arch	+ ; CP	Hypocalcemia	75
9	12;10	F	De novo	VSD + tetralogy of Fallot	+ ; PP		78

Note. TOF: Tetralogy of Fallot; VSD: Ventrical Septum Defect; P.S.: pulmonary stenosis. CP: Cleft Palate; PP: pharyngoplasty. VUR: vesico-ureteral reflux.

- Reading-comprehension – Bel 0, 1, 2a, 3a (Moenaert, 1985, 1987)
- Mathematics – Kortrijk Arithmetic Test (KRT) (Cracco et al., 1994);
- Spelling – Praxis (Van den Heuvel, 1983)

12. Psychosocial functioning – Child Behaviour Checklist (CBCL, Achenbach & Edelbrock) (Dutch version: Verhulst, Koot, Akkerhuis, & Veerman, 1990). Validity and reliability of all the tests of the battery are sufficient.

Raw scores obtained on each of the tests were standardized using published age-based norms. Z-scores (with a mean of 0 and a standard deviation of 1) were calculated in order to compare the results of the different tests. A z-score of < -1 is considered to be deficient. Group profiles were established to make an abstraction of the individual profiles. Therefore group means were calculated in z-scores. Those profiles make it possible to look for tendencies within the group and to compare these tendencies with those of children with NLD. Comparison of the mean scores with the age-based control group was made to demonstrate which skills are deficient ($z \leqslant -1$), normal or better than their peers.

RESULTS

Intellectual Profile

Mean FSIQ was 74 ($SD = 3.70$).

Profile analysis revealed a non-significant ($t(8) = 2.098; p = .692^{1}$) difference between VIQ ($M = 80.11$) and PIQ ($M = 72.78$) for the group. Seven children (77.8%) had better results on verbal tasks relative to visuo-spatial tasks, but only two of them had a statistically significant (.05) discrepancy (see Table 2). A difference of at least 10 points was considered clinically significant (Rourke, 1971, 1973, in Rourke, 1989). Three children (3/9) had a clinically significant VIQ-PIQ discrepancy of 10 points. The remaining six children (6/9) did not have a clinically significant VIQ-PIQ discrepancy of 10 points.

Analysis of the IQ factor scores, showed a non-statistically ($t(8) = 2.982; p = .181$) but a clinically significant difference (difference >10 IQ-points) between the verbal comprehension factor F1IQ

---

[1] To avoid the risk for type 1 error, Bonferonni correction was done (p-value was multiplied by 10)

Table 2. Intelligence Results (WISC-R) of the Group Studied (*n* = 9).

Subject n°	Age (y;m)	Sex	TIQ	TVIQ	TPIQ	F1IQ	F2IQ	F3IQ
1	6;10	F	81	93	74	95	76	82
2	7;1	F	75	82	73	91	67	82
3	7;9	M	73	73	79	79	82	68
4	10;2	M	71	76	70	75	70	77
5	11;6	F	70	73	71	80	69	79
6	12;0	M	70	76	68	79	70	72
7	12;5	M	73	73	77	71	75	86
8	12;6	F	75	81	75	90	74	74
9	12;10	F	78	94	68	93	59	98
M	10;5		74	80.11	72.78	83.66	71.33	79.77
(*SD*)				(3.70)	(8.28)	(3.86)	(8.67)	(6.48)	(8.81)

F1IQ - F2IQ

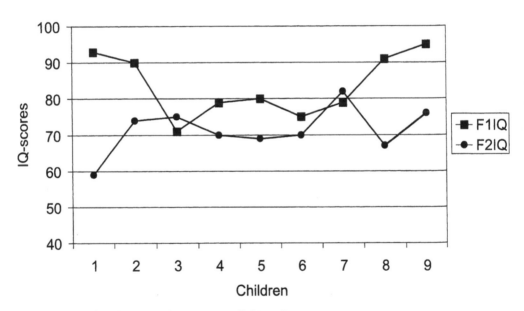

Fig. 1. F1IQ > F2IQ discrepancy in the group studied (*n* = 9).

(*M* = 83.67) and the perceptual-organizational factor F2IQ (*M* = 71.33) (see Fig. 1). Five children had an F1IQ more than 10 points higher than the F2IQ; four of them had F1IQ's that were significantly (.05) better.

The third factor, the freedom from distractibility factor F3IQ (*M* = 79.77) was not significantly lower than the verbal comprehension F1IQ factor or the perceptual-organizational F2IQ factor.

Academic Skills

Seven children were able to do an arithmetic (KRT) and reading test at their school level. At the time of the testing, the two youngest children did not reach a sufficient reading and arithmetic level to perform the tests. Likewise, only six children were able to do the spelling test. Five children were also presented a reading comprehension test. Mean scores for the school assessment battery are given in Table 3.

Table 3. Mean Scores on the School Assessment Battery.

Test	Group Mean (M)-z-score	Standard Deviation (SD)
Arithmetic (KRT) ($n = 7$)	−1.429	(0.45)
Reading (test 1 – Brus) ($n = 7$)	0.043	(0.911)
Reading (test 2 – Klepel) ($n = 7$)	−0.05	(0.881)
Reading Comprehension (Bel) ($n = 5$)	0.19	(0.589)
Spelling (Praxis) ($n = 6$)	−0.5	(1)

Comparing mean results on the Arithmetic test and those of reading (decoding), the discrepancy is obvious. The difference between the mean results of the KRT and the Brus ($p = .036$[1]) and of the KRT and the Klepel ($p = .018$[1]) is more than 1 standard deviation and can be rated clinically and statistically significant. All children ($n = 7$) had better scores on reading tests in comparison to the arithmetic test. Six of them (6/7) had a discrepancy of at least one standard deviation, in favor of the reading tests.

Only five children were tested on both reading-comprehension and decoding skills. Mean z-scores are better for reading-comprehension than for decoding, but the difference is negligible.

A comparison of the Spelling and Arithmetic results shows a better group mean for spelling. The difference is nearly one standard deviation. The spelling results of three children of the group ($n = 6$) were at least one standard deviation better than the results on an arithmetic test. The results on the Praxis (Spelling) were statistically not significantly better ($p = .327$[1]) than those on the KRT (Arithmetic).

Concerning Spelling, Arithmetic and decoding-skills, the results of the group are similar to those of children with NLD. There is an obvious difficulty in completing Arithmetic tests, while their reading and spelling skills are quite normal (see Fig. 2). On the other hand, in contrast with children with NLD, the children with VCFS in our study group did not have better results on the reading-decoding test than on the reading-comprehension test.

Tactile Perception

Eight out of nine children (8/9) had a total finger localization score within the borderline or clinical range. The 4 youngest children of the group had a percentile 0. Group results were statistically significant, with a p-value of <.001 on the z-test.

The tactile perception was obviously deficient. Their problems are even worse when children are younger. Correlation between total raw scores and age of the children was .921.

Six children had better raw scores on the right-hand side compared to the left-hand side. Two children scored similarly on both sides. Group mean raw scores were also better on the right-hand side. The difference between the right and the left-hand side is statistically significant ($p = .033$[1]). Tactile perceptual problems seem therefore to be more obvious on the left side of the body.

The lowest raw scores were on the most complex part of the test (simultaneously touching two fingers behind a box, when the child cannot see his fingers). The difference between the first part (touching one finger while the child is seeing his fingers) and the third and most complex part of the test is statistically significant ($p = .003$[1]) as is the difference between the second part (touching one finger while the child cannot see his finger) and the third part ($p = .007$[1]).

Visual Perception

Three subtests of the TVPS were presented: Visual Form Constancy, Figure–Ground and Visual Closure. Mean scores of the three subtests of all the children ($n = 9$) were calculated. Only one child had a mean z-score of at least 0. All the other children had a negative score, of which three (3/9) scored below −1. Group mean z-score of the three subtests was −.79 which means a weak but not deficient score.

Psychomotor Skills

All children had very weak psychomotor skills on the Bruininks-Oseretzky test of motor proficiency. Each child had a total z-score of −1 or less.

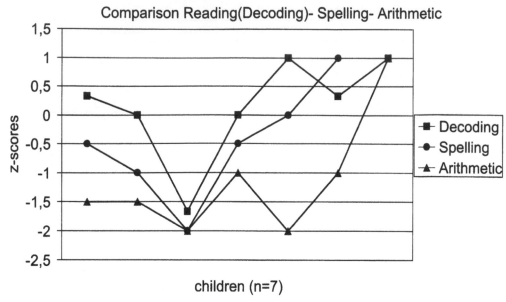

Fig. 2. Comparison between reading (decoding), spelling, and arithmetic in the group studied ($n = 7$).

The highest total motor percentile reached was percentile 12. Three children had a percentile 1 or even less. Five children (5/9) had a lower score on gross motor skills in comparison to fine motor skills.

On the Visual-motor Integration test, the mean group z-score ($z = -.093$) was situated within the normal range. Six children (6/9) had a standard score below one standard deviation of what could be expected according to their age. The visuo-motor integration skills are deficient for the majority of children with VCFS. Problems with visuo-motor skills increased with age.

Executive Function

Fisher, DeLuca, & Rourke (1997) mentioned that deviations of at least one standard deviation for perseverative errors and categories completed can be rated significant. The mean group z-score for perseverative errors in our study group was $-.18$ ($SD = 0.92$) which falls within the normal range. Only one child was making more perseverative errors than could be expected according to age. The other eight children were able to use new strategies if necessary.

Results for categories completed, on the contrary, were weak. Six children (6/9) were not able to fulfill as many categories as their peers. The

mean group z-score was -2 ($SD = 2.2$): we conclude the children had difficulties in finding correct solution strategies.

Attention

The "Bourdon-Vos dots test" is a visual attention test. Each child is evaluated for speed and for correctness. There are five speed (-2 to $+2$) and six correctness (-3 to $+2$) categories. A category score of -1 or less, can be called deficient. Z-scores are available.

With regard to correctness, the mean category-score is -1.843 ($SD = 1.855$). Six children (6/9) have category-scores of -1 or less. In the speed categories, seven children (7/9) have a z-score of -1 or -2.

Even when the children work slower, they are not working more correctly. Only three children had correctness categories of 0 or better. The other children score in the -1, -2 or -3 category. Four of them were working very impulsively, e.g., not starting at the beginning of the lines, or skipping parts. They all score category -3.

Memory

The "15 words of Rey", is an auditory memory test. Each child listens to 15 words being read five times and has to repeat as many words as possible after each time. Z-scores are available for each time and a total z-score can be calculated.

Z-scores for the first time they hear the words are variable: 3/9 have a score below -1, 3/9 score normal and 3/9 have scores above 1. The mean group z-score ($z = 0.48$; $SD = 1.764$) is within the normal range.

The mean z-score for the total group ($z = 0.08$; $SD = 1.764$) is also situated within the normal range. Only one child has a result that deviates more than one standard deviation from the age-related mean. All the other children (8/9) have normal to above normal results.

Language

The 9 children of our study group have scores within the normal range on each subtest of the TVK (Language Tests for Children). Group mean z-scores on each subtest were $-.6$; $-.06$; $-.095$; $-.045$; $-.16$.

Psychosocial Functioning

The Child Behavior Checklist (CBCL), the Teacher Report Form (TRF) and the Youth Self Report (YSR) each consist of 112 behavior patterns (problem items), and these score as follows: 0 if the item is "not true" for the child; 1 if the item is "somewhat or sometimes true"; and 2 is "very true or often true".

T-scores ($M = 50$, $SD = 10$) were calculated for each child. For the total problem score, the internalizing (withdrawn, somatic complaints, anxious/depressed) and externalizing (aggressive behavior and delinquent behavior) subscores, a total t-score of 63 or higher (90th percentile or more) is considered to be in the clinical range. T-scores of 71 or higher (98th percentile or more) for the 8 "small band syndromes" (withdrawn, somatic complaints, anxious/depressed, social problems, thought problems, attention problems, aggressive behavior, delinquent behavior) are found in children with severe behavioral and emotional problems. T-scores of 66 or higher (>93rd percentile) are considered to be "of concern".

All parents filled out the CBCL. The mean group t-score was 62.6 ($SD = 9.30$), which is at the border of the clinical range ($t > 63$). Two-thirds of the parents (6/9) score the behavior of their

children within the clinical range. The majority of children have internalizing problems: the mean t-score for internalizing behavior problems is 62.7 ($SD = 6.946$), which is almost 10 points higher than the mean t-score for externalizing behavior problems ($t = 54.8$; $SD = 14.03$). Most problems found concerned social skills (problems in relationships with peers), attention problems and withdrawal. Only one child had more externalizing than internalizing problems. She is the youngest girl of the group studied.

Seven teachers filled out the TRF. The mean group t-score on the TRF is 59 ($SD = 5.88$). According to the teachers, the children with VCFS had more internalizing problem behavior ($t = 56.43$; $SD = 17.93$) than externalizing problem behavior ($t = 52.43$; $SD = 6.68$). 4/7 of the teachers rated the internalizing problem behavior of their pupils within the clinical range; none of the pupils (0/7) had a clinical score for externalizing problem behavior. The two highest scores on the small band syndromes are on "withdrawn" ($t = 64.428$; $SD = 9.18$) and on "social problems" ($t = 62.857$; $SD = 7.081$).

All six children of 11 years and older, filled out the YSR. The mean group t-score on the YSR was 55 ($SD = 5.138$). All had higher scores for internalizing problem behavior patterns (mean t-score $= 54.33$; $SD = 8.04$) than for externalizing problem behavior (mean t-score $= 46.5$; $SD = 6.28$). The two highest scores on the small band syndromes were on "social problems" ($t = 66.83$; $SD = 10.048$) and on "attention problems" ($t = 60$; $SD = 7.924$). Four of the six adolescents (4/6) had a score within the borderline or clinical range for "social problems", two scored within the borderline range for "attention problems".

DISCUSSION

Before interpreting the results of the current investigation, two important considerations should be noted. First, it is interesting to note that all children in this study had the 22q11 deletion *de novo*. In an earlier study (Swillen et al., 1997) we have shown that the incidence of intellectual disability/mental retardation is correlated with the mode of inheritance: mental retardation is more frequent in the group of children who inherited the deletion from one of their parents. Second, the mean FSIQ of our study group is 74 (range 70–81; $SD = 3.70$). In most other studies on children with NLD, the intelligence range is 70–100. Our study group is therefore at the border of the intelligence range. We believe that it is important to keep this in mind when interpreting the results of the current study.

Although Fuerst et al. (1995) have speculated on the relationship of VCFS (22q11 deletion) and NLD, this study is the first to provide in depth systematic data on this issue. In the earlier study (Swillen et al., 1997) we reported that the IQ scores of 11 school-aged (7–16 years old) children with a mean full-scale IQ score in the 70s with verbal IQ scores were significantly higher than the performance IQ scores. These data confirmed a report by Moss et al. (1995) of a verbal/performance "split". The same researchers (1999) recently reported data on the psychoeducational profile of 33 children and adolescents with the 22q11 deletion and concluded that the IQ and academic profiles are reminiscent of NLD although achievement was not inconsistent with IQ. The results of our study are summarized in Table 4 and show that for many neuropsychological functions, VCFS and NLD have the same deficiencies.

Analysis of the total group shows a clear NLD profile. Like children with NLD, children with VCFS show a VIQ-PIQ discrepancy in their *intelligence profile* in favor of the verbal IQ. When we compare the verbal comprehension factor (F1IQ; $M = 83.67$) with the perceptual-organizational factor (F2IQ; $M = 71.33$), this discrepancy is clinically significant.

With regard to *academic achievement*, we found, as with NLD-children, a statistically significant difference (.05 level) between the reading (decoding) skills and arithmetic. Also, the children with VCFS in the group studied performed better on spelling compared to arithmetic. Therefore, as in children with NLD, primary school age children with VCFS exhibited severe difficulties in mechanical arithmetic and average to above-average single-word reading and spelling skills. However, we noted two differences in the learning profile of children with VCFS in comparison to children with NLD. First, we did not find significantly better results for reading (decoding) in comparison to reading comprehension. It would be interesting to explore the reading comprehension skills of NLD children further. It is our hypothesis that scores of NLD children on a reading comprehension test may depend on the way the test is constructed. We think that NLD children will fail on a reading comprehension test only if the child has to infer the answers from the text. In other words, if the NLD child can find the answers literally in the text, he will perform on the same level as his decoding skills and this may explain the good scores of our group. Second, the children with VCFS did not spell hyperphonetically. Several studies (Sweeny & Rourke, 1978, 1985) have found that children with NLD tend to make phonetically accurate spelling mistakes. These studies were conducted with English-speaking subjects. However the native language of our group was Dutch, a language with a spelling that is phonetically much more accurate than English. It is our clinical experience that the dimension of phonetic accuracy is not as significant in the assessment of

Table 4. Comparison of NLD-VCFS.

Domains	NLD	VCFS
Intelligence	VIQ > PIQ (10 points or >)	VIQ > PIQ (n.s.)
Academic Skills	R and S > Arithmetic	R and S > Arithmetic (.05)*
Visual-Perceptual-Organizational Skills	Deficient	Weak but not deficient
Psychomotor Skills	Deficient	Z-scores of −1 or more*
Complex and New Material	Problematic	Problematic: Z-scores of −2*
Tactile-Perceptual Skills	Left side of the body	Right > left hand side(.05)*
Psychosocial Skills	Poor social and interactive skills	Withdrawal, poor social skills, internalizing problems*

Note. *Criteria are met.

Dutch speaking children with NLD, and we believe that this may be accounted for by the different spelling systems of the two languages.

We found the following pattern of strengths and weaknesses for our group on the *neuropsychological* test battery: deficient tactile-perceptual skills (more problems on the left-hand side of the body), weak but not deficient visual-perceptual abilities, deficient visual-spatial skills, extremely poor psychomotor skills (complex motor skills more deficient than simple motor skills), problems with processing of new and complex material (WCST), poor visual attention, good auditory memory and relatively good language skills. These findings correspond to the pattern of neuropsychological assets and deficits that has been described for the NLD syndrome (Rourke, 1987, 1988b, 1989). It seems, however, that the deficiencies in psychomotor skills of children with VCFS are more pronounced, compared to children with NLD (Cracco, personal communication). Certain medical complications of VCFS such as a congenital heart defect (Tetralogy of Fallot, conotruncal heart defect) or the hypotonia, may in part explain the deficient gross motor skills. The finding of poorer tactile performance for the left than the right hand could suggest that the right hemisphere is more compromised by this condition than the left. However, until now, there are no data from brain imaging studies in children with VCFS that confirm this hypothesis. To date, most structural neuroimaging studies of VCFS individuals have been qualitative and reported the presence of an agenesis of the corpus calosum, a small cerebellum, periventricular white matter abnormalities, white matter hyperintensities, cavum septum pellucidum, smaller total brain volume, and enlarged Sylvian fissures (Mitnick et al., 1994; Lynch et al., 1995; Chow et al., 1999; Bingham et al., 1997).

The *psychosocial profile* of children with VCFS seems to be similar to that of children with NLD. Parents, teachers and youngsters themselves report more internalizing problem behavior than externalizing problem behavior. All three sets of informants most frequently report social problems (especially problems in relationships with peers), withdrawn behavior, and attention problems. Children with NLD are particularly

vulnerable to psychosocial problems. These problems tend to get worse when they grow older and extend well into adulthood with a higher prevalence of psychiatric disorders (Rourke, Young, & Leenaars, 1989). Previous reports (Goldberg et al., 1993; Shprintzen et al., 1992) in adolescents and adults with VCFS found that at least 10% of them will develop psychiatric disorders: symptoms most frequently described are those associated with depression, anxiety disorders and psychotic disorders (including schizophrenia). A good follow-up with special concern for the development of social skills and self-image of VCFS children is indispensable, and parents, teachers and professionals must be alert for behavioral changes.

Because of the small sample, and the lack of a control group, the data from this study should be treated with caution. For future research, multicenter studies on learning problems in VCFS are needed including control groups (children with velopharyngeal insufficiency and learning problems, children with a congenital heart disease and learning problems). However, an exploratory study like the present one, can be the first step in unraveling the underlying complex mechanisms by which the learning problems arise in this syndrome.

In future, studies on the relationship between cognitive function, behavior, psychiatric disorder and abnormalities in brain anatomy in young people with VCFS will be highly needed.

In clinical practice, it is worthwhile exploring in greater depth the neuropsychological functions of children with VCFS to rule out NLD, since they may benefit from specific remediation following the learning principles of the NLD-treatment as described by Rourke (1995).

REFERENCES

Aarnoutse, C.A.J., & Roelofs, E.C. (1994). *Deel IV: Samenvattingstest*. Nijmegen: Berkhout B.V.

Achenbach, T., & Edelbroch (1983). *The Child Behavior Checklist:* Manual. University of Vermont.

Beery, K.E. (1982). *Revised Administration, Scoring and Teaching Manual for the Developmental Test of Visual-Motor Integration*. Cleveland: Modern Curriculum Press.

Benton, A. (1955). Development of the finger-localisation capacity in school children. *Development*, 26, 225–230.

Benton, A., Sivan, A., de S Hansher, K., Varney, N., & Spreen, O. (1994). *Contributions to Neuropsychological Assessment: A Clinical Manual* (2nd edition). New York: Oxford University Press.

Bingham, P.M., Zimmerman, R.A., & McDonald-McGinn, D. (1997). Enlarged sylvian fissures in infants with interstitial deletion of chromosome 22q11. *American Journal of Medical Genetics (Neuropsychiatric Genetics)*, 74, 538–543.

Bleichrodt, N., Drenth, P.J.D., Zaal, J.H., & Resing, W.C.M. (1984). *Rakit: Instructie, Normen, Psychometrische Gegevens*. Lisse: Swets & Zeitlinger.

Bruininks, R.H. (1978). *Bruininks–Oseretsky Test of Motor Deficiency: Examiner's Manual*. Circle Pines: American Guidance Device.

Brus, B.T., & Voeten, M.J.M. (1979). *Eén Minuut Test, Vorm A en B: Verantwoording en Handleiding*. Nijmegen: Berkhout.

Chow, E., Zipursky, R.B., & Mikulis, D. (1999). MRI findings in adults with 22q11 deletion syndrome and schizophrenia, *Schizophrenia Research, 138 (1–3)*, 89.

Cracco, J., Baudonck, M., Debusschere, A., Dewulf, B., Samyn, F., & Vercaemst, V. (1994). *Handleiding bij de Kortrijkse Rekentest*. Kortrijk: Revalidatiecentrum Overleie.

Devriendt, K., Swillen, A., & Fryns, J.P. (1996). Het Velo-Cardio-Faciaal syndroom: een frequent genetische aandoening veroorzaakt door microdeleties in chromosoom 22q11. *Tijdschrift voor Geneeskunde*, 52, 511–521.

Devriendt, K., Mortier, G., Van Thienen, M., Keymolen, K., & Fryns, J.P. (1998). The annual incidence of DG/VCFS syndrome. *J. Med. Genetics*, 35, 9, 789–790.

Fisher, N.J., DeLuca, J.W., & Rourke, B.P. (1997). Wisconsin card sorting test and Halstead category performances of children and adolescents who exhibit the syndrome of nonverbal learning disabilities. *Child Neurology*, 3, 61–7.

Fuerst, K.B., Dool, C.B., & Rourke, B.P. (1995). Velocardiofacial syndrome. In B.P. Rourke (Ed.), *Syndrome of Nonverbal Learning Disabilities: Neurodevelopmental manifestations*. New York: Guilford Press.

Gardner, M. (1982). *TVPS Test of Visual Perceptual Skills (Non-Motor): Manual*. Seattle: Special Child Publications, pp. 119–137.

Goldberg, R., Motzkin, B., Marion, R., Scambler P., & Shprintzen, R. (1993). Velo-cardio-facial syndrome: a review of 120 patients. *American J. of Med. Genet.*, 45, 313–319.

Golding-Kushner, K.J., Weller, G., & Shprintzen, R.J. (1985). Velo-Cardio-Facial syndrome: language and

psychological profiles. *Journal of Craniofacial Genetics and Developmental Biology*, 5, 259–266.

Harnadek, M.C.S., & Rourke, B.P. (1994). Principal identifying features of the syndrome of nonverbal learning disabilities in children. *Journal of Learning Disabilities*, 27, 144–154.

Heaton, R.K. (1981). *Wisconsin Card Sorting Test Manual*. Odessa: Florida: Psychological Assessment resources.

Kelly, D., Goldberg, R., Wilson, D., Lindsay, E., Carey, A., Goodship, J., Burn, J., Cross, I., Shprintzen, R.J. & Scambler, P.J. (1993). Confirmation that the velo-cardio-facial syndrome is associated with haplo-insufficiency of genes at chromosome 22q11. *American Journal of Medical Genetics*, 32, 612–618.

Lynch, D.R., McDonald-McGinn, D., & Zackai E.H. (1995). Cerebellar atrophy in a patient with velo-cardio-facial syndrome. *Journal of Medical Genetics*, 32, 561–563.

Mitnick, R.J., Bello J.A., & Shprintzen R.J. (1994). Brain anomalies in velo-cardio-facial syndrome. *American Journal of Medical Genetics*, 54, 100–106.

Moenart, H. (1985). *Onderzoek van het Technisch en Begrijpend Lezen in De Eerste Graad. Instructies en Onderzoeksverslag bij Zes Gestandardiseerde Tests*. Brussel: C.S.B.O.

Moenart, H. (1987). *Onderzoek van het Technisch en Begrijpend Lezen in de Tweede Graad. Instructies en Onderzoeksverslag bij Vijf Gestandardiseerde Tests*. Brussel: C.S.B.O.

Moss, E.M., Wang, P.P., McDonald-McGinn, D.M., Gerdes, M., DaCosta, A.M., & Christensen, K.M. (1995). Characteristic cognitive profile in patients with a 22q11.2 deletion: verbal IQ exceeds non-verbal IQ. *American Journal of Human Genetics*, 57 (Suppl.), A20.

Moss, E.M., Batshaw, M.L., Solot, C.B., Gerdes, M., McDonald-McGinn, D., Driscoll, D.A., Emanuel, B.S., Zackai, E.H., & Wang, P.P. (1999) Psychoeducational profile of the 22q11.2 deletion: a complex pattern. *Journal of Pediatrics*, 134, 193–198.

Rey, A. (1958). *L'Examen Clinique en Psychologie*. Paris: Presses Universitaires de Frances.

Rourke, B.P. (1987). Syndrome of nonverbal learning disabilities. The final common pathway of white-matter disease/dysfunction? *The Clinical Neuropsychologist*, 1, 209–234.

Rourke, B.P. (1988). Syndrome of nonverbal learning disabilities. Developmental manifestations in neurological disease, disorder, and dysfunction. *The Clinical Neuropsychologist*, 2, 293–330.

Rourke, B.P., Young, G., & Leenaars, A. (1989). A childhood learning disability that predisposes those afflicted to adolescent and adult depression. *Journal of Learning Disabilities*, 22, 169–175.

Rourke, B.P. (1989). *Nonverbal Learning Disabilities: The Syndrome and the Model.* New York: Guilford Press.

Rourke, B.P. (Ed.) (1995). *Syndrome of Nonverbal Learning Disabilities: Neurodevelopmental Manifestations.* New York: Guilford Press.

Scambler, P.J., Kelly, D., & Lindsay, E. (1992). Velo-cardio-facial syndrome associated with chromosome 22 deletions encompassing the DiGeorge locus. *Lancet, 339,* 1138–1141.

Shprintzen, R.J., Goldberg, R.B., Lewin, M.D., Sidoto, E.J., Berkman, M.D., Argamaso, R.V., & Young, D. (1978). A new syndrome involving cleft palate, cardiac anomalies, typical facies, and learning disabilities: Velo-cardio-facial syndrome. *Cleft Palate Journal, 5,* 56–62.

Shprintzen, R., Goldberg, R., Golding-Kushner, K., & Marion, R. (1992). Late-onset psychosis in the velo-cardio-facial syndrome. *American Journal of Medical Genetics, 42,* 141–142.

Sweeny, J.E., & Rourke, B. (1978). Neuropsychological significance of phonetically accurate and phonetically inaccurate spelling errors in younger and older retarded spellers. *Brain and Language, 6,* 212–225.

Sweeny, J.E., & Rourke, B. (1985). Spelling disability subtypes. In B.P. Rourke (Ed.), *Neuropsychology of Learning Disabilities: Essentials of Subtype Analysis.* New York: Guilford Press, pp. 147–165.

Swillen, A., Devriendt, K., Legius, E., Eyskens, B., Dumoulin, M., Gewillig, M., & Fryns, J.P. (1997). Intelligence and psychosocial adjustment in velo-cardio-facial syndrome: a study of 37 children and adolescents with VCFS. *Journal of Medical Genetics, 34,* 453–458.

Swillen, A., Devriendt, K., Vantrappen, G., Vogels, A., Rommel, N., Eyskens, B., Gewillig, M., & Fryns, J.P. (1998). Letter to the editor: Familial deletions in chromosome 22q11: the Leuven experience. *American Journal of Medical Genetics, 80,* 531–532.

Van Bon, W.H.J. (1982). *Taaltests voor Kinderen. Handleiding:* Lisse: Swets & Zeitlinger.

Van den Bos, K.P., Spelberg, H.C.L., Scheepstra, A.S.M., & De Vries, J.R. (1994). *De Klepel: Pseudowoordentest.* Nijmegen: Berkhout.

Van den Heuvel, F. (1983). *Spellingtoetsen voor het Basisonderwijs.* Den Bosch: Malmberg.

Van Haasen, P., De Bruyn, E., Pijl, Y., Poortinga, Y., Spelberg, H., Vander Steene, G., Coetsier, P., Spoelders-Claes, R., & Stinissen, J. (1986). *WISC-R: Handleiding.* Lisse: Swets & Zeitlinger.

Van Haasen, P., De Bruyn, E., Pijl, Y., Poortinga, Y., Spelberg, H., Vander Steene, G., Coetsier, P., Spoelders-Claes, R., & Stinissen, J. (1986). *WISC-R: Scoring en Normen.* Lisse: Swets & Zeitlinger.

Verhulst, F.C., Koot, J.M., Akkerhuis, G.W., & Veerman, J.W. (1990). *Praktische Handleiding voor de CBCL.* Assen: Van Gorcum.

Vos, P.G. (1988). *Bourdon Vos Test: Handleiding.* Lisse: Swets & Zeitlinger.

Journal of Clinical and Experimental Neuropsychology
1998, Vol. 20, No. 2, pp. 211–220

Validation of the Warrington Theory of Visual Processing and the Visual Object and Space Perception Battery

Lisa J. Rapport[1], Scott R. Millis[2], and Patricia J. Bonello[1]

[1]Wayne State University, Detroit, MI, and [2]Department of Psychology and Neuropsychology, Rehabilitation Institute of Michigan, Detroit

ABSTRACT

Competing hypotheses regarding the nature of visual processing were examined using the performance of 111 healthy older persons on the Warrington and James (1990) Visual Object and Space Perception Battery (VOSP). Confirmatory factor analysis indicated that a two-factor model corresponding to the Warrington theory of object and space perception as discrete domains showed excellent congruence with the data, despite limitations in the VOSP space perception tests that may have resulted in underestimation of model fit. Moreover, compared to a unidimensional model of visual processing, the Warrington model demonstrated a superior fit to the data. These findings add to the bodies of evidence supporting a dissociation between object- and space-perception abilities and defining the construct validity of the VOSP battery.

The evaluation of object and space perception is an integral part of a comprehensive neuropsychological assessment. Both object and space perception may present as selective deficits, even among patients with normal visual acuity (McCarthy & Warrington, 1990). Unfortunately, common neuropsychological tests often fail to assess these abilities separately. Instead, many tests combine several aspects of visual processing, as well as motoric demands such as constructional abilities. Although complex tasks are useful as screening measures for impairment in broad domains of functioning, they provide little insight into the specific nature of abilities. This, in turn, limits both the theoretical and clinical insights that may be obtained from the assessment. Even in the absence of impairment, distinctions between related cognitive abilities are useful in enhancing our understanding of relative strengths and weaknesses in the assessment profile. For example, the phenomenon of general intellectual functioning is examined in terms of relative

abilities in verbal and nonverbal (i.e., performance) domains, and language functioning is described in terms of expressive versus receptive abilities.

Warrington and colleagues (McCarthy & Warrington, 1990; Warrington & James, 1988; Warrington & Rabin, 1970) have proposed that object and space perception are functionally independent domains of visual processing. They devised a series of tasks to represent the components of each domain and compiled them into a battery designed to measure these abilities. The theoretical foundation on which the Visual Object and Space Perception Battery (VOSP; Warrington & James, 1991) was based is described briefly below.

Object perception

Object perception is a requisite to object recognition, which represents the successful integration of sensory, perceptual, and representational information. Lissauer (1890; as cited in Warrington & James, 1988) first proposed a two-stage model of

Address correspondence to: L. Rapport, Department of Psychology, 71 West Warren, Wayne State University, Detroit, MI 48202, USA. E-mail: rapport@sun.science.wayne.edu
Accepted for publication: January 14, 1998.

object recognition: *apperception*, which reflects the conscious awareness of a sensory impression (i.e., sensory and perceptual processes combined), and *association*, which reflects the connection of meaning to the content of apperception. This is conceptually similar to Marr's paradigm of object recognition, which maintains that a three-dimensional model of representation (i.e., geometry and volume) precedes the assignment of meaning (Marr, 1982). In contrast, the Warrington model of object recognition allows for both a postsensory stage of visual analysis, as well as presemantic influences (Warrington & James, 1988). Because perceptual categorization becomes optional as opposed to a mandatory phase, this model explains better than does Marr's serial model the occurrence of these deficits in the absence of impairments in visual semantic knowledge.

The Warrington tripartite model distinguishes between three subtypes of impaired object recognition: (1) disorders of visual sensory discrimination, which reflect selective deficits affecting sensory processing, including acuity, shape discrimination, and color discrimination; (2) apperceptive agnosia, which refers to disorders of object perception; and (3) associative agnosia, which refers to disorders in deriving the meaning of visually presented objects, even in the presence of normal sensory and perceptual abilities (McCarthy & Warrington, 1990).

In the phenomenon of apperceptive agnosia, impairments are observed on tasks that manipulate the perceptual dimensions of a stimulus, such as altering the angle from which an object is viewed or changing lighting conditions. These impairments are associated with right hemisphere brain damage and are most severe following damage to the right parietal lobe (Warrington & Taylor, 1973). Tasks that degrade, distort, or obscure salient features of an image are especially vulnerable to right posterior lesions, yet these patients may retain the ability to achieve form discrimination (Warrington & James, 1988). For example, a case study of a right-hemisphere-injured patient reported by Humpreys and Riddoch (1984) demonstrated that, despite difficulty recognizing objects from an unusual view, the abilities to determine relative length, size, and position of objects in space may remain intact.

Space Perception

McCarthy and Warrington (1990) provide a detailed discussion of the clinical and anatomical considerations involved in spatial perception. In brief, *visual disorientation* refers to an impairment in localizing the position of objects in space with intact function in visual acuity. This disorder is commonly observed following bilateral damage at the occipitoparietal boundary. The ability to determine single-point localization is considered a prerequisite to higher-order functions of spatial perception. Therefore, patients with this impairment show profound deficits on many spatial tasks. *Visuospatial agnosia* is a disorder of spatial analysis observed on more complex tasks such as position discrimination (e.g., matching the locations of stimuli), stimulus orientation, and stimulus enumeration (e.g., cube analysis). Visuospatial agnosia includes impairments frequently associated with unilateral neglect, such as problems in spatial discrimination (e.g., line bisection) and spatial search (e.g., detection and cancellation tasks). In general, these abilities are linked to the right hemisphere, with posterior lesions producing the most severe and longlasting impairment.

Dissociation of Abilities in Object and Space Perception

Although patients with right posterior lesions frequently are impaired on both spatial analysis and object perception tasks, there appears to be little relationship between these problems (Newcombe, 1969; Warrington & James, 1988; Warrington & Rabin, 1970). For example, a patient may be impaired in identifying objects from an unusual view, but may test within normal limits on position discrimination tasks. Kartsounis and Warrington (1991) reported the case of a woman with well-preserved shape discrimination and impaired figure-ground discrimination who was unable to perceive stimuli requiring minimal spatial organization. According to McCarthy and Warrington (1990), it is common for patients with right posterior damage to perform poorly on both object perception and spatial analysis tasks; however, it is not possible to predict one set of impairments from the other.

There is also evidence for the anatomical separateness of object and space perception. Mishkin and Manning (1978) found that lesions of the principal sulcus in rhesus monkeys trained on delayed object matching tasks yielded severe deficits on spatial memory tasks, but only small and transient deficits on nonspatial tasks. Lesions of the inferior frontal convexity produced severe and lasting deficits on object perception tasks. Mishkin, Ungerleider, and Macko (1983) suggested that there are different cortical pathways for object and spatial vision: Identification of objects is associated with a pathway connecting the striate, prestriate, and inferior temporal areas, whereas spatial processing is linked to a pathway connecting the striate, prestriate, and inferior parietal areas. Similarly, Livingstone and Hubel (1988) suggested that the monkey has independent pathways selective for form in the parvocellular geniculate subdivisions and for depth in the magnocellular subdivisions. A dissociation of object and spatial abilities associated with working memory has been observed in neuroimaging studies of the human brain (Courtney, Ungerleider, Keil, & Haxby, 1996); however, there have been mixed findings in studies of visual working memory in this regard (Owen, Evans, & Petrides, 1996).

In sum, there is evidence that object and space perception are both functionally and anatomically discrete. The types of tasks representing these abilities are fairly specific, and exemplars of these tasks are included in the Visual Object and Space Perception Battery (VOSP; Warrington & James, 1991).

Validation of the Warrington Theory of Visual Processing

The present study addresses both theoretical and psychometric issues regarding the model of object and space perception as proffered by Warrington and colleagues. Research examining the validity of this theory has focused on clinical populations. An impressive collection of evidence indicates that a two-factor model, in which object and space perception dissociate, accurately describes the disordered brain (see Humpreys & Riddoch, 1984; Kartsounis & Warrington, 1991; McCarthy & Warrington, 1990; Postle et al., 1997; Warrington & James, 1988; 1991). However, among normal individuals, abilities in domains sharing similar features tend to be highly related. Thus, the functional

distinction between object and space perception as proposed by Warrington and colleagues may not exist or may be so subtle as to be irrelevant in the absence of selective deficit. A parsimonious model might posit that visual processing is a unidimensional phenomenon in the normal brain, and that this general rule of functioning may be disrupted by brain insult to result in selective sparing of visual processing abilities.

Validation of a test purported to measure a construct is itself evidence for the theory of the construct, and this should be demonstrated through multiple methods and measures (Campbell & Fiske, 1950; Cronbach & Meehl, 1955). The validity of the VOSP battery in detecting right hemisphere damage has been demonstrated in numerous studies finding expected performance differences between these patients and left-hemisphere-damaged patients, as well as normal controls (see Warrington & James, 1991). However, no research has examined the congruence of the VOSP battery dimensional structure with the theoretical structure on which it was developed. Confirmatory factor analysis provides one method to evaluate this essential aspect of validity.

Purpose

The present investigation examines competing hypotheses regarding the nature of visual processing in a sample of healthy older persons. Two models of visuoperceptual and visuospatial functioning were specified a priori using the subtests from the VOSP and evaluated using confirmatory factor analysis: (1) a first-order, one-factor model postulating that object and space perception are best understood as a unitary process; and (2) a first-order, two-factor model representing Warrington's concept of separate and discrete object perception and space perception constructs. Statistical incongruence between the theoretical model of visual processing and the VOSP may reflect problems with the construct validity of the test, due to inadequate representation of a valid theory, or problems with the theory, were it assumed that the test battery represents an adequate assessment of visual processing abilities. Conversely, evidence for the independence of abilities on VOSP tests of object and space perception would lend powerful support for the two-factor theory of visual processing.

METHOD

Participants

The sample consisted of 111, healthy older adults (66 females and 45 males) aged 50 to 84 years (M = 68.2, SD = 9.5). Mean level of education was 13.3 years (SD = 2.2; range = 4–18). Volunteers for the study were recruited from senior citizen activity centers and churches. These participants held or had held jobs classified as unskilled (7.2%), service work (6.3%), craftsperson (11.7%), managerial/clerical (50.5%), and professional (16.2%), or they were not employed outside the home (8.1%).

Exclusionary criteria included significant health problems in the past 5 years, history of neuropsychologic risk factors, or use of prescription drugs that may adversely affect cognitive functioning (see Measures). The present sample excludes 4 persons who reported use of prescription drugs that have known effects on cognitive functioning, as well as 1 person with a history of stroke. The Shipley-Hartford Vocabulary Test was used to obtain an estimate of IQ (Zachary, 1986). The standard score on the Shipley-Hartford (M = 112.5, SD = 26.17) suggests that the verbal IQ of the present sample was equivalent to that of the original normative sample; however, this suggests also that the sample demonstrated an above-average level of functioning.

Measures

The Physical Health domain of the Philadelphia Geriatric Center Multilevel Assessment Instrument (MAI; Lawton, Moss, Fulcomer, & Kleban, 1982).

The MAI was used to assess the health status of the participants. According to Hultsch, Hammer, and Small (1993), self-reported health status is an excellent predictor of actual health status and performance on cognitive tasks. Physical health is assessed by the MAI in three subdomains: (1) ratings of health status; (2) health-related behaviors, such as number of physician visits, days hospitalized, and days bedridden at home; and (3) a checklist that screens for 22 medical conditions, including neuropsychologic risk factors such as stroke, hypertension, heart disease, head injury, Parkinson's disease, tumor, and diabetes. Participants in the present study were excluded for history of any of these conditions. Normative data for healthy older individuals indicate an expected value of 63.65 (SD = 4.79; Lawton et al., 1982). This compares favorably to the mean health rating of 64.49 (SD = 4.20) observed in the present sample, and it indicates that the sample was in good health.

Visual Object and Space Perception Battery (VOSP; Warrington & James, 1991)

The VOSP consists of a screening test to establish requisite sensory acuity and eight clinical tests. According to the test authors, object perception is measured by the Incomplete Letters, Silhouettes, Object Decision, and Progressive Silhouettes tests, whereas space perception is measured by the Dot Counting, Position Discrimination, Number Location, and Cube Analysis tests. Detailed descriptions of the tests are included in the manual (Warrington & James, 1991), and the reliabilities of the tests when used with older persons have been described elsewhere (Bonello, Rapport, & Millis, 1997).

VOSP Tests of Object Perception: *Incomplete Letters* assesses the ability to identify shapes with degraded perceptual clarity. The test includes 20 stimulus cards, each depicting a letter degraded by 70%, and examinees are asked to identify the letters. *Silhouettes* assesses the ability to identify common objects depicted from atypical perspectives. The test consists of 30 silhouette drawings created by rotating the objects on the lateral axis. *Object Decision* requires examinees to select the silhouette drawing of a real object from among a distractor set of three nonsense objects (20 trials). *Progressive Silhouettes* requires the identification of objects rotated from frontal view so that the defining features of the object are obscured. The task consists of two series of stimulus cards (a gun and a trumpet), each consisting of 10 silhouette drawings, with each successive drawing revealing progressively more details of the object. Examinees attempt to identify the object as each drawing in the series is presented.

VOSP Tests of Spatial Perception: The *Dot Counting* test requires examinees to identify the number of stimuli presented in a random array (10 trials). Both the Position Discrimination and Number Location tests require the ability to discriminate relative spatial positions. The *Position Discrimination* test presents two squares, each containing a black dot, and examinees discern which of the squares contains the centered dot (20 trials). In *Number Location*, the stimulus cards also consist of two squares: one square presents a random array of numbers and the other contains a black dot. Examinees determine the number in the upper square that corresponds most closely with the position of the dot in the bottom square (10 trials). The *Cube Analysis* test assesses the ability to interpret three-dimensional space represented in two dimensions. Examinees are asked to determine the number of blocks represented in line drawings, including blocks that may be hidden from view (10 trials).

Procedure

Following informed consent procedures, participants completed a brief demographic questionnaire, as well as the MAI, Shipley-Hartford, and the VOSP battery. All measures were administered using the standardized methods described in the test manuals. Each volunteer received $5 for participating in the study. The data were collected initially for a study examining the normative and psychometric properties of the VOSP when used with older persons native to North America, and the results of this investigation have been published (Bonello et al., 1997).

RESULTS

Table 1 presents the correlations, means, and standard deviations used in the analysis. As described above, the cognitive functions described by Warrington were proposed to represent a two-factor

model: object perception measured by the Incomplete Letters, Silhouettes, Object Decision, and Progressive Silhouettes tests; and space perception measured by the Dot Counting, Position Discrimination, Number Location, and Cube Analysis tests. The one-factor model represented the unidimensional hypothesis that the eight VOSP tests measured only one latent construct of visual processing.

The primary estimation technique used in the confirmatory factor analysis was the SCALED χ^2 technique with robust standard errors (Bentler, 1993). The maximum likelihood (ML) estimator was used as a secondary method. The SCALED χ^2 statistic was chosen as the primary estimator because the data in this study evidenced significant nonnormality. Tests for multivariate normality revealed the following statistics for skewness ($z = 28.77$), kurtosis ($z = 12.28$), and for third and fourth moments considered jointly ($\chi^2 = 978.26$). Most of the VOSP subtests were negatively skewed, showing a ceiling effect with participants making low numbers of errors on the procedures. An important assumption underlying the ML estimator is that the data are multivariate normal. Violation of this assumption can lead to an inadequate evaluation of the model: the χ^2 goodness-of-fit test tends to reject too many true models and parameter estimates may be biased, yielding too many significant results (Browne, 1984; West, Finch, & Curran, 1995).

Table 1. Correlations, Means, and Standard Deviations of Visual Object and Space Perception Battery (VOSP) Subtests.

	LETT	SIL	OBJ	PROG	DOT	LOC	CUBE	POS
LETT	1.00							
SIL	.33	1.00						
OBJ	.14	.50	1.00					
PROG	.22	.60	.53	1.00				
DOT	−.03	.29	.11	.11	1.00			
LOC	.33	.33	.27	.23	.18	1.00		
CUBE	.24	.44	.25	.32	.34	.29	1.00	
POS	.22	.05	.13	.20	−.02	.17	.15	1.00
M	19.28	17.81	16.51	10.90	9.72	8.04	9.01	19.37
(*SD*)	(1.12)	(4.53)	(2.39)	(2.60)	(0.65)	(2.48)	(1.66)	(1.18)

Note. LETT = Incomplete Letters; SIL = Silhouettes; OBJ = Object Decision; PROG = Progressive Silhouettes; DOT = Dot Counting; LOC = Number Location; CUBE = Cube Analysis; POS = Position Discrimination.

Table 2. Summaries of Fit for Measurement Models.

Model	SCALED χ^2 (df)	P	Robust CFI	χ^2	p	GFI	AGFI	NNFI	IFI	CFI	RMSEA	90% CI RMSEA	p-close	ECVI
One-Factor	31.36 (20)	.05	.88	38.54	.01	.92	.86	.84	.89	.89	.09	.05–.13	.06	.64
Two-Factor	27.55 (19)	.09	.91	31.49	.04	.93	.87	.89	.93	.92	.08	.02–.12	.17	.56
One-Factor Respecified	28.18 (19)	.08	.91	33.45	.02	.93	.87	.87	.92	.91	.08	.03–.13	.12	.61
Two-Factor Respecified	23.69 (18)	.17	.94	26.06	.10	.95	.89	.92	.95	.95	.06	.00–.11	.31	.56

Note. CFI = Comparative Fit Index; GFI = Goodness of Fit Index; AGFI = Adjusted Goodness of Fit Index; NNFI = Non-normed Fit Index; IFI = Incremental Fit Index; RMSEA = Root Mean Square Error of Approximation; ECVI = Expected Cross-validation Index.

One-Factor Model

Table 2 is a summary of fit measures for all models. The one-factor model was associated with 20 degrees of freedom (36 observed variances and covariances, 16 estimated parameters). According to overall fit criteria, the one-factor model resulted in relatively poor fit on the basis of the absolute indexes (SCALED χ^2 = 31.36, p = .051, ML χ^2 = 38.54, p = .008), as well as on selected Type-2 and Type-3 indexes, measures based on the population discrepancy, and information-theoretic measures (see Table 2). The component fit measures also indicated misspecification. Although the individual parameter estimates were in the expected direction and there was no evidence of Heywood cases, the structural coefficient for Position Discrimination was not statistically significant. In addition, several of the standardized structural coefficients (i.e., "factor loadings") were of low magnitude (Position Discrimination = .18, Dot Counting = .29, Incomplete Letters = .37), as were some of the squared multiple correlations, R^2 (Position Discrimination = .03, Dot Counting = .08, Incomplete Letters = .14). As Bollen (1989) demonstrated, the squared multiple correlation coefficient is a measure of reliability, whereas the structural coefficients assess aspects of validity in determining which measures are strong indicators of the latent construct.

In considering both global and component indicators of model fit, it appeared that problems with this one-factor model stemmed from both model misspecification and poor psychometric properties of some VOSP subtests, particularly Position Discrimination and Incomplete Letters. The subtests having the largest structural coefficients were those that purportedly measure object perception: Silhouettes, Object Decision, and Progressive Silhouettes. In contrast, the subtests proposed to measure space perception had smaller coefficients. Taken together, these results suggest the presence of more than one latent construct.

Two-Factor Model

The two-factor model was associated with 19 degrees of freedom (36 observed variances and covariances, 17 estimated parameters). This model fit the data significantly better than did the one-factor model: ΔSCALED χ^2 (1) = 3.81, p = .05,

$\Delta\chi^2$ (1) = 7.05, p = .008. According to overall fit criteria, the two-factor model resulted in a more reasonable fit on the basis of the absolute indexes (SCALED χ^2 = 27.55, p = .09, ML χ^2 = 31.49, p = .04) and Type-2 and Type-3 indexes (see Table 2). In contrast to the one-factor model, the structural coefficients were consistent with the model's hypothesis: object perception measures had loadings that ranged from .62 to .85 except for Incomplete Letters (.36), whereas space perception measures had loadings that ranged from .41 to .68 except for Position Discrimination (.21). The pattern of R^2 values for the two-factor analysis was consistent with that observed for the one-factor model; that is, Position Discrimination and Incomplete Letters again appeared to be unreliable measures, and the structural coefficient for Position Discrimination was nonsignificant. Although model misspecification and psychometric weaknesses of some VOSP subtests appeared to account for model misfit in the one-factor model, subtest psychometric shortcomings seemed predominant in the two-factor model. The object and space perception factors were significantly correlated (r = .72) in the two-factor model.

Model Respecification

A conservative strategy for respecification to improve model fit was employed, based on guidelines suggested by Hoyle and Smith (1994). These authors assert that post hoc added correlated errors of measurement frequently capitalize on idiosyncratic characteristics of the sample; therefore,

justification for post hoc estimations of these covariances should be based on theoretical criteria rather than statistical criteria alone.

The Lagrange Multiplier (LM) procedure was used to determine whether previously fixed parameters in both the one- and two-factor models could be freed to be estimated in order to improve model fit. For both models, the multivariate LM test indicated that allowing the following measurement errors to correlate would significantly improve fit: Object Decision and Progressive Silhouettes, Silhouettes and Position Discrimination, Incomplete Letters and Number Location.

It is noteworthy that the latter two covariances were based on the least reliable VOSP measures and were unrelated to the theoretical constructs tested in the present study. Consequently, it did not appear justifiable to estimate these covariances. In contrast, allowing the errors of Object Decision and Progressive Silhouettes to correlate made substantive sense. These two subtests showed sound reliability and theoretically share some degree of method variance in that both subtests employ shadowed stimuli.

Table 2 contains a summary of the fit indexes for the respecified models and Table 3 presents standardized structural coefficients and squared multiple correlations. Although both respecified models yielded improved fit, the two-factor model appeared superior: ΔSCALED χ^2 (1) = 4.48, p = .03, $\Delta\chi^2$ (1) = 7.40, p = .007. Again, in the one-factor model, the R^2 values and structural coefficients for the space perception measures

Table 3. Standardized Structural Coefficients and Squared Multiple Correlations for Respecified Models.

Subtest	One-Factor Model-Respecified		Two-Factor Model-Respecified		
	Visuoperception	R^2	Object Perception	Spatial Perception	R^2
LETT	.38	.15	.36		.13
SIL	.87	.75	.92		.85
OBJ	.56	.31	.54		.30
PROG	.67	.45	.65		.43
DOT	.31	.10		.43	.19
LOC	.42	.18		.47	.22
CUBE	.53	.28		.69	.48
POS	.15	.02		.18	.03

Note. LETT = Incomplete Letters; SIL = Silhouettes; OBJ = Object Decision; PROG = Progressive Silhouettes; DOT = Dot Counting; LOC = Number Location; CUBE = Cube Analysis; POS = Position Discrimination.

were lower than were the corresponding values for the object perception measures. In addition to better overall fit, the structural coefficients of the two-factor model were larger and theoretically consistent with the proposed model of separate latent components comprising the VOSP.

DISCUSSION

The present findings provide support for the Warrington theory of visual processing. A two-factor model of object and space perception as discrete domains showed good congruence with the performance patterns of healthy older persons and fit the data better than did a unidimensional model of visual processing. Moreover, the difference between the one- and two-factor models may have been greater were it not for the low psychometric reliability of the VOSP space perception measures. The object perception measures were stronger and more reliable indicators of their respective latent construct than were the space perception measures; consequently, detection of a spatial construct was hampered. Indeed, it is striking that a spatial construct could be measured in this context.

Although a two-factor model described the structure of the visual processing data well, the object and space perception factors were strongly related. With this degree of association, higher-order factor models frequently are proposed because a second-order general factor is able to account more fully for the relationships among the factors than is a first-order factor model (Rindskopf & Rose, 1988). That is, specific constructs can be highly correlated with each other because they are related to a general construct, yet these constructs may retain a significant amount of unique variance that is unrelated to the general construct. Higher-order models provide a method for evaluating both common and unique variance represented by the factors (Hull, Tedlie, & Lehn, 1995). It is theoretically plausible to propose a higher-order model in the present investigation; however, such a model would be statistically infeasible to test due to problems with underidentification. In essence, among the two first-order factors there are two variances and one covariance, but a higher-order model would require the estimation of four parameters (two second-order factor loadings and two error variances for the first-order factors). Were the factor loadings constrained to be equal, the model is just-identified and no new information is obtained. Thus, more than two first-order factors are needed for a higher-order model to yield meaningful information (S. Mulaik, personal communication, December 2, 1997).

Although the age range of the participants spanned 34 years and the participants were in good health, generalizability of the present conclusions are limited to older persons. Based on current knowledge of the effects of aging on object and space perception in the normal brain, it is unclear whether a different result would be obtained with younger adults. There is substantial evidence of changes in visual ability with age, including alterations in acuity, accommodation, adaptation to darkness, color and peripheral vision, and convergence, as well as depth perception and object size (see Bennett & Eklund, 1983). In addition, evidence suggests that there is slowing of visual processing with age (Clancy Dollinger, 1995; Hale, Myerson, Faust, & Fristoe, 1995). It is unclear, however, whether normal aging disproportionately affects object versus space perception. The stability of object and space perception performance patterns associated with aging in the normal brain would best be addressed through replication with a longitudinal design.

In many aspects, the VOSP exemplifies a good test: It began as a theory-driven approach to assessment, and studies of both group differences and the latent structure of the battery are consistent with the theory on which it was based. From a psychometric perspective, the VOSP object perception subtests show considerable promise in measuring visuoperception; however, the space perception subtests of the battery appear weak. Different or modified space perception measures may enhance the description of a discrete space perception construct.

These findings add to the bodies of evidence supporting a dissociation between object and space perception abilities and defining the construct validity of the VOSP battery. Future research should focus on the clinical utility of the object-space dissociation in both normal aging and disease states.

REFERENCES

Bennett, E.S., & Eklund, S.J. (1983). Vision changes, intelligence, and aging. *Educational Gerontology*, *9*, 255–278.

Bentler, P.M. (1993). *EQS: Structural equations program manual*. Los Angeles: BMDP Statistical Software.

Bollen, K.A. (1989). *Structural equations with latent variables*. New York: Wiley and Sons.

Bonello, P.J., Rapport, L.J., & Millis, S. (1997). Psychometric properties of the visual object space perception battery in normal older adults. *The Clinical Neuropsychologist*, *11*, 436–442.

Browne, M.W. (1984). Asymptotically distribution-free methods for the analysis of covariance structures. *British Journal of Mathematics and Statistical Psychology*, *37*, 62–83.

Campbell, D., & Fiske, D. (1959). Convergent and discriminant validation by the multitrait-multimethod matrix. *Psychological Bulletin*, *56*, 81–105.

Clancy-Dollinger, S.M. (1995). Effect of degraded viewing on visual asymmetry patterns in older adults. *Experimental Aging Research*, *21*, 47–57

Courtney, S.M., Ungerleider, L.G., Keil, K., & Haxby, J.V. (1996). Object and spatial visual working memory activate separate neural systems in human cortex. *Cerebral Cortex*, *6*, 39–49.

Cronbach, L., & Meehl, P. (1955). Construct validity in psychological tests. *Psychological Bulletin*, *52*, 281–302.

Hale, S., Myerson, J., Faust, M., & Fristoe, N. (1995). Converging evidence for domain-specific slowing from multiple nonlexical tasks and multiple analytic methods. *Journals of Gerontology: Series B: Psychological Sciences & Social Sciences*, *50B*, P202–P211.

Hoyle, R., & Smith, G. (1994). Formulating clinical research hypotheses as structural equation models: A conceptual overview. *Journal of Consulting and Clinical Psychology*, *62*, 429–440.

Hull, J.G., Tedlie, J.C., & Lehn, D.A. (1995). Modeling the relation of personality variables to symptoms complaints. In R. H. Hoyle (Ed.), *Structural equation modeling: Concepts, issues, and applications* (pp. 217–235). Thousand Oaks, CA: Sage.

Hultsch, D.F., Hammer, M.E., & Small, B.J. (1993). Age differences in cognitive performance in later life: relationships to self-reported health and activity life style. *Journal of Gerontology*, *48*, P1–P11.

Humphreys, G.W., & Riddoch, M.J. (1984). Routes to object constancy: Implications from neurological impairments of object constancy. *Quarterly Journal of Experimental Psychology*, *26A*, 383–415.

Kartsounis, L., & Warrington, E.K. (1991). Failure of object recognition due to a breakdown of figure-ground discrimination in a patient with normal acuity. *Neuropsychologia*, *29*, 969–980.

Lawton, M.P., Moss, M., Fulcomer, M., & Kleban, M.H. (1982). A research and service oriented multilevel assessment instrument. *Journal of Gerontology*, *37*, 91–99.

Livingstone, M., & Hubel, D. (1988). Segregation of form, color, movement, and depth: Anatomy, physiology, and perception. *Science*, *240*, 740–749.

Marr, D. (1982). *Vision: A computational investigation into the human representation and processing of visual information*. San Francisco: W.H. Freeman.

McCarthy, R.A., & Warrington, E.K. (1990). *Cognitive neuropsychology*. San Diego, CA: Academic Press.

Mishkin, M., & Manning, F.J. (1978). Non-spatial memory after selective prefrontal lesions in monkeys. *Brain Research*, *143*, 313–323.

Mishkin, M., Ungerleider, L.G., & Macko, K. (1983). Object vision and spatial vision: Two cortical pathways. *Trends in Neuropsychology*, *6*, 414–417.

Newcombe, F. (1969). *Missile wounds of the brain: A study of psychological deficits*. London: Oxford Press.

Owen, A., Evans, A., & Petrides, M. (1996). Evidence for a two-stage model of spatial working memory processing within the lateral frontal cortex: A positron emission tomography study. *Cerebral Cortex*, *6*, 31–38.

Postle, B.R., Jonides, J., Smith, E.E., Corkin, S., & Growdon, J.H. (1997). Spatial, but not object, delayed response is impaired in early Parkinson's disease. *Neuropsychology*, *11*, 171–179.

Rindskopf, D., & Rose, T. (1988). Some theory and applications of confirmatory second-order factor analysis. *Multivariate Behavioral Research*, *23*, 51–67.

Warrington, E.K., & James, M. (1988). Visual apperceptive agnosia: A clinico-anatomical study of three cases. *Cortex*, *24*, 13–32.

Warrington, E.K., & James, M. (1991). *The Visual Object and Space Perception Battery*. Bury St. Edmunds UK: Thames Valley Test Company.

Warrington, E.K., & Rabin, P. (1970). Perceptual matching in patients with cerebral lesions. *Neuropsychologia*, *8*, 475–487.

Warrington, E.K., & Taylor, A.M. (1973). Contribution of the right parietal lobe to object recognition. *Cortex*, *9*, 152–164.

West, S.G., Finch, J.F., & Curran, P.J. (1995). Structural equation models with nonnormal variables. In R. H. Hoyle (Ed.), *Structural equation modeling: Concepts, issues, and applications* (pp. 56–75). Thousand Oaks, CA: Sage.

Zachary, R.A. (1986). *The Shipley Institute of Living Scale-Revised Manual*. Los Angeles: Western Psychological Services.

Chapter IX

GENERAL CONCLUSIONS AND FUTURE DIRECTIONS

This book was intended as an updating of its predecessor (Rourke et al., 1992). Topics included: distinguishing between statistics and biostatistics; differentiating parametric from nonparametric approaches to data analysis; critically examining and updating Stevens' quadripartite classification of scales of measurement; and discussing in some detail a wide range of possible reliability and validity assessments. These were followed by a large number of biostatistical and methodologic articles on most of these topics, as well as some unusual variations on these themes, such as: using base rates to study the validity of brain–behavior relationships; controlling for practice effects as threats to the reliability and validity of reported study results; examining the roles of both meta-analysis and moderator variables in biobehavioral research; as well as the role of validity assessments in the broader context of null hypothesis significance testing and power and precision issues; and a series of articles focusing on model building and model testing in clinical and experimental neuropsychology.

Emphasis throughout has been on a conceptual rather than a mathematical approach to these ideas. We have tried to present biostatistical techniques in terms of their advantages as well their limitations. We have also sought to connect major multivariate techniques, such as structural equation modeling and individual growth curve analysis, to their less complex and more standard univariate predecessors. This was done in the hope that these techniques would not be utilized in an uncritical or haphazard manner, simply because they are here and rather widely accessible.

The book also points to the need for further critical thinking on the part of clinical neuropsychologists, such as the lack of use of randomized clinical trials that can, in specified circumstances, have distinct advantages over other techniques that might be applied. Finally, we have alluded to many other references in the literature, including a variety of other textbooks that the interested researcher and consumer of research may wish to consult in order to broaden knowledge of methodological and biostatistical issues as they impinge upon clinical neuropsychology and biobehavioral research more generally.

It is our hope that this volume can be used for a course on research methodology; as an adjunct to a biostatistical text, by consumers of research; and for clinical research scientists in clinical neuropsychology or in any of the other behavioral and medical disciplines.

There are numerous ways in which the ideas presented in this text can be utilized in a course on biobehavioral research methodology either in clinical neuropsychology or in any other related health disciplines. The most obvious and straightforward option would be to teach a conceptually oriented methodology course using the text as is.

A second would be to use the concepts herein expressed to teach students to become better consumers of published research. As Grimm and Yarnold (1995) correctly note: "It is unnecessary to master multivariate analyses to understand the Results section of an article that uses such analyses. What is essential, however, is that the consumer of research findings be able to follow the statistical reasoning used by the investigators" (p. 18).

A third option, should the course be one offered to medical students, is to use this text in conjunction with an outstanding biomedical biostatistical text such as that published recently by Feinstein (2002).

A fourth option would involve giving a two-semester course on biobehavioral methodology for advanced students. One suggestion would be to use the current text the first semester as a conceptual foundation, and then to offer a more mathematically sophisticated course the following semester that could utilize methods and research examples given in, say, Sheskin (2000) for univariate statistical applications, and, for multivariate applications to perhaps use a combination of the Little, Schnabel, and Baumert (2000) text on the modeling of multilevel and longitudinal data and the Raudenbush and Bryk (2002) updated text on hierarchical linear modeling.

A fifth option would be to teach a course on single subject research by a comprehensive investigation of the important role it has had in advancing both science (e.g., clinical neuropsychology and medicine) and biostatistics (e.g., the work of R.A. Fisher on the lady tasting tea).

The overarching theme could be cast under the framework of the nomothetic (group-oriented) versus the ideographic (single-subject) approach to scientific inquiry in biobehavioral research, with emphasis on the latter. A very useful text by Kazdin (2003) could be used, especially Chapter 10, "The Case Study and Single-Case Research Designs," and Chapter 11, "Evaluation of the Single Case in Clinical Work."

The section on reliability and validity assessments for the single case can be drawn from the current text, with Wilson's (1999) excellent text as an example of the knowledge gained in the research evaluation of the effectiveness of neuropsychological rehabilitation programs carefully designed for individual patients with neuropsychological impairments. Her book is also valuable in the major contribution it makes in linking theory and research to advances in clinical knowledge. Relevant portions of Salsburg's (2001) and Holschuh's (1980) writings, as well as the original work of R.A. Fisher (1935), can further amplify and elucidate the contributions to knowledge about single-subject or single-case research designs in biostatistics. Finally, Blampied's (2000) commentary on the importance of single-case research designs deserves high praise. He correctly observes the following:

> The many virtues of single-case research designs deserve much more favorable attention in graduate training programs and in textbooks on methodology. It is also necessary to ensure that faculty can teach, demonstrate, and mentor the use of such designs. Gatekeeping practices within research funding agencies, editorial boards, and publication manuals also need modification to accompany single-case research designs. This will help psychologists eliminate what Valsiner (1986) referred to as psychology's "double standard (p. 1) in its treatment of individuals: claiming to be able to apply science to individual persons while working exclusively with group-aggregate data" (p. 960).

Additional supplementary texts, as well as others to which we have alluded in various parts of the text are now described briefly in order to provide further ideas for developing courses in research methodology at both an undergraduate and graduate level.

Sheskin's (2000) handbook of parametric and nonparametric statistical procedures has the distinct advantage of presenting basic biostatistical concepts in the context of hypothetical research questions and hypotheses. This valuable text can also serve as a refresher 'course' on fundamental univariate and multivariate techniques, along with their respective formulae for the mathematically inclined. The aforementioned review published by Cicchetti (2002) can provide more insight into the potential value of this handbook in the context of preparing a course on clinical research methodology in any specific area of biobehavioral focus.

Feinstein's (2002) reader friendly text on principles of medical statistics is long on biostatistical problems and their resolution as they appear in numerous medical research contexts.

Raudenbush and Bryk's (2002) updated text on hierarchical linear models is a natural, necessary, and comprehensive updating of the earlier Bryk and Raudenbush (1992) text in the light of the many technologic, methodologic and biostatistical advances since the publication of the earlier edition.

Little, Schnabel, and Baumert's (2000) text on the modeling of longitudinal and multilevel data makes for an insightful conceptual and mathematical contribution to the field.

The Grimm and Yarnold (1995) text provides for a well written, conceptual, nonmathematical approach to the understanding of a number of multivariate data analytic strategies—multiple regression and correlation, path analysis, principal-components analysis and exploratory and confirmatory factor analysis—multidimensional scaling, logistic regression, multivariate analysis of variance (MANOVA), discriminant analysis, and meta-analysis.

Salsburg (2001) has published a very readable and very informative conceptual approach to the role of statistics as a force that revolutionized scientific thought in the twentieth century. It is a must-read written by a very knowledgeable biostatistician who shares his own personal experiences with some of the great names in the field.

Louis Menand (2001) shares with the reader a provocative and insightful historical description of the development of the 'law of errors' that originated in the seventeenth century, was conceptually linked to statistics and probability theory, had early application in astronomy, and appears to have formed the basis of empirical knowledge about how any series of repeated measurements of a stationary object, when plotted, will form the familiar normal distribution or bell-shaped curve. This critical discovery underlies the interpretation of probability levels in the application of statistical tests to data deriving from an almost infinite number of areas of empirical inquiry in clinical and experimental science.

Abelson's (1995) thoughtful and provocative text conceives of statistics as 'principled argument' and provides multiple examples of his own unique and very imaginative approaches to data analysis and interpretation. As just one example, he has made a major and most original contribution to our understanding of the meaning of and differentiation between main effects and interactions deriving from the application of analysis of variance techniques in numerous research applications in the field of social psychology. These valuable insights have broader application to biobehavioral research more generally.

Four more specialized texts are also notable for making major contributions to their respective areas of inquiry: one on an incisive and rather comprehensive, albeit simple and lucid conceptual approach to power analysis, by Kraemer and Thiemann (1987); another a comprehensive treatment of multiple comparison methods for researchers by Toothaker (1991); and a third on statistical strategies for small sample research that was edited by Hoyle in 1999. We have also alluded to some useful computer programs, for performing various reliability and validity procedures, meta-analyses, and various types of power and precision analyses. Dan Zelterman's (1999) lucid text *"Models for Discrete Data"* represents a comprehensive guide to research in which the outcome variable is a classification of individuals into two (dichotomous) or more (polychotomous) discrete categories. Among other important contributions, Zelterman provides a comprehensive, in-depth analysis of sample size and power issues in the context of discrete data analysis. The text is also rich in the integration of statistical theory with the necessary computer software required to provide answers to a multitude of research questions. The text is also replete with exercises that appear at the end of each chapter and range in level of complexity from 'abstract mathematical' to what Zelterman refers to as "the practical how-to variety" (p. vi). Given this range of coverage, it can be used by both advanced and less knowledgeable consumers of research, depending specifically upon the topics of interest. It can also serve as a general reference to a wide range of issues that confront the research scientist in the context of discrete data analysis. The author himself best summarizes the usefulness of the text:

What do I ask of my readers? At a minimum, the reader should know about such elementary statistical concepts as sample means and variances, the Pearson chi-squared, and statistical distributions such as the binomial and Poisson. The reader with a basic knowledge of SAS will understand the computing examples. In order to more fully appreciate all of the theory, the reader should have had a one-year level course in mathematical statistics at the level of Hogg and Craig (1970) and a single semester course in linear models covering topics such as orthogonal contrasts. This advanced reader should also be familiar with matrix multiplication, maximum likelihood estimation, sufficient statistics, moment generating functions, and hypothesis tests. The small amount of linear algebra needed is reviewed in Section 5.1 (p. vi).

Finally, in two earlier reports Rourke and Adams (1984) and Rourke and Brown (1986) discuss a number of methodological issues we have identified and alluded to in the text, this in a rich clinical neuropsychological research context.

A number of possible future directions for research in clinical neuropsychology were expressed in Rourke (1991) and in Rourke et al. (1992). These included, among others, the continued powerful role of the computer, the improvement of statistical computer paradigms and programs, a wide array of analytic and graphic programs, and a continued multi-disciplinary collaboration in clinical neuropsychology, at the level of research, clinical and educational endeavors.

One issue that we have discussed only briefly in this volume is an increased usage of computer simulation techniques. These have been developed and applied successfully in a number of critical areas, such as: for determining an optimal number of scale points to utilize in biobehavioral research when the researcher has insufficient a priori knowledge to make this decision (Cicchetti, Showalter, & Tyrer, 1985); for developing a better understanding of how to appropriately apply analysis of covariance techniques (Adams et al., 1985, 1992); and the empirical testing of various imputation techniques to handle the problem of missing data.

These latter approaches have tended to rely upon the technique of removing data from a known and complete data set; and then utilizing different imputation algorithms to determine which technique comes closest to reproducing the original data set (e.g., Graham & Shafer, 1999). One critical issue that needs to be examined here is the set of assumptions pertaining to the missingness of the data. Some programs such as NORM assume that the data are missing at random, an assumption that may not be warranted. The plausibility of this assumption is discussed in Schafer (1997) and Graham, Hofer, Donaldson, Mackinnon, and Schafer (1997). Computer simulation methodology has also been utilized successfully in the development and testing of small sample strategies to be utilized with multivariate techniques such as confirmatory factor analysis (Marsh & Hau, 1999) and structural equation modeling (SEM) (Chin & Newsted [1999]).

But, as was the case in Rourke et al. (1992), perhaps the most important phenomenon boding well for producing major and hopefully groundbreaking advances in clinical neuropsychology and other biobehavioral areas is the continued and increasing trend toward multi-disciplinary research collaboration. As part of our own research enterprise, we continue to publish in collaboration with scientists in other fields of psychology, neurology, internal medicine, pediatrics, psychiatry, genetics, biochemistry, speech and language, biostatistics and computer science. We predict that in the foreseeable future, this valuable research activity will become more the rule than the exception.

And finally, as we expressed in Rourke et al. (1992) "... the neuropsychological community will become more methodologically adept and sophisticated as graduate programs increasingly update their aims, curricula, and faculty. They will prepare students for the years ahead as innovative methods become available to study questions old and new. The editors and authors hope this volume has provided the reader with some of this promise and excitement" (p. 547).

REFERENCES

Abbott, R.D. (2002). Statistics at square two: Understanding modern statistical applications in medicine. *The American Statistician, 56*, 331.

Abelson, R.P. (1995). *Statistics as principled argument*. Hillside, NJ: Lawrence Erlbaum Associates.

Adams, K., Brown, G., & Grant, I. (1985). Analysis of covariance as a remedy for demographic mismatch of research subject groups: Some sobering simulations. *Journal of Clinical and Experimental Neuropsychology, 7*, 445–462.

Adams, K., Brown, G., & Grant, I. (1992). Covariance is not the culprit: Adams, Brown, and Grant reply. *Journal of Clinical and Experimental Neuropsychology, 14*, 983–985.

Baca-Garcia, E., Blanco, C., Saiz-Ruiz, J., Rico, F., Diaz-Sastre, C., & Cicchetti, D.V. (2001). Assessment of reliability in the clinical evaluation of depressive symptoms among multiple investigators in a multicenter clinical trial. *Psychiatry Research, 102*, 163–173.

Bartko, J.J. (1966). The intraclass correlation coefficient as a measure of reliability. *Psychological Reports, 19*, 3–11.

Bartko, J.J. (1976). On various intraclass correlation reliability coefficients. *Psychological Bulletin, 83*, 762–765.

Bentler, P.M., & Stein, J.A. (1992). Structural equation models in medical research. *Statistical Methods in Medical Research, 1*, 159–181.

Berkson, J. (1958). Smoking and lung cancer: Some observations on two special reports. *Journal of the American Statistical Association, 53*, 28–38.

Blampied, N.M. (2000). Single-case research designs: A neglected alternative. *American Psychologist, 55*, 960.

Bolanowski, S.J., & Gescheider, G.A. (Eds.) (1991). *Ratio scaling of psychological magnitude: In honor of the memory of S.S. Stevens*. Hillsdale, NJ: Lawrence Erlbaum Associates.

Boneau, C.A. (1960). The effects of violations of assumptions underlying the *t* test. *Psychological Bulletin, 57*, 49–64.

Boneau, C.A. (1962). A comparison of the power of the U and *t* tests. *Psychological Review, 69*, 246–256.

Borenstein, M. (1998). The shift from significance testing to effect size estimation. In A.S. Bellak & M. Hersen (Series Eds.) & N. Schooler (Vol. Ed.), *Research and methods. Vol. 3, Comprehensive clinical psychology* (pp. 313–349). New York, NY: Pergamon.

Borenstein, M., & Rothsteinn, H. (1999). *Comprehensive meta-analysis: A computer program for research synthesis*. Mahwah, NJ: Lawrence Erlbaum Associates.

Borenstein, M., Rothstein, H., & Cohen, J. (1997). *Power and precision: A computer program for statistical power analysis and confidence intervals*. Englewood, NJ: Biostat, Inc.

Borenstein, M., Rothstein, H., & Cohen, J. (2001). *Power and precision: A computer program for statistical power analysis and confidence intervals.* Englewood, NJ: Biostat, Inc.

Bradley, J.V. (1968). *Distribution-free statistical tests.* Englewood, NJ: Prentice-Hall.

Brand, J.L. (2002). Why chance is a good theory. *American Psychologist, 57,* 66–67.

Bryk, A.S., & Raudenbush, S.W. (1992). *Hierarchical linear models: Applications and data analysis methods.* Newbury Park, CA: Sage Publications.

Buchler, J. (1940). *Philosophical writings of Pierce.* New York, NY: Dover.

Campbell, M.J. (2001). *Statistics at Square One: Understanding Modern Statistical Applications in Medicine.* London, BMJ Books.

Chase, J.M. (1970). Normative criteria for scientific publication. *The American Sociologist, 5,* 262–265.

Chin, W.W., & Newsted, P.R. (1999). Structural equation modeling analysis with small samples using partial least squares. In R.H. Hoyle (Ed.), *Statistical strategies for small sample research* (pp. 307–341). Thousand Oaks, CA: Sage Publications.

Chow, S.L. (1998). Statistical significance: Rationale, validity, and utility. *Behavioral and Brain Sciences, 21,* 169–239.

Chow, S.L. (2000). The Popperian framework, statistical significance, and rejection of chance. *Behavioral and Brain Sciences, 23,* 294–298.

Cicchetti, D.V. (1972). Extension of multiple-range tests to interaction tables in the analysis of variance: A rapid, approximate solution. *Psychological Bulletin, 77,* 405–408.

Cicchetti, D.V. (1976). Assessing inter-rater reliability for rating scales: Resolving some basic issues. *British Journal of Psychiatry, 129,* 452–456.

Cicchetti, D.V. (1981). Testing the normal approximation and minimal sample size requirements of weighted kappa when the number of categories is large. *Applied Psychological Measurement, 5,* 101–104.

Cicchetti, D.V. (1988). When diagnostic agreement is high, but reliability is low: Some paradoxes occurring in joint independent neuropsychology assessments. *Journal of Clinical and Experimental Neuropsychology, 10,* 605–622.

Cicchetti, D.V. (1994a). Guidelines, criteria, and rules of thumb for evaluating normed and standardized assessment instruments in psychology. *Psychological Assessment, 6,* 284–290.

Cicchetti, D.V. (1994b). Multiple comparison methods: Establishing guidelines for their valid application in neuropsychological research. *Journal of Clinical and Experimental Neuropsychology, 16,* 155–161.

Cicchetti, D.V. (1998). Role of null hypothesis significance testing (NHST) in the design of neuropsychologic research. *Journal of Clinical and Experimental Neuropsychology, 20,* 293–295.

Cicchetti, D.V. (1999). Sample size requirements for increasing the precision of reliability estimates: Problems and proposed solutions. *Journal of Clinical and Experimental Neuropsychology, 21,* 567–570.

Cicchetti, D.V. (2001). The precision of reliability and validity estimates re-visited: Distinguishing between clinical and statistical significance of sample size requirements. *Journal of Clinical and Experimental Neuropsychology, 23,* 695–700.

Cicchetti, D.V. (2002a). A comprehensive review of the biostatistical landscape: A review of D.J. Sheskin (2000), *Handbook of parametric and nonparametric statistics* (2nd ed.). New York, NY: Prentice-Hall. In *Contemporary Psychology: APA Review of Books, 47,* 449–452.

Cicchetti, D.V. (2002b). Reliability and validity assessments for multiple independent judgments on a single case: State-of-the-art biostatistical methodologies and applications. Presented at First Hawaii International Conference on Statistics, Honolulu, HI.

Cicchetti, D.V., Aivano, S.L. & Vitale, J. (1976). A computer program for assessing the reliability and systematic bias of individual measurements. *Educational and Psychological Measurement, 36*, 761–764.

Cicchetti, D.V., Aivano, S.L. & Vitale, J. (1977). Computer programs for assessing rater agreement and rater bias for qualitative data. *Educational and Psychological Measurement, 37*, 195–201.

Cicchetti, D.V., & Feinstein, A.R. (1990). High agreement but low kappa: II. Resolving the paradoxes. *Journal of Clinical Epidemiology, 43*, 551–568.

Cicchetti, D.V., & Fleiss, J.L. (1977). Comparison of the null distributions of weighted kappa and the C ordinal statistic. *Applied Psychological Measurement, 1*, 195–201.

Cicchetti, D.V., & Heavens, R. (1979). RATCAT (Rater Agreement/Categorical Data). *The American Statistician, 33*, 91.

Cicchetti, D.V., & Heavens, R., Jr. (1981). A computer program for determining the significance of the difference between pairs of independently derived values of kappa or weighted kappa. *Educational and Psychological Measurement, 41*, 189–193.

Cicchetti, D.V., Heavens, R., Didriksen, J., & Showalter, D. (1984). A computer program for assessing the reliability of nominal scales using varying sets of multiple raters. *Educational and Psychological Measurement, 44*, 671–675.

Cicchetti, D.V., Kaufman, A.S., & Sparrow, S.S. (in press). The relationship between pre-natal exposure to polychlorinated biphenyls (PCBs) and cognitive neuropsychological and behavioral deficits. *Psychology in the Schools.*

Cicchetti, D.V., Lee, C., Fontana, A.F., & Dowds, B.N. (1978). A computer program for assessing specific category rater agreement for qualitative data. *Educational and Psychological Measurement, 38*, 805–813.

Cicchetti, D.V., & Nelson, L.D. (1994). Re-examining threats to the reliability and validity of putative brain behavior relationships: New guidelines for assessing the effect of patients lost to follow-up. *Journal of Clinical and Experimental Neuropsychology, 16*, 339–343.

Cicchetti, D.V., Rosenheck, R., Showalter, D., Charney, D., & Cramer, J. (1999). Interrater reliability levels of multiple clinical examiners in the evaluation of a schizophrenic patient: Quality of life; level of functioning; and neuropsychological symptomatology. *The Clinical Neuropsychologist, 13*, 157–170.

Cicchetti, D.V., & Showalter, D. (1988). A computer program for determining the reli-ability of dimensionally scaled data when the numbers and specific sets of exam-iners may vary at each assessment. *Educational and Psychological Measurement, 48*, 717–720.

Cicchetti, D.V., & Showalter, D. (1997). A computer program for assessing interexaminer agreement when multiple ratings are made on a single subject. *Psychiatry Research, 72*, 65–68.

Cicchetti, D.V., Showalter, D., & McCarthy, P. (1990). A computer program for calculat-ing subject-by-subject kappa or weighted kappa coefficients. *Educational and Psychological Measurement, 50*, 153–158.

Cicchetti, D.V., Showalter, D., & Rosenheck, R. (1997). A new method for assessing interexaminer agreement when multiple ratings are made on a single subject: Applications to the assessment of neuropsychiatric symptomatology. *Psychiatry Research, 72*, 51–63.

Cicchetti, D.V., Showalter, D., Rourke, B.P., & Fuerst, D. (1992a). A computer program for analyzing ordinal trends with dichotomous outcomes: Application to neuro-psychological research. *The Clinical Neuropsychologist, 6*, 458–463.

Cicchetti, D.V., Showalter, D., & Tyrer, P. (1985). The effect of number of rating scale cat-egories upon levels of interrater reliability: A Monte Carlo investigation. *Applied Psychological Measurement, 9*, 31–36.

Cicchetti, D.V., Showalter, D., & Wexler, B.E. (1993). A computer program for per-forming meta-analyses when the outcome variable is dichotomous: Relevance to neuropsychology and biomedical research. *The Clinical Neuropsychologist, 7,* 454–459.

Cicchetti, D.V., & Sparrow, S.S. (1981). Developing criteria for establishing interrater reliability of specific items: Applications to assessment of adaptive behavior. *American Journal of Mental Deficiency, 86,* 127–137.

Cicchetti, D.V., Volkmar, F., Klin, A., & Showalter, D. (1995). Diagnosing autism using ICD-10 criteria: A comparison of neural networks and standard multivariate procedures. *Child Neuropsychology, 1,* 26–37.

Cicchetti, D.V., Volkmar, F., Sparrow, S.S., Cohen, D., Fermanian, J., & Rourke, B.P. (1992b). Assessing the reliability of clinical scales when the data have both nominal and ordinal features: Proposed guidelines for neuropsychological assessments. *Clinical and Experimental Neuropsychology, 14,* 673–686.

Cohen, J. (1960). A coefficient of agreement for nominal scales. *Educational and Psychological Measurement, 23,* 37–46.

Cohen, J. (1965). Some statistical issues in psychological research. In B.B. Wolman (Ed.), *Handbook of clinical psychology* (pp. 95–121). New York, NY: McGraw-Hill.

Cohen, J. (1968). Weighted kappa: Nominal scale agreement with provision for scaled disagreement or partial credit. *Psychological Bulletin, 70,* 213–220.

Cohen, J. (1988). *Statistical power analysis for the behavioral sciences* (2nd ed.). Hillsdale, NJ: Lawrence Erlbaum Associates.

Cohen, J. (1994). The earth is round ($p < .05$). *American Psychologist, 49,* 997–1003.

Cohen, J. (1997). *Much ado about nothing.* Invited Address: Master Lecture Series. Annual Meeting of American Psychological Association, Chicago, Illinois.

Coombs, C.H. (1953). Theory and methods of social measurement. In L. Festinger & D. Katz (Eds.), *Research methods in the behavioral sciences* (pp. 471–535). Hillside, NJ: Erlbaum.

Cortina, J.M., & Dunlap, W.P. (1997). On the logic and purpose of significance testing. *Psychological Methods, 4,* 161–172.

Coyle, S.L., Boruch, R.F., & Turner, C.F. (1991). *Evaluating AIDS prevention programs.* Washington, DC: National Academy Press.

Cronbach, L.J. (1951). Coefficient alpha and the internal structure of tests. *Psychometrika, 16,* 297–334.

de Leeuw, J. (2002). Series editor's introduction to hierarchical linear models. In S.W. Raudenbush, & A.S. Bryk (2002), *Hierarchical linear models: Applications and data analysis methods* (p. xxiv). Thousand Oaks, CA: Sage Publications.

Detre, K.M., Wright, E., Murphy, M.L., & Takaro, T. (1975). Observer agreement in evaluating coronary angiograms. *Circulation, 52,* 979–986.

Embretson, S.E., & Hershberger, S.L. (Eds.) (1999). *The new rules of measurement: What every psychologist should know.* Mahwah, NJ: Lawrence Erlbaum Associates.

Feinstein, A.R. (1973). Clinical biostatistics XX. The epidemiologic trohoc, the ablative risk ratio, and retrospective research. *Clinical Pharmacology and Therapeutics, 14,* 291–307.

Feinstein, A.R. (1977). *Clinical biostatistics.* St. Louis, MO: C.B. Mosby Co.

Feinstein, A.R. (2003). *Principles of medical statistics.* Boca Raton, FL: Chapman & Hall/CRC.

Feinstein, A.R., & Cicchetti, D.V. (1990). High agreement but low kappa: I. The problem of two paradoxes. *Journal of Clinical Epidemiology, 43,* 543–549.

Fisher, R.A. (1935). *The design of experiments.* Edinborough, Scotland: Oliver & Boyd.

Fitzpatrick, A. (1983). The meaning of content validity. *Applied Psychological Measurement, 7,* 3–13.

Fleiss, J.L. (1971). Measuring nominal scale agreement among many raters. *Psychological Bulletin, 76,* 378–382.

Fleiss, J.L. (1975). Measuring agreement between two judges on the presence or absence of a trait. *Biometrics, 31,* 651–659.

Fleiss, J.L. (1981). *Statistical methods for rates and proportions* (2nd ed.). New York, NY: Wiley.

Fleiss, J.L., & Cicchetti, D.V. (1978). Inference about weighted kappa in the non-null case. *Applied Psychological Measurement, 2,* 113–117.

Fleiss, J.L., & Cohen, J. (1973). The equivalence of weighted kappa and the intraclass correlation coefficient as measures of reliability. *Educational and Psychological Measurement, 33,* 613–619.

Fleiss, J.L., Cohen, J., & Everitt, B.S. (1969). Large sample standard errors of kappa and weighted kappa. *Psychological Bulletin, 72,* 323–327.

Fleiss, J.L., Levin, B., & Cho Paik, M. (2003). *Statistical Methods for Rates and Proportions* (3rd ed.). New York, NY: Wiley.

Fleiss, J.L., Nee, J.C.M., & Landis, J.R. (1979). The large sample variance of kappa in the case of different sets of raters. *Psychological Bulletin, 86,* 974–977.

Francis, D.J. (1988). An introduction to structural equation models. *Journal of Clinical and Experimental Neuropsychology, 10,* 623–639.

Francis, D.J., Fletcher, J.M., Stuebing, K., Davidson, K.C., & Thompson, N.M. (1991). Analysis of change: Modeling individual growth. *Journal of Consulting and Clinical Psychology, 59,* 27–37.

Fuerst, D.R., Fisk, J.L., & Rourke, B.P. (1990). Psychosocial functioning of learning-disabled children: Relations between WISC verbal IQ-performance IQ discrepancies and personality types. *Journal of Consulting and Clinical Psychology, 58,* 657–660.

Garcia, C., Rosenfield, N.S., Markowitz, R.I., Seashore, J.H., Touloukian, R.J., & Cicchetti, D.V. (1987). Appendicitis in children: Accuracy of the barium enema. *American Journal of Diseases of Children, 141,* 1309–1312.

Graham, J.W., Hofer, S.M., Donaldson, S.I., MacKinnon, D.P., & Schafer (1997). Analysis with missing data in prevention research. In K. Bryant, M. Windle, & S. West (Eds.), *The science of prevention: Methodological advances from alcohol and substance abuse research* (pp. 325–366). Washington, DC: American Psychological Association.

Graham, J.W., & Shafer, J.L. (1999). On the performance of multiple imputation for multivariate data with small sample size. In R.H. Hoyle (Ed.), *Statistical strategies for small sample research* (pp. 1–29). Thousand Oaks, CA: Sage Publications.

Greenwald, A.G., Gonzalez, R., Harris, R.J., & Guthrie, D. (1993). *Using p values and effect sizes to evaluate novel findings: Significance vs. replicability and demonstrability.* Unpublished manuscript, University of Washington, Seattle, WA.

Grimm, L.G., & Yarnold, P.R. (1995). *Reading and understanding multivariate statistics.* Washington, D.C.: American Psychological Association.

Guenther, R.K. (2002). How probable is the null hypothesis? *American Psychologist, 57,* 67–68.

Guion, R.M. (1976). Recruiting, selection, and job placement. In M.D. Dunnette (Ed.), *Handbook of industrial and organizational psychology.* Chicago: Rand McNally.

Guion, R.M. (1977). Content validity: Three years of talk—What's the action? *Public Personnel Management, 6,* 407–414.

Haig, B.D. (2000). Statistical significance testing, hypothetico-deductive method, and theory evaluation. *Behavioral and Brain Sciences, 23,* 292–293.

Heavens, R.H., Jr., & Cicchetti, D.V. (1978). A computer program for calculating rater agreement and bias statistics using contingency table input. Proceedings of the *American Statistical Association (Statistical Computing Section), 21,* 366–370.

Hebben, N. (*in press*). Polychlorinated biphenyls (PCBs), toxins, and neuropsychological deficits: Good science is the antidote. *Psychology in the Schools.*

Hedeker, D., Gibbons, R.D., & Waternaux, C. (1999). Sample size estimation for longitudinal designs and attrition: Comparing time-related contrasts between two groups. *Journal of Educational and Behavioral Statistics, 24,* 70–93.

Hoenig, J.M., & Heisey, J.M. (2001). The abuse of power: The pervasive fallacy of power calculations for data analysis. *The American Statistician, 55,* 19–24.

Hofman, S.G. (2002). Fisher's fallacy and NHST's flawed logic. *American Psychologist, 57,* 69–70.

Hogg, R.V., & Craig, A.T. (1970). *Introduction to Mathematical Statistics* (3rd ed.). New York, NY: Macmillan.

Holschuh, N. (1980). Randomization and design: I. In S. Fienberg, & D.V. Hinkley (Eds.), *R.A. Fisher: An appreciation* (pp. 36–39). New York, NY: Springer-Verlag.

Hoyle, R.H. (Ed.) (1999). *Statistical strategies for small sample research.* Thousand Oaks, CA: Sage Publications.

Hoyle, R.H., & Smith, G.T. (1994). Formulating clinical research hypotheses as structural equation models: A conceptual overview. *Journal of Consulting and Clinical Psychology, 62,* 429–440.

Hsiao, J.K., Bartko, J.J., & Potter, W.Z. (1989). Diagnosing diagnoses: Receiver operating characteristic methods and psychiatry. *Archives of General Psychiatry, 46,* 664–667.

Jonckheere, A.R. (1970). Techniques for ordered contingency tables. In J.B. Riemersma, & H.C. van der Meer (Eds.), *Proceedings of the NUFFIC International Summer Session in Science "Het Oude Hof"*, The Hague.

Kaufman, A., & Kaufman, N. (1993). *Kaufman Adolescent and Adult Intelligence Test (KAIT).* Circle Pines, MN: American Guidance Service (AGS).

Kazdin, A.E. (2003). *Research design in clinical psychology* (4th ed.). Boston, MA: Allyn and Bacon.

Kraemer, H.C. (1982). Estimating false alarms and missed events from interobserver agreement: Comment on Kaye. *Psychological Bulletin, 92,* 749–754.

Kraemer, H.C., Kazdin, A.E., Offord, D.R., Kessler, R.C., Jensen, P.S., & Kupfer, D.J. (1997). Coming to terms with the concept of risk. *Archives of General Psychiatry, 54,* 337–343.

Kraemer, H.C., Kazdin, A.E., Offord, D.R., Kessler, R.C., Jensen, P.S., & Kupfer, D.J. (1999). Measuring the potency of risk factors for clinical or policy significance. *Psychological Methods, 4,* 257–271.

Kraemer, H.C., Periyakoil, V., & Noda, A. (2002). Tutorial in biostatistics: Kappa coefficients in medical research. *Statistics in Medicine, 21,* 2109–2129.

Kraemer, H.C., & Thiemann, S. (1987). *How many subjects? Statistical power analysis in research.* Newbury Park, CA: Sage publications.

Krantz, D.H. (1999). The null hypothesis controversy in psychology. *Journal of the American Statistical Association, 44,* 1372–1381.

Kreft, I.G.G., de Leeuw, J., & van der Leeden, R. (1994). Review of five multilevel analysis programs: BMDP-5V, GENMOD, HLM, ML3, VARCL. *The American Statistician, 48,* 324–335.

Krueger, J. (2001). Null hypothesis significance testing: On the survival of a flawed method. *American Psychologist, 56,* 16–26.

Krueger, J. (2002). Bayes rules. *American Psychologist, 57,* 70–71.

Landis, J.R., & Koch, G.G. (1977). The measurement of observer agreement for categorical data. *Biometrics, 33,* 159–174.

Laor, N., Wolmer, L., & Cicchetti, D.V. (2001). The comprehensive assessment of defense style: Measuring defense mechanisms in children and adolescents. *Journal of Nervous and Mental Disease, 189,* 360–368.

Leach, C. (1979). *Introduction to statistics: A nonparametric approach for the social sciences.* New York, NY: John Wiley & Sons.

Littell, R.C., Milliken, G.A., Stroup, W.W., & Wolfinger, R.D. (1996). *SAS system for mixed models.* Cary, NC: SAS Institute Inc.

Little, T.D., Lindenberger, U., & Maier, H. (2000). Selectivity and generalizability in longitudinal research: On the effects of continuers and dropouts. In T.D. Little,

K.U. Schnabel, & J. Baumert (Eds.), *Modeling longitudinal and multilevel data: Practical issues, applied approaches and specific examples* (pp. 187–200). Mahwah, NJ: Lawrence Erlbaum Associates.

Little, T.D., Schnabel, K.U., & Baumert, J. (Eds.) (2000). *Modeling longitudinal and multilevel data: Practical issues, applied approaches and specific examples.* Mahwah, NJ: Lawrence Erlbaum Associates.

Marcus, K.A. (2002). Beyond objectivity and subjectivity. *American Psychologist, 57,* 68–69.

Marsh, H.W., & Hau, K.-T. (1999). Confirmatory factor analysis: Strategies for small sample sizes. In R.H. Hoyle (Ed.), *Statistical strategies for small sample research* (pp. 251–284). Thousand Oaks, CA: Sage Publications.

Mayes, L.C., & Cicchetti, D.V. (1995). Prenatal cocaine-exposure and neurobehavioral development: How subjects lost to follow-up bias study results. *Child Neuropsychology, 1,* 128–139.

Mayes, L.C., Cicchetti, D.V., Acharyya, S., & Zhang, H. (2003). The developmental trajectories of cocaine-and-other-drug exposed and non-cocaine-exposed children. *Journal of Developmental Behavioral Pediatrics, 24,* 323–335.

McCarthy, P., Walls, T., Cicchetti, D.V., Mayes, L., Rizzo, J., Lopez-Benitez, J., Sadek, S., Baron, M., Fink, H., Anderson, R., Little, T., LaCamera, R., & Freudigman, K. (2003). Prediction of resource use during acute pediatric illnesses: A structural evaluation model. *Archives of Pediatrics and Adolescent Medicine, 157,* 990–996.

McCarthy, P.L., Sznajderman, S.D., Lustman-Findling, K., Baron, M.A., Fink, H.D., Czarkowski, N., Bauchner, H., & Cicchetti, D.V. (1990). Mothers' clinical judgment: A randomized trial of the acute illness observation scales. *Journal of Pediatrics, 116,* 200–206.

Menand, L. (2001). *The metaphysical club: A story of ideas in America.* New York, NY: Farrar, Strauss, and Giroux.

Messick, S.M. (1980). Test validity and the ethics of assessment. *American Psychologist, 35,* 1012–1027.

Nelson, L.D., & Cicchetti, D.V. (1991). Validity of the MMPI Depression Scale for outpatients. *Psychological Assessment, 3,* 55–59.

Nunnally, J.C. (1978). *Psychometric theory* (2nd ed.). New York, NY: McGraw-Hill.

Oud, J.H.L., Jansen, R.A.R.G., & Haughton, D.M.A. (1999). Small samples in structural equation state space modeling. In R.H. Hoyle (Ed.), *Statistical strategies for small sample research* (pp. 285–306). Thousand Oaks, CA: Sage Publications.

Pepe, M.S. (2000). Receiver operating characteristic methodology. *Journal of the American Statistical Association, 95,* 308–311.

Petrinovich, L.F., & Hardyck, C.D. (1969). Error rates for multiple comparison methods: Some evidence concerning the frequency of erroneous conclusions. *Psychological Bulletin, 71,* 43–54.

Preston, C.C., & Colman, A.M. (2000). Optimal number of response categories in rating scales: Reliability, validity, discriminating power, and respondent preferences. *Acta Psychologica, 104,* 1–15.

Raudenbush, S.W., & Bryk, A.S. (2002). *Hierarchical linear models: Applications and data analysis methods* (2nd ed.). Thousand Oaks, CA: Sage Publications.

Rice, L.N., & Wagstaff, A.K. (1967). Client voice quality and expressive style as indexes of productive psychotherapy. *Journal of Consulting Psychology, 31,* 557–563.

Rosenfield, N.S., Ablow, R.C., Markowitz, R.I., DiPietro, M., Seashore, J.H., Touloukian, R.J., & Cicchetti, D.V. (1984). Hirschsprung Disease: Accuracy of the barium enema examination. *Radiology, 150,* 393–400.

Rosenthal, R. (1991). *Meta-analytic procedures for social research* (Revised edition, Applied Social Research Methods Series, Vol. 6). Newbury Park, CA: Sage Publications.

Rosenthal, R., & Rubin, D.B. (1979). A note on percent variance explained as a measure of the importance of effects. *Journal of Applied Social Psychology, 9,* 395–396.

Rosenthal, R., & Rubin, D.B. (1982). A simple, general purpose display of magnitude of experimental effect. *Journal of Educational Psychology, 74,* 166–169.

Rourke, B.P. (1991). Neuropsychology in the 1990s. *Archives of Clinical Neuropsychology, 6,* 1–14.

Rourke, B.P., & Adams, K.M. (1984). Quantitative approaches to the neuropsychological assessment of children. In R.E. Tarter, & G. Goldstein (Eds.), *Advances in clinical neuropsychology* (Vol. 2, pp. 79–108). New York: Plenum.

Rourke, B.P., & Brown, G.G. (1986). Clinical neuropsychology and behavioral neurology: Similarities and differences. In S.B. Filskov, & T.J. Boll (Eds.), *Handbook of clinical neuropsychology* (Vol. 2, pp. 3–18). New York: Wiley.

Rourke, B.P., Costa, L., Cicchetti, D.V., Adams, K.M., & Plasterk, K.J. (1992). *Methodological and biostatistical foundations of clinical neuropsychology.* Lisse, The Netherlands: Swets & Zeitlinger.

Rubin, H. (June, 2002). *Psychometrics or Psycho Metrics? Alpha abuse.* Paper presented at First Annual Hawaii International Conference on Statistics. Honolulu.

Salsburg, D. (2001). *The lady tasting tea: How statistics revolutionized science in the twentieth century* (Chapter 1, pp. 1–8). New York, NY: W.H. Freeman and Co.

Schafer, J.L. (1997). *Analysis of incomplete multivariate data.* New York, NY: Chapman and Hall.

Scheffé, H.A. (1959). *The analysis of variance.* New York, NY: Wiley.

Schmidt, F., & Hunter, J. (2002). Are there benefits from NHST? *American Psychologist, 57,* 65–66.

Schonfeld, D.J., O'Hare, L.L., Perrin, E.C., Quackenbush, M., Showalter, D.R., & Cicchetti, D.V. (1995). A randomized, controlled trial of a school-based multifaceted AIDS education program in the elementary grades: The impact on comprehension, knowledge and fears. *Pediatrics, 95,* 480–486.

Scott, W.A. (1955). Reliability of content-analysis: The case of nominal scale coding. *Public Opinion Quarterly, 19,* 321–325.

Sheskin, D. (2000). *Handbook of parametric and nonparametric statistics* (2nd ed.). New York, NY: Prentice-Hall.

Shoemaker, M.R., Schonfeld, D.J., O'Hare, L.L., Showalter, D.R., & Cicchetti, D.V. (1996). Children's understanding of the symptoms of AIDS. *AIDS Education and prevention: An Interdisciplinary Journal, 8,* 403–414.

Sohn, D. (2000). Does the finding of statistical significance justify the rejection of the null hypothesis? *Behavioral and Brain Sciences, 23,* 293–294.

Sparrow, S.S., Balla, D.A., & Cicchetti, D.V. (1984). *The Vineland Adaptive Behavior Scales: A revision of the Vineland Social Maturity Scale by Edgar A. Doll: I. Survey Form.* Circle Pines, MN: American Guidance Service (AGS).

Sparrow, S.S., & Cicchetti, D.V. (1989). *The Vineland Adaptive Behavior Scales.* In C.S. Newmark (Ed.), *Major psychological assessment instruments* (Chapter 8, pp. 199–231). Boston, MA: Allyn and Bacon.

Steinberg, M., Rounsaville, B., & Cicchetti, D.V. (1991). Detection of dissociative disorders in psychiatric patients: A comparison of a screening instrument and a structured diagnostic interview. *American Journal of Psychiatry, 148,* 1050–1054.

Stevens, S.S. (1946). On the theory of scales of measurement. *Science, 103,* 677–680.

Stevens, S.S. (1951). Mathematics, measurement, and psychophysics. In S.S. Stevens (Ed.), *Handbook of Experimental Psychology* (pp. 1–49). New York, NY: Wiley.

Stevens, S.S. (1968). Measurement, statistics, and the schemapiric view. *Science, 161,* 849–856.

Swinscow, T.D.V. (1980). *Statistics at square one* (6th ed.). London, England: British Medical Association.

Tenopyr, M.L. (1977). Content-construct confusion. *Personnel Psychology, 30,* 47–54.

Toothaker, L.E. (1991). *Multiple comparisons for researchers*. Newbury Park, CA: Sage Publications.

Tryon, W.W. (2002). Network models contribute to cognitive and social neuroscience. *American Psychologist, 57,* 728.

Valsiner, J. (1986). Where is the individual subject in scientific psychology? In J. Valsiner (Ed.), *The individual subject and scientific psychology* (pp. 1–16). New York, NY: Plenum.

Venter, A., Maxwell, S.E., & Bolig, E. (2002). Power in randomized group comparisons: The value of adding a single intermediate time point to a traditional pretest-posttest design. *Psychological Methods, 7,* 194–209.

Volkmar, F.R., Carter, A.S., Sparrow, S.S., & Cicchetti, D.V. (1993). Quantifying social development in autism. *Journal of the American Academy of Child and Adolescent Psychiatry, 32,* 627–632.

Volkmar, F.R., Cicchetti, D.V., Dykens, E., Sparrow, S.S., Leckman, J.F., & Cohen, D.J. (1988). An evaluation of the Autism Behavior Checklist. *Journal of Autism and Developmental Disorders, 18,* 81–97.

Wainer, H. (1999). One cheer for null hypothesis significance testing. *Psychological Methods, 4,* 212–213.

Wexler, B.E., & Cicchetti, D.V. (1992). The outpatient treatment of depression: Implications of outcome research for clinical practice. *Journal of Nervous and Mental Disease, 180,* 277–286.

Wilson, B.A. (1987). Single-case experimental designs in neuropsycholgical rehabilitation. *Journal of Clinical and Experimental Neuropsychology, 9,* 527–544.

Wilson, B.A. (1999). *Case Studies in Neuropsychological Rehabilitation*. New York, NY: Oxford University Press.

Youden, W.J. (1950). Index for rating diagnostic tests. *Cancer, 3,* 32–35.

Zelterman, D. (1999). *Models for discrete data*. New York, NY: Oxford University Press.

INDEX